Palliative Care Nursing

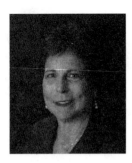

Marianne Matzo, PhD, APRN-CNP, AOCNP, ACHPN, FPCN, FAAN, is the director of research for the Hospice and Palliative Nurses Association in Pittsburgh, Pennsylvania. In 2012, she pioneered the development of the Supportive Care Center at the Peggy and Charles Stephenson Cancer Center in Oklahoma City and continues to counsel patients there for sexual health following their cancer diagnosis. She is an oncology nurse practitioner at the VA Medical Center and is a clinical professor at the Department of Family Medicine, University of Oklahoma College of Medicine. She was the first nurse to be awarded the prestigious Project on Death in America Faculty Scholars Fellowship, funded by the Soros Foundation. Dr. Matzo was awarded a doctorate in gerontology from the University of Massachusetts—Boston and a master's degree in nursing from the Gerontological Nurse Practitioner program at the University of Massachusetts—Lowell. She has presented educational programs regionally, nationally, and internationally on many topics related to care of the dying person, gerontological nursing, and curriculum development. She has authored four books, including two published by Springer Publishing; is a member of several nursing and palliative care editorial boards; and has published numerous data-based and scholarly articles.

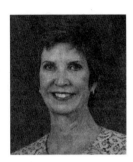

Deborah Witt Sherman, PhD, APRN, ANP-BC, ACHPN, FAAN, is a professor with tenure at Florida International University and has a strong career in education, research, clinical practice, leadership, and administration. Dr. Sherman is certified as an adult nurse practitioner and a palliative care nurse practitioner. She was awarded the Prestigious Project on Death in America Faculty Scholars Fellowship, funded by the Soros Foundation, to start palliative care in the United States along with 11 other PhD nurses and 74 physicians. In 2009, she received the Hospice and Palliative Care Nurses Association's "Leading the Way Award," which is the highest honor recognizing her implementation of the first Palliative Care Nurse Practitioner Program in the United States and the first national certification examination in Advanced Palliative Care Nursing. In November 2011, Dr. Sherman was awarded the Lifetime Achievement Award in Nursing from MD Anderson Cancer Center in Houston, Texas. Dr. Sherman also serves as a professor at Tenshi College in Hokkaido, Japan, where she implemented Japan's first Palliative Care Master's Program in Nursing. Besides serving as the coeditor of this award-winning textbook, she has published several other books related to palliative care, over 35 book chapters, and 80 peer-reviewed research and clinical practice publications. Dr. Sherman has been a keynote speaker and presenter on topics regarding nursing, interprofessional collaboration, and palliative care at over 190 local, regional, national, and international conferences.

Dr. Sherman served for 7 years as the codirector and faculty of the Bronx VA Medical Center Interprofessional Palliative Care Fellowship Program. She has been a faculty for the End-of-Life Nursing Education Consortium (ELNEC) and served as a member of the steering committee in developing the National Consensus Guidelines for Quality Palliative Care.

Dr. Sherman has a strong clinical background in palliative care, serving as nurse attending at Mount Sinai Medical Center, the Bronx VA Medical Center, the University of Maryland Medical Center, and several hospice organizations. She is currently a palliative care practitioner at Miami Jewish Health Systems.

Dr. Sherman received a predoctoral research fellowship by the Langer Foundation and a Postdoctoral Research Fellowship Award from the Aaron Diamond Foundation. Dr. Sherman has received funding for palliative care research by the National Institutes of Health. She is a member of several nursing and palliative care editorial boards and is currently an associate editor of the *Journal of Palliative Medicine*. Dr. Sherman completed the American Association of Colleges of Nursing Leadership Program as well as the Florida International University (FIU) Leadership Program and is also serving in FIU's Center for Academic Advancement and Teaching.

Dr. Sherman's education includes a diploma degree in nursing from Beth Israel School of Nursing, New York; a BSN from Mount Saint Mary's College, Newburgh, New York; a master's degree from Pace University, Tarrytown, New York; a doctoral degree in nursing from New York University; and a post-master's certificate as an adult nurse practitioner from New York University.

Palliative Care Nursing

Quality Care to the End of Life

Fifth Edition

Marianne Matzo, PhD, APRN-CNP, AOCNP, ACHPN, FPCN, FAAN
Deborah Witt Sherman, PhD, APRN, ANP-BC, ACHPN, FAAN

Editors

SPRINGER PUBLISHING COMPANY

Springer Publishing Company, LLC
11 West 42nd Street
New York, NY 10036
www.springerpub.com

Acquisitions Editor: Elizabeth Nieginski
Managing Editor: Cindy Yoo
Compositor: S4Carlisle Publishing Services
Cover photograph: Jimmy C. McDonald

ISBN: 978-0-8261-2712-9
e-book ISBN: 978-0-8261-2719-8
Instructor's Test Bank ISBN: 978-0-8261-3549-0
Instructor's PowerPoints ISBN: 978-0-8261-3557-5

Instructor's Materials: Qualified instructors may request supplements by emailing textbook@springerpub.com.

18 19 20 21 22/5 4 3 2 1

The author and the publisher of this Work have made every effort to use sources believed to be reliable to provide information that is accurate and compatible with the standards generally accepted at the time of publication. Because medical science is continually advancing, our knowledge base continues to expand. Therefore, as new information becomes available, changes in procedures become necessary. We recommend that the reader always consult current research and specific institutional policies before performing any clinical procedure. The author and publisher shall not be liable for any special, consequential, or exemplary damages resulting, in whole or in part, from the readers' use of, or reliance on, the information contained in this book. The publisher has no responsibility for the persistence or accuracy of URLs for external or third-party Internet websites referred to in this publication and does not guarantee that any content on such websites is, or will remain, accurate or appropriate.

Library of Congress Cataloging-in-Publication Data

Names: Matzo, Marianne, editor. | Sherman, Deborah Witt, editor.
Title: Palliative care nursing : quality care to the end of life / [edited
   by] Marianne Matzo, Deborah Witt Sherman.
Other titles: Palliative care nursing (Matzo)
Description: Fifth edition. | New York : Springer Publishing Company, [2019]
   | Includes bibliographical references and index.
Identifiers: LCCN 2018016745| ISBN 9780826127129 | ISBN 9780826127198
   (e-book) | ISBN 9780826135490 (Instructor's Test Bank) | ISBN
   9780826135575 (Instructor's PowerPoints)
Subjects: | MESH: Hospice and Palliative Care Nursing | Critical
   Illness--nursing | Terminal Care | Quality of Health Care
Classification: LCC RT87.T45 | NLM WY 152.3 | DDC 616/.029--dc23 LC record available at https://lccn.loc
.gov/2018016745

Printed in the United States of America.

When this book was conceived in 1998, I would never have envisioned that 20 years later we would be writing the fifth edition. We never would have been able to do this work without the commitment of our chapter authors, most of whom have grown and developed their body of work through each iteration of this book. Therefore, this book is dedicated to these authors for their commitment to educating others about the art and science of palliative nursing.

To Dr. Betty Ferrell, an ongoing influence and friend who is appreciated and valued. To Dr. Deb Sherman, who maintains our energy and motivation. And, lastly, to my daughters, LeaRose and Giuliana LaPorte, I wouldn't trade a second of the last 20 plus years with the two of you. I am so proud to be your mom.

—Marianne Matzo

We speak of the circle of life and of its seasons. We wonder who we are and what we are becoming. We search for meaning and purpose in our lives. Well, a place in my heart held forever dear is for Heloise Gruneberg, my spiritual mother and life mentor, who died last June. Within the last 2 years, I have faced the incremental loss of my dear mother, Mary, who is coming toward the end of her time on earth as well. As her primary family caregiver, I am amazingly challenged despite all I know regarding palliative care and my years of experience. I thank God for my sister, Kathy, who absolutely shares my pain.

But in life, with loss, there may also be gains with dying and birth on two ends of a continuum. Into the world was born my beautiful baby granddaughters, Sasha Marie and Kiran Witt, and her newborn sister, Lila Ray. My sweet grandson, Austin, who is now 9 years old, loves his little girl cousins, and is my computer wizard. My amazing son, Ben, and his lovely wife, Meera; my dedicated and loving daughter, Rachael; and my fantastic son, Joe, and his beautiful wife, Alexandra, are each making a tremendous difference as health professionals in improving the quality of lives of their patients and families across our country. My life is coming full circle. My children are holding the torch and taking the lead in healthcare in America. My dear friends, especially my closest friend, Laurie, and sweetheart, Andrew, also bring much valued support, love, and joy.

I thank God for all blessings in my life, and importantly for the wonderful nursing students and colleagues, who have shared a dedication to palliative and hospice care, and who will lead our profession forward and who I will count on for their knowledge and compassion in the autumn and winter of my life. For all my colleagues at Springer Publishing, who have made this fifth edition possible, I send you my deepest thanks. And dear Marianne, who said, "Deb, let's do it," here we are almost 20 years later publishing this fifth edition. I send you all love—now and always!

—Deborah Witt Sherman

Contents

Contributors

Maritza C. Alencar, DNP, ANP-BC, BMTCN
Advanced Practice Provider Supervisor & Co-Director
  of Oncology Nurse Practitioner Fellowship Program
University of Miami, Sylvester Comprehensive Cancer
  Center
Miami, Florida

Elizabeth A. Ayello, PhD, RN, CS, CWOCN, ETN,
  MAPWCA, FAAN
Faculty member at Excelsior College School of
  Nursing, Albany, New York
Clinical Editor, Advances in Skin and Wound Care
Executive Editor Emeritus, WCET Journal
Faculty, Excelsior College, School of Nursing
Vice President, World Council of Enterostomal
  Therapists (WCET)
Senior Adviser, Hartford Institute for Geriatric
  Nursing
President, Ayello, Harris & Associates, Inc.
Copake, New York

Cynthia Reno Balkstra, PhD(c), RN, ACNS
Case Manager
PruittHealth Hospice
Dahlonega, Georgia

Raymond R. Blush III, DNP, ACNP-BC
Clinical Assistant Professor
University of Michigan School of Nursing
Ann Arbor, Michigan

Marilyn Bookbinder, PhD, RN, FPCN
Director of Quality and Performance Improvement
Metropolitan Jewish Health System
Institute of Innovation in Palliative Care
New York, New York

Kristi L. Bratkovich, PhD
Psychologist
VAMC-Oklahoma City
Oklahoma City, Oklahoma

Mary M. Brennan, DNP, ACNP-BC, GNP-BC, ANP,
  CNS, RN
Clinical Associate Professor
Coordinator, Adult and Gerontology Acute Care
  Nurse Practitioner Program
New York University College of Nursing
New York, New York

Constance M. Dahlin, MS, APRN, BC, PCM, FAAN
Advanced Practice Nurse—Palliative Care Services
  Consultant
Boston, Massachusetts

Lucie B. Dlugash, PhD, ARNP
Clinical Associate Professor and Adult-Gerontology
  Nurse Practitioner Program Leader
Florida International University
Miami, Florida

David C. Free, DNP, MHA, FNP-BC, ACHPN
Executive Director, Lisaard and Innisfree Hospice
Kitchener, Ontario, Canada
Professor (Adjunct)
Brock University School of Nursing
St. Catharines, Ontario, Canada

Melody Hope Gallamore, MS, RN
University of Oklahoma Health Sciences Center
Fran and Earl Ziegler College of Nursing
Oklahoma City, Oklahoma

*Debra J. Hain, PhD, ARNP, AGPCN-BC, FAANP,
    FNKF*
Professor
Florida Atlantic University College of Nursing
Coconut Creek, Florida

Kathrine Hammill, PhD, BAppSc(Hons)
Lecturer in Occupational Therapy
School of Science and Health
Western Sydney University
Penrith, New South Wales, Australia

Lissi Hansen, PhD, RN
Professor and Faculty Member
School of Nursing
Oregon Health & Science University
Portland, Oregon

Jane A. Hill, MS, RN
OU Physicians
Oklahoma City, Oklahoma

Rose Anne Indelicato, DNP, ANP-BC, ACHPN, OCN
Nurse Practitioner, Palliative Care
Montefiore New Rochelle Hospital
New Rochelle, New York

Patrick Kenny, ACRN, RN-BC, NE-BC, APRN-PMH
Nursing Faculty, Jersey College
President-Elect of HIV/AIDS Certifying Organization
Newtown, Pennsylvania

Carl A. Kirton, DNP, RN, MBA
Chief Nursing Officer, University Hospital
Newark, New Jersey
Adjunct Clinical Professor of Nursing, New York
    University
New York, New York
Adjunct Lecturer, Saint Peter's University
Jersey City, New Jersey

Anna Krakowski, MS, AGPCNP-BC, CHPN
Palliative Care Nurse Practitioner
New York Presbyterian/ Lower Manhattan Hospital
New York, New York

Mary Layman-Goldstein, RN, MS, ANP-BC, ACHPN
Nurse Practitioner, Pain and Palliative Care Service
Memorial Sloan-Kettering Cancer Center
New York, New York

Nicole G. Loving, MS, AGPCNP-BC, ACHPN
Nurse Practitioner
Mount Sinai Hospital
New York, New York

Carla Mariano, EdD, RN, AHN-BC, FAAIM
Professor
Pacific College of Oriental Medicine
Adjunct Associate Professor
New York University Rory Meyers College of Nursing
New York, New York

*Marianne Matzo, PhD, APRN-CNP, AOCNP,
    ACHPN, FPCN, FAAN*
Clinical Professor
Department of Family Medicine
University of Oklahoma Health Sciences Center
Oklahoma City, Oklahoma

Tonie Metheny, MS, RN
Clinical Instructor
Fran and Earl Ziegler College of Nursing at the
    University of Oklahoma Health
    Sciences Center
Oklahoma City, Oklahoma

Kathleen O. Perrin, PhD, RN, CCRN
Saint Anselm College
Manchester, New Hampshire

Mertie L. Potter, ND, APRN, DC
Professor Emerita
Massachusetts General Hospital Institute
    of Health Professions
Boston, Massachusetts
Nurse Practitioner, MVCA
Nashua, New Hampshire

John P. Rosenberg, PhD, RN
Queensland University of Technology
Kelvin Grove, Queensland, Australia

Anna Sasaki, MD, PhD
VA Portland Health Care System
Portland, Oregon

Deborah Witt Sherman, PhD, APRN, ANP-BC,
 ACHPN, FAAN
Professor
Florida International University
Nicole Wertheim College of Nursing and Health
 Sciences
Miami, Florida

R. Gary Sibbald, BSc, MD, M.Ed, FRCPC (Med),
 FRCPC (Derm), MACP, FAAD, MAPWCA
Professor of Medicine and Public Health
Faculty of Medicine and Dalla Lana Faculty
 of Public Health
University of Toronto
Program Director
Wound Prevention and Care
MScCh, University of Toronto
Women's College Hospital
Director
International Interdisciplinary Wound Care Course
 (IIWCC)
Toronto, Ontario, Canada

Kristen H. Sorocco, PhD
Psychologist
VAMC-Oklahoma City
Oklahoma City, Oklahoma

Anita J. Tarzian, PhD, RN
Associate Professor
University of Maryland School of Nursing
Baltimore, Maryland

Anne M. Wilkinson, MS, PhD
Chair in Palliative and Supportive Care
School of Nursing and Midwifery
Edith Cowan University
Joondalup, Western Australia, Australia

Brendan P. Wynne, DNP
Psychiatric Nurse Practitioner
Medication Clinic
Lahey Health Behavioral Services
Beverly, Massachusetts

Foreword: Compassion and Competence

Many years ago I had the opportunity to attend a lecture given by Dame Cicely Saunders as she visited a hospice in the United States. It was an overwhelming privilege for me to hear Dame Cicely, known throughout the world as the founder of the hospice movement. Following her presentation, she accepted questions from the eager audience. Several questions were asked, all of which focused on psychosocial aspects of care, presence, and compassion. After several questions, I sensed in Dame Cicely a rising tension, and then quite suddenly and with great conviction she halted the questions, acknowledged how all of the questions were focused on one dimension of care, and then with the great force she was well known for, she proclaimed, "Let me remind you—your patients need your compassion but they also need your competence!" What followed was what I can only describe as "Act Two" of the lecture, in which she challenged the audience to be equally committed to physical aspects of care and building evidence-based practice.

It has likely been 20 years since that lecture, but Dame Cicely's words have remained close to me—"compassion and competence." Those words remain as the challenge of our still evolving field of palliative nursing.

This fifth edition of the *Palliative Care Nursing* textbook is an excellent response to the charge of compassion and competence. The editors and authors have again created a timely text that indeed captures both the science and the art of palliative nursing. This edition also mirrors an important new development, that is, the growing recognition of the importance of interdisciplinary practice. The case studies and commentaries remind us of the many opportunities for nursing not only to advance our clinical practice, but to also work collaboratively with our colleagues to improve care for patients and families.

This fifth edition is an important achievement; it is a symbol of commitment to the field of palliative nursing, where we have been and where we are going.

Dame Cicely would be very proud.

Betty R. Ferrell, PhD, RN, FAAN, FPCN, CHPN
Professor
City of Hope Medical Center

Preface

The world is changing with increasing complexity and periods of obvious chaos juxtaposed to order. Natural disasters, wars, societal violence, and political discord permeate our lives. On a personal or family level, health may deteriorate for physical, emotional, social, or spiritual reasons, wreaking havoc on well-being and creating the circumstances that are the prelude to illness, sickness, and death.

This is the story of humankind, a story that reflects the nature of life, living, death, and dying over centuries. But what is different today is the level of interconnectedness due to technology that transports horror experienced in all parts of the world into the protective enclave of our homes. Schools are no longer safe havens for children to learn and grow to their full potential. Music events, which inspire and elevate the spirit, may become the sites of carnage and death in this all-too-violent world. It appears that in many cases, children and adults are more committed to their phones or tablets with an ever-increasing lack of social and interpersonal skills. The irony is that they are "connected" and "not connected" all at once.

Yet on the positive side, the medical system is translating new scientific discoveries into emergent targeted treatments to save or extend lives. The emergence of immunotherapy, advanced medical procedures or surgical approaches, and precision medicine, which matches treatments with the genetic profile of a person, has extended the life span. The question is, "Has advanced technology improved the quality of life?" Perhaps the benefit may be that another day is possible to see the sun rise, hear the birds, and smell the flowers or learn of the birth of a new grandchild or great grandchild, all joys to be cherished. But as people are living to be centennials or beyond, the only thing people may recognize as they look in the mirror may be their eyes. Over many, many years their bodies have aged, and their spirits are trapped, while the world around them is also less and less familiar. There is the suffering of loneliness as they may be the only one left of family and friends of their generation. Sequestered in their homes or nursing homes due to extreme frailty, life as they knew it has already passed away. The positives of living remain in question as life is no longer the same and families also come to recognize that life will be different when their loved one passes on if it is not different already.

There is a struggle at any age when faced with chronic, debilitating, and painful conditions about whether prolonging the suffering through advanced medical technology is what should be done. Perhaps allowing a natural death, with loved ones around the bed, reminiscing about the happy times and moments of life, holding hands, and kissing the last kiss may be a patient's wish. When is the right time to die? The question is asked but the pondering of such a question leads to discomfort and can only be answered by the person whose life is in question. Is living more painful than dying? Nevertheless, the distress comes from the fact that whereas a person knows life—the good and bad—death remains an unknown and hence death is feared.

Life is intense on every level because every life experience beckons new questions. Medical choices and decisions are made through a partnership of patients, families, and healthcare professionals. What can be done, what should be done, and what do I want done are questions proposed regarding the treatment options available. Suffering remains the constant. Relief of suffering has emerged as an imperative of patients, families, and healthcare providers. We cannot cut out the cancer, but can we cut out the pain of an amputation, of the disfigurement of a body that was once whole? What are the medical risks that patients and families are willing to take given the age of the person afflicted? How can we heal the physical, emotional, or spiritual pain? Medicalization affords us the technology and tools to save lives but where do clinical judgment and the patient's wishes and preferences fit into the culture of healthcare today?

It has been nearly 20 years since this textbook was conceptualized. Early in 2000, Marianne and I, as co-editors, were immersed in the vision and mission of the Soros Foundation as Project on Death in America Faculty Scholars. Soros experienced the painful death of his mother, and along with her he suffered. He vowed to change the culture of death in America, to reform the healthcare system through research on end-of-life care and to embolden physicians, nurses, and social workers to bring palliative care to America to assuage the pain of patients and families experiencing critical life events. Great Britain, Canada, and Australia had already recognized that the hospice model of end-of-life care was of value as patients and families were the unit of care, and an interprofessional approach to care was essential to address the physical, emotional, and spiritual suffering of those with life-threatening conditions. Soros realized that moving the principles of hospice "upstream" in the illness trajectory to earlier than the last 6 months of life was needed to humanize rather than medicalize the illness experience for patients and families.

Through Soros' efforts and the efforts of the Robert Wood Johnson Foundation in the period from 1995 to 2010, Palliative Care was conceptualized and defined and now has become mainstream in the culture of the American healthcare system. Early on, oncologists and other specialists knew their specialty well, but many are focused almost exclusively on the organ system of their concern. What about the whole person? What about the physical and emotional symptoms such as pain, dyspnea, anxiety, fear, and depression that patients were experiencing in the context of cancer, end-stage organ disease, neurodegenerative disorders, or life-threatening infections such as HIV/AIDS? What was being done to relieve their spiritual suffering, their fears, their losses on many levels, and their death anxiety? How can the best of people emerge in the face of overwhelming illness and impending death? How can their resiliency be strengthened, and how can they continue to find meaning and purpose in life despite the challenges and life's transitions?

Can one health profession do this work alone, such as one doctor, one nurse, or one social worker? The answer is that it takes the expertise of an interprofessional team of colleagues, including physicians, advanced practice nurses, and registered nurses, as well as chaplains, pharmacists, occupational therapists, physical therapists, music therapists, and others to guide the patient in living life fully even as death approaches or to adjust to a "new normal" in the face of chronic illness. The interprofessional collaboration of healthcare experts brings the best of minds and hearts to focus on the needs of patients and their family. Indeed, they will cure what can be cured, relieve symptoms even as illness progresses, and show love and compassion to comfort aching hearts of lives being changed forever.

Palliative care is considered a subspecialty of medicine and nursing, with certifications offered to ensure the highest quality of care that can be offered to those with acute, chronic, progressive, life-altering, or life-threatening diseases. If we think about the conception and birth of a newborn, there is a family focus as a child is welcomed into the world. If we think about the nearing death of our grandparents or great grandparents, they are leaving rather than coming into our world. The transitions from home to hospital, to rehabilitative centers, independent living, assisted living, and nursing homes are settings where palliative care practitioners attend to the comprehensive, holistic needs of patients and families. Whether for young parents facing the death of their newborn or adult children facing the death of their parents or siblings, the pain of grief is present. Palliative care practitioners have the courage, sensitivity, and advanced knowledge and skills to help not only the seriously ill or dying but also those who remain behind and must face life without their loved one.

Palliative and hospice care are on the same continuum. Hospice care is offered in the last 6 months of life, whereas palliative care is offered earlier, at the time of diagnosis, with any diagnosis that can eventually lead to death. Palliative care is not only comfort and supportive care, but also aggressive management of uncomfortable to unbearable symptoms. If the symptoms of illness are not alleviated, the path to death is extremely turbulent. Families and friends reciprocally suffer, not knowing how to help and therefore become the secondary victims of the disease. Palliative care practitioners understand that they must care for patients and their families. Although they do not manage the physical and emotional symptoms of the family member, they offer love, care, concern, counseling, education, and referrals for treatment, which are the much needed "therapies" to support caregivers in their role. With aggressive management of physical symptoms, the emotional and spiritual work that needs to be done by patients and families can occur as death approaches. Healing or "to be made whole" can happen even in the face of loss and eventual death. Family members and palliative care practitioners are the companions of the seriously ill or dying in their journey.

The fifth edition of *Palliative Care Nursing: Quality Care to the End of Life* will give you as palliative care and hospice nurses the advanced knowledge you need, beyond your undergraduate and graduate nursing education, to incorporate advanced empirical, aesthetic, ethical, and personal knowledge into your nursing practice. Empirical knowledge, which is the science of nursing, emphasizes the importance of evidence-based practice. Aesthetic knowledge, which is the art of nursing, helps you recognize the meaning of any life experience. Ethical knowledge, which is doing what is right and just, as well as personal knowledge in which we understand from our own lived experiences, the joys and sorrows of life, are also extremely important to our work in palliative and hospice care. We can recognize these ways of knowing throughout the sections of this textbook.

Section I of this book articulates the purpose and value of palliative care and hospice nursing and the revolution across America and the world, which demands the relief of suffering and every effort to promote quality of life until its end. The chapters on ethical and legal aspects of palliative care will enlighten you to act on the basis of your ethical principles and help patients and families discuss the goals of care and to make decisions regarding treatment options that are consistent with their cultural and personal values, wishes, and preferences.

In Section II of the book, the care for the whole person and family is emphasized. The chapters on culture and spirituality and on sexuality will help you to recognize that a person is more than a physical body, exploring the interface of the mind, body, and spirit. The art of communication, the promotion of health, and holistic therapies are taught, as well as ways of facing loss, dealing with grief, and moving to a stage of acceptance.

Section III focuses on advancing your knowledge of life-threatening diseases, including their incidence, prevalence, etiology, pathophysiology, and treatment management. Each disease can create a high level of symptom burden for patients and families. Effective management of symptoms by pharmacologic, nonpharmacologic, and complementary therapies allows emotional and spiritual work to be done as patients and families move across the illness and dying trajectory. In the peri-death chapter, nurses will learn how their presence at the deathbed can imprint a memory that replaces fear with calm, suffering with relief, and sorrow with abundant appreciation and love.

Marianne and I have dedicated the last 20 years of our nursing careers to palliative care and hospice nursing. It is important that as we age, we embrace the upcoming generation of expert nurse practitioners, educators, and nurse researchers who will take the next steps to move forward palliative and hospice care as a nursing specialty. We emphasize that people are more than the sum of their parts; they are transcendent beings who also leave their legacy to the world. They do this through their families, through their music or art, through their written words, through their professional work, and through the day-to-day joy that they share, which creates positive and loving energy in the world. We hope that our work has made a difference to you, for that difference will be shared with the thousands of lives that you will touch over your nursing careers in palliative and hospice nursing. Marianne and I are hopeful that this book is responsive to your educational needs as you offer your wisdom, love, and care to all people, everywhere.

Marianne Matzo
Deborah Witt Sherman

Understanding Palliative Care

Anne M. Wilkinson, Deborah Witt Sherman,
Tonie Metheny, & Marianne Matzo

Palliative Care Nursing

CHAPTER

1

KEY POINTS

- Palliative care (PC) and hospice nursing reflect a holistic philosophy of care implemented across the life span and in diverse health settings. PC and hospice nurses relieve suffering along the course of illness, through the death of the patient, and into the bereavement period of the family.
- The focus of PC is on the prevention and early identification of serious, progressive, chronic, or life-threatening illness and relief of pain and other physical, psychological, or spiritual problems.
- PC and hospice nursing are provided for patients and their families in a variety of care settings, including, but not limited to acute care hospital units; long-term care facilities; assisted-living facilities; inpatient, home, or residential hospices; PC clinics or ambulatory settings; private practices; and prisons.
- As demonstrated by the nursing process, the standards of practice in PC and hospice nursing describe a competent level of generalist and advanced practice registered nursing care involving assessment, diagnosis, outcome identification, planning, implementation, and evaluation.
- The standards of professional performance require the integration of specific core competencies aimed at ensuring the delivery of safe, quality patient-centered care, including the demonstration of competent professional role behaviors in practice, education, research, and leadership.
- Hospice and palliative nurses' professionalism is enhanced through membership in their professional organizations, certification in their specialty, and professional development through academic and continuing education.
- Family-centered care is the foundation for PC philosophy and PC nursing, meaning the patient and family, rather than the disease, are the primary focus.
- PC nursing embraces cultural, ethnic, and faith differences and preferences, while interweaving the principles of ethics, humanities, and human values into every patient and family-care experience.
- PC nurses collaborate with all members of the interprofessional team to ensure quality and continuity of care in meeting the needs of patients and their families.

CASE STUDY

In May 2017, Rachael graduated from an accredited master's-level program as a family nurse practitioner and became certified by the American Nurses Credentialing Center (ANCC). After the death of her grandmother from colon cancer, Rachael decided to enroll in a post-master's palliative care (PC) program and became a member of the Hospice and Palliative Nurses Association (HPNA). With 500 clinical hours in PC, Rachael had achieved the required hours of practice in PC; thus, she sought the opportunity to become certified in hospice and PC nursing by the National Board for Certification of Hospice and Palliative Nursing. One patient that Rachael will never forget was J. L., a divorced 45-year-old woman with metastatic colon cancer who had a 12-year-old son and a 14-year-old daughter. J. L. was transitioning out of the hospital to home. Rachael was a member of the Palliative Care Consult team when J. L. was readmitted to the hospital 3 weeks after discharge with nausea, projectile vomiting, and severe abdominal pain. She was diagnosed with a partial bowel obstruction, secondary to recurrence of her cancer, and initially treated with a nasogastric (NG) tube, intravenous octreotide, and opioids for pain. On day four, J. L. requested removal of the NG tube because "the tube hurts worse than my stomach pain did." After much discussion with the interprofessional team, Rachael was able to advocate for J. L.'s desire to have the NG tube removed and receive palliative medication. Rachael told J. L. that the team was concerned that she would begin frequent vomiting again after the tube removal, but J. L. wanted to continue only the medication.

On her next assessment, Rachael asked J. L. what else she needed. J. L. said, "I need to get home as soon as possible." When asked about her sense of urgency, as the vomiting was still not under control, J. L. replied, "I don't have much time left, and want to be home with my children. They need me and I have to make plans so my family knows my wishes. I need to make funeral arrangements and talk to my family about caring for my children. My former husband is in the army and so he won't be able to raise them."

The scope of hospice and palliative care (PC) nursing continues to evolve as the science and art of PC develop in response to changes in society, including the aging of the population, changes in the trajectory of dying, and the rise in advanced chronic illnesses as the major causes of death. In contrast to the acute, disease-focused model of nursing care, in which there is less emphasis on the individuality of the patient and the relationship between the nurse and the patient and family, PC and hospice nursing focuses on the individual (and family) and on the nurse, whose responsibility involves the active, total care of patients and their families to promote and improve their quality of life (QOL; B. R. Ferrell, Coyle, & Paice, 2015; World Health Organization [WHO], 2017). The focus of PC is on the prevention and early identification of serious, progressive, chronic, or life-threatening illness and relief of pain and other physical, psychological, or spiritual problems. PC is not an alternative to other care. It is a complementary and vital part of management that should be integrated in people with advanced illness, alongside appropriate care to reverse illness or prolong life (Faull, 2012). Although hospice nursing and PC are similar in goals and intent, B. R. Ferrell et al. (2015) have indicated that the basic difference between the two is that "hospice can best be described as a program through which palliative care is intensified as an individual moves closer to death," whereas PC is ideally delivered to "patients living with a chronic, debilitating, and progressive disease and their families … throughout the course of the patients' disease and its treatment." As patients move closer to death, they should be able to transition seamlessly into a hospice program of care (B. R. Ferrell et al., 2015, p. 4).

PC and hospice nursing reflect a holistic philosophy of care implemented across the life span in diverse health settings. PC and hospice nurses relieve suffering along the course of illness, through the death of the patient, and into the bereavement period of the family (Hospice and Palliative Nurses Association [HPNA], 2017b).

Although PC builds upon the template of hospice care, the latter is now recognized as a type of PC that is offered toward the end of life. PC is the combination of active and compassionate therapies intended to comfort and support individuals who are living with and dying from life-threatening illness. The rise in hospice programs in the United States from 1 program in 1979 to more than 6,100 programs in 2014, including 1,500 hospital-based PC programs, along with a rise in the number of patients and families served from 128,000 in 1985 to approximately 1.65 million in 2014, supports the projection of future needs for hospice/PC services (B. R. Ferrell et al., 2015; Morrison, Augustin, Souvanna, & Meier, 2011; National Hospice and Palliative Care Organization [NHPCO], 2015).

PC and hospice nursing are provided to patients and their families in a variety of care settings, including, but not limited to acute care hospital units; long-term care facilities; assisted-living facilities; inpatient, home, or residential hospices; PC clinics or ambulatory settings; private practices; and prisons. Practice settings for PC and hospice nursing are changing in response to the dynamic nature of today's healthcare environment. For example, although the majority of hospice care is provided in private residences (nursing homes, homes, and residential facilities), an increasing percentage of care is being provided in hospice inpatient facilities (21.9% in 2010 vs. 26.1% in 2011; NHPCO, 2015). Fulfilling the goals of PC and hospice nursing requires the provision of a wide range of care and services by members of an interprofessional team of experts (Munday & Charlton, 2012).

PC and hospice nurses are licensed, registered nurses who are educationally prepared and qualified for specialty practice at two levels: generalist and advanced. These levels are differentiated by educational preparation, complexity of practice, and performance of certain nursing functions. Palliative and hospice-licensed practical/vocational nurses are also educationally prepared and licensed, but at a different level of complexity in their practice. PC and hospice nursing assistants are educationally prepared through local- and state-mandated processes to meet the requirements of the specific setting in which they function. These requirements differ significantly across the United States, although hours-of-education requirements are specifically defined in the home care, hospice, and long-term care settings on a national basis. There are no licensure requirements for the nursing-assistant level of palliative and hospice caregiver.

According to an article titled "History of the Hospice Nurses Association, 1986–1996" (Amenta, 2001), the founding of the Hospice Nurses Association (HNA) occurred as follows:

> [I]n spring 1986 a group of nurses attending the Third Western Hospice Nursing Conference sponsored by the Hospice Organization of Southern California in San Diego, frustrated by the failure of national groups to develop adequate standards and networking structures for hospice nurse, put out the call to start a national hospice nursing organization. (p. 13)

Membership in the organization grew rapidly. In 1998, the word "palliative" was added to the organization's name, now known as the HPNA. By the year 2000, 2,800 nurses had joined this growing organization. With a pattern of continued growth, membership to date has reached more than 11,000 across the 45 national chapters (HPNA, 2017a). In 2014, the HPNA

came together with the Hospice and Palliative Nurses Foundation (HPNF) and the Hospice and Palliative Credentialing Center (HPCC) to form a partnership with a synergized mission. The three distinct organizations form Advancing Expert Care (AEC) and share a joint mission to "advance expert care in serious illness" and a shared vision to "transform the care and culture of serious illness" (Advancing Expert Care [AEC], 2016, p. 1).

■ EVOLUTIONARY PERSPECTIVE OF HOSPICE AND PALLIATIVE CARE NURSING

In the early years of the specialty of PC, Billings and Block (1997) identified the following forces that increased national attention regarding PC:

1. A growing interest in death and dying
2. The development of hospice programs
3. Increasing integration of pain and symptom management into conventional care
4. Concern about the high cost of dying
5. Increasing national focus on pain management
6. Greater attention to the role of medicine in caring rather than curing
7. National debates on physician-assisted suicide and euthanasia

These factors combined to create a dramatically increased demand for healthcare providers, including nurses, who are educated at all levels to provide expert, comprehensive palliative and hospice care.

In addition, the landmark "Study to Understand Prognoses and Preferences for Outcomes and Risks of Treatment" (SUPPORT; SUPPORT Study Investigators, 1995) highlighted an urgent need for healthcare professionals who were prepared and committed to improving the QOL of seriously ill and dying patients and their families. The findings indicated a lack of communication between patients and their providers, particularly related to end-of-life (EOL) preferences, aggressiveness of medical treatments, and a high level of reported pain by seriously ill and dying patients. The SUPPORT Study Investigators (1995) believed that improving the experience of seriously ill and dying patients requires an individual and collective commitment of healthcare providers, as well as proactive efforts at shaping the caregiving process.

In 1997, the Institute of Medicine (IOM) released a significant report entitled *Approaching Death: Improving Care at the End of Life* (Field & Cassel, 1997). This report identified gaps of knowledge regarding the care of the seriously ill or dying. Based on this report, Field and Cassel reiterated that "the need for consensus and action to improve care for those approaching death is growing more urgent" (p. 17). On average, Americans live longer than they did in the 19th century, with more than 70% of the population dying after the age of 65 years. According to the National Center for Health Statistics (NCHS), the average life expectancy in the United States in 2016 was 78.6 years, 76.4 years for males and 81.2 years for females (Kochanek, 2017). Over the past 100 years, the leading causes of death have changed from primarily infectious diseases to chronic illnesses experienced by an increasingly aging population. In 2014, the 10 leading causes of death were heart disease, cancer, chronic lower respiratory diseases, unintentional injuries, stroke, Alzheimer's disease, diabetes, influenza and pneumonia, kidney disease, and suicide. These 10 causes of death accounted for 74% of the 2.6 million deaths in 2014 (Xu, Murphy, Dochanek, & Arias, 2016). Although some people will die suddenly and unexpectedly, the dying process for many has been extended, with some individuals, such as those with cancer, facing a steady and fairly predictable decline, whereas others will have long periods of chronic illness punctuated by crises and increasing disability that are often fatal (Gill, Gahbauer, Han, & Allore, 2010; Lage & Crombet, 2011; Lunney, Lynn, Foley, Lipson, & Guralnik, 2003). The result is a national increase in the number of individuals who require PC.

Although hospice and PC have been delivered mainly to patients with cancer, other patients with incurable diseases are also candidates for these services, including the growing number of older adults, those suffering from chronic diseases such as cardiovascular, pulmonary, neurological, and renal disease, as well as patients with AIDS (Boland & Johnson, 2013; Haley, 2013; Mitchell, Noble, Finlay, & Nelson, 2012; NHPCO, 2015; Stiel et al., 2014). In addition, the IOM collaborated with the National Cancer Policy Board and the National Research Council to release a follow-up report called *Improving Palliative Care for Cancer* (Foley & Gelband, 2001), which further supported the need for changes in care of the dying. The report details the undertreatment of distressing symptoms resulting from continued deficiencies in the training of healthcare professionals.

In the report titled *Crossing the Quality Chasm: A New Health System for the 21st Century* (Foley & Gelband, 2001), the IOM argued that professional associations should commit to professional development and competency enhancement by developing curricula, disseminating information, and promoting practice guidelines and standards related to hospice and PC. In April 2004, the standards and guidelines of PC were defined by the National Consensus Project (NCP) Steering Committee in its *Clinical Practice Guidelines for Quality Palliative Care*. This document was the culmination of 2 years of collaboration by 20 representatives from five leading national hospice and PC organizations, specifically the American Academy of Hospice and Palliative Medicine, Center to Advance Palliative Care, HPNA, NHPCO, and the former Last Acts organization. A need for consensus had been defined by practitioners to

provide credible, broad-based guidelines for practice in an effort to standardize and improve the quality of PC in the United States. That need was affirmed when, in the first 2 weeks following publication, 90,000 copies of the guidelines were downloaded from the NCP website (www.nationalconsensusproject.org). More recent, the American Society of Clinical Oncologists (ASCO; Smith et al., 2012) issued a provisional clinical opinion (PCO) calling for the seamless integration of PC into standard oncology practice at the time a person is diagnosed with metastatic or advanced cancer. Although PC is frequently misconstrued as synonymous with EOL care, PC is actually focused on the relief of suffering, in all of its dimensions, throughout the course of a patient's illness. The authors state that "although the use of hospice and other palliative care services at the end of life has increased, many patients are enrolled in hospice less than 3 weeks before their death, which limits the benefit they may gain from these services" (Smith et al., 2012, p. 1094). Strong evidence from a phase III randomized controlled trial (RCT; Temell et al., 2010, 2011) demonstrated that patients with metastatic non–small-cell lung cancer and their families significantly benefited from early PC involvement in their standard cancer care.

Based on the NCP guidelines, the National Quality Forum (NQF, 2012) released *Palliative Care and End-of-Life Care* in recognition of the services increasingly being rendered within the healthcare system. This report endorsed the framework of preferred practices to improve hospice and PC and has been utilized as the first step in developing quality measures (NQF, 2012). Both documents attempt to formalize the concept of PC by providing extended descriptions and definitions differentiating PC from other types of care, and each structures the theory and practice of PC into eight domains: (1) structure and processes of care; (2) physical aspects of care; (3) psychological and psychiatric aspects of care; (4) social aspects of care; (5) spiritual, religious, and existential aspects of care; (6) cultural aspects of care; (7) care of the imminently dying patient; and (8) ethical and legal aspects of care (NCP, 2013). The guidelines are for all settings in which the NQF framework has implications for reimbursement, development of quality measures, and accreditation. These documents are companion pieces serving to complement the process of improving PC quality (NCP, 2013). One of the baseline assumptions of the NCP guidelines is that the qualifications of caregivers are determined by the organizations that grant professional credentials and programmatic accreditation. As a specialty organization, the Hospice and Palliative Care Nurses Association has identified the scope and standards of hospice and PC nursing and the competencies at all levels of nursing practice, specifically nursing assistants, licensed vocational nurses, professional registered nurses, and advanced practice nurses (APNs).

■ EDUCATIONAL PREPARATION

It has been recognized that educational preparation for EOL care is inconsistent at best and neglected for the most part, in both undergraduate and graduate medical and nursing curricula (American Association of Colleges of Nursing [AACN], 1997; Chiu et al., 2015; Paice et al., 2006a, 2006b; Shea, Grossman, Wallace, & Lange, 2010). In addition, there is a lack of role models for students in clinical settings as well as a lack of PC content in medical and nursing textbooks (Maani-Fogelman & Bakitas, 2015, p. 30). In accordance with the International Council of Nurses' (ICN) mandate that nurses have a unique and primary responsibility for ensuring the peaceful death of patients, the American Association of Colleges of Nursing (AACN), supported by the Robert Wood Johnson Foundation, convened a roundtable of expert nurses to discuss and initiate educational change related to PC. It was concluded that precepts underlying hospice care are essential principles for all EOL care. Such precepts include the assumptions that persons are living until the moment of death; that coordinated care should be offered by a variety of professionals with attention to the physical, psychological, social, and spiritual needs of patients and their families; and that care should be sensitive to patient and family diversity. It was proposed that these precepts be foundational to the educational preparation of nurses. Based on these precepts, the document entitled *Peaceful Death* was developed, which outlined baccalaureate competencies for palliative and hospice care and content areas where competencies can be taught (AACN, 1997).

Emphasizing the role of nursing in EOL care, the American Nurses Association (ANA) formulated a position statement regarding the promotion of comfort and relief of pain of dying patients, reinforcing nurses' obligation to promote comfort and ensure aggressive efforts to relieve pain and suffering. Specialized PC educational initiatives began in medicine and nursing, such as Education for Physicians on End-of-Life Care (EPEC), and the nursing initiative End-of-Life Nursing Education Consortium (ELNEC). The original goal of ELNEC was to train nurse educators from associate and baccalaureate programs. The ELNEC curriculum has also been modified and specialized for graduate education, geriatrics, pediatrics, oncology, and for use with veterans.

■ DEVELOPING THE SCOPE, STANDARDS, AND COMPETENCIES OF PALLIATIVE AND HOSPICE NURSING PRACTICE

By developing and articulating the scope and standards of professional nursing practice, the specialty defines its boundaries, informs society about the parameters of nursing practice, and guides the development of rules and regulations for the specialty. As in all nursing specialties, PC nurses must accept professional practice accountability and ensure that their practice remains within the scope of their state's nurse practice act, their professional code of ethics, and professional practice standards.

To ensure provision of quality hospice and palliative nursing care, standards have been defined by a credible body of peers who were charged with this responsibility. The standards of hospice care were defined by the NHPCO in 1986. The standards of hospice and palliative nursing practice were first defined by the HNA in 1995, with subsequent revisions to the name of the organization to include PC. Scope and standards of hospice and palliative nursing care define the body of knowledge needed in terms of the standards of practice and performance. Standards of practice refer to the basic level of care that should be provided to all hospice and PC patients and families. Standards of performance for palliative and hospice care nurses describe the standards for activities related to quality of care, performance appraisal, education, collegiality, ethics, collaboration, participation in research, and resource utilization. Documents, such as agency standards, guidelines, policies, procedures, and protocols, may further direct the individual's performance. Standards are defined in broad terms to specify the scope of the specialty of palliative and hospice care nursing.

The standards of palliative and hospice care nursing practice are authoritative statements described by the HPNA for the nursing profession, which identifies the responsibilities for which palliative and hospice care nurses are accountable. Standards reflect the values and priorities of PC nursing and provide a framework for the evaluation of practice. The standards are written in measurable terms and define palliative and hospice care nurses' accountability to the public and the individual and family outcomes for which they are responsible. Standards remain stable over time, as they reflect the philosophical values of the profession; however, the criteria should be revised to incorporate advancements in scientific knowledge, technology, and clinical practice. Criteria must be consistent with current nursing practice and must reflect evidence-based practice.

Standards of Practice

Standards of practice (ANA and HPNA, 2014) describe a competent level of generalist and advanced practice registered nursing care as demonstrated by the nursing process, involving assessment, diagnosis, outcome identification, planning, implementation, and evaluation. The development and maintenance of a therapeutic nurse–patient and family relationship is essential throughout the nursing process, which forms the foundation of clinical decision making and encompasses all significant actions taken by hospice and PC nurses in providing care to individuals and families. The precepts of nursing practice include the following:

1. Providing age-appropriate and culturally, ethnically, and spiritually sensitive care and support
2. Maintaining a safe environment
3. Educating patients and families to identify appropriate settings and treatment options
4. Ensuring continuity of care and transitioning to the next appropriate setting
5. Coordinating care across settings and among caregivers
6. Managing information and protecting confidentiality
7. Communicating promptly and effectively

A fundamental practice focus for hospice and PC is the *plan of care*, which is developed with the patient and family as the unit of care and members of the interprofessional team. At the very minimum, the interprofessional team includes the physician, nurse, social worker, and clergy. Care responsibilities extend beyond the death of the patient and offer bereavement care to families for a minimum of 1 year. Relief of suffering and QOL for individuals and families are enhanced by:

■ Providing effective pain and symptom management
■ Addressing psychosocial and spiritual needs of patient and family
■ Incorporating cultural values and attitudes in developing a plan of care
■ Creating a healing environment to promote a peaceful death
■ Supporting those who are experiencing loss, grief, and bereavement
■ Promoting ethical and legal decision making
■ Advocating for personal wishes and preferences
■ Utilizing therapeutic communication skills in all interactions
■ Facilitating collaborative practice
■ Ensuring access to care and community resources through influencing and developing health and social policy
■ Contributing to improved quality and cost-effective services
■ Creating opportunities and implementing initiatives for PC education for patients, families, colleagues, and community
■ Participating in the generation, testing, and evaluation of PC knowledge and practice

Registered nurses at the generalist level have completed a nursing program and passed the state licensure examination for registered nurses. Registered nurses who practice in PC settings may provide direct patient and family care, and may function as educators, case managers, and administrators as well as in other nursing roles. Advanced practice registered nurses (APRNs), those with postgraduate education in nursing, including advanced didactic and clinical education, knowledge, skills, and scope of practice in a nursing specialty, are in a unique position to substantially contribute to the improvement of care provided to dying patients and patients with advanced chronic illness (Shea et al., 2010). APRNs develop and implement advanced plans of care based on the synthesis of complex health-assessment data. APNs are expert clinicians, leaders, educators, consultants, and researchers. The standards apply to both generalists and APNs. There is specific notation of standards that apply only to the APN.

Standard 1: **Assessment.** The hospice and palliative registered nurse collects comprehensive data pertinent to the patient's health or the situation.
Standard 2: **Diagnosis.** The hospice and palliative registered nurse analyzes the assessment data to determine nursing diagnoses or issues.
Standard 3: **Outcome identification.** The hospice and palliative registered nurse, in partnership with the interprofessional healthcare team, identifies the expected outcome for a plan of care individualized to the patient or the situation.
Standard 4: **Planning.** The hospice and palliative registered nurse develops a plan of care that describes strategies and alternatives to attain expected outcomes.
Standard 5: **Implementation.** The hospice and palliative registered nurse implements the identified plan of care.
Standard 5A: **Coordination of care.** The hospice and palliative registered nurse coordinates care delivery.
Standard 5B: **Health teaching and health promotion.** The hospice and palliative registered nurse employs strategies to promote health and a safe environment.
Standard 5C: **Consultation.** The hospice and palliative registered nurse and the nursing- role specialist provide consultation to influence the identified plan, enhance the abilities of others, and effect change.
Standard 5D: **Prescriptive authority and treatment.** The advanced practice hospice and palliative registered nurse uses prescriptive authority, procedures, referrals, treatments, and therapies in accordance with state and federal laws and regulations.
Standard 6: **Evaluation.** The hospice and palliative registered nurse evaluates progress toward attainment of outcomes.

Standards of Professional Performance

Standards of professional performance (ANA and HPNA, 2014) and the associated measurement criteria describe professional role behaviors, including those related to ethics, education, evidence-based practice and research, quality of practice, communication, leadership, collaboration, professional practice evaluation, resource utilization, and environmental health. Hospice and palliative nurses must be self-directed and purposeful in seeking necessary knowledge and skills to develop and maintain their competency. Hospice and palliative nurses' professionalism is enhanced through membership in their professional organizations, certification in their specialty, and professional development through academic and continuing education.

Standard 7: Ethics. The hospice and palliative registered nurse integrates ethical provisions in all areas of practice.

Standard 8: Education. The hospice and palliative registered nurse attains knowledge and competency that reflects current hospice and palliative nursing practice.

Standard 9: Evidence-based practice and research. The hospice and palliative registered nurse integrates research findings into practice and generates new knowledge related to the specialty.

Standard 10: Quality of practice. The hospice and palliative registered nurse systematically enhances the quality and effectiveness of nursing practice.

Standard 11: Communication. The hospice and palliative registered nurse communicates effectively with members of the interprofessional team and contributes to the professional development of peers and colleagues.

Standard 12: Leadership. The hospice and palliative registered nurse provides leadership in the professional practice setting and the profession.

Standard 13: Collaboration. The hospice and palliative registered nurse collaborates with the patient, the family, the interprofessional team, and others in the conduct of nursing practice.

Standard 14: Professional practice evaluation. The hospice and palliative registered nurse evaluates one's own nursing practice in relation to professional practice standards and guidelines, relevant statutes, rules, and regulations.

Standard 15: Resource utilization. The hospice and palliative registered nurse considers factors related to safety, effectiveness, cost, and impact on practice in the planning and delivery of nursing services.

Standard 16: Environmental health. The hospice and palliative nurse promotes a healthy environment.

Standards of practice and standards of professional performance are also written for palliative- and hospice-licensed practical/vocational nurses and for palliative and hospice nursing assistants. Variations to each standard are made to adapt to scopes of practice and statutory regulations.

Competencies

Practice in the current healthcare system presents nurses with increasingly complex issues and situations arising from a multitude of factors, including advances in medical technology, greater acuity of patients in hospital and community settings, aging populations and complex disease processes, as well as ethical and multicultural issues. Nursing competencies must reflect and address these new challenges. According to ANA and HPNA (2014), competencies represent the "quantifiable knowledge, attitudes, and skills that practitioners demonstrate in the performance of safe, consistent, compassionate, state-of-the-art, evidence-based EOL care, which conforms to the patients' and their families' wishes" (p. 1). This definition applies to all levels of nursing practice, although the specific clinical judgments and core competencies vary with each level. The competencies for the palliative and hospice generalist and APN were initiated in 2001. Subsequently, competencies for the palliative- and hospice-licensed practical/vocational nurse and nursing assistant were also written.

The basic competencies of PC nursing represent the knowledge, skills, and attitudes demonstrated when providing evidence-based physical, emotional, psychosocial, and spiritual care. The care is provided in a collaborative, interprofessional manner across the life span in diverse settings to individuals and families experiencing progressive illness. The generalist-level competencies and the related general statements are written to the text that follows with special notation only for APNs when applicable.

■ **Clinical Judgment.** Critical thinking is a multidimensional skill involving a cognitive or mental set of processes or procedures involving reasoning and thoughtful, systematic, reflective, rational, outcome-directed thinking based on a body of knowledge, as well as examination and analysis of all available information and ideas (M. Ferrell, 2017). At the generalist level, the palliative and hospice nurse demonstrates critical thinking, analysis, and clinical judgment in all aspects of palliative and hospice care of patients and families experiencing life-limiting illness through the use of the nursing process to address the physical, psychosocial, and spiritual/existential needs of patients and families. At the advanced practice level, the palliative and hospice nurse must be able to respond to all disease processes with advanced clinical skills.

■ **Advocacy and Ethics.** The use of sophisticated medical technology, precision medicine, and genetics/genomics has created new challenges for nurses in all settings, but with implications for the appropriateness of advanced technological care with advanced illness or those at the end of life. Understanding the role of the professional nurse in ethical decision making helps the nurse articulate her or his own ethical positions and also develops the skills needed to make ethical decisions in the development of care plans (M. Ferrell, 2017). The palliative and hospice nurse incorporates ethical principles and professional standards in the care of patients and families who are experiencing life-limiting illnesses or progressive illness, as well as identifying and advocating for their wishes and preferences. Promoting ethical and legal decision making, advocating for personal wishes and preferences, and ensuring access to care and community resources through influencing or developing health and social policy are ways for the nurse to incorporate ethical principles and professional standards in the care of patients and their families.

■ **Professionalism.** *Professional conduct in nursing* refers to the manner in which a person behaves while acting in a professional capacity. It is generally accepted that when performing their duties and conducting their affairs, nursing professionals will uphold exemplary standards of conduct, commonly taken to mean standards not generally expected of laypeople or the "ordinary person in the street." The palliative and hospice nurse demonstrates knowledge, attitude, behavior, and skills that are consistent with the professional standards, code of ethics, and scope of practice for palliative and hospice nursing.

■ **Collaboration.** Interprofessional collaborative practice involves employing multiple health professionals to work together with patients, family, and communities to deliver best practices and to ensure the best patient outcomes (M. Ferrell, 2017). The palliative and hospice nurse actively promotes dialogue with patients and families, the healthcare team, and the community to address and plan for issues related to living with and dying from chronic, life-limiting progressive illness.

■ **Systems Thinking.** A systems approach applied to health is one that employs scientific insights to understand the elements that influence health outcomes; models the relationships between those elements; and alters the design, processes, or policies based on the resultant knowledge to produce better health at a lower cost. By understanding how these elements operate independently, as well as how they depend on one another, a systems approach can help with the design and integration of people, processes, policies, and organizations and can be useful at all levels of the health system—patient–clinician interaction, healthcare unit, organization, and community (Kaplan et al., 2013). The palliative and hospice nurse utilizes resources necessary to enhance QOL for patients and families experiencing life-limiting progressive illness through knowledge and negotiation within the healthcare system.

■ **Cultural Competence.** *Culture* is defined as the learned patterns of behavior, beliefs, and values that can be attributed to a particular group of people, including such elements as manner of dress, language spoken, rules and norms of behavior, dietary practices, and even health beliefs, all of which guide a person's thinking, decisions, and actions (M. Ferrell, 2017). Most countries today are extremely culturally diverse, and as such, nurses need the knowledge and skills to interact with a variety of individuals and groups of similar and dissimilar cultural backgrounds. The palliative and hospice nurse demonstrates cultural competence by respecting and honoring the unique diversity and characteristics of patients, families, and colleagues in palliative and hospice care.

■ **Facilitation of Learning.** The palliative and hospice nurse facilitates learning of patient, family, self, members of the healthcare team, and the community through the development, implementation, and evaluation of formal and informal education related to living with and dying from life-limiting progressive illnesses.

■ **Communication.** Many nursing professionals feel unprepared or uncomfortable in communicating with patients and families facing a life-limiting illness, particularly when delivering bad news. However, it is important that nurses become skilled in PC communication. Reflection, obtaining education, reading, and talking with PC professionals and colleagues can assist the individual in considering his or her own attitudes and values pertaining to the end of life, but also improve his or her skills in communicating with others, including members of interprofessional teams. The palliative and hospice nurse demonstrates the use of effective verbal, nonverbal, and written communication with patients and families, members of the healthcare team, and the community to address therapeutically and convey accurately the palliative and hospice care needs of patients and families.

Advanced practice hospice and palliative nurses are held to the same competencies, but at an advanced level, because they exercise a high degree of critical thinking, analysis, and independent judgment, within the framework of autonomous and collaborative interprofessional practice. APNs are distinguished by their ability to synthesize complex data, implement advanced plans of care, and provide leadership in palliative and hospice care. The roles of the advanced practice hospice and palliative nurse include, but are not limited to expert clinician, leader, or facilitator of interprofessional teams; educator; researcher; consultant; collaborator; advocate; and administrator. Advanced practice palliative and hospice nurses who have fulfilled the requirements established by their state's nurse practice act may be authorized to assume autonomous responsibility for clinical role functions, which may include prescription of controlled substances, medications, or therapies. To practice as an advanced practice palliative and hospice nurse, national certification in advanced practice palliative and hospice nursing is recommended, although it is recognized that the advanced practice palliative and hospice nurse may have concurrent advanced practice certification in another specialty.

Competencies for the licensed practical nurse focus on decision making instead of clinical judgment. For the nursing assistant, clinical judgment is rooted in observation and reporting. Although the core competencies are very similar in all four levels of nursing, the criteria are specific to the various scopes of practice.

■ CERTIFICATION IN HOSPICE AND PALLIATIVE CARE NURSING

Incorporated in 1987, the HNA became the first professional nursing organization dedicated to promoting excellence in the practice of hospice nursing. In March 1994, the National Board for the Certification of Hospice Nurses (NBCHN) offered the first certification examination and the credential of Certified Registered Nurse Hospice (CRNH). In 1999, the NBCHN became the National Board for Certification of Hospice and Palliative Nurses (NBCHPN), offering a new designation to recognize base competence in hospice and palliative nursing: the certified hospice and palliative nurse (CHPN). The NBCHPN is now known as the *HPCC*. For the licensed generalist, a minimum of 2 years of clinical experience in palliative and hospice care is recommended. By 2015, nearly 11,000 registered nurses were certified as CHPNs.

Recognizing the need to offer an examination for advanced practice hospice and palliative nurses, in 2000 the NBCHPN began discussions with New York University and the ANCC to collaborate for this purpose. In an effort to expand the portfolio of examinations, NBCHPN successfully negotiated a buy out of the partnership with ANCC effective December 2004 and has been successfully certifying nurses as advanced certified hospice and palliative nurses (ACHPNs). Eligibility for this level includes having a current unrestricted registered nurse license, graduating from an accredited institution granting graduate-level academic credit for a master's or higher degree in nursing, and having a minimum of 500 hours of supervised advanced practice in PC as a clinical nurse specialist or nurse practitioner. As of 2015, nearly 1,200 individuals were certified ACHPNs (HPNA, 2017a).

Through a commitment to a strategic plan to provide certification for all levels of caregivers, NBCHPN began certifying nursing assistants in hospice and PC in 2001 as certified hospice and palliative nursing assistants (CHPNAs). To be eligible for the examination, the nursing assistant must have a minimum of 2,000 hours in palliative and hospice care as validated by the nursing supervisor. By 2013, nearly 4,000 nursing assistants were certified as CHPNAs. Continuing with the strategy of providing certification for all levels of caregivers, in 2002 NBCHPN began the process of developing the scope, standards, and competencies for the licensed practical/vocational hospice and palliative nurse. To be eligible for the examination, the certified hospice and palliative

licensed practical/vocational nurse (CHPLN) must be licensed and recommended to have logged 2,000 clinical hours in the prior 2 years. In 2017 (HPNA, 2017a), more than 811 CHPLNs had successfully completed the certification requirements.

Certification, as defined by the American Board of Nursing Specialties (ABNS, 2017), is "the formal recognition of the specialized knowledge, skills, and experience demonstrated by the achievement of standards identified by a nursing specialty to promote optimal patient care." Certification is valued for the following reasons:

- Certificates achieve a tested and proven competency across the spectrum of hospice and PC.
- Certificates increase nurses' knowledge of hospice and PC by seeking and maintaining certification.
- Certificates demonstrate a commitment to one's specialty practice through pursuit of certification.
- Certificates demonstrate dedication to professional development by attaining the credential.
- Certificates are assets in themselves because the commitment to certification improves patient outcomes, provides compensation incentives, and gains industry-wide recognition for nurses.
- Certified nurses are assets to their employers because, in an atmosphere of increasing awareness regarding quality in healthcare and appropriate utilization of services, certification is a recognized marker of quality by patients, physicians, providers, quality-improvement organizations, insurers, credentialers, and the federal government.

■ PRINCIPLES OF PALLIATIVE CARE AND RELEVANT CONCEPTUAL FRAMEWORKS

A core principle of PC across the entire disease spectrum and in all settings is the concept that the patient and family constitute the unit of care. The patient and family, rather than the disease, are the primary focus of care. The constructs of family-centered care form the foundation of the PC philosophy. PC addresses the meaning of disease, suffering, life, and death within the context of each family unit (NCP, 2013). PC recognizes that each family member will experience the disease process and all of its implications within the context of his or her particular worldview, and individual care plans are developed to reflect these worldviews. Another core PC principle is the commitment to collaborate through an interprofessional team process (Cairns & Yates, 2003; Leslie, Adams, & Kutner, 2002; Meier & Beresford, 2008; NCP, 2013; Oliviere & Hargreaves, 2017). So as to assist a family in crisis to establish and then achieve mutually agreed-upon goals, the PC team integrates and coordinates the assessment and interventions of each team member and creates a comprehensive plan of care.

Good PC is significant in the manner in which it embraces cultural, ethnic, and faith differences and preferences while interweaving the principles of ethics, humanities, and human values into every patient- and family-care experience (Dy, Lupu, & Seow, 2012; Morrison & Meier, 2004; Oliviere & Hargreaves, 2017). Furthermore, clinical ethics is an essential footprint for the provision of palliative and EOL care. Although clinicians often learn the theoretical principles behind ethics (Beauchamp, 2003; Dy et al., 2012; Morrison & Meier, 2004), PC necessitates that these principles be incorporated into the practice or "put into motion" 24 hours a day, 7 days a week (Block, 2007; Bruera & Hui, 2012). PC embodies this concept of ethics in motion, as each interprofessional team member, including patient and families, contemplates the ethical questions in advanced disease and in EOL decision making. Ethical challenges present themselves to the PC interprofessional team on an hourly basis.

Several conceptual frameworks or middle-range theories in nursing or related health disciplines provide a lens in both the assessment and treatments of PC patients and their families. The founder of St. Christopher's Hospice in London, Dame Cicely Saunders, put forth a conceptual model of "whole-person" suffering. Saunders espoused that whole-person suffering has four dimensions: physical, psychological, spiritual, and social (De Lima & Pastrana, 2016; Mount, Hanks, & McGoldrick, 2006; Oliviere & Hargreaves, 2017; WHO, 2007). Under this concept, suffering affects each domain of the biopsychosocial–spiritual aspects of care. This conceptual model forms the basis for the description of PC nursing practice. Also relevant is the Calkin model of advanced nursing practice (Bryant-Lukosius, Dicenso, Browne, & Pinelli, 2004), which serves as an excellent model on which to base PC advanced practice nursing. Calkin defines the clinical judgment abilities of three nursing practice levels as novice, expert by experience, and the master's-prepared nurse. The following case study illustrates Saunders's four dimensions of human suffering within the context of Calkin's model. The case study also demonstrates the APN subroles of expert clinician, educator, consultant, researcher, and collaborator (Callaway, 2012; Chulk, 2008).

CASE STUDY *Conclusion*

Once a decision was reached that J. L. would pursue palliative treatment, Rachael insured that the interdisciplinary team met with J. L. and her family members to include them in planning and to discuss home care. J. L. was able to verbalize her desire that she spend her remaining time at home, even if she was vomiting. The coordination of care between the PC nurse practitioner and the home care team was extremely important. J. L.'s sister assumed responsibility for her home care and J. L. agreed to enroll in hospice. All family members agreed that this was the best course of action as it adhered to their cultural and religious beliefs. J. L. felt secure given the expertise of the PC nurse practitioner and valued the person- and family-centered approach to care that would also be offered by interprofessional members of the hospice team. J. L. stated, "I'm so grateful that I can spend it at home surrounded by my family and friends and I know the nurses will care not only for me but my family. The nurses have helped to relieve not only my pain and other symptoms, but have helped me find strength to make peace with my life."

The Advance Practice Nurse's Role in Palliative Care

The following case example is that of an APN bringing a specific and well-defined set of qualities, knowledge, and judgments to caring for individuals and families facing serious, progressive, or life-threatening illness. This includes advanced scientific and biophysical knowledge, analytical skills, and mastery of a broad repertoire of communication and interpersonal skills. Specialized knowledge and proficiency in the ability to incorporate ethics; humanities; cultural diversity; family, spiritual, and psychological issues into care are also demanded (Bruera & Hui, 2012; Coyne, 2003; Kuebler, 2003; Meier & Beresford, 2006). The Calkin model of advanced nursing practice (Bryant-Lukosius et al., 2004) serves as an excellent model on which to base PC advanced practice nursing. The following case study illustrates Dame Cicely Saunders's four dimensions of human suffering within the context of Calkin's model, while demonstrating the APN subroles of expert clinician, educator, consultant, researcher, and collaborator (Callaway, 2012).

CASE STUDY *An Exemplar Relevant to Advanced Practice Nursing*

Mrs. S. is a 52-year-old woman who has been suffering from the sequelae of stage 4 metastatic breast cancer for the past 3 years. All curative interventions, including surgical resection, chemotherapy, radiotherapy, hormone therapy, and experimental therapy, have failed to halt the progression of her disease, which now affects her lungs, liver, and bones, most notably her spine. Mrs. S.'s major distressing physical symptom is severe neuropathic pain, which radiates around her back to her abdomen. This pain has limited her ability to bathe, cook, eat, get dressed, and walk. Essentially all activities of daily living have been stripped from her, and she is now confined to bed under the care of her husband. Prior to her cancer, she prided herself on being extremely independent. Currently, her neuropathic pain is being managed by steroids, tricyclic antidepressants, neuroleptics, and methadone. Mrs. S. has two teenage children and has been on disability from her job as a television personality for the past several months. She is Baptist and is an active member of her church.

ASSESSMENT OF THE PATIENT AND FAMILY

Through daily interactions with Mrs. S. and her family, the APN on the PC unit built a therapeutic relationship that focused on all dimensions of human suffering: physical, psychological, spiritual, and psychosocial. Despite the aggressive titration of pharmacotherapy being used to treat Mrs. S.'s pain, she continued to suffer from intense neuropathic discomfort. Her pain rating consistently was eight or above out of 10 on a visual analog scale, and over time, her sense of despair about dying in such agony was increasing. In consultation with other interprofessional team members, the APN was analyzing current research and consulting with other pain experts for novel approaches in treating neuropathic pain. The use of intravenous lidocaine has been successful in similar scenarios, and after critical analysis by the APN, the interprofessional team decided to try this therapy. The APN presented all the literature regarding the use of intravenous lidocaine in refractory neuropathic pain to the hospital's quality committee. The committee granted permission for immediate use and requested that the APN develop an evidence-based guideline to be used in future for patients with neuropathic pain. The APN quickly developed an evidence-based guideline as the neuropathic pain was escalating daily. The next step was to educate all team members, specifically, the nursing and pharmacy staff, as well as the patient and family, about the etiology, sequelae, and rationale for choosing this intervention. Mrs. S. received a test dose of the lidocaine and her pain decreased about 10% within 1 hour. Thus, the intravenous lidocaine was deemed appropriate to continue. Over the next days, her pain level decreased to two out of 10. Respecting the value of nonpharmacological measures in relieving pain, the APN assisted in having Mrs. S. offered massage and music therapy. She declined guided imagery.

While Mrs. S. was experiencing her pain crisis, the APN spent a lot of time with her, thus allowing an opportunity for Mrs. S. to express her feelings and fears. She revealed that she felt close to death and was struggling with guilt about one of her desires upon dying—that of spending her last minutes alone, if possible. She was fearful that this request would offend her very protective and involved family. But she had lived a very independent life and wanted to die that way. The APN listened, reflected, and assessed the situation and reported her findings to the interprofessional team. Based on the APN's observations and recommendations, the interprofessional team members set forth a plan to help Mrs. S. and her family deal with these very important issues. Social work and chaplaincy intensified their involvement.

Through interventions by the interprofessional team, Mrs. S.'s family was learning to become more comfortable with respecting her request and were working through their feelings of "abandoning" their wife and mother in time of need. This would continue to be a process.

With in-depth knowledge of family systems theory, the APN identified the need for the interprofessional team to address the already actualized loss of Mrs. S.'s role within the family, including that of mother and wife. The APN consulted the bereavement counselor as an early intervention for high-risk grief status, as Mrs. S.'s family was still dealing with their loved one's request of dying alone.

Progressively, Mrs. S. showed signs and symptoms of nearing death. As her pain increased, the APN adjusted Mrs. S.'s pain regimen so that she would remain comfortable. The APN and the interprofessional team increased support to Mrs. S.'s family to help them honor her wish for privacy at the time of death.

By maintaining a consistent presence with the patient and family and among the interprofessional team members, the APN helped to minimize decision-making conflicts. With advanced knowledge in the humanities, the APN, through language and image, gave expression to the experience of illness, death, grief, and human suffering.

DISCUSSION OF THE ADVANCED PRACTICE NURSE'S ROLE

Clinician. The APN utilized sophisticated and appropriate assessment strategies to evaluate pain and symptoms. The APN interfaced with other interprofessional team members to develop and implement a comprehensive plan of care. The APN identified novel approaches to the treatment of neuropathic pain and developed hospital-based standards of practice to reflect and support this treatment strategy and then executed the interventions. Advanced clinical knowledge of complex pain syndromes and comfort measures used to address symptoms was demonstrated through utilization of innovative, ethically sound, and scientifically based practice.

Educator. The APN facilitated complex philosophical, ethical, and clinical management discussions that assisted the patient, family, and all interprofessional team members in achieving a positive outcome. The APN assessed the learning needs of Mrs. S. and her family and the entire staff. The APN presented scientifically based education on the following issues: (a) the management of neuropathic pain, (b) the potential for role conflict, (c) the actual loss/anticipatory grief, and (d) the potential for high-risk bereavement. The APN also educated other disciplines; for example, she influenced the quality committee and pharmacy staff through in-service activities and guidelines on the philosophy of PC and developed individualized treatment strategies, most notable, the use of intravenous lidocaine for intractable neuropathic pain.

Researcher. The APN generated new knowledge through research and the translation of evidence into practice. The APN investigated and integrated PC research strategies, for example, the use of intravenous lidocaine, to formulate an individualized plan of care for Mrs. S.

Collaborator. The APN mentored staff in biopsychosocial and spiritual assessments and interventions. The APN built and preserved collaborative relationships and identified resources and opportunities to work with PC colleagues. The APN facilitated the development and implementation of staff forums, in-service training, physician–nurse collaboration, and quality committee consultation. The APN demonstrated the value of collaboration with the patient and family, the interprofessional team, and other healthcare professionals to facilitate the best possible outcome.

Consultant. The APN consulted with the PC physician, PC colleagues, and quality-committee representatives to determine the appropriate treatment strategies for meeting the needs of the patient and family. Also, the bereavement counselor was consulted after the APN identified the actualized loss experienced by Mrs. S.'s family. As a consultant, the APN was consistently available to the patient and family, interprofessional team members, and other healthcare professionals to discuss and explain issues surrounding the PC philosophy.

■ CONCLUSIONS

Generalist nurses and APNs in PC and hospice care bring a specific and well-defined set of qualities, knowledge, and judgments to caring for individuals and families facing serious, progressive, or life-threatening illness. This includes advanced scientific and biopsychosocial–cultural–spiritual knowledge, analytical skills, and mastery of a broad repertoire of communication and interpersonal skills.

Evidence suggests that early interventions of PC improve QOL, cost of care, and even survival in patients with metastatic cancer. Until recently, data from RCTs demonstrating the benefits of PC in patients with metastatic cancer who are also receiving standard oncology care have not been available (Smith et al., 2012). PC is an emerging specialty within healthcare and nursing. The philosophy and delivery of PC transcends all areas of nursing where suffering accompanies illness. The PC nurse is a true leader within the interprofessional team and hence is in an ideal position to establish standards for consistent practice, foster education, and promote research. It is a professional privilege to be in the field of PC nursing as it brings hopefulness to areas of EOL care that traditionally have been avoided—for example, ethics, pain, and human suffering. Equally applicable to the art of PC nursing practice is Thoreau's (1854) statement: "It is something to be able to paint a picture, or to carve a statue, and to make a few objects beautiful. But it is far more glorious to carve and paint the atmosphere in which we work, to affect the quality of the day—this is the highest of the arts" (p. 90).

CASE STUDY

AN INTERPROFESSIONAL PERSPECTIVE

Mackenzie Frederick, BS in Nutrition Sciences, Dietetic Technician, Registered (DTR)

Although Mrs. S. is suffering from severe pain, her other major distressing physical problem was malnutrition. The role of the dietician in the PC interdisciplinary team is to assess patients for adequate dietary and fluid intake, recommend interventions that will increase QOL, and evaluate the patient's nutritional status. Most cancer patients who are receiving PC pass away from malnutrition, so measures to maintain an adequate dietary intake preserve life and increase QOL. As such, nutrition goals are directed at these measures rather than increasing weight.

The dietician should remove all dietary restrictions placed on the patient and should not impose calorie or protein goals. Any dietary intake is encouraged. The dietician will assess the patient for intake by performing a 24-hour recall, and help the patient to determine what types of foods he or she would enjoy eating or previously have enjoyed. The patient's activity tolerance would be evaluated to identify tasks that can be performed in the kitchen, such as peeling vegetables while sitting at a kitchen table. The family will be coached to involve the patient in any way so as to increase QOL by participating in tasks that are enjoyable.

A particular area of focus for the dietician who is on the interprofessional PC team is assessment of bowel patterns, gastrointestinal (GI) disturbances, and fluid intake. Patients with cancer experience a range of GI problems secondary to chemotherapy and pain medications. These problems include early satiety, loss of appetite, loss of or altered taste, nausea, vomiting, constipation, and dehydration. A patient like Mrs. S. is at a high risk for dehydration, which is the number one reason for hospitalization in patients receiving PC. If the risk is identified early, the patient can be coached on strategies that encourage fluid intake or the patient can receive IV fluids several times a week in a clinic or treatment facility to avoid hospitalization.

The dietician who recognizes opioid-induced constipation will recommend stool softeners or laxatives to be added to the medication regimen.

Patients can experience loss of appetite secondary to depression, and in the event that depression is disclosed to the dietician, a referral to counseling or social services would be made. Patients who may also express interest in regaining strength lost from muscle atrophy secondary to malnutrition are referred to physical therapy.

Evidence-Based Practice

McCorkle, R., Jeon, S., Ercolano, E., Lazenby, M., Reid, A., Davies, M., … Gettinger, S. (2015). An advanced practice nurse coordinated multidisciplinary interventions for patients with late-stage cancer: A cluster randomized trial. *Journal of Palliative Medicine, 18*(11), 962–969. doi:10.1089/jpm.2015.0113

ABSTRACT

Background
It has been demonstrated that patient health outcomes improve when the PC team is consulted. There are few studies that document patient's self-reported clinical outcomes when PC is integrated within comprehensive cancer care.

Objective

To evaluate the effects of a multidisciplinary coordinated intervention by APNs at the oncology clinic level, as compared with patients newly diagnosed with advanced cancer seen by the usual multidisciplinary oncology care team.

Methods

Clustered RCT of 146 patients who were enrolled with late-stage cancer from four disease-specific multidisciplinary oncology clinics (gynecology, lung, head and neck, and gastrointestinal) and randomized to a 10-week standardized intervention or usual oncology care. The intervention was delivered by different members of the multidisciplinary oncology team, but was coordinated by an APN. The intervention included monitoring patient's status, providing symptom relief, teaching patients and their family caregivers, coordinating care, responding to questions, and executing complex care procedures. The usual oncology care group also involved multidisciplinary care but was not coordinated by an APN. Patient's self-reported health, health distress, symptoms, depression, anxiety, uncertainty, self-efficacy, functional status, and QOL were recorded at baseline and at 1 and 3 months.

Results

There was no statistically significant difference between the intervention group directed by an APN and the usual disease-specific multidisciplinary oncology care groups at 1 and 3 months postbaseline. However, physical and emotional symptoms remained stable or significantly improved for both groups.

Conclusions

For patients with advanced cancer, their self-reported clinical outcomes remained stable or improved in both the intervention and the usual care groups over time. A multidisciplinary approach to cancer care with the integration of PC into disease-specific comprehensive oncology care results in stable or improved patient outcomes.

■ REFERENCES

Advancing Expert Care. (2016). Shared mission, vision and pillars. Retrieved from http://advancingexpertcare.org/about/shared-mission-vision-pillars

Amenta, M. O. (2001). History of the Hospice Nurses Association. *Journal of Hospice and Palliative Nursing, 3,* 128–136. doi:10.1097/NJH.0b013e3182331160

American Association of Colleges of Nursing. (1997). Peaceful death: Recommended competencies and curricular guidelines for end-of-life nursing care. Retrieved from https://files.eric.ed.gov/fulltext/ED453706.pdf

American Board of Nursing Specialties. (2017). About us. Retrieved from http://www.nursingcertification.org/about

American Nurses Association and Hospice and Palliative Nurses Association. (2014). *Palliative nursing: An essential resource for hospice and palliative nurses.* Silver Spring, MD: American Nurses Association. Retrieved from https://www.hpna.org/FileMaintenance_View.aspx?ID=2157

Beauchamp, T. L. (2003). Methods and principles in biomedical ethics. *British Medical Journal, 29,* 269–274. doi:10.1136/jme.29.5.269

Billings, J. A., & Block, S. (1997). Palliative care in undergraduate medical education. Status report and future directions. *Journal of the American Medical Association, 278*(9), 733–738. doi:10.1001/jama.1997.03550090057033

Block, S. D. (2007). Clinical and ethical issues in palliative care. *Focus, 5,* 393–397. doi:10.1176/foc.5.4.foc393

Boland, J., & Johnson, M. (2013). End-of-life care for non-cancer patients. *BMJ Supportive and Palliative Care, 3,* 2–3. doi:10.1136/bmjspcare-2013-000446

Bruera, E., & Hui, D. (2012). Conceptual models for integrating palliative care at cancer centers. *Journal of Palliative Medicine, 15*(11), 1261–1269. doi:10.1089/jpm.2012.0147

Bryant-Lukosius, D., Dicenso, A., Browne, G., & Pinelli, J. (2004). Advanced practice nursing roles: Development, implementation and evaluation. *Journal of Advanced Nursing, 48*(5), 519–529. doi:10.1111/j.1365-2648.2004.03234.x

Cairns, W., & Yates, P. M. (2003). Education and training in palliative care. *Medical Journal of Australia*, *179*(6 Suppl.), S26–S28.

Callaway, C. (2012). Timing is everything: When to consult palliative care. *Journal of the American Academy of Nurse Practitioners*, *24*(11), 633–639. doi:10.1111/j.1745-7599.2012.00746.x

Chiu, N., Cheon, P., Lutz, S., Lao, N., Pulenzas, N., Chiu, L., … Chow, E. (2015). Inadequacy of palliative training in the medical school curriculum. *Journal of Cancer Education*, *30*, 749–753. doi:10.1007/s13187-014-0762-3

Chulk, P. (2008). Clinical nurse specialists and quality patient care. *Journal of Advanced Nursing*, *26*, 501–506. doi:10.1046/j.1365-2648.1997.t01-9-00999.x

Coyne, P. J. (2003). The evolution of the advanced practice nurse within palliative care. *Journal of Palliative Medicine*, *6*(5), 769–770. doi:10.1089/109662103322515275

De Lima, L., & Pastrana, T. (2016). Opportunities for palliative care in public health. *Annual Review of Public Health*, *37*, 357–374. doi:10.1146/annurev-publhealth-032315-021448

Dy, S. M., Lupu, D., & Seow, H. (2012). Progress towards systems of quality measurement that capture the essence of good palliative care. *Palliative Medicine*, *26*(4), 291–293. doi:10.1177/0269216312444796

Faull, C. (2012). Context and principles of palliative care. In C. Faull, S. de Caestecker, A. Nicholson, & F. Black (Eds), *The handbook of palliative care* (3rd ed.). London, England: Wiley Blackwell.

Ferrell, B. R., Coyle, N., & Paice, J. A. (2015). *Oxford textbook of palliative nursing* (4th ed.). Oxford, England: Oxford University Press.

Ferrell, M. (2017). *Smeltzer & Bare's textbook of medical surgical nursing*. Philadelphia, PA: Wolters Kluwer.

Field, M. J., & Cassel, C. K. (1997). *Approaching death: Improving care at the end of life* (The Institute of Medicine Consensus Study Report). Washington, DC: National Academies Press.

Foley, K. M., & Gelband, H. (Eds). (2001). *Improving palliative care for cancer*. Washington, DC: National Academies Press.

Gill, T. M., Gahbauer, E. A., Han, L., & Allore, H. B. (2010). Trajectories of disability in the last year of life. *New England Journal of Medicine*, *362*(13), 1173–1180. doi:10.1056/NEJMoa0909087

Haley, W. (2013). Family caregiving at the end-of-life: Current status and future directions. In R. C. Talley & R. J. V. Montgomery (Eds), *Caregiving across a lifespan* (pp. 157–175). New York, NY: Springer Publishing.

Hospice and Palliative Nurses Association. (2017a). Membership map. Retrieved from http://www.hpna.org/hpna_map.aspx

Hospice and Palliative Nurses Association. (2017b). *Value of the professional nurse in palliative care*. Pittsburgh, PA: Author.

Hospice and Palliative Nurses Association and American Nurses Association. (2007). *Hospice and palliative nursing scope & standards of practice*. Silver Spring, MD: American Nurses Association.

Institute of Medicine, Committee on Quality of Healthcare in America. (2001). *Crossing the quality chasm: A new health system for the 21st century*. Washington, DC: National Academies Press.

Kaplan, G., Bo-Linn, P., Carayon, P., Pronovost, W., Rouse, P., & Saunders, R. (2013). *Bringing a systems approach to health* (Discussion Paper). Washington, DC: Institute of Medicine and National Academy of Engineering. Retrieved from https://nam.edu/perspectives-2013-bringing-a-systems-approach-to-health

Kochanek, K. D., Murphy, S. L., Xu, J. Q., & Arias, E. (2017). *Mortality in the United States, 2016*. NCHS Data Brief, no. 293. Hyattsville, MD: National Center for Health Statistics.

Kuebler, K. K. (2003). The palliative care advanced practice nurse. *Journal of Palliative Medicine*, *6*(5), 707–714. doi:10.1089/109662103322515211

Lage, A., & Crombet, T. (2011). Control of advanced cancer: The road to chronicity. *International Journal of Environmental Research and Public Health*, *8*(3), 683–697. doi:10.3390/ijerph8030683

Leslie, B., Adams, L., & Kutner, J. S. (2002). Integrating an end-of-life curriculum into the internal medicine clerkship. *Journal of Palliative Medicine*, *5*(5), 752–753. doi:10.1089/109662102320880615

Lunney, J. R., Lynn, J., Foley, D. J., Lipson, S., & Guralnik, J. M. (2003). Patterns of functional decline at the end of life. *Journal of the American Medical Association*, *289*, 2387–2392. doi:10.1001/jama.289.18.2387

Maani-Fogelman, P., & Bakitas, M. A. (2015). Hospital-based palliative care. In B. R. Ferrell, N. Coyle, & J. A. Paice (Eds), *Oxford textbook of palliative nursing* (4th ed., pp. 41–57). New York, NY: Oxford University Press.

Meier, D. E., & Beresford, L. (2006). Advanced practice nurses in palliative care: A pivotal role and perspective. *Journal of Palliative Medicine*, *9*(3), 624–627. doi:10.1089/jpm.2006.9.624

Meier, D. E., & Beresford, L. (2008). The palliative care team. *Journal of Palliative Medicine*, *11*(5), 677–681. doi:10.1089/jpm.2008.9907

Mitchell, H., Noble, S., Finlay, I., & Nelson, A. (2015). Defining the palliative care patient: Its challenges and implications for service delivery. *BMJ Supportive & Palliative Care*, *5*, 46–52. doi:10.1136/bmjspcare-2012–000220

Morrison, R. S., Augustin, R., Souvanna, P., & Meier, D. E. (2011). America's care of serious illness: A state-by-state report card on access to palliative care in our nation's hospitals. *Journal of Palliative Medicine*, *14*(10), 1094–1096. doi:10.1089/jpm.2011.9634

Morrison, R. S., & Meier, D. E. (2004). Clinical practice: Palliative care. *New England Journal of Medicine*, *350*(25), 2582–2590. doi:10.1056/NEJMcp035232

Mount, B., Hanks, G., & McGoldrick, L. (2006). The principles of palliative care. In M. Fallon & G. Hanks (Eds), *ABC of palliative care* (2nd ed., pp. 1–4). Oxford, England: Blackwell.

Munday, D., & Charlton, R. (2012). Palliative care in the community. In C. Faull, S. de Caestecker, A. Nicholson, & F. Black (Eds), *The handbook of palliative care* (3rd ed.). London, England: Wiley Blackwell.

National Center for Health Statistics. (2016). *Health, United States, 2015: With special feature on racial and ethnic health disparities*. Hyattsville, MD: Author.

National Consensus Project. (2013). *Clinical practice guidelines for quality palliative care* (3rd ed.). Pittsburgh, PA: National Consensus Project for Quality Palliative Care. Retrieved from https://www.nationalcoalitionhpc.org/ncp-guidelines-2013

National Hospice and Palliative Care Organization. (2015). *NHPCO facts and figures: Hospice care in America.* Alexandria, VA: Author.

National Quality Forum. (2012). Palliative care and end-of-life care. Retrieved from www.qualityforum.org/Projects/Palliative_care_and_end-of-life_care.aspx

Oliviere, D., & Hargreaves, R. (2017). *Good practices in palliative care: A psychosocial perspective.* Aldershot, England: Ashgate (Routledge).

Paice, J. A., Ferrell, B. R., Virani, R., Grant, M., Malloy, P., & Rhome, A. (2006a). Appraisal of the graduate end-of-life nursing education consortium training program. *Journal of Palliative Medicine, 9*(2), 353–360. doi:10.1089/jpm.2006.9.353

Paice, J. A., Ferrell, B. R., Virani, R., Grant, M., Malloy, P., & Rhome, A. (2006b). Graduate nursing education regarding end-of-life care: Solutions to an urgent need. *Nursing Outlook, 54*(1), 45–52. doi:10.1016/j.outlook.2005.04.003

Shea, J., Grossman, S., Wallace, M., & Lange, J. (2010). Assessment of advanced practice palliative care nursing competencies in nurse practitioner students: Implications for the integration of ELNEC curricular modules. *Journal of Nursing Education, 49*(4), 183–189. doi:10.3928/01484834-20090915-05

Smith, T. J., Temin, S., Alesi, E. R., Abernethy, A. P., Balboni, T. A., Basch, E. M., … Von Roenn, J. H. (2012). American Society of Clinical Oncology provisional clinical opinion: The integration of palliative care into standard oncology care. *Journal of Clinical Oncology, 30*(8), 880–887. doi:10.1200/JCO.2011.38.5161

Stiel, S., Matthies, D. M. K., Seub, D., Walsh, D., Lindena, G., & Ostagthe, C. (2014). Symptoms and problem clusters in cancer and non-cancer patients in specialized palliative care: Is there a difference? *Journal of Pain and Symptom Management, 48*(1), 26–35. doi:10.1016/j.jpainsymman.2013.08.018

SUPPORT Study Investigators. (1995). A controlled trial to improve care for seriously ill hospitalized patients: The study to understand progress and preference for outcomes and risks for treatments (SUPPORT). *Journal of the American Medical Association, 274,* 1591–1598. doi:10.1001/jama.1995.03530200027032

Temel, J. S., Greer, J. A., Admane, S., Gallagher, E. R., Jackson, V. A., Lynch, T. J., … Piri, W. F. (2011). Longitudinal perceptions of prognosis and goals of therapy in patients with metastatic non-small-cell lung cancer: Results of a randomized study of early palliative care. *Journal of Clinical Oncology, 29*(17), 2319–2326. doi:10.1200/JCO.2010.32.4459

Temel, J. S., Greer, J. A., Muzikansky, A., Gallagher, E. R., Admane, S., Jackson, V. A., … Lynch, T. J. (2010). Early palliative care for patients with metastatic non-small-cell lung cancer. *New England Journal of Medicine, 363,* 733–742. doi:10.1056/NEJMoa1000678

Thoreau, H. D. (1854). *Walden; or, life in the woods.* Boston, MA: Ticknor and Fields.

World Health Organization. (2017). WHO definition of palliative care. Retrieved from http://www.who.int/cancer/palliative/definition/en

Xu, J., Murphy, S. L., Dochanek, K. D., & Arias, E. (2016). *NCHS Data Brief, No. 267: Mortality in the United States, 2015.* Hyattsville, MD: National Center for Health Statistics.

Deborah Witt Sherman & Marilyn Bookbinder

Palliative Care: Responsive to the Need for Healthcare Reform in the United States

CHAPTER

2

Hospice care originated in the 11th century and was afforded to weary travelers on religious pilgrimages; later it was identified as the care of the sick and dying. By the 14th century, the term "palliate" was coined, which meant "to cloak" or "soothe" the symptoms associated with illness or its treatment (Connor, 1998). The principles of hospice care embrace holistic patient- and family-centered care, offered by an interprofessional team of practitioners. Built on the foundation of hospice care, palliative care (PC) addresses care of the mind, body, and spirit as health practitioners develop the most effective and appropriate plan of care for and with patients and families experiencing serious, life-threatening, progressive, or chronic illnesses. The difference between hospice care and PC is that PC begins at the time of diagnosis with such illnesses and continues until the death of the patient and into the bereavement period for families, whereas hospice care is provided during the last 6 months of life. Unlike hospice care, PC is not dependent on prognosis and can be provided in the context of curative treatments, curing what can be cured, but with the concurrent attempt to alleviate symptoms caused by the disease or its treatment. Both palliative and hospice care can be the main focus of care when solely comfort and supportive interventions are desired to promote quality of life (QOL) until its end (Sherman et al., 2016–2020). Currently, palliative and hospice care are considered on a continuum of care, with PC beginning earlier in the illness trajectory and potentially continuing until death, as compared to hospice care, which is at the end of the illness trajectory, supporting patients and families in the last stages of life. However, not all patients who are dying choose hospice, nor do they meet the eligibility criteria to be enrolled in hospice care, which is a Medicare benefit. Where hospice strives to maximize comfort for the patient, PC can provide patients with disease-modifying or supportive treatments regardless of their diagnoses even when they are living with chronic and serious illnesses (Kelley & Meier, 2015).

CASE STUDY

Mr. H. is an 89-year-old male with mild dementia, advanced heart disease, chronic constipation, and rheumatoid arthritis. He lives alone in a small apartment outside the city. His wife died 1 year ago and his two children live in the suburbs, about 2 hours away. His sight and balance have progressively worsened within the last 6 months, and he constantly has extreme edema in his lower extremities. He depends on home delivery from a fast-food restaurant near his apartment that was arranged by his children. The children bring canned and processed foods during their monthly visits. Recently, Mr. H. had a fall in his apartment in the middle of the night on route to the bathroom. He couldn't get up and couldn't reach his phone to call for help. His neighbor heard his call for help and dialed 911.

At the hospital, Mr. H. was treated for acute pain as well as fluid overload. Following an abdominal x-ray, the doctors also discovered that he had a large bowel obstruction from what appeared to be a tumor. He was in a lot of pain and overwhelmed by being in the hospital setting. He had trouble comprehending the healthcare team who were discussing his treatment options.

His daughter arrived at the hospital and asked whether she could speak with the hospitalist caring for her father. After some discussion, the hospitalist consulted the PC team at the hospital. Mr. H.'s daughter informed the PC team that Mr. H. had been experiencing moderate to severe chronic pain and had fallen multiple times in his apartment. He also had a long history of constipation. Working together, the PC team, including a nurse practitioner, worked with Mr. H. and his daughter to discuss a plan of care for him both in the hospital and after discharge. Mr. H.'s daughter was concerned that he had no one to care for him once he got home because she lived so far away. The PC team recommended home-health PC to help manage Mr. H.'s pain and constipation, as well as a home-safety and fall-risk evaluation, and physical therapy. His children were not yet prepared to enroll their father in hospice.

Mr. H. was discharged home. His daughter arranged a private aid to assist him with activities of daily living and him to receive weekly visits from his PC team, including a nurse and a physical therapist, who helped him with pain management, comfort measures, and mobility. However, after 6 months he could not walk without two people assisting him; he lost his appetite, lost weight, and was asking for his children all the time. The PC team made recommendations to reconsider hospice enrollment, which would provide additional services to support both Mr. H. and his family. Mr. H.'s daughter took time off from work to stay with him in the apartment and agreed to hospice care for her father. Within a week, Mr. H. passed away peacefully at home with his children present; he had the support of the hospice nurse and team, and his symptoms were alleviated.

■ PALLIATIVE CARE: MOVING INTO THE MAINSTREAM OF HEALTHCARE

PC is moving into the mainstream of healthcare as a highly structured and organized system of care (National Consensus Project for Quality Palliative Care, 2013). PC addresses the physical, emotional, social, and cultural needs of patients and their families. It embraces an inherent philosophy of comprehensive and patient- or family-centered care, which matches treatments with the values and preferences of the patient and family (Meier, 2010). PC promotes positive health outcomes, such as alleviation of pain and other symptoms, optimization of function, and social support, as well as spiritual and personal growth (National Consensus Project for Quality Palliative Care, 2013). The World Health Organization (WHO, 2015) describes PC as "an approach that improves the quality of life of patients and their families through the prevention and relief of suffering."

PC is offered to patients experiencing a wide range of illnesses, including neonates with congenital anomalies or intrauterine health conditions; individuals with progressive, chronic, or debilitating illness or life-limiting injuries; and those with advancing diseases, such as cancers, end-stage organ diseases, HIV/AIDS, neurodegenerative disorders, and dementia (National Consensus Project for Quality Palliative Care, 2013). PC allows practitioners of various health disciplines to bring their specialized competencies and expertise to focus on serious and complex health problems. PC practitioners combine their clinical expertise and judgment with the best evidence available through research and an understanding of the preferences of patients and families, known as *evidence-based care* (Sherman et al., 2016–2020). At the various stages of disease, PC provides relief of pain and symptoms, increases communication about care and continuity of care, offers support for family caregivers, improves survival, and reduces healthcare costs (Meier & Beresford, 2009).

There are several clinical models of PC, including programs offered by consultation services within a hospital or on a designated PC unit, as well as in assisted-living facilities, nursing homes, community home-based programs, or ambulatory clinics. Similarly, hospice care is most often offered in the home, but can be provided in hospitals, assisted-living facilities, nursing homes, or residential hospices (Kamal, Currow, Ritchie, Bull, & Abernethy, 2013; Sherman et al., 2016–2020). In addition, with a greater need for PC, some institutions have unit-based PC teams, such as those in intensive care units, in addition to hospital-based teams.

■ PALLIATIVE CARE AND HEALTHCARE REFORM IN AMERICA

Seminal data provided by the SUPPORT study (1995) constituted the failing report card of U.S. hospitals in the care of the seriously ill and dying. Yet, 10 years later, Teno et al. (2004) reported that 25% of patients continued to report inadequate pain management, 33% of families reported inadequate emotional support, and 33% of patients indicated that they were not educated about the treatment of their symptoms nor were arrangements for follow-up care provided upon hospital discharge. The Joint Commission now recognizes the value of PC with a voluntary process of PC accreditation, and there is evidence that PC services improve pain management and provide continuity of care, as well as emotional and spiritual support, to patients and their families (Teno et al., 2004). Within the context of healthcare reform, it is realized that PC promotes quality health outcomes, providing added value while lowering costs.

In the United States, the federal government has estimated that the population of individuals aged 85 and older will grow from 5.3 million in 2006 to nearly 21 million by 2050 (Federal Interagency Forum on Aging Related Statistics, 2016b). In 2030, the number of people age 65 and over is projected to more than double from the year 2000, growing from 35 million to 74 million and representing 21% of the total U.S. population (Federal Interagency Forum on Aging Related Statistics, 2016a). Furthermore, the U.S. per capita spending on healthcare is greater than anywhere else in the world. It is reported that $2.4 trillion was spent on healthcare in 2008 (Medicare Payment Advisory Commission, 2009). National Health Expenditure (NHE) grew 5.8% to $3.2 trillion in 2015, or $9,900 per person, and accounted for 17.8% of gross domestic product (GDP; National Health Expenditure [NHE], 2016a). In 2013 the United States spent $2.9 trillion and, by 2040, "one out of every three dollars spent in the United States will be spent on healthcare" (Kelley & Meier, 2015, p. 212). There is also a rapid growth in the eligible nursing home population, which represents 6% to 7% of the Medicaid population and more than half of all Medicaid expenditures (Huskamp, Stevenson, Chernew, & Newhouse, 2010; Kaiser Family Foundation, 2011; Meier, Lim, & Carlson, 2010; Mitchell et al., 2009). In response to current economic crises and the escalating costs of healthcare, hospitals are responding by reducing services and staffing, creating mergers with other institutions, and divesting assets, all of which have significant implications for quality healthcare (American Hospital Association, 2008). It is also realized that increased healthcare costs do not necessarily result in better care. This is supported by data indicating that the highest mortality rates are associated with regions with highest utilization, the highest number of specialists, and the greatest number of ICU patients and hospital days (Fisher, Wennberg, Stukel, & Gottlieb, 2004; Fisher et al., 2003; Mitka, 2006).

As a new paradigm of healthcare, PC is responsive to the need for healthcare reform in America and globally (Sherman & Cheon, 2012). With Medicare, hospice can be restricted to only those who qualify with a specific diagnosis of less than 6 months to live and a daily total of $156 per day for costs. PC can address the comprehensive needs of patients and families who do not meet hospice eligibility criteria or do not wish to enroll in hospice (Kelley & Meier, 2015). It is positioned to become a universally accepted approach to healthcare with the imperative of improving QOL and quality of dying across the illness/dying trajectory and into the bereavement period of families.

Given the current political climate in the United States after the presidential election of 2016, there is contentious debate regarding the repeal and replace of the Affordable Care Act passed by the Obama Whitehouse, which insured healthcare for millions of uninsured Americans and insurance to those with preexisting medical conditions. Although both the House and the Senate, as well as the executive branch, are Republican, there is intense disagreement on the passage of any healthcare plan. As of July 2017, if no agreement can be reached among the Republican Party, leader of the Senate indicates that Republicans must reach across the isle and work with Democrats to create a new healthcare plan or reform the Affordable Care Act. The passage of the Affordable Care Act in March 2010 expanded the access to healthcare for more than 30 million Americans (Pelosi, 2010). Individuals were to be guaranteed insurance coverage for preexisting conditions, along with the expansion of Medicaid to include more low-income Americans (Foster, 2009; Keehan et al., 2011). There was also a projected reduction of $400 billion in Medicare expenditures over a 10-year period (Pelosi, 2010). Under the Affordable Care Act of 2010, the Centers for Medicare and Medicaid Services (CMS) were required to implement a 3-year demonstration project. This project allowed patients to receive aggressive treatment and palliative/hospice care concurrently (Office of the Legislative Counsel, 2010). This would require an evaluation of the current hospice eligibility criteria; the current criteria may need to be relaxed regarding the current requirement of a less than 6-month prognosis (Casarett, 2011). Additional project outcomes to be measured were the cost saving of palliative home healthcare programs and evaluation of patients' and families' QOL. A hypothesis of this project was that there will be improved survival rates, as compared to usual care, when PC is offered in addition to life-sustaining treatments (Temel et al., 2010). Meier and Beresford (2009) emphasize that PC is extremely relevant in promoting healthcare reform and ensuring effective, quality, and consistent healthcare delivery. Data indicate that when PC is offered in conjunction with aggressive disease treatment, there is a reduction in healthcare utilization and costs (Brumley et al., 2007; Temel et al., 2010).

■ THE VALUE OF PALLIATIVE CARE IN THE UNITED STATES

PC not only lowers the cost of healthcare but also improves health-related outcomes for patients and families. As more and more individuals express their desire to remain at home during an illness and to die at home, PC allows the shift of care from hospital to home (Brumley et al., 2007). The result is fewer hospital days, fewer emergency department or physician office visits, and fewer days in a skilled nursing facility. Kamal et al. (2013) report that community PC programs result in the reduction of symptoms, improved QOL, increased survival, and improved patient and family satisfaction. PC–hospice partnerships create a commonsense allocation of healthcare resources as patients move across the illness trajectory and approach the end of life. Morrison et al. (2011) reported that PC, when compared to usual care, reduced the total costs of ICU admissions by $2,642, lowered the cost per day by $279, lowered the direct costs per admission by $1,696, and also reduced laboratory costs. It was further indicated that for a hospital with 400 beds, annual cost savings from PC is more than $1.3 million per year. May et al. (2015) found that among patients with a cancer diagnosis, early intervention with PC during hospital admission lowered cost equal to a 14% to 25% reduction in overall hospital costs during a hospital stay. Based on a report by the Health and Medicine Division (of the National Academies of Sciences, Engineering, and Medicine), if PC were fully integrated into the nation's hospitals, there would be a projected total cost savings of greater than $6 billion per year (Morrison et al., 2011). More recent, Kain and Eisenhauer (2016) reported that compared with no PC consultation, a PC consult within 2 days of hospital admission reduced inpatient care costs by 24%. The early intervention of PC assists patients and families in discussing the goals of care and the use of advanced technology in the face of incurable cancer.

Research by Penrod et al. (2010) indicated that for patients who receive PC on the hospital units, 44% are less likely to be admitted to an ICU when compared to usual-care patients. Furthermore, the length of stay was shortened by 3.5 days ($p < .01$) for those patients who received PC consults while still in the emergency department before transferring to an inpatient hospital unit (Wu, Newman, Lasher, & Brody, 2013). Overall, studies conclude that PC reduces the overuse of marginally effective, ineffective, and unnecessary treatments and results in fewer hospital readmissions, allowing greater continuity of care and the development of safe transition plans upon initial discharge (Penrod et al., 2006, 2010; Smith et al., 2003).

Additional positive health outcomes of PC include better

- Management of pain and other symptoms
- Emotional, spiritual, and social support of patients and families
- QOL for patients and families
- Patient/family satisfaction
- Handling of time-intensive family/patient/team meetings
- Coordination of care

- Specialty-level assistance to attending physicians
- Support for discharge planning staff
- Nurse and physician satisfaction (National Consensus Project for Quality Palliative Care, 2013)

Based on the National Palliative Care Research Center's (2015) state-by-state report card, PC has grown rapidly in the U.S. health system, with 90% of large hospitals with 300 or more beds now having a PC team. PC programs are most prevalent in the New England (88% of hospitals), Pacific (77% of hospitals), and Mid-Atlantic (77% of hospitals) areas, and least prevalent in the western south central (43%) and eastern south central (42%) states. In contrast, only 26% of for-profit hospitals, 37% of community hospitals, and 54% of public hospitals offered PC (National Palliative Care Research Center, 2015). In 2017, two thirds of hospitals across the nation had PC programs as compared to only 53% in 2008; currently, 90% of hospitals with 300 or more beds have palliative programs (Dumanovsky et al., 2016; National Palliative Care Registry, 2017). Furthermore, a study done by Rabow, O'Riordan, and Pantilat (2014) showed that outpatient and community-based PC services are dramatically less common compared to inpatient PC. Only 18% of 136 hospitals with an adult PC program had outpatient PC as well.

Although 92% of people polled believe that palliative services should be available at all hospitals, access to PC remains elusive for millions of Americans. Despite a 164% increase in the number of PC programs over the last 12 years (National Palliative Care Registry, 2017), there is state-to-state and region-to-region variability in accessibility and availability of PC (National Palliative Care Research Center, 2015). This remains an issue even into 2018.

In examining the gap between recommendations and practice of PC and hospice in cancer patients in the Department of Veterans Affairs (VA) and VA Purchased Care, Gidwani et al. (2016) reported that most veterans received hospice care (71%), whereas 52% received PC. Eligible Veterans and their dependents can get a range of healthcare services external to VA facilities through Purchased Care at Health Administration Center (www.ebenefits.va.gov/ebenefits/CHAMPVADashboard). However, there was variation with hospice enrollment based on the type of cancer; specifically, patients with prostate and hematological cancer were least likely to be enrolled. Fifty-nine percent of veterans were enrolled in hospice in the last 3 days of their lives, whereas the median number of days before death was 20. It was concluded that a gap remains between the timing of supportive services and that difficulties in prognosticating death were not fully responsible for underenrollment in hospice.

More promising are survey results from 2008 to 2011, which indicate that there has been an overall improvement in the PC grade of institutions (Center to Advance Palliative Care, 2015). Grades have improved from a grade of C to a grade of B, showing that by 2011, most states exceeded the minimal standards of quality PC. The overall grade received for PC programs in the United States was a B for 2015, which was the same grade as that in 2011 (Center to Advance Palliative Care, 2015). In fact, the number of states with an A grade increased from 3% in 2008 to 17% in 2015 (Center to Advance Palliative Care, 2015).

Issues related to the availability of PC may rest in part with a shortage of trained professionals in PC, particularly in public and community provider hospitals, which serve Americans who are without healthcare insurance or those who live in geographically isolated areas. Spetz et al. (2016) reviewed data from the 2012 to 2013 annual surveys of the National Palliative Care Registry, which indicate that only one quarter of participating PC programs have physicians in funded positions, whereas the majority of PC programs are lead by advanced practice and registered nurses. In addition, Aldridge et al. (2016) identified "a lack of awareness of palliative care services among respondents, the tendency of clinicians to equate palliative care with end-of-life (EOL) care and lack of adequate reimbursement for palliative care services by insurers" (p. 225) as further reasons for why there are multiple obstacles in relation to PC implementation. The current voluntary certification in PC, as recommended by The Joint Commission, as well as the expectation for hospitals to achieve Magnet status, supports the mandate for healthcare reform in America and the provision of PC for patients and families.

■ AN EXEMPLARY PALLIATIVE CARE ACTION PLAN DEVELOPED IN MARYLAND

In 2016, the State of Maryland focused on promoting healthcare reform in America by convening an interprofessional taskforce to update the Maryland Cancer Control Plan for Palliative and Hospice Care. The goal was to promote quality and affordable healthcare in the state (2016–2020 Maryland Comprehensive Cancer Control Plan, 2016; CDC Cooperative Agreement Number 5 U58 DP003919-04, https://ftp.cdc.gov/pub/publications/cancer/ccc/maryland_ccc_plan.pdf). This "Blueprint for Success in Palliative and Hospice Care" came at a time when citizens of the United States most needed a complement to cancer care. This comprehensive "all hands on deck" approach to healthcare is critical given an aging population, an increase in the number of cancer diagnoses, and an increase in the number of survivors of cancer and other life-threatening illnesses who live with their disease as chronic conditions, often with ongoing physical and emotional symptoms (Sherman et al., 2016–2020).

The blueprint endorses the belief that quality and affordable healthcare is important during any stage of the illness trajectory, particularly as disease progresses and death approaches, and necessitates the active involvement and the ongoing, collaborative efforts of patients,

families, communities, healthcare professionals, institutions, healthcare policy makers, legislators, and payers. These key stakeholders can ensure quality of care and QOL, lowered cost, increased access to cancer care and PC, greater coordination and continuity of care, and the reduction in health disparities (Sherman et al., 2016–2020).

The key stakeholder groups in palliative and hospice care include:

1. Patients, families, and communities
   - *Patients:* Individuals with a diagnosis of cancer at any phase of the illness experience
   - *Family:* Any individual who provides direct or indirect support to a patient experiencing cancer
   - *Community:* A group of interacting people living in a common location who share common values or interests
2. Healthcare professionals and associated staff
   - *Healthcare professionals:* All members of the PC and hospice interprofessional team, including physicians, nurses, social workers, psychologists, chaplains, pharmacists, and physical or occupational therapists, as well as the patient's oncologist or primary care physician
   - *Associated staff:* All individuals involved in the caring process who offer direct or indirect support in the care of oncology patients and their families across all healthcare settings
3. Institutions
   - All healthcare delivery systems that provide palliative or hospice care, such as medical centers, hospitals, rehabilitation hospitals, subacute and long-term care facilities, assisted-living facilities, hospices (inpatient, home, or residential), or related office/outpatient clinics
4. Healthcare policy makers, legislators, and payers
   - State and congressional legislators, the state executive branch of government, the CMS and the Centers for Disease Control and Prevention (CDC), insurers, philanthropists, caregiver advocacy organizations, as well as the business community, including employers (Sherman et al., 2016–2020)

Sherman et al. (2016–2020) proposed that Maryland's Action Plan for Palliative and Hospice Care highlight the critical need to achieve what they have identified as the "four As"—awareness, acknowledgment, access, and action—by each of the identified stakeholder groups, as identified in Table 2.1.

Each of the identified stakeholder groups need to develop an awareness of PC, acknowledge its value, promote access to quality palliative and hospice care, and take action to implement a standard of practice in palliative and hospice care (Sherman et al., 2016–2020).

According to Maryland's Action Plan, the education of patients, families, and communities regarding palliative and hospice care, including advanced care

TABLE 2.1 The "Four As" of Maryland's "Blueprint for Success" Action Plan

Awareness implies knowledge and appreciation gained through one's perceptions or by means of information about palliative and hospice care.
Acknowledgment is the recognition and acceptance of the value of palliative and hospice care.
Access is the right, privilege, or ability to make use of resources and information related to palliative and hospice care.
Action is the development, implementation, and evaluation of initiatives to promote palliative and hospice care, which will lead to inclusion of palliative and hospice care in the standards of care and setting of future goals.

planning, is imperative. Such knowledge will result in further conversations with healthcare providers, hospital administrators, policy makers, and insurers, as PC becomes consumer driven. With increased awareness and improved communication, there will also be the expectation that patients and families will be involved in personal healthcare decisions, with consideration of their wishes and preferences and greater assurance of individualized and patient- and family-focused care (Sherman et al., 2016–2020).

In addition, healthcare professionals must be educated to insure adequate staffing of PC programs, particularly given the increase in the number of programs. To increase the preparation of PC practitioners, medical, nursing, and social work schools are not only integrating PC into their curriculums, but are also creating graduate programs with a focus on PC. In addition, several interprofessional fellowship programs in PC are offered across the country, which reinforce the importance of interprofessional collaboration and teamwork. The development of PC and hospice competencies for health professionals requires the advancement of research in PC so that the knowledge from science, as well as the art of healing, can be integrated into clinical education and practice (Sherman et al., 2016–2020). Despite these efforts, there is still a significant barrier to the implementation of PC in the United States: the need for education. Because of a lack of sufficient training and satisfactory education of medical professionals and a misunderstanding of what PC entails by both providers and the public, PC is limited in effectiveness (Aldridge et al., 2016).

At the institutional level, administrators are important stakeholders as they acknowledge national priorities, incorporate PC goals and tactics into the institution's strategic plan, and provide substantial budgetary resources to ensure appropriate utilization of PC. With acknowledgment of the PC outcomes of cost savings, cost avoidance, quality care, and patient and family satisfaction, administrators must work to secure philanthropic contributions for hiring skilled and credentialed interprofessional health professionals (Sherman et al., 2016–2020).

As an important group of stakeholders, healthcare legislators, policy makers, and payers must be informed of barriers to accessing PC and the importance of

incorporating access to quality PC within the Patient's Bill of Rights. These stakeholder groups can facilitate change in quality standards, health policy, reimbursement, and incentives, which promote PC education and quality care across the illness trajectory (Aldridge et al., 2016). State governments can also promote the development of Centers of Excellence in PC, which support community provider hospitals and the care offered in urgent care centers and clinics. As data are tracked regarding the number of PC consults, patient and family outcomes, healthcare professional outcomes, and financial and economic outcomes, legislative agendas can be developed to further expand access to quality PC and address complex issues related to reimbursement for PC services. The time has also come for studies that focus on the comparative effectiveness of PC and hospice with traditional hospital care, bundled payments, and the funding of demonstration projects that test the integration of comprehensive PC in the care of patients with complex medical needs (Sherman et al., 2016–2020). As a stakeholder group, legislators, policy makers, and payers can ensure the implementation of PC initiatives that will slow the nation's total healthcare expenditures while improving the quality of healthcare in America (Sherman et al., 2016–2020).

Cornerstones of Maryland's Blueprint for Success Action Plan for palliative and hospice care include identified goals, objectives, and strategies related to palliative and hospice care, which have been described in relation to each of the "four As" (Table 2.2) for each of the stakeholder groups.

■ PALLIATIVE CARE AS A GLOBAL IMPERATIVE

PC arose from a movement outside of medicine as a response to what was recognized by some as "bad dying" (Gallagher & Baldwin, 2016, p. 256). The discipline of PC has developed exponentially over the last 40 years or so. Starting in the 1960s in the United Kingdom, through the pioneering work of Dame Cicely Saunders, expert care of the dying is now evident in many parts of the world (O'Connor & Gwyther, 2014). The *Global Atlas of Palliative Care at the End of Life* estimated that every year greater than 20 million patients need PC (WHO, 2014). Six percent of these patients are children. According to the *Atlas*, in 2011, approximately 3 million patients received PC and only one in 10 people in need is currently receiving it. Although most PC is provided in high-income countries (HIC), almost 80% of the global need is in low- and middle-income countries (LMIC). Only 20 countries have PC well integrated into their healthcare systems (De Lima, 2015). WHO and the International Association for Hospice and Palliative Care (IAHPC) are examples of associations that support and guide PC at an international level. IAHPC has representatives from more than 1,000 countries and has a vision of access to high-quality PC, which is integrated into all levels of healthcare systems and offered within the continuum of care and includes disease prevention, early diagnosis and treatment, and relieves suffering to the greatest extent possible. Adequate PC in a country requires "the four components of the WHO palliative care public health strategy: 1) adequate healthcare policies; and 2) education

---

TABLE 2.2   Goals, Objectives, and Strategies of the Maryland Blueprint for Success

Goal: To implement a blueprint for success for palliative and hospice care for patients and families experiencing cancer in the state of Maryland

Objective 1 (Awareness): To develop an awareness campaign to educate Maryland citizens about palliative and hospice care within 50% of Maryland jurisdictions

Strategies (by stakeholder group):

1) *Patients/families/communities* should seek information on palliative and hospice care and advanced care planning from their healthcare providers, public library, national and local cancer agencies, and local health department.
2) *Healthcare professionals* and associated staff should increase communication related to PC issues in patient conversations, healthcare publications, and media/marketing.
3) *Institutions* should initiate PC activities with the goal of obtaining buy-in from various constituencies.
4) *Healthcare legislators/policy makers/payers* should conduct an internal education effort on strategies to reduce barriers that Maryland residents face in regard to quality palliative and hospice care. The education effort should include widespread distribution, discussion, and the development of an action plan based on:
   ■ The 2009 *Workgroup Report on Hospice Care, Palliative Care, and End of Life Counseling*, released by the Maryland Attorney General's Counsel for Health Decisions Policy workgroup
   ■ Reports of the Maryland State Advisory Council on quality of care at the end of life

Objective 2 (Acknowledging the value): To increase the participation in and support for palliative and hospice care initiatives by stakeholders as outlined in the strategies

Strategies (by stakeholder group):

1) *Patients/families/communities* should participate in campaigns that support/promote palliative and hospice care and advanced care planning.
2) *Healthcare professionals and associated staff* should actively participate in palliative education and PC initiatives as demonstrated by attendance at national conferences, increase in certification and credentialing rates, and referral to PC services and hospice care.
3) *Institutions* should develop a strategic plan that incorporates goals and related tactics to institutionalize PC as it relates to ongoing professional education, implementing and maintaining supportive services for patient/families, supporting research and evidence-based practice, and driving healthcare policy and legislative initiatives that promote PC.
4) *Healthcare legislators/policy makers/payers* should conduct outreach efforts via email, town halls, and focus groups to educate constituents about the knowledge as well as financial and administrative barriers Maryland cancer patients and their families face in regard to palliative and hospice care and get their input on options to reduce them.

Objective 3 (Access): To increase access to palliative and hospice care services in Maryland

Strategies (by stakeholder group):

1) *Patients/families/communities* should request access to palliative and hospice services.
2) *Healthcare professionals and associated staff* should develop and implement educational programs (formal and informal) related to palliative and hospice care.
3) *Institutions* should
   ■ Develop a mechanism to track the percentage of PC consultations for hospital patients admitted with cancer.
   ■ Ensure clinical support through hiring a skilled and credentialed/certified team of interprofessional PC professionals and associated support staff in order to implement a PC consult service or other delivery models (such as an inpatient unit, an outpatient clinic, and a homecare program and/or establishing partnerships with community hospices).
4) *Healthcare legislators/policy makers/payers* should explore legislative options for expanding access to and payment for palliative and hospice care, building on best practices.

(continued)

TABLE 2.2   Goals, Objectives, and Strategies of the Maryland Blueprint for Success (*continued*)

Objective 4 (Action): For stakeholders to take ownership of the Blueprint for Success and act on 70% of the strategies recommended for each stakeholder group

Strategies (by stakeholder group):

1) *Patients/families/communities* should advocate for effective and compassionate PC across healthcare settings to ensure that the goals of care are achieved.

2) *Healthcare professionals and associated staff* should incorporate the National Quality Forum Preferred Practices of Palliative Care as a standard of care within the institution (National Quality Forum, 2006).

3) *Institutions* should initiate quality-improvement studies to evaluate the provision of quality PC by tracking the following:

   ■ Requests for PC consults
   ■ Patient/family and community outcomes
   ■ Healthcare professional outcomes
   ■ Economic outcomes

4) Healthcare legislators/policy makers/payers should support pilot programs that test the following:

   ■ The feasibility and impact of training lay workers to serve as palliative and hospice care counseling coaches and navigators
   ■ Reimbursement models for providing EOL care counseling
   ■ The impact of innovative clinical–financial models of palliative and hospice care for cancer patients and their families designed to reduce knowledge, financial, and administrative barriers to their use

Note: A more detailed version of the goals/objectives/strategies can be found on the Palliative and Hospice Care page of the Maryland Cancer Plan website: www.marylandcancerplan.org.

EOL, end-of-life; PC, palliative care.

Source: Sherman, D. W., Evans, S., Halstead, L., Kelleher, C., Kenworthy, C., Olson, L., & Piet, L. (2016–2020). Maryland comprehensive cancer control plan: Palliative and hospice care (pp. 8–9). Retrieved from https://phpa.health.maryland.gov/cancer/cancerplan/plan2011/Chapter15Palliative.pdf

of health providers, legislators, and the public; 3) availability of medications, and 4) implementations of services at all levels of care" (De Lima et al., 2017, p. 9). "At the end of the first decade of the 21st century, the provision of PC is beginning to feature in the political and policy agendas of many different countries as they seek to respond to the challenges of epidemiological and sociodemographic change, particularly given aging populations" (Seymour, 2011, p. 18).

In many countries, access to PC is being considered a human right (Sherman & Cheon, 2012). Wright, Wood, Lynch, and Clark (2008) have described the typology of PC globally by mapping its availability, specifically (a) no identified hospice/PC activities; (b) the capacity for developing PC, with no palliative services available; (c) the provision of localized PC; and (d) countries where PC is being integrated with mainstream healthcare services. Based on this mapping, PC services were reported in 115 of 234 countries. However, there was no identified activity in 78 (33%) countries; 41 (18%) countries had the capacity to build PC services; 80 (34%) countries had only localized provision of PC; and 35 (15%) countries approached integration. As nearly half of the world's countries do not have PC, there are many challenges to improve awareness of PC through education, to increase access to opioid medications for the management of pain and other symptoms, and secure institutional and political support for PC. A study on implementation of PC programs reveals that most hospitals does not meet the requirements per The Joint Commission standards. More funding and more education are needed

urgently. PC should be added to prelicensure programs and continuing-education programs to reach out to all healthcare personnel (Spetz et al., 2016).

Gidwani et al. (2016) report that "per WHO recommendations and a World Health Assembly Resolution, national governments must ensure access to palliative care and to essential medicines, including immediate release of oral morphine, for relief of pain and suffering. Failure to do so violates the right to health and freedom from cruel, inhumane, and degrading treatment" (De Lima et al., 2017, p. 10).

In day centers, such as those available in Great Britain, or for use with mobile PC teams, there is also a need to implement differing models of PC service delivery that go beyond traditional PC or hospice consultations or inpatient units (Centeno et al., 2007). Globally, there are recommendations to sustain, optimize, and expand the 8,000 dedicated PC services that currently exist in the world (Gomes, Harding, Foley, & Higginson, 2009).

International Recommendations for the Advancement of Palliative Care

"The WHO PHS [Public Health Service] suggests a measured approach and four essential elements to assist the successful implementation of palliative care. The four elements include: 1) engaging policymakers and governments so that palliative care is incorporated into national health policies and plans; 2) ensuring drug availability in relation to the issues of prescribing, costs, and distribution; 3) educational activities like public advocacy and developing palliative care content in the curricula of health disciplines; and 4) developing appropriate services for palliative care and utilizing opinion leaders and clinical leaders to develop resources, infrastructure and standards of care" (O'Connor & Gwyther, 2014, p. 7). To direct the international future of PC, a meeting of clinicians, health economists, researchers, policy makers, and advocates was convened with the identification of seven recommendations: (a) the importance of shared definitions of PC; (b) recognition of the strengths and weaknesses of different payment systems; (c) identification of country-specific and international research priorities; (d) determination of appropriate economic evaluation methods; (e) evaluation of PC costs; (f) the imperative to support interprofessional PC education and training programs; and (g) the development of national standards to regulate and determine PC planning and development (Gomes et al., 2009; Lynch et al., 2009). As leaders of healthcare globally, the United States, the United Kingdom, Canada, and Australia are at the forefront of providing quality palliative and hospice care and addressing these international recommendations.

Australia, as a world leader in hospice and PC, has been visionary in overcoming funding and financing issues, as there are shared responsibilities for managing the healthcare system for both the state and its territories (Gordon, Eagar, Currow, & Green, 2009). It rests on the premise that because there is no national model for funding inpatient or community PC services, states and territories must fund PC services. PC funding varies by the type of care offered and whether those who offer it are generalist providers, specialist providers, or those offering support services in nongovernment, private, and public sectors. PC continues to evolve rapidly as a healthcare service in Australia with flexible evidence-based models of care delivery that consider not only the type of provider but also diverse patient groups (Gordon et al., 2009).

To reduce discrepancies in the field of PC development, a web initiative called "ehospice" has been developed internationally. Ehospice is a collaborative venture in which national and regional PC organizations from around the world, including Africa, Australia, Canada, India, Kenya, South Africa, and the UK, provide information for specific counties or regions. Latin America and U.S. editions will be initiated soon. In addition, "the Worldwide Palliative Care Alliance and International Children's Palliative Care Network produce international editions for the adult and children's palliative care communities" (Ward & Jackson, 2013, p. 109).

■ PALLIATIVE AND HOSPICE CARE NURSES: LEADERS OF HEALTHCARE REFORM

Nursing is the world's largest and most trusted profession, with approximately 19.4 million nurses working globally (WHO, 2012). The integration of scientific,

aesthetic, personal, and ethical knowledge in nursing supports the leadership of nursing in reshaping societal perspectives regarding illness, dying, and death. Indeed, nurses who are educated in PC nursing "facilitate the caring process through a combination of science, presence, openness, compassion, mindful attention to detail, and teamwork" (Coyle, 2006, p. 5). In the 2014 report, *Dying in America* by the Health and Medicine Division of the National Academies of Sciences, Engineering, and Medicine, a committee of experts reported that improving the quality and availability of healthcare services for patients and their families could not only enhance QOL through the end of life, but may also contribute to a more sustainable care system. The Health and Medicine Division (of the National Academies of Sciences, Engineering, and Medicine) committee believes a person-centered, family-oriented approach that honors individual preferences and promotes QOL through the end of life should be a national priority (Institute of Medicine [IOM], 2015, p. 1, 4). Indeed, an interdisciplinary team of specialist nurses, counselors, spiritual care workers, PC doctors, bereavement counselors, trained volunteers, and other allied care support ensures a holistic rather than a medical model approach to care (O'Connor & Cowan, 2014). Professional nurses play a leading role as members of PC and hospice teams across the continuum of care. Professional PC nursing is grounded in the positive traditions of past practices while shaping care for the future to meet the evolving needs of chronically ill and dying patients. The professional nurse establishes and supports the methods and means to respond to these changing needs within organizations and communities (Hospice and Palliative Nurses Association [HPNA], 2015a, 2015b). As members of the interprofessional PC team, nurses, along with colleagues from other professions, create an effective and compassionate plan of care for patients and families facing serious, chronic, or life-threatening illness, which improves the quality of their lives.

In both generalist and specialist roles in palliative and hospice care, nurses are leaders of healthcare reform in the United States as they combine knowledge, experience, and commitment to advancing the specialty and promoting quality palliative and EOL care. Certified at the basic level of competency, the nurse may be licensed as a licensed practical nurse or registered professional nurse who has gained competencies in palliative and hospice care through general educational programs, professional work experiences, and ongoing continuing education. By virtue of graduate education and related clinical expertise, the advanced practice PC nurse is a specialist who demonstrates greater depth and breadth of knowledge and skill in theory, research, and practice reflected in the standards of care of PC and hospice nursing (HPNA, 2015a, 2015b).

The standards of care reflect the values and priorities of PC nursing and provide a framework with which to evaluate practice. The standards of care are written at both the basic and the advanced practice levels and reflect the nursing process, which involves assessment, diagnosis, outcome identification, planning, implementation, and evaluation. Foundational to the standards of care are the following tenets (Hospice and Palliative Care Nurses Association, 2017):

▪ Care should be age appropriate and culturally sensitive.
▪ A safe environment should be maintained.
▪ Education of patients and families is essential.
▪ Coordination and continuity of care across settings and caregivers must occur.
▪ Communication and the management of information must be effective.

Nurses in palliative and hospice care consider not only the physical and emotional needs of patients and families but also their cultural and spiritual beliefs and values, which may influence the patient's preference for treatment options. With consideration of developmental needs, PC and hospice nurses empower patients and families to remain in control of their lives by being active participants in determining the plan of care. By discussing the expectations related to the illness trajectory, anticipated symptoms, and associated pharmacological and nonpharmacological treatments, advanced practice nurses, who have prescriptive authority, can take into account not only the best evidence available through science and their own clinical judgment, but also the patients' and families' preferences, with optimal communication to health professionals across all care settings. PC and hospice nurses discuss the risks and benefits of tests, procedures, and treatments, considering the negative and positive impact on the patient's QOL and its economic implications (Meier & Brawley, 2011).

▪ THE ROLES OF ADVANCED PRACTICE PALLIATIVE CARE NURSES

Advanced practice nurses, specifically nurse practitioners, work in a variety of settings, including acute care. They have the assessment skills and clinical knowledge to incorporate palliative care into treatment for all of their patients. In the media, conversations often arise about the high costs of health care, the low number of physicians available to care for patients in the primary care role, and a lack of available specialists, such as oncologists, in the acute care setting. Advanced practice nurses are educated and well positioned to have a large impact on these issues. The "role of palliative care nurse practitioners varies, not only state to state, but among practice settings within the state" (Fox, 2014, p. 41). Advanced

practice registered nurses represent a valuable resource in national efforts to improve healthcare and increase access to quality PC for all Americans and their families living with serious illness, whether life-limiting illness or chronic progressive illness (Hospice and Palliative Nurses Association, 2015a).

Meier and Beresford (2006) emphasize that "advanced practice nurses often embody in a single person PC's focus on the whole person and the medical practitioner's ability to diagnose conditions, prescribe medications and order treatment interventions—while recouping salary costs through billing for consultations." (p. 624). Advanced practice nurses in PC often spearhead the development, implementation, and evaluation of PC services, assuming pivotal leadership roles not only as clinicians, but also as administrators, researchers, educators, advocates, and health policy makers.

Advanced practice nurses are often the health professionals who make the case to the hospital administration to implement a palliative care program and develop the business plan with consideration of interprofessional resources, feasibility and accessibility, cost control, revenue generation, integration and leveraging of existing services, and decisions regarding the structure and model of the programs (Center to Advance Palliative Care, 2011). They put forth to the administration the operational plan for implementation of PC programs, such as space needs, staffing roles and requirements, basic policies and procedures, and projections of patient volumes and program capacity, as well as consideration of financial and strategic planning issues. The advanced practice nurse makes the case to the administration regarding the hospital's financial viability, including the value of the program regarding length of stay at the hospital, daily census, hospital billing revenues, estimated cost savings, and potential contributions by philanthropy (Center to Advance Palliative Care, 2011). Given their advanced clinical knowledge and expertise related to healthcare systems, advanced practice nurses provide a futuristic perspective as to how PC can meet the expectations of quality care within the context of cost-effectiveness and reform. Nurse practitioners provide PC in a holistic manner, collaborate with other healthcare providers, provide consultation and support when needed to optimize PC practices, work within the organization to build capacity and help others learn about their role in PC to better integrate it within the team, and improve system outcomes, such as the accessibility of care and the number of hospital visits (Donald et al., 2013). Fox (2014) identified the role of the acute care nurse practitioner (ACNP) in implementing PC within the context of oncology care and in accordance with the American College of Surgeons Commission on Cancer. The ACNP skills improve PC by educating patients and families about their disease, prognosis, and treatment options; having difficult conversations regarding goals of care; managing transitions of care; identifying barriers to PC in the acute care setting; becoming involved in legislation to promote nurse practitioner practice; educating hospitalists and intensivists about PC; and using healthcare efficiently, with reduction in expensive and unwanted tests (Fox, 2014). Schreibeis-Baum et al. (2016) interviewed 22 professional state- and federal-level advocates who work in geriatrics or PC. It was clear from their interviews that the challenges to advancing PC policies are knowledge about PC in healthcare settings, cultural beliefs and public understanding about PC, and payment/reimbursement for PC services. Clearly, the advanced practice nurse is excellently positioned to address these barriers and increase the recognition of the role of PC in healthcare delivery.

PC nursing research generates basic and applied knowledge to improve the care of patients and families with serious and life-threatening illness in areas of symptom management, psychological responses to illness, and the family caregiver experience (Ferrell, 2010). Nurse researchers who conduct qualitative studies in palliative and hospice care seek to develop theories based on the subjective experiences of patients and their families. PC nurse researchers also conduct quantitative studies to test theories as well as to examine the incidence, prevalence, and severity of symptoms; evaluate models of care; and test the effectiveness of PC and hospice interventions.

Since the establishment of the National Institutes of Nursing Research as an institute within the U.S. National Institutes of Health in 1997, there has been increased funding of PC research and significant contributions made to science by PC nurse researchers. In addition, the Hospice Nurses Foundation in the United States has become a funding agency for PC nursing research. The Hospice Nurses Foundation agenda for 2009 to 2012 focused on funding studies that investigate the symptoms of dyspnea, constipation, and fatigue (HPNA, 2012).

The Hospice and Palliative Nurses Association (HPNA) research agenda for 2012 to 2015 was based on the Clinical Practice Guidelines for Quality Palliative Care, and addressed the first three domains of the guidelines. The first domain focused on the structure and processes of care, considering the optimal membership of interprofessional teams, the focus on the patient and family as the unit of care, and the locations and models of care delivery. In relation to research, the second domain focused on the physical aspects of care, including symptom management and disease progression in patients with multiple comorbid conditions, as well as the physical care of patients in special populations. The third domain involved psychological and psychiatric care, with a particular focus on the needs of individuals with serious mental illness (HPNA, 2012). Other funding agencies are interested in ways of promoting interprofessional education, the value of professional specialty certification, the integration of PC concepts into standard care across health communities, the value of concurrent curative care with PC, and the use of research findings to shape health policy (HPNA, 2012). At the 2017 HPNA meeting, there was significant discussion regarding continuation of the prior research agenda, which has not been completed. There was discussion regarding the rethinking of the research priorities of the organization that move beyond research on specific symptoms to a more focused research approach on processes related to PC, such as interprofessional collaboration. HPNA's new research agenda is in progress.

All nurses have the opportunity to participate in research by identifying clinical problems specific to palliative and hospice care, participating in data collection, and critiquing research findings to determine the application of findings, particularly in the development of clinical standards of care and the development of policies (Lunney, 2011). As principal investigators nurse researchers often lead the interprofessional research team. In collaboration with other nurses who are doctors of nursing practice (DNP), and other health practitioners and scientists, nurse researchers develop new knowledge related to the specialty and facilitate the translation of this PC and hospice knowledge into clinical practice.

Another key role in the advancement of PC nursing is that of educator. A survey conducted among acute care nurses in an inpatient unit revealed that nurses lack the knowledge and confidence to discuss PC options as well as to use nonpharmacological measures to alleviate the suffering of patients (Ashley & Fasolino, 2016). In the academic setting, PC nurses advance the specialty through curriculum development and the inclusion of PC content within the curriculum. Through programs, such as the End of Life Nursing Education Consortium (ELNEC) Train-the-Trainer, there is further dissemination of knowledge related to PC as it is integrated within undergraduate and graduate nursing curricula both domestically and internationally (Paice, Ferrell, Coyle, Coyne, & Callaway, 2008). At the graduate level, PC can be offered as a component of the adult nurse practitioner, geriatric nurse practitioner, or family nurse practitioner curricula or as a post-master's certification. Modification of public perceptions of PC is central to improving the knowledge of and access to services, empowering individuals, and involving communities in EOL care. Nurses, as educators, must focus on achieving comprehensive knowledge of the public regarding PC. This requires early discussion of PC upon diagnosis with a serious illness like cancer (McIlfatrick et al., 2013). As health educators in clinical settings, palliative nurses integrate PC concepts into the generalist setting, where most EOL care occurs. This includes providing patients and families with information regarding pain and symptom management, self-care, and other interventions. As members of an interprofessional team, PC nurses further mentor and teach other members of the team regarding evidence-based approaches in PC.

PC nurses also serve in the role of public health advocates. By virtue of their numbers, experience, education, time spent at the bedside, and insight into the lived experiences of patients and families, nurses play a prominent role as public health advocates for PC at the local, national, and global levels (Payne, Ingleton, Sargeant, & Seymour, 2009). With shifts in population, disease demographics, and the aging of the population, particularly given the health needs of the baby boom generation, nurses lead the much-needed healthcare reform to ensure quality care across generations (Gott, Ingleton, Bennett, & Gardiner, 2011). As advocates, nurses inform key decision and policy makers about the importance and effectiveness of quality, accessible, and equitable PC, as well as its outcomes and cost-effectiveness (Morrison et al., 2008; Penrod et al., 2010).

In their advocacy role, PC and hospice nurses focus on the following:

■ Coordinating and ensuring continuity of care across settings and caregivers
■ Educating patients, families, and providers
■ Promoting and upholding PC as a basic human right
■ Establishing networks of providers
■ Increasing equity and access to palliative and EOL care in developed countries, particularly in underdeveloped or resource-poor countries
■ Developing and enhancing PC delivery models
■ Increasing access to opioids and other symptom management modalities
■ Increasing public and political awareness
■ Developing integrated care pathways
■ Actively participating in public policy development, engagement, and social/political activism levels (Payne et al., 2009)

In their multiple roles in PC, nurses strive to influence the societal changes occurring at international, national, regional, and local levels, which promote health and well-being across the life continuum. Nurses are a valuable resource in national efforts to improve care and QOL for patients and their families living with advanced, life-limiting illness. It is through collaborative efforts that the roles of hospice and PC nurses will be fully actualized. Professional organizations in nursing, medicine, hospice, and PC are called upon to engage in dialogue about the role of advanced practice nurses and opportunities and strategies to enhance and empower the role. The Program of Experience in the Palliative Approach (PEPA) offers an appropriately trained and skilled primary care workforce that can complement specialist providers by providing the right service in the right place at the right time to people with serious healthcare or EOL needs. PEPA "offers professional development opportunities in palliative care to general practitioners, registered nurses, enrolled nurses, assistants in nursing and allied health professionals" (*Australian Nursing and Midwifery Journal*, 2014, p. 43).

■ CONCLUSIONS

"PC ensures that the person is viewed in his or her entirety, not as a collection of organs and medical problems" (National Palliative Care Research Center, 2015, p. 12). PC reduces high levels of suffering and distress of patients with serious illness at any age and at any stage of disease; improves communication; addresses the needs of family caregivers; reduces unwanted, unnecessary, and painful interventions; and improves patient, family, and staff satisfaction, while also improving survival (National Palliative Care Research Center, 2015). PC is also an economic imperative in reducing the cost of healthcare. But, even more important, PC is a humanistic imperative to ensure that QOL is promoted during all phases of the illness experience for both patients and their family caregivers (Sherman & Cheon, 2012).

Early integration of PC has been demonstrated to improve QOL; avoid unnecessary ER visits, hospitalization, and aggressive treatments; and thereby reduce healthcare costs. In fact, these "savings should be directed towards investing on integrating early palliative care with terminal illness diagnoses, as well as to educating the patient, family, society, and healthcare personnel about the difference between palliative care and hospice care" (Kain & Eisenhauer, 2016, p. 377).

The three dominant PC delivery models in the United States are hospital PC, community PC, and hospice. There remain significant barriers to palliative and hospice care both within the United States and internationally. A literature on review of PC education, implementation of programs, and policy barriers indicates a lack of adequate education/training and perception of PC as EOL care; inadequate size of the PC-trained interprofessional workforce; the challenge of identifying patients appropriate for PC referral; the fragmented healthcare system in the United States and other nations; lack of adequate reimbursement for PC; regulatory barriers, particularly in the nursing home setting; and lack of funding for PC and hospice research (Aldridge et al., 2016).

PC nurses advance the science and art of PC through clinical practice, administration, research, education, and advocacy. With a focus on ensuring quality care within the context of a changing healthcare environment, palliative and hospice care nurses promote the awareness of palliative and hospice care, acknowledge its value to patients and families and the healthcare community, and find ways of promoting access to care and actions to ensure the integration of PC into the healthcare system. As leaders of healthcare, PC nurses have the knowledge and skills to bring together patients, families, communities, health institutions and practitioners, legislators, payers, and insurers to move our world ahead by advancing local, national, and global PC initiatives. PC is responsive to healthcare reform in the United States, and PC nurses play a leading role in ensuring QOL for patients and families across the illness trajectory.

CASE STUDY

INTERPROFESSIONAL PERSPECTIVE

Myra Glajchen, DSW

The case of Mr. H. highlights several important issues, including the impact of medical and social isolation for elderly patients facing advanced and terminal illness; the burden of care coordination as symptom burden and medical management increase in complexity; and family fragmentation, which is endemic in many developed countries. The hospital setting often serves as the gateway to needed services for such patients. Ideally, Mr. H. and his daughter would have benefited from a psychosocial assessment by a trained social worker to identify areas of unmet need and anticipate areas of risk such as environmental safety within the home, food insufficiency, and loneliness. A family meeting could have helped the H. family discuss goals of care and make treatment decisions that honored Mr. H.'s wishes. Ensuring that the patient's voice is heard in decision making is an essential part of patient-centered care, as the PC team helps the patient make an informed decision and communicate those wishes to others, rather than allowing family members to decide on the patients behalf. Although Mr. H. was referred to hospice so late, both he and his children benefited from high-quality symptom management and psychosocial support at end of life. This gave his children a great deal of comfort after he died and afforded them the benefit of free bereavement counseling for 13 months.

A significant barrier to PC is the shortage of trained PC professionals in all disciplines. As the number of Medicare beneficiaries doubles over the next 20 years, and the number of PC programs grow, there will be an unmet need for staff specifically trained in PC who are prepared to meet the full range of medical, psychosocial, and spiritual needs of patients and families with serious illness. Because PC is delivered by an interdisciplinary care team, interprofessional education has gained popularity in many areas. Such training does not take the place of discipline-specific education and training, but rather focuses on a base of common knowledge and skills across disciplines, including advance care planning, communication, patient-centered care, and conducting a family meeting.

The federal Palliative Care and Hospice Education and Training Act (PCHETA) was developed to expand the PC workforce. The bill establishes PC and hospice education and training centers, academic career awards, career incentive awards, and workforce development for advanced practice nurses, physicians, clinical social workers, pharmacists, and psychology students. If passed, this bill would support PC training across disciplines using previously validated training models to retain midcareer staff and attract new students to the field. It is hoped this bill will gain traction as the need for PC services is increasingly recognized.

Patients like Mr. H. and his family deserve the highest quality care as they face the challenges of life-threatening illness. However, the highest quality of care does not necessarily mean the latest in medical technology. Rather, it means care that is consistent with the goals, values, and preferences of the patient and family. An interprofessional team, including physicians, advanced practice nurses, and social workers, through multiple conversations can identify the plan of care that addresses the physical, emotional, social, and spiritual needs of the patient and her or his family. The clarion call is to prepare a workforce of trained health professionals who can provide palliative and hospice care across the illness experience and bereavement care to families as they adjust to life in the face of their serious loss.

Evidence-Based Practice

May, P., Garrido, M., Cassel, J. B., Kelley, A., Meier, D., Normand, C., ... Morrison, R. S. (2017). Cost analysis of a prospective multi-site cohort study of palliative care consultation teams for adults with advanced cancer: Where does the cost savings come from? *Palliative Medicine, 31*(4), 378–386.

Purpose/Background

Research suggests that utilizing a PC team in an acute hospital setting is beneficial in producing cost savings, but the analysis of where savings occur is historically obscured. This study analyzes the cost in using a hospital-based PC team compared to usual care by looking at differences in the intensity of care, length of admission, and the overall cost of hospitalization. The study also analyzed differences in cost between "early" versus "late" intervention of PC teams.

Methods

This was a multisite prospective cohort study. The sample contained 863 patients from three U.S. hospitals with established PC teams. Inclusion criteria were adults who received an advanced-stage cancer diagnosis between 2007 and 2011 and who were discharged from the hospital while alive. Early PC was defined as the first consultation with the PC team within 2 days of admission.

Results/Conclusions

The study demonstrated that when patients who have an advanced cancer diagnosis receive a PC team consultation within 2 days of hospital admission, the length and intensity of stay are reduced, suggesting cost savings.

■ REFERENCES

Aldridge, M. D., Hasselaar, J., Garralda, E., van der Eerden, M., Stevenson, D., McKendrick, K., ... Meier, D. E. (2016). Education, implementation, and policy barriers to greater integration of palliative care: A literature review. *Palliative Medicine, 30*(3), 224–239. doi:10.1177/0269216315606645

American Hospital Association. (2008, November). Rapid response survey, the economic crisis: Impact on hospitals. Retrieved from https://www.aha.org/system/files/content/00-10/081119econcrisisreport.pdf

Ashley, J. L., & Fasolino, T. K. (2016). Palliative and Hospice Care: Educational needs of inpatient registered nurses. *Creative Nursing, 22*(2), 114–120. doi:10.1891/1078-4535.22.2.114

Australian Nursing and Midwifery Journal. (2014). Making palliative care everyone's business. *Australian Nursing and Midwifery Journal, 21*(10), 43.

Brumley, R., Enguidanos, S., Jamison, P., Seitz, R., Morgenstern, N., Saito, S., ... Gonzalez, J. (2007). Increased satisfaction with care and lower costs: Results of a randomized trial of in-home palliative care. *Journal of the American Geriatrics Society, 55*(7), 993–1000. doi:10.1111/j.1532-5415.2007.01234.x

Casarett, D. J. (2011). Rethinking hospice eligibility criteria. *Journal of the American Medical Association, 305*(10), 1031–1032. doi:10.1001/jama.2011.271

Centeno, C., Clark, D., Lynch, T., Racafort, J., Praill, D., De Lima, L., ... Giordano, A.; EAPC Task Force. (2007). Facts and indicators on palliative care development in 52 countries of the WHO European region: Results of an EAPC task force. *Palliative Medicine, 21*(6), 463–471. doi:10.1177/0269216307081942

Center to Advance Palliative Care. (2011). Building a hospital-based palliative care program. Retrieved from http://www.capc.org/building-a-hospital-based-palliative-care-program

Center to Advance Palliative Care. (2015). *America's care of serious illness 2015 state-by-state report card on access to palliative care in our nation's hospitals.* New York, NY: Author. Retrieved from https://reportcard .capc.org/wp-content/uploads/2015/08/CAPC-Report-Card-2015.pdf

Connor, S. R. (1998). *Hospice: Practice, pitfalls, and promise.* Washington, DC: Taylor & Francis.

Coyle, N. (2006). Introduction to palliative care nursing care. In B. R. Ferrell & N. Coyle (Eds), *The textbook of palliative nursing* (pp. 5–12). New York, NY: Oxford University Press.

De Lima, L. (2015). Palliative care and pain treatment in the global health agenda. *Pain, 156*, S115–S118. doi: 0.1097/01.j.pain.0000460349.23083.0b

De Lima, L., Woodruff, R., Pettus, K., Downing, J., Buitrago, R., Munyoro, E., … Radbruch, L. (2017). International association for hospice and palliative care position statement: Euthanasia and assisted suicide. *Journal of Palliative Medicine, 20*(1), 8–14. doi:10.1089/jpm.2016.0290

Donald, F., Martin-Misener, R., Carter, N., Donald, E. E., Kaasalainen, S., Wickson-Griffiths, A., … DiCenso, A. (2013). A systematic review of the effectiveness of advanced practice nurses in long-term care. *Journal of Advanced Nursing, 69*(10), 2148–2161. doi:10.1111/jan.12140

Dumanovsky, T., Augustin, R., Rogers, M., Lettang, K., Meier, D., & Morrison, R. S. (2016). The growth of palliative care in U.S. hospitals: A status report. *Journal of Palliative Medicine, 19*(1), 8–15. doi:10.1089/jpm.2015.0351

Federal Interagency Forum on Aging Related Statistics. (2016a). Aging stats. Retrieved from https://agingstats.gov

Federal Interagency Forum on Aging-Related Statistics. (2016b, August). Older Americans 2016: Key indicators of well-being. Washington, DC: U.S. Government Printing Office. Retrieved from https://agingstats.gov/docs/latestreport/older-americans-2016-key-indicators-of-wellbeing.pdf

Ferrell, B. R. (2010). Palliative care research: Nursing response to emergent society needs. *Nursing Science Quarterly, 23*, 221–225. doi:10.1177/0894318410371842

Fisher, E. S., Wennberg, D. E., Stukel, T. A., & Gottlieb, D. J. (2004). Variations in the longitudinal efficiency of academic medical centers. *Health Affairs (Suppl.)*, VAR19–32. doi:10.1377/hlthaff.var.19

Fisher, E. S., Wennberg, D. E., Stukel, T. A., Gottlieb, D. J., Lucas, F. L., & Pinder, E. L. (2003). The implications of regional variations in Medicare spending. Part 2: Health outcomes and satisfaction with care. *Annals of Internal Medicine, 138*(4), 288–298. doi:10.7326/0003-4819-138-4-200302180-00007

Foster, R. S. (2009). Estimated financial effects of the "Patient Protection and Affordable Care Act of 2009," as proposed by the Senate Majority Leader on November 18, 2009. Retrieved from https://www.cms.gov/ActuarialStudies/Downloads/S_PPACA_2009-12-10.pdf

Fox, K. (2014). The role of the acute care nurse practitioner in the implementation of the Commission on Cancer's standards on palliative care, *Clinical Journal of Oncology Nursing, 18*(1), 39–44. doi:10.1188/14.CJON.S1.39-4

Gallagher, R., & Baldwin, C. (2016). Palliative care: Therapy for the living. *British Columbia Medical Journal, 58*(5), 256–261.

Gidwani, R., Joyce, N., Kinosian, B., Faricy-Anderson, K., Levy, C., Miller, S. C., … Mor, V. (2016). Gap between recommendations and practice of palliative care and hospice in cancer patients. *Journal of Palliative Medicine, 19*(9), 957–963. doi:10.1089/jpm.2015.0514

Gomes, B., Harding, R., Foley, K. M., & Higginson, I. J. (2009). Optimal approaches to the health economics of palliative care: Report of an international think tank. *Journal of Pain and Symptom Management, 38*(1), 4–10. doi:10.1016/j.jpainsymman.2009.04.008

Gordon, R., Eagar, K., Currow, D., & Green, J. (2009). Current funding and financing issues in the Australian hospice and palliative care sector. *Journal of Pain and Symptom Management, 38*(1), 68–74. doi:10.1016/j.jpainsymman.2009.04.002

Gott, M., Ingleton, C., Bennett, M., & Gardiner, C. (2011). Transitions to palliative care in acute hospitals in England. *BMJ Supportive & Palliative Care, 1*, 42–48. doi:10.1136/bmj.d1773

Hospice and Palliative Nurses Association. (2012). *2012–2015 research agenda*. Pittsburgh, PA: Author.

Hospice and Palliative Nurses Association. (2015a). HPNA position statement: Value of the advanced practice registered nurse in palliative care. Retrieved from http://hpna.advancingexpertcare.org/wp-content/uploads/2015/08/Value-of-the-Advanced-Practice-Registered-Nurse-in-Palliative-Care.pdf

Hospice and Palliative Nurses Association. (2015b). HPNA position statement: Value of the professional nurse in palliative care. Retrieved from http://hpna.advancingexpertcare.org/wp-content/uploads/2015/08/Value-of-the-Professional-Nurse-in-Palliative-Care.pdf

Huskamp, H. A., Stevenson, D. G., Chernew, M. E., & Newhouse, J. P. (2010). A new Medicare end-of-life benefit for nursing home residents. *Health Affairs, 29*(1), 130–135. doi:10.1377/hlthaff.2009.0523

Institute of Medicine. (2015). *Dying in America: Improving quality and honoring individual preferences near the end of life*. Washington, DC: National Academies Press.

Kain, D. A., & Eisenhauer, E. A. (2016). Early integration of palliative care into standard oncology care: Evidence and overcoming barriers to implementation. *Current Oncology, 23*(6), 374–377. doi:10.3747/co.23.3404

Kaiser Family Foundation. (2011). Medicaid's long-term care beneficiaries: An analysis of spending patterns across institutional and community-based settings. Retrieved from http://www.kff.org/medicaid/upload/7576-02.pdf

Kamal, A. H., Currow, D. C., Ritchie, C. S., Bull, J., & Abernethy, A. P. (2013). Community-based palliative care: The natural evolution for palliative care delivery in the U.S. *Journal of Pain and Symptom Management, 46*(2), 254–264. doi:10.1016/j.jpainsymman.2012.07.018

Keehan, S. P., Sisko, A. M., Truffer, C. J., Poisal, J. A., Cuckler, G. A., Madison, A. J., … Smith, S. D. (2011). National health spending projections through 2020: Economic recovery and reform drive faster spending growth. *Health Affairs, 30*(8), 1594–1605. doi:10.1377/hlthaff.2011.0662

Kelley, A. S., & Meier, D. E. (2015). The current and potential role of palliative care for the medicare population. *Generations, 39*(2), 112–118.

Lunney, J. (2011). Hospice and palliative nursing research: 25 years of progress. *Journal of Hospice and Palliative Nursing, 13*(6), S3–S7. doi:10.1097/NJH.0b013e31822f98d2

Lynch, T., Clark, D., Centeno, C., Rocafort, J., Flores, L. A., Greenwood, A., … Wright, M. (2009). Barriers to the development of palliative care in the countries of central and eastern Europe and the commonwealth of independent states. *Journal of Pain and Symptom Management, 37*(3), 305–315. doi:10.1016/j.jpainsymman.2008.03.011

McIlfatrick, S., Hasson, F., McLaughlin, D., Johnston, G., Roulston, A., Rutherford, L., … Kernohan, W. G. (2013). Public awareness and attitudes toward palliative care in Northern Ireland. *BMC Palliative Care, 12*(1), 34. doi:10.1186/1472-684X-12-34

Medicare Payment Advisory Commission. (2009, March 17). Report to Congress: Medicare payment policy. Retrieved from http://www.medpac.gov/docs/default-source/reports/march-2009-report-to-congress-medicare-payment-policy.pdf

Meier, D. E. (2010). The development, status and future of palliative care. In D. E. Meier, S. L. Isaacs, & R. Hughes (Eds.), *Palliative care: Transforming the care of serious illness*. San Francisco, CA: Jossey-Bass. Retrieved from http://www.rwjf.org/files/research/4558.pdf

Meier, D. E., & Beresford, L. (2006). Advanced practice nurses in palliative care: A pivotal role and perspective. *Journal of Palliative Medicine, 9*(3), 624–627. doi:10.1089/jpm.2006.9.624

Meier, D. E., & Beresford, L. (2009). Palliative care seeks its home in national health care reform. *Journal of Palliative Medicine, 12*(7), 593–597. doi:10.1089/jpm.2009.9596

Meier, D. E., & Brawley, O. W. (2011). Palliative care and the quality of life. *Journal of Clinical Oncology 29*(20), 2750–2752. doi:10.1200/JCO.2011.35.9729

Meier, D. E., Lim, B., & Carlson, M. D. (2010). Raising the standard: Palliative care in nursing homes. *Health Affairs, 29*(1), 136–140. doi:10.1377/hlthaff.2009.0912

Mitchell, S. L., Teno, J. M., Kiely, D. K., Shaffer, M. L., Jones, R. N., Prigerson, H. G., … Hamel, M. B. (2009). The clinical course of advanced dementia. *New England Journal of Medicine, 361*(16), 1529–1538. doi:10.1056/NEJMoa0902234

Mitka, M. (2006). Less may be more when managing patients with severe chronic illness. *Journal of the American Medical Association, 296*(2), 159–160. doi:10.1001/jama.296.2.159

Morrison, R. S., Dietrich, J., Ladwig, S., Quill, T., Sacco, J., Tangeman, J., & Meier, D. E. (2011). Palliative care consultation teams cut hospital costs for Medicaid beneficiaries. *Health Affairs, 30*(3), 454–463. doi:10.1377/hlthaff.2010.0929

National Consensus Project for Quality Palliative Care. (2013). *Clinical practice guidelines for quality palliative care* (2nd ed.). Pittsburgh, PA: Author. Retrieved from http://www.nationalcoalitionhpc.org/ncp-guidelines-2013

National Palliative Care Registry. (2017). Research in the field. Retrieved from https://registry.capc.org/metrics-resources/research-in-the-field

National Palliative Care Research Center. (2015). America's care of serious illness: A state-by-state report card on access to palliative care in our nation's hospitals. Retrieved from https://reportcard.capc.org

National Quality Forum. (2006). *A national framework and preferred practices for palliative and hospice care quality*. Washington, DC: Author. Retrieved from https://www.qualityforum.org/Publications/2006/12/A_National_Framework_and_Preferred_Practices_for_Palliative_and_Hospice_Care_Quality.aspx

O'Connor, M., & Cowan, G. (2014). Home-based palliative care and interdisciplinary teamwork [online]. *Australian Nursing and Midwifery Journal, 21*(9), 40–41. Retrieved from https://search.informit.com.au/documentSummary;dn=191184101714997;res=IELHEA

O'Connor, M., & Gwyther, L. (2014). Strengthening International networks to advance global palliative care. *Illness, Crisis and Loss, 22*(1), 3–10. doi:10.2190/IL22.1.b

Office of the Legislative Counsel. (2010, May 1). Compilation of Patient Protection and Affordable Care Act of 2010, S 3140, 111th Congress, 2nd Session. Retrieved from http://docs.house.gov/energycommerce/ppacacon.pdf

Paice, J. A., Ferrell, B. R., Coyle, N., Coyne, P., & Callaway, M. (2008). Global efforts to improve palliative care: The international End-of-Life Nursing Education Consortium Training Programme. *Journal of Advanced Nursing, 61*(2), 173–180. doi:10.1377/hlthaff.2010.0929

Payne, S., Ingleton, C., Sargeant, A., & Seymour, J. (2009). The role of the nurse in palliative care settings in a global context. *Cancer Nursing Practice, 8*(5), 23–28. **doi:**10.7748/cnp2009.06.8.5.21.c7085

Pelosi, N. (2010, March 20). *Letter to the Honorable Nancy Pelosi providing estimates of the spending and revenue effects of the reconciliation proposal*. Washington, DC: Congressional Budget Office. Retrieved from https://www.dpc.senate.gov/healthreformbill/healthbill04.pdf

Penrod, J. D., Deb, P., Dellenbaugh, C., Burgess, Jr., J. F., Zhu, C. W., Christiansen, C. L., … Morrison, R. S. (2010). Hospital-based palliative care consultation: Effects on hospital cost. *Journal of Palliative Medicine, 13*(8), 973–979. doi:10.1089/jpm.2010.0038

Penrod, J. D., Deb, P., Luhrs, C., Dellenbaugh, C., Zhu, C. W., Hochman, T., … Morrison, R. S. (2006). Cost and utilization outcomes of patients receiving hospital-based palliative care consultation. *Journal of Palliative Medicine, 9*(4), 855–860. doi:10.1089/jpm.2006.9.855

Rabow, M. W., O'Riordan, D. L., & Pantilat, S. Z. (2014). A statewide survey of adult and pediatric outpatient palliative care services. *Journal of Palliative Medicine, 17*(12), 1311–1316. doi:0.1089/jpm.2014.0144

Schreibeis-Baum, H., Xenakis, L., Chen, E., Hanson, M., Ahuwailia, S., Ryan, G., & Lorenz, K. (2016). A qualitative inquiry on palliative and end of life policy reform. *Journal of Palliative Medicine, 19*(4), 400–407. doi:10.1089/jpm.2015.0296

Seymour, J. (2011). Changing times: Preparing to meet palliative needs in the 21st century. *British Journal of Community Nursing, 16*(1), 18. doi:10.12968/bjcn.2011.16.1.18

Sherman, D. W., & Cheon, J. (2012). Palliative care: a paradigm of care responsive to the demands for health care reform in America. *Nursing Economics*. Retrieved from https://www.highbeam.com/doc/1G1-291496699.html

Sherman, D. W., Evans, S., Halstead, L., Kelleher, C., Kenworthy, C., Olson, L., & Piet, L. (2016–2020). Maryland comprehensive cancer control plan: Palliative and hospice care (pp. 1–10). This publication was supported by CDC Cooperative Agreement Number 5 U58 DP003919-04, funded by the Centers for Disease Control and Prevention. Its contents are solely the responsibility of the authors and do not necessarily represent the official views of the Centers for Disease Control and Prevention or the Department of Health and Human Services. Retrieved from https://ftp.cdc.gov/pub/publications/cancer/ccc/maryland_ccc_plan.pdf

Smith, T. J., Coyne, P., Cassel, B., Penberthy, L., Hopson, A., & Hager, M. A. (2003). A high-volume specialist palliative care unit and team may reduce in-hospital end-of-life care costs. *Journal of Palliative Medicine, 6*(5), 699–705. doi:10.1089/109662103322515202

Spetz, J., Dudley, N., Trupin, L., Rogers, M., Meier, D. E., & Dumanovsky, T. (2016). Few hospital palliative care programs meet national staffing recommendations. *Health Affairs, 35*(9), 1690–1697. doi:10.1377/hlthaff.2016.0113

SUPPORT Principal Investigators. (1995). A controlled trial to improve care for seriously ill hospitalized patients: The Study to Understand Prognoses and Preferences for Outcomes and Risks of Treatments (SUPPORT). *Journal of the American Medical Association, 274*, 1591–1598. doi:10.1001/jama.1995.03530200027032

Temel, J. S., Greer, J. A., Muzikansky, A., Gallagher, E. R., Admane, S., Jackson, V. A., … Lynch, T. J. (2010). Early palliative care for patients with metastatic non-small-cell lung cancer. *New England Journal of Medicine, 363*(8), 733–742. doi:10.1056/NEJMoa1000678

Teno, J. M., Clarridge, B. R., Casey, V., Welch, L. C., Wetle, T., Shield, R., & Mor, V. (2004). Family perspectives on end-of-life care at the last place of care. *Journal of the American Medical Association, 291*(1), 88–93. doi:10.1001/jama.291.1.88

Ward, D., & Jackson, K. (2013, March). Ehospice: Palliative care news, views and inspiration from around the world. *International Journal of Palliative Care Nursing, 19*(3), 109. doi:10.12968/ijpn.2013.19.3.109

World Health Organization. (2012). World health statistics annual, 2011. Retrieved from http://www.who.int/entity/whosis/whostat/EN_WHS2011_Full.pdf

World Health Organization. (2014). Global atlas of palliative care at the end of life. Retrieved from http://www.who.int/nmh/Global_Atlas_of_Palliative_Care.pdf

World Health Organization. (2015). World health statistics annual, 2015. Retrieved from http://www.who.int/gho/publications/world_health_statistics/en

Wright, M., Wood, J., Lynch, T., & Clark, D. (2008). Mapping levels of palliative care development: A global view. *Journal of Pain and Symptom Management, 35*(5), 469–485. doi:10.1016/j.jpainsymman.2007.06.006

Wu, F. M., Newman, J. M., Lasher, A., & Brody, A. A. (2013). Effects of initiating palliative care consultation in the emergency department on inpatient length of stay. *Journal of Palliative Medicine, 16*(11), 1362–1367. doi:10.1089/jpm.2012.0352

Deborah Witt Sherman & Anne M. Wilkinson

Interprofessional Collaboration   C H A P T E R

3

KEY POINTS

- Patients and families facing a life-threatening illness have needs that are best addressed through an interprofessional palliative care team model.
- Interprofessional collaboration and coordination of care has been underemphasized in professional training.
- The Institute of Medicine Report (IOM) suggests that healthcare professionals work collaboratively with a spirit of team cooperation, and to practice to the fullest extent of their education and training.
- The first domain of the National Consensus Project for Quality Palliative Care is "Structure and Processes," which emphasizes interprofessional training and ongoing collaboration in providing coordinated assessments and interventions for patients and families across healthcare settings.
- Research suggests that interprofessional learning is essential for patient-centered, cost-effective, efficient, safer, timelier, and more equitable healthcare.
- An effective interprofessional team will attend to these particular needs and will include specialists as warranted by the distinctive illness and needs of the patient and family.
- With a comprehensive palliative care program, the interprofessional team works with the patient and family in a coordinated and collaborative manner to achieve mutually established goals.
- An interprofessional team approach integrates separate disciplines into a single consultation, discussing the patient history, assessment, diagnosis, intervention, and short- and long-term care management.
- A dynamic and outcome-oriented interprofessional team requires collaboration, leadership, coordinated decision making, and conflict resolution.
- The Center for Advancement of Interprofessional Education (IPE) emphasizes the unique as well as shared competencies of health professionals, as well as the importance of having a champion of interprofessional collaboration, who may assume a leadership role, and engages all team members.
- Interprofessional palliative care teams ideally consist of a team leader (usually the advanced nurse practitioner or the physician), nurses, social workers, and a chaplain.
- Interprofessional education is key to developing a workforce of the future that will provide comprehensive, compassionate, cost-effective, continuous, and evidence-based healthcare for varying patient populations, families, and communities.

CASE STUDY

M. K. is a 69-year-old woman of Haitian descent who suffered a massive thrombotic right hemisphere (RH) cerebrovascular accident (CVA) in June 2017. M. K.'s husband of 38 years was killed in the 2010 Haitian earthquake, and their long-time residence outside of Port-au-Prince was destroyed. M.K. and her husband were shopkeepers in Haiti, maintaining and running a hardware and appliance shop for 25 years. The shop also was destroyed in the earthquake. M. K. and her husband have three children, the oldest of whom is a son, age 46, who lives in the Little Haiti section of Miami. M. K. migrated to the United States in 2011 and has lived with this son and his family in a two-bedroom apartment on the third floor of a three-story walkup building. M. K.'s son owns and maintains a commercial and residential floor-polishing business in the Miami area and her daughter-in-law is a licensed practical nurse (LPN) at a local nursing facility. They have two children, aged 14 and 11. With her son's assistance, M. K. was able to obtain a green card, indicating permanent residency in the United States, and she became a U.S. citizen last year.

Prior to the stroke, M. K.'s health was generally adequate, although she is overweight (5'4", 190 lbs) and has a 10-year history of type II diabetes, high blood pressure, and hypertension. M. K. has been taking medication for control of blood pressure for the past 3 years with vacillating results. Within a year of arriving in Miami, she was able to secure employment as a seamstress at a local dry cleaning and alteration shop and worked at this facility until her stroke in June 2017. As a result of her U.S. citizenship and consistent employment, M. K. was able to obtain health insurance, which she has had for the last year.

For the first 2 weeks after the CVA, M. K. was at a stroke ward in a large public hospital, not far from the family residence in downtown Miami. As her condition stabilized and a placement was secured and approved, M. K. was transferred to a rehabilitation facility in the southern part of Miami-Dade County for 6 weeks. Although this location made it difficult for her son and his family to visit on a regular basis, M. K. was able to receive an intense interprofessional plan of care, which included excellent round-the-clock nursing follow-up, daily physical and occupational therapy, speech–language pathology services, dietetic consultation, neuropsychological evaluation, social work assessment and planning, and primary practice and neurological medical treatment. However, at release from the rehabilitation center, the stroke continued to result in numerous residual deficits, including dense left hemiplegia, more significant in the arm than the leg; moderate left-sided visual neglect; mild–moderate dysphagia for both liquids and solids; and mild–moderate cognitive deficits that have included significant working memory and attentional impairments, orientation deficits, and high-level language problems disrupting abstract thinking and pragmatic interactions. Furthermore, although M. K. has lost some weight (15 lbs), stabilizing her diabetes and hypertension continues to be problematic.

Since September 2017, M. K. has been back in Little Haiti, living with her son and his family. As a result of her continuing physical and cognitive deficits, M. K. has been confined primarily to her son's apartment and needs daily supervision. The left-sided hemiplegia makes it almost impossible for M. K. to walk up and down the stairs to the apartment, although she began using a four-pronged walker for about 2 months. However, the persisting left-sided neglect interferes with using the walker to even navigate the apartment. She is unable to prepare any meals for herself as a result of the left arm hemiplegia and her cognitive difficulties, particularly the working memory and attentional impairments. She continues to need a pureed diet, which must be prepared for her, because of the persisting dysphagia. Furthermore, she is unable to return to work because of her physical and cognitive deficits. These outcomes have appeared to contribute to M. K.'s current depression, anxiety, and aggression, which consequently have negatively impacted both her blood pressure and her hypertension. M. K.'s weight loss aided in stabilizing her diabetes; however, due to her frustration in being unable to care for herself and prepare her meals, M. K. often "sneaks" foods that are not optimum for her and is regaining weight. Her daughter-in-law wants to place M. K. in a nursing facility; she is trying to encourage her husband to consider placement in the facility where she works. However, her son prefers to keep M. K. at home, utilizing home-health services for his mother's care. At present, there is medical concern of M. K. suffering another CVA due to her current physical and mental status.

Patients and families facing a life-threatening illness have needs that are diverse, complex, multidimensional, and dynamic that are best addressed through an interprofessional palliative care (PC) team model. *PC* is "family and patient centered care that optimizes quality of life by anticipating, preventing, and treating suffering while addressing physical, intellectual, emotional, social, and spiritual needs and to facilitate patient autonomy, access to information, and choice" (National Consensus Project for Quality Palliative Care, 2013, p. 10). As Mitra and Vadivelu (2012) emphasize, PC patients' needs extend the established narrow bounds of the traditional disease-focused model of care with a focus on body organ systems, lab tests, and procedures (e.g., heart failure, white blood cell [WBC] counts, CT scans) to encompass the aggressive management of physical and emotional symptoms (e.g., pain, depression, etc.) and multiple overlapping dimensions of physical, emotional, intellectual, social, cultural, and spiritual well-being. PC requires a comprehensive and holistic approach to care that cannot be addressed by just one person, or even one team of professionals from a single discipline. Hence, the essential need is for an "interprofessional" approach in PC (Bowen, 2014; Sherman et al., 2017).

Although healthcare has historically been delivered by multiple health professionals working together to optimize patient outcomes, interprofessional collaboration and coordination of care have been underemphasized in professional training (O'Leary, Shegal, Terrell, & Williams, 2012). The landmark publications of *To Err Is Human: Building a Safer Health System* (Kohn, Corrigan, & Donaldson, 2001) and *Crossing the Quality Chasm: A New Health System for the 21st Century* (IOM, 2001) have focused attention on the development of effective healthcare teams to improve patient safety and outcomes, and put forth the recommendation of establishing interdisciplinary teams.

With recognition of the need to reduce morbidity and mortality rates, improve care coordination, provide patient-centered care, reduce healthcare costs, and enhance group accountability for the quality of healthcare, the Institute of Medicine report (IOM, 2001) suggested that healthcare professionals work collaboratively with a spirit of team cooperation and practice to the full extent of their education and training. They emphasized the need to redesign healthcare education, retrain health professionals already in the workforce, as well as reform the overall healthcare system. For this to occur, education in academic institutions and healthcare centers needs to change in order for professionals to develop the knowledge and skills to practice interdependently, rather than independently (IOM, 2001). Research suggests that interprofessional learning is essential for patient-centered, cost-effective, efficient, safer, timelier, and more equitable healthcare (Karstadt, 2012). For patients and family members, interprofessional practice can decrease total patient complications and reduce the length of hospital stay; outpatient visits; and mortality rates, including suicide rates (World Health Organization [WHO], 2010).

Since the first publication of the National Consensus Project (NCP) guidelines for quality palliative care (NCP) in 2004, there has been increasing recognition of the importance of interprofessional collaboration and teamwork. The first domain of the NCP is "Structure and Processes," which emphasizes interprofessional training and ongoing collaboration in providing coordinated assessments and interventions for patients and families across healthcare settings. According to the World Health Organization (WHO, 2010), interprofessional collaboration occurs "when multiple health workers from different professional backgrounds work together with patients, families, and communities to deliver the highest quality care" (p. 7).

■ PALLIATIVE CARE AS A MODEL OF CARE REQUIRING INTERPROFESSIONAL EXPERTISE

Each health profession has a unique body of knowledge that guides its clinical practice. It is also recognized that health professions have shared common knowledge of the physical and social sciences and humanities. PC, as a model of care, encourages the integration of knowledge, expertise, and skills of various health professionals to address the needs of the patient and family (Sherman et al., 2017).

Within the traditional medical model of care lies a perceived dichotomy between curative/death-defying care and PC, which offers aggressive symptom management and supportive care. For many years, the goal of care of medicine was *first* and *only* cure, and then, only if unable to cure, to relieve suffering. Still today, this perceived dichotomy prevents or delays the introduction of PC measures for patients and their families. For provision of quality, comprehensive, and whole-person care, the goals of curative care and PC can be integrated. In PC, it is appropriate to relieve suffering *at the same time* as pursuing curative life-prolonging therapies (De Lima & Pastrana, 2016; Ferrell, 2015).

PC starts with the initial diagnosis of serious illness, at which time the whole-person approach to care becomes extremely important, as is maximizing function and quality of life. PC culminates in the management of complex physical, psychological, social, and spiritual issues that patients and members of their families will experience during the final phase of life and will include bereavement care for the family (Dy, Lupu, & Seow, 2012; Oliviere & Hargreaves, 2017).

The principles and tenets of PC are applicable throughout the life span. From the neonate to the older adult, each group faces unique circumstances as they endure a life-threatening or life-limiting illness (Haley, 2013; Kapo, Morrison, & Liao, 2007; Malloy, Sumner, Virani, & Ferrell, 2007; Oliviere & Hargreaves, 2017). An effective interprofessional team will attend to these particular needs and will include specialists as warranted by the distinctive illness and needs of the patient and family. For example, in the setting of pediatrics, in addition to the core interprofessional team members, the interprofessional team may consist of pediatric specialists such as child life specialists, pediatric advanced practice nurses (APNs), and chaplains trained in pediatrics, whereas an elderly patient's interprofessional team may include, among others, physical and occupational therapists trained in the aging population, a geriatrician, and a geriatric nurse practitioner. It is the responsibility of the interprofessional team to determine the need to seek referral with other specialists or health professionals as the condition and needs of the patient and family change across the illness experience.

With the recognition that PC is a distinct medical and nursing specialty, more hospitals and providers have developed training programs related to enhancing PC within the acute care setting. An increasing number of hospitals offer an inpatient PC unit, PC consultation teams, outpatient PC clinics, and home hospice programs (Dumanovsky et al., 2016). By providing a continuum of care, patients with advanced progressive disease and their families have access to PC expertise in all healthcare settings. With a comprehensive PC program, the interprofessional team will work with the patient and family in a coordinated and collaborative manner to achieve mutually established goals. PC's reliance upon the interprofessional team is a key factor for successful patient and family outcomes.

■ UNDERSTANDING THE DISTINCTION BETWEEN MULTIDISCIPLINARY AND INTERPROFESSIONAL PRACTICE

Although the terms "multidisciplinary" and "interdisciplinary" are often used interchangeably, there are differences as well as similarities between them. Most recent, the term "interdisciplinary" has been replaced with the term "interprofessional."

Multidisciplinary teams utilize the skills and experience of individuals from different disciplines in which each professional approaches the patient from his or her own professional perspective, often involving separate consultations and a sequential process (Bruera & Hui, 2012). Although multidisciplinary team members may discuss their findings and plans or care, there is minimal integration in which all aspects of care are presented. In the traditional multidisciplinary team, the physician primarily directs care of the patient, and the family needs may or may not be considered. The primary mode of communication among disciplines is the medical chart. The result is often incomplete communication among professions, lack of accountability, and the tendency for each discipline to develop its own patient-care goals. Family needs are often unidentified and most often are not incorporated into the overall plan of care. As a result,

care may be uncoordinated and independent (Bruera & Hui, 2012).

In contrast, an interprofessional team approach integrates separate disciplines into a single consultation, discussing the patient history, assessment, diagnosis, intervention, and short- and long-term care management. The goals of care are established by the team, together with the patient and the family, who are "intimately involved" in making healthcare decisions. The team provides the patient and family with important information regarding the diagnosis, prognosis, and treatment options with recognition of their values and preferences. This interprofessional approach to care allows health professionals to "step out of their discipline silos" to work together for the best outcome for the patient and family (Jessup, 2007). The identity of the interprofessional team supersedes personal identities and agendas (O'Connor & Fisher, 2011), and the concept of the "whole is greater than the sum of its parts" is valued and respected. In the PC model, leadership is filled by the member of the interprofessional team who is best educated and qualified to address and focus on specific patient or family goals and lead the decision-making process. An advantage of this interprofessional model of care is that leadership, communication, and decision making is shared with the goal of meeting the patient/family's needs and goals (O'Connor & Fisher, 2011; Oliviere & Hargreaves, 2017). The interprofessional model facilitates team members to (a) directly interact with the patient and family, (b) share information among team members, (c) provide consultation to one another, and (d) work interdependently together to provide comprehensive, continuous care across the healthcare settings.

■ THE COMPOSITION OF INTERPROFESSIONAL TEAMS

Interprofessional PC teams ideally consist of a team leader (usually the advanced nurse practitioner or the physician), nurses, social workers, and chaplain. Beyond this core of team members, the interprofessional team can have other healthcare professionals, such as nutritionists, massage therapists, music therapists, pharmacists, physical therapists, and occupational therapists (NCP, 2013). Table 3.1 lists the most common members of the PC interprofessional team, explains their function within the team, and discusses their interrelationship with the PC APN.

To determine team membership, the following questions should be considered: Who has the information necessary to make the decision? Who needs to be consulted before the decision is made? Who needs to be informed of a decision after it is made (O'Conner & Fisher, 2011)? Certain levels of decision making may be done by individual members of the team (e.g., titrating a pain medication based on patient needs), whereas

TABLE 3.1   The Interprofessional Team Member's Function and Interrelationships

Registered Nurse

Function: Conducts a comprehensive assessment of patients' and families' physical, emotional, and spiritual needs and intervenes through therapeutic presence and communication, use of nursing interventions, and administration of medical treatments to improve quality of life.
Interrelationship: Collaborates with all members of the interprofessional team in developing and implementing an effective and compassionate plan of care.

Advanced Practice Nurse

Function: Incorporates the role of advanced clinician, educator, researcher, and consultant to families, staff, colleagues, and communities.
Interrelationship: Acts as a consultant, educator, role model, and mentor to the PC nurse to synergistically achieve quality outcomes for patients and families.

Bereavement Counselor

Function: Through interprofessional team assessment, identifies high-risk family members for bereavement and provides anticipatory grief counseling. Coordinates bereavement services for families, including counseling sessions, grief support groups, memorial services, and community outreach programs.
Interrelationship: Relies on the PC nurse's assessment of the family upon a patient's death in order to begin bereavement care. Values the PC nurse's role in identifying high-risk family members for grief and bereavement.

Patient/Family

Function: The patient/family are the focus of care of the interprofessional team. The goals identified by the patient/family direct the participation of other members of the team.
Interrelationship: The patient/family understand that the PC nurse is the coordinator of interprofessional care and continuously confers with the PC nurse regarding patient/family needs.

Palliative Care Physician

Function: Consults with the primary care physician and collaborates with the interprofessional team to provide expertise in pain management, communication, and treatment decisions at the end of life for patients and families.
Interrelationship: Understands that the PC nurse has the greatest prolonged contact with the patient and family and relies upon the holistic assessment and interventions of the nurse to develop a comprehensive medical care plan in collaboration with the interprofessional team

Pastoral Care Counselor

Function: Provides in-depth assessment of the spiritual needs of patient/family, including search for the meaning and purpose of life. Acts as a liaison with community clergy and a resource for the interprofessional team regarding ethical questions, faith traditions, and world religions.
Interrelationship: Respects the spiritual assessment of the PC nurse and is consulted when family issues require advanced assessment and intervention. Acts as a resource for the PC nurse when a debriefing is required after a difficult death or experience.

Primary Care Physician

Function: Initiates a relationship with the PC team with referral of a new patient/family. Provides a medical history of the patient's illness and any other pertinent medical and psychosocial information; continues to be the primary physician or transfers the role to the PC physician.
Interrelationship: Coordinates assessments and interventions of the PC nurse and those of the interprofessional team to establish a comprehensive plan of care for the patient and family.

Social Worker

Function: Provides history (via genogram) regarding the strengths, resources, and realities of patient/family system. Interventions include emotional support through individual, family, high-risk, and bereavement counseling. Provides referrals for families to the community as needed for social services.
Interrelationship: Provides delivery of care, which involves ongoing collaboration with the PC nurse, who is continuously identifying psychosocial needs and outcomes of the patient and family.

(continued)

TABLE 3.1 The Interprofessional Team Member's Function and Interrelationships (*continued*)

Therapies (Pharmacy, Occupational, Physical, Dietary, Speech, Art, Music, Touch, Massage)

Function: Provides education and/or "hands-on" therapy of specialized discipline to maximize independence and quality of life of patient and family.
Interrelationship: Participates in plan of care when consulted by PC nurse and reports outcomes of interventions through collaboration with the PC nurse.

Volunteer

Function: Gives time freely to contribute to patient and family needs by direct service, administrative support of the PC program, public relations, and community education.
Interrelationship: Reports observed family dynamics to the PC nurse to facilitate the revision of plan of care if needed.

Volunteer Coordinator

Function: Recruits, screens, educates, supervises, and retains volunteer staff to provide supportive services to patients and families.
Interrelationship: Plans assignments of volunteers based on identified needs of family by the PC nurse; involves the PC nurse in volunteer training.

PC, palliative care.

other levels will require input from the team as a whole (e.g., developing a care plan). Poor, fragmented decision making results from failure to include appropriate team members in the decision-making process (O'Connor & Fisher, 2011).

■ THE IMPORTANCE OF COLLABORATION OF INTERPROFESSIONAL TEAM MEMBERS AND THE MANAGEMENT OF CONFLICT

A dynamic and outcome-oriented interprofessional team requires collaboration, leadership, coordinated decision making, and conflict resolution. *Collaboration,* as defined by the Merriam-Webster dictionary (2017), is the ability to work with others, especially on intellectual endeavors. It is the process of collaboration that empowers team members to act as decision makers within the group. For example, if a question on pain arises, various members of the team may provide observations and opinions in an effort to maximize the relief of all dimensions of pain. Using a true collaborative process, the ultimate decision maker regarding this aspect of care would not come to a conclusion solely benefiting one member or one member's own perspective, but rather would make a decision reflecting the team's total input. Through collaboration, effective patient- and family-driven quality outcomes are achieved (Bruera & Hui, 2012; Dobrof, Heyman, & Greenberg, 2011; Oliviere & Hargreaves, 2017; Porter-O'Grady, Alexander, Blaylock, Minkara, & Surel, 2006).

As with any close working situation, health professionals may have differing perspectives regarding the clinical issue, the priority of the issue, the best treatment plan, and who should be involved in providing the care. Because of the interdependency among interprofessional team members, professional conflict may arise, which can be, under the right circumstances and with guidance from leadership and the team, beneficial to team growth and collaboration. Team climate and performance are significantly impacted by the respect and trust in each team member's knowledge, skills, expertise, and motivation, as well as by the available leadership (Klarare, Hagelin, Fürst, & Fossum, 2013). Lack of respectful team communication may stifle the creativity and the professional advancement and development of team members. Diverse ideas and opinions can be the impetus for innovative solutions for patient care problems and, in the process, may deepen the professional dialogue within the team. However, conflict becomes destructive when it is personalized or viewed as a threat to a member's role. Thus, the art in managing conflict is not to avoid it, but to manage it effectively so that team members and patients benefit (Klarare et al., 2013).

■ A CLOSER LOOK AT THE ROLE OF NURSES ON INTERPROFESSIONAL TEAMS

Although the composition of interdisciplinary teams in hospice and PC varies depending on the needs of the patient/family unit and the resources available to the patient in his or her community, at a minimum, the team includes a nurse (registered nurse or APN) and a physician. No matter what the configuration of the team, the nurse's personal relationship with the patient and family is seen as crucial. This relationship, together with the nurse's clinical knowledge and skills, is "the essence of palliative care nursing" (Ferrell, 2015) and represents not only the combination of the science and art of nursing, but a valuing of interprofessional collaboration. PC nursing is recognized as a specialty, and certification can be obtained as certified nursing assistants, licensed practical nurses, registered nurses, and APNs.

As a coordinator of care and a core member of the interprofessional team, the nurse has the responsibility to spearhead the development of therapeutic relationships, not just between himself/herself and the patient and family, but also with all pertinent members of the team. The nurse's role, in turn, ensures effective and goal-driven supportive communication and quality patient outcomes. The PC nurse needs to continually reassess the goals of the patient and family, and their treatment preferences, and offer support. A hallmark of quality PC is the collaborative role that the nurse develops with the physician. Often, the physician has had a long-term relationship with the patient and family, and as the needs for traditional medical model of curative care lessen, the physician may feel a sense of loss. The collaborative relationship with the physician may also be a source of support for the physician both personally and professionally.

The nurse is also a primary conduit within the interprofessional team for information, critical assessments, and evaluation of the goals of patient and family. A critical aspect of PC involves the identification and subsequent resolution of often divergent goals of the patient, family, or the healthcare team. The PC nurse is in the ideal position to be instrumental in coordinating and implementing a comprehensive family-focused plan of care.

Health professionals, including APNs, bring a specific and well-defined set of qualities, knowledge, and judgments to caring for individuals and families facing serious, progressive, or life-threatening illness. This includes advanced scientific and biophysical knowledge, analytical skills, and mastery of a broad repertoire of communication and interpersonal skills. Specialized knowledge and proficiencies also include the ability to incorporate ethics and cultural diversity, and offer spiritual and psychological care (Bruera & Hui, 2012; Coyne, 2003; Kuebler, 2003; Meier & Beresford, 2008; Rodin, et al., 2015).

■ INTERPROFESSIONAL EDUCATION AND OUTCOMES

According to the WHO (2010), "interprofessional education occurs when students from two or more professions learn about, from, and with each other to enable effective collaboration and improve health outcomes" (p. 35). There is recognition of shared values and codes of conduct with an appreciation for interdependence, rather than a focus on independence. Through interprofessional education, the goal is to augment one another's roles and competencies by association with each other, rather than to dilute well-established health professions and their identity (Karstadt, 2012). The Center for Advancement of Interprofessional Education (IPE; 2009) emphasizes

the unique and shared competencies of health professionals, as well as the importance of having a champion of interprofessional collaboration, who may assume a leadership role, but engages all team members (Sherman et al., 2017).

To achieve interprofessional competence, it is important for health professionals to learn the underlying principles of interprofessional healthcare, specifically, (a) patient centered and community/population focused rather than profession centered; (b) relationship focused; (c) process oriented; (d) linked to educational strategies and learning activities that are developmentally appropriate and integrated across the learning continuum; (e) applicable across the professions by acquiring an essential combination of knowledge, attitudes, values, and skills that allow for team-based problem solving and brainstorming; (f) sensitive to the systems context with applicability across practice settings; and (g) outcomes driven (Interprofessional Education Collaborative [IPEC], 2011; WHO, 2010).

Research indicates that interprofessional collaboration benefits the members of the healthcare team. A qualitative study conducted in Sweden concluded that "interprofessional education giving clarity on one's own professional role and knowledge of other professions would most likely benefit patients and family caregivers" (Klarare et al., 2013). Sinha and colleagues (2015) conducted a pilot study titled the "Heart of Medicine (HOM)." This study consisted of three workshops to enhance interprofessional knowledge, comfort, and collaboration in the end-of-life care of medical and nursing student participants. Based on the results of pre- and posttests, the workshop increased student's understanding of the roles of other professionals and increased their sense of collaboration. These findings are consistent with a study by Doll et al. (2012). They reported that a one-time IPE experience that is well structured by faculty with expertise in IPE can effectively foster the competencies in students of all health professions. They suggest that repeated exposure to these sorts of activities may be even more beneficial.

A prospective comparative pilot study was conducted by Younho, Bainbridge, and Hsien (2015) to determine the effectiveness of a nurse specialist-led PC team versus a usual-care team in a rural setting. To identify the perceptions regarding collaboration, a total of 29 physicians, nurses, nurse practitioners, and case managers completed the Modified Index of Interdisciplinary Collaboration Scale (MIIC), which consists of four subscales (interdependence and flexibility, newly created professional activities, collective ownership of goals, and reflection on the process), and the Interprofessional Collaboration Scale (IPCS), which consists of three subscales (communication, accommodation, and isolation). The results indicated a trend of higher levels of interprofessional collaboration based on the MIIC Scale for the specialist team, as well as a similar trend with the IPCS (Younho et al., 2015). There is a need for well-designed studies to examine the experience and outcomes of interprofessional education.

◼ IDENTIFYING THE ASSUMPTIONS, GROUP PROCESSES, AND EXPERIENCE OF INTERPROFESSIONAL COLLABORATION

Understanding the assumptions and processes of interprofessional collaboration is an important first step in promoting interprofessional care in both clinical and academic settings. Led by a nurse champion in interprofessional collaboration, a group of eight interprofessional colleagues in the College of Nursing and Health Sciences was formed to develop a simulated case study of a combat veteran with a traumatic brain injury and to explore the assumptions, group processes, and the experience of interprofessional collaboration (Sherman et al., 2017). The interprofessional group included colleagues from nursing, occupational therapy, physical therapy, communication science disorders (speech pathology), athletic trainers, and health services administration.

Before the work on the simulated case study began, the group explored their *assumptions regarding interprofessional collaboration*, which included the following:

- Interprofessional team members must recognize their own abilities and limitations.
- Interprofessional team members must learn to "dance with a different partner" so as not to step on toes.
- Expertise of the interprofessional teams is dependent on variability in team culture, including disciplines represented, ethnicity/race, gender, and age.
- Expertise of the interprofessional team is dependent on the length of time the group has worked together and group dynamics as members move in and out of the team.
- Interprofessional collaboration changes as patient populations change and teams are subject to external forces, such as changes in the healthcare system, educational system, or society at large (Sherman et al., 2017).

Written documentation of all meetings was kept by the group leader and shared by email with team members. As the development of an interprofessional case study emerged, a reflective process by the group leader led to the identification of seven steps of the group collaborative process. These include:

1. Recognize the champion who brought the group together and then engage in group discussion to determine the leadership of the group going forward. It was agreed that the leadership of the group may change depending on the clinical issue to be addressed.
2. Determine the group process that promotes commitment and accountability, such as establishing the best day and time to meet or using technology to conduct meetings, as well as strategies for communicating through email.
3. Share group responsibility in reviewing the health sciences literature regarding the care of the specific patient population, with each member contributing findings from his or her disciplinary perspective during group discussion.
4. Outline the components of the comprehensive health history and physical examination from an interprofessional perspective and develop case-specific details for the combat veteran with traumatic brain injury.
5. Review the case findings with identification and prioritization of clinical diagnoses (overarching diagnoses as well as discipline-specific diagnoses/ clinical problems).
6. Develop holistic interventions, including discipline-specific and complementary interventions from an interprofessional perspective to address diagnoses/ clinical problems.
7. Involve all team members in the evaluation of health outcomes (Sherman et al., 2017).

The development of an interprofessional simulated case study not only highlighted the processes of interprofessional collaboration, as identified previously, but was an opportunity for team members to *reflect on their experience of interprofessional collaboration*. Following the development of a simulated case study, the group leader conducted individual debriefing interviews with the eight participants.

Overall, what was learned from developing the case study was that there are shared and unique areas of clinical assessment depending on the discipline in the determination of a diagnosis and treatment plan. Interprofessional collaboration included brainstorming during the assessment as details about the patient's history or physical examination were discussed.

In reflecting on the experience of interprofessional collaboration, the participants selected such words as "united," "respectful," "compromising," and "interactive" to describe the group process. They believed that the simulation exercise changed their perspective, stating that it improved their outlook on teamwork, increased their recognition of alternative approaches, and provided a new frame of reference and approach to patient care. This resulted in an evaluation of personal values, knowledge, and skill, and an appreciation of shared and unique values and competencies (Sherman et al., 2017).

The interviews indicated that collaboration is promoted when an individual facilitates the process, shares responsibility and accountability, and shows respect for what each team member offers to the process. With a sense of shared purpose, there was enthusiasm and enjoyment in the collaborative work. Equally important was listening with openness and a willingness to "agree to disagree" at times (Sherman et al., 2017).

The challenges related to interprofessional collaboration were high workloads with competing demands, coordinating times to meet, and, for some participants, finding their niche within the team. One team member felt that it is sometimes easier to just work alone rather than try to find an agreeable schedule. Another team member indicated that at times interprofessional collaboration necessitates that you "wear even more hats," referring to the need for shared responsibility. Yet, several members agreed that despite the challenges, it is important to "step out of our silos" and "establish a collective identity" (Sherman et al., 2017, p. 229).

■ CONCLUSIONS

Interprofessional education is key to developing a workforce of the future that will provide comprehensive, compassionate, cost-effective, continuous, and evidence-based healthcare for varying patient populations, families, and communities (Sherman et al., 2017). What is needed is a simultaneous top-down and bottom-up approach involving commitment from university and college administration, chairs and directors of departments and programs, faculty and students, and colleagues from affiliated healthcare institutions. With the leadership of a champion of interprofessional collaboration, the group

of professionals benefit from identifying their values and assumptions related to collaboration. With recognition of a collective set of values and sense of accountability, internal and external challenges to the process can be overcome. Sharing or rotating group leadership is of value in equalizing power and responsibility and acknowledging and appreciating the expertise of all members of the interprofessional group.

Both in the use of simulated case studies in academia and in the discussion of patient cases in the healthcare setting, each member of the healthcare team can provide a new lens regarding the questions asked in a comprehensive health history, a more detailed physical examination, and insights into beneficial treatments. The synergy of team members is very comforting to patients as they are sent the same message of clinical options and feel that their health and lives are in the hands of a group of experts who have their best interest at heart and will provide the most effective treatments. For the health professionals, the best thinking of colleagues is also of value as there is a sense of shared responsibility in ensuring the best patient and family healthcare outcomes.

Transformative change in education and clinical practice involves interprofessional networking of colleagues within, across, and beyond the university and those within healthcare systems and agencies. Further research into the structure, processes, and outcomes related to interprofessional collaboration is needed as it relates to patients/families, healthcare providers, and institutional outcomes.

CASE STUDY

INTERPROFESSIONAL PERSPECTIVE

Monica Strauss Hough, PhD, CCC/SLP, ASHA Fellow

In the case of M. K., several issues need to be addressed to enhance the quality of M. K.'s life as well as that of her family. An interprofessional collaborative approach to working with M. K. and her family is paramount to positive changes in the current situation. Nursing services are pivotal to the assessment of medical issues and working with nutrition services to monitor diabetes, weight gain, and blood pressure. A specific diet that addresses glucose and sodium intake should be implemented and monitored closely by family members. It is encouraged that M. K. be instructed to monitor her glucose on a daily basis if it is determined that she has the ability to complete this task. Speech–language pathology services will be helpful in working with these disciplines to evaluate M. K.'s cognitive abilities relative to following directions, abstract thinking, and working memory, and thus ensure that M. K. can participate in self-help goals. Furthermore, speech–language pathology should coordinate with nursing and nutrition services relative to dietary issues with regard to M. K.'s current swallowing status and tolerance for liquids and solid foods. Occupational therapy would be valuable to instruct and guide M. K. in self-feeding skills.

As indicated, M. K. is confined to the apartment she shares with her son's family due to hemiplegia and directed attention problems as the result of visual spatial neglect. It is essential that physical and occupational therapy services address mobility and coordination. Specifically, physical therapy should address gait and improved walker use to navigate the environment with input from occupational therapy and speech–language pathology services to remediate neglect and visual attentional difficulties as they impact gait and mobility.

The family is divided relative to M. K.'s living environment. Social work services are critical to managing this issue to ensure the best care for M. K. Obviously, the living situation for M. K. and her family, even under the best circumstances prior to M. K.'s CVA, have resulted in very close quarters for all involved. However, since M. K.'s stroke, her limited mobility, inability to work, and need for continuous supervision, the living environment has been more congested and the tension among all family members has significantly increased. Thus, placing M. K. in a skilled nursing facility that includes therapy services previously mentioned may be a viable option that should be considered. Input from all disciplines in conjunction with family discussion, which is coordinated by social work services, will continue until an agreed-upon placement is finalized.

Given the value and expertise of an interprofessional team of healthcare providers, many institutions provide comprehensive, holistic, and quality care for patients, such as M. K. and her family, by initiating a PC consult. The PC team works closely with the primary care team to coordinate physical, emotional, social, and spiritual care across healthcare settings. PC team members discuss the goals of care with patients and families to determine their needs, wishes, and preferences. Collaborating with other members of the healthcare team is important to M. K. achieving as successful a recovery as possible, with consideration of the illness experience and needs of the family, as the patient and family are considered the "unit of care" in PC.

Evidence-Based Practice

Gaudet, A., Kelly, M. L., & Williams, A. M. (2014). Understanding the distinct experience of rural interprofessional collaboration in developing palliative care programs. *Rural and Remote Health*, 14(2), 1–14.

Introduction
Interprofessional collaboration in PC is an important component of a rural generalist practice. The literature suggests core competencies for interprofessional practice; however, it is not documented whether there are differences in rural practices. The purpose of this study is to examine the working operations of rural PC teams and highlight the elements that are important to collaborative practice.

Methods
This is a qualitative, naturalistic, and ethnographic study that uses purposive sampling to recruit key informants of members of four rural PC teams in Ontario, Canada. A preliminary analytic framework that identified seven essential elements of interprofessional collaboration, specifically, responsibility and accountability, coordination, communication, cooperation, assertiveness, autonomy, and mutual trust and respect, was used to explore the experience. Inductive analysis was used to reduce the data and provide a description of the story.

Results
The core team of rural PC practitioners consisted of nurses, physicians, social workers, and hospice volunteers. Each of the key elements of interprofessional collaboration

was confirmed in rural PC, supporting the preliminary analytic framework used. Interprofessional collaboration is an automatic and informal process in rural PC, which can be facilitated between members of different clinical backgrounds and experiences.

Conclusions

Recruiting and preparing practitioners in rural communities is challenging, but the education of practitioners is important. Understanding the processes of how interprofessional collaboration occurs in rural areas will help the successful functioning of interprofessional PC-teams.

■ REFERENCES

Bowen, L. (2014). The multidisciplinary team in palliative care: A case reflection. *Indian Journal of Palliative Care*, *20*(2), 142–145. doi:10.4103/0973-1075.132637

Bruera, E., & Hui, D. (2012). Conceptual models for integrating palliative care at cancer centers. *Journal of Palliative Medicine*, *15*(11), 1261–1269. doi:10.1089/jpm.2012.0147

Centre for the Advancement of Interprofessional Education. (2009). Retrieved from https://www.caipe.org/about-us

Coyne, P. J. (2003). The evolution of the advanced practice nurse within palliative care. *Journal of Palliative Medicine*, *6*(5), 769–770. doi:10.1089/109662103322515275

De Lima, L., & Pastrana, T. (2016). Opportunities for palliative care in public health. *Annual Review of Public Health*, *37*, 357–374. doi:10.1146/annurev-publhealth-032315-021448

Dobrof, J., Heyman, J. C., & Greenberg, R. M. (2011). Building on community assets to improve palliative and end-of-life care. *Journal of Social Work in End-of-Life and Palliative Care*, *7*(1), 5–13. doi:10.1080/15524256.2011.548044

Doll, J., Packard, K., Furze, J., Huggett, K., Jensen, G., Jorgensen, D., … Maio, A. (2012). Reflections from an interprofessional education experience: Evidence for the core competencies for interprofessional collaborative practice. *Journal of Interprofessional Care*, *27*(2), 194–196. doi:10.3109/13561820.2012.729106

Dumanovsky, T., Augustin, R., Rogers, M., Lettang, K., Meier, D., & Morrison, R. S. (2016). The growth of palliative care in U.S. hospitals: A status report. *Journal of Palliative Medicine*, *19*(1), 8–15. doi:10.1089/jpm.2015.0351

Dy, S. M., Lupu, D., & Seow, H. (2012). Progress towards systems of quality measurement that capture the essence of good palliative care. *Palliative Medicine*, *26*(4), 291–293. doi:10.1177/0269216312444796

Ferrell, B. R. (2015). General principles. In B. R. Ferrell, N. Coyle, & J. A. Paice (Eds), *Oxford textbook of palliative nursing* (4th ed., pp. 4–5). Oxford, UK: Oxford University Press.

Haley, W. (2013). Family caregiving at the end-of-life: Current status and future directions. In *Caregiving across a lifespan* (pp. 157–175). New York, NY: Springer Publishing.

Institute of Medicine, Committee on Quality of Healthcare in America. (2001). *Crossing the quality chasm: A new health system for the 21st Century*. Washington, DC: National Academies Press.

Interprofessional Education Collaborative. (2011). *Core competencies for interprofessional collaborative practice: Report of an expert panel*. Washington, DC: Author.

Jessup, R. L. (2007). Commentaries: Interdisciplinary versus multidisciplinary care teams: Do we understand the difference? *Australian Health Review*, *31*(3), 330–331. doi:10.1071/AH070330

Kapo, J., Morrison, L. J., & Liao, S. (2007). Palliative care for the older adult. *Journal of Palliative Medicine*, *10*(1), 185–209. doi:10.1089/jpm.2006.9989

Karstadt, L. (2012). Does interprofessional education provide a global template? *British Journal of Nursing*, *21*(9), 522. doi:10.12968/bjon.2012.21.9.522

Klarare, A., Hagelin, C. L., Fürst, C. J., & Fossum, B. (2013). Team interactions in specialized palliative care teams: A qualitative study. *Journal of Palliative Medicine*, *16*(9), 1062–1069. doi:10.1089/jpm.2012.0622

Kohn, L. T., Corrigan, J., & Donaldson, M. S. (2001). *To err is human: Building a safer health system*. Washington, DC: National Academies Press.

Kuebler, K. K. (2003). The palliative care advanced practice nurse. *Journal of Palliative Medicine*, *6*(5), 707–714. doi:10.1089/109662103322515211

Malloy, P., Sumner, E., Virani, R., & Ferrell, B. (2007). End-of-life nursing education consortium for pediatric palliative care (ELNEC-PPC). *American Journal of Maternal Child Nursing*, *32*(5), 298–302; quiz 303. doi:10.1097/01.NMC.0000288000.87629.de

Meier, D. E., & Beresford, L. (2008). The palliative care team. *Journal of Palliative Medicine*, *11*(5), 677–681. doi:10.1089/jpm.2008.9907

Merriam-Webster. (2017). *Merriam-Webster's collegiate dictionary* (10th ed.). Springfield, MA: Author.

Mitra, S., & Vadivelu, N. (2012). *Multidisciplinary approach and coordination of care*. New York, NY: Springer Publishing.

National Consensus Project. (2013). *Clinical practice guidelines for quality palliative care* (3rd ed.). Pittsburg, PA: National Consensus Project for Quality Palliative Care. Retrieved from http://www.nationalconsensusproject.org

O'Connor, M., & Fisher, C. (2011). Exploring the dynamics of interdisciplinary palliative care teams in providing psychosocial care: "Everybody thinks that everybody can do it and they can't." *Journal of Palliative Medicine, 14*(2), 191–196. doi:10.1089/jpm.2010.0229

O'Leary, K. J., Shegal, N. L., Terrell, G., & Williams, M. V. (2012). Interdisciplinary teamwork in Hospitals: A review and practical recommendations for improvement. *Journal of Hospital Medicine, 7*(1), 48–54. doi:10.1002/jhm.970

Oliviere, D., & Hargreaves, R. (2017). *Good practices in palliative care: A psychosocial perspective.* Aldershot, UK: Ashgate/Routledge.

Porter-O'Grady, T., Alexander, D. R., Blaylock, J., Minkara, N., & Surel, D. (2006). Constructing a team model: Creating a foundation for evidence-based teams. *Nursing Administration Quarterly, 30*(3), 211–220. doi:10.1097/00006216-200607000-00005

Rodin, D., Balboni, M., Mitchell, C., Smith, P. T., VanderWeele, T. J., & Balboni, T. A. (2015). Whose role? Oncology practitioners' perception of their role in providing spiritual care to advanced cancer patients. *Supportive Care Cancer, 23*(9), 2543–2550. doi:10.1007/s00520-015-2611-2

Sherman, D. W., Maitra, K., Hough, M., Restrepo, J., Barbera, S., Olenick, M., ... Singh, A. (2017). Illustrating and analyzing the processes of interprofessional collaboration: Lessons learned from palliative care in deconstructing the concept. *Journal of Palliative Medicine, 20*(3), 227–234. doi:10.1089/jpm.2016.0332

Sinha, P., Murphy, S. P., Becker, C. M., Poarch, H. J., Gade, K. E., Wolf, A. T., ... Brashers, V. (2015). A novel interprofessional approach to end-of-life care education: A pilot study. *Journal of Interprofessional Care, 29*(6), 643–645. doi:10.3109/13561820.2015.1041585

World Health Organization. (2010). *Framework for action on interprofessional education & collaborative practice.* Geneva, Switzerland: Author.

Younho, H., Bainbridge, D., & Hsien, S. (2015). Measuring interprofessional collaboration between two palliative care teams. *Journal of Hospice and Palliative Nursing, 17*(3), 229–234. doi:10.1097/NJH.0000000000000153

Anita J. Tarzian

Ethical Aspects of Palliative Care

C H A P T E R

4

KEY POINTS

■ Ethics address right and wrong actions, decisions, character, and ends, and is influenced by one's core values.

■ *Nursing ethics* is a form of applied ethics that addresses questions of right and wrong in the practice of nursing.

■ *Moral residue* involves feelings of regret, guilt, or uncertainty when resolving an ethical concern or dilemma resulting in compromising a core value; *moral distress* involves knowing the right thing to do but not being able to do it.

■ The "ethics of being" involves cultivating one's character to act with integrity; the "ethics of doing" involves applying theoretical analytical approaches to clarify moral uncertainty, address ethical questions, and resolve moral dilemmas.

■ Two major approaches to theoretical ethical analysis are deontological (duty based) and utilitarian (consequence based).

■ Ethical principles of significance to nurses include respect for persons and autonomy, beneficence, nonmaleficence, justice, and fidelity.

■ Decision-making capacity is situation specific and differs from the concept of mental competence.

■ Surrogate decision makers should strive to make a "substituted judgment" of what an incapacitated patient would have wanted. A "best interest" standard is used if it is unknown what the patient would have wanted.

■ Advance directives may be helpful in identifying what a patient would have wanted when he or she no longer has decision-making capacity.

■ Minors have the right to be included in end-of-life (EOL) decision making, depending on their decision-making capacity and maturity.

■ Parents or legal guardians of minors must make decisions within the medical standard of care.

■ There is no moral distinction between withholding or withdrawing life-sustaining treatment.

■ Decisions to withhold or withdraw life-prolonging interventions, such as ventilators or artificial nutrition and hydration, are not considered forms of assisted suicide.

■ Nurses should identify resources available to them to support ethical decision making, including decision-making frameworks, ethics committees, the Code of Ethics for Nurses, and expert colleagues.

CASE STUDY

Mrs. S. is a 78-year-old woman who has resided in a nursing home for the past 5 years. Due to end-stage dementia, she is totally dependent on the nursing home staff for all activities of daily living, is noncommunicative, and receives nutrition through a feeding tube. She has no family, but has received consistent visits from Mrs. J., a close friend and former neighbor. Mrs. S. has a living will stipulating that if she were terminally ill, she should be kept comfortable rather than be treated with aggressive life-prolonging medical technology. However, Mrs. S. checked off on her living will that she would want artificial nutrition through tube feedings to keep her alive. Mrs. J. served as a witness when Mrs. S. signed the living will document. Mrs. J. tells the nurse that Mrs. S. would never have wanted to be kept alive in the state she is currently in—contracted into a fetal position, unable to meaningfully interact with others. She says that the lawyer did not fully explain what getting nutrition through a feeding tube might entail for someone with end-stage dementia. Instead, the lawyer presented this as something that might be implemented if Mrs. S. was "hungry and couldn't eat." Mrs. J. asks whether the tube feedings could be stopped and Mrs. S. allowed to die in peace.

Some decisions nurses make when providing EOL care seem particularly difficult. Even experienced nurses may feel uncertain about whether they made the "right" decision in these situations. When the issue is what, all things considered, is the *right* thing to do, a moral or ethical question is asked. It is often exquisitely difficult to determine what the right response is when, for example, a terminally ill and suffering patient pleads with you to help speed her or his dying. You want to help without causing her or him harm and without violating your professional duty. What should you do? An ethically hard case is one in which the good that you want to bring about can be realized only if the harm you seek to avoid is also brought about, that is, when benefiting the patient cannot be disentangled from harm (Cavanaugh, 1996).

Advances in scientific knowledge and developments in medical technology far exceed any social consensus about the circumstances for their appropriate use. The process of dying can now be prolonged almost indefinitely; this technological imperative (*can do* implies *ought to*) has given rise to an unprecedented array of professional, moral, and legal questions within healthcare. Many Americans fear the possibility of dying a painful, protracted, or undignified death, in an institutional setting, absent personal control or meaning (Pew Research Center, 2013). Studies indicate that nurses also have concerns about how best to provide care for dying patients. Beckstrand, Wood, Callister, Luthy, and Heaston (2012) identified ED nurses' perceptions of ways to improve EOL care. These included increasing the time ED nurses are given to care for dying patients, allowing family presence during resuscitation, providing comfortable patient rooms that preserve privacy, and providing family grief rooms. Aslakson et al. (2012) conducted focus groups with surgical ICU nurses and identified 34 barriers to optimal communication regarding prognosis, summarized into the following four domains: logistics, clinician discomfort with discussing prognosis, inadequate skill and training, and fear of conflict. Focus group analysis revealed 24 barriers to optimal EOL care summarized into four domains as well: logistics, inability to acknowledge an EOL situation, inadequate skill and training, and cultural differences relating to EOL care.

Ethical aspects of EOL decision making pose compelling challenges for nurses because they frequently involve conflicts among values, principles, and priorities of care; such conflicts require reasoned deliberation for their resolution. This chapter provides practicing nurses with the tools needed to identify and address the ethical issues in EOL care. To identify ethically relevant aspects of complex cases, nurses are encouraged to engage in values clarification and personal reflection. To address the ethical issues in EOL care effectively, nurses should use a decision-making framework that incorporates ethical theories, clearly defined moral concepts, and an understanding of the *Code of Ethics for Nurses* (American Nurses Association [ANA], 2015).

Ethical and legal issues often seem intertwined in many EOL decisions. For example, the selection of who is permitted to speak for a person who is decisionally incapable is a legally determined question, but which treatment the decision maker chooses is often a moral issue. Often the most difficult clinical conflicts occur at the junction of law and ethics, where an act that is illegal may seem morally required, or one that is legally required may seem morally inappropriate. Many of these cases resist satisfactory solutions. Although ethics and law function similarly in society in that they both sanction and guide behavior, they also differ in important ways. This chapter focuses on ethical issues in nursing care for patients approaching death.

■ ETHICS AND ETHICAL THEORY

Ethics is a branch of philosophy that considers and examines the moral life. The word "ethics" comes from the Greek "ethos," and originally meant "character" or "conduct"; the word "moral " comes from the Latin "mores," which means "customs" or "habit" (Davis, Aroskar, Liaschenko, & Drought, 1997). "Ethics" and "morals" are frequently used interchangeably in nursing ethics to refer to conduct, character, and motivations involved in moral acts, although distinctions are sometimes made between these terms.

The concept of morality is often used to refer to personally embraced concepts of duty, obligation, and principles of conduct. "Morals" is frequently used interchangeably with "values " and refers in particular to values or principles of conduct to which one is personally and actually committed (Jameton, 1984). Use of the word "ethics" is distinguished by reflective thinking and practical reasoning, and often includes overarching, publicly stated sets of rules or principles, such as those found in professional ethics codes. Stanley and Zoloth-Dorfman (2001) note that ethics seek to logically justify choices for right behavior and rules—particularly in situations that challenge established norms of behavior or in those that require a new paradigm for judging behavior. These authors add that ethical inquiry—which seeks to interpret acts and to answer such questions as "What is the right thing to do?"—traditionally includes an evaluation of (a) the moral agent and his or her character, (b) the motive for the act itself, and (c) the effect of the action on others. A focus on character may be referred to as the "ethics of being," whereas justifications of decisions or actions by applying ethical principles or theories may be referred to as the "ethics of doing." *Normative* ethics seeks ways to answer questions about right and wrong, or good or bad in situations that call for a moral decision (i.e., identifying what *should* be done). Nursing ethics is both normative and practical, in that it makes use of ethical theory and analysis to examine and resolve what *ought to be done* in situations involving moral conflict in nursing practice. "Bioethics" refers to the application of ethics and ethical analysis to moral and practical problems in biological sciences, medicine, and healthcare. Although the term "morality" refers to right and wrong as determined by an individual situated within a particular culture or religious group, and "ethics" refers to theories of right and wrong applied across groups, in everyday language the terms are used interchangeably.

Values and Value Clarification

Values have been called the cornerstone of nursing's moral art (Uustal, 1987). Few aspects of our personal or professional lives are value free. Values are ubiquitous, although often unspoken and frequently unexamined; they determine the nature of our moral choices. Values are foundational to our notions of good and bad, and inform our understanding of what constitutes benefit and harm; thus, they are instrumental to the ethical decisions we make. Because our values influence the choices we make, they may also bias our judgments about the worth of our own view and negatively influence our judgments about the merits of others' choices, hence the need for values clarification. In the absence of reflection, we may simply assume that others believe and would (should) do as we do.

Bill Peace is a paraplegic (he prefers the term "cripple") who writes a blog about disability rights (badcripple.blogspot.com). In an essay, he wrote about a botched attempt by a hospitalist to speak with him about his EOL preferences. Peace had a wound that had become infected with antibiotic-resistant bacteria. The hospitalist explained the seriousness of the situation and offered him the option of foregoing antibiotics and other life-sustaining interventions and switching to comfort care. Peace (2011) declined the offer and described the fear he felt during his long recovery:

> My fear was based on the knowledge that my existence as a person with a disability was not valued. Many people—the physician I met that fateful night included—assume disability is a fate worse than death. Paralysis does not merely prevent someone from walking but robs a person of his or her dignity. In a visceral and potentially lethal way, that night made me realize I was not a human being but rather a tragic figure. Out of the kindness of the physician's heart, I was being given a chance to end my life.

Perhaps, if the hospitalist had reflected on his own values, beliefs, and attitudes and how these influenced his recommendations for Mr. Peace, he might have approached this patient differently. The topic of death (the clinician's, his or her loved ones', and his or her patients') can emotionally trigger clinicians in many ways. Clinicians' unexamined emotional triggers thwart effective communication about EOL care. This can bias their recommendations for patients or cause them to avoid such conversations altogether, which fails both the patients and the loved ones who will grieve for them.

Values clarification is a process of self-reflection that helps individuals identify, consider, and articulate the belief, purposes, and attitudes they prize and that drive their actions. Beliefs about death and what makes life worth living, our conclusions about the nature and significance of truth, and the meaning of paths not chosen are all moral values. For example, observant Orthodox Jews, who value saving life, may not agree that permanent loss of brain function ("brain death") constitutes the death of the *person*. However, this same value may direct them to donate their organs even if declared brain dead if it means saving others' lives. Clarifying what their values are and how those values inform medical decisions often requires consulting other experts, such as clinicians and religious advisors. Fowler (1987) states that the purpose of values clarification is to assist individuals to identify those personal and professional values that influence their behavior and moral decision making. It is recognized that the essence of ethical conflict is the clash of values, principles, legal rules, and personal perspectives (Dubler & Liebman, 2011). The need for values clarification is an essential first step in moral decision making.

Every nursing intervention in the life of a patient has at least the possibility of enhancing or transgressing some value cherished by that patient. In situations of moral uncertainty or when encountering a true ethical dilemma, questions of values conflicts will always be foundational. *Moral uncertainty* occurs when nurses are uncertain *whether* a moral problem exists, are unsure about its nature, and are unclear which values conflict and which principles might facilitate clarification. These situations often occur in nursing practice. Moral uncertainty may occur when a patient seems to be suffering unnecessarily or is refusing pain medication, but is unwilling or unable to explain the reason for refusing your efforts to help. *An ethical dilemma* occurs less frequently and is understood as a situation in which two or more clear ethical principles apply that support mutually inconsistent courses of action. Each alternative course of action can be justified by an ethical rule or principle, but one can choose or satisfy only one course of action at the expense of *not* satisfying the other. The nurse who believes he or she is duty bound both to preserve life and to reduce suffering may experience a dilemma when preserving life causes intense suffering or when suffering can be reduced only by interventions that may shorten life. There is no truly satisfying "right" answer to an ethical dilemma, but one should utilize reasoned (principled) thinking to provide a rationale for the decision reached.

The third type of moral problem is the experience of *moral distress,* an emotion that occurs when nurses have identified and know what right response is called for, but institutional or other constraints make it almost impossible to pursue the right course of action (Jameton, 1984). Hamric (2012) found that moral distress can emerge from factors present in unit cultures, in institutions, and in the larger healthcare environment, as well as from factors internal to the individual and specific to a given clinical situation. Nurses surveyed by Varcoe, Pauly, Storch, Newton, and Makaroff (2012) identified a variety of situations they found morally distressing, including witnessing unnecessary suffering and being forced to provide care that compromised values. Kayser, Nault, and Ostiguy (2012) describe how nurses resolved moral distress when caring for patients who continued to smoke while using home oxygen therapy. Nurses who experience moral distress from institutional constraints on their ability to practice as morally autonomous clinicians

should seek support from colleagues and from other institutional and professional resources such as institutional ethics committees and state nursing associations.

Resources to assist the nurse in managing ethical concerns or dilemmas effectively are included in subsequent sections of this chapter. However, whatever the conflict, knowing one's own values and being sensitive to the values of others is an essential first step in ethically grounded nursing practice.

■ ETHICAL THEORIES

Moral theories are methods of determining what counts when a decision must be made, and to offer a method for weighing or ranking considerations identified as morally relevant to that decision. More succinct, an ethical theory provides a framework of principles within which an agent can determine morally appropriate actions (Beauchamp & Childress, 2012).

It should be noted that nurses regularly explore and resolve ethical questions in their practices without recourse to ethical theories and without a formal consideration of the nature of their foundational moral values. Yet, people hold different foundational views, which sometimes can heighten moral conflict and diminish the options for resolution. The following scenario related by Benjamin and Curtis (1992) illustrates the role that ethical theories can play in facilitating or hampering decision making. The case involves the question of whether everything should be done to prolong the life of an elderly gentleman in a nursing home who lacks decision-making capacity. The staff must make the decision because there are no friends or family and no prior indication of the gentleman's wishes. Person A argues that he should be treated because not to do so would violate the duty to protect and preserve life. Person B agrees that the man should be treated, but for a different reason. B argues that he should be treated because he is not in any pain, and although he is significantly cognitively impaired, he seems fairly content. In B's view, what one ought to do above all is to maximize happiness, and therefore the man's life should be prolonged. As presented, the question about whether to continue treatment can be answered without agreement about the nature of basic ethical values and with the use of dissimilar ethical theories.

Suppose the facts are changed a little, so that the gentleman is experiencing intractable pain and distress. In this case, with her foundational commitment to maximizing happiness, B would revise her judgment and conclude that they should no longer strenuously attempt to extend the man's life. But this change in facts would be irrelevant to A, and her judgment that the patient's life should be prolonged would remain the same. This conflict is not likely to be resolved without further questions about the nature and justification of ethical principles that are the foundation to approaches of making ethical decisions.

Within bioethics, there are two major approaches to theoretical considerations—deontological and teleological systems of ethics. The deontological (from "deon," Greek for "duty"), or Kantian, approach to ethics focuses on duties and obligations. Teleological theories (from "telos," Greek for "end") base the determination of whether an action is right or wrong on the action's consequences. These two ethical theories have been subject to criticism for their overreliance on unrelated and often conflicting principles in dealing with moral problems in healthcare (Clouser & Gert, 1990) and by feminist moral theorists for their indifference to the particularity of relationships (Gadow, 1996). These theories continue to dominate the ethical arguments used to resolve moral problems in healthcare, and nurses must recognize them and be familiar with their use in decision making. These two theories are described below and contrasted to a decisional theory based on caring.

Deontological Moral Theory

A deontological, or Kantian, approach to decision making focuses on duty and obligations. Kantian deontology is attributed to the 18th-century moral philosopher Immanuel Kant. Deontologists maintain that whether an act is right or wrong depends on the nature of the act itself when considered in terms of its inherent moral worth. Kant argued further that consequences can never make an action right or wrong. Duty-based theories hold particular duties to be fundamental and make use of principles or their derivative rules to guide decision making. Examples of duty-based theories include natural law, which identifies a duty to obey God's will and requires that one not kill, and the rules of traditional medical morality derived from the Hippocratic tradition, which maintain that above all we should do no harm.

A deontological position requires commitment to the principle of universalizability, which means that once a moral decision is made, that same decision must be made in all similar situations. The essence of this position is that morality requires that we cannot make exceptions for ourselves. Thus, if the proposed action is one that would be wrong if done generally, then the particular action is also wrong—even when the specific action has no harmful consequences. Such rules as "it is always wrong to directly take innocent human life" are considered valid when they meet certain conditions, identified by Kant as *categorical imperatives*. Proposed by Kant as a means to resolve conflicts between rules and principles, a categorical imperative means that for a rule to be valid it must be applicable to everyone universally. This principle can be illustrated as follows: If it is morally acceptable for me to act as I do for my patient (e.g., not charging for services, stealing medications for his or her use, skipping home visits, etc.), so must it also be acceptable for every other nurse to act similarly for his or her patients.

Another form of this categorical imperative requires that persons should always be treated (and valued) as ends in themselves, and never solely as means. Thus, nurses are required to respect individuals and their beliefs regardless of consequences, and they are similarly obliged to respect persons' autonomous choices. Kant identified these categorical imperatives as unconditional commands that are morally required and obligatory under any circumstances (Davis et al., 1997). Within this theoretical perspective, it is simply one's duty to obey categorical imperatives without any exceptions, without reference to the consequences of the act and in the absence of external or guiding authority. The moral standard includes keeping promises, avoiding or preventing harm, and respecting persons; these are principles that are morally required and are consistent with the rules provided in our professional code of ethics. Fiester (2007) cautions that the trend to approach ethical decision making using a "four principles" approach (i.e., weighing obligations toward beneficence, nonmaleficence, respect for persons, and justice) predisposes clinicians to overlook other ethical obligations toward patients, such as the obligation to acknowledge another's suffering and to apologize and make amends when clinicians make mistakes.

Teleological Moral Theories

Teleological theories determine an action to be right or wrong based on the consequences of the action. The most important teleological theory for contemporary healthcare is utilitarian ethics (Steinbock, Arras, & London, 2012). Utilitarianism is best understood as a moral theory that asserts there is only one basic principle in ethics, the principle of utility, which declares that we ought always to produce the greatest possible balance of value over disvalue for the greatest number of persons (Beauchamp & Childress, 2012). This position assumes that one can weigh and measure harms and benefits and arrive at the greatest possible balance of good over evil for the most people.

Utilitarians are disinterested in considerations of the agent's intentions, feelings, or convictions; all are viewed as irrelevant to the question of "What is the right thing to do?" In the same fashion, utilitarians regard the question of whether a proposed action conforms to established social norms or ethical codes as relevant only to the extent that conforming (or not) has a bearing on the production of happiness or value over unhappiness (Steinbock et al., 2012). At least in principle, utilitarians are able to provide definite answers to specific questions about how one ought to act. The question of whether it is ever morally permissible to be untruthful depends upon context and circumstances. For example, in those situations in which telling a lie would produce, overall, more happiness or value than unhappiness, then telling a lie would be morally justified.

As with deontological theories, there are two versions of this theory: An act-utilitarian is primarily concerned with the consequences of particular acts, whereas a rule-utilitarian is more concerned about the consequences of general policies. To illustrate the difference between these versions, imagine that a nurse is trying to decide whether it would be morally right to help a terminally ill patient die. An act-utilitarian would try to determine which alternative in this particular situation would maximize happiness or minimize suffering or both. The considerations included in making that determination would be the nature of the disease and the certainty of prognosis, the presence of a treatable depression, whether the patient really wanted to die or needed better palliative care (PC), the impact on the patient's family, and the professional repercussions for the nurse. In contrast, a rule-utilitarian uses the principle of utility to formulate and justify moral rules, viewing the correct moral rules as those that promote the greatest happiness for the greatest number (Steinbock et al., 2012). In this particular case, the nurse would ask whether a general rule permitting physician-assisted death (PAD) would maximize happiness. Important considerations of this approach include questions about whether such a practice would put us on a slippery slope and threaten the lives of other terminally ill patients who do not really want to die but might feel obliged or are susceptible to being coerced. Thus, a rule-utilitarian might agree that although helping this particular patient to die might maximize happiness (or minimize suffering) for the individual, it would still be wrong because of the larger negative consequences of a general policy permitting PAD (Steinbock et al., 2012).

How would a Kantian resolve this nurse's problem? Steinbock et al. (2012) suggest that the categorical imperative gives less guidance—it functions only to tell us what *cannot* be done, and not what *should* be done. The principle of universalizability is just one value in Kantian ethics; the other mandate is respect for persons. The question would then be reframed: Does a policy of PAD promote respect for persons, or would such a policy lead to the devaluing of human life and to nonvoluntary killing of the weak, the vulnerable, and the poor? Each of these theories has strengths and limitations, but neither ethical theories nor principles alone will provide a formula for resolving specific ethical questions. What they do provide is a framework for trying to reach workable solutions to complex and difficult questions (Steinbock et al., 2012).

Focus on Caring

An ethic of caring that focuses on relationships and responsibility is one aspect of the broader field of feminist ethics. This ethic stems in part from a criticism of traditional ethical theories as being biased in their representation of the experiences of men rather than women. Another dimension of feminist ethics is the consideration of oppression and dominance within relationships and social institutions. It is certain that power differentials among nurses (who are more often women), physicians, patients, administrators, and payers illustrate just some of the relational inequalities that exist in most healthcare organizations (Davis et al., 1997). *Caring*, within the context of an *ethics of care*, refers to "care for, emotional commitment to, and willingness to act on behalf of persons with whom one has a significant relationship. Noticeably downplayed are Kantian universal rules, impartial utilitarian calculations, and individual rights" (Beauchamp & Childress, 2008, p. 369).

The idea of an ethic of caring is particularly appealing to nurses because caring is considered to be the very foundation of their practice. Sara Fry, a nurse philosopher, proposed caring as a fundamental value for the development of a theory of nursing ethics (Fry, 1989). Care for others is a core notion in an ethic of care and is evident in the ANA *Code of Ethics for Nurses* (2015), which mandates respectful care of the individual as its core tenet. Wright and Brajtman (2011, p. 26) acknowledge that "nursing is unique in how it cares; what is unique about nursing is the nature of the work that nurses do." They describe the importance of maintaining relationships in healthcare encounters by acknowledging the power of narrative and "embodied knowing," writing: "Nurses' moral identities are dialogical, narrative, relational, and contextual, where moral responsibility in nursing involves striving to do good in situations that are never the same twice" (p. 26).

Fry, Killen, and Robinson (1996) maintain that

the actions and judgments made using care-based reasoning must be measured against what it means to be "caring" within the context of the responsibilities the decision maker has to others. . . . [C]are-based reasoning does not involve the application of abstract ethical principles to the situation or impartiality on the part of the decision maker. (p. 42)

Critics of the ethics of care posit that it is not clearly defined and distinguished from other approaches (Edwards, 2009). Thus, an ethic of care is not yet adequately developed to function as a conceptual theory for identifying "right" actions in morally troubling situations.

■ ETHICS OF DOING VERSUS BEING

One way of framing ethical theories is to consider whether they focus primarily on actions and decisions (i.e., "ethics of doing") or on an individual's character attributes and virtues (i.e., "ethics of being"). To be sure, resolving ethical dilemmas requires figuring out "what to do." But nurses should keep in mind that although ethical theories are often used to figure out what is the right thing "to do" in a particular situation, it's also important to consider the impact of actions and decisions on who we are as moral actors and how we relate to one another. One example of this that nurses frequently confront in acute care settings is the issue of whether it is ethically acceptable to attempt cardiopulmonary resuscitation (CPR) on patients for whom it is not expected to provide a benefit, but whose surrogate decision maker insists be done. Some clinicians and bioethicists, using a utilitarian justification, may argue that if a patient is dying and experiences cardiac arrest, attempting CPR to assuage the family's grief is justified because the unconscious patient won't suffer and the family would benefit from knowing that "everything was done." Others may argue (assuming the patient hadn't expressed prior wishes to forego CPR attempts) that this demonstrates lack of respect for a dying body and misuse of medical resources, and perhaps misses an opportunity to provide more effective interventions with loved ones to minimize their future regrets. Regardless of whether a decision is made to allow CPR attempts that are not expected to benefit the patient, clinicians at the bedside who would provide CPR attempts are impacted by this decision. An "ethics of being" approach addresses how to care for not just the patient and family members, but also the staff involved, to minimize regrets and moral distress for all.

▪ ETHICAL PRINCIPLES AND CONCEPTS

The major ethical principles of significance to nurses are respect for persons and autonomy, beneficence, nonmaleficence, and justice. The duties of veracity, fidelity, and confidentiality are moral rules derived from these principles that further guide and direct nursing actions. These moral rules are embedded in the provisions of the *Code of Ethics for Nurses* (ANA, 2015). One particular rule that resonates for nurses who care for patients at the end of life is the proscription that "nurses may not act with the sole intent to end life" in the process of relieving "pain and other symptoms in the dying patient" (ANA, 2015, p. 3). There may be occasions when moral agents feel obliged to question these rules and their appropriateness in particular circumstances, and they may wish to "appeal" to a higher level of moral authority (Veatch & Fry, 1995). Perhaps a nurse may question whether it is *always* wrong to "act with the sole intent of ending a patient's life" and to ask whether other duties, such as mercy and compassion, might sometimes prevail. This higher level of authority within a moral framework consists of ethical principles.

Respect for Persons and the Principle of Autonomy

The most fundamental ethical principle within nursing practice is the principle of respect for persons. The first provision in the *Code of Ethics for Nurses* (ANA, 2015)

calls for nurses to "respect the dignity and rights of all human beings regardless of the factors contributing to the person's health status. The worth of a person is not affected by illness, ability, socioeconomic status, functional status, or proximity to death" (p. 1). The principle of respect for persons is broader and more abstract than the principle that addresses individual autonomy and self-determination. Respect for persons requires that each individual be treated as unique and entitled to treatment that is respectful of his or her human dignity. It is this principle of respect for persons that requires particular justification before we are permitted to interfere with the plans, privacy, or behavior of autonomous adult persons, and specifically constrains *paternalistic* decisions made by health professionals for patients with decision-making capacity.

The concept of autonomy is multidimensional and in its broadest sense incorporates the following: having a minimum of relevant information, self-determined choice, freedom to act on the basis of one's choices, and self-governance (Yeo, Moorhouse, & Dalziel, 1996). Autonomous (or decisionally capable) persons determine their own course of action in accordance with a plan they chose. An autonomous action is understood as one done intentionally, with the understanding of relevant information and without controlling influences that determine the action (Beauchamp & Childress, 2012).

How are nurses to understand and apply this principle? This principle guides nursing actions in that nurses are duty bound to respect patients' autonomous choices in all situations unless this principle is overridden by another moral principle of greater weight or standing (Fry, 1987). Such would be the case when questions are raised about whether the choice is truly autonomous, whether the choice is perceived as harmful to the individual or others, and in other situations in which autonomous choice is not possible. In these situations, the nurse's obligation to prevent harm to others or to benefit the patient may be determined to have greater moral weight. The example of intervening to prevent a suicide motivated by depression or mental illness is often cited. Orentlicher, Pope, and Rich (2016) and Wittwer (2013) present arguments to exempt "rational" suicide in the case of dying individuals ending their lives through access to lethal prescription. Consider another example of a patient who writes an advance directive (AD) stipulating that he not be fed—either artificially or by spoon feeding—in the event that he develops dementia and does not recognize family and friends. Imagine that he develops Alzheimer's disease that is in an advanced stage. The staff members at the nursing home where he is living may argue that to withhold freely accepted oral feedings from this patient would cause a greater harm to him than overriding his prior wishes that he not be fed, and may be construed as negligence on their part.

It is the principle of respect for persons and autonomy that is the foundation of informed consent. According to this rule, persons must be given sufficient, accurate, and complete information necessary to make informed decisions about treatment choices. This includes decisions to accept, refuse, or terminate treatments, whether or not these treatments are necessary for sustaining or prolonging life.

Limiting Autonomy

Nurses who care for patients at the end of life may sometimes wonder whether they ought to intervene to prevent harm that they fear may result from a patient's decision. When are clinicians justified in limiting or interfering with a person's autonomy? The two most frequently occurring ways that healthcare professionals infringe upon patient autonomy are through control of information (e.g., withholding, deceiving, or equivocating) or through preventing a patient from acting upon his or her choice (e.g., refusing to comply or assist, constraining, or forcing treatment; Yeo, Moorhouse, & Dalziel, 1996). This type of interference, known as *paternalism* or *parentalism*, occurs often in healthcare and is done with the best of intentions; indeed, by definition it is understood as an intervention that is imposed for the patient's good or benefit.

In fact, paternalistic actions, such as deception, breaking promises, or interfering with adult choices, are violations of moral rules that are never morally permitted unless an adequate reason is provided. To justify such violations, philosophers Culver and Gert (1982) assert: "If all rational persons would agree that the evil prevented by universally allowing this violation would be greater than the evil caused by universally allowing it, the violation is strongly justified" (p. 149). In other words, we must determine whether we would publicly advocate this kind of violation in all similar situations. This would be a difficult standard to meet for those who presume that justification exists for telling a lie based solely on the belief that doing so would benefit another. A classic example of meeting such a standard is the case of a Dutchman who hid a Jewish family during World War II and lied to a Nazi officer to protect the Jewish family. In considering circumstances when limitations on autonomy may be justified, "weak" paternalism is sometimes accepted to prevent persons from causing themselves serious harm. In this view, one would be justified in interfering to prevent a significant harm from occurring, but only when the person's conduct is substantially nonvoluntary or nonautonomous (Yeo, Moorhouse, & Dalziel, 1996). An example would be stopping a patient about to jump out of a hospital window. To justify this type of interference, one would have to demonstrate that the presumption of autonomy or self-determination is no longer held and that the person's choices were in fact no longer autonomous or freely elected.

"Strong" paternalism, in contrast, involves limiting or interfering with the self-determination of someone whose autonomy is not in question (i.e., an adult capable of rational decision making), and thus is very rarely justified. For example, a decisionally capable person who at the end of his or her life makes a thoughtful and considered decision to stop eating and drinking would be seriously wronged or harmed if a clinician were to override his or her decision and insert a feeding tube or intravenous line to prolong life. Paternalistic behavior, regardless of how good the motives or the size of the benefit gained or the harm avoided, violates the right of an adult to be treated as a person. To disregard a person's life plans and values in such a fashion is to show contempt for the individual as a person, or in Kant's terms, it is to treat the person as a mere means to an end, rather than as an end in himself or herself.

Before an act of paternalism can be considered justified, each of the following conditions must be present (Benjamin & Curtis, 1992):

1. The patient's capacity for rational reflection must be significantly impaired. This (*autonomy* condition) must be clinically determined and substantiated.
2. The patient is likely to be significantly harmed if no one interferes (the *harm* condition).
3. It is reasonable to assume that the patient will, at a later time, with recovery of capacity for rational reflection, ratify or agree to the decision made to interfere (the *ratification* condition).

Questions About Capacity for Autonomous Choice

Patients should be assumed to have the capacity to make decisions for themselves unless there is clear evidence to the contrary (Beauchamp & Childress, 2012). Clinical judgments about a person's decision-making capacity play a gatekeeping role in healthcare by distinguishing those whose decisions should be solicited and honored from persons whose decisions need not or should not be solicited or accepted (Beauchamp & Childress, 2012). Patient capacity is often neither completely present nor totally absent, as is particularly the case in some elderly persons who may evidence a level of capacity that waxes and wanes. When capacity waxes and wanes, caregivers should take advantage of opportunities to engage the patient in decision making and advance care planning when the patient's capacities are at their best (Lynn et al., 1999). Capacity is best understood as task specific, in that a higher level of decision-making capacity is required for decisions associated with serious consequences (e.g., whether to consent to enroll in a research study testing an investigational cancer drug) and a lower level is required for decisions associated with less serious consequences (e.g., choosing meals or where to eat them; Mezey, Mitty, & Ramsey, 1997). This "sliding scale" for decision-making capacity is justified by the principle of respect for persons, which requires a clinician to assess the harms associated with a particular decision (especially high-stakes decisions) to determine whether the clinician is obligated to override a patient's choice based on evidence that the patient does not have sufficient cognitive capacity to understand the pros and cons associated with that choice. For example, a patient who *consents* to a life-saving leg amputation would generally be subject to less questioning to ensure his or her decision-making capacity than a patient who *refuses* it. Although some staff members think this presents a double standard, the different approach is ethically justified by the risk–benefit analysis associated with life-saving leg amputation surgery. A capacity determination is a clinical judgment made by caregivers who know the patient best. When the stakes of a capacity determination are particularly high or the determination is contentious, clinicians may wish to seek a psychiatric consultation to assist in the capacity determination. In these instances, it is important to distinguish between a decision-making capacity assessment, which is situation specific, and a mental competency assessment, which is global. For example, individuals may lack the decision-making capacity to complete a living will while retaining the decision-making capacity to appoint a healthcare agent.

There are occasions when nurses may question whether a treatment choice reflects what the patient truly wants or whether the patient's decision was informed and autonomous. Nurses may want to know whether the patient is capable of making an informed and autonomous choice and whether they should comply with a decision that seems inconsistent with previously stated wishes or values.

Assessing Decision-Making Capacity

A decisionally capable person is able to understand a proposed intervention (or its termination), deliberate regarding major risks and benefits, make a decision in light of that deliberation, and communicate the choice to others (whether verbally or nonverbally). The following is information that decisionally capable patients should understand:

- The condition for which the intervention is recommended
- The nature of the recommended intervention
- The risks and benefits of the recommended intervention, and of alternative interventions, including no intervention or treatment

Healthcare providers should determine that

- The patient acknowledges that treatment is recommended.
- The patient understands how the proposed treatment or lack of treatment can affect his or her quality of life (QOL).
- The patient's decision is not substantially based on a delusional belief (Yeo, Moorhouse, & Dalziel, 1996).

These criteria are intended to establish whether the patient is capable of making a rational choice, not whether the choice being made is right or wrong in itself.

Deciding for Others

If a patient lacks the capacity to make informed choices, other means must be identified for surrogate decision making. There are three standards for surrogate decision making: written ADs (e.g., living wills), substituted judgment, and best interest. These three standards are ordered so that ADs have priority over the other two and substituted judgment has priority over the best-interest standard (Lynn et al., 1999). The best of all situations is a thoughtfully drafted AD applied by a surrogate decision maker who knows the patient's values and wishes.

Substituted judgment is a subjective standard that is ideally based on knowledge of the patient's wishes, values, views about particular interventions, and QOL determinations. If a patient has completed an AD, this should inform the surrogate's substituted judgment assessments. Realistically, a surrogate's knowledge about the patient's goals and values is typically not entirely clear and decisive regarding a particular choice of treatment. Lynn et al. (1999) state that "in practice, surrogate decision-making for incompetent patients often has to draw on all three standards for decisions about an incompetent patient's care" (p. 273). Some in the disability rights community prefer the term "best supported decision-making" over "substituted judgment," as experiences with guardians who make decisions for adults with developmental or intellectual disabilities have revealed overly paternalistic approaches that fail to represent the voice of those served (see jennyhatchjusticeproject.org). The best-interest standard is used when the patient's treatment wishes, or values, are unknown. Under these circumstances, the decision maker must objectively weigh the expected benefits and burdens associated with the treatment recommended by the healthcare team and determine what would be best for this patient.

Nurses have an important role to play in supporting surrogate decision making. The surrogate must be encouraged to focus on what the now noncommunicative patient would want if he or she were able to communicate. It is often difficult for grieving family members to put aside their own distress about the implications of honoring their loved one's preferences, especially when the decision involves withholding or withdrawing life-sustaining treatments (LSTs). This is especially true in ICUs, where increasingly complex life-prolonging interventions are initiated without clear communication regarding when such interventions would be stopped (e.g., left ventricular assist devices, continuous dialysis, extra-corporeal membrane oxygenation). Family members who spend weeks or months hoping their loved one will "beat the odds" are often unprepared for what stopping treatment feels like after such emotional investment in the patient's hoped-for recovery. In these situations, it is helpful for loved ones to know something about the patient's preferences in such a situation. Thus, although the patient retains capacity, he or she should be encouraged and guided by nurses to discuss EOL choices with family members or other potential surrogate decision makers. Nurses are well positioned to describe to patients and their loved ones the actual risks and benefits that are known to be associated with the use of interventions such as CPR, tube feedings, and mechanical ventilation. Use of "certified decision aids" (Cardona-Morrell, et al., 2017) and AD software programs (www.mydirectives. com) may be useful resources. As Perrin (1997) notes, "Advance directives are unlikely to have an effect on care if a health care provider, proxy, or family member does not support and advocate for following the person's wishes" (p. 25). Yet, ADs often are unavailable or not applicable in many of the clinical situations faced by seriously ill adults (Fagerlin & Schneider, 2004). It is hoped that the rise of AD online registries will address the former shortcoming (Jones, Sabin, & Torma, 2016).

■ **Use of Advance Directives.** Researchers investigating how ADs actually function in various clinical settings have explored whether the presence of an AD ensures compliance with patients' EOL wishes. A number of commentators agree that there are persistent difficulties associated with the use of *written* directives; these include incomplete information, the inability to anticipate future medical conditions, and uncertainty regarding the meaning and intent of written instructions (Fagerlin & Schneider, 2004; Peryakoil, Neri, & Kraemer, 2017). These problems of interpretation require clinicians to seek information from others in their attempt to determine what the patient "really meant" (Tonelli, 1996). Although some argue that having individuals complete ADs promotes advance care planning conversations between patients and clinicians, Lewis, Cardona-Morrell, Ong, Trankle, & Hillman, K. (2016) found that increased AD completion was not associated with better healthcare provider engagement in EOL discussions with patients. Tonelli (1996) and Dexter, Wolinsky, Gramelspacher, Eckert, and Tierney (2003) conclude that because of the limitations associated with the use of written directives, it is preferable to recommend that adults appoint a durable power of attorney for healthcare. Yet, surrogates also have difficulties accurately predicting their loved one's EOL treatment preferences and often experience distress when deciding to withdraw LST from a loved one who lacks decision-making capacity in the absence of an AD (Tilden, Tolle, Nelson, & Fields, 2001). Shalowitz, Garrett-Mayer, and Wendler (2006) reviewed 16 studies on surrogate accuracy published between 1966 and 2005 and found that, overall, surrogates are inaccurate 32% of the time (Shalowitz et al., 2006). Perkins (2007) argues that ADs promise more control over future care and EOL decisions than is possible to achieve. He concludes that

"advance care planning must refocus from completing ADs to preparing patients and families for the uncertainties and difficult decisions of future medical crises" (p. 51).

Recently, the focus has shifted from merely completing an AD to adults engaging in advance care planning (ACP) *conversations* with their healthcare provider(s) and loved ones, and documenting their preferences for care at the end of life (Norals & Smith, 2015). In the absence of a thoughtful discussion that includes general EOL values and specific preferences about use of interventions such as artificial nutrition and hydration (ANH), the legally appointed surrogate may be poorly prepared to identify or implement treatment decisions that conform with the patient's actual EOL preferences (Kelly, Rid, & Wendler, 2012). When ADs are informed by ACP conversations, they are more likely to be of value.

Some have advocated for better methods of approaching EOL care planning. Waldrop and Meeker (2012) identify types of ACP and barriers to effective communication about EOL preferences, including lack of physician education; inadequate methods for providing information; lack of protocols for such communication; reluctance to discuss death; difficulty discussing the unknown; and inadequate shared understanding about values and implications among the patient, family, and care provider. The Respecting Choices Model (respectingchoices.org) has been shown to achieve higher AD completion rates, based reportedly on better staff training in discussing EOL care planning. Hickman, Keevern, and Hammes (2015) provide evidence that Physician Orders for Life-Sustaining Treatment (POLST) transportable resuscitation orders are effective complements to traditional ADs to achieve EOL care that coheres with patients' preferences (www.polst.org).

Beneficence and Nonmaleficence

"Beneficence," known generically as *doing good*, is often hard to separate from "nonmaleficence," or the duty not to inflict harm. Some philosophers argue that the principle of beneficence includes four rules (Frankena, 1973):

1. One ought not to inflict evil or harm (what is bad).
2. One ought to prevent evil or harm.
3. One ought to remove evil.
4. One ought to do good or promote good.

These rules are prioritized in that the first takes precedence over the second, which is in turn more compelling than the third, which takes moral precedence over the fourth, all things being equal (Frankena, 1973). Although it can seem difficult in clinical practice to distinguish preventing harm from providing benefit, Benjamin and Curtis (1992) believe that it is easier to get agreement on what constitutes harm than on what constitutes a benefit. When the duty not to inflict harm conflicts with the duty to provide benefit, there is agreement that, all things being equal, there is a greater obligation not to injure others than to benefit them (Beauchamp & Childress, 2012).

In healthcare, the principle of nonmaleficence is understood as requiring clinicians to avoid intentionally causing patients unnecessary harm or pain, whether psychological or physical. Neither the principle of nonmaleficence nor any of its derived moral rules are absolute. We often do harm to patients to benefit them or to prevent a greater harm from occurring—administering chemotherapy to treat cancer is an obvious example. What is morally relevant is whether causing the harm is morally justified. Under most circumstances, death is considered a major harm; the question of whether causing death is ever justified is an issue of significance to nurses who provide care at the end of life.

Patients at the end of their lives may be particularly vulnerable to harm. They are harmed when they receive unwanted or unnecessary interventions, when they are overtreated with burdensome technological interventions that serve only to prolong dying, and also when treatments are unjustifiably withdrawn without their consent or agreement. Most certain, they are harmed when their pain or air hunger is not managed adequately due to the nurse's fear that the patient's death might be hastened as a result of giving appropriate doses of opiates. The *Code of Ethics for Nurses* (ANA, 2015) not only stipulates that nurses should "not act with the sole intent to end life," but also requires that "the nurse should provide interventions to relieve pain and other symptoms in the dying patient consistent with palliative care practice standards" (p. 3).

Balancing Good and Evil: The Principle of Double Effect

Any discussion that includes attempts to distinguish between harming and benefiting patients often includes the principle of double effect. Developed by Roman Catholic moral theologians in the Middle Ages, this principle is applied to situations in which it is impossible to avoid all harmful action and a decision must be made about whether one potentially harmful action is preferable to another (Quill, Dresser, & Brock, 1997). This principle is used to justify claims that the results of an act that would be morally wrong if caused intentionally are permissible if foreseen but unintended. The principle is often cited to explain why certain forms of care at the end of life that result in death are morally permissible and others are not (Coyle, 1992; Latimer, 1991; Quill, Lo, & Brock, 1997; Schwarz, 2004b, Truog et al., 2008).

The traditional formulation of this principle stipulates that the following four conditions be met before an act with both good and bad consequences may be morally justified (Schwarz, 2004b):

1. The action itself must be good or at least morally indifferent.
2. The individual must sincerely intend only the good effect and not the evil.

3. The evil effect cannot be the means to the good effect.
4. There must be a proportionately valid reason for permitting the evil effect; that is, there must be a favorable balance between the good and evil effects of the action.

The first condition determines whether the potential action is ever permissible, whereas the second and third conditions are used to determine whether the potential harm is intentional or unintentional, either as a means or as an end in itself. The fourth condition requires the agent to compare the net good and bad effects of the potential act to determine which course produces an effect of proportionally greater good (Quill, Dresser, & Brock, 1997).

Nurses may appeal to this principle in morally difficult situations in which it is not possible to benefit a patient by an action without causing harm at the same time. An example is that of a dying patient on a ventilator, for whom a decision is made to withdraw the ventilator, and death is expected. Medications like opioids given to avoid respiratory distress during the process of stopping the ventilator might also hasten the patient's death. The nurse has a moral duty to prevent and remove evil (respiratory distress) that appears to conflict with the duty to benefit patients (protect and preserve life). The answer to the question of whether the nurse may administer opioids is clearly yes. Applying the criteria of double effect illustrates why this is so (Schwarz, 2004b):

1. The action of giving opioids is itself morally indifferent.
2. The intended effect is to relieve respiratory distress, not to depress the respirations.
3. Respiratory depression is not the means by which the respiratory distress is palliated.
4. The relief of respiratory distress and the related reduction of suffering combine to provide a sufficiently important reason, or proportionately greater good than the harm that is incurred—respiratory depression and likely death.

Although this moral analysis is consistent with the position found within the *Code of Ethics for Nurses* (ANA, 2015), some question the clinical usefulness of this principle as a guide to ethical decision making (Beauchamp & Childress, 2012). In particular, some clinical experts in PC challenge the purported "double effect" of opiate use in terminally ill patients and describe the likelihood of a secondarily associated hastened death as an "overblown myth" (Manfredi, Morrison, & Meier, 1998, p. 139). Indeed, some studies have shown that opioids do not hasten death in terminally ill patients, particularly in patients who are not opioid naïve, because individuals develop a tolerance to an opioid's respiratory depressant effect (Bakker, Jansen, Lima, & Kompanje, 2008; Portenoy et al., 2006). Macauley (2012) found that some ethics educators mistakenly believe that opioids are likely to cause significant respiratory depression that hastens death in terminally ill patients, and others who do not believe this still rely on the principle of double effect to justify this possibility, which may contribute to clinical misperceptions and underuse of opioids at the end of life.

Experienced PC nurses recognize that death sometimes occurs secondarily as an unintended, though foreseen, side effect of medications used to manage refractory symptoms in dying patients. Despite the clear legal and moral consensus supporting the appropriateness of such interventions, when a patient dies immediately after a nurse provides an opioid, it can *feel* to the nurse that he or she is causing the patient's death. However, ethics is based on providing well-reasoned justifications to support a given action, rather than relying on feelings alone. Nurses must be well versed in the ethical justification supporting actions to reduce patients' suffering at the end of life, even if such actions hasten a patient's death. Nurses are encouraged to consult the ANA (2013) position statement on euthanasia, assisted suicide, and aid in dying, which states, "The provision of medications with the intent to promote comfort and relieve suffering is not to be confused with the administration of medication with the intent to end the patient's life" (p. 6).

Justice

The last principle that may facilitate nurses' decisions about EOL care is justice, which is understood broadly as fairness. Justice involves the determination of what someone or some group is owed, merits, deserves, or otherwise is entitled to something (Yeo, Moorhouse, & Donner, 1996). At the societal (macro) level of resource allocation, the concept of justice includes questions of how scarce resources ought to be distributed and what should "count" as morally relevant differences between individuals to justify differences in treatment. Microallocation issues involve determining which particular person will receive a specific and limited resource. A number of criteria for making such selections include likelihood of medical benefit and present and future QOL criteria (Yeo, Moorhouse, & Donner, 1996). It is generally agreed that if a medical intervention will not benefit a patient, it is considered medically futile or "nonbeneficial," and as such its use is morally and professionally unwarranted. In other words, it is outside the medical standard of care. The Society of Critical Care Medicine's ethics committee recommends replacing the term "futile" with "potentially inappropriate" when referring to interventions that are unlikely—rather than unable—to achieve an intended goal (Kon et al., 2016). Medically futile interventions should not be proposed or offered to patients or families. As an illustration of how questions of futility have been clinically addressed, the Texas Advance Directive Act (TADA) provides a process to address situations in which clinicians believe that particular interventions are medically futile but whose surrogate decision maker insists that such interventions be provided. The process requires consultation with an ethics or medical committee; the option of family participation in the committee deliberations; and whether the committee concludes that treatment is medically inappropriate or "futile," giving the family 10 days to transfer the patient, appeal to the courts, or accept that the interventions will be withheld or withdrawn (usually resulting in the patient's death). The concept of "medically inappropriate" treatment is broader than the concept of "medically futile" treatment (Kon et al., 2016). Both, however, involve analyzing probabilities of achieving a desired goal and weighing proposed benefits against imposed burdens. For example, when considering whether CPR attempts would be medically futile, Westphal (2008) reported survival data to hospital discharge for patients with advanced cancer in the 6% to 7% range. This rate does not meet the criterion of medical futility that Schneiderman and Jecker (1995) proposed—that a treatment should be considered medically futile if it has not achieved its intended goal in the last 100 cases. Nevertheless, Varon and Marik (2007) argue that obtaining do-not-resuscitate (DNR) orders for patients with advanced cancer is medically *inappropriate*, whether or not it fits the definition for being medically *futile*. Still, others question whether we have become so reliant on medical technology that we should view CPR attempts as a kind of EOL ritual to assuage the grief of survivors (Mohammed & Peter, 2009). If a patient for whom CPR is not expected to achieve its medical goal remains a "full code" merely to honor the patient's wishes or assuage survivors' grief, those clinicians who may be called on to attempt CPR should be involved ahead of time to weigh in on what is expected during such CPR attempts and allowed to opt out. For example, physicians have been known to offer nonstandard resuscitation options to patients or surrogates, such as "one round of Advanced Cardiac Life Support (ACLS)" to reassure patients or survivors that "everything was done." This is questionable practice, as the person making such a promise can't translate this into actionable orders, because "one round of ACLS" is not the medical standard of care, and the physician promising this option is most likely not the clinician who will provide this intervention. Tarzian (1995, p. 3) proposed that the euphemism of "doing everything" to refer to attempting CPR and other interventions to delay the moment of death be redefined to include "standing firm on decisions of CPR futility and offering family members the image of a less invasive death—one supported and guided by those who know meaningful rituals other than medical interventions to make that death less burdensome for all."

At the bedside level, clinicians cite justice to support all individuals who are terminally ill and receiving access to high-quality PC. In the current era of cost containment and social injustice, some fear that those who are already marginalized and disadvantaged by poverty, chronic or terminal illness, old age, cultural and racial status, or gender may feel a duty to die to spare families financial or emotional strain (Bergner, 2007). Individual nurses or other healthcare professionals will not resolve these complex issues at the bedside. However, many who advocate for U.S. healthcare reform agree that cost must be considered in the allocation of healthcare resources (Donley & Danis, 2011; Emanuel, 2008). Kahn et al. (2015) point to the expanding category of "chronic critical illness" in the United States—that is, patients requiring ICU-level interventions as destination therapy. How to fairly weigh such costs and associated burdens against benefits requires interprofessional understanding and cooperative effort among all affected parties within society (American College of Physicians, 2008; Scheunemann & White, 2011). Meanwhile, the *Code of Ethics for Nurses* (ANA, 2015) stresses that the nurse's commitment is to particular patients, unaffected by "illness, ability, socioeconomic status, functional status, or proximity to death" (p. 1). The challenge for caregivers is to reach ethically supportable decisions that are fair to individual patients while using available resources responsibly and to treat comparable cases alike. Kon et al. (2016) present strategies for more effective shared decision making in ICU settings.

■ ELEMENTS OF A DECISION-MAKING FRAMEWORK

When nurses must choose between alternative courses of action that seem equally unattractive, they experience an ethical dilemma. Deciding what to do in such cases has significant implications for the well-being of the patient, involved family members, and others affected by the choice. The nurse's ability to provide an ethically defensible rationale for decisions is recognized as foundational to professional practice and the integrity of individual nurses (Davis et al., 1997). Rushton and Reigle (1993) argue in support of a shared decision-making model that promotes patient well-being and self-determination. According to this model, the healthcare team offers expert knowledge, treatment recommendations, and advice about medically available and appropriate options to the patient ("patient" being understood as the patient/family unit). The patient decides which option will best promote his or her life goals and values. The nurse is particularly well positioned to understand the values that inform patients' choices and to appreciate the context of a patient's whole life, including the patient/family unit; their cultural, religious, and spiritual affiliations; and other unique preferences. The nurse is a vitally important member of this decision-making team.

When a clinical problem is identified as having ethical dimensions (i.e., conflicts in moral values or ethical principles are present), the following steps will assist the nurse to discuss, analyze, and successfully develop an ethically supportable decision:

1. Review the overall situation—identify what is going on in this case.
2. Gather all relevant facts about the patient and his or her contextual situation, including:
   ■ Significant medical and social history
   ■ Decision-making capacity
   ■ Existence of any advance treatment directives—written, appointed, or verbal—and any pertinent institutional policies
3. Identify the parties or stakeholders involved in the situation, including those who will be affected by the decision(s) made.
4. Identify relevant legal data, including both state and federal laws.
5. Identify specific conflicts of ethical principles or values. Identify and consider nursing guidelines and the profession's code of ethics and position statements.
6. Identify possible choices, their purpose, and their probable consequences to the welfare of the patient, who is the focus of primary concern. Identify and make use of interprofessional and institutional resources such as institutional ethics committees, ethics consultants, chaplains, social workers, and other experienced colleagues.
7. Identify practical constraints to decision making (e.g., institutional, legal, organizational, political, and economic).
8. Take action if you are the decision maker and implementer of the decision(s). If not, support the authorized decision maker.
9. Review and evaluate the situation after action is taken to determine what was learned that will help in the resolution of similar situations in patient care and policy development (Cassells & Gaul, 1998; Davis et al., 1997).

■ CONCEPTUAL CONFUSION AND DIFFICULT DECISIONS IN END-OF-LIFE CARE

The final segment of this chapter explores issues of patient autonomy and decisions about EOL interventions that range from instances of allowing or permitting death to hastening or intentionally causing death, and how these decisions are understood by nurses.

Autonomy and the Refusal of Life-Sustaining Treatment

If the concept of autonomy means anything at all, it means the right to accept or refuse medical treatments. Decisions about the use or withdrawal of LSTs are often complex and value laden, in part because such decisions may forestall or hasten the time of death. Decisions regarding the use of LST may also influence the patient's experience of the final stage of life by determining where death occurs, who is present, and whether the patient is able to communicate with loved ones.

The concept of LSTs includes any medical or nursing intervention, procedure, or medication, no matter how simple or complex, that is necessary for continued life. In the past, some treatments were considered ordinary and morally required, whereas others were called *extraordinary* and considered optional. This distinction between ordinary and extraordinary treatments has a prominent history within the Roman Catholic tradition and was used to determine whether a patient's refusal of treatment should be classified as suicide. Within that faith tradition, refusal of ordinary means was considered by some to be an unacceptable decision that was morally equivalent to an act of suicide (Beauchamp & Childress, 2012).

Optional or *nonburdensome* treatments include all medications, treatments, and operations that offer a reasonable hope of benefit and can be obtained and used without excessive expense, pain, or other inconvenience from the patient's perspective. *Extraordinary* (or *burdensome*) treatments are those that are very costly, unusual, difficult, or dangerous or do not offer a reasonable hope of benefit to the patient (Davis et al., 1997). What should be of moral concern for nurses is not what the intervention is, but whether the benefits of its continued use outweigh its associated burdens, as determined by the patient or surrogate decision maker.

Withholding and Withdrawing Life-Prolonging Treatments

Many healthcare professionals and family members are more comfortable not initiating LSTs than stopping them once begun. However, the question to be answered is whether this psychological fact has any moral significance (Beauchamp & Childress, 2012). Some clinicians regard withdrawing LST as "letting die," an act previously referred to as *passive euthanasia*, whereas others view withdrawing LST as an *act* that feels more like causing death, or killing. Withdrawing LSTs may be experienced as morally problematic for some nurses, particularly those who emphasize the "sanctity of life" and believe that continued life is an intrinsic good, regardless of burdens imposed by illness. However, nurses should be familiar with the legal and moral consensus that recognizes no moral distinction between withholding and withdrawing LSTs.

This consensus began to emerge in the early 1980s when a presidential commission was created to explore significant ethical issues in healthcare (President's Commission, 1983). One of their reports, entitled "Deciding to Forego Life-Sustaining Treatment," maintains that "neither criminal nor civil law—if properly interpreted and applied … forces patients to undergo procedures that will increase their suffering when they wish to avoid this by foregoing life-sustaining treatments" (p. 89). The commission further held that "the distinction between failing to initiate and stopping therapy—that is, withholding versus withdrawing treatment—is not in itself of moral (or legal) importance. A justification that is adequate for not commencing a treatment is also sufficient for ceasing it" (p. 61).

There is a clear ethical consensus that LST may be withheld or withdrawn under certain circumstances—in particular, when its use is against the patient's wishes (provided the patient is or was fully informed and not coerced or unduly influenced), when it will or has begun to harm the patient, or when it does not or will not benefit the patient (Beauchamp & Childress, 2012). The ANA (2013) position statement on assisted suicide similarly encourages nurses to honor the refusal of treatments by an informed patient, either because they are deemed overly burdensome or because they will not benefit the patient. This position statement specifically notes that when nurses participate in decisions to forego LSTs or provide other interventions aimed at relieving suffering that have an associated risk of hastening death, these acts are ethically acceptable and do not constitute assisted suicide. One might argue that the ethical permissibility of withdrawing life support allows a "prolife" position enabling the use of limited trials of life-prolonging interventions. For example, imagine a situation in which a patient is critically ill and the prognosis is grave. There is a small chance that the use of continuous renal replacement therapy (CRRT) could restore kidney function and help achieve hemodynamic stability. Clinicians recommend a trial of this therapy with a plan to stop it after 3 days if it doesn't achieve its intended goal. For those who believe that once an LST is started, it can't (ethically) be stopped, then this potentially life-prolonging intervention would not be an option because they would not agree to stopping the CRRT if it didn't achieve its intended effect. However, more attention is needed on ways to emotionally prepare surrogates for stopping LST after limited trials like these, as there is often substantial emotional investment by members of the healthcare team and patient's loved ones to have LST interventions not be "all for nothing" if the patient ends up dying.

Withdrawing Artificial Nutrition and Hydration

Often the most difficult decisions about withholding treatments are those that involve simple noninvasive therapies, such as the use of antibiotics, and those that are symbolically linked to caring and nurturing interventions, such as providing food and fluids. "Artificial" or technologically provided ANH must be distinguished from the oral provision of food and water. Although dying patients typically experience a decline in appetite as death nears, nurses should continue to offer fluids and food as long as patients indicate any interest or derive pleasure in eating or in drinking fluids. The administration of ANH is viewed differently. A moral and legal consensus concludes that ANH is a medical treatment that may be refused or withdrawn on the same grounds as any other medical intervention, that is, on an estimation of its expected benefit or burden to the patient (Beauchamp & Childress, 2012). Ethical difficulties arise when it is unclear whether continued provision of nutrition is more beneficial or harmful to the patient.

Evidence suggests that routine use of ANH in the care of terminally ill persons is unwarranted and that providing ANH is unlikely to achieve the clinical outcomes for which it is most often employed, for example, to enhance comfort, prolong survival, and improve QOL (Choi & Billings, 2002; Ersek, 2003; Suter, Rogers, & Strack, 2008). However, disability rights advocates argue that bias toward associating ANH with reduced QOL may reveal an underlying disability bias (Johnson, 2006).

In cases in which a patient is unable to make his or her wishes known, or is unable to evaluate the benefits or harms of refusing ANH, a surrogate decision maker should help inform the healthcare staff regarding the patient's stated wishes or known values or beliefs relevant to a decision about whether to provide ANH based on a substituted judgment or best-interest standard. Nurses should know whether their state's legislative policy restricts or limits surrogates' rights to decide about the administration of ANH.

From Letting Die to Assisted Dying

Nurses who regularly care for dying patients may experience requests for assistance in dying (AID) from patients or family members. Interest in clinician-provided assisted dying is thought, in part, to reflect an American public increasingly fearful of the process of dying, particularly the possibility of dying a painful, protracted, and undignified death that lacks personal control or meaning (Schwarz, 2004a). Gallup's 2015 annual survey on values and beliefs found that 68% of Americans believe that "doctor-assisted suicide" is morally acceptable, a dramatic rise from previous years, likely due to media attention surrounding Brittany Maynard's publicized access to a lethal prescription by way of Oregon's Death with Dignity Act (Bever, 2014). As of this writing, five states in the United States have legalized physician-assisted suicide (i.e., providing a lethal prescription to terminally ill adults who meet certain criteria). Although interest in such legislation is growing, some suggest that the option of voluntarily stopping eating and drinking (VSED) may

be a preferable alternative to physician-assisted dying when suffering patients seek information about hastening death (Berry, 2009; Terman, 2007). Although those unfamiliar with VSED consider it to entail unjustified suffering, with references to the dying person "starving" herself or himself, it's relevant to know that such a death is hastened not by malnutrition but by dehydration, and that generally the sensation of thirst (which occurs during the first 24 to 48 hours, until the patient becomes comatose) is alleviated with oral mouth swabbing (Menzel, 2016). Other PC clinicians consider VSED to be an option of last resort for those whose suffering is intractable (Quill & Byock, 2000). Schwarz (2008, citing 42 U.S.C. § 5106g [6]) argues that nurses ought to respond to dying patients' questions about EOL options that may permit them to control their own dying; VSED is one such option that patients may legally choose.

Rakatansky (2017) points out the importance of having state laws and institutional policies conform to consensus on allowing VSED if it's a patient's informed choice—for example, Rhode Island's Medical Orders for Life-Sustaining Treatment (MOLST) form states, "Offer food by mouth if feasible and desired" (p. 1), whereas Maryland's Health Care Decisions Act, states, "A health care provider shall make reasonable efforts to provide an individual with food and water by mouth and to assist the individual as needed to eat and drink voluntarily" (Maryland Office of the Attorney General, n.d., p. 20). The latter wording may create confusion among hospice or long-term care facility staff caring for patients who choose VSED to hasten their death.

The Oregon Death With Dignity Act

Since 1997, physician-assisted dying has been a legally available EOL option in Oregon for terminally ill, decisionally capable citizens who make repeated, documented, and voluntary requests for such assistance. In Oregon, a physician may write a prescription for a lethal amount of medication following a 15-day waiting period, between the first and second oral requests for assistance, and after receiving a written request by the patient. The physician also must determine that the patient is terminally ill, decisionally capable, and making an informed and voluntary request for AID and that the patient has been informed about and referred to palliative and hospice care. A second consulting physician must confirm that the patient is in the terminal stage of disease and verify the absence of any impairment in judgment due to psychiatric or other psychological disorders such as untreated depression.

Oregon physicians are required by law to explore and document the reasons for their patient's request for aid in dying, and to submit that and other demographic data to the Oregon Department of Human Services, which publishes those data annually (Oregon Health Authority [OHA], 2018). Thus, we know the following about those who used the law in 2016 (133 deaths): approximately 79% of patients were diagnosed with cancer, most were 65 years and older (median, 73 years), most patients (89%) died at home, and most were enrolled in hospice and had some form of health insurance (89% and 99%, respectively). Each year, approximately two thirds of those who receive prescriptions actually use them, and only a small proportion of terminally ill Oregonians choose to hasten their deaths by using this law. Since the law was passed in 1997, a total of 1,749 patients have received lethal prescriptions and 1,127 have died using the Oregon Death With Dignity Act (ODWDA) (OHA, 2018).

Oregon physicians report that, although their patients often have multiple reasons for their decision to hasten death, the following three concerns are consistently reported: (a) loss of autonomy, (b) decreasing ability to participate in activities that make life enjoyable, and (c) loss of dignity. Disability rights advocates point to this finding as cause for concern that the growing endorsement of aid-in-dying statutes may have an unintended consequence of unwittingly legitimizing a pervasive disability bias (Golden & Zoanni, 2010). However, to date, data from Oregon show that terminally ill Oregonians who choose to hasten their death under the provisions of the ODWDA do so infrequently and only after thoughtful consideration and careful planning. Such measured and considered steps, in a process that requires at least 2 weeks to complete, seems to many to be distinct from acts of suicide that are frequently accompanied by impulsive, irrational, and often violent behavior. Perhaps, in recognition of that distinction, in October 2006, the Oregon Department of Human Services adopted a policy to stop using the terms "suicide" or "physician-assisted suicide" when referring to the death of persons who use the ODWDA. That policy is consistent with the actual language in the law specifically stating that actions taken in accordance with the Act shall *not* constitute suicide, assisted suicide, mercy killing, or homicide.

Increasingly, members of some professional organizations who work with dying patients have joined in the call for use of emotionally neutral language to describe the EOL choices made by decisionally capable, terminally ill persons who are considering hastening their deaths. In 2007, the American Academy of Hospice and Palliative Medicine (AAHPM) published a position statement on PAD that explained the reasons for their preferred use of the term "PAD," stating that PAD more accurately captures the essence of the process than the more "emotionally charged designation of physician-assisted suicide" (AAHPM, 2016, p. 1; http://aahpm .org/positions/pad). This organization also took a position of "studied neutrality" on the question of whether PAD should be legally regulated or prohibited. Also in 2007, the American Medical Woman's Association published a position statement supporting the right of physicians to provide a competent, terminally ill patient with—but not administer—a lethal dose of medication or medical knowledge, so that the patient can, without further assistance, hasten his or her own death. They call this practice "aid in dying."

No nursing organizations have taken a similar position. Indeed, in 2006, the Hospice and Palliative Nurses Association (HPNA) reconfirmed their opposition to the legalization of assisted suicide. The ANA revised its 1994 position statement in 2013, but continues with a position of opposition to a nurse's involvement in assisted suicide. This will likely evolve as public debate continues, given the majority public opinion favoring physician aid in dying and the growing number of nurses who support a patient's choice, particularly nurses in states where the practice is legally available.

Nurses hold varied views about nurse participation in assisted dying and often justify their position by referring to their own clinical experience (Schwarz, 1999). Crucial to most who argue in support of assisting in dying are duties of beneficence, compassion for irremediable suffering, and the obligation to respect the autonomy of competent persons (Daly, Berry, Fitzpatrick, Drew, & Montgomery, 1997). Some experienced hospice nurses argue for those "very occasional" patients who, despite receiving skilled PC, prefer death to the life with which they are left (Stephany, 1994). Most participants in the study by Schwarz (2003, 2004a) maintained that if patients were decisionally capable, had received good EOL PC, and made a voluntary and informed decision to end their own lives, they had the right to do that, but patients did not have the right to have a nurse's AID (Schwarz, 2004a).

The ANA opposes nurse involvement in both active euthanasia and assisted suicide; participation in either action is considered a breach of the *Code of Ethics for Nurses* (ANA, 2015) and the ethical traditions of the profession. Opposition to assisted suicide is based on the "ethical traditions and goals of the profession, and its covenant with society," which obligate nurses to "provide humane, comprehensive, and compassionate care that respects the rights of patients but upholds the standards of the profession in the presence of chronic, debilitating illness and at end of life" (ANA, 2013, p. 1). However, given that about two thirds of Americans support aid in dying and that five states have now legalized the practice, there is growing concern that a nonnegotiable position categorically forbidding nurses' involvement in aid in dying will be ultimately untenable. For example, Vogelstein (2016) argues that such a position discourages nurses from thinking thoughtfully and critically about this morally complex issue. It is this author's position that opposition to legalizing aid in dying is more justifiably grounded in a "slippery slope" argument than one centered on a breach of nursing's societal covenant. That is, although some individuals benefit from access to lethal prescriptions to control the timing of their death, and others are harmed by lack of access, concerns about unintended negative consequences to others of legalizing and sanctioning this practice—particularly before effective PC is readily accessible—may justify opposing clinicians' involvement *as policy*. In other words, the concern is that allowing healthcare providers to support patients who choose to end their lives through legally and professionally sanctioned access to a lethal prescription will accelerate a cultural shift that will lead some of our most vulnerable members of society to die "before their right time," a position that Philipa Foote argued many decades ago (Foote, 1977). So far, data out of Oregon show no evidence of this, but disability rights literature provides an alternative view (Stramondo, 2016). Clearly, nurses should consider this position from all angles. The Hospice and Palliative Nurses Association (HPNA, 2011, 2017) advises that nurses "guard against communicating a negative judgment against the patient because of his/her decision" to access a lethal prescription. The ANA (2013, p. 8) recommends that we "increase education for nurses in values clarification to promote nurses' understanding and clarify attitudes toward euthanasia and assisted suicide while at the same time supporting a patient's autonomous decision-making."

Ethical Issues in Gerontology

Medical research and technology have extended life spans, which, together with the aging baby boomer generation, have shifted the population age demographics toward the older adult. Indeed, the fastest growing age demographic in the United States is persons 85 years and older. Although on the one hand, this is a marker of success, on the other hand, it forces more complex decisions to be made about when, if ever, to place limits on the use of medical interventions for the older adult. Should the focus be on life prolongation regardless of QOL? How should decisions be made about allocating limited medical resources to older adults, who have less time to reap the benefits of expensive and potentially risky medical therapies? What obligations are owed to caregivers of the elderly, whose lives are often greatly affected by the choices elders make about their health and living situation? Although many embrace the *idea* of caring for their aging parents, the physical and emotional caregiving burden can be overwhelming, particularly when we consider the stressors experienced by the "sandwich generation"—those caring for both their own children and elder family members at the same time or in quick succession (Do, Cohen, & Brown, 2014).

In discussing ethics at the *end of life*, the term usually serves as a euphemism for the process of dying and death. It is generally reserved for those who are expected to die within a given time frame (e.g., less than 6 months) from an incurable, progressive disease.

By this definition, the end of life is not restricted to the older adult. Yet, as one ages and surpasses his or her estimated life expectancy, mortality looms closer regardless of health status, causing most to include the older adult in discussions of "ethics at the end of life." This is likely what prompted a healthy 90-year-old woman to tell her healthcare providers she was 10 years younger than she was to ensure that they would not "give up too easily" in providing her medical care.

However, although some fear that doctors may "give up" too easily on their elderly patients, others suggest that the overreliance on procedural, high-tech medical diagnostics and interventions is creating more burden than benefit among the elderly. Such concerns, backed by research findings, have led to a movement known as "slow medicine" (www.slowmedicine.info) and "minimally disruptive medicine" (minimallydisruptivemedicine.org) in which physicians stop to consider less aggressive alternatives before implementing high-risk medical interventions that may reap limited rewards for the elderly. In these approaches, patients and families must be re-educated to resist the default option of ED visits and hospitalizations if they are not likely to achieve the desired goal of improving QOL (Gross, 2008). Lynn and Goldstein (2003) also point out that the face of fatal illness has changed. Patients with chronic lung or heart disease, dementia, or even cancer typically face many years of chronic illness and waxing and waning health before they die from the disease. Hence, Lynn and Goldstein use the term "chronic fatal illness" instead of "terminal illness." They advocate adjusting our approach to caregiving and EOL planning to accommodate this longer, less predictable dying trajectory.

The question of rationing is often raised when discussing high-tech, expensive medical interventions that produce limited benefit. Could one conclude that individuals of a certain age should not be candidates for certain therapies, because they cannot reap enough benefit in their remaining years of life? It has been pointed out that age-based rationing already occurs in the United States through the Medicare program. That is, elders are *favored* in that they, unlike children in this country and the nonworking people who do not qualify for Medicaid, are assured of healthcare coverage. Some suggest that age-based rationing that would limit certain medical interventions (e.g., no renal dialysis or organ transplants, and certain other life-extending therapies, to those over a certain age) would be justified based on egalitarian and utilitarian arguments. The egalitarian argument is that individuals receive a greater investment of resources when they are young to allow them to be well-functioning citizens, with the understanding that as they get older, they will receive fewer resources to ensure that the next generation is able to enjoy the same investment of resources in their youth (Daniels, 1985). The problem with that argument is that not all citizens enjoy the same access to resources before they reach their senior years. Furthermore, Jecker (1991) argues that age-based rationing would unjustly disadvantage women, whose life opportunities may have been limited due to gender discrimination; who provide the bulk of child and family member caregiving; and who, because they comprise a greater percentage of older adults, would be subjected to age-based rationing more often than their male counterparts. Finally, there is evidence that age-based rationing already exists implicitly (Hurst et al., 2006; Ward, 2000) and would only further disadvantage older persons and erode their trust in the healthcare system (and further diminish the respect owed to them) if it were formalized through explicit rationing schemes.

A utilitarian argument for age-based rationing was constructed on poorer outcomes in older adults for certain medical interventions, established on available evidence such as "quality-adjusted life years" (QALY; Dolan, 2001). Critics of this approach argue that age alone is an insufficient predictor of healthcare outcomes, and that if rationing of medical interventions were to be based on outcomes, such decisions should be made on overall health indicators, rather than age alone.

Many have observed that the U.S. culture is youth oriented and does not afford the older adult the respect that other cultures bestow upon their elders. We are a death-denying culture that seeks to defy individual mortality and the aging process (Piers et al., 2012). A rapidly growing category of patients are those with "chronic critical illness," that is, those requiring ICU-level life support, which is being increasingly provided in subacute facilities providing interventions such as long-term ventilator support and renal dialysis. Such care is likely contributing to increasing EOL care costs—Medicare dollars pay for about 80% of deaths in the United States, and about 25% of Medicare dollars are spent in the patient's last year of life (HJK Family Foundation, 2016). Thus, some argue that elders have a duty to accept the limits of their natural life span and avoid requests beyond that point for expensive life-extending medical technology (Callahan, 2000). However, most agree that the healthcare reforms needed in this country cannot be achieved through strict age-based rationing (what some refer to as "hard rationing"). Rather, instead of placing no limits on aggressive, life-extending medical technology while price-rationing the more effective, efficient, and humanistic primary care, we should re-envision our healthcare priorities to focus on quality, justice, and caring rather than life extension alone. As Churchill wrote:

> Most patients would not bankrupt their family and deny their children a fair start in life by striving for a last, expensive extension of their own lives. Neither should we extend our lives at the margins if by so doing we deprive nameless and faceless others a decent provision of care. And such a gesture should not appear to us as a sacrifice, but as the ordinary virtue entailed by a just, social conscience. (Churchill, 1988, p. 647)

Clearly, decisions about withholding or withdrawing LST at the end of life can weigh heavily on healthcare providers. However, the more seemingly mundane decisions about resource allocation for elders in the clinician's office or clinic may be the more difficult ones on which to reach consensus about what is just. A step in the right direction would be to put healthcare decisions in the hands of healthcare professionals and the inevitable rationing decisions in public forums where they can be debated and approached rationally, transparently, and compassionately. However, others argue that rationing is already happening at the bedside and that clinicians must be part of the process rather than perpetuate the illusion that rationing is something that happens only at a macro level (Strech & Danis, 2014).

Ethical Issues in Pediatrics

A cornerstone of ethics in pediatrics is recognizing the patient's and parent's input into medical decision making throughout the developmental trajectory. From birth to the age of majority, pediatric patients' involvement in their medical care evolves as they grow and mature. Likewise, parents must respond to different obligations that accompany parenting an infant, a toddler, a child, and an adolescent.

In pediatrics, as in other subspecialties, many ethical issues and dilemmas are born out of the increasingly complex medical technology that has evolved over recent decades. A growing number of neonates, for example, require the special services of a neonatal intensive care unit (NICU). This is partly due to high-risk pregnancies of women who delay pregnancy until later in life and the increased reliance on artificial reproductive technologies that result in multiple gestation pregnancies (Goldenberg, Culhane, Iams, & Romero, 2008). Such pregnancies are more likely to result in premature births that require NICU support. The ensuing dilemmas were poignantly described in the seminal book *Playing God in the Nursery* (Lyon, 1985). Many point to the NICU babies who beat the survival odds as "miracle babies" whose survival provides proof that pushing the boundaries of neonatal viability is worth the money and resources. Others suggest that providing life-saving NICU technologies to some severely compromised, extremely low-birth-weight premature babies is tantamount to human experimentation (Chervenak, McCullough, & Levene, 2007). Parents and healthcare providers must consider several important questions when considering whether to pursue life-saving technology for an impaired neonate (National Association of Neonatal Nurses, 2006). These include the following:

- Is there a reasonable chance that the infant will survive?
- If the infant survives, will he or she have an acceptable QOL?
- Will future required medical care entail a net benefit or harm to the child?
- When, if ever, is a life of severe physical or cognitive impairment worse than death?
- Are resources available to support the future medical needs of the child?

In addition, parents must consider their own beliefs and values, and how their decision will impact other family members. For example, some parents may feel that subjecting a severely impaired infant to aggressive medical therapy that may likely result in neurological devastation and dependence on intensive medical interventions throughout childhood not only imposes undue suffering on that child, but would also place an unacceptable burden on other children in the family, who would be deprived of parental attention. In contrast, other parents may believe that it is their obligation to prolong their child's life no matter what the outcome. You can see here that the former example leans more toward *consequentialism*—deciding what to do based on outcomes, whereas the latter example leans more toward *deontology*—deciding what to do based on moral duty, regardless of outcomes.

In the unique settings of the NICU and labor and delivery ward, parents do not have the final say about whether infants receive life-saving interventions. In the early 1980s, a case gained national attention involving an infant born with Down syndrome and esophageal atresia. The parents refused a routine surgical procedure to correct the deformity, resulting in the infant's otherwise preventable death. In response, the federal "Baby Doe" regulations were adopted by the Department of Health and Human Services to protect against discriminatory treatment toward babies and children with disabilities. The courts soon struck down the regulations, which hospitals protested as being overly restrictive. In 1984, Congress amended the Child Abuse Protection and Treatment Act (CAPTA) to help discourage disability bias from influencing life-and-death decisions, while also avoiding mandating high-tech treatment for dying infants (Schwartz, 2008). According to CAPTA, a life-prolonging therapy may be withheld or withdrawn from an infant if it is considered to

- Merely prolong dying
- Not be effective in correcting all of the infant's life-threatening conditions
- Be futile in terms of the infant's survival

Because a baby's prognosis for survival may not be known immediately at birth, depending on state law, if an infant is born breathing, the healthcare providers may be legally obligated to administer life-saving interventions. However, despite the restrictions on foregoing life support at birth, palliative comfort care should always be an option for any neonate whose prognosis for survival is poor (Catlin & Carter, 2002; Kain, 2006).

For the most part, the same process for ethical decision making applies to pediatric patients as to adults: Consider the likely benefits and burdens of available choices and act to minimize harm and maximize benefit. Children in general are considered to be "vulnerable persons" who must be protected. Generally, this involves a parent or legal guardian ("parent") making medical decisions for the child, with assent from the child obtained if he or she is capable. Ethical concerns in pediatrics often involve differences of opinion among providers, parents, and patients about the patient's course of treatment. Consider the case of Katie Wernecke. Katie was diagnosed with Hodgkin's lymphoma when she was 13 years old. Her oncologist gave her an 80% chance of survival with chemotherapy followed by radiation. However, Katie's parents wanted to forego the radiation to pursue an alternative treatment of vitamin C infusions. How did the healthcare team respond? Child Protective Services was involved, and Katie was placed with foster parents while she continued with her radiation. Ultimately, a judge ruled that Katie should be allowed to return to her parents and pursue the alternative treatment, but only after she finished the recommended course of radiation. Some might advocate for a less adversarial way to resolve this conflict, to maintain Katie's family integrity and harmony at a time when she most needed it. However, such decisions are difficult when lives are at stake.

As you can see, neither Katie nor her parents had boundless autonomy rights. The state intervened to ensure that Katie received the medical standard of care, which provided a good chance of putting Katie's cancer into remission. This is different from how the state handles a competent adult who refuses life-saving therapy. In that case, forced treatment would be considered a form of battery. The state recognizes a competent adult's right to refuse life-saving therapy, but usually considers the state's interest in preserving life to trump autonomy rights when a child's life is at stake. Therefore, if a parent's request falls outside an acceptable medical standard of care, healthcare providers may be obligated to override the parent's request. Whenever possible, this should be approached using open channels of communication between the parents and the healthcare team to avoid the need to involve the courts.

Conflicts may also ensue when the wishes of the parent and the child differ. Consider a 14-year-old child who has advanced cancer with no chance of cure, but whose life may be prolonged with another course of chemotherapy. The patient tells the nurse that she does not want the chemotherapy, is tired of fighting the cancer, and prefers to focus on being as comfortable as possible. The parents insist that the chemotherapy be started as soon as possible. In such a situation, the healthcare team has an ethical obligation to resolve this conflict and not proceed without the patient's assent to chemotherapy (Jacobs, 2005).

In rare cases, the rights of a "mature minor" to forego LST are recognized. For example, if a 15-year-old Jehovah's Witness demonstrates a clear and consistent commitment to forego blood products, an ethical argument could be made that this young person's autonomous choice should be respected, even if the risk of death is high. However, in most situations in which death is likely and reasonably avoidable, and in which parents refuse life-saving interventions for their minor child, healthcare providers opt to petition the court to mandate life-saving treatments.

Pediatric staff should familiarize themselves with their state's law regarding "emancipated minors." These are persons recognized by the courts as able to make their own medical decisions, even though they have not reached the legal age of majority (18 years in most states). Criteria for emancipation vary from state to state, but typically include living independently from parents, having a child, and being on active duty in the armed forces. Minors are also allowed to obtain medical treatment for certain conditions without parental permission (e.g., birth control and certain types of mental healthcare). The rationale for allowing these exceptions is that many teens may not seek needed medical intervention if they know a parent must be notified. Here, healthcare providers must continually weigh the dueling obligations that the principle of *respect for persons* demands—respecting a decisionally capable person's wishes and protecting a vulnerable person from harm. Because a teenager's ability to make well-reasoned, mature decisions evolves over time, the degree to which his or her wishes and privacy should be respected is situation specific. Regardless of who makes the final medical decision, children and adolescents should always be included in medical decision making to the extent that their developmental level allows.

Barriers in the Practice Environment to Sound Ethical Practice

Nurses need to find ways to talk to each other and validate their experiences, tell their stories of despair or triumph, and share their experiences of moral uncertainty. Nurses may experience conflict between their own moral values and the values of the profession, and

they have the right to remain true to their conscientious moral and religious beliefs. Although prohibited from compromising legitimate patient choices or imposing their values on others, nurses who are ethically opposed to certain patient interventions will find support for their position in the *Code of Ethics for Nurses* (ANA, 2015). They have the right to withdraw from providing interventions that run counter to their core beliefs, assuming that arrangements can be made for the patient's safe transfer to the care of another.

It is undoubtedly true that some of the barriers that constrain nurses from participating in ethical decision making are situations over which the nurse has no control. For example, most nurses practice as employees in healthcare organizations whose goals are business oriented and whose focus is utilitarian (institutional values providing the greatest good for the greatest number). Nurses, by virtue of their education, experience, and moral commitment to caring, are focused on doing good for individual patients. Conflict inevitably arises between nurses' roles as caregivers and patient advocates, institutional employees, and clinicians expected to implement physicians' orders (Epstein & Hamric, 2009; Hamric & Blackhall, 2007; Wiegand & Funk, 2012). The experience of being the nurse in the middle combined with the moral distress of being unable to do the right thing may result in nurses perceiving that they are unable to act as morally autonomous agents. In such cases, nurses must learn how to address individual, interpersonal, and systemic issues that impede their moral agency and ability to advocate for ethically supportable patient care (Huffman & Rittenmeyer, 2012). Georgina Morley (2016a, 2016b) describes the role of the nurse ethicist in helping nurses identify and better manage moral distress in the workplace. Rushton and Carse (2017) call for moving from recognizing moral distress to cultivating resiliency and supporting professional integrity at an organizational level.

Ethics Committees and Ethics Consultation Services

Ethical issues in clinical practice often involve life-or-death decisions, and such decisions give rise to a host of emotions and concerns. Just as physicians and patients turn to medical specialists and subspecialists for advice and consultations on questions of medicine, healthcare professionals and patients may need to consult an ethics committee or ethics consultant(s) to discuss today's perplexing ethical issues. The overall role of an ethics committee is threefold. First, the committee may educate itself, the hospital administration, and the hospital staff about ethical issues occurring in our current healthcare environment. Second, the committee may participate in policy development. Third, the committee provides ethics consultations, which are more timely, less adversarial, and more flexible than court proceedings as a way to resolve disputes. Fox, Myers, and Pearlman (2007) found that 81% of U.S. hospitals (and all hospitals with more than 400 beds) have an ethics consultation service. Ethics consultation is one mechanism by which a hospital may satisfy The Joint Commission's requirement to have a mechanism to address ethical issues that arise in patient care.

Different goals may be sought by an ethics consultation. The American Society for Bioethics and Humanities (ASBH; 2011, p. 3; Tarzian, 2013) identifies the general goal of ethics consultation as improving "the quality of healthcare through the identification, analysis, and resolution of ethical questions or concerns." This is achieved through intermediary goals, such as helping staff to identify and understand the specific ethical issues the case raises; improving communication among the patient, family, and healthcare team; providing emotional support to the healthcare team members involved in a difficult case; offering "ethically justifiable" recommendations for how to resolve an ethical question or a dilemma; and improving patient care by preventing patient care decisions that run counter to ethical guidelines and standards. In addition, Dubler and Liebman (2011) focus on the goal of conflict resolution through ethics consultation.

Another goal of ethics consultation may be, as Margaret Urban Walker (1993) suggests, to "protect moral spaces" within the healthcare setting. According to this view, burgeoning high-tech, expensive medical technology—along with our fragmented healthcare system—has increased the complexity and burden of medical decision making. Yet, healthcare providers have less time to grapple with this increasing complexity. Ethics consultations may provide one countermeasure to this trend toward fast-paced decision making by allowing patients, families, and healthcare providers to take a step back and reflect on the ethical issues involved before rushing to judgment about a particular case.

One issue of concern is that a majority of ethics committee members have been found to lack formal training in ethics (Fox et al., 2007). The ASBH (2011; Tarzian, 2013) has identified core skills and knowledge competencies that ethics consultants (or consult services, collectively) should possess to effectively respond to consultation requests. ASBH also adopted a code of ethics for healthcare ethics consultants, signifying recognition of this evolving professional role (Tarzian, 2015). Nurses should be knowledgeable about who serves on the ethics consultation service at their facility, how their competence is ensured, and how to access the service. Nurses should develop their own ethics knowledge and skills competencies to effectively advocate for their patients. This might involve collaborating with an institution's ethics committee to provide education and mentoring in

ethics. The National Center for Ethics in Health Care's Integrated Ethics program through the Department of Veterans Affairs provides excellent resources (available via open access at www.ethics.va.gov/integratedethics).

Preventing Burnout

Nurses who care for dying patients often may find themselves in situations of ethical conflict; burnout is one potential consequence. To avoid the experience of burnout, nurses should seek support from peers, share experiences of uncertainty, and seek ethics advice and support for the development of skills in identifying and resolving ethical problems in clinical practice (Hlubocky, Back, & Shanafelt, 2016). It is most important for nurses to acknowledge their own suffering and sense of frustration in caring for patients at the end of life. For example, it can be very upsetting and discouraging to identify a treatment approach that appears to be in a patient's best interest but then be unable to implement it (perhaps due to disagreements among team members or family members about what is in the patient's best interests). Sometimes, with reflection, a morally acceptable compromise can be identified, one that preserves the underlying values of the concerned parties. Agreement to a trial of therapy and to reassess within a specified time can help resolve some of the uncertainty.

Hospitals and healthcare organizations that provide nurse support systems that encourage and facilitate moral growth and understanding will employ nurses who are less likely to succumb to moral passivity. Nurses should be encouraged to create their own opportunities for support regarding EOL issues and may consider the following interventions:

1. Use of an ethics consultant can be a source of guidance and help nurses acquire the necessary skills for future application. When requesting an ethics consultation, nurses should clarify the role they would like the ethics consultant(s) to play. For example, are they looking to clarify information about ethical standards, or do they also want the ethics consultant(s) to be actively involved in mediating conflict and communicating with a patient or family members? It is important for nurses to remain engaged in ethical decision making when an ethics consultation is requested. This is an excellent way for nurses to improve their ethics knowledge, skills, and abilities.
2. Multidisciplinary and nursing ethics committees should be available to nurses for case consultation regarding ethical conflicts. Nurses should be members of these committees and should work in concert with professional colleagues. Multidisciplinary institutional ethics committees also develop institutional policies and guidelines and plan programs to educate staff about ethics.

3. Activities, such as Schwartz Rounds (2018; www .theschwartzcenter.org) and nurse resilience programs (www.humanmedia.org), are excellent mechanisms to proactively address factors that can lead to moral distress and burnout. Interprofessional ethics rounds also present an opportunity for individuals working in different patient care disciplines to discuss regularly troubling cases that may not require an immediate decision. Such meetings allow for analysis, exploration, and sharing of different points of view. Thus, when ethical problems do occur, a foundation exists to provide guidance about the most effective way to respond. Wocial and colleagues' "unit-based ethics conversations" hold promise to improve nurses' ethics proficiency and encourage a workplace culture where moral distress does not thrive (Wocial, Hancock, Bledsoe, Chamness, & Helft, 2010).

■ CONCLUSIONS

Healthcare providers justifiably look for definitive answers when asking what is the "right" thing to do in a given situation. Sometimes, after sorting through the facts and stakeholder viewpoints of a troubling case, the right way to handle the uncertainty or conflict becomes apparent. But often, there is no one "right" answer. Sometimes more than one response can be ethically justified (as in the example of responding to a dying patient's request for assistance in hastening death). Other times, whatever course of action is taken requires compromising a core ethical principle, such as abiding by a patient's prior wish to be kept alive with aggressive medical technology, despite the pain and suffering it invokes with little apparent gain. Nurses should be encouraged to continue to provide compassionate care and a caring presence as they struggle, together with patients, family members, and professional colleagues, in the attempt to identify what, all things considered, ought to be done in situations of moral conflict. In doing so, we are reminded that "to the extent that care of the dying draws us into their lives, we experience the gifts and deprivations of their own deaths and painfully anticipate the death of our loved ones and even ourselves" (Dixon, 1997, p. 297).

Nurses should continually seek to improve their ethics knowledge base by looking for learning opportunities. At a minimum, they should be familiar with ethical theories of deontology (duty-based ethics) and teleology (consequence-based ethics), ethical principles, and the concepts of decision-making capacity, surrogate decision making, ADs, mature minors, consent versus assent, moral justifications for withholding and withdrawing LSTs, and responding to requests for a hastened death. Nurses should access resources to assist them in ethical decision making and in nurturing their moral agency, such as institutional ethics committees, colleagues, and the *Code of Ethics for Nurses* (ANA, 2015).

CASE STUDY *Conclusion*

How does one start in addressing the question of whether Mrs. S.'s tube feedings should be continued? Cassells and Gaul's Ethical Assessment Framework (1998) offers a guide. One of the first steps is to gather the relevant facts. What exactly does the living will document state? Was it properly witnessed and thereby legally valid? Why is it that Mrs. J. thinks Mrs. S. would benefit from having her tube feedings stopped at this time? Does she think that this has caused Mrs. S. to suffer? One should involve other experts, as needed, to provide input in this fact-finding phase. In determining which options are ethically justifiable, one should consider how different ethical principles apply to the case. The two components of the principle of *respect for persons* are relevant—protecting vulnerable persons and respecting the autonomy of competent adults. Regarding the latter, in considering whether Mrs. S.'s tube feedings should be continued, the nursing home staff is obligated to provide medical care that is consistent with Mrs. S.'s prior stated wishes. Mrs. J. has cast doubt on the validity of Mrs. S.'s living will as it relates to tube feedings. However, given that stopping Mrs. S.'s tube feedings would hasten her death, and assuming that the living will is legally valid, Mrs. J.'s request alone would be insufficient to warrant stopping the feedings. This exemplifies the obligation to protect Mrs. S. as a vulnerable person. One would need a good justification for withdrawing a medical treatment that would result in hastening a patient's death. This does not mean that Mrs. S.'s tube feedings should be continued beyond the point where they are no longer achieving their intended goal. If the tube feedings are considered medically ineffective (e.g., they are no longer providing nutrition as evidenced by continued weight loss and increased residual gastric content and fluid backup), it would be ethically justifiable for a clinician to order them to be stopped based on this criterion, if in accordance with local laws and policies (Pope, 2016). Whether or not a decision is made to continue Mrs. S.'s tube feedings, the nurse should discuss with Mrs. J. what is being done to maximize Mrs. S.'s comfort and dignity. If Mrs. S. meets hospice admission criteria, hospice could be involved to help manage her EOL care. Just because Mrs. S. has a feeding tube, keeping her alive does not change the fact that she is dying from end-stage dementia and deserves all the best that PC has to offer.

CASE STUDY

AN INTERPROFESSIONAL PERSPECTIVE

Thaddeus Mason Pope, PhD, JD
Mitchell Hamline School of Law

This case study raises at least two different issues. First, what is the source of Mrs. J.'s decision-making authority? Second, what is the scope of Mrs. J.'s decision-making authority? Specifically, may she refuse artificial nutrition despite the request in Mrs. S.'s living will?

Mrs. S. has a "living will." That term refers to a document that provides only healthcare instructions. Unlike an AD, a living will does not appoint a healthcare agent. Plus, we have additional confirmation that Mrs. J. is not a healthcare agent. Mrs. J. witnessed the living will. Because agents may not witness their own appointment, Mrs. S. did not appoint Mrs. J. as her healthcare agent.

If Mrs. J. did not get decision-making authority from Mrs. S., then from where did she get it? Only around half of U.S. states would recognize Mrs. J. as a default surrogate because of her "close friend" relationship to Mrs. S. (DeMartino et al., 2017). In the remaining states, Mrs. S. would be legally "unbefriended" (Farrell et al., 2017). Even in the absence of state law, some institutions might still permit Mrs. J. to make healthcare decisions for Mrs. S. Some might help Mrs. J. obtain guardianship. These approaches are desirable. Given Mrs. J.'s obvious involvement in Mrs. S.'s life, she appears to be the best available surrogate decision maker.

But we still have an ethical challenge. Even if the healthcare provider recognizes Mrs. J.'s authority to make healthcare decisions for Mrs. S., it remains unclear whether she may directly contradict instructions in the living will. Living wills constitute clear and convincing evidence of the patient's preferences. Because surrogates are supposed to exercise substituted judgment, they are normally constrained by the patient's own instructions.

Yet, although the presumption is strong, it is rebuttable. Bruce et al. (2016) propose four ethical considerations for determining whether it is ethically justifiable to allow a surrogate to override treatment preferences stated in a patient's living will: (1) Would the expected benefit of the surrogate's requested intervention outweigh the anticipated harms? (2) Is the surrogate's judgment of what the patient really wanted plausible? (3) Is there any evidence that the patient would have allowed the surrogate to make this decision? (4) Is there any evidence that the patient misunderstood the nature of the living will?

The first two conditions are satisfied here. Overwhelming evidence demonstrates that tube feedings in end-stage dementia provide no benefit and probably just do harm (American Geriatrics Society, 2014). Had Mrs. S. been properly advised, it is extremely unlikely that she (or anyone) would want tube feedings in end-stage dementia. In the absence of documented use of a patient decision aid (UNC School of Medicine, 2012) or articulated reasons for the request, it is safe to conclude Mrs. S. would not have wanted artificial nutrition in her current state.

Evidence-Based Practice

Matthews, E. A., Magid-Bernstein, J., Presciutti, A., Rodriguez, A., Roh, D., Park, S., ...
Agarwal, S. (2017). Categorization of survival and death after cardiac arrest. *Resuscitation*,
114, 79–82.

Methods

Data Sources: Retrospective medical record review 2008 to 2015.

Study Selection and Assessment: Adults (N = 385) treated for cancer at Columbia
University's ICUs between 2008 and 2015 were retrospectively categorized into various
modes of survival and death based on documented goals-of-care (GOC) discussions.
Cerebral performance category (CPC) was calculated at hospital discharge based on
medical record documentation and at 1-year post-arrest based on detailed phone
interviews with patients or family members. CPC greater than 2 was defined as a poor
outcome at discharge and 1-year post-arrest.

Outcomes

Information on GOC conversations, physician prognostication, and families' subsequent decisions was collected from daily chart reviews. Patients were then categorized
as follows: (a) survival after early recovery without any GOC discussions, (b) survival
due to physician–family agreement of good prognosis, (c) survival due to family wishes
despite the physician predicting poor neurological prognosis, (d) survival despite withdrawing LST (WLST), (e) WLST due to ADs, (f) WLST after physician–family agreement,
(g) death after ICU treatment was capped (e.g., "no escalation of treatment" barring
new life-prolonging interventions), (h) death despite full support before any GOC
conversation, (i) death despite full support after GOC conversation, and (j) brain death.

Main Results

Among 385 patients meeting inclusion criteria, 118 survived and 267 died. Survivors
were younger, with lower (i.e., "good") baseline CPC scores, a lower out-of-hospital
cardiac arrest rate, shorter time to return of spontaneous circulation, and higher incidence of ventricular tachycardia/fibrillation on presentation (versus asystole or pulseless
electrical activity). Most survivors had a poor neurological outcome (i.e., CPC score
of 5 at discharge and 1 year later (69% and 79%, respectively). Fourteen percent of
survivors had good neurological outcomes (i.e., CPC score of 1–2) at discharge (about
the same 1 year later at 13%). Seventy-two percent of patients had a GOC discussion,
but most survivors (57%, n = 67) did not. One fifth of survivors (n = 24) were predicted by physicians as having a poor neurological prognosis but their family members
requested continuation of LST—only two of these patients had good neurological outcomes (CPC 1–2) at discharge and 1 year later. About 17% (n = 20) of survivors had
family member and physician agreement to continue LST, and more of these patients
had good neurological outcomes (30% and 40%, respectively, at discharge and 1 year
later). About 6% of survivors had LST withdrawn but survived without it.

Conclusions

About a third (31%) of patients with cancer who experienced cardiac arrest were successfully resuscitated and discharged from the hospital, but most had poor neurological

outcomes at hospital discharge (85%) and 1 year later (87%). Neurological outcomes were better for patients whose physician and family agreed to continue LST in anticipation of good neurological recovery, compared with patients whose physician gave them a poor recovery prognosis. Nevertheless, a small number of patients ($n = 2$) not predicted by physicians to achieve favorable neurological recovery whose family requested continuation of LST achieved a good neurological recovery, demonstrating that clinicians cannot always accurately predict when CPR will be ineffective in achieving its intended goal.

Commentary

Originally promoted as a first-aid technique for the public to learn, CPR techniques were introduced as a medical procedure in the early 1960s. The originators cautioned physicians that the procedure was not meant to be used for all patients; rather, it should be applied selectively to patients who were likely to benefit from it. However, their caution was not heeded (Santonocito, Ristagno, Gullo, & Weil, 2013). The implementation of CPR on all patients who suffer cardiopulmonary arrest (in the absence of a do-not-attempt-resuscitation [DNAR] order) has given way to efforts to reduce the indiscriminate use of CPR. For example, the Patient Self-Determination Act of 1990 and state out-of-hospital orders for life-sustaining treatment initiatives encouraged the use of ADs and discussions about EOL care planning between patients and physicians. The challenge healthcare providers face today is that survival rates *overall* for witnessed in-hospital cardiopulmonary arrest have improved, likely due to improved techniques. For example, studies that Reisfield et al. (2006) identified before 1990 showed that resuscitation to hospital discharge was unsuccessful for all patients with metastatic cancer but had improved to 7.8% after 1990 (although survival rates in the ICU [2.2%] were much lower than those in the wards [10.1%]). Although Gershengorn, Li, Kramer, and Wunsch (2012) study found that 15.7% of resuscitated ICU patients survived to discharge, the authors do not report what percentage of these patients had advanced cancer. The same is true for Matthews and colleagues' study—these were all patients treated for cancer, with no indication of the stage of their illness. Statistics like these complicate the process of EOL decision making. Clinicians may be reluctant to definitively state that CPR attempts for a particular patient would be medically futile, because the success rates Gershengorn et al. report are above the futility threshold that was established of less than 1%. For patients facing death, a 15% or 7% or even a 2% chance of surviving to hospital discharge may be worth the associated burdens. What is harder to discern is whether surrogates making such decisions are accurately representing what the patient would have wanted or making decisions based on their own emotions (i.e., not wanting to let go or "give up"). Thus, some have argued that for subsets of patients for whom CPR is unlikely to achieve its intended goal, offering them (or their surrogate decision maker) the false choice of CPR attempts is disingenuous and overly burdensome. These clinicians may write DNR orders for patients based on medical futility criteria (Fritz & Fuld, 2010), or based on their recommendation and nondissent from the patient or surrogate (Kon, 2011).

Unfortunately, some clinicians interpret "communicating about EOL preferences" to mean "getting the patient to agree to a DNR order." This puts the focus on what the team will *not* do for the patient, rather than on what the team *will* do, based on the patient's GOC. Whether or not it is possible to extend a patient's life through CPR, clinicians should always "do everything" to ensure that dying patients receive compassionate care that is consistent with their wishes, if known, and within the scope of ethically acceptable healthcare practices. Nurses are in a good position to support such efforts.

■ REFERENCES

American Academy of Hospice and Palliative Medicine. (2016). Statement on physician-assisted dying, Approved by the AAHPM board of directors on June 24, 2016. Retrieved from http://aahpm.org/positions/pad

American College of Physicians. (2008). Achieving a high-performance health care system with universal access: What the United States can learn from other countries. *Annals of Internal Medicine, 148*, 55–75. doi:10.7326/0003-4819-148-1-200801010-00196

American Geriatrics Society Ethics Committee and Clinical Practice and Models of Care Committee. (2014). American Geriatrics Society feeding tubes in advanced dementia position statement. *Journal of the American Geriatrics Society, 62*(8), 1590–1593. doi:10.1111/jgs.12924

American Nurses Association. (2013). *Position statement on euthanasia, assisted suicide, and aid in dying.* Washington, DC: Author.

American Nurses Association. (2015). *Code of ethics for nurses with interpretive statements.* Washington, DC: Author.

American Society for Bioethics and Humanities' Core Competence Update Task Force. (2011). *Core competencies for health care ethics consultation: The report of the American Society for Bioethics and Humanities* (2nd ed.). Glenview, IL: American Society for Bioethics and Humanities.

Aslakson, R. A., Wyskiel, R., Thornton, I., Copley, C., Shaffer, D., Zyra, M., ... Pronovost, P. J. (2012). Nurse-perceived barriers to effective communication regarding prognosis and optimal end-of-life care for surgical ICU patients: A qualitative exploration. *Journal of Palliative Medicine, 15*(8), 910–915. doi:10.1089/jpm.2011.0481

Bakker, J., Jansen, T. C., Lima, A., & Kompanje, E. J. (2008). Why opioids and sedatives may prolong life rather than hasten death after ventilator withdrawal in critically ill patients. *American Journal of Hospice and Palliative Care, 25*(2), 152–154. doi:10.1177/1049909108315511

Beauchamp, T., & Childress, J. (2008). *Principles of biomedical ethics* (6th ed.). New York, NY: Oxford University Press.

Beauchamp, T., & Childress, J. (2012). *Principles of biomedical ethics* (7th ed.). New York, NY: Oxford University Press.

Beckstrand, R. L., Wood, R. D., Callister, L. C., Luthy, K. E., & Heaston, S. (2012). Emergency nurses' suggestions for improving end-of-life care obstacles. *Journal of Emergency Nursing, 38*(5), e7–e14. doi:10.1016/j.jen.2012.03.008

Benjamin, M., & Curtis, J. (1992). *Ethics in nursing* (3rd ed.). New York, NY: Oxford University Press.

Bergner, D. (2007, December 2). Death in the family. *New York Times Magazine.* Retrieved from http://www.nytimes.com/2007/12/02/magazine/02suicide-t.html

Berry, Z. S. (2009). Responding to suffering: Providing options and respecting choice. *Journal of Pain and Symptom Management, 38*(5), 797–800. doi:10.1016/j.jpainsymman.2009.09.001

Bever, L. (2014). How Brittany Maynard may change the right-to-die debate. *Washington Post.* Retrieved from https://www.washingtonpost.com/news/morning-mix/wp/2014/11/03/how-brittany-maynard-may-change-the-right-to-die-debate-after-death/

Bruce, C. R., Bibler, T., Childress, A. M., Stephens, A. L., Pena, A. M., & Allen, N. G. (2016). Navigating ethical conflicts between advance directives and surrogate decision-makers' interpretations of patient wishes, *Chest, 149*(2), 562–567. doi:10.1378/chest.15-2209

Callahan, D. (2000). *The troubled dream of life.* Washington, DC: Georgetown University Press.

Cardona-Morrell, M., Benfatti-Olivato, G., Jansen, J., Turner, R. M., Fajardo-Pulido, D., & Hillman, K. (2017). A systematic review of effectiveness of decision aids to assist older patients at the end of life. *Patient Education and Counseling, 100*(3), 425–435. doi:10.1016/j.pec.2016.10.007

Cassells, J., & Gaul, A. (1998, January). An ethical assessment framework for nursing practice. *Maryland Nurse, 6*(1), 9–12.

Catlin, A., & Carter, B. (2002). Creation of a neonatal end-of-life palliative care protocol. *Journal of Perinatology, 22*(3), 184–195. doi:10.1038/sj.jp.7210687

Cavanaugh, T. A. (1996). The ethics of death-hastening or death-causing palliative analgesic administration to the terminally ill. *Journal of Pain and Symptom Management, 12*(4), 248–254. doi:10.1016/0885-3924(96)00153-4

Chervenak, F. A., McCullough, L. B., & Levene, M. I. (2007). An ethically justified, clinically comprehensive approach to peri-viability: Gynaecological, obstetric, perinatal and neonatal dimensions. *Journal of Obstetrics and Gynaecology, 27*(1), 3–7. doi:10.1080/01443610601133605

Choi, Y. S., & Billings, J. A. (2002). Changing perspectives on palliative care. *Oncology, 16*(4), 515–522; discussion 522.

Churchill, L. (1988). *Rationing health care in America.* South Bend, IN: Notre Dame University Press.

Clouser, K. D., & Gert, B. (1990). A critique of principlism. *Journal of Medicine and Philosophy, 15*(2), 219–236. doi:10.1093/jmp/15.2.219

Coyle, N. (1992). The euthanasia and physician-assisted suicide debate: Issues for nursing. *Oncology Nursing Forum, 19*(7 Suppl.), 41–46.

Culver, C., & Gert, B. (1982). *Philosophy in medicine: Conceptual and ethical issues in medicine and psychiatry.* New York, NY: Oxford University Press.

Daly, B. J., Berry, D., Fitzpatrick, J. J., Drew, B., & Montgomery, K. (1997). Assisted suicide: Implications for nurses and nursing. *Nursing Outlook, 45*(5), 209–214. doi:10.1016/S0029-6554(97)90067-1

Daniels, N. (1985). *Just health care.* Cambridge, UK: The Press Syndicate of the University of Cambridge.

Davis, A. J., Aroskar, M. A., Liaschenko, J., & Drought, T. S. (1997). *Ethical dilemmas and nursing practice* (4th ed.). Stanford, CT: Appleton & Lange.

DeMartino, E. S., Dudzinski, D. M., Doyle, C. J., Sperry, B. P., Gregory, S. E., Siegler, M., ... Kramer, D. B. (2017). Who decides when a patient can't? Statutes on alternate decision makers. *New England Journal of Medicine, 376*(15), 1478–1482. doi:10.1056/NEJMms1611497

Dexter, P. R., Wolinsky, F. D., Gramelspacher, G. P., Eckert, G. J., & Tierney, W. M. (2003). Opportunities for advance directives to influence acute medical care. *Journal of Clinical Ethics, 14*(3), 173–182.

Dixon, M. D. (1997). The quality of mercy: Reflections on provider-assisted suicide. *Journal of Clinical Ethics, 8*, 290–302.

Do, E. K., Cohen, S. A., & Brown, M. J. (2014). Socioeconomic and demographic factors modify the association between informal caregiving and health in the Sandwich Generation. *BMC Public Health, 14*, 362–374. doi:10.1186/1471-2458-14-362

Dolan, P. (2001). Utilitarianism and the measurement and aggregation of quality-adjusted life years. *Health Care Analysis, 9*(1), 65–76. doi:10.1023/A:1011387524579

Donley, G., & Danis, M. (2011). Making the case for talking to patients about the costs of end-of-life care. *Journal of Medical Law and Ethics, 39*(2), 183–193. doi:10.1111/j.1748-720X.2011.00587.x

Dubler, N. N., & Liebman, C. B. (2011). *Bioethics mediation: A guide to shaping shared solutions* (rev. & expanded ed.). Nashville, TN: Vanderbilt University Press.

Edwards, S. D. (2009). Three versions of an ethics of care. *Nursing Philosophy, 10*(4), 231–240. doi:10.1111/j.1466-769X.2009.00415.x

Emanuel, E. J. (2008). The cost-coverage trade-off: "It's health care costs, stupid." *Journal of the American Medical Association, 299*(8), 947–949. doi:10.1001/jama.299.8.947

Epstein, E. G., & Hamric, A. B. (2009). Moral distress, moral residue, and the crescendo effect. *Journal of Clinical Ethics, 20*(4), 330–342.

Ersek, M. (2003). Artificial nutrition and hydration: Clinical issues. *Journal of Hospice and Palliative Nursing, 5*, 221–230. doi:10.1097/00129191-200310000-00019

Fagerlin, A., & Schneider, C. E. (2004). Enough: The failure of the living will. *Hastings Center Report, 34*(2), 30–42. doi:10.2307/3527683

Farrell, T. W., Widera, E., Rosenberg, L., Rubin, C. D., Naik, A. D., Braun, U., … Shega, J.; For Ethics, Clinical Practice and Models of Care, and Public Policy Committees of the American Geriatrics Society. (2017). AGS position statement: Making medical treatment decisions for unbefriended older adults. *Journal of the American Geriatrics Society, 65*(1), 14–15. doi:10.1111/jgs.14586

Fiester, A. (2007). Viewpoint: Why the clinical ethics we teach fails patients. *Academic Medicine: Journal of the Association of American Medical Colleges, 82*(7), 684–689. doi:10.1097/ACM.0b013e318067456d

Foote, P. (1977). Euthanasia. *Philosophy and Public Affairs, 6*(2), 85–112.

Fowler, M. D. (1987). Introduction to ethics and ethical theory. In M. D. Fowler & J. Levine-Ariff (Eds.), *Ethics at the bedside: A source book for the critical care nurse* (pp. 24–38). Philadelphia, PA: Lippincott.

Fox, E., Myers, S., & Pearlman, R. A. (2007). Ethics consultation in United States hospitals: A national survey. *American Journal of Bioethics, 7*(2), 13–25. doi:10.1080/15265160601109085

Frankena, W. K. (1973). *Ethics* (2nd ed.). Englewood Cliffs, NJ: Prentice-Hall.

Fritz, Z., & Fuld, J. (2010). Ethical issues surrounding do not attempt resuscitation orders: Decisions, discussions and deleterious effects. *Journal of Medical Ethics, 36*(10), 593–597. doi:10.1136/jme.2010.035725

Fry, S. T. (1987). Autonomy, advocacy, and accountability: Ethics at the bedside. In M. D. Fowler & J. Levine-Ariff (Eds.), *Ethics at the bedside: A source book for the critical care nurse* (pp. 39–49). Philadelphia, PA: Lippincott.

Fry, S. T. (1989). Towards a theory of nursing ethics. *Advances in Nursing Science, 11*(4), 9–22. doi:10.1097/00012272-198907000-00005

Fry, S. T., Killen, A. R., & Robinson, E. M. (1996). Care-based reasoning, caring, and the ethic of care: A need for clarity. *Journal of Clinical Ethics, 7*(1), 41–47.

Gadow, S. (1996). Aging as death rehearsal: The oppressiveness of reason. *Journal of Clinical Ethics, 7*(1), 35–40.

Gershengorn, H. B., Li, G., Kramer, A., & Wunsch, H. (2012). Survival and functional outcomes after cardiopulmonary resuscitation in the intensive care unit. *Journal of Critical Care, 27*(4), 421.e9–e17. doi:10.1016/j.jcrc.2011.11.001

Golden, M., & Zoanni, T. (2010). Killing us softly: The dangers of legalizing assisted suicide. *Disability and Health Journal, 3*(1), 16–30. doi:10.1016/j.dhjo.2009.08.006

Goldenberg, R. L., Culhane, J. F., Iams, J. D., & Romero, R. (2008). Epidemiology and causes of preterm birth. *Lancet, 371*(9606), 75–84. doi:10.1016/S0140-6736(08)60074-4

Gross, J. (2008, May 5). For the elderly, being heard about life's end. *New York Times*, A1. Retrieved from http://www.nytimes.com/2008/05/05/health/05slow.html

Hamric, A. B. (2012). Empirical research on moral distress: Issues, challenges, and opportunities. *HEC Forum: An Interdisciplinary Journal on Hospitals' Ethical and Legal Issues, 24*(1), 39–49. doi:10.1007/s10730-012-9177-x

Hamric, A. B., & Blackhall, L. J. (2007). Nurse-physician perspectives on the care of dying patients in intensive care units: Collaboration, moral distress, and ethical climate. *Critical Care Medicine, 35*(2), 422–429. doi:10.1097/01.CCM.0000254722.50608.2D

Hickman, S. E., Keevern, E., & Hammes, B. J. (2015). Use of the physician orders for life-sustaining treatment program in the clinical setting: A systematic review of the literature. *Journal of the American Geriatrics Society, 63*, 341–350. doi:10.1111/jgs.13248

HJK Family Foundation. (July 20, 2016). The facts on medicare spending and financing. Retrieved from http://kff.org/medicare/issue-brief/the-facts-on-medicare-spending-and-financing

Hlubocky, F. J., Back, A. L., & Shanafelt, T. D. (2016). Addressing burnout in oncology: Why cancer care clinicians are at risk, what individuals can do, and how organizations can respond. *American Society of Clinical Oncology Educational Book, 35*, 271–279. doi:10.14694/EDBK_156120

Hospice and Palliative Nurses Association. (2011). Position statement on legalization of physician assisted suicide. Retrieved from http://hpna.advancingexpertcare.org/wp-content/uploads/2014/09/HPNA-Legalization-of-Assisted-Suicide-Position-Statement-080311.pdf

Hospice and Palliative Nurses Association. (2017). Guidelines for the role of the registered nurse and advanced practice registered nurse when hastened death is requested. Retrieved from http://advancingexpertcare.org/wp-content/uploads/2017/07/Guidelines-for-RN-and-APRN-When-Hastened-Death-Requested.pdf

Huffman, D. M., & Rittenmeyer, L. (2012). How professional nurses working in hospital environments experience moral distress: A systematic review. *Critical Care Nursing Clinics of North America, 24*(1), 91–100. doi:10.1016/j.ccell.2012.01.004

Hurst, S. A., Slowther, A. M., Forde, R., Pegoraro, R., Reiter-Theil, S., Perrier, A., ... Danis, M. (2006). Prevalence and determinants of physician bedside rationing: Data from Europe. *Journal of General Internal Medicine*, *21*(11), 1138–1143. doi:10.1111/j.1525-1497.2006.00551.x

Jacobs, H. H. (2005). Ethics in pediatric end-of-life care: A nursing perspective. *Journal of Pediatric Nursing*, *20*(5), 360–369. doi:10.1016/j.pedn.2005.04.016

Jameton, A. (1984). *Nursing practice: The ethical issues*. Englewood Cliffs, NJ: Prentice-Hall.

Jecker, N. S. (1991). Age-based rationing and women. *Journal of the American Medical Association*, *266*(21), 3012–3015. doi:10.1001/jama.1992.03490140126048

Johnson, M. (2006). Terri Schiavo: A disability rights case. *Death Studies, 30*, 163–176. doi:10.1080/07481180500455640

Jones, F. M., Sabin, T. L., & Torma, L. M. (2016). Improving the advance directive request and retrieval process in critical access hospitals: Honoring the patient's wishes. *Journal of Nursing Care Quality, 31*(3), 275–281. doi:10.1097/NCQ.0000000000000168

Kahn, J. M. Le, T., Angus, D. C., Cox, C. E., Hough, C. L., White, D. B., ... Carson, S. S. (2015). The epidemiology of chronic critical illness in the United States. *Journal of Critical Care Medicine, 43*(2), 282–287. doi:10.1097/CCM.0000000000000710

Kain, V. J. (2006). Palliative care delivery in the NICU: What barriers do neonatal nurses face? *Neonatal Network*, *25*(6), 387–392. doi:10.1891/0730-0832.25.6.387

Kayser, J. W., Nault, D., & Ostiguy, G. (2012). Resolving moral distress when caring for patients who smoke while using home oxygen therapy. *Home Healthcare Nurse, 30*(4), 208–215. doi:10.1097/NHH.0b013e31824c2892

Kelly, B., Rid, A., & Wendler, D. (2012). Systematic review: Individuals' goals for surrogate decision-making. *Journal of the American Geriatrics Society, 60*(5), 884–895. doi:10.1111/j.1532-5415.2012.03937.x

Kon, A. A. (2011). Informed non-dissent: A better option than slow codes when families cannot bear to say "let her die." *American Journal of Bioethics, 11*(11), 22–23. doi:10.1080/15265161.2011.603796

Kon, A. A., Davidson, J. E., Morrison, W., Danis, M., & White, D. B. (2016). Shared decision making in ICUs: An American College of Critical Care Medicine and American Thoracic Society Policy Statement. *Journal of Critical Care Medicine, 44*(1), 188–201. doi:10.1097/CCM.0000000000001396

Kon, A. A., Shepard, E. K., Sederstrom, N. O., Swoboda, S. M., Marshall, M. F., Birriel, B., & Rincon, F. (2016). Defining futile and potentially inappropriate interventions: A policy statement from the Society of Critical Care Medicine ethics committee. *Critical Care Medicine, 44*(9), 1769–1774. doi:10.1097/CCM.0000000000001965

Latimer, E. J. (1991). Ethical decision-making in the care of the dying and its applications to clinical practice. *Journal of Pain and Symptom Management, 6*(5), 329–336. doi:10.1016/0885-3924(91)90058-C

Lewis, E., Cardona-Morrell, M., Ong, K., Trankle, S., & Hillman, K. (2016). Evidence still insufficient that advance care documentation leads to engagement of healthcare professionals in end-of-life discussions: A systematic review. *Palliative Medicine, 30*(9), 807–824. doi:10.1177/0269216316637239

Lynn, J., & Goldstein, N. E. (2003). Advance care planning for fatal chronic illness: Avoiding commonplace errors and unwarranted suffering. *Annals of Internal Medicine, 138*(10), 812–818. doi:10.7326/0003-4819-138-10-200305200-00009

Lynn, J., Teno, J., Dresser, R., Brock, D., Nelson, H. L., Nelson, J. L., ... Itakura, H. (1999). Dementia and advance-care planning: Perspectives from three countries on ethics and epidemiology. *Journal of Clinical Ethics, 10*(4), 271–285.

Lyon, J. (1985). *Playing God in the nursery*. New York, NY: W. W. Norton.

Macauley, R. (2012). The role of the principle of double effect in ethics education at US medical schools and its potential impact on pain management at the end of life. *Journal of Medical Ethics, 38*(3), 174–178. doi:10.1136/medethics-2011-100105

Manfredi, P. L., Morrison, R. S., & Meier, D. E. (1998). The rule of double effect. *New England Journal of Medicine*, *338*(19), 1389–1391. doi:10.1056/nejm199805073381917

Maryland Office of the Attorney General. (n.d.). The Health Care Decisions Act, §5–611 (d). Retrieved from www.marylandattorneygeneral.gov/Pages/HealthPolicy/hcda.aspx

Menzel, P. T. (2016). Merits, demands, and challenges of VSED. *Narrative Inquiry in Bioethics, 6*(2), 121–126. doi:10.1353/nib.2016.0029

Mezey, M., Mitty, E., & Ramsey, G. (1997). Assessment of decision-making capacity. Nursing's role. *Journal of Gerontological Nursing, 23*(3), 28–35. doi:10.3928/0098-9134-19970301-13

Mohammed, S., & Peter, E. (2009). Rituals, death and the moral practice of medical futility. *Nursing Ethics, 16*(3), 292–302. doi:10.12968/bjon.2016.25.1.36

Morley, G. (2016a). Efficacy of the nurse ethicist in reducing moral distress: What can the NHS learn from the USA? *British Journal of Nursing, 25*(1), 36–39. doi:10.12968/bjon.2016.25.1.36

Morley, G. (2016b). Efficacy of the nurse ethicist in reducing moral distress: What can the NHS learn from the USA? Part 2. *British Journal of Nursing, 25*(3), 156–161. doi:10.12968/bjon.2016.25.3.156

National Association of Neonatal Nurses. (2006). Position statement #3015: NICU nurse involvement in ethical decisions. Retrieved from http://nann.org/uploads/About/PositionPDFS/1.4.12_Nurse%20Involvment%20in%20Ethical%20Decisions.pdf

Norals, T. E., & Smith, T. J. (2015). Advance care planning discussions: Why they should happen, why they don't, and how we can facilitate the process. *Oncology, 29*(8), 567–571.

Oregon Health Authority. Death With Dignity Act. (2018, February 9). Death with Dignity Act annual reports 2017 data summary. Public Health Division, Center for Health Statistics. Retrieved from http://www.oregon.gov/oha/PH/PROVIDERPARTNERRESOURCES/EVALUATIONRESEARCH/DEATHWITHDIGNITYACT/Documents/year20.pdf

Orentlicher, D., Pope, T. M., & Rich, B. A. (2016). Clinical criteria for physician aid in dying. *Journal of Palliative Medicine, 19*(3), 259–262. doi:10.1089/jpm.2015.0092

Peace, W. (2011, March 6). Conference day. [Web log post] Retrieved from http://badcripple.blogspot.com/search?q=conference+day

Perkins, H. S. (2007). Controlling death: The false promise of advance directives. *Annals of Internal Medicine*, *147*(1), 51–57. doi:10.7326/0003-4819-147-1-200707030-00008

Perrin, K. O. (1997). Giving voice to the wishes of elders for end-of-life care. *Journal of Gerontological Nursing*, *23*(3), 18–27. doi:10.3928/0098-9134-19970301-12

Peryakoil, V. S., Neri, E., & Kraemer, H. (2017). A randomized controlled trial comparing the letter project advance directive to traditional advance directives. *Journal of Palliative Medicine, 20*(9), 954–965. doi:10.1089/jpm.2017.0066

Pew Research Center. (2013). Views on end-of-life medical treatments. Retrieved from http://www.pewforum.org/2013/11/21/views-on-end-of-life-medical-treatments

Piers, R. D., Van den Eynde, M., Steeman, E., Vlerick, P., Benoit, D. D., & Van Den Noortgate, N. J. (2012). End-of-life care of the geriatric patient and nurses' moral distress. *Journal of the American Medical Directors Association, 13*(1), 80. e7–80.13e. doi:10.1016/j.jamda.2010.12.014

Pope, T. M. (2016). Introduction: Voluntarily stopping eating and drinking. *Narrative Inquiry in Bioethics, 6*(2), 75–77. doi:10.1353/nib.2016.0034

Portenoy, R. K., Sibirceva, U., Smout, R., Horn, S., Connor, S., Blum, R. H., … Fine, P. G. (2006). Opioid use and survival at the end of life: A survey of a hospice population. *Journal of Pain and Symptom Management, 32*(6), 532–540. doi:10.1016/j.jpainsymman.2006.08.003

President's Commission for the Study of Ethical Problems in Medicine and Biomedical and Behavioral Research. (1983). *Deciding to forego life-sustaining treatment*. Washington, DC: U.S. Government Printing Office.

Quill, T. E., & Byock, I. R. (2000). Responding to intractable terminal suffering: The role of terminal sedation and voluntary refusal of food and fluids. *Annals of Internal Medicine, 132*(5), 408–414. doi:10.7326/0003-4819-132-5-200003070-00012

Quill, T. E., Dresser, R., & Brock, D. W. (1997). The rule of double effect: A critique of its role in end-of-life decision-making. *New England Journal of Medicine, 337*(24), 1768–1771. doi:10.1056/NEJM199712113372413

Quill, T. E., Lo, B., & Brock, D. W. (1997). Palliative options of last resort: A comparison of voluntarily stopping eating and drinking, terminal sedation, physician-assisted suicide, and voluntary active euthanasia. *Journal of the American Medical Association, 278*(23), 2099–2104. doi:10.1001/jama.1997.03550230075041

Rakatansky, H. (2017). Complexities to consider when patients choose VSED (voluntarily stopping eating and drinking). *Rhode Island Medical Journal, 100*(2), 12–13.

Reisfield, G. M., Wallace, S. K., Munsell, M. F., Webb, F. J., Alvarez, E. R., & Wilson, G. R. (2006). Survival in cancer patients undergoing in-hospital cardiopulmonary resuscitation: A meta-analysis. *Resuscitation, 71*, 152–160. doi:10.1016/j.resuscitation.2006.02.022

Rushton, C. H., & Carse, A. (2017). Harnessing the promise of moral distress: A call for re-orientation. *Journal of Clinical Ethics, 28*(1), 15–29.

Rushton, C. H., & Reigle, J. (1993). Ethical issues in critical nursing. In M. Kinney, D. Packa, & S. Dunbar (Eds.), *AACN's clinical reference for critical care* (pp. 8–27). St. Louis, MO: Mosby.

Santonocito, C., Ristagno, G., Gullo, A., & Weil, M. H. (2013). Do-not-resuscitate order: A view throughout the world. *Journal of Critical Care, 28*(1), 14–21. doi:10.1016/j.jcrc.2012.07.005

Scheunemann, L. P., & White, D. B. (2011). The ethics and reality of rationing in medicine. *Chest, 140*(6), 1625–1632. doi:10.1378/chest.11-0622

Schneiderman, L. J., & Jecker, N. S. (1995). *Wrong medicine: Doctors, patients, and futile treatment*. Baltimore, MD: Johns Hopkins University Press.

Schwarz, J. (2008). I can't help you with that. *American Journal of Nursing, 108*, 11. doi:10.1097/01.NAJ.0000330239.52465.34

Schwarz, J. K. (1999). Assisted dying and nursing practice. *Image: The Journal of Nursing Scholarship, 31*(4), 367–374. doi:10.1111/j.1547-5069.1999.tb00522.x

Schwarz, J. K. (2003). Understanding and responding to patients' requests for assistance in dying. *Journal of Nursing Scholarship, 35*(4), 377–384. doi:10.1111/j.1547-5069.2003.00377.x

Schwarz, J. K. (2004a). Responding to persistent requests for assistance in dying: A phenomenological inquiry. *International Journal of Palliative Nursing, 10*(5), 225–235; discussion 235. doi:10.12968/ijpn.2004.10.5.13071

Schwarz, J. K. (2004b). The rule of double effect and its role in facilitating good end-of-life care: A help or a hindrance? *Journal of Hospice and Palliative Nursing, 6*, 125–133. doi:10.1097/00129191-200404000-00017

Schwartz, J. (2008, Spring). Considering Baby Doe rules. *Mid-Atlantic Ethics Committee Newsletter*.

Schwartz Rounds. (2018). The Schwartz Center. Retrieved from http://www.theschwartzcenter.org/supporting-caregivers/schwartz-center-rounds

Shalowitz, D. I., Garrett-Mayer, E., & Wendler, D. (2006). The accuracy of surrogate decision makers: A systematic review. *Archives of Internal Medicine, 166*(5), 493–497. doi:10.1001/archinte.166.5.493

Stanley, J. K., & Zoloth-Dorfman, L. (2001). Ethical considerations. In B. R. Ferrell & N. Coyle (Eds.), *Textbook of palliative nursing* (pp. 663–681). New York, NY: Oxford University Press.

Steinbock, B., Arras, J., & London, A. (2012). *Ethical issues in modern medicine: Contemporary readings in bioethics* (8th ed.). Columbus, OH: McGraw-Hill.

Stephany, T. M. (1994). Assisted suicide: How hospice fails. *American Journal of Hospice and Palliative Care, 11*(4), 4–5. doi:10.1177/104990919401100403

Stramondo, J. A. (2016). Why bioethics needs a disability moral psychology. *Hastings Center Report, 46*(3), 22–30. doi:10.1002/hast.585

Strech, D., & Danis, M. (2014). How can bedside rationing be justified despite coexisting inefficiency? The need for "benchmarks of efficiency." *Journal of Medical Ethics, 40*(2), 89–93. doi:10.1136/medethics-2012-100769

Suter, P. M., Rogers, J., & Strack, C. (2008). Artificial nutrition and hydration for the terminally ill: A reasoned approach. *Home Healthcare Nurse, 26*(1), 23–29. doi:10.1097/01.NHH.0000305551.55467.24

Tarzian, A. J. (1995). Last rites. *Hastings Center Report, 25*(6), 3. doi:10.2307/3527832

Tarzian, A. J.; the ASBH Core Competencies Update Task Force. (2013). Health care ethics consultation: An update on core competencies and emerging standards. *American Journal of Bioethics, 13*(2), 3–13. doi:10.1 080/15265161.2012.750388

Tarzian, A. J., & Wocial, L. D.; the American Society for Bioethics and Humanities' Clinical Ethics Consultation Affairs Committee. (2015). A code of ethics for healthcare ethics consultants: Journey to the present & implications for the field. *American Journal of Bioethics, 15*(5), 38–51. doi:10.1080/15265161.2015.1021966.

Terman, S. A. (2007). *The best way to say goodbye: A legal peaceful choice at the end of life.* Carlsbad, CA: Life Transitions Publications.

Tilden, V. P., Tolle, S. W., Nelson, C. A., & Fields, J. (2001). Family decision-making to withdraw life-sustaining treatments from hospitalized patients. *Nursing Research, 50*(2), 105–115. doi:10.1097/00006199-200103000-00006

Tonelli, R. R. (1996). Pulling the plug on living wills: A critical analysis of advance directive. *Chest, 110,* 816–822. doi:10.1378/chest.110.3.816

Truog, R. D., Campbell, M. L., Curtis, J. R., Haas, C. E., Luce, J. M., & Rubenfeld, G. D.; American Academy of Critical Care Medicine. (2008). Recommendations for end-of-life care in the intensive care unit: A consensus statement by the American College of Critical Care Medicine. *Critical Care Medicine, 36*(3), 953–963. doi:10.1097/CCM.0B013E3181659096

UNC School of Medicine. (2012). Improving decision-making about feeding options in dementia. Retrieved from http://www.med.unc.edu/pcare/resources/feedingoptions

Uustal, D. B. (1987). Values: The cornerstone of nursing's moral act. In M. D. Fowler & J. Levine-Ariff (Eds.), *Ethics at the bedside: A source book for the critical care nurse* (pp. 136–170). Philadelphia, PA: Lippincott.

Varcoe, C., Pauly, B., Storch, J., Newton, L., & Makaroff, K. (2012). Nurses' perceptions of and responses to morally distressing situations. *Nursing Ethics, 19*(4), 488–500. doi:10.1177/0969733011436025

Varon, J., & Marik, P. E. (2007). Cardiopulmonary resuscitation in patients with cancer. *American Journal of Hospice and Palliative Care, 24*(3), 224–229. doi:10.1177/1049909107301485

Veatch, R. M., & Fry, S. T. (1995). *Case studies in nursing ethics.* Boston, MA: Jones & Bartlett.

Vogelstein, E. (2016). Professional hubris and its consequences: Why organizations of health-care professions should not adopt ethically controversial positions. *Bioethics, 30*(4), 234–243. doi:10.1111/bioe.12186

Waldrop, D. P., & Meeker, M. A. (2012). Communication and advanced care planning in palliative and end-of-life care. *Nursing Outlook, 60*(6), 365–369. doi:10.1016/j.outlook.2012.08.012

Walker, M. U. (1993). Keeping moral space open. *Hastings Center Report, 23*(2), 33–40. doi:10.2307/3562818

Ward, D. (2000). Ageism and the abuse of older people in health and social care. *British Journal of Nursing, 9*(9), 560–563. doi:10.12968/bjon.2000.9.9.6292

Westphal, C. (2008). Is cardiopulmonary resuscitation medically appropriate in end stage disease? Review of the evidence. *Journal of Hospice and Palliative Nursing, 10*(3), 128–132. doi:10.1097/01.NJH.0000306749.33506.bb

Wiegand, D. L., & Funk, M. (2012). Consequences of clinical situations that cause critical care nurses to experience moral distress. *Nursing Ethics, 19*(4), 479–487. doi:10.1177/0969733011429342

Wittwer, H. (2013). The problem of the possible rationality of suicide and the ethics of physician-assisted suicide. *International Journal of Law and Psychiatry, 36*(5–6):419–426. doi:10.1016/j.ijlp.2013.06.009

Wocial, L. D., Hancock, M., Bledsoe, P. D., Chamness, A. R., & Helft, P. R. (2010). An evaluation of unit-based ethics conversations. *JONA'S Healthcare Law, Ethics and Regulation, 12*(2), 48–54; quiz 55. doi:10.1097/NHL.0b013e3181de18a2

Wright, D., & Brajtman, S. (2011). Relational and embodied knowing: Nursing ethics within the interprofessional team. *Nursing Ethics, 18*(1), 20–30. doi:10.1177/0969733010386165

Yeo, M., Moorhouse, A., & Dalziel, J. (1996). Autonomy. In M. Yeo & A. Moorhouse (Eds.), *Concepts and cases in nursing ethics* (2nd ed., pp. 91–138). Peterborough, ON, Canada: Broadview Press.

Yeo, M., Moorhouse, A., & Donner, G. (1996). Justice. In M. Yeo & A. Moorhouse (Eds.), *Concepts and cases in nursing ethics* (2nd ed., pp. 211–266). Peterborough, ON, Canada: Broadview Press.

Kathleen O. Perrin

Legal Aspect of Palliative Care and Advance Care Planning

CHAPTER

5

KEY POINTS

- An adult is presumed to have the ability to make his or her own healthcare decisions—including termination of life-sustaining technology—unless he or she is shown to be incapacitated by clinical examination or ruled incompetent by a court of law.
- Advance care directives are legal vehicles used by people to provide guidance to their healthcare providers concerning the care they would desire in the event they become incapacitated and cannot make their own decisions.
- Common forms of advance directives are living wills, do-not-resuscitate (DNR) directives, and durable powers of attorney for healthcare purposes.
- Problems with advance directives may arise when they do not seem to apply to the patient's situation, so the healthcare team may be reluctant to follow them.
- In general, courts are hesitant to enforce advance directives.
- Conflicts among healthcare providers, patients, and/or families about a patient's end-of-life (EOL) care may be resolved by the development of consensus about goals for care through listening, thoughtful discussion, multidisciplinary rounds, and ethics consultation.
- Many states now have intractable legislation for pain management either as part of their natural death acts or as separate legislation that affirms dying patients' rights to adequate pain management.
- Nurses play essential roles in helping patients receive ethically and legally appropriate EOL care. These roles include educating the patient and family about the patient's condition and legal EOL choices, identifying the patient's and family's wishes for EOL care, articulating the patient's and family's desires to other members of the healthcare team, and assisting the patient and family to obtain necessary and appropriate EOL care.

CASE STUDY

Harriet, a 76-year-old retired nurse, developed endocarditis and mitral valve dysfunction from an infected pacemaker lead. Harriet's past history included a 3-month hospital stay following mitral valve surgery 7 years earlier. She is overweight and has long-standing chronic lung disease, but is precise in managing all her medications. Harriet has lived alone for the past year following the death of her husband. She recently updated her advance directive and durable power of attorney for healthcare, reaffirming that she wanted to be intubated, have hemodialysis, and have cardiopulmonary resuscitation, if they were necessary. In addition, she gave her brother power to make healthcare decisions for her if she became incapacitated.

Harriet was awake and able to understand what was happening to her when the cardiac surgeon at her local hospital explained that her chances of surviving a second operation on the valve while she had endocarditis were slim. He stated that the infection was not responding to antibiotics, so surgery was necessary but was more risky than could be performed locally. He informed her that she had two choices: Recognize that she was not likely to recover and forego surgery or transfer to a teaching hospital and see whether they were willing to operate. Harriet chose to transfer and have surgery.

Initially, the surgery went well; Harriet was extubated 5 days after surgery and transferred to a step-down unit. Then, Harriet had respiratory arrest, was resuscitated, and required reintubation. Following her cardiac arrest, Harriet developed renal failure and was started on hemodialysis with her consent. When it became apparent that Harriet was not going to tolerate extubation, she was asked whether she wanted a tracheostomy to which she immediately responded, "yes." Harriet's brother and some of her friends asked the nurses, "Why are you still doing all this? She's been through it once already, isn't that enough?"

Lay and professional communities throughout the world are struggling with bioethical and legal dilemmas brought about by the proliferation of medical technology. A heightened sense of self-determination and the decision making associated with the use of available life-sustaining technology, termination of life-prolonging treatment, patient-requested euthanasia, and assisted suicide have engendered bioethical and legal dilemmas in end-of-life (EOL) care. Although these dilemmas have different ramifications for different people, a patient's well-being can best be served when healthcare professionals are able to collaborate with each other, the patient, and the family to set goals for patient care as the EOL approaches.

For nurses in particular, EOL decision making is a moral issue as well as a legal one. The moral question of what is "right" or "best" for the patient, what ought to be done, and who is the person best suited to do the "right" or "best" thing evokes strong personal sentiments when discussing EOL care. These questions have the potential to provoke conflict among those involved in patient care—physicians, nurses, social workers, and others—and the questions for each are clouded by the individual's personal and professional ethics.

EOL questions pose a different dilemma for the family. Many times, families are faced with discussions regarding whether to stop treatment and allow the patient to die a natural death. Family members or patients may not understand that there are limits to how long and how well medical technology can sustain life. For example, most people do not realize how unlikely a person is to survive cardiopulmonary resuscitation (CPR). More important, family members may not be certain of what the patient would have wanted if she or he had been able to make the decision.

Knowledge of the patient's wishes is important; legal and ethical scholars agree that decisions about care at the EOL ought to be made in accordance with an individual's wishes, preferences, beliefs, and values. No one should be subject to medical care against his or her wishes. For the past 20 years in the United States, autonomy and self-determination have been the foundation for such decisions.

Nursing faculty, nursing students, and practicing nurses address ethical and legal issues, including EOL care, with patients and family members in clinical practice daily. With increased medical technology and competing interests of dying patients, their families, and significant others, fulfilling the wish of many to die with dignity is a concern for healthcare professionals. Nurses are in a key position to address the escalation of bioethical dilemmas that result in wrenching situations for patients, families, providers, and the courts. Since the landmark cases of Karen Ann Quinlan (*In re Quinlan*, 1976) and Nancy Beth Cruzan (*Cruzan v. Director*, 1990), nurses, physicians, and other healthcare professionals have shaped public policy regarding patient and surrogate participation in EOL decision making even when the patient is incapacitated and unable to make decisions.

■ LAW AND ETHICS: SAME OR DIFFERENT?

Law and *ethics* are similar in that they have developed in the same historical, social, cultural, and philosophical soil (Davis, Aroskar, Liaschenko, & Drought, 1997). *Black's Law Dictionary* defines "law as" "that which is laid down, ordained, or established; a body of rules of action or conduct prescribed by controlling authority and having binding legal forces; and that which must be obeyed and followed by citizens subject to sanctions or legal consequences" (Garner, 2009, pp. 884–885). The law may be defined better as the sum total of rules and regulations by which a society is governed. "Ethics," in contrast, refers to informal or formal standards that guide how individuals or groups of people believe they ought to behave.

Law and ethics may differ in what they allow or require a person to do. For example, some actions may be legal yet not ethical. A historical example is the legality of slavery in the United States until the Civil War. More recent, a nurse in Oregon might legally have assisted a patient to commit suicide, although the American Nurses Association (ANA) declared that such assistance was unethical. Other actions may be ethical but not legal. A historical example would be the development of the Underground Railroad to assist slaves fleeing to Canada. This dichotomy can occur because legal rights are grounded in the law and ethical rights are grounded in ethical principles and values. The law establishes rules that define a person's rights, obligations, and the appropriate penalty for those who violate it. Moreover, the law describes how the government will enforce the rules and penalties. There are many laws that affect the practice of nursing, and nurses must be able to differentiate between ethical claims that suggest how a nurse should act and legal requirements for the nurse to act in specific ways or potentially incur sanctions.

■ NURSING AND THE LAW

Legal and moral obligations are not new to nurses. Each state's nurse practice act, a legal statute regulating nursing, and the professional code of ethics followed by nurses are the foundations of nursing practice. Similarly, nurses are confronted with complex moral and legal questions on a regular basis when caring for dying patients: When does death occur? Does an individual have a right to choose death? Is there a difference between letting a person die and taking measures to hasten death? Do you disclose a terminal diagnosis to a patient? These are just a few of the ethical and legal issues in contemporary nursing.

Decision making at the EOL has been at the heart of many ethical dilemma discussions and legal cases in bioethics in the past 25 years. Because nurses are legally responsible and accountable for the healthcare that patients and their families receive, nurses can no longer afford to view the questions of ethics and law as solely an academic exercise, nor should ethical and legal considerations of today's healthcare issues remain solely in the purview of the organization's ethics committee or risk management departments. Nurses must understand the basic concepts of ethical decision making and know the relevant laws that address the current controversies to ensure that individual and societal rights and values are protected.

■ INFORMED CONSENT

Informed consent is not only a legal requirement, but also a moral imperative. The legal requirement of informed consent is based on the value of patient autonomy and self-determination. Every human being of adult years and sound mind has a right to determine what shall be done with his or her own body (*Schloendorff v. Society of New York Hospital*, 1914). In accordance, the fundamental goals of informed consent are patient autonomy and self-determination (*In re Farrell*, 1987). This goal is effectuated by allowing patients to make their own decisions about their healthcare based on their own values for as long as they are able.

A second goal of informed consent is to empower patients to exercise their right to autonomy rationally and intelligently (Meisel & Cerminara, 2001). There is no guarantee that providing patients relevant information about treatment will result in patients making intelligent decisions, nor does it guarantee that they will use the information provided; however, without such a requirement, the likelihood of rational decision making diminishes (Meisel & Cerminara, 2001). The patient's right to consent presumes that the patient has sufficient information to make a reasonable decision.

Consent to treatment is valid only when the patient has the capacity to consent (Meisel & Cerminara, 2001). *Competence* is not the same as *capacity*, yet they are frequently considered to be synonymous. A competent individual is able to comprehend the nature of a potential action and understand its significance. The law presumes that all adults are competent and have the ability to make their own decisions, including those about healthcare, and that assumption is ordinarily correct (Meisel & Cerminara, 2001). Therefore, incompetence is determined only in a court of law. However, a patient need not be adjudicated incompetent to lack the capacity to consent to medical treatment (Meisel & Cerminara, 2001).

Capacity is determined not by the courts, but rather by clinicians who assess functional capabilities to determine whether the capacity to make a specific decision is lacking. Incapacity is not determined solely by a medical or psychiatric diagnosis. Rather, decisional capacity within healthcare is determined via clinical assessment and the ability of the patient to give valid consent (Cooney, Kennedy, Hawkins, Hurme, & Balch, 2004).

The basic elements of a valid consent—the determination that a patient has sufficient decisional capacity to consent or refuse treatment—are based on the observation of a specific set of abilities. In order to have decision-making capacity, the patient must be able to understand the relevant information, appreciate the situation and its consequences, reason about treatment options, and communicate a choice (Appelbaum, 2007). Appelbaum notes that the use of standardized questions can increase the reliability of raters determining a patient's capacity.

He recommends the McArthur Competence Assessment Tool, which takes approximately 20 minutes to administer and score. However, he also suggests questions that are normally included when assessing each criterion to determine whether a patient has the capacity to make a healthcare decision. Examples of the questions include the following:

- Would you please tell me in your own words what your doctor told you about your current problem and its treatment?
- What is the treatment likely to do for you?
- What makes this treatment a good choice for you? Why is it better than any other one?
- Please tell me what you have decided to do.

Not all health decisions require the same level of decision-making capacity in order to make a valid decision. Decision-making capacity is not an "on–off switch" (Mezey, Mitty, & Ramsey, 1997), meaning a patient either has it or does not have it. Rather, capacity is usually viewed as task specific; an individual may be able to perform some tasks adequately and may have the ability to make some decisions, but may still be unable to perform all tasks or make all decisions. The notion of "decision-specific capacity" assumes that an individual has or lacks capacity for a particular decision at a particular time and under a particular set of circumstances (Mezey, Mitty, et al., 1997; Mitty & Mezey, 2004).

Special Concerns With Children: Assent Rather Than Consent

In contrast to adults, children younger than 18 years of age are not considered to be legally competent and usually are not considered to be capable of giving fully reasoned consent. Therefore, in most cases, parents and healthcare providers make healthcare decisions for children without the child's consent. Instead of giving consent, a child is asked to assent, which means to freely express an opinion in favor of a treatment. The child's assent about EOL care is deeply affected by the child's developmental and chronological age, because young children have limited understandings of illness and death.

Over the past 40 years, the thinking about children and medical decision making has evolved. Although at one time the decision was made for the child without explanation of the illness or consultation, now there is more likely to be a shared decision-making process, in which children have more autonomy as they develop greater cognitive maturity. This change in emphasis from making decisions for children to giving children a voice promotes their dignity and quality of life (QOL), but presents many challenges (Whitty-Rogers, Alex,

MacDonald, Gallant, & Austin, 2009). Preschool children are usually considered too young to make clearly rational decisions, so their parents are asked to make decisions for them based on the best-interests standard. This can be problematic, because parents' emotional distress may prevent them from realizing what is in the child's best interests.

When children reach school age, they are usually provided with information about their condition in a manner that they can understand. Although school-age children may express a preference and assent to treatment, parents and healthcare providers usually continue to be the primary decision makers, because the child is not thought to have the capacity to make an informed decision yet. In contrast to this common belief and practice, a study by Hinds et al. (2005) found that children as young as 10 years dying from brain tumors could understand the potential treatment options and recognize that their death could be the consequence of their decision. Hinds et al. (2005) noted that these children usually based their decisions on their relationships with others and the risks that the treatment imposed on themselves and others.

Once a child enters adolescence, there is less controversy. Some cultures actually assume that adolescents will make their own decisions (Whitty-Rogers et al., 2009), because they are expected to have the decision-making capacity of adults. Harrison, Kenny, Sidarous, and Rowell (1997) recommend that the decision-making capacity of adolescents be examined in the light of their

- Ability to understand and communicate relevant information
- Ability to think and choose with some independence
- Ability to assess the potential for benefit, risk, or harm, as well as to consider consequences and multiple options
- Achievement of a fairly stable set of values

Nurses' Roles in the Informed-Consent Process

Nurses can make a valuable contribution by ensuring that the informed-consent process is accurately carried out (Virani & Sofer, 2003). Nurses must become proficient in assessing decisional capacity and take an active role when the multidisciplinary team is determining decisional capacity. When nurses and other healthcare professionals assess capacity objectively, two types of mistakes can be avoided: first, the mistake of preventing persons who have the capacity to make healthcare decisions from directing the course of their treatment is avoided; and second, there is no failure to protect incapacitated persons from the harmful effects of their decisions (President's Commission, 1982). It is easy when a patient is very ill to let someone take over decision making for the person. However, as long as an adult patient has the capacity to make the decision, it is her or his right to do so.

Nurses must be certain that their patients have the capacity to make an informed decision. In addition, nurses should be certain that their patients were offered appropriate and understandable information that would help them to make the decision. Finally, nurses should ensure that their patients are aware that they have a right to either refuse or accept treatments—that their patients were actually offered options and were not coerced into one decision over another (Sims, 2008). Sometimes, this can be ascertained by expanding Appelbaum's (2008) questions to include, "How did you reach your decision?" or "Who else had input into your decision?" Nurses should make efforts to meet their legal and ethical obligations so that patients retain their rights to make decisions for as long as they are able.

CASE STUDY *Continued*

Harriet was aware of her surroundings, recognized that she would die if she were extubated, and had experienced 2 months of ventilation in the past. Although she was too weak to write and did not tolerate a speaking valve, she made her wishes clearly known. She wished to have a tracheostomy and continue both ventilation and dialysis. She was not ready to die. Because all those involved in her care were convinced that Harriet was competent and had the capacity to make decisions for herself, neither her medical directive nor her durable power of attorney for healthcare came into effect. The care that she was receiving, although extensive, was believed to have the potential to benefit her and was not deemed to be futile. Thus, Harriet continued to make her own decisions about the amount and type of healthcare she desired.

■ THE SUPPORT STUDY

Although in the case study, Harriet Billings wanted to continue to receive life-sustaining therapy, in many instances patients wish to discontinue interventions. Unfortunately, even with the increased attention to EOL issues in lay and medical publications, physicians are often unaware of their patients' preferences concerning EOL care. The Study to Understand Prognoses and Preferences for Outcomes and Risks of Treatment (SUPPORT) and its companion study, the Hospitalized Elderly Longitudinal Project (HELP), both studies of seriously ill hospitalized patients, documented the lack of communication between physicians and their very ill patients about EOL issues (Knaus et al., 1995; SUPPORT Principal Investigators, 1995). The original SUPPORT study (SUPPORT Principal Investigators, 1995) and its offshoots documented the ineffectiveness of advance directives (Teno et al., 1994; Teno, Licks et al., 1997; Teno, Lynn et al., 1997), the effect of serious illness on patients and their families (Covinsky et al., 1994, 1996), the lack of cost-effectiveness of life-extending interventions at the EOL (Hamel et al., 1997), and the influence of patient age and race on decision making (Hamel et al., 1996, 1999; Phillips et al., 1996).

However, most important, the SUPPORT study (SUPPORT Principal Investigators, 1995) suggested that because physicians did not understand their patients' preferences about EOL care, they often continued aggressive, painful life-sustaining treatment beyond the time patients and their families believed was appropriate. Because of that, families indicated that patients spent a considerable amount of time during their last days and hours in pain. One of the reasons offered for such aggressive care at the EOL in the SUPPORT study was that it was not clear to the healthcare providers that patients were definitely dying until less than 48 hours before the patients' deaths. How, then, should a healthcare provider know when to counsel palliative care (PC)? How should a provider know when care is excessive for a patient?

■ NATURAL DEATH ACTS

Natural death acts sprang from the belief that medical technology had made possible the artificial prolongation of patients' lives beyond their natural limits. Another underlying assumption of the acts was that adults in the United States have the right to control decisions about how they live their lives as well as how they die. The California Natural Death Act was one of the first in the country. Originally enacted in 1975 and revised in 1992, it authorized people to sign a declaration directing that life-sustaining treatment be withheld or withdrawn if they become terminally ill or permanently unconscious if the administration of life-sustaining procedures would only prolong their dying process or unconscious condition.

Now, every state has a natural death act explicitly allowing patients to refuse excessive medical care at the EOL. In addition, the natural death acts in some states, such as Washington, specifically state that "physicians and nurses should not withhold or unreasonably diminish pain medication for patients in a terminal condition where the primary intent of providing such medication is to alleviate pain and maintain or increase the patient's comfort" (Washington Natural Death Act, 1992, Chapter 70. 122 RCW). Finally, most states also include in their natural death act a provision that a person's right to control his or her healthcare may be exercised by an authorized representative who validly holds the person's durable power of attorney for healthcare (DPAHC).

However, as shown by the SUPPORT study (SUPPORT Principal Investigators, 1995), the presence of natural death acts did not ensure that patients and their families were able to obtain the EOL care they desired. Guido (2006) states that the case of Nancy Cruzan, a young woman who remained in a persistent vegetative state following an automobile accident and whose family maintained that she would never have desired such technologically driven care, motivated Congress to enact federal legislation that would require states to make patients aware of their rights to have advance directives and to decide about their own care (*Cruzan v. Director*, 1990).

■ THE PATIENT SELF-DETERMINATION ACT

The Patient Self-Determination Act (PSDA), which became effective on December 1, 1991, was the first federal law to focus on the rights of adults to refuse life-sustaining treatment. The Act was motivated by concerns that in the absence of clear directives regarding their views on life-sustaining treatment, patients' views would not be respected when they became incapacitated. The PSDA requires that facilities participating in the Medicare and Medicaid program provide written information to individuals about their right to participate in medical decision making and formulate advance directives. The key provisions of the legislation are touched on here.

With regard to the PSDA, facilities must provide the following:

1. *Written information* to each adult individual concerning "an individual's rights under State law (whether statutory or as recognized by the courts of the State) to make decisions concerning such medical care, including the right to accept or refuse medical or surgical treatment and the right to formulate advance directives"
2. *Written policies* of the provider or organization respecting the implementation of such advance directives
3. *Inquiry* as to whether a person has an advance directive
4. *Documentation* in the patient's medical records whether the individual has executed an advance directive
5. *Nondiscrimination,* that is, not conditioning the provision of care or otherwise discriminating against an individual based on whether the individual has executed an advance directive

6. *Compliance* with requirements of state laws respecting advance directives at facilities of the provider or organization
7. *Education* for staff on issues concerning advance directives and provision for community education regarding advance directive

■ PURPOSE AND TYPES OF ADVANCE DIRECTIVES

Since the PSDA was enacted, all states have passed natural death acts and/or advance directive legislation. However, the specific types of advance directives, the formalities for executing a directive, and the requirement to alleviate pain and promote comfort at the EOL sometimes included within the directive vary from state to state. Despite these state-to-state variations, advance directives have become an important tool to determine patients' desires for EOL care (Duke, Yarbrough, & Pang, 2009) because determining patient preferences and documenting them in advance directives result in improved EOL care for patients with serious illnesses (Detering, Silveira, Arnold, & Savarese, 2017). Benefits from advance care planning and directives include

■ An increased likelihood that both healthcare providers and family members comply with a patient's wishes
■ A reduction in hospitalizations at the EOL
■ A reduction in risk, stress, anxiety, and depression in surviving relatives
■ An increased likelihood that a person will die where she or he would prefer
■ An increase in the utilization of hospice services (Detering et al., 2017)
■ An increase in out-of-hospital expenditures for provision of comfort for patients (Brinkman-Stoppelenburg, Rietjens, & van der Helde, 2014)

Advance directives have several major purposes (Meisel & Cerminara, 2001). The first and perhaps most important purpose is that advance directives are a mechanism by which individuals who are currently competent indicate the type of healthcare they would desire if they lack decision-making capacity at some time in the future. Directives provide guidelines to healthcare providers and family about the kind of medical care the person would like to receive in advance of the need for that care. Advance directives generally are discussed in the context of the right to forego life-sustaining treatments. However, they also may be used to direct the administration of specific treatments, as they were in the case of Harriet Billings. Advance directives pertain to decision making about any kind of healthcare, and they may be executed by any adult as long as he or she possesses the requisite decision-making capacity.

The second purpose of advance directives is to provide guidance, especially to healthcare professionals, regarding how to proceed with decision making about life-sustaining treatment for a patient with diminished capacity. When patients lack decision-making capacity, a great deal of confusion can arise as to how healthcare decisions are to be made, who has the authority to make them, and what the treatment should be. Teno, Gruneir, Schwartz, Nanda, and Wetle (2007) found that bereaved family members of patients with advance directives did report fewer concerns with communication with healthcare providers about treatment decisions and believed that the directives had facilitated the process.

The third purpose of advance directives is that they provide immunity from civil and criminal liability to healthcare providers when they act in good faith and in accordance with state statutes respecting advance directives (Meisel & Cerminara, 2001). Most litigated right-to-die cases end up in court because of the healthcare provider's fear of liability. Statutory immunity provisions provide an impetus for clinical decision making by protecting healthcare professionals who comply with an advance directive. However, a healthcare provider who fails to comply with a directive or a family member's interpretation of the directive may be subject to professional sanctions or civil litigation (Duke et al., 2009).

Despite the potential benefits of advanced directives, rates of completion vary markedly among Americans. Although approximately 70% of older Americans complete an advance directive prior to their death, only about 37% of patients with advanced cancer engage in advance care planning with their healthcare provider (Detering et al., 2017). Patient characteristics associated with a higher likelihood of completion of an advance directive include older age, Caucasian race, a history of chronic disease, higher education or socioeconomic level, and prior knowledge about advance directives and EOL care. Minority groups have significantly lower rates of completion of advance directives (Detering et al., 2017). There are two broad types of advance directives. The first is the instructional directive, which has several subtypes, including the living will, the medical directive, and the DNR order. Instructional directives usually give guidance about the type and amount of care the person desires if she or he becomes incapacitated. The second type of advance directive is the DPAHC, also known as the healthcare proxy. DPAHC documents usually identify an agent to serve as a surrogate for decision making. This section discusses each of these as well as other relevant issues pertaining to advance directives.

Instructional Directives

■ **Living Wills.** Instructional directives identify the amount and type of care a patient would wish to receive if certain conditions are met. In the case of the living will, the patient affirms that if she or he is terminally ill, she or he does not wish to receive life-sustaining treatment(s). There are two major problems with the living will. First, it is not always clear when a person is dying. In the SUPPORT (1995) study of seriously ill patients, many of the patients were still predicted to have a 50% chance of surviving at least 2 months, 2 days before they died. Also, healthcare providers are reluctant to recognize that patients with some diagnoses, particularly heart failure, are dying (Forbes, 2001). Furthermore, the patient does not usually have the opportunity to refuse specific treatments. Despite these problems, older patients with living wills are more likely to have their desires for EOL care met. They are more likely to die in their place of residence than in a hospital (Degenholtz, Rhee, & Arnold, 2004). In addition, they are less likely to have aggressive treatment and more likely to have a priority placed on comfort care (Silveira, Kim, & Langa, 2010).

■ **Medical Directives.** Medical directives are more specific, and they allow patients to specify their desires for or refusals of specific treatments under certain circumstances if the patient becomes incapacitated. For example, patients might indicate that they do not wish to be resuscitated or would not want to be intubated, be ventilated, receive nasogastric feedings, or be dialyzed under specific circumstances, such as becoming comatose. The major problem with medical directives that are not specific to a patient's illness is that the patient's situation may not be similar enough to the circumstance described in the advance directive for anyone to determine how the patient would wish to be treated. Teno, Lynn, et al. (1997) realizes that directives were specific enough in only 3% of actual circumstances to guide decision making. Healthcare providers voice concern with the accuracy of medical directives because they do not allow for advances in medical treatment or for the patient to change his or her mind about one of the interventions or situations without changing or destroying the directive (Olick, 2012). In addition, the medical directive may represent the patient's desires for treatment only at the time the directive was completed, not at the time treatment is being planned. In contrast, health proxies and family decision makers tend to interpret medical directives literally and find these directives useful in determining what care ought to be provided. When medical directives were utilized, family members found comfort believing that the patients' wishes had been fully realized (Leder et al., 2015).

■ **Do-Not-Resuscitate Directives.** In the United States, about 60% of adults over the age of 65 have completed some type of advance directive (Griffin, Cubanski, Neumann, Jankiewicz, & Rousseau, 2016). Although in long-term care facilities three fourths or more of the residents may have a DNR order, DNR orders represent the most common type of advance planning done for adults in this country (Jones, Moss, & Harris-Kojetin,

2011) They are also often viewed as a "practical place to start" (Smith, Desch, Hackney, & Shaw, 1997) and are often the first step in considering treatment limitation at the EOL. When a DNR order is written, the patient or proxy designate and healthcare providers concur that if the patient is dying, the healthcare team will not make any attempt to stop the process or bring the patient back to life.

Originally, CPR was established to be used with witnessed cardiac arrests, sudden death in the young, drowning, and predictable arrests, such as in anesthesia and cardioversion (Hall, 1996). In 1988, New York became the first state to enact DNR legislation stating that consent for CPR was presumed, and if physicians did not want to resuscitate patients, they had to obtain the patients' consent before writing an order not to resuscitate (Swidler, 1989). Many other states have enacted DNR legislation since New York did. The American Medical Association (1991) mandates that patients and families be consulted before a DNR order is written. Since then, all patients who have a cardiopulmonary arrest—for any reason, of any age, or with any condition—will have CPR performed unless there is a specific order written to the contrary (the DNR decision). With a policy of automatic resuscitation, obtaining a DNR order is critical if the patient wishes to avoid cardiopulmonary resuscitation at the EOL.

Most healthcare providers believe that it is quite reasonable for people, especially older adults, to forego CPR because CPR is rarely successful when attempted on older adults. Buchanan (1998) estimated that two long-term care residents out of every 100 who receive CPR survive to hospital discharge, and they both would most likely have significant neurological impairments. Murphy, Murray, Robinson, and Campton, in a 1989 study of older adults receiving CPR in hospital, rehabilitation, and long-term care settings, found that 22% of patients survived the initial resuscitation attempt, but only 3.8% of the patients survived to hospital discharge. Banja and Bilsky (1993) had no patients survive to hospital discharge after resuscitation in a rehabilitation hospital. Survival rates after CPR for all age groups have stayed consistent for three decades at about 13% to as high as 18% (Schneider, Nelson, & Brown, 1993). Marik and Craft (1997) found that patients who survived to hospital discharge following CPR had one reversible condition, were otherwise healthy, and had suffered a sudden, unexpected dysrhythmia. Bishop, Brothers, Perry, and Ahmad (2010) argue that the widespread use of CPR has outlived its utility because it "obscures what is known to all: Resuscitation although able to stay death in a limited number of cases is a pseudo-option that will not resort in a satisfactory restoration of health" (p. 61). Thus, it seems very reasonable for adults with multiple chronic illnesses to forego CPR.

It is essential that healthcare providers offer information about what exactly is entailed in CPR and what a DNR means because only 48% of adults can accurately define "DNR" (Pirinea, Simunich, Wehner, & Ashurt, 2016). If they understand the process, the majority of clearly competent elders living in community or long-term-care facilities would prefer not to be resuscitated if they were gravely ill and probably dying (Diamond, Jernigan, Moseley, Messina, & McKeown, 1989; Eun-Shim & Resnick, 2001; Wagner, 1984). However, elders who have moderate to severe impairment in daily decision-making skills but are still alert and conversant may prefer CPR (O'Brien et al., 1995). Molloy et al. (1996) stated that there was no "gold standard" for determining when an older adult has the capacity to make decisions about EOL care and there is a lack of consensus about what tool ought to be used to measure capacity and who ought to administer the assessment. Eun-Shim and Resnick (2001) state that capacity must be clinically determined, because the person must be shown to be able to understand and appreciate the consequences of the EOL treatment plan.

What nurses need to know about DNR directives is that patients have a right to refuse CPR and may request DNR orders, when they have the capacity to make the decision, after they have been informed of the risks and benefits involved. Moreover, nurses need to know which patients have a DNR directive, the institutional policy and law governing the use of directives, the patient's wishes regarding interventions to be withheld, and their own values regarding the decision to withhold treatment. The medical record should clearly indicate the terms of the directive and whether the terms accurately reflect the patient's current stated preferences.

Recently, a number of healthcare providers have begun advocating for changes in approaches to DNR and CPR. Bishop et al. (2010) advocate that to the extent permissible by law, healthcare providers consider the term "DNR" obsolete and replace it with the term "do not attempt resuscitation" (DNAR). They believe that such a change in terms is the first step to acknowledging that resuscitation might not occur with CPR. Daly (2008) has called for nurses to be actively involved in advocating for the end of "automatic" CPR. Daly reviewed the likelihood of success of CPR (most recent an 18% survival with only 14% having a favorable neurological outcome) and noted the difficulties of explaining to a patient and/or family that they are being required to refuse a treatment that is still required even though it is not likely to be of benefit. She proposes that the use of CPR should be restricted to "those patients who provide adequate informed consent and for whom CPR has a reasonable chance of success" (Daly, 2008, p. 378). Both Bishop et al. (2010) and Daly (2008) agree that all patients should have their CPR status assessed on admission, and, in the absence of informed consent and a physician's order, CPR should not be attempted. Such a proposal would bring the use of CPR more clearly into the realm of other treatments and directives, and patients would be giving consent for treatment rather than nontreatment.

Durable Power of Attorney for Healthcare

The other broad category of advance directives are DPAHC documents. These documents permit individuals to designate another person to make healthcare decisions for them if they lose decision-making capacity. The person who is appointed by the patient to make decisions is called a *healthcare proxy, healthcare agent, surrogate,* or (in some states) a *durable power of attorney.* Shapiro (2015) found that surrogate decision makers participated in the decision-making process for all but 18% of critically ill patients with a DPAHC directive. This stands in contrast to a finding from the same study that even when medical directives were readily available, they were not usually consulted and made very little difference in the care provided.

DPAHC directives allow greater flexibility and more relevance to the patient's specific situation than instructional directives, as a DPAHC does not require that an individual know in advance all the decisions that may be needed for every situation that might arise. In fact, a healthcare proxy can interpret the patient's wishes as medical circumstances change and can make treatment decisions as the need arises. Although competent, the person should be encouraged to provide his or her proxy with guidance concerning the type of treatment he or she would like to receive. The advocacy group Aging with Dignity (2011) has promoted the five wishes public information campaign so that individuals have a format to use to discuss their wishes related to EOL care. The organization maintains a Five Wishes online secure site to guide people through completing the form.

The five wishes are as follows:

1. The person I want to make care decisions for me when I can't
2. The kind of medical treatment I want or don't want
3. How comfortable I want to be
4. How I want people to treat me
5. What I want my loved ones to know

Interactive e-planning advance directive tools, such as those offered through the Five Wishes online campaign, are assisting people to think about and articulate their wishes. The electronic format helps some people to convey their thoughts in a more systematic way than they would have been able to achieve verbally or on paper. Green and Levi (2012) believe that the electronic forms may actually help people to explore their values and articulate their wishes in ways that are more logically consistent than they otherwise would have been.

However, some patients do not have the capacity to answer these questions, or envision EOL scenarios, no matter how much assistance they receive. An advantage of a DPAHC noted by Molloy et al. (1996) is that the capacity required to designate a proxy is considerably less than that needed to envision scenarios and complete

a medical directive. Thus, proxy designations may be more appropriate for people who, although competent, are having difficulty understanding options and making decisions about EOL care.

Moreover, there are disadvantages to a DPAHC. The proxy designate may not realize all the responsibility that being a healthcare proxy entails and may have difficulty making a decision. The proxy may also confound his or her interests with those of the patient and fail to act in the patient's best interests (Perrin, 1997).

How should a proxy make an EOL decision for a patient? First and most important, the proxy should leave the decision to the patient until the appropriate time. Advance directives become effective only when it is determined that the individual is incompetent, lacks decision-making capacity, or requests that the proxy make the decisions for him or her. As long as the patient retains decision-making capacity and wishes to make the decision, his or her decisions govern. When the patient is deemed to lack decision-making capacity, the healthcare proxy is authorized to make treatment decisions on behalf of the patient. There are two ethically and legally acceptable ways by which a proxy might make a healthcare decision for an incapacitated patient: substituted judgment and the best-interests standard.

When considering *In re Quinlan* (1976), the courts recognized the use of substituted judgment for a family member declining the further use of mechanical ventilation for an incompetent patient. In such circumstances, the proxy makes the decision that he or she believes the patient would have made for himself or herself if he or she had the ability to do so. Sometimes the decision is clear because the patient has discussed the matter with the proxy or commented about what she or he would want to do under those circumstances. Overall, studies show that even if flawed, patients' wishes and decisions expressed by healthcare proxies more closely approximate the patient's own treatment preferences than do decisions of physicians or others (Danis, Garrett, Harris, & Patrick, 1994; Emanuel, Emanuel, Stoeckle, Hummel, & Barry, 1994). However, the patient preferences as expressed by proxies are not always followed. When physicians are surveyed concerning how they make treatment decisions for their incompetent patients, 81% state that they consider patients' preferences as expressed by the proxy, but only 29% of them consider it to be the most important factor in the decision about what care to provide (Torke, Moloney, Siegler, Abalos, & Alexander, 2010).

In situations in which there is no clear and convincing evidence of what the person would have wanted or the patient has never been competent, the proxy will be called on to make decisions on the basis of what he or she believes to be in the best interests of the patient. Under this approach, it is impossible to analyze the proxy's decision based on the patient's right to self-determination. However, Pope (2012) has identified a number of factors that the responsible surrogate should take into account when deciding what is in the patient's best interest. These factors include the patient's (a) level of cognitive functioning, (b) QOL, (c) treatment options, (d) current level of pain and suffering, (e) likelihood of pain and suffering if treatment is continued versus withdrawn, and (f) benefits and burdens from treatment. Although these factors seem objective, surrogate decision makers often find the factors difficult to consider and the surrogates' intense emotions may make it difficult for them to deliberate carefully (White, 2011).

Shapiro (2015) notes that even the most diligent and responsible surrogates experienced a lack of clarity and were unsure about how to weigh the risks and benefits to the patients. It was difficult for the surrogates to extrapolate from incomplete information and to appreciate the uncertainty of a prognosis. Shapiro states that "many surrogates know the right outcome, it is the process that haunts and paralyzes them" (2015, p. 520).

Intractable Pain Legislation

Some states, such as Washington, contain a mandate in their natural death acts for patient comfort and alleviation of pain at the EOL. Others have separate legislation regarding the management of pain at the EOL. Yet, all patients who suffer from pain, not just those who are dying, should be treated. The debate about patient-requested euthanasia and assisted suicide has drawn national and international attention to the fact that appropriate interventions can eliminate or drastically reduce the pain and suffering that many people experience. The need for appropriate types and amounts of pain medications was made clear in the U.S. Supreme Court ruling in *Vacco v. Quill* (1997). There is a relationship between pain and symptom management and requests for assisted suicide (Foley, 1991).

Through federal regulation on intractable pain, the government in 1974 clarified the federal law that prohibits physicians from prescribing opioids to detoxify or maintain an opioid addiction. The regulation stated, in part, that the prohibitive regulations are "not intended to impose any limitation on a physician … to administer or dispense narcotic drugs to persons with intractable pain in which no relief or cure is possible or none has been found after reasonable effort" (Institute of Medicine [IOM], 1997, p. 235). Similarly, some courts explicitly recognize that a patient's "right to be free from pain … is inseparable from his or her right to refuse medical treatment" (Meisel & Cerminara, 2001), and have granted immunity to healthcare providers who treat pain with strong doses of analgesic medications that inadvertently end the patient's life (*McKay v. Bergstedt*, 1990). Moreover, several states have enacted intractable pain statutes to encourage those who treat patients who are terminally ill and have intractable pain to manage the pain without threat of legal liability if the treatment results in the patient's death.

The 1997 IOM report *Approaching Death: Improving Care at End of Life*, coupled with other PC literature,

asserts that change must occur at many levels if we are to improve care for the dying. The development of intractable pain statutes is a good first step to the undertreatment of pain. However, they are imperfect. Problems associated with intractable pain statutes include the following:

1. They do not, in all cases, mark a clear area of medical practice in which physicians feel free to manage their patients' pain. The more specific laws—for example, those that set out detailed prescription practices—may actually afford physicians *less* leeway in the practice of medicine. In addition, by carving out an area of pain treatment that is immune from discipline, there may be an implication that other forms of pain treatment should be subject to disciplinary review. However, physicians did obtain some measure of comfort that they would not be prosecuted for appropriate prescription of pain medications by the *Gonzales v. Oregon* (2006) decision that limited the Drug Enforcement Agency's (DEA) jurisdiction to actions involving drug trafficking (Kollas & Boyer-Kollas, 2007).
2. Even the strongest intractable pain law is still limited by the term "intractable." Many cases are ambiguous, and physicians may believe that they must delay opioid treatment until pain is far enough along to be called "intractable."
3. Finally, legal affirmations in these laws of the importance of pain control do not, in themselves, correct practice patterns or improve physician training. Laws could, however, encourage patients to expect diligence in pain relief, including use of generally effective medications. Medical boards could consider disciplining physicians who fail to apply proven methods of pain control (IOM, 1997). In addition, Kollas and Boyer-Kollas (2007) observed that case law may be strengthening the requirement to relieve a patient's pain by establishing a new tort, failure to adequately manage pain. Not only have judges and juries repeatedly viewed pain in the dying patient as a compensatable injury, but recently plaintiffs have been able to "argue the tort of failure to appropriately manage pain by applying reasoning from *James v. Philhaven*[1] and *Gaddis v. U.S.*"[2] (Kollas & Boyer-Kollas, 2007, p. 1399).

Thus, changes in the healthcare system are needed to improve access to care and to eliminate barriers to effective treatment. Nurses need to educate patients and families about their right to adequate PC. In states that have intractable pain statutes, the PSDA requires all covered facilities to inform patients of their legal right to adequate PC (Meisel & Cerminara, 2001). Healthcare providers need to "add the assessment of pain as the fifth vital sign"

---

[1] Martin (James) v. Smith (Edward C.), Walmer (John D.), Philhaven Hospital, Shank (Rowland), 968 F.2d 13 (3d Cir. 1992)
[2] Gaddis v. US 549 US, 1266, 127 S. Ct. 1497—Supreme Court, 2007

(Meisel & Cerminara, 2001), and national pain management standards ought to be followed (Phillips, 2000).

Combination Directives

A number of states have a single advance directive statute that combines elements of an instructional directive, a DPAHC, and possibly a pain management directive or a values history into a single document. A combination of different advance directive documents may help to avoid ambiguity inherent in one document alone. If the instructions are too general, the healthcare proxy has the authority to determine whether instructions should be applied under the specific circumstances. If the instructions are too specific and do not address the particular situation at hand, the healthcare proxy has the discretion to apply them or not. One element that is often included in a combination advance directive is instruction about what the patient desires if she or he is unable to take food or fluids by mouth near the EOL or is in a persistent vegetative state. In some states (even if a designated surrogate is making the decision), artificial hydration and nutrition may be withheld only if the patient has previously completed a medical directive statement authorizing foregoing artificial feeding (Olick, 2012). In any case, a discussion between the patient and the healthcare proxy should occur regardless of whether there is a DPAHC or a combination directive. Communication is the most effective way to ensure that the patient's wishes are known and that the healthcare proxy is prepared to follow the patient's directives.

Oral Advance Directives

Although a written advance directive is preferable, especially in the case of an emergency, courts view oral advance directives favorably, especially living wills. The courts either have enforced them per se or have heavily relied upon them in deciding whether to forego life-sustaining treatment. Although state statutes recognize written advance directives, oral directives have been found to be legally operative in a number of jurisdictions. The more specific the oral advance directive, the more likely it is to be enforced and have clinical and legal significance.

When made by individuals with full decision-making capacity, courts have considered patients' statements when making a decision to terminate life-prolonging treatments. Criteria for weighing these statements include the following (Furrow, Greaney, Johnson, Jost, & Schwartz, 2001):

■ Whether the statements were made on serious occasions or were solemn pronouncements (were brought up when the parties were together)
■ Whether they were consistently repeated
■ Whether they were made by a mature person who understood the underlying issues

■ Whether they were consistent with values demonstrated in other aspects of the patient's life (including the patient's religion)
■ Whether they were made shortly before the need for the treatment decision
■ Whether they addressed, with some specificity, the actual condition of the patient

In accordance, such statements should be considered and documented by the healthcare providers when discussing advance directives with patients.

Family Consent Laws

Many people are under the impression that their family members will be allowed to make the proper decisions for them if the need arises and therefore see no need to execute a formal advance directive (Furrow et al., 2001). Healthcare professionals and the courts traditionally relied on families to make healthcare decisions for family members throughout the years, despite their lack of any legal authority to do so. In 1982, the President's Commission concluded that given this practice, family decision making had gained legitimacy and should be accorded legal acceptance. The commission pointed out five reasons why deference to family members is appropriate when done in consultation with the physician and other healthcare professionals:

1. The family is generally most concerned about the good of the patient.
2. The family usually is the most knowledgeable about the patient's goals, preferences, and values.
3. The family deserves recognition as an important social unit that, within limits, ought to be treated as a responsible decision maker in matters that intimately affect its members.
4. Especially in a society in which many other traditional forms of community have eroded, participation in a family often is an important dimension of personal fulfillment.
5. Because a protected sphere of privacy and autonomy is required for the flourishing of this interpersonal union, institutions and the state should be reluctant to intrude, particularly regarding matters that are personal and on which there is a wide range of opinion in society.

Motivated by concern over the formal legal status of family decision making in the 1980s, state legislatures recognized this and began to regulate family decision making by statute. In 1995, with the exception of New York and Missouri, the courts authorized family members and others close to the patient to make decisions (New York State Task Force on Life and the Law, 1995). In fact, the District of Columbia and 24 other states have statutes that explicitly grant family members and others close to the patient the right to make decisions for patients who lack capacity. Family consent statutes vary from state to state. Some have been added to state living-will statutes to provide an alternative mechanism for making life-sustaining treatment decisions for individuals who do not have an advance directive, whereas others are free-standing statutes that apply either to life-sustaining treatment or to healthcare decisions generally.

▪ Preference of Elders for Family Decision Makers.
Elders are more likely to speak with a family member about EOL care than with a healthcare provider. This does not mean that they have completed a healthcare proxy or DPAHC. Rather, most elders have simply discussed their preferences for EOL care with at least one family member (High, 1993). When asked whom they believe knows them well enough and whom they would trust to make a healthcare decision for them, elders overwhelmingly (94%) choose family members, primarily spouses or adult children. Confidence and trust in family members to make any necessary decision for them may be a major reason older adults do not complete advance directives (High, 1994).

High (1994) believes that elders prefer family decision makers for a variety of significant and appropriate reasons. The family member has an inherent knowledge of the culture, values, and expectations of the patient and is usually concerned with the patient's welfare. In most instances, High believes family members choose appropriately based on the patient's values and best interests. High suggests that too much emphasis has been placed on disagreement and abuse within families and not enough on family empowerment and good faith decision making. He suggests that elders' preferences for family decision makers ought to be recognized and advance directives should be encouraged only for those who "have very specific or unusual preferences, do not want family to serve as substitute decision makers, or have disagreements with family or have no family" (High, 1994, p. S17).

Elders say that they have thought at least a "moderate amount" about who they would want to make healthcare decisions for them if they became incapacitated. Overwhelmingly, they would choose to have their families make such decisions without the benefit of a written directive (High, 1994; Nolan & Bruder, 1997). Although the elders in one study realized that having a written advance directive would help their families to know their wishes and possibly prevent guilt among family members over the decision, most elders still did not complete advance directives (Nolan & Bruder, 1997). These elders wanted their families to decide about EOL care based on their families' best judgments in the specific situation. Perhaps this is because these elders put their trust in their families and not in a piece of paper (High, 1993). Or it might be because elders believe that the family is the center of their lives (Blustein, 1999) and no individual can be completely autonomous; any decision made for one individual affects the entire family. In High's (1993) study, none of the elders stated that he or she always expected to make his or her own decisions. Most elders realize that their families will be profoundly affected by providing or paying for their healthcare. Thus, elders may believe their families ought to have a significant role in determining what the most appropriate EOL care is.

Martin, Emanuel, and Singer (2000) emphasize that making a decision about EOL care ought to be done in a family context. They believe discussion with patients about EOL care "helps a patient prepare for death, is influenced by personal relationships, is a social process, and occurs within the context of family and loved ones" (p. 1672). They assert that the primary value of EOL care planning is to allow the patient and family to prepare for death and dying and to find ways to cope with the impending death. Thus, they believe one reason patients may communicate about EOL issues with families more often than with healthcare providers is that the discussion may help the family to resolve any outstanding issues and become ready for the patient's death.

▪ HEALTHCARE PROVIDER INVOLVEMENT IN END-OF-LIFE DECISION MAKING

Although most adults have had discussions about EOL care preferences with at least one family member, few patients have had such discussions with their physicians (Emanuel, Barry, Stoeckle, Ettelson, & Emanuel, 1991; Griffin et al., 2016; O'Brien et al., 1995). Although patients are willing and eager to engage in such a discussion, they believe that it is not their role to initiate the discussion (Emanuel et al., 1991). Thus, they wait for their physicians to start the conversation; unfortunately, the physician usually does not.

Reasons physicians may be reluctant to initiate such conversations include the following:

- Personal discomfort with discussing death and dying (Ventres, Nichter, Reed, & Frankel, 1992). If the physician believes that the patient is dying because the physician has failed and there is no more that she or he can do, the physician is less likely to discuss CPR preference with the patient.
- Lack of physician education and experience in conducting such a conversation (Tulsky, Chesney, & Lo, 1995). Resident physicians learn early in the course of their education that various attending and older residents have differing views on how and when EOL discussions should occur. Unfortunately, according to Tulsky et al., resident physicians receive very little education in how to conduct a discussion about EOL preferences, and consequently they "often did not provide essential information" (p. 436).
- Fear that the patient will believe the physician has "given up on and is abandoning the patient" (Cotton,

1993). Some doctors say that they have difficulty discussing EOL care without conveying a sense of hopelessness to the patient. Kohn and Menon (1988) state that physicians may be unwilling to bring up the issue until a crisis develops, because they are afraid of unnecessarily alarming the patient.

- The physician may feel legally or morally bound to treat until death is proximate (Hanson, Tulsky, & Danis, 1997). About 10% of physicians believe that they must treat all patients with maximal interventions and that to limit treatment is morally and ethically unacceptable. Another larger group of physicians believes that it is inappropriate to discuss treatment limitation until the patient is certainly going to die. Unfortunately, if discussion waits until the patient is definitely dying, the patient frequently no longer has the capacity to participate in decision making about her or his EOL care.

- Concern about the amount of time such a conversation will require (Emanuel et al., 1991). Some physicians fear that having discussions about EOL care planning may be very time-consuming. Studies indicate that it takes approximately 10 to 16 minutes of physician time to discuss care preferences with a patient and/or family for a DNR decision to be reached; this is often the first in a series of EOL decisions (Smith et al., 1997; Tulsky et al., 1995).

Although they do not tend to initiate EOL conversations with patients, most physicians (82%) believe that it is their responsibility to begin the discussion (Markson et al., 1997) and to write the appropriate orders. Some physicians (Reckling, 1997) report that they prefer nurses and other healthcare providers not to discuss these issues with patients. The result is that healthcare providers and patients and families talk among themselves about appropriate EOL care, but do not talk with each other (Kohn & Menon, 1988). Less than one tenth of patients have spoken with their physicians when planning an advance directive, and the majority of patients with advance directives have never been asked by or told their physicians that they have advance directives (Teno, Licks, et al., 1997). Thus, unfortunately, conversations about EOL care among physicians, patients, and families usually do not occur until a crisis develops.

Researchers have documented concerns with how physicians engage in EOL care discussions in crisis situations. In Tulsky and colleagues' 1995 study, conversations about resuscitation lasted about 10 minutes and the resident physicians dominated the speaking time. Researchers did not believe that the information the residents provided to patients/families was adequate for them to make decisions about CPR. For example, only 13% of physicians mentioned the futility of CPR and the chance of the patient surviving. In addition, residents did not allow patients or families many opportunities to ask questions and elicit information about the patient's values and goals in EOL care less than 10% of the time.

Hanson et al. (1997) reported similar findings. They noted that because physicians tended to focus on treatment descriptions rather than listening to patient concerns, their understandings of patient preferences remained poor even after face-to-face discussions. They stated that physicians tended to be coercive in forcing their opinions. Markson et al. (1997) surveyed physicians who admitted that they would attempt to persuade patients to change decisions that they believed were not well informed (91%), medically reasonable (88%), or in the patient's best interest (88%). Ventres et al. (1992) concluded: "Physicians' presentation of opinions to patients are not neutral. Options are often presented in such a way as to influence DNR decision making" (p. 163) and communication strategies "may work to distance physicians from their patients at times when it is imperative for them to explore the values and wishes of the patient" (p. 165).

According to Ventres et al. (1992), there are three common prototypes physicians use to approach the discussion of DNR with patients and families. The first might be described as legalistic or technical. In this situation, the physician might ask, once the patient has become incapacitated, whether the patient has an advance directive or has a healthcare proxy and whether someone can produce the appropriate papers. In the second approach, the physician might admit that there were no further medical treatments that might lead to a cure and ask the patient or family what the patient would want for EOL care. In the third approach, the physician might mention that there were legal requirements that CPR be attempted at the EOL unless a DNR order was written. The physician would next ask the patient's and/or family's opinion about the appropriateness of administering a painful and probably useless treatment.

Nurse practitioners also experience challenges when facilitating advance care planning. They indicate that it requires courage and sensitivity to begin the discussion. Like their physician counterparts, most nurse practitioners try to form a relationship with their patients and look for cues that the patient is ready before initiating a discussion about advance planning (Boot & Wilson, 2014). The two cues that they used most often were discussion of a DNR order and preparation for patient discharge.

Detering et al. (2017) advocate a practical approach to advance care planning for healthcare providers. They recommend that if possible the planning occur at a routine outpatient visit with a trusted healthcare provider. If that is not possible, they suggest other appropriate times are at hospital admission or when a patient is experiencing clinical deterioration and may require additional treatment. Detering states that before proceeding with the planning, an assessment of the patient's decision-making capacity should be performed by the provider and the provider should consider whether others (e.g., family members) should also be involved.

To begin the discussion, Detering et al. (2017) recommend that the provider ask for permission to discuss the patient's current condition and possible future medical care. Next, the provider should assess the patient's understanding of his or her medical condition and its management. If the patient is unclear or has a misunderstanding, Detering suggests providing unambiguous information about the current health and the likely future choices for care. Once the patient and family understand the health issues and possible choices for management accurately, then a discussion of risks and benefits, dilemmas in care, and values and beliefs can occur. Only then should the patient's specific preferences for care be elicited. A healthcare surrogate should also be identified at this time. Finally, the provider should document the patient's preferences in writing and the patient should prepare an advance directive.

■ CONTROVERSIES IN END-OF-LIFE DECISION MAKING

When decision making involves withholding or withdrawing interventions that are prolonging a patient's life, it is not surprising that difficulties may arise. Some of the issues include the following:

■ When is it certain that the patient is dying and further intervention is of limited benefit?
■ Is the patient able to clearly identify what she or he would like done, either by speaking herself or himself or by the presence of instructions in an advance directive?
■ If the patient has not spoken, is it possible to identify who the patient would want to speak for her or him?
■ Does the patient, or her or his proxy, desire interventions that members of the healthcare team believe are futile?

As noted earlier, the first issue is quite problematic for the members of the healthcare team, patient, and family. It is usually not absolutely apparent that a patient is dying, even to experienced hospice nurses, until 24 to 48 hours before the patient's death. When the daughter of an elderly woman asked her mother's physician how much longer her mother might live, she was told, "Your mother is a determined woman. Any other person might only live 2 hours but she could live 2 hours, 2 days, 2 weeks, or 2 months." Three months later, the woman was still alive. It can be difficult to decide what care is most appropriate when time frames are so unclear.

It is also sometimes difficult to determine for certain what the patient really wants. Patients who are awake and aware, like Harriet in the case study, can be depressed,

as she most likely was. The healthcare team was able to believe that she had the capacity to make an authentic decision by giving her a trial of an antidepressant. Sometimes there is no such easy resolution, and family, patient, and healthcare team members disagree about treatment.

Problems With Advance Directives

Advance directives were intended to clarify EOL decision making. However, there are a variety of problems with them. First, the public has not embraced the use of advance directives and most Americans do not have one even though surveys demonstrate strong support for them (Larson & Tobin, 2000). The low numbers of patients who complete advance directives are alarming and are one of the factors that prevent them from being used effectively to guide EOL decisions. The literature suggests that more patients would complete advance directives if they had more information and assistance in completing them (Emanuel et al., 1991; Mezey, Ramsey, Mitty, & Rappaport, 1997). To that end, a number of educational interventions have been implemented to address these issues. Notwithstanding, few interventions increased advance directive completion by more than 20% (Hare & Nelson, 1991; Rubin, Strull, Fialkow, Weiss, & Lo, 1994; Sachs, Stocking, & Miles, 1992) and many did not increase completion at all (Robinson, DeHaven, & Koch, 1993; Stiller et al., 2001). Sim, Zimmerman, and Krzyanowska (2016) concluded from a systematic review that although a multitude of interventions to enhance completion of advance directives have been studied, none were ready for wide-scale adoption.

Fears that an advance directive permits providers to withhold care or will lead to substandard care may be at the root of the rejection of advance directives by some patients. People may be concerned that once an advance directive is completed and it contains a statement to withhold treatment, providers will devote less attention to their care and may withhold more treatment than was desired (Caralis, Davis, Wright, & Marcial, 1993; Patel, Sinuff, & Cook, 2004). In a study by Elder, Schneider, Zweig, Peters, and Ely (1992), some individuals feared that an advance directive might allow care to be withheld too soon and could result in a shirking of societal duties. One person commented that he would not want to hear, "Sorry, we don't have the time or money to treat you." This fear is not present among patients alone; nurses and other healthcare providers hold similar beliefs (Davidson, Hackler, Caradine, & McCord, 1989; Louw, 2004).

Although there is no evidence that healthcare providers are purposefully withholding care, there is evidence that some providers do not understand the differences between types of advance directives and are not appropriately interpreting a directive resulting in care patients do not want. Mirarchi, Hite, Cooney, Kisiel, and Henry (2008) concluded, "A majority of caregivers at a level II trauma center construed a living will with a DNR order which in turn was associated with EOL care. Such understandings may unnecessarily put a patient at risk" (p. 1). Similarly, Pirinea et al. (2016) found healthcare providers, patients, and families may all have misunderstandings of what a DNR and living will entail, making EOL decision making in acute situations even more difficult.

Socioeconomic and cultural factors substantially influence decisions to complete an advance directive. Multiple studies confirm that people with less education and lower income or who are African American or Hispanic are less likely to formulate advance directives (High, 1993; Huang, Neuhaus, Choing, 2016; Mezey, Leitman, Mitty, Bottrell, & Ramsey, 2000; Phipps et al., 2003; Robinson et al., 1993). Several explanations are plausible. Individuals with these sociodemographic characteristics are less likely to have regular access to care. For them, limiting any medical care would seem unnecessary because they already have too little, not too much. They are also less likely to have exposure to the concept of advance directives (Mezey, Mitty, et al., 1997).

The location and timing of when a patient receives information about advance directives is also important. It is well recognized that an acute episode or emergency admission is an inappropriate time to receive this information, yet this is the point at which most hospitals fulfill their responsibilities under the PSDA. Information may be better utilized during the preadmission period when patients can discuss advance directives in the comfort of their own homes. Alternatively, information can be presented as part of the discharge process when the impact of hospitalization is still new, but without the distraction of acute symptoms.

Even when a patient has completed an advance directive, the directive may not be utilized because the healthcare team has not been made aware of its existence. A study of recently discharged hospital patients with advance directives documented that fewer than 15% were asked about an existing advance directive during their hospitalization, 60% of patients did not disclose to the hospital staff that they had a directive, and only 35% informed their physician about their advance directives (Mezey Ramsey, et al., 1997). Although failure to communicate this information might be attributed to the patient's presumption that the directive would not be relevant for the hospital stay, selective disclosure may reflect a patient's misunderstanding or fear about use of the advance directive.

There is increasing concern in the medical community that the problem with advance directives may not be the flawed implementation of a sound concept but rather that advance directives are a fundamentally flawed concept (Perkins, 2007). Although Perkins believes that there are some benefits of advance directives—primarily that people might consider what they would want at the EOL and that they remind physicians of the necessity of considering the patient's goals and desires at the EOL—he notes that there are a series of problems. First among them is how few people have completed them. In addition, he notes that healthcare providers, such as Jacobson et al. (1994), have expressed concerns about the patient's understanding of treatment options and thus the validity of the treatment choices the patient makes in the directive. A third problem Perkins identifies is physician nonadherence. He notes that physicians may disregard directives because they conflict with hospital policy or family preferences, or because they do not appear to pertain to the current situation.

Most important, though, Perkins (2007) believes that the use of advance directives is flawed because the "outcomes have consistently frustrated expectations" (p. 54). He believes that most people do not have the experience to envision a wide variety of scenarios at the EOL and merely know that they would want a death with dignity. He also believes that advance directives promise a degree of control that is not possible when a patient is critically ill and it is not certain if the patient is dying. Decisions in such situations must be made quickly. Finally, he believes that advance directives may engender rather than limit disagreements between family members or family members and healthcare providers, as the directives may be unclear and the proxy may be unprepared.

An Alternative to Advance Directives in End-of-Life Care: Physician Orders for Life-Sustaining Treatment

Because advocacy groups have spent considerable effort promoting advance directives without appreciable success, an alternative effort to ensure that EOL care is congruent with patient preferences has developed (Meier & Beresford, 2009). Physician Orders for Life-Sustaining Treatment (POLST) are *not* an advance directive; rather, they are a set of medical orders for a patient with a serious, life-threatening condition. The physician discusses predictable future events for a patient with a life-threatening condition (such as cardiac arrest in the patient with severe heart failure) and determines in conjunction with the patient or surrogate how the patient should be treated if/when the events arise. A document is created that specifies the treatment the physician has prescribed. The document is usually brightly colored so that it is easy to identify and it accompanies the patient across healthcare settings, ensuring continuity of care. It is designed to provide quick, clear guidance to healthcare providers about the care that the patient desires and the primary healthcare provider has prescribed.

The categories for choices on POLST forms vary from state to state. Physicians, after consultation with their patients or surrogates, prescribe either "attempt resuscitation" or DNAR at the start of the document. Other categories on the documents used in most states provide places for the physician to prescribe or to withhold a range of medical interventions from comfort measures only to full treatment, the use of antibiotics, and the administration of artificially administered nutrition.

Advocates for the use of POLST state that POLST allows greater individuation in the care of terminally ill patients and appears to be effective in preventing unwanted treatments (Hickman et al., 2009). In fact, Hickman et al. note that their study is remarkable for the extent to which the patients' preferences were respected. No patient in their study received unwanted CPR, ventilation, ICU admission, or feeding tubes, far exceeding anything recorded in studies of advance directives and suggesting a distinct advantage to the use of POLST. In a study directly comparing the effectiveness of POLST with durable powers of attorney for healthcare advance directives, Hammes, Rooney, Gundrum, Hickman, and Hager et al. (2012) found that POLST forms were consistent with treatment across a variety of settings 94% of the time. In contrast, Mirarchi, Doshi, Zerkle, and Cooney (2015) found that emergency department physicians could not consistently interpret POLST forms. They noted that in multiple scenarios, physician responses reflected confusion about how to interpret the patient's wishes from the form. The confusion about interpretation occurred even when physicians had received education about the POLST form. Mirarchi et al. concluded, "Additional training and/or safeguards are needed to allow patient choice as well as protect their safety" (p. 1).

POLST has been available since 1991, when it was developed in Oregon, and is currently available in 42 states in various forms. Hickman, Sabatino, Moss, and Nester (2008) believe that there may be legal barriers to its full implementation in some states. The most problematic barriers include the detailed out-of-hospital DNR forms required in some states, the witnessing requirements for healthcare decisions in some states, and limitations placed by some states on withholding some types of life-sustaining treatments. Despite these barriers, the POLST paradigm is gaining support and traction nationwide because it appears to offer severely ill people of any age a greater likelihood of having their desires for EOL care followed.

Conflict in End-of-Life Decision Making

Although it is infrequent, there are times when the healthcare team, patient, and family are not able to come to agreement about how to care for the dying patient and conflict develops (Luce, 2010). The patient, a member of the patient's family, or a member of the healthcare team may want to continue some or all of the life-saving treatments even though the others involved in treatment decision making believe that the patient is dying and treatments should be withheld or withdrawn (Perrin & Matzo,

2009). Sometimes the family believes that the treatment a physician is proposing is inappropriate (Luce, 2010) or that the patient is being lost in a healthcare system that favors system-wide cost effectiveness over providing the care an individual patient needs (Bailey, 2011).

When healthcare professionals ensure careful communication, instill trust, and listen to the voices of the people involved in the decision, most of the time, when death is imminent, consensus can be reached about which life-sustaining interventions should be provided and which withheld, so that the patient is able to die with dignity. However, sometimes consensus cannot be reached and conflict develops. One reason why conflict may develop is that trust was not established among the members of the multidisciplinary healthcare team, patient, and family early in the hospitalization. If lack of trust is the primary reason the patient and family want to continue life-sustaining care, the healthcare team should act to reestablish trust before proceeding with a decision about EOL care. Disagreement about treatment may also result when decision makers do not share a common understanding of the patient's prognosis. Sometimes the conflict may result from a family member or a healthcare provider experiencing guilt about the care of the patient; in other instances, there may be secondary gains for a family member from the patient remaining alive, or the patient may come from a religious tradition that does not permit the withdrawal of life-sustaining therapy. In such situations, it may not be possible to reach a consensus about limiting care (Perrin & Matzo, 2009).

Futile Care

The situation becomes especially complex when the patient or a family member demands an intervention that the healthcare team considers to be futile. Futility can be exceedingly difficult to define. In fact, one healthcare provider is said to have stated, "I can't define it but I know it when I see it." One possible definition is any treatment that is without any benefit to the patient. Because most treatments have the potential to provide at least minimal benefit, futility is not always apparent to all members of the healthcare team, the family, and the patient (Pfeifer & Kennedy, 2006). Bailey (2011) argues that some patients and surrogates demand more care because they feel so insecure about the quality of their healthcare. They fear that they are "stuck in a one-size-fits-all system" (p. 177) where their individual needs and preferences are not respected and they are not being treated fairly. Chwang (2009) argues that there is disagreement about what futile care is because we cannot agree or are not clear on what the goal of the treatment or the anticipated outcome is. This was the situation with Harriet Billings, the patient in the case study.

CASE STUDY *Continued*

Harriet had a tracheostomy tube inserted and continued on dialysis. She began to improve, was gradually weaned from the ventilator, and no longer required dialysis. After a 3½-month hospitalization, she was transferred to a rehabilitation center near her home. Three days after her transfer, when the aide went to awaken her in the morning, she was unresponsive. The rehabilitation facility had a copy of her durable power of attorney and immediately contacted a neurologist, the medical center from which she had been referred, and her brother. Because her advance directive clearly indicated that she wanted everything done, they anticipated her immediate transfer back to the medical center where she had been hospitalized.

Instead, Harriet was transferred to her local hospital, where she was examined by the neurologist. On examination, Harriet was unresponsive, decorticate on her right side, and flaccid on her left. Her blood pressure had increased to 200/120 mmHg and she was hyper-ventilating. A CT scan revealed a large cerebral bleed. When the neurologist consulted with the medical center, they decided that there was little that the center could do that would benefit Harriet and she would not be transferred. Harriet's brother arrived and wondered why she was not being transferred and whether she needed to be intubated since she was breathing erratically.

Ethics Consultation

When the healthcare team, patient, and family cannot reach a consensus about the continuation of life-sustaining treatment, the issue should be referred to the hospital's ethics committee. The Joint Commission requires hospitals to have an ethics committee for discussion and consultation to aid in the resolution of such difficult issues. The consultation may be with a member or member(s) of the ethics committee or the case may be presented before the entire committee. The goal of case consultations by ethics committees is to suggest ways to resolve disagreements in difficult situations.

Bernard Lo (1995) identifies five goals of ethics case consultations. First, the ethics committees can help the healthcare team identify and understand the specific ethical issues the case raises: for example, cases that involve questions about advance directives, surrogate decision making, or disputes over life-sustaining treatments. Healthcare providers need to think carefully and critically through the ethical issues themselves before they try to resolve disagreements with the patient or family. Second, the ethics committee can suggest how healthcare providers might improve communications with the patient and family. Poor communications and lack of communication among the healthcare providers and members of the team may be a problem that the ethics committee can identify and help resolve. Third, the committee may provide emotional support to the physician, nurses, and other healthcare team members in a case. Fourth, the committee may offer specific recommendations to help resolve the dilemma. Most committees or consultants help the healthcare team analyze the ethical issues and facilitate discussions with patients and families rather than offer specific recommendations for resolving the

dilemmas. Finally, the committees or consultants have a role in improving patient care. Patient care decisions do not necessarily have to change after consultations, nor is there a mandate that they must change. However, by participating in consultation, healthcare providers, patients, and families may feel that their concerns have been addressed and they may better understand the rationale for the treatment decision that is being proposed.

Unfortunately, not all cases can be resolved with an ethics consultation. In fact, a situation, such as Harriet's, when an individual is requesting futile treatment, is one common reason why the healthcare team, family, and patient might not be able to come to consensus about goals for EOL care. Some states, such as Texas, have laws that delineate procedures that must be followed prior to, during, and after ethics committee deliberations about futile treatment. After reviewing the case, the ethics committee might recommend either supporting the continuation of life-sustaining therapy or limiting treatment. In Texas, if the ethics committee recommends discontinuation of life-sustaining treatment, the patient and proxy must receive written notification of a 10-day treatment limit with an option to request transfer to another facility. If they cannot find another facility to accept the patient, then the life-sustaining treatment is discontinued after the 10th day (Pfeifer & Kennedy, 2006). Jacobs (2009) reviewed the Texas model on its 10-year anniversary. He concluded that despite requiring some modification to correct flaws, it was a model that reduced the morally unjustifiable treatment of dying patients.

■ **Role of the Courts.** There are times when disagreements concerning life-sustaining treatments give rise to litigation. Then, the institution's lawyer is well suited to advise and educate the healthcare team about litigation and should be available to answer questions about the legal process that the staff may encounter during litigation or to avoid litigation. Discussions with the lawyer may ease some of the fears and dispel some of the misconceptions that healthcare providers have about the law and litigation in this area. In addition, discussion with the lawyer may address the potential liability for members of the committee and available immunities.

In general, the courts are hesitant to become involved in litigation surrounding EOL care, in part because they are reluctant to become involved in disputes about dying (Schneider, 2004). Schneider offers several reasons for this. First, the judicial process is not tailored to address issues with the speed required, and by the time a decision to litigate is reached, the patient may have already died. In addition, such cases are usually very complex medically and the judicial process may not be able to untangle the complexity. Finally, "a suit to enforce a living will is usually a sign that horrible and irreconcilable differences polluted efforts to make decisions for a patient" (Schneider, 2004, p. 11). Or, as he summarizes, "in love and death alike, not all wrongs can be righted, and yet fewer can be righted by the law" (p. 11). Thus, for the most part, the courts have allowed and occasionally encouraged the process in which healthcare providers, patients, and families work together to come to a consensus about what type of EOL care should be provided.

■ THE ROLE OF THE NURSE IN END-OF-LIFE DECISION MAKING

What, then, should be nurses' involvement in EOL decision making? According to the ANA, in a position statement revised in 1995, nurses have a responsibility to facilitate informed decision making about EOL care, including but not limited to the discussion of advance directives. The ANA also recognizes that nurses have roles as educators about EOL care and as patient advocates to ensure that appropriate EOL care is provided. Thus, nursing responsibilities in EOL decision making may predominate at two times: when a plan for EOL care is being developed and when a plan for EOL care is being implemented.

The nurse may be involved in assisting a patient or resident to consider or plan for EOL care when the patient is admitted to a hospital or long-term care facility. Alternatively, nurses, in their roles as educators, may encounter people in the community who wish to discuss EOL care planning. For example, some critical care nurses are actively promoting EOL planning through television programming, group discussions, and community meetings. Most patients agree that it is when they are relatively well, which most believe they are even on

hospital admission, that they ought to be considering EOL care planning (Nolan & Bruder, 1997).

The ANA concurs that nurses need not focus on completion of an advance directive during such discussions but instead ought to provide education about possibilities at the EOL and explore patients' values, wishes, and preferences. Davison and Degner (1998) suggest that a logical place to begin the discussion is determining how much control the person wishes to exert over his or her EOL care. They utilize a card sort that establishes three categories of patient decision making. The three categories are as follows:

1. Active. The person might select "I prefer to make the final selection about which treatment I will receive." The patient might also choose to have the family make the final decision; a definitive choice for the family to decide is also seen as an active decision by the patient.
2. Collaborative. The person would choose from the card sort: "I prefer that my doctor and I (or my family and my physician) share the responsibility for deciding which treatment is best for me."
3. Passive. The person would select a choice such as "I prefer to leave all decisions concerning my treatment to my physicians." The person might suggest that the physician consult with the person or family for an opinion, but in this selection, the final decision is the physician's alone.

Davison and Degner (1998) suggest that once it has been determined what role the patient wishes to assume in decision making and whom the patient wishes to include in the decision making, it is the nurse's role to initiate appropriate discussion and education among decision makers.

Because most patients desire that they and their families have at least some input into EOL decisions, Davison and Degner (1998) recommend that the nurse next focus on identifying the patient's and family's goals and values, as well as their understanding of the possibilities and results of the use of life-sustaining technologies at the EOL. The nurse might begin such a discussion by saying:

I want you to imagine that you were diagnosed as having a terminal illness. By that I mean you are dying from the illness and will not be likely to get better no matter what treatment your doctor prescribes. What would matter to you? How would you like to be cared for at that time?

This is the step that many physicians avoid. Although difficult, it is imperative that the healthcare provider listen actively to the patient's and family's concerns, questioning and clarifying what they desire without the healthcare provider imposing his or her own values and goals. What the nurse is attempting to learn is what this person and his or her family believe they will value as the EOL approaches. Most elders have a strong tendency to favor limitation of treatment when they are unlikely to return to their baseline functioning or are probably dying (Gillick & Mendes, 1996), but this is not always true and some elders wish to continue to live until specific events occur or goals are reached. This is the nurse's opportunity to learn what the elder and family believe will probably be important as the EOL approaches.

After the patients' and families' goals and values have been explored, the nurse should assess what they understand about the use of life-sustaining treatment. According to Silveira, DiPiero, Gerrity, and Feudtner (2000), a significant proportion of outpatients misunderstand options at the EOL. This is not particularly surprising as many Americans obtain their information about life-sustaining technology and EOL care from television. Diem, Lantos, and Tulsky (1996) documented that in reality-based television medical shows, nearly all patients survive CPR. However, in fictional shows, such as *ER*, approximately 75% of patients survive CPR. This serious misinformation often has to be corrected and misperceptions dispelled before patients and families consider what types of life-sustaining interventions they would desire at the EOL.

According to the ANA, nurses have an important role in educating patients and their families about their options at the EOL. This includes a discussion of the experience and outcomes of such treatments as CPR and ventilation. The description of CPR should be accurate and include all of the elements of resuscitation (aeration with intubation, chest compressions, defibrillation, etc.). However, it is important the nurse allow the patient and family to develop their own opinions and come to their own conclusions. Just as physicians can color their discussions to patients and families with their perspectives on life-sustaining interventions, so can nurses. Many nurses have very negative remembrances of CPR (Page & Meerabeau, 1996), and it is quite possible for nurses to convey these impressions to their patients and the families. Nurses might begin discussion of specific preferences for life-sustaining treatments in a manner similar to the way in which they began discussion of the patient's values and goals for EOL care, such as:

> I want you to imagine that you are very close to dying and would not be likely to get better no matter what treatment your doctor prescribed. What type of medical interventions would you want us to try in an attempt to prolong your life and delay your death?

The final step in the development of an EOL plan should involve multidisciplinary development of a plan. The meeting (or preferably meetings) should involve at least the patient and physician, but also family and other healthcare providers as possible and appropriate. At the meetings, the patient and family can clarify any questions they might have about EOL care options and develop a plan, possibly a written directive. It is to be hoped that the final plan will include the extent to which the patient desires to be involved in the decision making, the role she or he wishes her or his family or physician to play, the patient's goals or values for EOL care, any specific desires the patient has for specific interventions to be utilized or withheld at EOL, and a choice of healthcare proxy, if appropriate. The more physicians and other healthcare providers are involved in developing a plan for EOL care for a patient, the more likely the plan is to be followed when the patient becomes ill and a decision needs to be made.

Once the person becomes ill and enters the healthcare system, the ANA recommends that the nurse assume the role of advocate for the patient's EOL care preferences. On admission to a healthcare institution, the patient and family must be asked whether the patient has an advance directive and, if a directive exists, whether they can produce a copy of the directive. Before assuming that the directive should come into effect, the nurse or another healthcare provider needs to inquire whether the patient still wants the directive to take effect. As previously noted, many patients change their minds about portions of their advance directive as they age and their health status changes. However, only one member of the healthcare team needs to inquire of the patient about the patient's current thoughts and feelings. The spouse of one patient who had declined all life-sustaining technologies recalled his wife being asked by 13 healthcare providers in 24 hours if she had changed her mind. Communication among healthcare providers about advance directives is essential.

Communication between healthcare institutions is also essential. One major problem with existing advance directives is that they are lost when the patient is transferred from one institution to another. If, as healthcare providers, we are asking people to complete advance directives prior to the development of an illness, we ought to be able to arrange for communication regarding the directive between facilities.

When a directive exists, the nurse may use it to help families to understand and follow the choices laid out in the directive for a family member who has become gravely ill and is incapacitated. When a patient has stated in a directive that she or he wishes to have life-sustaining interventions, such as CPR or intubation withheld, the family often feels relieved to know that they are not making the choice. Some families experience guilt over depriving a family member of even the smallest possibility of continued survival.

However, even when a directive exists, it is much more likely when a patient suddenly becomes gravely ill that the patient's choices will not be clearly related to the specific circumstances the patient is experiencing. Most likely of all is that no advance directive exists. When the patient is gravely ill, it is often the nurse who first notices that death is approaching. Clear communication to the family and physician is essential at this time because the family frequently has not considered death as an alternative (Caswell & Omery, 1990). Families need adequate, consistent information in terms that they can understand. Norton and Talerico (2000) caution that families need healthcare providers to use words such as "death" and "dying"; vague language confuses families. It is especially important, Norton and Talerico state, that healthcare providers not use terms like "better" when a patient's condition has temporarily stabilized but the overall prognosis is unchanged, because this leads to conflicting impressions among family members and family disagreement about treatment. Another term that confuses family members is "hope." Healthcare providers often use the term when there is hope for a good death or pain control; however, for family members, hope primarily means survival. Norton and Talerico (2000) recommend that nurses be specific in identifying that they are hoping for a good death or pain control for the patient, not continued life.

If death appears imminent and there has been no decision about EOL expectations, nurses may introduce the discussion of withholding or withdrawing of life-sustaining interventions, such as CPR, intubation, and ventilation. There are two common ways that nurses begin a discussion of these interventions (Norton & Talerico, 2000). One of them is to inform the family that the state requires that all people receive CPR (even when it is unlikely to be of any benefit to the person) unless a DNR order is written. This is often an easier way to begin the discussion if the family has not completely acknowledged that the patient is probably dying. However, it may prevent the family from acknowledging and discussing the nearness of the patient's death. Another common approach is to acknowledge that the patient is gravely ill, probably dying, and ask the family which vision of the patient's death would be in the patient's best interests: one in which they were surrounded by family with the lights lowered and were receiving medication for pain and symptom relief, or one in which they were surrounded by healthcare personnel who were providing CPR. A discussion of the likelihood of survival following CPR should also be included.

Most patients and families want to discuss EOL care with their nurse, but they need to hear the same message from the patient's physician. Thus, the nurse must be in communication with the physician about the patient's prognosis and the patient and family's preferences about EOL care. Hanson et al. (1997) note that one reason for delays in the withdrawal of patient treatments is that although patient preferences are documented, they are not communicated to physicians so that the physicians actually appreciate the patient's wishes. When there are differences in expectations of patient outcome or confusion over the appropriateness of various therapies, multidisciplinary patient care conferences are very important.

The nurse can assist a surrogate or family member to understand her or his role in the multidisciplinary team and to help make the decision about the patient's EOL care. To begin with, White (2011) believes that the nurse must educate the person about what the role of the surrogate entails as well as how important it is. Next, the nurse should ensure that there is not just one meeting, but regular meetings between the surrogate or family member and the multidisciplinary team. The nurse should prepare the surrogate before each meeting so that she or he is ready with questions, support the surrogate during the meeting, and debrief the surrogate following the meeting to ensure that the surrogate has an accurate understanding of the discussion (White, 2011).

Discussion about EOL care with families or patients in crisis cannot come as a barrage of questions all at once from multiple healthcare providers. It is best if the patient or family has some time to consider EOL care. Thus, withholding CPR is often discussed first and gradually questions concerning withholding or withdrawal of other life-sustaining interventions are introduced.

As the ANA has stated in its position statement, it is the responsibility of nurses to facilitate informed decision making for patients at the EOL. This responsibility begins when the nurse has a patient consider what would be important to him or her at the EOL, continues with the nurse educating the person about EOL care options, and is completed when the nurse advocates for and delivers the type of care the patient desires at the end of her or his life. However, this process of communication about EOL care is not solely the responsibility of the patient and the nurse; it is an interprofessional process that includes at least the physician and family in addition to the patient and nurse.

■ CONCLUSIONS

Numerous factors make it likely that EOL decision making will continue to raise difficult issues for healthcare professionals, patients, and patients' families. The reasons that people do not complete advance directives and discuss EOL care, even after educational interventions, seem much more compelling than the reasons for completing them. Healthcare providers often do not have enough regular ongoing contact with patients, so patients do not feel comfortable discussing EOL issues or completing advance directives.

Instead of focusing on the actual number of advance directives completed, we should look at whether our activities are encouraging discussions of EOL care with patients and families. The evidence to date indicates that simply providing information encourages patients to talk about their preferences with family members and friends, that is, the people who will be making decisions in the event the patient loses decision-making capacity. Anything that encourages such conversations enhances patient autonomy and self-determination.

Advance directives, DNR orders, court actions, and legislative actions are all important mechanisms for nurses to consider when seeking ways to resolve the dilemmas that exist when caring for patients at the EOL. Nurses must have opportunities to think critically and articulate their views and positions on the dilemmas they face as individuals and as professionals. Ethics rounds, grand rounds, ethics colloquia, courses in basic nursing education, continuing-education offerings, and conferences all provide forums for nurses, students, faculty, and clinicians to enhance their ethical and legal awareness. The American Nurses Association Center for Ethics and Human Rights is one rich resource for nurses who seek consultation and ethics information.

CASE STUDY *Conclusion*

Harriet was admitted to the ICU of the local hospital. Her nurse remembered Harriet and her brother from Harriet's previous admissions. She recognized that the brother was unsure about what ought to be done for Harriet. She said to him, "Despite all that we have done for her, Harriet is dying now. There is nothing we can do to stop the dying process. However, we can keep her comfortable, and I think that she would realize we have tried very hard to follow her directions. She asked you to be her health care proxy because she trusted you to know when the time had come to say, 'It is time to stop doing things that will not help her and time to keep her comfortable instead.'"

Harriet's brother agreed, and she died peacefully an hour later.

CASE STUDY *Commentary*

James McGhee, PhD
Professor Emeritus, Saint Anselm College
Member of ethics committees of several New Hampshire hospitals and hospices

This case depicts quite comprehensively the final chapter in the life of Harriet Billings. Over a lengthy period of months, she becomes very ill and close to death on several occasions. In accord with her own directive, every medical effort was made to keep her alive. Finally, when she had lapsed into a comatose state, her brother, who was her chosen attorney for healthcare, in consultation with others, decided that a limit had been reached in what could be done for her and agreed to take her off life support. With palliative treatment, she died peacefully soon after.

Clearly, the ethical issue here centers on the decisions made by Harriet and her brother. Her instructions to prolong her life by all available means, be they heroic, costly, or extraordinary, were carried out by medical personnel. When she was unconscious, her brother's decision to terminate treatment and allow her to die was also implemented. From an ethical standpoint, it could be argued that both acted well.

Two further relevant issues can be raised. First, the principle of totality urges us to treat patients comprehensively, not just physically, but also to care for their spiritual well-being. There is no mention of this concern in the presentation of this case. Second, the term "indirect euthanasia" might be used to describe Harriet's death. Indirect or passive euthanasia refers to the withdrawal of life support when there is no hope left from the treatment. Direct euthanasia, now legal in some western states like Oregon and California, is a direct intervention to bring about the death of a terminally ill person.

Evidence-Based Practice

Mirarchi, F., Doshi, A., Zerkle, S., & Cooney, T. (2015). How well do emergency physicians understand Physicians Orders for Life-Sustaining Treatment (POLST) forms? *Journal of Patient Safety, 11*(1), 1–8.

Q: How accurately can emergency department (ED) physicians interpret POLST forms so they provide the care that the patient wished to receive?

Methods

Data Sources: This study was an Internet survey composed of six scenarios in which critically ill patients with POLST documents were admitted to the ED. In each scenario, participants were required to review the POLST documents, which portrayed several levels of intervention; select a code status; and determine how to intervene.

Study Selection and Assessment: Participants were members of the Pennsylvania chapter of the American College of Emergency Physicians who were contacted via the Internet and asked to participate anonymously in the survey. Eight hundred fifty-five physicians were invited to participate and 223 provided responses (a 26% response rate).

OUTCOMES

Main Results

Six patient scenarios with POLST documents were provided for the physicians to review. There was consensus on the code status of the patient in only 13% of the scenarios, whereas only 17% of the questions about intervention led to consensus.

Conclusions

"Significant confusion exists among members of the Pennsylvania chapter of the American College of Emergency Physicians regarding the use of POLST in critically ill patients. This confusion poses risk to patient safety. Additional teaching and training are needed to allow patient choice as well as to protect their safety" (Mirarchi et al., 2015, p. 1).

Commentary

POLST forms were developed in response to concerns about misinterpretation of advance directives especially during acute illnesses or emergency situations. POLST forms have been documented in many settings to be less prone to misinterpretation about the healthcare a patient desires, thus facilitating the delivery of appropriate care. However, this study demonstrates that in emergent situations, POLST forms may be prone to the same sort of misinterpretation as advance directives. The authors of the study recommend further education for healthcare providers about how to interpret POLST forms and suggest the use of a resuscitation pause patient safety checklist before emergency measures are instituted even when a POLST document or an advance directive is available. The resuscitation pause proposed by the authors includes the following steps:

1. Ask the patient or surrogate to be clear about the intentions of the document (advance directive or POLST).
2. Be clear about whether this will be a terminal condition despite sound medical treatment.

3. Communicate clearly if you believe the condition is irreversible.
4. Design a plan and discuss next steps.
5. Explain that it's okay to withhold or withdraw life-sustaining treatment as long as it is in conjunction with the perceived patient's wishes.

■ REFERENCES

Aging with Dignity. (2011). *Five wishes online*. Tallahassee, FL: Author. Retrieved from https://fivewishesonline .agingwithdignity.org

American Medical Association Council on Ethical and Judicial Affairs. (1991). Guidelines for the appropriate use of DNR orders. *Journal of the American Medical Association, 265*, 1868–1871. doi:10.1001/ jama.1991.03460140096034

Appelbaum, P. S. (2007). Clinical practice: Assessment of patients' competence to consent to treatment. *New England Journal of Medicine, 357*(18), 1834–1840. doi:10.1056/NEJMcp074045

Bailey, M. (2011). Futility, autonomy, and cost in end-of-life care. *Journal of Law, Medicine and Ethics, 39*(2), 172–182. doi:10.1111/j.1748-720X.2011.00586.x

Banja, J. D., & Bilsky, G. S. (1993). Discussing cardiopulmonary resuscitation with elderly rehabilitation patients: Ethical and clinical considerations toward the formation of policy. *American Journal of Physical Medicine and Rehabilitation, 72*(3), 168–171. doi:10.1097/00002060-199306000-00013

Bishop, J. P., Brothers, K. B., Perry, J. E., & Ahmad, A. (2010). Reviving the conversation around CPR/DNR. *American Journal of Bioethics, 10*(1), 61–67. doi:10.1080/15265160903469328

Blustein, J. (1999). Choosing for others as continuing a life story: The problem of personal identity revisited. *Journal of Law, Medicine and Ethics, 27*(1), 20–31. doi:10.1111/j.1748-720X.1999.tb01432.x

Boot, M., & Wilson, C. (2014). Clinical nurse specialists' perspectives on advance care planning conversations: A qualitativie study. *International Journal of Palliative Nursing, 20*(1), 9–14. doi:10.12968/ijpn.2014.20.1.9

Brinkman-Stoppelenburg, A., Rietjens, J., & van der Helde, A.,(2014). The effects of advance care planning on end-of-life care: A systematic review. *Palliative Medicine, 28*(8), 1000–1025. doi:10.1177/0269216314526272

Buchanan, S. F. (1998). Guardians of care: Geriatrics and the law. *Clinical Geriatrics, 6*(12), 79–81.

Caralis, P. V., Davis, B., Wright, K., & Marcial, E. (1993). The influence of ethnicity and race on attitudes toward advance directives, life-prolonging treatments, and euthanasia. *Journal of Clinical Ethics, 4*(2), 155–165.

Caswell, D., & Omery, A. (1990). The dying patient in the critical care setting: Making the critical difference. *AACN Clinical Issues in Critical Care Nursing, 1*(1), 179–186. doi:10.4037/15597768-1990-1018

Chwang, E. (2009). Futility clarified. *Journal of Law, Medicine and Ethics, 37*(3), 487–95. doi:10.1111/j.1748-720X.2009.00409.x

Cooney, L. M., Kennedy, G. J., Hawkins, K. A., Hurme, S. B., & Balch, J. D. (2004). Who can stay at home? Assessing the capacity to choose to live in the community. *Archives of Internal Medicine, 164*(4), 357–360. doi:10.1001/archinte.164.4.357

Cotton, P. (1993). Talk to people about dying—they can handle it, say geriatricians and patients. *Journal of the American Medical Association, 269*(3), 321–322. doi:10.1001/jama.269.3.321

Covinsky, K. E., Goldman, L., Cook, E. F., Oye, R., Desbiens, N., Reding, D., ... Phillips, R. S. (1994). The impact of serious illness on patients' families: SUPPORT Investigators [Study to Understand Prognoses and Preferences for Outcomes and Risks of Treatment]. *Journal of the American Medical Association, 272*(23), 1839–1844. doi:10.1001/jama.272.23.1839

Covinsky, K. E., Landefeld, C. S., Teno, J., Connors, A. F., Dawson, N., Youngner, S., ... Phillips, R. S. (1996). Is economic hardship on the families of the seriously ill associated with patient and surrogate care preferences? SUPPORT Investigators *Archives of Internal Medicine, 156*(15), 1737–1741. doi:10.1001/archinte.1996.00440140177019

Cruzan v. Director, Missouri Dep't. of Health, 497 U.S. 261, 110 S. Ct. 2841 (1990).

Daly, B. J. (2008). An indecent proposal: Withholding cardiopulmonary resuscitation. *American Journal of Critical Care, 17*(4), 377–380.

Danis, M., Garrett, J., Harris, R., & Patrick, D. L. (1994). Stability of choices about life-sustaining treatments. *Annals of Internal Medicine, 120*(7), 567–573. doi:10.7326/0003-4819-120-7-199404010-00006

Davidson, K. W., Hackler, C., Caradine, D. R., & McCord, R. S. (1989). Physicians' attitudes on advance directives. *Journal of the American Medical Association, 262*(17), 2415–2419. doi:10.1001/jama.262.17.2415

Davis, A., Aroskar, M., Liaschenko, J., & Drought, T. (1997). *Ethical dilemmas and nursing practice* (4th ed.). Stanford, CT: Appleton & Lange.

Davison, B. J., & Degner, L. F. (1998). Promoting patient decision making in life-and-death situations. *Seminars in Oncology Nursing, 14*(2), 129–136. doi:10.1016/S0749-2081(98)80018-1

Degenholtz, H. B., Rhee, Y., & Arnold, R. M. (2004). Brief communication: The relationship between having a living will and dying in place. *Annals of Internal Medicine, 141*(2), 113–117. doi:10.7326/0003-4819-141-2-200407200-00009

Detering, K., Silveira, M., Arnold, R., & Savarese, D., (2017). Advance care planning and advance directives. *UpToDate*. Retrieved from http://www.uptodate.com/contents/advance-care-planning-and-advance-directives

Diamond, E. L., Jernigan, J. A., Moseley, R. A., Messina, V., & McKeown, R. A. (1989). Decision-making ability and advance directive preferences in nursing home patients and proxies. *The Gerontologist, 29*(5), 622–626. doi:10.1093/geront/29.5.622

Diem, S. J., Lantos, J. D., & Tulsky, J. A. (1996). Cardiopulmonary resuscitation on television: Miracles and misinformation. *New England Journal of Medicine, 334*(24), 1578–1582. doi:10.1056/NEJM199606133342406

Duke, G., Yarbough, S., & Pang, K. (2009). The Patient Self-Determination Act: 20 years revisited. *Journal of Nursing Law, 13*(4), 114–123. doi:10.1891/1073-7472.13.4.114

Elder, N. C., Schneider, F. D., Zweig, S. C., Peters, P. G., & Ely, J. W. (1992). Community attitudes and knowledge about advance care directives. *Journal of the American Board of Family Practice, 5*(6), 565–572. doi:10.3122/jabfm.5.6.565

Emanuel, L. L., Barry, M. J., Stoeckle, J. D., Ettelson, L. M., & Emanuel, E. J. (1991). Advance directives for medical care: A case for greater use. *New England Journal of Medicine, 324*(13), 889–895. doi:10.1056/NEJM199103283241305

Emanuel, L. L., Emanuel, E. J., Stoeckle, J. D., Hummel, L. R., & Barry, M. J. (1994). Advance directives: Stability of patients' treatment choices. *Archives of Internal Medicine, 154*(2), 209–217. doi:10.1001/archinte.154.2.209

Eun-Shim, N., & Resnick, B. (2001). End-of-life treatment preferences among older adults. *Nursing Ethics, 8*(6), 533–543. doi:10.1177/096973300100800607

Foley, K. M. (1991). The relationship of pain and symptom management to patient requests for physician-assisted suicide. *Journal of Pain and Symptom Management, 6*(5), 289–297. doi:10.1016/0885-3924(91)90052-6

Forbes, S. (2001). This is Heaven's waiting room: End of life in one nursing home. *Journal of Gerontological Nursing, 27*(11), 37–45. doi:10.3928/0098-9134-20011101-10

Furrow, B., Greaney, T., Johnson, S., Jost, J. T., & Schwartz, R. (2001). *Hornbook on health law* (2nd ed.). Eagan, MN: West Group.

Garner, B. A. (2009). *Blacks Law Dictionary* (9th ed.).New York, NY: Thomson West.

Gillick, M. R., & Mendes, M. L. (1996). Medical care in old age: What do nurses in long-term care consider appropriate? *Journal of the American Geriatrics Society, 44*(11), 1322–1325. doi:10.1111/j.1532-5415.1996.tb01402.x

Green, M. J., & Levi, B. H. (2012). The era of "e": The use of new technologies in advance care planning. *Nursing Outlook, 60*(6), 376–383.e2. doi:10.1016/j.outlook.2012.08.005

Griffin, S., Cubanski, J., Neumann, T., Jankiewicz, A., & Rousseau, D. (2016). Medicare and end of life care: Visualizing health policy. *Journal of the American Medical Association, 316*(17), 1754. doi:10.1001/jama.2016.15577

Gonzales v. Oregon, 546 U.S. 243 (2006).

Guido, G. (2006). *Legal and ethical issues in nursing* (3rd ed.). Upper Saddle River, NJ: Pearson/Prentice Hall.

Hall, J. (1996). *Nursing ethics and law.* Philadelphia, PA: Saunders.

Hamel, M. B., Phillips, R. S., Davis, R. B., Desbiens, N., Connors, A. F., Teno, J. M., … Tsevat, J. (1997). Outcomes and cost-effectiveness of initiating dialysis and continuing aggressive care in seriously ill hospitalized adults. SUPPORT Investigators. *Annals of Internal Medicine, 127*(3), 195–202. doi:10.7326/0003-4819-127-3-199708010-00003

Hamel, M. B., Phillips, R. S., Teno, J. M., Lynn, J., Galanos, A. N., Davis, R. B., … Goldman, L. (1996). Seriously ill hospitalized adults: Do we spend less on older patients? SUPPORT Investigators. *Journal of the American Geriatrics Society, 44*(9), 1043–1048. doi:10.1111/j.1532-5415.1996.tb02935.x

Hamel, M. B., Teno, J. M., Goldman, L., Lynn, J., Davis, R. B., Galanos, A. N., … Phillips, R. S. (1999). Patient age and decisions to withhold life-sustaining treatments from seriously ill, hospitalized adults. SUPPORT Investigators. *Annals of Internal Medicine, 130*(2), 116–125. doi:10.7326/0003-4819-130-2-199901190-00005

Hammes, B. J., Rooney, B. L., Gundrum, J. D., Hickman, S. E., & Hager, N. (2012). The POLST program: A retrospective review of the demographics of use and outcomes in one community where advance directives are prevalent. *Journal of Palliative Medicine, 15*(1), 77–85. doi:10.1089/jpm.2011.0178

Hanson, L. C., Tulsky, J. A., & Danis, M. (1997). Can clinical interventions change care at the end of life? *Annals of Internal Medicine, 126*(5), 381–388. doi:10.7326/0003-4819-126-5-199703010-00007

Hare, J., & Nelson, C. (1991). Will outpatients complete living wills? A comparison of two interventions. *Journal of General Internal Medicine, 6*(1), 41–46. doi:10.1007/BF02599390

Harrison, C., Kenny, N. P., Sidarous, M., & Rowell, M. (1997). Bioethics for clinicians: 9. Involving children in medical decisions. *Canadian Medical Association Journal, 156*(6), 825–828.

Hickman, S. E., Nelson, C. A., Moss, A. H., Hammes, B. J., Terwilliger, A., Jackson, A., & Tolle, S. W. (2009). Use of the Physician Orders for Life-Sustaining Treatment (POLST) paradigm program in the hospice setting. *Journal of Palliative Medicine, 12*(2), 133–141. doi:10.1089/jpm.2008.0196

Hickman, S. E., Sabatino, C., Moss, A., & Nester, J. (2008, Spring). The POLST (Physician Orders for Life-Sustaining Treatment) paradigm to improve end-of-life care: Potential state legal barriers to implementation. *Journal of Law, Medicine, and Ethics, 36*(1), 120–140. doi:10.1111/j.1748-720X.2008.00242.x

High, D. M. (1993). Advance directives and the elderly: A study of intervention strategies to increase use. *The Gerontologist, 33*(3), 342–349. doi:10.1093/geront/33.3.342

High, D. M. (1994). Families' roles in advance directives. *Hastings Center Report, 24*(6), S16–S18. doi:10.2307/3563476

Hinds, P. S., Drew, D., Oakes, L. L., Fouladi, M., Spunt, S. L., Church, C., & Furman, W. L. (2005). End-of-life care preferences of pediatric patients with cancer. *Journal of Clinical Oncology, 23*(36), 9146–9154. doi:10.1200/JCO.2005.10.538

Huang, I., Neuhaus, J., & Chiong, W. (2016). Racial and ethnic differences in advance directive possession; Role of demographic factors, religious affiliation, and personal health values in a national survey of older adults. *Journal of Palliative Medicine,19*(2), 149–156. doi:10.1089/jpm.2015.0326

Institute of Medicine, Committee on End of Life Care. (1997). Directions for research to improve care at the end of life. In M. Field & C. Cassel (Eds.), *Approaching death: Improving care at the end of life* (pp. 235–256). Washington, DC: National Academies Press.

In re Farrell, 108 N.J. 335, 529 A.2d 404 (1987).

In re Quinlan, 70 N.J. 10, 355 A.2d 647 (1976).

Jacobs, H. C. (2009). The Texas Advance Directives Act: Is it a good model? *Seminars in Perinatology, 33*(6), 384–390. doi:10.1053/j.semperi.2009.07.006

Jacobson, J. A., White, B. E., Battin, M. P., Francis, L. P., Green, D. J., & Kasworm, E. S. (1994). Patients' understanding and use of advance directives. *West Journal of Medicine, 160*(3), 232–236.

Jones, A., Moss, A., & Harris-Kojetin, L. (2011). *Use of advance directives in long-term care populations* (NCHS Data Brief No. 54). Hyattsville, MD: National Center for Health Statistics.

Knaus, W. A., Harrell, F. E., Lynn, J., Goldman, L., Phillips, R. S., Connors, A. F., ... Wagner, D. P. (1995). The SUPPORT prognostic model: Objective estimates of survival for seriously ill hospitalized adults [Study to Understand Prognoses and Preferences for Outcomes and Risks of Treatments]. *Annals of Internal Medicine, 122*(3), 191–203. doi:10.7326/0003-4819-122-3-199502010-00007

Kohn, M., & Menon, G. (1988). Life prolongation: Views of elderly outpatients and health care professionals. *Journal of the American Geriatrics Society, 36*(9), 840–844. doi:10.1111/j.1532-5415.1988.tb04270.x

Kollas, C. D., & Boyer-Kollas, B. (2007). Evolving medicolegal issues in palliative medicine. *Journal of Palliative Medicine, 10*(6), 1395–1401. doi:10.1089/jpm.2007.0092

Larson, D. G., & Tobin, D. R. (2000). End-of-life conversations: Evolving practice and theory. *Journal of the American Medical Association, 284*(12), 1573–1578. doi:10.1001/jama.284.12.1573

Leder, N., Schwarzkopf, D., Reinhart, K., Witte, E., Pfeifer, R., & Hartog, C. (2015). The validity of advance directives in acute situations-a survey of doctors' and relatives' perceptions from the intensive care unit. *Deutshes Arzteblatt International, 112,* 723–729. doi:10.3238/arztebl.2015.0723

Lo, B. (1995). *Resolving ethical dilemmas: A guide for clinicians.* Baltimore, MD: Lippincott Williams, & Wilkins.

Louw, S. (2004). Cultural issues in end-of-life decision making. *Age and Ageing, 33,* 212–213. doi:10.1093/ageing/afh033

Luce, J. M. (2010). A history of resolving conflicts over end-of-life care in intensive care units in the United States. *Critical Care Medicine, 38*(8), 1623–1629. doi:10.1097/CCM.0b013e3181e71530

Marik, P. E., & Craft, M. (1997). An outcomes analysis of in-hospital cardiopulmonary resuscitation: The futility rationale for do not resuscitate orders. *Journal of Critical Care, 12*(3), 142–146. doi:10.1016/S0883-9441(97)90044-7

Markson, L., Clark, J., Glantz, L., Lamberton, V., Kern, D., & Stollerman, G. (1997). The doctor's role in discussing advance preferences for end-of-life care: Perceptions of physicians practicing in the VA. *Journal of the American Geriatrics Society, 45*(4), 399–406. doi:10.1111/j.1532-5415.1997.tb05162.x

Martin, D. K., Emanuel, L. L., & Singer, P. A. (2000). Planning for the end of life. *Lancet, 356*(9242), 1672–1676. doi:10.1016/S0140-6736(00)03168-8

McKay v. Bergstedt, 106 Nev. 808, 801 P.2d 617 (1990).

Meier, D. E., & Beresford, L. (2009). POLST offers next stage in honoring patient preferences. *Journal of Palliative Medicine, 12*(4), 291–295. doi:10.1089/jpm.2009.9648.

Meisel, A., & Cerminara, K. L. (2001). *The right to die: Vols. 1 and 2: 2001 cumulative supplement.* New York, NY: Aspen Law & Business.

Mezey, M. D., Leitman, R., Mitty, E. L., Bottrell, M. M., & Ramsey, G. C. (2000). Why hospital patients do and do not execute an advance directive. *Nursing Outlook, 48*(4), 165–171. doi:10.1067/mno.2000.101772

Mezey, M. D., Mitty, E. L., & Ramsey, G. C. (1997). Assessment of decision-making capacity: Nursing's role. *Journal of Gerontological Nursing, 23*(3), 28–35. doi:10.3928/0098-9134-19970301-13

Mezey, M. D., Ramsey, G. C., Mitty, E. L., & Rappaport, M. (1997). Implementation of the Patient Self-Determination Act (PSDA) in nursing homes in New York City. *Journal of the American Geriatrics Society, 45*(1), 43–49. doi:10.1111/j.1532-5415.1997.tb00976.x

Mirarchi, F., Doshi, A., Zerkle, S., & Cooney, T. (2015). How well do emergency physicians understand physicians orders for life sustaining treatment (POLST) forms? *Journal of Patient Safety, 11*(1), 1–8. doi:10.1097/PTS.0000000000000165

Mirarchi, F. L., Hite, L. A., Cooney, T. E., Kisiel, T. M., Henry, P. (2008). TRIAD I-The Realistic Interpretation of Advanced Directives. *Journal of Patient Safety, 4*(4), 235–240. doi:10.1097/PTS.0b013e31818ab16f

Mitty, E. L., & Mezey, M. D. (2004). Advance directives: Older adults with dementia. In M. Matzo & D. Sherman (Eds.). *Gerontological palliative care nursing* (pp. 118–131). St. Louis, MO: Mosby.

Molloy, D. W., Silberfeld, M., Darzins, P., Guyatt, G. H., Singer, P. A., Rush, B., ... Strang, D. (1996). Measuring capacity to complete an advance directive. *Journal of the American Geriatrics Society, 44*(6), 660–664. doi:10.1111/j.1532-5415.1996.tb01828.x

Murphy, D. J., Murray, A. M., Robinson, B. E., & Campion, E. W. (1989). Outcomes of cardiopulmonary resuscitation in the elderly. *Annals of Internal Medicine, 111*(3), 199–205. doi:10.7326/0003-4819-111-3-199

New York State Task Force on Life and the Law. (1995). *A message about the Family Health Care Decisions Act of 1995.* New York, NY: Author.

Nolan, M. T., & Bruder, M. (1997). Patients' attitudes toward advance directives and end-of-life treatment decisions. *Nursing Outlook, 45*(5), 204–208. doi:10.1016/S0029-6554(97)90066-X

Norton, S. A., & Talerico, K. A. (2000). Facilitating end-of-life decision-making: Strategies for communicating and assessing. *Journal of Gerontological Nursing, 26*(9), 6–13. doi:10.3928/0098-9134-20000901-05

O'Brien, L. A., Grisso, J. A., Maislin, G., LaPann, K., Krotki, K. P., Greco, P. J., ... Evans, L. K. (1995). Nursing home residents' preferences for life-sustaining treatments. *Journal of the American Medical Association, 274*(22), 1775–1779. doi:10.1001/jama.1995.03530220041030

Olick, R. S. (2012). Defining features of advance directives in law and clinical practice. *Chest, 141*(1), 232–238. doi:10.1378/chest.11-1520

Page, S., & Meerabeau, L. (1996). Nurses' accounts of cardiopulmonary resuscitation. *Journal of Advanced Nursing, 24*(2), 317–325. doi:10.1046/j.1365-2648.1996.18413.x

Patel, R. V., Sinuff, T., & Cook, D. J. (2004). Influencing advance directive completion rates in non-terminally ill patients: A systematic review. *Journal of Critical Care, 19*(1), 1–9. doi:10.1016/j.jcrc.2004.02.002

Perkins, H. S. (2007). Controlling death: The false promise of advance directives. *Annals of Internal Medicine, 147*(1), 51–57. doi:10.7326/0003-4819-147-1-200707030-00008

Perrin, K. O. (1997). Giving voice to the wishes of elders for end-of-life care. *Journal of Gerontological Nursing, 23*(3), 18–27. doi:10.3928/0098-9134-19970301-12

Perrin, K. O., & Matzo, M. (2009). Caring for the ICU patient at the end of life. In K. Perrin (Ed.), *Understanding the essentials of critical care nursing.* Upper Saddle River, NJ: Pearson/Prentice Hall.

Pfeifer, G. M., & Kennedy, M. S. (2006). Understanding medical futility. *American Journal of Nursing, 106*(5), 25–26. doi:10.1097/00000446-200605000-00016

Phillips, D. M. (2000). JCAHO pain management standards are unveiled. Joint Commission on Accreditation of Healthcare Organization. *Journal of the American Medical Association, 284*(4), 428–429. doi:10.1001/jama.284.4.428

Phillips, R. S., Hamel, M. B., Teno, J. M., Bellamy, P., Broste, S. K., Califf, R. M., … Connors, A. F. (1996). Race, resource use, and survival in seriously ill hospitalized adults. SUPPORT Investigators. *Journal of General Internal Medicine, 11*(7), 387–396. doi:10.1007/BF02600183

Phipps, E., True, G., Harris, D., Chong, U., Tester, W., Chavin, S. I., & Braitman. L. E. (2003). Approaching the end of life: Attitudes, preferences, and behaviors of African-American and white patients and their family caregivers. *Journal of Clinical Oncology, 21*(3), 549–554. doi:10.1200/JCO.2003.12.080

Pirinea, H., Simunich, T., Wehner, J., & Ashurt, D. (2016). Patient and health care provider interpretation of do not resuscitate and do not intubate. *Indian Journal of Palliative Care, 22*(4), 432–436. doi:10.4103/0973-1075.191784

Pope, T. M. (2012). Legal fundamentals of surrogate decision making. *Chest, 141*(4), 1074–1081. doi:10.1378/chest.11-2336

President's Commission for the Study of Ethical Problems in Medicine and Biomedical and Behavioral Research. (1982, March). *Deciding to forego life-sustaining treatment.* Washington, DC: U. S. Government Printing Office.

Reckling, J. B. (1997). Who plays what role in decisions about withholding and withdrawing life-sustaining treatment? *Journal of Clinical Ethics, 8*(1), 39–45.

Robinson, M. K., DeHaven, M. J., & Koch, K. A. (1993). Effects of the Patient Self-Determination Act on patient knowledge and behavior. *Journal of Family Practice, 37*(4), 363–368.

Rubin, S. M., Strull, W. M., Fialkow, M. F., Weiss, S. J., & Lo, B. (1994). Increasing the completion of the durable power of attorney for health care. A randomized, controlled trial. *Journal of the American Medical Association, 271*(3), 209–212. doi:10.1001/jama.271.3.209

Sachs, G. A., Stocking, C. B., & Miles, S. H. (1992). Empowerment of the older patient? A randomized, controlled trial to increase discussion and use of advance directives. *Journal of the American Geriatrics Society, 40*(3), 269–273. doi:10.1111/j.1532-5415.1992.tb02081.x

Schloendorff v. Society of New York Hospitals, 211 N.Y. 125, 105 N.E. 92 (1914).

Schneider, A. P., Nelson, D. J., & Brown, D. D. (1993). In-hospital cardiopulmonary resuscitation: A 30-year review. *Journal of the American Board of Family Practice, 6*(2), 91–101.

Schneider, C. (2004). Liability for life. *Hastings Center Report, 34*(4), 10–11. doi:10.2307/3528684

Shapiro, S. (2015). Do advance directives direst? *Journal of Health, Politics, Policy, and Law, 40*(3), 487–520. doi:10.1215/03616878-2888424

Silveira, M. J., DiPiero, A., Gerrity, M. S., & Feudtner, C. (2000). Patients' knowledge of options at the end of life: Ignorance in the face of death. *Journal of the American Medical Association, 284*(19), 2483–2488. doi:10.1001/jama.284.19.2483

Silveira, M. J., Kim, S. Y., & Langa, K. M. (2010). Advance directives and outcomes of surrogate decision making before death. *New England Journal of Medicine, 362*(13), 1211–1218. doi:10.1056/NEJMsa0907901

Sim, H., Zimmerman, C., & Krzyzanowska, M. (2016). Systematic review of interventions to facilitate advance care planning (ACP) in cancer patients. *Journal of Clinical Oncology, 34*(29), 21. doi:10.1200/jco.2016.34.26_suppl.21

Sims, J. M. (2008). Your role in informed consent: Part 1. *Dimensions of Critical Care Nursing, 27*(2), 70–73. doi:10.1097/01.dcc.0000311599.25216.90

Smith, T. J., Desch, C. E., Hackney, M. H., & Shaw, J. E. (1997). How long does it take to get a "do not resuscitate" order? *Journal of Palliative Care, 13*(1), 5–8.

Stiller, A., Molloy, D. W., Russo, R., Dubois, S., Kavsak, H., & Bedard, M. (2001). Development and evaluation of a new instrument that measures barriers to implementing advance directives. *Journal of Clinical Outcomes Management, 8*(4), 26–31.

SUPPORT Principal Investigators. (1995). A controlled trial to improve care for seriously ill hospitalized patients: The Study to Understand Prognoses and Preferences for Outcomes and Risks of Treatment (SUPPORT). *Journal of the American Medical Association, 274,* 1591–1598. doi:10.1001/jama.1995.03530200027032

Swidler, R. N. (1989). The presumption of consent in New York State's do-not-resuscitate law. *New York State Journal of Medicine, 89*(2), 69–72.

Teno, J. M., Gruneir, A., Schwartz, Z., Nanda, A., & Wetle, T. (2007). Association between advance directives and quality of end-of-life care: A national study. *Journal of the American Geriatrics Society, 55*(2), 189–194. doi:10.1111/j.1532-5415.2007.01045.x

Teno, J. M., Licks, S., Lynn, J., Wenger, N., Connors, A. F., Phillips, R. S., … Knaus, W. A. (1997). Do advance directives provide instructions that direct care? SUPPORT Investigators. *Journal of the American Geriatrics Society, 45*(4), 508–512. doi:10.1111/j.1532-5415.1997.tb05179.x

Teno, J. M., Lynn, J., Phillips, R. S., Murphy, D., Youngner, S. J., Bellamy, P., ... Knaus, W. A. (1994). Do formal advance directives affect resuscitation decisions and the use of resources for seriously ill patients? SUPPORT Investigators. *Journal of Clinical Ethics, 5*(1), 23–30.

Teno, J. M., Lynn, J., Wenger, N., Phillips, R. S., Murphy, D. P., Connors, A. F., ... Knaus, W. A. (1997). Advance directives for seriously ill hospitalized patients: Effectiveness with the Patient Self-Determination Act and the SUPPORT intervention. SUPPORT Investigators. *Journal of the American Geriatrics Society, 45*(4), 500–507. doi:10.1111/j.1532-5415.1997.tb05178.x

Torke, A. M., Moloney, R., Siegler, M., Abalos, A., & Alexander, G. C. (2010). Physicians' views on the importance of patient preferences in surrogate decision-making. *Journal of the American Geriatrics Society, 58*(3), 533–538. doi:10.1111/j.1532-5415.2010.02720.x

Tulsky, J. A., Chesney, M. A., & Lo, B. (1995). How do medical residents discuss resuscitation with patients? *Journal of General Internal Medicine, 10*(8), 436–442. doi:10.1007/BF02599915

Vacco v. Quill, 521 U.S. 793, 117 S. Ct. 2293 (1997).

Ventres, W., Nichter, M., Reed, R., & Frankel, R. (1992). Do-not-resuscitate discussions: A qualitative analysis. *Family Practice Research Journal, 12*(2), 157–169.

Virani, R., & Sofer, D. (2003). Improving the quality of end-of-life care. *American Journal of Nursing, 103*(5), 52–60; quiz 61. doi:10.1097/00000446-200305000-00020

Wagner, A. (1984). Cardiopulmonary resuscitation in the aged. A prospective survey. *New England Journal of Medicine, 310*(17), 1129–1130. doi:10.1056/NEJM198404263101732

Washington Natural Death Act, ch. 98, § 1; 1979, ch. 112, § 2 (1992).

White, D. B. (2011). Rethinking interventions to improve surrogate decision making in intensive care units. *American Journal of Critical Care, 20*(3), 252–257. doi:10.4037/ajcc2011106

Whitty-Rogers, J., Alex, M., MacDonald, C., Pierrynowski Gallant, D., & Austin, W. (2009). Working with children in end-of-life decision making. *Nursing Ethics, 16*(6), 743–758. doi:10.1177/0969733009341910

Caring for the Whole Person and His or Her Family

Deborah Witt Sherman & David C. Free

Culture and Spirituality as Domains of Quality Palliative Care

KEY POINTS

- Culture and spirituality structure human experience, values, and behaviors.
- Spirituality provides a sense of connection to self, others, nature, and God and is important in crisis and illness.
- Cultural competence involves knowledge of your own and of other cultural groups.
- Cultural assessment has several areas to be addressed.
- Spirituality and religiosity help individuals to cope with serious illness and play a role in the dying process.
- Suffering is a part of the human condition and is experienced in physical, emotional, and spiritual ways.
- Suffering is reciprocal, involving not only the patient but also his or her family.
- Hope plays a role in promoting spiritual well-being.
- Health professionals must learn how to conduct a spiritual assessment and have conversations about spiritual and religious issues.
- Spiritual care discovers, reveres, and tends to the human spirit.
- Knowledge of cultural and spiritual perspectives on death informs care.
- Culturally and spiritually competent care requires self-reflection and self-care of health professionals.
- Palliative care (PC) addresses the cultural and spiritual needs of patients and families.

CASE STUDY

Mr. J. is an 82-year-old African American man who was diagnosed with heart failure and end-stage renal disease secondary to hypertension and diabetes. He is on several cardiovascular medications to manage his condition. He is currently receiving dialysis treatments 3 days a week and is on the organ-donation list awaiting a kidney transplant. Mr. J. has been experiencing chest pain intermittently for the past few days. He has a history of angina (chest pain) and is prescribed medication for management. Three days ago Mr. J. was found at home unresponsive by his daughter, who called 911 and immediately began cardiopulmonary resuscitation (CPR). Mr. J. was taken to the nearest hospital and admitted to the ICU. He suffered a massive heart attack resulting in a lack of oxygen delivery to his brain. Due to the unwitnessed heart attack, Mr. J. was not a candidate for therapeutic hypothermia management. He is currently intubated on ventilatory support and continuous renal replacement therapy. During neurological assessments, there is minimal response from Mr. J.

The interdisciplinary team caring for Mr. J. has arranged a conference with his family to discuss his current status and prognosis. Mr. J. has a large, close-knit family and, despite his illness, has been an active member of his church for the past 30 years. The conference consisted of his wife, six children, two younger siblings, and the pastor and his wife. Taking into account his cultural and spiritual beliefs, the team carefully discussed his current status, prognosis, and advanced directives with his family. Despite medical treatment, Mr. J.'s condition is worsening. The family expresses that Mr. J. does not have an advance directive, but they do not feel that one is required because they are strong believers in the power of God and believe that death is part of God's plan for us all and that it will happen in God's time. The team requests a PC consult to assist the family with decision making.

Culture and spirituality are among the most important factors that structure human experience, values, behaviors, and illness patterns. As a system of shared symbols and beliefs, culture supports a person's sense of security, integrity, and belonging and provides a prescription for how to conduct life and approach death (End-of-Life Nursing Education Consortium [ELNEC], 2013). Every culture has a worldview or construct of reality that defines the individual within that reality. Patients' cultural backgrounds are therefore fundamental in defining and creating their reality and determining their purpose in life. A transformation of identity begins when an individual is diagnosed with a fatal illness. Cultural rituals provide the sacred elements that support patients and families during times of illness and transition. Specific rituals assist individuals and families in coping with death, which is the final transition in life. The rituals of death change the identity of the patient from the living to the dead, and also the identity of the family member, for example, from spouse to widow or widower (Kagawa-Singer & Blackhall, 2001). Culture provides a framework of expectations about communication with others, including health professionals, and the role of family, and influences the dynamics of decision making regarding health issues and the dying process itself (Barclay, Blackhall, & Tulsky, 2007).

Spirituality plays a vital role in times of crisis and illness, as it provides a sense of connection to self, others, nature, and God, and is a means to cope with loss, grief, and death (Weaver, Flannelly, & Flannelly, 2001). Life-threatening illness is a crisis on many levels: physical, psychological, familial, social, and spiritual (Rome, Luminais, Bourgeois, & Blais, 2011). Given the uniqueness and individuality of each person, even people of the same culture and spirituality may have different backgrounds, experiences, needs, concerns, and interpretation of illness. In addition to the individuality of the person, the nature of the life-threatening illness may be different and the person may be at different points in adapting to the reality of the disease. Spiritual and cultural concerns may permeate the illness experience or may arise at any point across the illness/dying trajectory. For patients and families who are experiencing life-threatening illness, the concerns may be of suffering that may take multiple forms relative to the mind–body–spirit. It is now recognized that the uncertain and long-term nature of many life-threatening illnesses poses the potential for pain, alterations in body image, and confrontation with death, which may lead to spiritual distress. The renewed focus on incorporating spiritual care into nursing practice is congruent with nursing's commitment to holistic practice and the renewed valuing of human experiences that defy scientific description and explanation. Within the past few years, research has shown that religious beliefs and spiritual practices affect the meaning of illness, physical and emotional well-being, coping with illness, and healthcare decisions, particularly for individuals facing life-threatening illness (Puchalski & Ferrell, 2010).

Spiritual and cultural competences are central tenets of PC. As a philosophy of care, PC combines active and compassionate therapies to support and comfort individuals and families who are living with life-threatening illness. PC strives to meet their physical, psychological, social, and spiritual expectations and needs, while remaining sensitive to personal, cultural, and religious beliefs and practices (National Consensus Project, 2013). Undergraduate-prepared nurses and advanced practice nurses must become spiritually and culturally competent in the care they offer across the illness/dying trajectory. Such care is critical to enhancing the quality of life (QOL) and quality of dying, and to supporting the intrinsic dignity of patients and their families.

■ UNDERSTANDING CULTURE

"Culture" is defined as a way of life, which provides a worldview that is fundamental in defining and creating a person's reality, determining his or her meaning and purpose in life, and providing guidelines for living. As cultural perspectives evolve, changes are evident in the beliefs, values, and attitudes of a cultural group or its members. Cultures are not monolithic; rather there is a range of potential responses to each issue in every cultural group. Thus, there may be within-group variations, such as those attributed to acculturation differences, as well as to differences related to age, education, geographic location, and social context (Barclay et al., 2007; Kagawa-Singer & Blackhall, 2001). It is important to inquire whether an individual patient adheres to the beliefs and practices of his or her cultural group, rather than assuming that he or she holds the same values and beliefs (Crawley, Marshall, Lo, & Koenig, 2002).

Although culture is often identified with ethnicity, it is a far broader concept, which encompasses the components of gender, age, sexual orientation, differing abilities, educational level, employment, and place of residency (ELNEC, 2013). As examples, cultures may value male children more than female; the young more than the old; heterosexuals rather than homosexuals; the educated and employed more than the uneducated or unemployed; individuals with stable domiciles more than the homeless; and the healthy more than the physically, emotionally, or intellectually challenged. The diversity of the population with regard to many of these factors may increase its vulnerability in terms of perceived cultural status. Concepts of culture and ethnicity may be useful for making generalizations about populations; however, if they limit appreciation of the unique differences of people and are used to predict individual behavior, they may lead to stereotyping (Koenig, 2002).

Cultural background also relates to issues of power, decision making, language and communication, sources of support within the community, degree of fatalism or activism in accepting or controlling death, maintaining hope, and also views of the patient and family about death (Sherman, 2001). Cultural differences are further evident in terms of the relationship between the older adult and his or her family. In certain cultures, the older person is viewed as the patriarch or matriarch of the family and therefore has the final word in personal and family matters. In other cultures, the older person defers decision making to members of the family, as interdependence among the family and community members is more valued than individual autonomy (Ersek et al., 1998). Depending on cultural expectations, families may believe that it is their duty to protect the patient from bad news, which is believed to burden the individual or cause emotional distress or harm. Therefore, full disclosure of diagnosis and prognosis to the patient may be considered harmful by families (Barclay et al., 2007). As the cultural diversity of patients and practitioners in the United States continues to increase, there is a risk for cross-cultural misunderstanding surrounding care at the end of life. Cross-cultural understanding and communication techniques increase the likelihood that both the process and the outcome of healthcare are satisfactory for all involved (Kagawa-Singer & Blackhall, 2001).

■ CULTURAL PERSPECTIVES IN HEALTHCARE

Healthcare practitioners should get involved in spiritual health and expand their cultural competence to provide proper care and help their patients have better health outcomes (Wilson, 2012). Understanding the cultural backgrounds of patients is fundamental to the development of a trusting and supportive relationship among patient, family, and healthcare professionals, and is essential in developing a plan for healthcare that is consistent with their cultural expectations and health beliefs, as many health belief systems are culturally constructed (Herselman, 2004). Andrews and Boyle (2016) discussed three types of health belief systems: magico-religious, biomedical, and holistic. In the magico-religious paradigm, a person believes that God or supernatural forces control health and illness. In the biomedical paradigm, to which most Americans subscribe, it is believed that illness is caused by a disruption in physical or biochemical processes that can be manipulated by healthcare. In the holistic paradigm, health results from a balance or harmony among the elements of nature and illness is produced by disharmony. Examples of the magico-religious system are a Haitian patient who believes that his symptoms are caused by spirits, or the Mexican American who uses herbs, oils, incense, or religious figurines to drive away evil spirits or to relieve gastric pains. In the biomedical system, seek cure of illness through advanced medical technology and pharmacological management. Based on the holistic belief system, a Chinese woman may attribute her headache to a stagnation of *qi*, believing in the need for balance between *yin* and *yang*; a Native American patient may wear a bag of herbs blessed by the medicine man around his neck to maintain his strength (Grossman, 1996).

Recognition of these health belief systems is evident in the healthcare practices of many cultures. The health beliefs of African American, Chinese, Asian Indians, Latinos and Hispanics, and Native Americans are discussed on the basis of recent studies or cultural inquiries and provide a framework for offering culturally competent hospice and PC to members of these cultural groups. The only truly accurate way that one may know what individuals believe in or the effect that their culture or religion plays in their lives is to ask them. The following information will guide the nurse regarding areas to be assessed.

Cultural Perspectives of African Americans

The term "African Americans" refers to a diverse group of people from varied cultural backgrounds (Yancu, Farmer, Graves, Rhinehardt, & Leahman, 2015). Despite their diversity, research suggests that African Americans share a set of beliefs regarding spirituality and end-of-life (EOL) care. The first of these beliefs is that spirituality affects attitudes about death and dying, with God possessing control over life and death, including timing and circumstance. Second, emphasis is placed on the value of a long life and fighting for survival. Third, pain is a test of faith and there is redemption in suffering. Fourth, EOL decisions are entrusted to close family members rather than the individual (Yancu et al., 2015). Within the African American culture, there is a strong sense of community and of the importance of family, friends, and the church community as sources of support. The extended African American family consists of mother, father, children, grandparents, aunts, uncles, nieces, nephews, and cousins with a willingness to accept all relatives regardless of their circumstances (McDavis, Parker, & Parker, 1995). Older adults are prized in the African American family and they play key roles in the family, church, and community. Many grandparents accept the responsibility for rearing their grandchildren, while the parents of those children work or receive higher education. Children are taught to take care of their parents and to be devoted to them. In addition, older African American family members play a significant role in passing on cultural values, customs, and traditions to the children (McDavis et al., 1995).

African Americans are often distrustful of the healthcare system, given a history of oppression and mistreatment from slavery, racism, and even being subjected to medical experimentation in the United States, as seen in the infamous Tuskegee syphilis study conducted from 1932 to 1972 (Kennedy, Mathis, & Woods, 2007). Because of this distrust, African Americans may delay seeking EOL care in favor of aggressive treatment despite a poor prognosis (Yancu et al., 2015). Common themes of justice and respect have reinforced the importance of self-determination. In a study of attitudes, values, and questions of African Americans regarding participation in hospice programs, Taxis (2005) identified three main barriers: (a) a lack of information about hospice and inaccurate assumptions regarding hospice care, (b) cultural barriers resulting from an avoidance of discussions regarding EOL planning, and (c) institutional barriers resulting from a mistrust of the healthcare system. Bullock (2006) reported that even using a faith-based promotion model of advanced care planning, 75% of the 102 African American participants refused to complete advance directives. The participants' decisions were based on such factors as spirituality, view of suffering, dying and death, social support networks, and mistrust of the healthcare system. For African Americans, advance care planning conflicts with their beliefs and attitudes about fighting to the end, not giving up hope, and enduring suffering. In a study of 473 adults (220 Blacks and 253 Whites), Ludke and Smucker (2007) found that relative to Whites, near the end of life Blacks were significantly less likely to consider hospice even if their doctor recommended its use. However, Blacks who had a prior exposure to hospice and who trusted their doctor were more willing to consider hospice.

Yancu et al. (2015) conducted a study exploring the attitudes of African Americans toward death and dying. The study consisted of four focus groups from four predominantly African American churches. The researcher identified several themes during the focus groups. Death of older adults is easier to accept as they were seen to have lived a good life. The group viewed death as a release from suffering and pain; however, the journey of death was noted to be individual and based on personal salvation and spirituality. Contrary to previous research, it is never too early to have a conservation regarding death and dying in the African American community. Participants viewed advance directives and living wills as a gift to the dying individual's family. Nonetheless, similar to previous research, the use of PC and hospice was viewed as giving up and finding a place to die. Nevertheless, it was noted that it is acceptable to consider PC and hospice when the individual or family has accepted the prognosis. The focus groups agreed that the African American community needs to be better educated on hospice care (Yancu et al., 2015).

Because family is central to the care of the dying, and with the assistance of and supportive relationships established with church members and neighbors, there is a decreased need for outside support (Sherman, 2001). Given strong family loyalty, there is reluctance to hospitalize family members. As a measure of respect and devotion, elder African Americans are placed in nursing homes only as a last resort (Anderson & Turner, 2010). In the African American culture, death is integrated into the totality of life. Ancestor worship involves the communion with the living dead through memories, and the deceased are remembered by name. When living people no longer remember the deceased, they become part of the anonymous dead, but by this time, it is believed that their spirit has been reborn in a new child (Sherman, 2001).

To explore the meaning of death and the experience of grieving, Abrums (2000) conducted life-history interviews with nine church going women, ranging in age from 19 to 82 years, from a small Black storefront Baptist church in the Pacific Northwest. The findings indicated that the women in the church had been taught to be strong in the face of death and to handle their grief "head on." The women believed that they would one day be reunited with their loved ones. The terminology of dying used words such as "passed on," "passed away," or "died." Participants described many spirit visits for the purpose of offering warnings or as direct messages. Belief in an afterlife was sustained by day-to-day experiences of visions or messages from another world. It was believed that God spoke in many ways through premonitions perceived as the voice of God. There was strong emphasis on the journey of life in which there is a job to do on Earth and one's life has a purpose. No life is lived in vain. Time was needed to prepare for death and to make peace with God as a dying individual. Participants also described the importance of hope, acceptance, and responsibility to comfort the dying and the bereaved. Abrums (2000) concluded that health professionals should learn to value the spiritual beliefs and grieving behaviors of members of other cultures, rather than viewing them as maladaptive. Supporting dying patients and their families in their beliefs is important in providing spiritual care. Verbal recognition of specific actions taken by families to support the dying person provided a sense of comfort and support to the family in their grief. The people in this storefront church were often comforted by the recognition that God sustained them in times of adversity and God would protect their loved ones. This acknowledgment of the family's belief system by health professionals can augment the healing process during times of loss and grief.

Cultural Perspectives of the Chinese

In the Chinese culture, the primary theme of social structure is the centrality of the family. From the centrality of the family arises cultural expectations such as: (a) duty to family manifested by respect and reverence for parents; (b) conformance to family and societal norms, especially not bringing shame to the family; (c) family recognition through achievement; (d) emotional self-control manifested through reserved and formal public verbal and nonverbal communications; (e) family disagreement or demands are kept to a minimum; (f) collectivism is evidenced by people keeping a focus on the family and community over self; and (g) humility is manifested by a lack of striving for individual achievement, with emphasis on achievement that is related to the family (Kemp & Chang, 2002).

Given the traditionally hierarchical and patriarchal family structure of the Chinese, the oldest adult male is the primary decision maker. In family matters, elders have significant influence. Health decisions may be made by the family and are based on what is best not only for the elder patient but also for the family (Kemp & Chang, 2002). In general, yes and no questions should be avoided, as yes is considered to be the polite answer and is nearly always given.

In China, the primary religion is Buddhism. The essence of Buddhism is found in the Four Noble Truths: (a) all sentient beings suffer; (b) the cause of suffering is desire manifested by attachment to life, security, and others; (c) the way to end suffering is to cease to desire; and (d) the way to cease desire is to follow the Eightfold Path of knowledge of the Four Noble Truths: right intent, right speech, right action, right endeavor, right mindfulness, right meditation, and right concentration. It is believed that following the Eightfold Path leads to emancipation from rebirth (Kemp & Chang, 2002).

In the Chinese culture, it is also important to understand the significance of the balance of yin and yang, which are complementary forces. A second important concept is that of traditional Chinese medicine (TCM), which is based on channel (meridian) systems, in which various body channels carry vital or life energy called *chi* or *qi*. Imbalance or disruption of channels leads to illness, and the treatment goal of TCM is to restore balance. A third important concept in understanding Chinese approaches to health and illness is the use of allopathic medicine as well as TCM.

Issues central to the care of the Chinese at the EOL center around family and communications (Kemp & Chang, 2002). Symptom management may be complicated by the patient's and family's reluctance to complain because of respect for others in positions of authority. Concerns also center around fears of addiction, desire to be a good patient, and fear of distracting the physician from treating the disease. In some cases, elders may even deny symptoms when asked directly; however, a visual analog scale and numeric rating scale can be used to assess pain. For example, patients may want to keep warm during illness by wearing sweaters or socks in bed and drinking warm liquids and avoiding cold drinks. As death nears, the family may wish to call monks or nuns for ritual prayers (Kemp & Chang, 2002). Communications at the end of life are also complicated by reluctance to discuss prognosis and diagnosis. Chinese families often withhold information from patients and may pretend that they do not know what is happening. Families believe that discussing EOL issues is like wishing death upon the elder, or may lead to hopelessness, especially as terminal illness is not socially accepted. As death approaches, it is believed that a person's final days should be characterized by calm and the patient should not be involved in decision making. The best way to handle the conspiracy of silence is to ask patients how much they want to know, and, if they do not wish to know, then they should be asked to whom the information should be given and who should make decisions. Although a preference for nondisclosure of poor prognosis seems to have historically predominated in the Chinese culture, research with Chinese subjects is beginning to demonstrate a shift in attitudes with a preference for more direct and patient-centered disclosures of the prognosis (Ahalt et al., 2012; Yu et al., 2007; Yun et al., 2010). Families often feel it is their cultural obligation to care for the person who is dying, and therefore hospice services are often refused (Kemp & Chang, 2002).

Cultural Perspectives of Asian Indians

Among Asian Indians, living with extended family is prevalent and elders are highly respected. The husband's parents often move in with family after retirement, when the younger family decides to have children, or if there is illness. Elders are highly valued, as is their role as grandparents in helping to raise children. In Indian culture, value is placed on independence and privacy, and family issues are discussed within the immediate family before outside help is sought (Bhungalia & Kemp, 2002). Healthcare decisions usually require family input.

Many Indians are of the Hindu faith. The goal of Hinduism is to free the soul from endless reincarnation and the suffering inherent in existence. The endless reincarnations of the soul are the result of karma, or actions of the individual in this present life and the accumulation of actions from past lives.

The caste system is part of Hinduism. In this system, society is divided into four social classes: the highest class is the priest class, or Brahmans; and the lowest class is the laborer class, or Sudras. A person's class is inherited at birth based on his or her karma. Hindu beliefs that may affect patient care include the following:

■ Karma, or the consequences of one's actions or behaviors, influences the circumstances of life and may have caused an illness.
■ Meditation and prayer are important.
■ Hindus are vegetarians; many Hindus pray a specific prayer before eating to ask forgiveness for eating a plant or vegetable in which a soul may dwell.

The Indian system of medicine is known as *Ayurveda*, which means "knowledge of life." Indian medicine mixes religion and secular medicine, with more than 80% of people in India relying on herbal remedies to cure or prevent illness. In this system, the root of disease is not always considered to be inside the body, but may be related to the environment or other factors. In the Ayurvedic system, the body comprises three primary forces, called *dosha*: the *vata*, *pitta*, and *kapha*. Each represents characteristics derived from the five elements of space, air, fire, water, and earth; the balance between these forces is essential to health. Once there is imbalance among the forces, balance is sought using different therapies, which includes approximately 1,400 plants used in Ayurvedic medicine. Most Indians eat two to three meals a day, using the fingers of their right hand, and avoiding distractions while eating, such as watching television or excessive talking. Some foods are considered hot and others cold, and should not be eaten in combination, as this is believed to affect bodily functions.

With respect to EOL care, it is important for the ill individual to complete unfinished business and resolve relationships. Home is the preferred place of death, with many family members present when death is imminent. Symptoms may not be reported, as it is believed that suffering is inevitable and the result of karma. Many seek to be conscious during the dying process, not clouded by medications. As death approaches, the following Asian Indian rituals are valued:

■ A lamp may be placed near the patient's head; the body may be turned to face east, toward Mecca; sacred ash may be applied to the forehead.
■ A few drops of water from the sacred Ganges River may be placed in the dying person's mouth, while a mantra is softly chanted in the patient's right ear.
■ Prayer and incense are part of the rituals of the dying process.

After death, family members should be the only ones to touch the body, and ideally a family member of the same sex should clean the body. After the body is cleansed, a cloth is tied under the chin and over the top of the head, and the body is wrapped in red cloth. Embalming and organ donation are prohibited and cremation is preferred. Following the death, religious pictures at home are turned toward the wall and mirrors may be covered. It is believed that for 12 days the soul wanders in the home, trying to let go of life and the material world. During this time, the family prays and chants, and on the 12th day, the soul is reincarnated (Bhungalia & Kemp, 2002).

Cultural Perspectives of Latinos and Hispanics

The cultural group referred to as "Latinos" consists of individuals of Hispanic background. It is important to note that as with many cultural groups, not all Hispanics are the same nor do they originate from the same country; therefore, their cultural beliefs will vary. In general, this cultural group's healthcare is affected by obstacles they encounter due to language barriers, social issues, and economic hardships (O'Mara & Zborovskaya, 2016). Sullivan (2001) conducted 10 focus groups and interviews with 17 gatekeepers in Latino communities regarding EOL care and documented there can be difficult communications between Hispanics and healthcare practitioners. The results indicated that many Latinos felt that they could not communicate effectively with healthcare providers due to language barriers and were not able to understand informed consent even when interpreters were used. None of the Latino participants wanted to die in a nursing home, believing that it is the families' responsibility to care for its relatives. Most participants were also not aware of hospice services or had false information about hospice. Although participants expressed diverse views, one third of participants were against the use of life support, particularly if it prolonged the suffering of the patient. Participants also believed that their religious beliefs, especially fatalism and reliance on God, were central to their decision making regarding EOL care. There was division among the participants regarding the extent to which they wanted to be informed about a fatal diagnosis, citing that being informed may accelerate the illness. Many Latinos also perceived racial discrimination and cultural insensitivity as barriers to quality care and healing (Sullivan, 2001).

In the Hispanic culture, there are several considerations that relate to quality care at the EOL (Sherman, 2001). It is recognized that in Hispanic culture, there is strong family support and a belief that the dying person should be protected from his or her prognosis. Women show extreme grief or hysteria, whereas men show little or no grief. Death is often confronted with humorous sarcasm and is viewed as an equalizer (DeSpelder & Strickland, 1999). Mexican Americans, as well as other Hispanics, are likely to call a priest for the sacrament of the sick, and the bereaved may take turns being with the deceased person. There is strong support of family as a unit. The funeral is the single most important family ceremony and goes on for several days, as there is the belief that it takes time to grieve. Individuals are prohibited from speaking ill of the person who has died, and the bereaved visit the grave frequently. The Day of the Dead is celebrated in November and coincides with All Saints' Day, the feast of the commemoration of the dead. Although death is viewed as an adversity, references to dying and death are common in the culture, as children play with toys symbolizing death, and the funeral is an important family ceremony. It is a time of celebration with special foods, music, and the decoration of graves. It is believed that the dead return to the world of the living for this special celebration, and families are scorned if they neglect their responsibilities. The bereaved are discouraged from crying too many tears, as excessive grief may make the pathway traveled on by the dead slippery and burden them in the journey (DeSpelder & Strickland, 1999).

A clinical study of Latino immigrants at least 21 years old and living in the United States for less than 10 years (Selsky et al., 2012) used validated Spanish-language instruments to assess the hospice knowledge and intent of the 331 study subjects. Only 29% of the subjects intended to choose hospice and an additional 6% would choose hospice once it was explained. Greater knowledge of hospice was correlated with a higher education level. Subjects who believed that prognosis should remain a secret were 19% less likely to choose hospice. Higher degrees of social acculturation were associated with greater intent to use hospice. The study suggests that knowledge helps to increase the intent to use hospice among recent Latino immigrants (in the U.S. less than 10 years); however, the importance of social networks and acculturation were highlighted by the findings (Selsky et al., 2012).

Cultural Perspectives of Native Americans

For Native Americans the focus of one's identity is the tribe, rather than the Native American ancestry. This is important because values and beliefs vary among tribes and among the different bands of "First Nations." There

may be similarities in nations originating in the same region, but there are also tribal distinctions (Brokenleg & Middleton, 1993). For many Native Americans, however, life and death are a part of life, and death is accepted when caused by accident or war. However, when the death is caused by illness, many American Indians struggle to accept it. Death and end of life are topics that this culture avoids and are considered taboo. Native Americans believe that talking about death attracts evil spirits and brings negative feelings to them (Yoshiko Yamashita & Brown, 2014).

For many Native Americans, however, life and death are viewed as a natural part of the life cycle. Death is not the end of life but rather a transition in the life cycle (Gebauer et al., 2016). Death is seen as a fundamental part of nature and human existence that requires "no manipulation or anticipation" (Hepburn & Reed, 1995). In Navajo culture, however, it is believed that talking about death may precipitate it, and the appropriateness of such discussions should be assessed and, if problematic, should be avoided. Time is considered a recurring cycle rather than a linear process. Native Americans are concerned with how this cycle affects people in this life, and death is viewed as a motivation to treat people kindly and to lead a good life (Brokenleg & Middleton, 1993; Sherman, 2001).

From a cultural perspective, Native Americans avoid eye contact and are stoic regarding the expression of pain and suffering, and traditional tribal medicines are used (Sherman, 2001). Prayer is a medium through which one might accept the outcome of a situation, and it is not appropriate to question "why" something is happening, as there is an acceptance of the natural order of things (Brokenleg & Middleton, 1993). Death may be forecast by unusual spiritual or physical events. As examples, the sign of an owl may signify that someone close will soon die, and a blue light seen coming from the direction of a dead relative's home or room indicates death (Brokenleg & Middleton, 1993).

Given their reverence for the body in life and death, autopsies and cremation are not acceptable to Native Americans (Sherman, 2004a). Native Americans tend to stay within their own environment, practicing their own beliefs and religion to deal with EOL and death; the ideal way of death for this culture is to recognize oneself as a proud Indian (Yoshiko Yamashita & Brown, 2014). Funerals are usually performed at home, with members of the community expected to stay with the mourners. A death song is sung that represents the summary of a person's life and acknowledgment of death. The dead are considered guardian spirits. After death, the spirit lingers near the site of the death for several days. Native Americans use a funeral pyre and adorn the corpse with flowers, feathers, and animal skins. For 6 months to 1 year, the name of the deceased is not called in order to confirm their separation from the living. All material possessions of the deceased are given away so that the family can begin its new life without the presence of that person (Brokenleg & Middleton, 1993). In the Cocopa tribe, violent grief is expressed until cremation, at which time spirits are invited to join them in celebration. In the Hopi tribe, death is kept at a distance because it threatens order and control. The expression of grief remains limited and funerals are attended by few and held privately. For Native Americans, hallucinations in which they see and converse with the dead are regarded as a part of mourning (DeSpelder & Strickland, 1999).

Based on focus groups representing many Native American tribes and conducted by Native American nurses, Lowe and Struthers (2001) identified seven themes representing core principles relevant to healthcare: (1) caring, which embodies characteristics of health, relationships, holism, and knowledge, and is characterized as a "partnership in healing"; (2) traditions, which refer to valuing and connecting with heritage; (3) respect, which includes characteristics of honor, identity, and strength and compassion; (4) connection, which honors all people, including those past, present, and future as well as harmony with nature; (5) holism, which includes balance and culture; (6) trust, which is characterized through relationship, presence, and respect; and (7) spirituality, which includes unity, honor, balance, healing as well as healing touch, learning, and utilizing traditions to recognize oneness and unity with others.

■ DEVELOPING CULTURAL COMPETENCE

A culturally competent healthcare system "acknowledges and incorporates at all levels the importance of culture, the assessment of cross-cultural relations, vigilance toward the dynamics that result from cultural differences, and the expansion of cultural knowledge, and adaptation of services to meet culturally unique needs" (Cort, 2004, p. 68). Achieving cultural competence is a dynamic state in which health professionals gain knowledge of their own cultural and social backgrounds and become aware of the history, traditions, and values of other groups, including understanding the history, food, and lifestyles of people from other countries (Cort, 2004). According to Doorenbos and Schim's (2004) cultural competence model, there are four components of cultural competence:

1. Cultural diversity, which is reflected in every aspect of the healthcare system in the United States and recognizes diverse populations with unique values, beliefs, and customs
2. Cultural awareness, which implies knowledge and information exchange regarding health, beliefs, and practices specific to various communities, and cultural variations within groups
3. Cultural sensitivity, which requires the recognition of individual attitudes and beliefs and a refinement of communication skills related to active listening,

use of silence and touch, conversational distance, language patterns, and the effective use of translators
4. Cultural competence, which is the ultimate goal and incorporates diversity (fact), awareness (knowledge), and sensitivity (attitude) into everyday practice and behaviors

"Cultural diversity" refers to differences between people based on treasured beliefs, shared teachings, norms, customs, language, and meaning that influence the individual's and family's response to illness, treatment, death, and bereavement (Ballard-Reisch & Letner, 2003). Cultural diversity is evident in the perception of pain, ways of coping with life-threatening illness, and the behavioral manifestations of grief, mourning, and funeral customs (DeSpelder & Strickland, 1999). The acknowledgment of such concepts and their relationships may provide a framework for cultural assessment and an opportunity to provide quality care respectful of differences with regard to cultural expectations and needs. Failure to take culture seriously means that health professionals elevate their values above the values of others, which is culturally destructive rather than culturally skilled (Kagawa-Singer & Blackhall, 2001). Therefore, it is important to support trusting and effective patient and provider interactions through respect, and acknowledgment of cultural diversity and avoidance of misperceptions.

For those experiencing life-threatening illness, several issues are relevant with respect to cultural awareness. One such issue is patient autonomy, which emphasizes the rights of patients to be informed about their condition, its treatments, and the right to choose or refuse life-prolonging care. However, this reflects the American beliefs regarding independence and individual rights, which may not be shared by patients and families from other cultures (Kagawa-Singer & Blackhall, 2001). For example, those from Asian cultures may believe that the family as a whole should make decisions regarding an aged individual. This is an example of a "family-centered" rather than a "patient-centered" decision-making style (Barclay et al., 2007).

Another issue influenced by culture awareness is responses to inequities in care. When not addressed, this issue may lead to feelings of mistrust regarding the intentions of healthcare providers and a lack of cooperation and collaboration among the patient, family, and healthcare provider. Discussions of the cost of technology and the ineffectiveness of treatment may be perceived by the patient as a devaluation of his or her life (Crawley et al., 2002). As a result, there may be an increased desire for futile aggressive care at the EOL and dissatisfaction with care. This issue is relevant to the care of African American patients and families, who are more likely to want aggressive medical care at the EOL and less likely to have do-not-resuscitate (DNR) orders. To address this issue, practitioners can ask directly whether the individual trusts someone who is not from his or her same background. Practitioners can work toward addressing inequities in care, or can attempt to understand and accommodate desires for more aggressive care (Kagawa-Singer & Blackhall, 2001).

Furthermore, communication or language barriers may lead to bidirectional misunderstanding and unnecessary physical, emotional, social, or spiritual suffering. It is therefore important to avoid medical jargon, make language simple, check for understanding, or hire a trained interpreter. The use of family or untrained interpreters should be avoided, as they may misinterpret phrases, censor sensitive or taboo topics, or filter and summarize discussions rather than translating them completely (Crawley et al., 2002; Flores, 2005).

There may also be differences in religion and spirituality, which may create a lack of trust between the patient and professional from different backgrounds. To create a sense of connection, healthcare professionals need to ask about religious or spiritual beliefs and practices, and how the patient could be supported in addressing religious or spiritual needs.

Another issue, which may have to be negotiated, is truth-telling. Individuals from certain cultures may develop mistrust or anger if the healthcare team insists on informing patients about their diagnosis or prognosis against the wishes of the family. Families often believe that such knowledge will result in a sense of hopelessness for the patient, which contributes to suffering. In this situation, it would be appropriate for the healthcare provider to ask whether the patient would want to know everything about his or her illness, and be cognizant of nonverbal communication when discussing serious information (Kagawa-Singer & Blackhall, 2001).

Consideration should also be given to the issue of family involvement in decision making. Disagreement and conflict between family and healthcare professionals may occur when the family insists on making decisions for patients who have decisional capacity. As healthcare professionals, it is important to identify the key members of the family and involve them in the discussions as desired by the patient. If the patient is capable of making decisions for himself or herself, yet the family requests that information be withheld from the patient and that they make the decisions, it is helpful to conduct a family meeting in which the patient, family members, and healthcare professionals are present. This may provide an opportunity to clarify issues, address conflicts, and provide clarity about the decisions and preferences of the patient.

At the end of life, cultural differences may also exist regarding the desire to enroll in hospice care. Health professionals need to understand the feelings and perceptions of patients and families that have varying cultural perspectives and emphasize that hospice is not a replacement for the family, but a way of providing resources to support the QOL for patients and their families (Kagawa-Singer & Blackhall, 2001).

Although there may be diversity in terms of desires, preferences, and expectations across cultures, there are also similarities among cultures. In a study of the needs and experiences of non–English-speaking hospice patients and families in an English-speaking country, McGrath, Vun, and McLeod (2001) found, based on focus groups that included Indian, Filipino, Chinese, and Italian cultural groups and their caregivers, that participants from all groups expressed the same issues. These included the importance of support from families, the pressures on family members to care for relatives at the end of life, lack of knowledge about hospice and PC services, lack of choice in how they wished to care for their family member, difficulty in talking about dying, and desire to care for a family member at home.

In providing quality PC for patients and their families, consideration should also be given to the following principles of culturally sensitive care (Council on Social Work Education [CSWE] Faculty Development Institute, 2010). The first principle is to *be knowledgeable about cultural values and attitudes*. Healthcare professionals should attend to a patient's needs in a sensitive, understanding, and nonjudgmental way and respond with flexibility as much as possible. The second principle is for healthcare practitioners *to attend to diverse communication styles*, including spending time listening to the person's needs, views, and concerns. The third principle is to *ask the patient for his or her preferences for decision making* early in care. As a fourth principle, it is important to *recognize cultural differences and varying comfort levels* with regard to personal space, eye contact, touch, time orientation, learning styles, and conversation styles.

The fifth principle is to *use a cultural advisor from the patient's ethnic or religious background* to clarify cultural problems or concerns if communication with the patient or family is unclear. If necessary, ask the older adult to identify a family spokesperson and respect the appointment made by the patient, even if the person is not a family member or does not live nearby. If the elder's preference is for family involvement, family meetings are opportunities to identify family needs and concerns, and an opportunity for the family to understand the patient's goals of care and EOL wishes.

A sixth principle is to *get to know the community, its people, and resources* to identify the availability of social support and needed resources. Healthcare professionals may establish relationships with key community resources to assist the seriously ill older adult and his or her family.

As a seventh principle, health practitioners should *create a culturally friendly physical environment* by designing facilities with artwork or pictures valued by the cultural groups to whom care is most commonly provided. Written materials should be available in the patient's language to enhance his or her understanding of the disease and the treatment options and to provide a sense of partnership in making healthcare decisions.

As an eighth principle, it is appropriate for health professionals to *determine the acceptability of patients being physically examined by a practitioner of a different gender*. Patients should also be asked whether they would want to have a family member present during the physical examination. Recognize that symptom recognition, as well as its reporting and meaning, may vary based on the patient's cultural background.

A ninth principle is for health professionals to advocate *for availability of services, accessibility in terms of cost and location, and acceptability of services* that are compatible with cultural values and practices of the person.

Last, the 10th principle is for health professionals to *conduct a self-assessment of their own beliefs* about illness and death. This includes how one's beliefs influence one's attitudes, how culture and religion influence a health professional's personal attitudes toward death, what kind of death does the health professional prefer personally, what efforts do they believe should be made to keep a seriously ill person alive, how their bodies should be disposed of, as well as what rituals they have participated in to honor the dead.

Having considered the importance of a comprehensive cultural assessment, it is also valuable for health professionals to have knowledge of the principles of culturally sensitive care. With this knowledge and understanding, health professionals are able to develop a culturally appropriate plan of care. This plan should address the cultural needs and expectations of patients and their families and support their trust of health professionals and satisfaction with healthcare.

In providing culturally sensitive care, DeSpelder (1998) also suggests that health professionals listen for and mirror the language patterns based on an individual's culture. Small differences in language, such as saying "passed away" or "passed on," can indicate much about the speaker's experience. For example, "passed away" may describe the deceased from the survivor's perspective, whereas "passed on" may imply a belief in life after death. Nurses also can attend to the cultural needs of their patients by gathering information about distinctive rituals, practices, and beliefs, particularly an understanding of what is meaningful to the individual person. This assessment involves listening, observing, and asking about practices of patients and families that may be unfamiliar to the nurse. Furthermore, nurses can determine the strengths an individual draws on when encountering death, dying, or bereavement. These strengths may include internal resources provided by the individual's belief system or past experiences and external resources, such as the comfort provided by cultural customs (DeSpelder & Strickland, 1999). In caring for patients and families at the EOL, nurses can enhance the QOL and quality of dying by promoting a respectful and peaceful death through the recognition of their spiritual and cultural needs.

Cultural mistrust is a dynamic that has implications not only for individual healthcare providers, but also for administrators of healthcare systems (Cort, 2004). Measures carried out by hospices to overcome cultural mistrust may include (a) hiring competent African American staff and minority volunteers; (b) respecting differences in cultural preferences; (c) conducting public education campaigns by television or community and local organizations, newsletters, and church presentations; (d) involving African American pastors in capacities that permit them to serve as bridges of trust between their communities and the healthcare system; and (e) avoiding perceptions of injustice and inequality by promising only the services that can be delivered (Cort, 2004).

Cultural competency is a set of academic and personal skills that allow practitioners to increase understanding and appreciation of cultural differences among groups (American Medical Student Association, 2001). Practitioners need to appreciate and accept cultural differences, to learn to culturally assess a patient to avoid stereotyping, and to explain an issue from another's cultural perspective. Areas of dissonance between patients and healthcare providers include historical distrust, varying interpretations regarding disability, the influence of family structure on decision making, and differences in willingness to treat diseases without symptoms, such as high cholesterol, or appreciating illness even when there are no observable manifestations.

Cultural competence entails listening with sympathy and understanding, acknowledging and discussing differences and similarities between perceptions of illness and its treatment, recommending treatments while remembering the patient's cultural perspectives, and negotiating and compromising when worldviews are in conflict (American Medical Student Association, 2001; Crawley et al., 2002). In improving the relationship between the health professional and the patient across cultures, it is important to maintain nonjudgmental attitudes toward unfamiliar beliefs and practices and to determine what is appropriate and polite caring behavior. It is respectful to begin by being more formal with patients, addressing them by their surnames, rather than by first name. Recognize that it may be a sign of disrespect to look directly into another's eye or to ask questions regarding treatment. Shaking hands as a form of introduction, although valued in American culture, may be inappropriate if a female is introducing herself to an Orthodox Jewish or Muslim male (Grossman, 1996). Furthermore, a firm handshake may be interpreted as aggressive or rude by members of Native American tribes.

Asian Americans may tend to have subtle and indirect communication styles that rely heavily on nonverbal cues, such as facial expression, body movements, use of physical space, and tone of voice. For example, a patient may bow his head or may disengage from you if he is in disagreement with the plan of care (Grossman, 1996). Nodding of the head in Asian or Hispanic populations may be merely a social custom, showing politeness and respect for a person in authority rather than agreement. Given this possibility, the healthcare provider may then ask specific questions that require the patient to express his or her feelings and wishes (Crawley et al., 2002).

It is important to ask questions to explore the patients' beliefs about health, illness, and prevention. Accept the fact that many patients use complementary therapies as well as Western medicine, and do not discount the possible effects of the supernatural on health. As health professionals, it is important to have knowledge of the patient's family and kinship structure to help ascertain the values, differing gender roles, issues concerning authority and decision making within a household, and the value of involving the family in the treatment (Grossman, 1996). Discussion with patients and their families may also involve the importance of food and eating as potentially enhancing a sense of community and as a way of supporting customs and heritage. Such information can assist the healthcare team in providing appropriate dietary instructions. For examples, Islamic law forbids ingestion of alcohol or pork, or meat from animals that are not appropriately slaughtered. Jewish patients may observe the laws of *kashrut*, which prescribe specific ways of food preparation and prohibit the eating of pork, shellfish, and wild birds. Individuals from Cuban backgrounds may prefer a diet that is high in calories, starches, and saturated fats, and modification of such a diet may mean just adhering to a modest serving size of those foods (Grossman, 1996).

Nurses' Cultural Self-Awareness and Development of Cultural Competency

By being aware of their own feelings, attitudes, preferences, and biases, nurses can be more in touch with themselves, acknowledging their right to their own beliefs, but not allowing those values and beliefs to take precedence over those expressed by patients and families. In order for nurses to care effectively for patients from diverse cultural groups, they also must be willing to learn about the cultures and presuppositions of their patients. The first step is to find educational sources that provide information about various cultures, while recognizing that there are individual differences even within the same culture because of differences in social stratum, personal experiences with illness and death, and individual preferences and values. By asking someone of a particular culture to help them understand the taboos and meanings of experiences and events, nurses can actively learn about other cultures. Nurses must also recognize that losses have different meanings from person to person and culture to culture and may be viewed as major or minor.

The key to accommodating cultural diversity is for nurses to understand their own values, beliefs, and

customs related to the celebration of life and coping with illness and death. Irish, Lundquist, and Nelsen's (1993, p. 45) thoughts are still relevant today as they suggest that health professionals assess the degree to which they are proactive in their attitudes and activities toward diversity. They suggest that health professionals ask themselves the following questions:

■ Have I actively sought information to enhance my own awareness and understanding of multicultural diversity?
■ Have I consciously pondered my own attitudes and behaviors as they either enhance or hinder my relationships with others?
■ Have I evaluated my use of terms or phrases that may be perceived by others as degrading or hurtful?
■ Have I suggested or initiated workshops or discussions about multicultural diversity?
■ Have I openly disagreed with racial, cultural, or religious jokes, comments, or slurs?
■ Have I utilized appropriate occasions to discuss the multicultural climate in the organization with my colleagues and with institutional administrators?
■ Have I complained to the author when I see a broadcast, an advertisement, or a newspaper article that is racially, culturally, or religiously biased?

Furthermore, DeSpelder (1998) suggests that healthcare professionals develop EOL cultural competence when they reflect on their own attitudes, beliefs, and practices toward dying and death. Nurses may explore for themselves

■ Their own beliefs about death and what influenced these attitudes
■ How significant religion is in their attitudes toward death
■ What kind of death they would prefer
■ If diagnosed with a terminal illness, whom they would want to tell
■ What efforts should be made to keep a seriously ill person alive
■ How they would want their bodies to be disposed
■ What their experience is of participating in rituals to remember the dead

Cultural Assessment

Developing cultural competency requires that nurses listen carefully and gather cultural information. The patient's background may provide clues about a person's beliefs; however, these are only assumptions unless validated by asking patients about their beliefs, needs, expectations, and wishes. Knowledge about a person's cultural group should serve only as a starting point or guideline in assessing individual beliefs and behaviors (Lipson, Dibble, & Minarik, 1996).

In conducting a cultural assessment, there are several areas to be addressed:

■ Identify the birthplace of the patient.
■ Ask a patient about his or her immigration experience.
■ Determine his or her level of ethnic identity.
■ Evaluate the degree of acculturation as evidenced by his or her use of the English language, the length of time spent in the United States, and his or her adaptation to the current environment.
■ Determine his or her family structure.
■ Identify the use of informal networks and sources of support within the community.
■ Identify who makes decisions, such as the individual patient, the family, or another social unit.
■ Assess his or her primary and secondary languages.
■ Determine the person's verbal and nonverbal communication patterns.
■ Consider gender and power issues within relationships.
■ Evaluate the patient's sense of self-esteem.
■ Identify the influence of religion or spirituality on patients' and families' expectations and behaviors.
■ Ascertain the patient's perceptions regarding discrimination or racism.
■ Identify cooking and dining traditions and the meaning of food for the culture.
■ Determine the patient's educational level and socioeconomic status.
■ Assess attitudes, beliefs, and practices related to health, illness, suffering, and death.
■ Determine patients' and families' preferences regarding location of death.
■ Discuss expectations regarding healthcare.
■ Determine the degree of fatalism or activism in accepting or controlling care and death.
■ Evaluate the patient's knowledge and trust regarding the healthcare system.
■ Assess the value and use of pharmacological, nonpharmacological, and complementary therapies.
■ Discuss how hope is maintained (American Medical Student Association, 2001; ELNEC, 2013).

■ UNDERSTANDING SPIRITUALITY

Spirituality and religiosity are often fundamental to the way patients face chronic illness, suffering, loss, dying, and death. Spirituality and religiosity are integral to holistic care and are important considerations, particularly because spirituality may be foundational to the patient's understanding of his or her disease and way of coping. Religious convictions may also affect healthcare decision making (Puchalski, 2001). Spiritual ideas are fundamental to PC because both are concerned with nonabandonment, value interpersonal relationships, and recognize the value of transcendent support (Purdy, 2002).

Although "spirituality" and "religion" are often used interchangeably in common conversations, spirituality is a broader concept than religiosity. "Spirituality" comes from the Latin word *spiritus*, which refers to breath, air, and wind. Carroll (2001) has described several conceptual models of spirituality found in the literature, which all reflect the whole person and his or her dimensions, but in different ways. Spirituality has been described as the energy found in the deepest core of an individual that represents his or her fundamental nature. It is an integrating and interconnecting life force that gives ultimate meaning and purpose in life, and may allow us to transcend our physical selves. Spirituality represents the harmonious interconnectedness with self, others, nature, and God, and can also be communicated through art, music, and relationships with family or the community (Puchalski & Romer, 2000). Spirituality further involves a melding of the individual's past, present, and future (Hicks, 1999). Even individuals who have no specific religion or faith background are spiritual beings and can have spiritual needs.

Spirituality, as a concept, also includes references to the soul, as well as spiritual needs, perspectives, and spiritual well-being. Downey (1997) describes spirituality as the awareness that there are levels of reality not immediately apparent and that there is a quest for personal integration in the face of forces of fragmentation and depersonalization. Therefore, spirituality is that aspect of human beings that seeks to heal or be whole (Puchalski, 2001). LaRocca-Pitts (2015) describes spirituality as "a way of living in the world, which means being ensconced in a web of meaningful connections or relationships that include family, friends, faith, work, play, and aspirations. It is from this web of meaningful connections that a person derives a sense of purpose, of identity, and of place in the world" (p. 55).

Moore (1992) has discussed the individual's spiritual quest, which is a process of "re-sacralization" of the self and the world in which we live. Individuals are embarking on spiritual journeys to discover the transcendent in daily life and in interpersonal relationships. The spiritual need is one of finding the mystery and sacredness of daily existence. Wink (1999) believes that individuals are searching for meaning outside of the confines of their religion. This is particularly important for individuals who are aging and who may be experiencing a chronic, debilitating, or life-threatening illness and who are questioning the meaning of not only their lives but also their suffering. Within this context, the spirit of the person seeks to transcend suffering through the virtues of love, hope, faith, courage, acceptance, and a sense of meaning in the encounter with death (Arnold, 1989). Puchalski and Ferrell (2010) believe that spirituality can help people to transcend suffering by helping them to "tap into their own inherent abilities to heal and cope, find meaning and purpose and hope, and do well with whatever life offers them" (p. 113).

Throughout a person's lifetime, and particularly as people age, religion and spirituality assist them to confront their finitude and vulnerability; to uncover meaning, value, and dignity in illness and death; to establish connection with others and a higher life force; and to find hope, love, and forgiveness in the midst of fear and despair. As such, spirituality engenders serenity and transcendence, thereby buffering stress.

As a chaplain, Ryan (1997) emphasizes the five fundamental spiritual needs of all people: (a) the need to find meaning in life, particularly during adverse circumstances; (b) the need for a relationship with a higher life force or transcendent being; (c) the need to transcend the sources of suffering; (d) the need for hope no matter how difficult life can be; and (e) the need to have others who share our life journey and care for us. As one example, a 68-year-old woman with advanced breast cancer revealed her spiritual need when she stated, "I only wish there was one person in this world who could tell me that they love me."

Religiosity is one means of expressing spirituality (Puchalski, 1998a). "Religiosity" refers to beliefs and practices of different faiths and an acceptance of their traditions, such as Catholicism, Eastern perspectives, Islam, Judaism, and Protestantism. For many people, religion forms a basis for meaning and purpose in life, and provides the moral codes by which to live. As illness can call into question the person's purpose in life and work, spiritual and religious issues often arise. Seventy-eight percent of Americans indicate that they receive comfort and support through religious beliefs and have greater trust in health professionals who ask them about their spiritual or religious needs (Ehman, Ott, Short, Ciampa, & Hansen-Flaschen, 1999; Koenig, 2002).

Spirituality and Palliative Care

Even as the physical body declines, healing, which means to make whole, can occur as spiritual needs are identified and spiritual care is given to restore a person to wholeness. Healing can be accomplished through the spiritual journey of remembering, assessing, searching for meaning, forgiving, reconciling, loving, and maintaining hope (Puchalski, 1998a). Holistic care, including care of the soul or spirit, is important to quality PC, whose goal is to enhance a person's QOL across the illness trajectory. People do want their spiritual needs addressed at the EOL and feel that health professionals should speak to patients about their spiritual concerns (Gallop, 1997). Furthermore, elder individuals who are dying express the need for companionship and spiritual support, particularly human contact, and to have the opportunity to pray alone or with others (The Nathan Cummings Foundation and the Fetzer Institute, 1997).

When providing PC for patients and their families, it is important to remember the following principles (Doka & Morgan, 1993):

■ Each person has a spiritual dimension.
■ Illness and death can be opportunities for spiritual growth.

■ Spiritual care may be different for each individual, depending on his or her religious or cultural background.
■ Spirituality is supported through formal and informal ways, such as religious practices, secular practices, symbols, rituals, art, prayer, and meditation.
■ Care should be offered in settings that accommodate the needs of religious or spiritual practices and rituals, and promote spiritual work.

In addition to the preceding list, a series of recommendations to enhance the quality of spiritual care as a dimension of PC was published in 2009 after an interprofessional consensus conference (Puchalski et al., 2009). The recommendations are as follows:

1. The domain of spiritual care should be included in all PC programs, quality-improvement plans, and electronic medical records.
2. Spiritual care should be monitored and assessed with measurable quality and process outcomes and metrics. Assessment tools should be evaluated to determine which are most efficacious and clinically relevant and standardized across PC settings.
3. Quality-improvement frameworks should be developed based on National Consensus Project Guidelines that relate to the structure, process, and outcomes of spiritual care.
4. Quality-improvement models specific to spiritual care should be tested.
5. Research should be conducted that contributes to improving spiritual care outcomes for PC patients. Recognizing the complex definition of spirituality and its difficulty in measurement, studies should use quantitative and qualitative methods.
6. Funding should be sought to evaluate the current state of the science, establish a research agenda, and facilitate research opportunities for spiritual care research.

Spirituality and Health

Physicians, psychologists, and other professionals continue to research the role of spirituality in healthcare. Ongoing research indicates that spirituality is related to mortality, coping, and recovery, because people with regular spiritual practices tend to live longer; utilize health beliefs in coping with illness, pain, and life stress; and have enhanced recovery from illness and surgery (Puchalski, 2001). Based on 724 quantitative studies, a systematic review of the literature during the 20th century revealed a significant relationship between religious involvement and better mental health, greater social support, and less substance abuse (Koenig, Pargament, & Nielsen, 1998). In a study of religious coping in 850 hospitalized patients, a significant inverse correlation ($p < .001$) was found between religious coping and depressive symptoms (Koenig et al., 1998).

In a study of religiosity, Bergan and McConatha (2000) reported that religious affiliation and private religious devotion increased with age across the life span. Based on a sample of 2,025 community-dwelling elder residents, it was found that religious attendance provided a persistent protective effect against mortality, even after controlling for the most potential confounders, such as social support, health status, and physical functioning.

Studies also indicate that those who are religious or spiritual have lower blood pressure, fewer cardiac events, better result following heart surgery, and longer survival in general (Koenig, 2002). Furthermore, spirituality counteracts stress-related physiological states that impair healing and facilitate coping with chronic pain, disability, and serious illness by enhancing a sense of control that interrupts the cycle of anxiety and depression (Koenig, 2002). Those who participate in religious services express less loneliness and isolation as they receive support from others and believe that God is with them.

Religion or spirituality also facilitates coping with chronic pain, disability, and serious illness by providing an indirect form of control that helps to interrupt the cycle of anxiety and depression. For some individuals, prayer provides a form of control by believing that through prayer they can influence their medical outcome; in contrast, others deliberately turn over to God their health situation (Koenig, 2002). The belief that God is with them provides relief from loneliness and isolation. Individuals who attend religious services also have an opportunity for socialization and support from others, whereas praying for others in need often provides a distraction from one's own pain (Koenig, 2002). These findings are supported by Sinclair, Pereira, and Raffin (2006), who provide a thematic review of the spirituality literature regarding PC. Both articles provide comprehensive discussions related to differences between religion and spirituality, spiritual assessment, instruments to measure spirituality, correlates to health, and spiritual interventions.

In terms of health consequences, religious involvement has been associated with improved attendance at medical appointments, greater adherence to medical regimens, and improved medical outcomes. Furthermore, religious or spiritual practices are believed to influence sympathetic and parasympathetic nerve pathways connecting thoughts and emotions to circulatory and immune system changes, and counteracting stress-related physiological states that impair healing (Koenig, 2002).

Interested in religiosity and spirituality, Heintz and Baruss (2001) conducted a study based on a sample of 30 people whose mean age was 72.6 years. Although some religious behaviors, such as frequent religious practice, prayer, and church attendance, were correlated with some dimensions of spirituality, many of the scores on the Expressions of Spirituality Inventory were independent of self-reported religious behaviors. These results reinforced the differences between the concepts of religiosity and spirituality.

In a qualitative study of 41 male and female residents aged 66 to 92 years, most of the older adults believed that a higher power was present in their lives, which supported them constantly and was perceived as protecting, guiding, helping, teaching, and healing them (Mackenzie, Rajagopal, Meibohm, & Lavizzo-Mourey, 2000). God was perceived to work through the mundane world, such as through the work of physicians, loving friends, and helpful strangers. Many felt that their relationship with God formed the foundation of their psychological well-being. The authors concluded that the subjective experience of spiritual support may form the core of the spirituality–health connection for older adults.

The Role of Religiosity and Spirituality in Coping With Serious Illness

As patients are faced with chronic or serious illness and eventually near death, they may experience despair, with spiritual and religious concerns intensified or awakened (Lo et al., 2002). The patient may struggle with the physical aspects of the disease as well as the pain related to mental and spiritual suffering. They may ask (Puchalski, 2002), "Why did this happen to me?" "Why is God allowing me to suffer?" "What will happen after I die?" "Will I be remembered or missed?" "Will I be able to finish my life's work?" True healing requires an answer to these questions, as healing can be experienced as acceptance of illness and peace with one's life (Puchalski, 2001).

It is through spirituality that people find meaning in illness and suffering and are liberated from their despair. Spiritual care changes chaos to order, and seeks to discern what, if any, blessings might be revealed in spite of and even through tragedy (Purdy, 2002). As people are dying, they want to be listened to, to have someone share their fears, to be forgiven by God or by others, and to believe that they will live on in the hearts of others or through their good works (Puchalski, 2002).

In a study of 19 individuals with advanced cancer, Thomas and Retsas (1999) learned through in-depth interviews that people with cancer developed a spiritual perspective that strengthened their approach to life and death. As cancer progressed, participants described the transaction of self-preservation by discovering deeper levels of understanding self, which incorporates a higher level of spiritual growth, spiritual awareness, and spiritual experiences.

Individuals at EOL also express spiritual needs. Based on a qualitative study of nine hospice patients, Hermann (2000) reported these individuals' need for religion, companionship, involvement, the ability to complete unfinished business, to experience nature, and have a positive outlook. Participants perceived spirituality as a broad concept that may or may not involve religion, and spiritual needs were closely linked to the purpose in and meaning of life. In studying older patients approaching EOL from advanced heart disease, it was found that 24% of the variance in their global QOL was predicted by their spirituality (Beery, Baas, Fowler, & Allen, 2002).

Taylor and Outlaw (2002) conducted a qualitative study to understand the use of prayer among persons with cancer (*n* = 30) and recognized that individuals with cancer use prayer to cope with their illness. Participants viewed prayer as personal communication involving or allowing transcendence. The communication, or prayer, was initiative and receptive. The initiative aspect of praying was to talk to God, get in touch with God, or beseech God, whereas the receptive aspect of prayer was characterized by phrases like "being quiet," "being accessible," and "listening to God." For these individuals, prayer meant being constantly conscious of God and coming to that higher intention in life. Participants' illness increased their awareness of the inadequacy of relying on self and the need to rely on a greater power. They described prayer as an active cognitive process, whereas others described prayer as a more passive process or as "prayer of the heart." Assistive strategies for praying included constructing a prayer, writing a prayer, relaxing, and reading religious material, and how one prayed depended on the purpose of the prayer. Some individuals prayed about healing, or that "God's will be done." Many prayed for forgiveness or to be a better person. Most prayed for family and friends who needed peace and support, and also included thanks and praise in their prayers that they were given another day to live. Through the process of prayer, many individuals believed that they benefited, whether their prayer was answered or not. From prayer, they expected that the "best will happen," or that they will receive comfort, forgiveness, or salvation. As health professionals, the implications for prayer are that clinicians can help by fostering a condition and environment conducive to prayer and can facilitate patients' use of prayer, which is unique to individuals.

Through a qualitative study involving 28 African American and European American adult patients with cancer and their caregivers, Taylor (2003) examined participants' expectations of nurses in meeting their spiritual needs. Participants identified six approaches of nurses in addressing spiritual needs: (a) showing kindness and respect; (b) talking and listening; (c) praying, such as offering verbal prayer or saying, "You are in my thoughts and prayers"; (d) connecting with authenticity and genuineness; (e) providing quality temporal nursing care, such as coming back to check on the patient; and (f) mobilizing religious or spiritual resources. The authors concluded that nurses need to consider their role in spiritual care and educate the public about their role as holistic healthcare providers.

The effects of spirituality on the well-being of people with lung cancer were studied by Meraviglia (2004). Based on a sample of 60 adults who were predominately female

and Caucasian, it was found that higher meaning-in-life scores were associated with higher psychological well-being and lower symptom distress. Prayer was positively related to psychological well-being, explaining 10% of meaning in life variance. Regression analysis indicated that meaning in life mediated the relationship between functional status and physical responses to lung cancer and explained 9% of the variance in symptom distress. The author concluded that this study supported the importance of providing spiritual care for patients with cancer.

Lorenz et al. (2005) examined religiousness and spirituality among HIV-infected Americans. Based on a sample of 2,266 patients receiving care for HIV infection, 80% reported a religious affiliation and the majority indicated that they rely on religious or spiritual means when making a decision or confronting problems. Women, older patients, and non-Whites were more spiritual, but the clinical stage of the disease was not associated with religiosity or spirituality. It was concluded that religious or spiritual organizations should be used to support patients diagnosed with HIV infection.

Mako, Galek, and Poppito (2006) reported that of the 57 patients with advanced-stage cancer in a PC hospital, 96% reported spiritual pain due to intrapsychic conflict, interpersonal loss, or conflict in relation to the dying. Depression was correlated with the intensity of spiritual pain but not with physical pain or severity of illness. The authors conclude that unaddressed spiritual pain contributes to overall suffering.

Based on a study of 50 adult hospice patients, Prince-Paul (2008) also reported strong positive correlations among spiritual well-being, communicative acts, and QOL at EOL, when controlling for physical symptoms, explaining 53.5% of the variance. A multicenter, cross-sectional study of 580 chronic pain patients found that spirituality and religiosity went far beyond just a "fatalistic acceptance" of chronic pain, but was found to be an active, adaptive, and mitigating coping mechanism for patients (Büssing et al., 2009). In another study of 69 patients with advanced cancer receiving radiation therapy, 84% of the cross-sectional study participants indicated a reliance on religious and spiritual beliefs to cope with cancer. In multivariate analysis, patient spirituality and religious coping were associated with improved QOL (β = 10.57, p <.001 and β = 1.28, p =.01, respectively). Most patients considered attention to spiritual concerns by their providers as an important part of their cancer care (Vallurupalli et al., 2012).

Spirituality or Religiosity During the Dying Process

The attitudes an individual holds regarding death and the dying process are embedded in his or her cultural and religious values. Values affect the way individuals conceptualize death and behave in relation to death (Meagher & Bell,

1993). Many people return to the religious legacies of their childhood during the dying process as that may have been the first time that they heard about death and learned about Christian resurrection (Satterly, 2001). A study of 170 patients receiving PC at home showed a marginal increase in the strength of individual spiritual beliefs over the time of the study as patients approached death (King et al., 2013).

During the dying process, it is important to explore guilt as central to a person's religious pain as well as the concept of forgiveness from his or her religious perspective. Religious rituals for cleansing or religious doctrine may allay feelings of remorse and guilt, providing for renewal of the soul and redemption. In supporting elders in spiritual pain, it may also be helpful to consider the concept of love. Most religious traditions provide a hopeful belief in the unconditional love of God, as well as reinforce the way unconditional love is offered to all, especially when an individual may have previously engaged in self-criticism or self-hatred (Satterly, 2001).

As individuals approach death, Doka and Morgan (1993) identified the spiritual need of individuals to die in a way that is consistent with their self-identity. For example, if a person's approach to life has also been to remain in control and "not give up the fight," then it would be expected that this person may not want to forego aggressive therapies, even if the chances of cure or remission are low. His or her spiritual need may be to continue to fight the disease. For those who are dying, Doka and Morgan (1993) also emphasize the spiritual task of finding hope that extends beyond the grave, as one seeks a sense of symbolic immortality. Individuals often need to feel that they are leaving a legacy, whether through having children or being remembered through their contributions to community, or through artwork, music, or writings.

Suffering and Spirituality

Suffering is a part of life and the human condition, with suffering either personally experienced in a physical, emotional, social, or spiritual way, or experienced when one is witness to another's suffering. Suffering varies with the type of disease, type of personality, and the relationship between these factors. Cassell (1982) defined "suffering" as "the state of severe distress associated with events that threaten the intactness of a person" (p. 639). Suffering is usually psychological and represents an afflicted state "that happens to a particular person on whom has been [in]flicted unendurable pain or other symptoms, losses, enduring fear, hardship, injury, disaster, grief, sorrow or care and who has been changed as a result of the burden" (Cassell, 2004, p. 76). Cassell (1982) also believes that many aspects of a person can be sources of or be affected by suffering such as personality, character, the past, relationships, life experiences, roles, one's rights and responsibilities, family, and cultural background.

According to Kahn and Steeves (1996), suffering is a private-lived experience of a whole person, unique to each individual. As such, suffering cannot be assumed present or absent in any given clinical condition or situation because suffering is dependent on the meaning of the event or loss. The experience of suffering is also both intrapersonal and interpersonal because it involves the person's own coping with suffering and the caring of others (Kahn & Steeves, 1996). "Meaningless suffering can lead to spiritual disintegration. However, the finding of transcendent meaning in the suffering experience can be a profound attenuator of how the suffering is experienced" (Emblen & Pesut, 2001, p. 42). Although we may not find answers about why we suffer, as a part of the human family we build relationships, communities, and society to reach out to one another to relieve suffering and sustain us in our struggle (McGann, 1997).

As a chaplain, Millspaugh (2005a) describes suffering as spiritual pain that involves an awareness of death, loss of relationships, loss of self, loss of purpose, and loss of control, which can be lessened by life-affirming and life-transcending purpose and an internal sense of control. The loss of self involves fears about death, loss of independence, loss of body image, loss of a God who can be bribed, and loss of relationships to others. As spiritual pain is often marked by a sense of being alone, the task of the practitioner is to earn the person's trust and to walk with him or her by being present with the belief that a greater Spirit is at work—a joining of spirits, which provides the sufferer with a sense of being understood and feeling a sense of control in the situation (Millspaugh, 2005b).

Although "suffering" and "pain" often are referred to interchangeably, they are not identical. In some cases, they are both present; at times, one exists without the other. The transition from pain to suffering can occur when pain is unrelieved and out of control or when the source of pain is unknown. The persistence of pain and uncertainty therefore can increase suffering exponentially. Yet, suffering can continue even when pain is controlled. Adunsky, Aminoff, Arad, and Bercovitch (2007) found, based on a sample of 177 end-stage cancer patients who had an expected life expectancy of less than 1 month to live in a hospice and using the Mini-Suffering State Examination (Aminoff, Purits, Noy, & Adunsky, 2004), that there was a low level of suffering despite maintaining a constant rate (68%) of the use of opioids at admission and through the last week of life. The reduction in the level of suffering in EOL cancer patients, in the face of pain needs, may be attributed to the medical and nursing care offered through hospice care.

Health professionals may recognize spiritual pain as the person expresses sorrow or grief and verbalizes a sense of meaninglessness or emptiness to life, fear and avoidance of the future, sense of hopelessness and despair, anger toward God, as well as isolation of self and others (Matthews, 1999). It is important to realize that indications of spiritual pain can be both verbal and nonverbal, and that just as physical pain may change in nature and intensity over time, so, too, can spiritual pain change over time. As death approaches, new spiritual issues may arise, which may or may not be accompanied by spiritual pain (O'Connor, 1993). Furthermore, although health professionals may wish to alleviate spiritual pain, it is important to recognize the meaning and value of experiencing pain from the patient's perspective. Some individuals may believe that pain will lead to salvation or act as a way of coming closer to God. Others may find the experience of losing a loved one to be a source of anger toward God and, as a result, feel distanced from the support that their personal relationship with God might bring for them at a time when they need it most. A survey of hospice patient family members found that 44% of the 134 participants reported some degree of anger toward God. Anger toward God was also found to have a positive correlation with self-reported depressive symptoms, which may have implication for family assessment, support, and referral (Exline, Prince-Paul, Root, & Peereboom, 2013).

At the EOL, suffering may also be exacerbated because of protracted or chronic illness, multiple simultaneous diseases and comorbid conditions, recurrent disease, and awareness of mortality. Because suffering has to do with a personal understanding of the physical, emotional, and spiritual self and their interrelationships, we learn about suffering only by the ways in which an individual expresses an awareness of the threats to his or her personal wholeness (Smith, 1996). In validating the Dignity Model, based on 211 patients receiving PC, Chochinov et al. (2006) reported that "not being treated with respect or understanding" and "feeling a burden to others" were the issues most identified as having an influence on dignity. In a logistic regression model, "feeling life no longer had meaning or purpose" was the only variable that predicted overall sense of dignity. Addressing these issues is believed to be the cornerstone of dignity-conserving care.

Using heuristic research, Wayman and Gaydos (2005) explored the question, "What is the experience of self-transcendance through suffering?" Four people were interviewed who self-identified as self-transcending. The themes were presented linearly but participants were able to move freely among themes. Participants identified a *turning point* in their suffering when they turned from self-identification with suffering, as it became a part of their lives but not who they were. This was a wake-up call and invitation to change. Then there was a *pause*—a forced pause in all activity due to treatment. This pause was followed by *confrontation* with their experience of suffering and their response, accepting their suffering for what it was. Participants *surrendered* to a new truth, which led to *extraordinary experiences* of peace and interconnectedness. These experiences became the *touchstones* of change as they reminded themselves of the lessons of suffering and the changes they had made.

Participants were changed after transcending their suffering and valuing their lives more, and became truly who they really were. Their transcending encouraged an unfolding of the hidden, with their inner selves becoming more congruent with their outer selves. This led to the desire for meaningful work and a sense of gratitude for the experience. Their humility grew as they honestly assessed themselves. The experience of self-transcendance is part of the patient's struggle and life journey, which can be supported when nurses facilitate opportunities for pause and reflection, and give reassurance and compassion, which facilitate a patient's sense of wholeness and well-being.

In a study of terminally ill patients ($n = 96$) on PC units and hospice, Schroepfer (2007) identified four critical events as motivating individuals to consider hastening their death: perceived insensitive and uncaring communication of a terminal diagnosis, unbearable physical pain, unacknowledged feelings regarding treatment, and dying in a distressing environment. To address these issues, the authors recommended changes in policies and practices that promote time for communication by health professionals coupled with appropriate training in communication skills. It is further recommended that support be offered by members of the interprofessional team to reduce suffering and take a proactive rather than reactive approach to EOL care.

Inherent in the discussion of requests for a hastened death is the concept of refractory suffering. Although suffering continues to be explored from the perspective of patients and families, few studies have examined the effect that witnessing refractory suffering has on PC clinicians. A qualitative study of 17 Australian PC practitioners from medicine (5), nursing (10), social work (1), and pastoral care (1) identified four subthemes in clinicians' experiences with refractory suffering that have implications for practice improvement and health (Breaden, Hegarty, Swetenham, & Grbich, 2012):

■ Must change the approach from "fixing" to "being with"
■ Maintain perspective
■ Negotiate and maintain boundaries
■ Live the paradoxes (detachment and commitment, desensitization and compassion, accepting limits and trying to do everything)

Reciprocal Suffering of Patients and Family

Within the context of life-threatening illness, suffering, in the form of physical, emotional, social, and spiritual distress, often becomes an experience not only of the patient but also of the family caregivers, as the suffering of one amplifies the distress of the other (Foley, 1995). Family members, like patients themselves, are in transition from living with the disease to anticipating the death of their loved one from the disease (Davies, Reimer, & Martens,

1994). They fear that death will occur in their absence, and may therefore refuse to leave the patient's side for even a moment. There is also a strong compulsion to attend to the patient's every need with disregard for their own needs. As the patient's illness progresses, the needs of the family also intensify and change, with both the patient and family caregivers potentially experiencing a significant compromise in the quality of their lives (Sherman, 1998).

Although family members may express the rewards of caring for terminally ill relatives, such care can have major psychosocial and physical effects, including heightened symptoms of depression, anxiety, psychosomatic symptoms, restrictions of roles and activities, strain in relationships, and poor physical health (Higginson, 1998). As witnesses to the patient's pain and suffering, family caregivers may also experience a sense of powerlessness, and are often frightened and confused by the dramatic physical and emotional changes they perceive in their loved one as the disease progresses (Loscalzo & Zabora, 1998).

Coyle (1995) gives examples of suffering, such as when patients experience despair, loneliness, and vulnerability; feel trapped by fear and bewilderment; experience loss and worry about treatment decisions; worry about being a burden; have financial concerns; experience abandonment; or fear dying, yet are weary of life and experience pain or the loss of hope. Families suffer as they assume the responsibilities of caregiving, watch the patient's deterioration, become exhausted, neglect their own needs, experience uncertainty about goals of care, and become anxious about the place of care. The suffering of family members also occurs because of fear of the dying process and the experience of the loss of life as it was, of the person they knew, and of hope, as well as guilt in wanting death to come soon.

There are also many conflicting emotions and adjustment tasks, including conflict among feelings of loss, sadness, guilt, difficulty in knowing how to talk with the person who is dying, and worry about dying and death (Beeney, Butow, & Dunn, 1997). Furthermore, the family caregiver must adapt to changes in family roles and responsibilities while attempting to meet the increased emotional needs of other family members and performing standard family functions (Doyle, 1994). Given that 25% of caregivers lose their employment due to caregiver responsibilities and nearly one third of families lose their major source of income or their savings, families also experience significant financial burdens (Lederberg, 1998). This may lead to feelings of anger, jealousy, and an increase in the family caregiver's own needs because of heightened psychological distress. In addition, there is often a loss of social mobility, as well as social abandonment by friends, which negatively affect the QOL of family caregivers (Lederberg, 1998).

From a spiritual perspective, family members may question the meaning of the illness and suffering. They often spend considerable time reviewing painful aspects of the past with feelings of regret for disagreements, conflicts,

or failures and a wish that relationships with the patient and with each other were somehow different. Buck and McMillan's (2008) study of the unmet spiritual needs of caregivers of patients with advanced cancer emphasizes that, based on a sample of 110 caregivers of hospice home care patients, the highest spiritual needs of caregivers were related to outlook such as seeing smiles, thinking happy thoughts, laughing, and being with family. Caregivers' unmet total needs were predicted by caregivers' outlook, caregivers' religion, and the patient's distress score. To reduce caregiver suffering, it was concluded that healthcare providers must be aware of the needs for positive thinking and reminiscing about happier times through storytelling or the use of pictures, and that chaplains may offer comfort through the reading of religious texts and speaking with caregivers about spiritual issues.

With each family member's unique experience of the stress, families may find it difficult to come together to effectively cope with the imposed life changes (Sherman, 1998). In their search for meaning, patients and families affirm spiritual values, change life priorities, and examine how the experience of illness has contributed to their personal growth. Like their dying loved one, they live day to day to make the most of the present as they prepare for death on practical, cognitive, emotional, and spiritual levels (Davies et al., 1994). In a recent pilot study, family caregivers of patients with advanced pancreatic cancer often described the concept of reciprocity in both suffering and strengthening. Caregivers described a sense of being in sympathy with the "ups" and "downs" of the patient in terms of mood and functional status and being comforted by the strength of the patients themselves in dealing with their illness (Sherman, McGuire, Free, & Cheon, 2013).

The hope is that through palliative nursing care, both patients and family members can transcend their reciprocal suffering and experience growth as they face the challenges of life-threatening or terminal illness (Sherman, 1998).

The Care of Those Who Are Suffering

Cassell (1982) believes that the ways to relieve suffering are first through the assignment of meaning to the injurious condition or event and second, through transcendence, which is the most powerful way of restoring an individual's personhood to wholeness. Watson (1986) proposes four generic meanings of suffering, which include *correction*, in which an individual is being corrected of his or her wrongdoing; *affirmation*, in which a person is affirmed of his or her "rightdoing" and the ability to be a role model for others; *naturalism*, in which the individual experiences general human destiny; and *altruism*, in which an individual's suffering will have benefit to others. In caring for those who are suffering, health professionals may help individuals come to a healthy, maintainable higher understanding to their suffering. From a theological perspective, Smith (1996) discusses the religious response to suffering and the possibility of transcendence of suffering through intellectual, ethical, and experiential dimensions of religion. The intellectual dimension involves the realization of some transcendent meaning, which connects the suffering person with some greater reality and delivers the individual from the threat of meaninglessness that is raised by illness and pain. The ethical dimension of religious life provides a perspective regarding how to interpret and respond to suffering. Suffering may be seen as a test of one's virtue or fidelity to God, as a test of the worth of religious commitment, or as an opportunity of personal transformation. Within the experiential dimension of religion, the life of oneself and others and of the relationship of these lives to each other and to God are contemplated. The religious experience of suffering may therefore enable an individual to provide redemptive relationships with others, including God, and experience transcendence.

In caring for the suffering, Spross (1996) believes that the role of the nurse is one of coaching. "Coaching is an interpersonal intervention that requires the therapeutic use of the self, involving one's mind, past experience, words, heart, and hand to comfort those who suffer" (Spross, 1996, p. 201). In coaching, the nurse

■ Establishes a trusting partnership
■ Assesses those who are at risk for suffering or who are vulnerable
■ Reassures patients that although their suffering may not disappear, they will not be abandoned
■ Identifies factors that may be eliminated or modified to alleviate suffering
■ Intervenes to facilitate expression of feelings, find meaning in suffering, and help patients and families redefine the QOL

Spross (1996) states that the ability to alleviate suffering or find meaning in the experiences of suffering depend on the intrapersonal and interpersonal qualities of the nurse. The nurse must be self-accepting, be secure in his or her own self-concept, and feel confident in strengthening others. As coach, the nurse values others and communicates that the individual's feelings, goals, and opinions are respected, while conveying that the person is trustworthy, responsible, capable of self-direction, and able to identify relevant goals and find meaning in life.

Watson (1986) believes that nurses and other health professionals can relieve suffering in six ways: first, by being a companion to sufferers by identifying the pain of their losses, and exploring the circumstance and extent of the loss; second, by listening for statements of meaning from a sufferer and allowing natural instincts and energy to know when to bring the issue of higher meaning; third, by valuing any self-disclosure on meaning that a sufferer offers, by analyzing the meaning of the statements and learning what the statement reveals about the sufferer's view of himself or herself; fourth, by encouraging the sufferer's interpretation of his or her experience; fifth, by validating the sufferer's interpretation of his or her own experience while clarifying the meaning, seeking further definition of the meaning, and offering alternatives for reframing the meaning; and finally, by identifying supportive resources and hoping for the sufferer to extend his or her identity and meaning in the future.

In alleviating the suffering of others, Bird (1986) offers seven principles to be considered within the context of nursing practice:

1. Remember that institutions do not dehumanize patients; staff members do.
2. Assume responsibility for morale whenever you are in the chain of command.
3. Be a whole person yourself, with a healthy sense of humor and attitude.
4. Do not add clinical ineptitude to the further suffering of patients.
5. Be empathetic rather than sympathetic to patients' needs; otherwise, human suffering can emotionally devastate the nurse.
6. Offer holistic care and well-chosen words to allay suffering.
7. Determine to touch the life of at least one patient daily with some depth.

Halifax (1999) believes that healthcare providers, patients, and families can go to the root of their own suffering and transform the suffering into inherent wisdom. As a Buddhist, she reminds health professionals to come to the caregiving relationship with loving kindness, to bring compassion by being in touch with one's own and others' suffering, to see joy in the well-being of others, and to nurture equanimity in others.

The Role of Hope in Spiritual Well-Being

Cousins (1979) has said that death is not the ultimate tragedy of life; rather, that tragedy is being separated from our connection with others and separated from a desire to experience the things that make life worth living—to be separated from hope. Spirituality may help people to cope with their dying, as it may offer hope. In early illness, the hope may be for cure of the disease by treatment, and later on for hope of prolongation of life. When cure is not possible, hope may be to see a loved one, to have a day without pain, to celebrate a certain life event, or to have the time to travel or complete unfinished business. Eventually, hope may be for a peaceful death. It may be hope that allows seriously ill individuals to find courage and strength to transcend their suffering, and teach others how to die with dignity.

Mitchell (1997) offers a definition that hope is not a belief that something is going to go well, but rather a belief that whatever happens will make sense, no matter how it turns out. For patients who are dying, "hope" may be defined as "an inner life force that helps each dying person to live life until the moment of death" (Parker-Oliver, 2002, p. 115). Indeed, "hope" may be defined as the positive expectation for meaning attached to an event, recognizing that individuals shape their hopes by finding new meanings for living (Parker-Oliver, 2002). Hope allows a sense of control and promotes an active rather than passive participation in life's events. Even in dying, people have the hope to discover new meanings.

The challenge for healthcare professionals is therefore to help individuals find hope as they search for meaning in their illness, suffering, and death. This can happen as professionals assist individuals to identify key relationships, to facilitate caring relationships, and to encourage the opportunity to heal relationships and complete unfinished business. Byock (1997) encourages the completion of relationships by saying, "I forgive you," "forgive me," "I love you," "thank you," and "goodbye." Through the encouragement of short-term, attainable goals, hope can also be promoted by recognizing and encouraging a sense of determination and courage in the face of adversity. Gum and Snyder (2002) conclude that hope can be maintained when healthcare providers offer clear information, control symptoms, and maintain functionality.

Hope can also be found within the context of spirituality, as spiritual belief systems offer hope for happiness and a promise of an afterlife. Spirituality offers hope for living on in the world through a connection with others, traditions, and rituals and through establishing legacies. Hope can also be easily discovered by just asking patients what is meaningful to them and what they want to do with the remainder of their lives. Based on a study of 69 participants, aged 65 or older, Theris (2001) reported a significant difference in hope based on the religion of participants. Based on a one-way analysis of variance (ANOVA), Catholic participants expressed greater hope than those of the Jewish faith, and another significant difference existed between participants of the Protestant and Jewish faiths. There was also a significant, positive correlation between spirituality and level of hope ($r = .73$, $p = .000$). In a multiple-regression analysis, which was used to test for the combined contribution of spirituality and connectedness with others to levels of hope, only spirituality emerged as a significant predictor of hope. The authors concluded that connection with oneself and connection with a higher being was especially important in the maintenance of hope in nursing home residents. Such results are consistent with the findings of Buchanan (1993), who reported, based on a sample of 160 older adults who were depressed or not depressed, that higher levels of spirituality, hope, health, and social support were positively correlated with meaning in life and that there was an inverse relationship between meaning in life and depression.

Duggleby (2000) found that hope was a process of enduring suffering through trust in a higher power and making meaning of one's life. Despite the stage of illness and a situation of poor prognosis, practitioners can provide hope and a positive outlook by discussing goals of care, offering symptom control, providing supportive resources, and promising the patient that they will not abandon her or him (Barclay et al., 2007).

For those who are dying, the focus of hope changes from a hope in the future or a redefinition of the future, to a hope of living day to day. The focus of hope for those with advanced disease is also hope for no more suffering, for life after death, and for their families to not suffer when they are gone (Duggleby, 2001). At times, the most important way to provide hope is by listening attentively and being physically present, which convey a sense of value and affirmation of worth. Hope is then gained that the patient will not be abandoned and isolated (Duggleby, 2000). Guided by Parse's theory of human becoming, Hutchings (2007) conducted a qualitative study of eight people who were dying. The interviews illustrated that persons at the end of life still envision hopes and possibilities despite declining function and decreased energy. Such findings help health professionals understand that dying patients co-create meaning day by day while emphasizing the importance of bearing witness to the struggles, joys, and hope of dying persons.

Rawdin, Evans, and Rabow (2013) studied the association of hope, pain, distress, and spiritual well-being in 78 oncology outpatients using the Hearth Hope Index (HHI; Herth, 1992). As with previous published studies on hope and pain, there was a negative correlation of hope with average pain intensity ($p = .2$), worst pain intensity ($p < .01$), and pain interference with function ($p < .05$). However, this study demonstrated that the negative correlation is eliminated when depression and spiritual well-being are adjusted for in the multivariate linear regression model, suggesting that hope more strongly correlates to other psychospiritual factors than to pain.

Learning About Spiritual Assessment and Caregiving

Health professionals need to be attuned not only to their own cultural beliefs but also to their own spirituality before participating in spiritual care. Personal preparation for spiritual caregiving includes the professional self-evaluating his or her personal spirituality; reviewing personal beliefs, opinions, and biases; understanding the meaning of spirituality; becoming aware of how one's own religious beliefs influence caregiving; and establishing a trusting patient–provider relationship (Hermann, 2000; Saguil & Phelps, 2012).

As in the care of all patients and families, health professionals caring for dying patients and their families must learn the specific techniques for addressing spirituality in clinical practice, including how to conduct a spiritual assessment. This also requires that the health professional be totally present and open by listening actively to spiritual issues (Hermann, 2000). Learning spiritual assessment and caregiving can also occur through a combination of teaching/learning strategies, including small-group discussions; reflective writing; storytelling; use of poetry; case presentation and discussion; panel discussions with chaplains, patients, and healthcare practitioners; role-playing with standardized patients; and attending lectures on the role of spirituality in healthcare (Puchalski, 2001).

In providing spiritual care, healthcare professionals must remember that religion is only one way of enhancing spiritual well-being. Conversations about life, love, hope, trust, and forgiveness may renew the spirit of both patients and healthcare providers. Although the perspectives of health professionals are of personal value in one's role as a health practitioner, it is important to be nonjudgmental, never imposing one's own beliefs and values on the patient or family and always remembering that it is the spiritual or religious perspective of the patient or family that is important. Indeed, the therapeutic value of the self will be recognized through listening, being present, and being available.

Millspaugh (2005b) suggests that in providing spiritual care for individuals who are suffering, practitioners must be able to maintain boundaries, empathize, contain their own suffering, focus and attend to the sufferer's agenda, use theology as well as the social and behavioral sciences to inform assessments and interventions, and engender a sense of security and comfort.

Conversations About Spiritual or Religious Issues

Some factors might hinder conversations about spiritual or religious issues between the provider and the patient. Some of these factors include lack of experience with the subject, lack of time, and lack of spiritual-assessment tools incorporated into the professional practice (Saguil & Phelps, 2012). A study done in various medical centers regarding spiritual assessments found that out of 456 patients, "33% wanted their physician to inquire about religious beliefs, 19% wanted their physician to pray with them, and, if dying, 70% would want their physician to know their beliefs and 50% would want their physician to pray with them" (Saguil & Phelps, 2012).

Conversation regarding spiritual needs often begins with the use of open-ended questions such as, "Do you have any thoughts about why this is happening to you?" Practitioners can also encourage the patient to say more with such statements as, "Tell me more about that." When

exploring spiritual concerns, the practitioner should acknowledge and normalize the patient's concerns by making comments such as, "Many patients ask the same question" and responding with emphatic comments such as, "That sounds like a painful situation" (Lo et al., 2002).

Pitfalls in discussions about spiritual or religious issues near the end of life often occur by trying to solve the patient's problems or resolve unanswerable questions; going beyond the practitioner's expertise or role in providing spiritual care; imposing one's beliefs on the patient; or providing premature reassurance, which may appear superficial or deter the disclosure of other important issues or emotions (Lo et al., 2002). When patients inquire about the religious background of the practitioner, they may be inquiring to determine whether it is safe to talk about spiritual or religious issues, or they may prefer to talk to someone who shares the same religious faith. However, practitioners may answer the question regarding their religious background, but need not explicate or expound on their religious or spiritual beliefs (Lo et al., 2002). If the patient asks for details, it is appropriate to refocus the conversation back to the patient.

In addition to clarifying the patient's spiritual concerns and needs by following spiritual cues and exploring emotions with emphatic support, healthcare professionals may also do the following:

■ Make wish statements such as, "I also wish you were not ill."
■ Identify common goals for care and reach agreement on clinical decisions.
■ Mobilize support for the patient and family from family, church members, or the community (Lo et al., 2002).

In situations in which the patient or his or her family are praying for a miracle even in medically futile situations, the role of health professionals is to respect their beliefs and remain supportive by trying to understand their worldview and the role their beliefs have in coping. Criticism or confrontation will lead to distrust and close the dialogue between the healthcare professional and the patient. When older patients and their families feel that they can talk to health professionals about their religious or spiritual beliefs, there is greater chance that they will accept what the professional is saying. A response may be as follows: "Sometimes God answers our prayers for healing in interpersonal ways that may ultimately be more important than physical healing" (Koenig, 2002, p. 492).

Conducting a Spiritual Assessment

Holistic care involves assessment not only of physical, emotional, and social needs, but also of spiritual needs and expectations. A *spiritual history* is a history about a person's values or beliefs that explicitly opens the door to conversations about the role of spirituality and religion in the person's life (Puchalski & Romer, 2000). A spiritual history is important not only to identify ways individuals may cope with adverse life circumstances, but also to examine potential negative effects in which religious beliefs are a source of distress and emotional turmoil (Koenig, 2002). Religious pain is a condition in which the patient feels guilty over the violation of the moral codes or values of his or her religious tradition. This may arise due to major transgressions, such as abortion, adultery, overt cruelty, or from minor transgressions such as not seeking a second opinion or failing to take better care of one's self. As a result, the patient may feel that God is disappointed in his or her past or present behaviors, actions, or thoughts (Satterly, 2001). Feelings of guilt are often accompanied by a fear of punishment from God, that God does not love him or her, or that God has abandoned this person in a time of need.

Although it is not the health professional's responsibility to solve spiritual problems or provide answers, health practitioners need to conduct a spiritual assessment to identify when a patient or family member is experiencing spiritual distress. It is important to create an environment that nurtures the patient's exploration of spiritual needs and concerns and supports the patient in his or her search for answers. A spiritual history or assessment should be completed with each new patient visit and on annual examinations, as a part of routine history taking (Puchalski, 2001). When conducting a spiritual assessment, it is important to be aware that not everyone is spiritual or religious and this may be seen as offensive (Timmins & Caldeira, 2017). A spiritual history inquires about the role that religion or spirituality plays in the patient's ability to cope with illness. Affiliation with a religious or spiritual community is important for many individuals and often serves as an extended family for many adults, especially those who live alone or have limited family support (Koenig, 2002).

In taking a spiritual history, Puchalski (1998b) suggests that the acronym FICA be used:

- "F" refers to faith as identified by the question "What is your faith or beliefs and do you consider yourself religious or spiritual?"
- "I" refers to influence, which is assessed by the question, "How does your faith or spirituality influence your medical decisions?"
- "C" refers to community and is related to the question, "Are you a part of a spiritual or religious community?"
- "A" refers to addressing spiritual concerns as exemplified by the question, "Would you like someone to address your spiritual needs or concerns?"

As another approach, Highfield (2000) uses the letters from the word "spirit" to remember questions appropriate to a spiritual interview, specifically:

- S—Spiritual belief system (religious affiliation)
- P—Personal spirituality (beliefs and practices of affiliation that the patient and family accepts)
- I—Integration with a spiritual community (role of the religious/spiritual group; individual's role in the group)
- R—Ritualized practices and restrictions (beliefs that healthcare providers should remember during care)
- I—Implications for medical care
- T—Terminal-events planning (impact of beliefs on advance directives; contacting the clergy)

A more recently developed spiritual assessment approach is known by the acronym FACT (LaRocca-Pitts, 2009):

- F—Faith/beliefs: What is your faith or belief? Do you consider yourself a spiritual person or person of faith? What things give your life meaning and purpose?
- A—Active (or Available, Accessible, Applicable): Are you currently active in a faith community? Are you part of a religious or spiritual community? Is support for your faith available to you? Do you have access to what you need to apply your faith/beliefs? Is there a person or a group whose presence and support you value at a time like this?
- C—Coping (or Comfort), Conflicts (or Concerns): How are you coping with your medical situation? Is your faith (your beliefs) helping you cope? How is your faith (your beliefs) providing comfort in light of your diagnosis? Do any of your religious beliefs or spiritual practices conflict with medical treatment? Are there any particular concerns you have for us as your medical team?
- T—Treatment plan: This step of the FACT model sets it apart from the previous spiritual-history tools in that it asks the clinic to make an assessment of the patient's spiritual needs and coping, and to develop a treatment plan that may involve referral and/or interventions that may take the form of prayer, counseling, or scriptural reading recommendations (LaRocca-Pitts, 2009).

Four FACTs is a recently modified version of the original FACT spiritual assessment (LaRocca-Pitts, 2015):
- Facts: What are the facts of the patient's current medical or clinical situation?
- Feelings: How does the patient feel about his or her current medical or clinical situation?
- Family/Friends: Whom does the patient consider to be family and friends?
- Faith: What is the patient's faith, belief, worldview, or spiritual practice?

Spiritual assessment further includes assessment of personal beliefs, sources of meaning and hope, values, belief in an afterlife, and sense of connection to self, others, nature, and God. Although use of formal spiritual-assessment tools provides the basic framework for health practitioners, informal assessment allows for spiritual care to occur on a continuum. Creation of a trusting, therapeutic relationship with the individual may enhance the effectiveness of an informal assessment (Timmins & Caldeira, 2017). Health practitioners begin to address spirituality by asking such questions as, "How are your spirits?" "How do you define your spirit?" "What nourishes your spirit?" or "How have you relieved your spiritual pain in the past?" (O'Connor, 1993). For adults with life-limiting or life-threatening illness, valuable questions to explore include the following:

■ Are you suffering in physical, emotional, social, or spiritual ways?
■ What is the meaning of illness and suffering?
■ Do you see purpose in your suffering?
■ Are you able to transcend your suffering?
■ Are you at peace, or feeling hope and despair?
■ Do your personal beliefs help you to cope with anxiety about pain and death, and provide a way for achieving peace? (Puchalski & Larson, 1998)

Hermann (2000) further asks in a spiritual assessment such questions, as "What gives your life meaning and purpose?" "Do you have goals you would still like to achieve?" "How has your diagnosis changed the meaning of your life?" "What kinds of things do you hope for?" and "To whom do you turn for help?" Practitioners should also observe for objective data such as signs of depression; flat affect or refusal of treatment; presence of religious, spiritual, or inspirational books or other literature; or religious jewelry (Hermann, 2000).

Instruments to Measure Spirituality and Suffering

In the past several years, there has been a focus on the role of spirituality, as distinct from religion, in coping with illness. However, there remains a dearth of well-validated, psychometrically sound instruments to measure aspects of spirituality (Peterman, Fitchett, Brady, Hernandez, & Cella, 2002). One instrument that is a psychometrically sound measure of spiritual well-being is the Functional Assessment of Chronic Illness Therapy–Spiritual Well-Being (FACIT-Sp; Peterman, et al. 2002). This instrument comprises two subscales, one measuring a sense of meaning and peace, and the other assessing the role of faith in illness. The FACIT-Sp has convergent validity with five other measures of spirituality and religion in samples of early-stage and metastatic cancer diagnoses, as well as documented reliability. A total score can be obtained.

A second spirituality assessment instrument with clinical utility is the Paloutzian and Ellison (1982) Spiritual Well-Being Scale, which has also been administered to 70 family members caring for a relative with life-limiting

illness. This 20-item instrument yields three scores: a total score of spiritual well-being (overall score); an existential well-being score, which relates to feelings about meaning and purpose in life, feelings about the future, and sense of well-being; and a religious well-being score, which represents a sense of support and connection with God (Kirschling & Pittman, 1989).

Such instruments are of value in conducting research studies that explore the relationships of spirituality and QOL for patients on PC. By identifying a patient's or family member's sense of spiritual well-being or spiritual distress, spiritual interventions may be provided to maintain or improve spiritual well-being and, it is hoped, the QOL and quality of dying as perceived by patients and family members.

A relatively recent review identified 10 instruments specifically designed for the clinical assessment and research of suffering (Krikorian, Limonero, & Corey, 2013). Each instrument was assessed for ease of scoring; time to administer; and readability/comprehension; as well as for various psychometric properties, including content and construct validity, internal consistency, test–retest reliability, responsiveness, interpretability, agreement, and floor–ceiling effects. Of the available tools, PRISM (Pictorial Representation of Illness and Self Measure) is a validated, self-administered tool that is regularly used, is widely accepted, and was found to have the strongest psychometric properties of all the instruments studied (Krikorian et al., 2013).

Spiritual Caregiving

"Spiritual care is so much more than religious care. Spiritual care discovers, reverences, and tends the spirit—that is the energy or place of meaning and values—of another human being" (Driscoll, 2001, p. 334). In providing spiritual care, health professionals express the capacity to enter the world of others; respond to fears, concerns, and feelings with compassion; and bear witness to the physical, emotional, social, and spiritual dimensions of their suffering. As adults age, healthcare professionals can provide an opportunity to find intrinsic dignity, which comes from being a human being with inherent value and worth. By reviewing past life experiences, health professionals can assist individuals to reflect on their life accomplishments and the value of their relationships with others, to forgive or be forgiven by others, and to say goodbye. Support can be given to patients to complete unfinished tasks or goals and make peace with themselves or with God.

During hospitalizations, health professionals may ask whether the person would like to speak with the clergy or chaplain or have the opportunity to attend a hospital worship service. Patients may also be asked whether they would like someone to pray with or for them or to have spiritual reading materials. Prayer has been identified as the most frequently reported alternative treatment modality of elders, with women and Blacks using prayer as a coping strategy significantly more than men and Whites (Dunn & Horgas, 2000). At times, if the patient is of the same faith background as the health professional, the patient may request prayer. However, prayer is appropriate only when the patient wants it and will be comforted by it (Koenig, 2002). Prayer should not be prescribed because the risk is that the intention is not patient centered, but provider centered, and in that context prayers offered by health professionals may be viewed as coercive (Koenig, 2002). The existing religious or spiritual beliefs of the patient should be supported and encouraged, yet the EOL is not the appropriate time to introduce new or unfamiliar spiritual beliefs or practices (Koenig, 2002). In a study of 30 individuals with cancer, Taylor, Outlaw, Bernardo, and Roy (1999) reported that several individuals described hesitancies about petitionary prayers for particular things, for cure, or for themselves, and described inner conflicts about releasing control to God.

If a person is not religious or does not want a health professional to address religious issues, spiritual conversations around hope, love, courage, and forgiveness can occur in the provider–patient relationship (Koenig, 2002). Patients and health professionals of different faith backgrounds can appreciate the commonalties of basic human needs, such as love and hope, and explore issues of coping and what it means to live with an illness. Although health professionals can assess spiritual needs and address uncomplicated spiritual issues, caring and listening are the interventions needed, not giving advice or trying to address spiritual problems (Koenig, 2002).

As a member of the interprofessional team, addressing spiritual problems is often the role of the chaplain or clergy. The chaplain is a healthcare professional who has been trained to offer spiritual care to all people of any or no religious tradition and whose primary focus is the spiritual needs of patients, families, and staff (Driscoll, 2001). Like other members of the PC team, chaplains are alert to the expressed needs of the patient. As counselors, they take time to listen, discern the significance of the words spoken, intuit the importance of what is unspoken, and affirm the value of shared silence (Purdy, 2002). Often, spiritual support consists of listening to rhetorical questions from patients wanting an honest hearing of the question, rather than an answer. Patients may want to explore with chaplains whether God exists, the meaning of mortality, what Heaven is like, who goes to Hell, the integrity of doubt, the possibility of a miracle, the need to forgive, or the loneliness of suffering (Purdy, 2002). Patients and their families experience spiritual support when interprofessional team members actively listen to their anxiety and allow discussion of the question, "Are we doing the right thing here?" (Purdy, 2002). Health professionals can also provide support by silent witnessing, presence, as well as serving as a liaison with other

health professionals in addressing physical, emotional, and spiritual needs (Hicks, 1999).

A cross-sectional multihospice study of 66 hospice nurses found that the nurse participants deemed spiritual care to be highly important. Although generalist spiritual assessment and care is within the purview of nursing practice, participants acknowledged the importance of spiritual care performed by a chaplain or pastor (Tiew, Kwee, Creedy, & Chan, 2013).

Humor also has an effect on the spiritual aspect of healing, as many patients find humor "spiritually uplifting." As an element of spirituality and a coping method for spiritual growth and healing, humor can be transcendent, momentarily removing one from an isolated state to join in surprise at ludicrous human situations (Johnson, 2002). In a study of nine women with breast cancer, participants stated that they looked for meaning in their lives through spirituality and humor, as humor helped them to laugh at themselves and life. For some, it appeared that God had a sense of humor and that finding humorous moments was a step to recovery, as humor heals and gives hope to survive the moment (Johnson, 2002).

Health professionals can also encourage patients to socialize with friends, family, and children, as well as encouraging them to help others, even if only by active listening. Supporting others often preserves a person's meaning in life and sense of usefulness. Adults can also pass on their legacy to others by recording personal histories, telling stories, and reminiscing about the past. Conducting a life review by asking questions, such as tell me about tranquil times in your life, a chaotic time, what your childhood was like, what obstacle you overcame, what you have achieved, and what your fondest memories are, help individuals to recontextualize and reframe mistakes and failure, allow forgiveness of self and others, reclaim an unlived life, and take advantage of current opportunities to participate in enjoyed activities (Jenko, Gonzalez, & Seymour, 2007). If the person is isolated, the health practitioner can suggest his or her watching spiritual or religious television programs or provide an opportunity to enjoy his or her favorite sacred or secular music, or other forms of art (Hermann, 2000). Practitioners may encourage opportunities for patients to experience nature in whatever ways they can, such as a walk or wheelchair ride in the garden or courtyard, or as they sit outside feeling the air and warmth of the sun.

In the present moment, spiritual uplifting can also occur as the practitioner attempts to create meaning and a source of pleasure in the present moment. As one example, a bed-bound patient with parkinsonism found a moment of meaning and pleasure in his day by telling the nurse practitioner a story from his childhood while anticipating his family bringing him a favorite meal the following day. Spiritual care can also involve "making meaning" through other forms of life review, such as looking at old photographs or personal memorabilia, reading old letters or diary entries. By such efforts, health-care professionals can acknowledge the individuality of a person and promote his or her sense of connection to self, others, and nature, thereby supporting his or her spirits and sense of well-being.

Chochinov and Cann (2005) reinforce not only general approaches to spiritual care, such as those offered by PC and psychotherapeutic approaches, but also specific approaches, such as relief of symptoms, as well as exploring guilt, encouraging forgiveness of self and others, and using complementary practices that promote healing. Other supportive interventions include music and art and supportive–affective programs that focus on the spirit, emotions, and relationships.

Spiritual support may also be available through parish nursing, which expands home health and public health provider roles. Parish nursing uses the faith community as a cooperative means of successful health promotion and maintenance for the older adult (Boland, 1998).

■ SPIRITUAL AND RELIGIOUS PERSPECTIVES ON DEATH

Losses in life often challenge our faith and philosophical systems. Those who experience loss and grief may differ regarding the religious and spiritual perspectives from which they seek answers and search for meaning, and to which they turn for ritual, comfort, and support (Doka & Davidson, 1998). Understanding the ways that spirituality or religiosity facilitate or complicate the adjustment to loss and grief is a critical task for those involved in PC.

Death From a Jewish Perspective

Judaism began when the descendants of Abraham's grandson Israel were enslaved in Egypt. Moses led these descendants to Palestine. During this time, the law of God, known as *the Torah*, was divinely revealed to Moses. The Sabbath is celebrated from sunset on Friday to sunset on Saturday. It is the day of rest. The degree to which a Jew observes the Sabbath and other rituals depends on whether he or she is Orthodox, Conservative, or Reformed (Sherman, 2004a). For Jews, one's focus is on life and its preservation and in fostering and establishing religion in the life of people on Earth, rather than focusing on the world beyond. The Jewish faith offers consolation in death by affirmation of life. Sickness and death are viewed as neither punishment nor reward. Death is not considered evil but rather inevitable and natural, as it comes from God and should not be feared. Jewish teaching says that the soul exists before the body comes into existence and continues to live on after the body is dead. Although the Orthodox believe

in resurrection, this belief may be figurative rather than literal (Grollman, 1993).

Jewish death practices help the bereaved to realize that the loved one is dead and to learn to gradually fill the void he or she left in a constructive way. The memory of the deceased must be perpetuated. Although Jews are usually buried, cremations are also done. A religious rite is the rending of mourners' clothes, signified by the cutting of a black ribbon that is pinned to the mourners' clothing in the funeral chapel or cemetery. This signifies the loss of a loved one. The Jewish funeral is a rite of separation, in which the casket actualizes the experience. The rabbi recites prayers expressive of the spirit of Judaism and the memory of the deceased. *Shiva* refers to the 7 days of intensive mourning beginning right after the funeral. The bereaved remain at home and condolence calls are made to pay respects to the family. A shiva candle burns for 7 days and the family prepares the meal of consolation held after the funeral, known as *seudat havra'ah*. Following shiva come the 30 days of *sloshim*. During this time, normal activities are resumed but entertainment is avoided. If a parent dies, the mourning continues for an entire year. The mourner's prayer is called the *Kaddish*, which is recited during the weekly Sabbath as a pledge to dedicate one's life to God, acknowledge the reality of death, and affirm life. The anniversary of the death is called *yahrzeit*. The Kaddish prayer is recited and yahrzeit candles are again kindled (Grollman, 1993).

Death From the Roman Catholic Perspective

Catholics believe that Jesus experienced suffering, grief, death, and resurrection. Jesus's death and the death of all is viewed as a part of God's divine providence. As sinners, human beings experience the tragedy of death, yet are beneficiaries of forgiveness and liberation. Resurrection is integral to death in Catholicism. Catholics believe that Christ died and rose from the dead, and that faith will allow them to see death as an entry into life with God. Confession and communion are important rituals conducted by priests. The sacrament of the anointing of the sick provides bodily and spiritual renewal, and has replaced the term "the last rites," which was viewed as a harbinger of death.

Since the second Vatican Council, the contemporary Catholic view places emphasis on risen life. There is a move from a preoccupation with sin and death toward an orientation of blessing for a Christian life. Christians follow Jesus into the mystery of death in order to find a life like his own (Miller, 1993). The funeral becomes a time of thanksgiving and consolation; the funeral Mass is offered on behalf of the deceased, aiding him or her to the other side of death and giving the bereaved the consolation of hope. It is believed that Christ accompanies the dying person to heaven and that dying is an act of faith in God (Miller, 1993).

Death From the Protestant Perspective

In Protestantism, spirituality is viewed as a dimension of humanness, a process of interaction, and an awareness of relationship. Spirituality cannot be lived in the abstract, but rather is lived through one's religion, which is regarded as a cultural institution (Klass, 1993). God is viewed as a single being who spoke to His people through the Bible; God protects, but also judges. Each Protestant has a direct and personal relationship with God, unmediated by priest or sacrament. The church is viewed as a voluntary association of believers. The Protestant community consists of the local congregation or particular denomination supporting interpersonal relationships, yet is often split along racial, ethnic, and social class lines (Klass, 1993). Anointing the sick is an accepted act by some groups and prayers are given to offer support to the sick and their family.

Death is a challenge because it raises the problem of evil and the meaningfulness of suffering. The experience of suffering and overcoming evil are core Protestant teachings. For Protestants, the focus is salvation, which depends on one's moral QOL on earth. Heaven is a hope, but not a guarantee. The belief in an afterlife is expressed through memory, a sense of presence, and shared community. Although Jesus is a model for physical, emotional, social, and spiritual suffering, the individual faces the cosmos alone. The issue is not how the individual can participate in Jesus's suffering, but rather accepting the gift of God's grace as revealed through Jesus's death (Klass, 1993).

Death From the Islamic Perspective

Islam means submission. *Muslim* means one who submits to *Allah*, the Arabic word for "God." The founder of Islam is Mohammad, who received a vision while meditating, the content of which later became the Koran. The Five Pillars of Islam are confession of faith daily in front of witnesses, prayer five times a day, fasting during the month of Ramadan, almsgiving, and a pilgrimage to Mecca. Fasting during Ramadan is not required of the sick. Second-degree male relatives (e.g., cousins or uncles) should be contacted when a person is sick. They determine whether a person or family should be told the diagnosis or prognosis. The Islamic teachings encourage Muslims to seek treatment when they are sick, including modern medicine, spiritual healing, and traditional healing practices such as recitation of verses of the Noble Qur'an. They believe in divine predestination and perceive suffering as atonement for one's sins. When asking about the life expectancy of a patient, they are more likely to be comfortable with less definitive answers such as "it is in the hands of God," as Allah determines the time of death (Zafiral-Shahri & Al-Khenaizan, 2005).

Death is viewed as the beginning of a different form of life in which there are blessings given from Allah. Discussions about death are not usually welcomed. Grief may be expressed by slapping or hitting the body. Same-sex Muslims should handle the body after death; otherwise the individual should wear gloves so as not to touch the body. Islam forbids cremation, and burial should happen as soon as possible (Zafiral-Shahri & Al-Khenaizan, 2005).

Death From Eastern Perspectives

Hinduism originated in India. Hindus believe in cycles of birth and death that occur in an infinite series of lives, or successive creations. Hinduism teaches about *karma*, which states that every act of a human being, even a thought, has an effect on who that person becomes; it is the sum of the person's actions in this and previous existences and decides one's fate in future existences. One becomes virtuous through good actions and bad by bad actions (Ryan, 1993).

Originating in India, Buddhism does not include a belief in a God or the soul. Buddhism teaches that suffering is a part of life and that in death there is a transference of consciousness out of the body (Smith-Stoner, 2006). Buddhists believe in karma and rebirth. Karma is a principle of cause and effect. Buddhists train their minds to remain calm and peaceful as death approaches. Buddha taught that a way to overcome ignorance and attain truth is through the path to enlightenment, or a changed state of awareness called *Nirvana*. Buddhists believe that the way to Nirvana is through meditation, whereas others believe that it can be attained through faith.

Another Eastern tradition is Confucianism, which has its origins in China and stresses the importance of improving human relationships. The proper relationship between the living and the dead is one of continuous remembrance and affection, through which one attains social immortality. The value of ritual is that it ties the living with the dead. Memories of parents and ancestors are honored through regular remembrance rituals, which also provide a vehicle for the expression of the human emotions of grief and affection.

Taoism also has its origins in China. In Taoism, the focus is on nature and remedying society's disorder and lack of harmony. One looks toward nature to discover the principles to follow in life. Life is viewed as the companion of death, and death is viewed as the beginning of life and part of the living–dying process. Taoism offers a way to transcend the limits of the world, as there are ceaseless transformations through which the person is not lost. Yin and yang are the basic principles for all natural change. The yang is the light half, which is characterized as masculine, active, hot, bright, dry, and hard. The yin is the dark half, which is characterized as feminine, passive, cold, dark, wet, and soft. They are viewed as complementary forces that transform into each other. There is no light without dark, evil without good, or life without death (Ryan, 1993).

Many Asian patients—Chinese, Japanese, Koreans—have an Eastern perspective, in which formal behaviors are valued. It is believed that to rebel against death reveals a fundamental lack of understanding about life. Therefore, sadness and grief are kept private. Such behavior sets a good example and contributes to one's good reputation (Ryan, 1993). Patients may seek comfort in images, such as Buddha, Krishna, or the Divine Mother, or in repeating holy mantras. Those with an Eastern perspective believe that a person's final dying thoughts may determine one's rebirth.

Spiritual Issues in Death and Dying for Those Who Have No Conventional Religious Beliefs

Religion traditionally has provided a context for understanding and interpreting death. However, individuals who are not religious can still find comfort and meaning through spirituality and by stepping back from the material world (Orion, 1993). Individuals with no conventional religious beliefs often interpret life on the basis of a sense of being a part of a larger whole and from a scientific worldview. There is belief that an individual's life has a beginning and an ending, but the life process is indefinite. Whether the process is defined in terms of social or biological continuity, the brevity of life does not suggest insignificance. A particular life is short and seemingly inconsequential but assumes value and importance as a significant element in the entire ongoing process. Even a brief life is viewed as a contribution to the life process.

Those without conventional religious beliefs often consider the present as the real world and take full responsibility for their decisions. There is the belief that immortality occurs by biological immortality such as living on in the genetic pool of one's descendants, or living on in the memories of others or one's contributions to the world (Orion, 1993). The focus is on actualizing human potential. From the naturalistic perspective, death is not avoided or denied. Death is viewed as real, final, and inevitable and a mark of humans' solidarity with nature and the evolutionary process. Naturalism leads an effort to place the death of an individual in a framework of the process of living and dying, emergence, and extinction. In this framework (Orion, 1993), death is:

- A working out of the natural law by which all living things die
- The absorption of the differentiated person in the natural process
- A contribution to the evolutionary process
- Cessation of life's potential for negative and positive contributions
- Reabsorption into new ways in nature

Fear of death can be overcome by remembering that everything dies but existence goes on. When death is seen as part of the natural order or part of the universal condition, it can be tolerated more easily. Life and death are continuous parts of the whole (Orion, 1993).

Given the dearth of studies regarding the perspectives of atheists in palliative medicine, Smith-Stoner (2007) conducted a study of 88 individuals who self-identified as atheists, defined as someone who does not accept that there are any gods, heaven, hell, devils, souls, miracles, an afterlife, or anything else supernatural. Based on an analysis of open- and closed-ended survey questions, the results of EOL preferences indicate that participants' idea of a good death included respect for nonbelief and the withholding of prayer or any other references to God. However, consistent with a definition of spirituality, which includes intrapersonal, interpersonal, and a natural focus, atheists expressed a deep desire to find meaning in their own lives (intrapersonal), to maintain connection with family and friends (interpersonal), and to continue to experience and appreciate the natural world.

■ NURSES' NEED FOR SELF-REFLECTION AND SELF-HEALING IN PALLIATIVE CARE

Doka and Morgan (1993) describe the caregivers' assumptions and principles of spiritual care. First, nurses represent diverse spiritual or cultural backgrounds and, like patients, have the right to expect respect for their belief systems. Second, nurses should be offered opportunities to explore their own values and attitudes about life and death and their meaning and purpose in life. Third, nurses should be aware that they have the potential for providing spiritual care, and should be encouraged to offer spiritual care to dying patients and their families as needed. Fourth, as with all caregivers, nurses should be flexible and realistic in setting spiritual goals. Fifth, ongoing care of the dying and bereaved may cause a severe drain of energy and uncover old and new spiritual issues for the caregiver. Therefore, spiritual growth and renewal are a necessary part of staff support and a personal priority for each caregiver.

Indeed, in caring for dying patients and bereaved families, nurses may have experiences that create a grief response of their own because they have lost someone in whom they have invested themselves emotionally. Nurses' grief responses, like those of their patients, will be influenced by their spiritual and cultural values and beliefs. If accumulated grief is not worked through, the nurse is vulnerable to the same manifestations of unresolved grief as any other individual who has had a loss but failed to complete the grief work (Sherman, 2004b). Nurses therefore need to resolve their own feelings of loss, with their spiritual convictions supported, sense of failure alleviated, and emotional strength replenished (Sherman, 2004b).

In coping with the stress of caring for the dying, Harper (1994) believes that professional caregivers progress through five stages of adaptation: (a) intellectualization, (b) emotional survival, (c) depression, (d) emotional arrival, and (e) deep compassion. It is essential that nurses work through these stages in order to reduce their anxiety about caring for dying patients, as well as to engender personal and professional growth and be able to adapt to comfortably care for patients and their families at the end of life. Other stressful life events, previous personal and professional experiences with death and dying, the presence or absence of social supports for the caregiver, the degree of engagement in healthy self-care behaviors, and the ability to pursue and live a balanced life can all affect a caregiver's ability to adapt and cope with the stress of caring for the dying (Arnold & Egan, 2004). Recently, a sixth stage of adaptation, the doer, has been suggested to reflect professional caregivers who have experienced and processed the previous five steps in a healthy way; who demonstrate a level of adaptation and integration of their knowledge, learning, and experiences in caring for dying patients. The result is a provider who is not only efficient and vigorous in the care given, but also possesses a deep understanding of the meaning of the care in the greater context (Egan-City & Labyak, 2010).

In developing awareness and supporting nurses' spiritual well-being, nurse educators may ask their students or nursing colleagues the following questions:

- What expectations do you have about yourself in caring for the dying and bereaved?
- What would define success in your work?
- What are the three most difficult aspects of your work in caring for patients with life-threatening illness?
- What are you doing to help yourself cope with stress and replenish yourself to avoid becoming overstressed?

"Nurses must recognize their stress reactions and symptoms and employ self-care strategies to replenish themselves in physical, emotional, mental, and spiritual ways to overcome the various sources of stress" (Sherman, 2004b, p. 53). In reducing burnout in PC nursing, *physical health* is promoted as nurses care for their bodies by eating well, engaging in restful and relaxing activities, and counterbalancing fatigue by making improvements in lifestyle. *Emotional* health is bolstered by developing a calm mind and peaceful thoughts through such activities as meditation or listening to quiet music, as well as consciously letting go of negative thoughts and emotions. *Mental health* is strengthened by making choices, setting priorities, letting go of conflict, and saying no, while remaining open to new opportunities and possibilities. *Intuitional health* is nurtured by listening to the soul's wisdom and recognizing the need for balance and wholeness.

In overcoming interpersonal stressors, particularly when relations with others are difficult, nurses may find it helpful to reflect on the rewards of their work and the moments in which they have made the greatest difference in the lives of their patients and families. To cope with feelings of grief and loss, nurses can take time to reflect on what happened at the time of the patient's death and the lessons learned, speak to colleagues or journal about feelings, perceptions, and experiences (Sherman, 2004b).

Within the context of EOL care, and given that spirituality has emerged as a vital component of health, it becomes necessary for nurses to acknowledge their own spiritual beliefs and values and to deal with their own spiritual and cultural issues. Based on a sample of 155 Israeli oncology nurses, Musgrave and McFarlane (2004) reported that nurses' attitudes toward spiritual care are influenced by their spiritual well-being, intrinsic and extrinsic religiosity, and education. In a descriptive, qualitative study of the spiritual care perspectives and practices of 204 hospice nurses, Belcher and Griffiths (2005) recognized that the majority of the sample stated that they personally expressed their spirituality by attending church and related activities, that there was an openness and level of comfort in being a spiritual caregiver, and that there was no role conflict in spiritual expression. The majority of hospice nurses learned of the spiritual needs of their patients and families through personal interactions and the support of pastoral counselors or learning from their own personal life experiences. As hospice nurses, most indicated that they conducted spiritual assessment and recognized the importance of addressing spiritual needs, although their basic educational programs did little to prepare them for this. It was clear that hospice nurses value education regarding spirituality, which they believe enhances the quality of care.

Clark et al. (2007) examined the spirituality of members of a hospice interprofessional team ($n = 215$). Based on the Jarel Spiritual Well-Being Scale (Hunglemann, Kenkel-Rossi, Klassen, & Stollenwerk, 1989), the Chamiec-Case Spirituality Integration Scale (Chamiec-Case, 2009), and the Job Satisfaction Scale (Spector, 1985), respondents reported high levels of spiritual well-being, self-actualization, and job satisfaction. Structural path analyses revealed that job satisfaction is more likely realized by a model that transforms one's spirituality into processes of integrating spirituality at work and self-actualization.

According to Hunnibell, Reed, Quinn-Griffin, and Fitzpatrick (2008), hospice, PC, and oncology nurses manifest self-transcendence, which is characterized by awareness of the spiritual self, one's relationship to others, a higher being, and finding meaning and purpose in life. Based on a sample of 563 nurses (244 hospice nurses and 319 oncology nurses), both groups of nurses scored high on the Self-Transcendence Scale, although hospice nurses had the highest scores. For both groups of nurses, the greater the level of self-transcendence, the lower the nurses' scores of burnout, as measured by the Maslach Burnout Inventory, as emotional exhaustion, depersonalization, and personal accomplishment (Maslach &

Jackson, 1979). Oncology nurses manifested higher levels of burnout than hospice nurses, particularly with respect to depersonalization. It was suggested that nurses should be encouraged to connect with other nurses and form support groups to share their experiences. Strategies, such as keeping a journal, sharing one's stories, and recognizing positive individual contributions to care, may increase sense of worth and reduce professional burnout.

The importance of spiritual care was emphasized in a position statement published by the Hospice and Palliative Care Nurses Association (2007). The statement emphasized the commitment of hospice and PC nursing to compassionate care at EOL, acknowledgment of the importance of spiritual care, encouragement of organizational support in the provision of spiritual care, commitment to education and resources to promote spiritual care, and recognition of the right of individuals to decline spiritual care.

In caring for people with life-threatening and progressive illness, nurses must remain in tune with their own spiritual needs, healing themselves as well as others. To do so, Halifax (1999) suggests a contemplative exercise for nurses to remain centered, renewed, and whole as they care for others: Sit in a relaxed position, with eyes closed and have an awareness of the rhythm of the breath, focus one at a time on each of five phrases, which are repeated twice slowly. The nurse then allows the phrase to pass into the background of her or his awareness, moving attention to the breath and to the next phrase. The phrases are as follows:

- May I offer my care and presence unconditionally, knowing that it may be met with gratitude, indifference, anger, or anguish.
- May I offer love, knowing that I cannot control the course of life's suffering or death.
- May I remain in ease and let go of my expectations.
- May I view my own suffering with compassion just as I do the suffering of others.
- May I be aware that my suffering does not limit my good heart.
- May I forgive myself for things left undone.
- May I forgive all who have hurt me.
- May those whom I have hurt forgive me.
- May all beings and I live and die in peace.

Coulehan and Clary (2005) suggest that poetry can play a role in healing, as the written word becomes an instrument of healing and an opportunity for practitioners to reframe negativity, learn to function in the face of uncertainty, and support a compassionate presence in the care of the seriously ill and dying. Writing and reading poetry assists practitioners in understanding their own beliefs, feelings, attitudes, and response patterns, and in the process fosters empathic connection and a relationship that heals both patients and practitioners.

A survey of 605 ELNEC conference participants asked nurses to rate themselves on self-care behaviors and activities. Overall, the participants rated taking vacation and having meaningful relationships outside work as their most common self-care activities. Relationships in the workplace were also seen as important. Participants rated the ability to emotionally debrief at work as the most challenging self-care activity. The current literature shows that nurses are well aware of the importance of self-care activities and the need for balance between one's professional and personal life in order to properly care for their patients and help prevent burnout; however, for a variety of reasons, this awareness is not always translated into self-care action (Vachon & Huggard, 2010).

Spiritually and culturally competent care, therefore, require self-reflection and self-care of nurses. Replenishing one's own vessel in spiritually and culturally renewing ways is important in supporting nurses' caregiving potential. Only by doing so will nurses come to the bedside with the strong healing presence and true compassion needed to alleviate the suffering of patients and their families.

■ CONCLUSIONS

Illness and dying are occurrences that take us to the very core of our being. Although they are intensely personal experiences, they occur within the context of our spiritual and cultural traditions. Culture and spirituality therefore cannot be separated from who we are, as they are often the very source of our nourishment and physical, emotional, social, and spiritual well-being. Through sensitive and competent cultural and spiritual care, nurses can protect patients and families from the ultimate tragedy of depersonalization. They will be able to sustain patients and families in a personalized environment that recognizes their individual needs, reduces their fears, and offers them hope and dignity. Sulmasy (1997) believes that "when patients collapse spiritually in the face of illness, a clinician with the right perspective will understand much more acutely how desperate their plight really is and will treat the wounds of such patients with even more liberal applications of the wine of fervent zeal and the oil of compassion" (p. 52).

Cultural and spiritual values, beliefs, and practices profoundly influence life and living, and death and dying. Identifying cultural and spiritual factors pertinent to a patient's health is critical to the development of a successful plan of care that supports a person's sense of worth, integrity, and the continued actualization of her or his potential. Within the context of culturally and spiritually diverse beliefs and practices, health professionals should preserve beliefs and practices of individuals that have beneficial effects on health, encourage the adaptation or adjustment of practices that are neutral or indifferent, and suggest the repatterning of those practices that are potentially harmful to health (Leininger, 1995).

Culturally and spiritually competent care requires self-reflection and self-care if healthcare professionals are to be therapeutic. Hence, healthcare professionals need to replenish their own vessels in culturally and spiritually renewing ways to actualize their caregiving potential. In doing so, healthcare practitioners can offer a strong healing presence, true compassion, and sensitivity to the cultural and spiritual needs of patients and their families (Sherman, 2001).

Consideration of the cultural and spiritual backgrounds of patients and attention to their cultural and spiritual needs often enables older patients to live as fully as possible until death, and to maintain or restore quality to their lives. Byock (1997) reminds us that through competent and compassionate EOL care, older adults and all other patients can achieve a sense of inner well-being even as death approaches, and that "when the human dimension of dying is nurtured, for many the transition from life can be as profound, intimate, and precious as the miracle of death" (p. 57).

CASE STUDY *Conclusion*

The PC team, consisting of the PC nurse practitioner, chaplain, and social worker, began the conference by having the family share stories about the man Mr. J. is beyond his illness. The team learns that Mr. J. is a man whose main goal is the happiness of others. He remains an active member of his church and is a father figure/mentor to several members of the church and his local community. His daughter describes him as a man willing to give his last dime to feed the less fortunate. Despite the progression of his condition in recent years, the family states that he has maintained a positive outlook and kept his faith in God. Having an understanding of who Mr. J. is, the PC team discusses Mr. J.'s QOL and EOL decisions. They explain that Mr. J. will need to undergo several procedures to stabilize his heart, which may be futile. The family requests more time to discuss among themselves and asks the chaplain to lead them in prayer before ending the meeting.

With a serious decline in his condition, the family decides to make Mr. J. a DNR. They decide to provide only comfort and supportive treatments. The family understands that he has only days to live and would like to give members of the church and extended family the opportunity to say their goodbyes. As the days went on, family and friends prayed and sang hymns. Mr. J. died surrounded by the love of his family, friends, and members of his church.

CASE STUDY *Commentary*

AN INTERPROFESSIONAL PERSPECTIVE

Chaplain Deborah Galtere

As a chaplain approaching Mr. J. and his family for the first time, I need to create an atmosphere that is warm and free of anxiety in spite of the circumstances. As Mr. J. is on a ventilator and unable to speak and only minimally neurologically responding, his family will be making decisions regarding advance directives and EOL choices. I must facilitate this family to freely explore the options before them. Their faith/religious background will weigh heavily in their decision-making process. As an interfaith chaplain, my role is to ensure that I possess the internal space and open heart to listen without prejudice, worry, or expectation of this family. As their pastor is present and involved in the decision-making process and very much a part of their lives, my role in spiritual intervention takes a secondary role to their pastor.

I will provide emotional and spiritual support as needed including providing education regarding DNR and explain it with the acronym AND (Allow Natural Death)—this terminology is used often with pediatric EOL issues, and families seem to be often more accepting of this term rather than DNR.

When the family strongly believes in the "power of God and that death is part of God's plan for us all and it will happen in God's time," this statement helps me as a chaplain to determine the potential for spiritual growth during this dying journey with their family member and also interventions that might be possible in spite of being a secondary spiritual presence as their pastor may be present. If the family is open to spiritual interventions such as prayer, hymn singing, encouragement by scriptural readings, and brief exhortation, this can be done by either their pastor, or the chaplain, or both depending upon the circumstances. As a chaplain on site, I would have internal benchmarks to help me ascertain if the interventions are effective. These internal benchmarks depend upon the chaplain comprehending that each person is on a unique path and will be transformed in his or her own way and not according to some preset schedule, structure, process, or program.

I would ask permission of the family if I, too, could be present at Mr. J.'s bedside to offer gentle therapeutic touch to his head, hand, arm, and so forth and also to speak to Mr. J., as it is a medical belief that a patient hears you, though they may not be able to respond, either because of their physical condition or because of the effects of medications.

The family's decision to sign the DNR but first allow family members, members of their church, and others to say their farewells will be honored by medical and psychosocial staff, including the chaplain. The chaplain can also be of comfort to those waiting to visit with Mr. J.

I will also help the family to understand the medical processes that would occur during extubation or in signing a DNR. Common questions often asked by family members include: Will it hurt my loved one? How long does it take to remove the tube? After the tube is removed, what will happen? How long will they stay in ICU before being moved to a room? Do I/We (family) need to be present when they remove the rube? Will they die right away? Will they be able to hear us? Will they be able to talk, open their eyes? Will God see this as killing or forgive me for killing?

As a chaplain, I am prepared to answer such questions. However, questions about how long will he live after extubation cannot be answered simply as it is dependent on the patient's physical condition and disease process. It is always important to invite people to talk about their image of God and what they believe. At the same time, there are occasions when the chaplain may need to gently offer other viewpoints to consider so any feelings of guilt can be relieved. Overall, the chaplain offers a calming presence and communication between the family and the medical staff, reducing any feelings of anxiety. The chaplain's active listening skills, ability to help a family reach consensus, expression of empathy, and gathering of valuable information make him a valuable resource for the family at this difficult time.

Evidence-Based Practice

LEVEL IV EVIDENCE: DESCRIPTIVE, CORRELATIONAL

Delgado-Guay, M., Parsons, H., Hui, D., De la Cruz, M., Thorney, S., & Bruera, E. (2013). Spirituality, religiosity, and spiritual pain among caregivers of patients with advanced cancer. *American Journal of Hospice and Palliative Care*, 30(5), 455–461. doi:10.1177/1049909112458030

Background
Caregivers of patients with advanced cancer often face physical, social, and emotional distress as well as spiritual pain. Limited research has focused on the spiritual aspects of caregivers' suffering.

Purpose
To assess spirituality, religiosity, and spiritual pain in caregivers of patients with advanced cancer.

Methods

Forty-three caregivers of patients with advanced cancer were interviewed in a PC outpatient clinic. Demographic characteristics, religious affiliation, and relationship to the patient were determined. Levels of spirituality, religiosity, and spiritual pain were self-reported using numeric rating scales (0 = lowest; 10 = highest). The participants completed various validated questionnaires to assess sleep disturbances, psychosocial distress, coping skills, and QOL.

Results

The median age was 52 years (range, 21–83); 29 (67%) were women; 34 (78%) were white, 7 (17%) were African American, and 2 (5%) were Hispanic; 39 (91%) were Christian, 1 (2%) was Jewish, and 1 (2%) was agnostic; 37 (86%) were married; 18 (42%) were working full-time; and 25 (58%) were spouses. All considered themselves spiritual, and 98% considered themselves religious. All the caregivers reported that spirituality and religiosity helped them cope with their loved one's illness, and many reported that spirituality and religiosity had a positive impact on their loved one's physical (58%) and emotional (76%) symptoms. Spiritual pain was reported by 23 (58%), with a median score of 5 (interquartile range, 2–8). Caregivers with spiritual pain had higher levels of anxiety (median 10 vs. 4; $p = .002$), depression (6 vs. 2; $p = .006$), and denial (3 vs. 2; $p = .01$); more behavioral disengagement (3 vs. 2; $p = .011$), more dysfunctional coping strategies (19 vs. 16; $p < .001$), and worse QOL (70 vs. 51; $p < .001$) than those who did not have spiritual pain.

Conclusions

The majority of caregivers of patients with advanced cancer considered themselves spiritual and religious. Despite this, there is high prevalence of spiritual pain in this population. Caregivers with spiritual pain experienced worse psychological distress and worse QOL. These findings support the importance of spiritual assessment of and spiritual support for caregivers in this setting.

■ REFERENCES

Abrums, M. (2000). Death and meaning in a storefront church. *Public Health Nursing (Boston, Mass.), 17*(2), 132–142. doi:10.1046/j.1525-1446.2000.00132.x

Adunsky, A., Aminoff, B. Z., Arad, M., & Bercovitch, M. (2007). Mini-Suffering State Examination: Suffering and survival of end-of-life cancer patients in a hospice setting. *American Journal of Hospice and Palliative Care, 24*(6), 493–498. doi:10.1177/1049909107307374

Ahalt, C., Walter, L. C., Yourman, L., Eng, C., Pérez-Stable, E. J., & Smith, A. K. (2012). "Knowing is better": Preferences of diverse older adults for discussing prognosis. *Journal of General Internal Medicine, 27*(5), 568–575. doi:10.1007/s11606-011-1933-0

American Medical Student Association. (2001). *Cultural competency in medicine.* Retrieved from https://www.amsa.org/advocacy/action-committees/reach/

Aminoff, B. Z., Purits, E., Noy, S., & Adunsky, A. (2004). Measuring the suffering of end-stage dementia: reliability and validity of the Mini-Suffering State Examination. *Archives of Gerontology and Geriatrics, 38*(2), 123–130. doi:10.1016/j.archger.2003.08.007

Anderson, J. R., & Turner, W. L. (2010). When caregivers are in need of care: African-American caregivers' preferences for their own later life care. *Journal of Aging Studies, 24*(1), 65–73. doi:10.1016/j.jaging.2008.06.002

Andrews, M., & Boyle J. (2016). *Transcultural concepts in nursing care.* Philadelphia, PA: Wolters Kluwer.

Arnold, E. (1989). Burnout as a spiritual issue: Rediscovering meaning in nursing practice. In V. Carson (Ed.), *Spiritual dimensions of nursing practice* (pp. 320–353). Philadelphia, PA: Saunders.

Arnold, R., & Egan, K. (2004). Suffering, loss, grief, and bereavement. In M. Matzo & D. Sherman (Eds.), *Gerontologic palliative care nursing* (pp. 148–164). St. Louis, MO: Mosby.

Ballard-Reisch, D. S., & Letner, J. A. (2003). Centering families in cancer communication research: Acknowledging the impact of support, culture and process on client/provider communication in cancer management. *Patient Education and Counseling, 50*, 61–66. doi:10.1016/S0738-3991(03)00082-X

Barclay, J. S., Blackhall, L. J., & Tulsky, J. A. (2007). Communication strategies and cultural issues in the delivery of bad news. *Journal of Palliative Medicine, 10*(4), 958–977. doi:10.1089/jpm.2007.9929

Beeney, L., Butow, P., & Dunn, S. (1997). Normal adjustment to cancer: Characteristics and assessment. In R. K. Portenoy & E. Bruera (Eds.), *Topics in palliative care* (Vol. 1, pp. 213–244). New York, NY: Oxford University Press.

Beery, T. A., Baas, L. S., Fowler, C., & Allen, G. (2002). Spirituality in persons with heart failure. *Journal of Holistic Nursing, 20*(1), 5–25; quiz 26. doi:10.1177/089801010202000102

Belcher, A., & Griffiths, M. (2005). The spiritual care perspectives and practices of hospice nurses. *Journal of Hospice and Palliative Nursing, 7*(5), 271–279. doi:10.1097/00129191-200509000-00014

Bergan, A., & McConatha, J. (2000). Religiosity and life satisfaction. *Activities, Adaptation & Aging, 24*(3), 23–24. doi:10.1300/J016v24n03_02

Bhungalia, S., & Kemp, C. (2002). (Asian) Indian health beliefs and practices related to end of life. *Journal of Hospice and Palliative Nursing, 4*(1), 54–58. doi:10.1097/00129191-200201000-00016

Bird, L. (1986). Suffering, thanatology, and whole-person medicine. In R. DeBellis, E. Marcus, A. Kutscher, C. Smith Torres, V. Barrett, & M. Siegel (Eds.), *Suffering: Psychological and social aspects in loss, grief, and care* (pp. 31–39). New York, NY: Haworth Press.

Boland, C. S. (1998). Parish nursing: Addressing the significance of social support and spirituality for sustained health-promoting behaviors in the elderly. *Journal of Holistic Nursing, 16*(3), 355–368. doi:10.1177/089801019801600305

Breaden, K., Hegarty, M., Swetenham, K., & Grbich, C. (2012). Negotiating uncertain terrain: A qualitative analysis of clinicians' experiences of refractory suffering. *Journal of Palliative Medicine, 15*(8), 896–901. doi:10.1089/jpm.2011.0442

Brokenleg, M., & Middleton, D. (1993). Native Americans: Adapting, yet retaining. In D. Irish, K. Lundquist, & V. Nelsen (Eds.), *Ethnic variations in dying, death, and grief* (pp. 101–112). Philadelphia, PA: Taylor & Francis.

Buchanan, D. (1993). *Meaning in life, depression, suicide in older adults: A comparative survey study* (Unpublished doctoral dissertation). Rush University, Chicago, IL.

Buck, H., & McMillan, S. (2008). The unmet spiritual needs of caregivers of patients with advanced cancer. *Journal of Hospice and Palliative Nursing, 10*(2), 91–105. doi:10.1097/01.NJH.0000306737.08850.71

Bullock, K. (2006). Promoting advance directives among African Americans: A faith-based model. *Journal of Palliative Medicine, 9*(1), 183–195. doi:10.1089/jpm.2006.9.183

Büssing, A., Michalsen, A., Balzat, H. J., Grünther, R. A., Ostermann, T., Neugebauer, E. A., & Matthiessen, P. F. (2009). Are spirituality and religiosity resources for patients with chronic pain conditions? *Pain Medicine, 10*(2), 327–339. doi:10.1111/j.1526-4637.2009.00572.x

Byock, I. (1997). *Dying well: The prospect for growth at the end of life.* New York, NY: Riverhead Books.

Carroll, M. M. (2001). Conceptual models of spirituality. *Social Thought, 20,* 5–21. doi:10.1080/15426432.2001.9960278

Cassell, E. (1982). The nature of suffering and the goals of medicine. *New England Journal of Medicine, 306,* 639–645. doi:10.1056/NEJM198203183061104

Cassell, E. J. (2004). When suffering patients seek death. In T. E. Quill & M. P. Battin (Eds.), *Physician-assisted dying: The case for palliative care and patient choice* (pp. 75–88). Baltimore, MD: Johns Hopkins University Press.

Chamiec-Case, R. (2009). Developing a scale to measure social workers' integration of spirituality in the workplace. *Journal of Religion & Spirituality in Social Work: Social Thought, 28*(3), 284--305. doi:10.1080/15426430903070228

Chochinov, H. M., & Cann, B. J. (2005). Interventions to enhance the spiritual aspects of dying. *Journal of Palliative Medicine, 8*(Suppl. 1), S103–S115. doi:10.1089/jpm.2005.8.s-103

Chochinov, H. M., Krisjanson, L. J., Hack, T. F., Hassard, T., McClement, S., & Harlos, M. (2006). Dignity in the terminally ill: Revisited. *Journal of Palliative Medicine, 9*(3), 666–672. doi:10.1089/jpm.2006.9.666

Clark, L., Leedy, S., McDonald, L., Muller, B., Lamb, C., Mendez, T., . . . Schonwetter, R. (2007). Spirituality and job satisfaction among hospice interdisciplinary team members. *Journal of Palliative Medicine, 10*(6), 1321–1328. doi:10.1089/jpm.2007.0035

Cort, M. A. (2004). Cultural mistrust and use of hospice care: Challenges and remedies. *Journal of Palliative Medicine, 7*(1), 63–71. doi:10.1089/109662104322737269

Coulehan, J., & Clary, P. (2005). Healing the healer: Poetry in palliative care. *Journal of Palliative Medicine, 8*(2), 382–389. doi:10.1089/jpm.2005.8.382

Council on Social Work Education Faculty Development Institute. (2010). Cultural competence. Retrieved from https://www.cswe.org

Cousins, N. (1979). *Anatomy of an illness.* New York, NY: Norton.

Coyle, N. (1995). Suffering in the first person. In B. R. Ferrell (Ed.), *Suffering* (pp. 21–32). Sudbury, MA: Jones & Bartlett.

Crawley, L. M., Marshall, P. A., Lo, B., & Koenig, B. A. (2002). Strategies for culturally effective end-of-life care. *Annals of Internal Medicine, 136*(9), 673–679. doi:10.7326/0003-4819-136-9-200205070-00010

Davies, B., Reimer, J. C., & Martens, N. (1994). Family functioning and its implications for palliative care. *Journal of Palliative Care, 10*(1), 29–36.

Delgado-Guay, M. O., Parsons, H. A., Hui, D., De la Cruz, M. G., Thorney, S., & Bruera, E. (2013). Spirituality, religiosity, and spiritual pain among caregivers of patients with advanced cancer. *American Journal of Hospice and Palliative Care, 30*(5), 455–461. doi:10.1177/1049909112458030

DeSpelder, L. (1998). Developing cultural competency. In K. Doka & J. Davidson (Eds.), *Living with grief* (pp. 97–106). Washington, DC: Hospice Foundation of America.

DeSpelder, L., & Strickland, A. (1999). *The last dance: Encountering death and dying.* Mountain View, CA: Mayfield.

Doka, K., & Davidson, J. (1998). *Living with grief.* Philadelphia, PA: Hospice Foundation of America.

Doka, K. J., & Morgan, J. D. (1993). *Death and spirituality.* Amityville, NY: Baywood.

Doorenbos, A. Z., & Schim, S. M. (2004). Cultural competence in hospice. *American Journal of Hospice and Palliative Care, 21*(1), 28–32. doi:10.1177/104990910402100108

Downey, M. (1997). *Understanding Christian spirituality.* Mahwah, NJ: Palest Press.

Doyle, D. (1994). *Caring for a dying relative: A guide for families.* New York, NY: Oxford University Press.

Driscoll, J. (2001). Spirituality and religion in end-of-life care. *Journal of Palliative Medicine, 4*(3), 333–335. doi:10.1089/109662101753123940

Duggleby, W. (2000). Enduring suffering: A grounded theory analysis of the pain experience of elderly hospice patients with cancer. *Oncology Nursing Forum, 27*(5), 825–831.

Duggleby, W. (2001). Hope at the end of life. *Journal of Hospice and Palliative Nursing, 3*(2), 51–57. doi:10.1097/00129191-200103020-00003

Dunn, K. S., & Horgas, A. L. (2000). The prevalence of prayer as a spiritual self-care modality in elders. *Journal of Holistic Nursing, 18*(4), 337–351. doi:10.1177/089801010001800405

Egan-City, K., & Labyak, M. (2010). Hospice palliative care for the 21st century: A model of quality end of life care. *Oxford Medicine.*

Ehman, J. W., Ott, B. B., Short, T. H., Ciampa, R. C., & Hansen-Flaschen, J. (1999). Do patients want physicians to inquire about their spiritual or religious beliefs if they become gravely ill? *Archives of Internal Medicine, 159*(15), 1803–1806. doi:10.1001/archinte.159.15.1803

Emblen, J., & Pesut, B. (2001). Strengthening transcendent meaning. A model for the spiritual nursing care of patients experiencing suffering. *Journal of Holistic Nursing, 19*(1), 42–56. doi:10.1177/089801010101900105

End of Life Nursing Education Consortium. (2013). *Module 5: Cultural considerations.* City of Hope Medical Center and American Association of Colleges of Nursing. Available from the American Association of Colleges of Nursing: www.aacn.nche.edu/elnec

Exline, J. J., Prince-Paul, M., Root, B. L., & Peereboom, K. S. (2013). The spiritual struggle of anger toward God: A study with family members of hospice patients. *Journal of Palliative Medicine, 16*(4), 369–375. doi:10.1089/jpm.2012.0246

Flores, G. (2005). The impact of medical interpreter services on the quality of health care: A systematic review. *Medical Care Research and Review, 62*(3), 255–299. doi:10.1177/1077558705275416

Foley, K. (1995). Pain, physician-assisted suicide, and euthanasia. *Pain Forum, 4,* 163–178. doi:10.1016/S1082-3174(11)80050-4

Gallop, G. (1997). *Spiritual beliefs and the dying process: A national survey conducted for the Nathan Cummings Foundation and the Fetzer Institute.* New York, NY: Nathan Cummings Foundation.

Gebauer, S., Knox Morley, S., Haozous, E. A., Finlay, E., Camarata, C., Fahy, B., . . . Marr, L. (2016). Palliative care for American Indians and Alaska Natives: A review of the literature. *Journal of Palliative Medicine, 19*(12), 1331–1340. doi:10.1089/jpm.2016.0201

Grollman, E. (1993). Death in Jewish thought. In K. Doka & J. Morgan (Eds.), *Death and spirituality* (pp. 21–32). Amityville, NY: Baywood.

Grossman, D. (1996). Cultural dimensions in home health nursing. *American Journal of Nursing, 96*(7), 33–36. doi:10.1097/00000446-199607000-00031

Gum, A., & Snyder, C. R. (2002). Coping with terminal illness: The role of hopeful thinking. *Journal of Palliative Medicine, 5*(6), 883–894. doi:10.1089/10966210260499078

Halifax, J. (1999, October). *Being with dying: Contemplations on death and dying.* Presentation at the Art of Dying III Conference: Spiritual, Scientific and Practical Approaches to Living and Dying by the New York Open Center and Tibet House, New York, NY.

Harper, B. (1994). *Death: The coping mechanism of the health professional.* Greenville, SC: Southeastern University Press.

Heintz, L. M., & Baruss, I. (2001). Spirituality in late adulthood. *Psychological Reports, 88*(3 Pt. 1), 651–654. doi:10.2466/pr0.2001.88.3.651

Hepburn, K., & Reed, R. (1995). Ethical and clinical issues with Native-American elders: End-of-life decision making. *Clinics in Geriatric Medicine, 11*(1), 97–111.

Hermann, C. (2000). A guide to the spiritual needs of elderly cancer patients. *Geriatric Nursing (New York, N.Y.), 21*(6), 324–325. doi:10.1067/mgn.2000.gn00324

Herselman, S. (2004). Anthropology of health. In A. Tjale & L. de Villiers (Eds.), *Cultural issues in health and health care.* Cape Town, South Africa: Juta.

Herth, K. (1992). Abbreviated instrument to measure hope: Development and psychometric evaluation. Journal of Advanced Nursing, 17, 1251–1259. doi:10.1111/j.1365-2648.1992.tb01843.x

Hicks, T. J. (1999). Spirituality and the elderly: Nursing implications with nursing home residents. *Geriatric Nursing (New York, N.Y.), 20*(3), 144–146. doi:10.1016/S0197-4572(99)70006-6

Higginson, I. J. (1998). Introduction: Defining the unit of care: Who are we supporting and how? In E. Bruera & R. K. Portenoy (Eds.), *Topics in palliative care* (Vol. 2, pp. 205–207). New York, NY: Oxford University Press.

Highfield, M. E. (2000). Providing spiritual care to patients with cancer. *Clinical Journal of Oncology Nursing, 4*(3), 115–120.

Hospice and Palliative Care Nurses Association. (2007). HPNA position paper: Spiritual care. *Journal of Hospice and Palliative Care Nursing, 9*(1), 15–16.

Hunglemann, J., Kenkel-Rossi, E., Klassen, L. & Stollenwerk, R. (1989). Development of the J.A.R.E.L. spiritual well-being scale, Classification of Nursing Diagnosis. In Proceedings of the 8th Conference, North American Diagnosis Association, J.B. Lippincott.

Hunnibell, L., Reed, P., Quinn-Griffin, M., & Fitzpatrick, J. (2008). Self-transcendence and burnout in hospice and oncology nurses. *Journal of Hospice and Palliative Nursing, 10*(3), 172–179. doi:10.1097/01.NJH.0000306742.95388.80

Hutchings, D. (2007). Struggling in change at the end of life: A nursing inquiry. *Palliative and Supportive Care, 5*(1), 31–39. doi:10.1017/S1478951507070058

Irish, D., Lundquist, K., & Nelsen, V. (1993). *Ethnic variations in dying, death, and grief.* Philadelphia, PA: Taylor & Francis.

Jenko, M., Gonzalez, L., & Seymour, M. (2007). Life review with the terminally ill. *Journal of Hospice and Palliative Nursing, 9*(3), 159–167. doi:10.1097/01.NJH.0000270002.74614.10

Johnson, P. (2002). The use of humor and its influences on spirituality and coping in breast cancer survivors. *Oncology Nursing Forum, 29*(4), 691–695. doi:10.1188/02.ONF.691-695

Kagawa-Singer, M., & Blackhall, L. J. (2001). Negotiating cross-cultural issues at the end of life: "You got to go where he lives." *Journal of the American Medical Association, 286*(23), 2993–3001. doi:10.1001/jama.286.23.2993

Kahn, D. L., & Steeves, R. (1996). An understanding of suffering grounded in clinical practice and research. In B. R. Ferrell (Ed.), *Suffering* (pp. 3–27). Sudbury, MA: Jones & Bartlett.

Kemp, C., & Chang, B. (2002). Culture and the end of life: Chinese. *Journal of Hospice and Palliative Nursing, 4*, 173–177. doi:10.1097/00129191-200207000-00017

Kennedy, B. R., Mathis, C. C., & Woods, A. K. (2007). African Americans and their distrust of the health care system: Healthcare for diverse populations. *Journal of Cultural Diversity, 14*(2), 56–60.

King, M., Llewellyn, H., Leurent, B., Owen, F., Leavey, G., Tookman, A., & Jones, L. (2013). Spiritual beliefs near the end of life: A prospective cohort study of people with cancer receiving palliative care. *Psycho-Oncology, 22*(11), 2505–2512. doi:10.1002/pon.3313

Kirschling, J. M., & Pittman, J. F. (1989). Measurement of spiritual well-being: A hospice caregiver sample. *Hospice Journal, 5*(2), 1–11. doi:10.1080/0742-969X.1989.11882644

Klass, D. (1993). Spirituality, Protestantism, and death. In K. Doka & J. Morgan (Eds.), *Death and spirituality* (pp. 51–73). Amityville, NY: Baywood.

Koenig, H. G. (2002). An 83-year-old woman with chronic illness and strong religious beliefs. *Journal of the American Medical Association, 288*(4), 487–493. doi:10.1001/jama.288.4.487

Koenig, H. G., Pargament, K. I., & Nielsen, J. (1998). Religious coping and health status in medically ill hospitalized older adults. *Journal of Nervous and Mental Disease, 186*(9), 513–521. doi:10.1097/00005053-199809000-00001

Krikorian, A., Limonero, J. T., & Corey, M. T. (2013). Suffering assessment: A review of available instruments for use in palliative care. *Journal of Palliative Medicine, 16*(2), 130–142. doi:10.1089/jpm.2012.0370

LaRocca-Pitts, M. (2009). In FACT, chaplains have a spiritual assessment tool. *Australian Journal of Pastoral Care and Health, 3*(2), 8–15. doi:10.1080/08854720802698350

LaRocca-Pitts, M. (2015). Four FACTs spiritual assessment tool. *Journal of Health Care Chaplaincy, 21*(2), 51–59. doi:10.1080/08854726.2015.1015303

Lederberg, M. (1998). The family of the cancer patient. In J. Holland (Ed.), *Psycho-Oncology* (pp. 981–993). New York, NY: Oxford University Press.

Leininger, M. (1995). *Transcultural nursing: Concepts, theories, research, and practice.* New York, NY: McGraw-Hill.

Lipson, J., Dibble, S., & Minarik, P. A. (1996). *Culture and nursing care: A pocket guide.* St. Louis, MO: Mosby.

Lo, B., Ruston, D., Kates, L. W., Arnold, R. M., Cohen, C. B., Faber-Langendoen, K., . . . Tulsky, J. A.; Working Group on Religious and Spiritual Issues at the End of Life. (2002). Discussing religious and spiritual issues at the end of life: A practical guide for physicians. *Journal of the American Medical Association, 287*(6), 749–754. doi:10.1001/jama.287.6.749

Lorenz, K. A., Hays, R. D., Shapiro, M. F., Cleary, P. D., Asch, S. M., & Wenger, N. S. (2005). Religiousness and spirituality among HIV-infected Americans. *Journal of Palliative Medicine, 8*(4), 774–781. doi:10.1089/jpm.2005.8.774

Loscalzo, M., & Zabora, J. (1998). Care of the cancer patient: Response of family and staff. In E. Bruera & R. K. Portenoy (Eds.), *Topics in palliative care* (Vol. 2, pp. 209–246). New York, NY: Oxford University Press.

Lowe, J., & Struthers, R. (2001). A conceptual framework of nursing in Native American culture. *Journal of Nursing Scholarship, 33*(3), 279–283. doi:10.1111/j.1547-5069.2001.00279.x

Ludke, R. L., & Smucker, D. R. (2007). Racial differences in the willingness to use hospice services. *Journal of Palliative Medicine, 10*(6), 1329–1337. doi:10.1089/jpm.2007.0077

Mackenzie, E. R., Rajagopal, D. E., Meibohm, M., & Lavizzo-Mourey, R. (2000). Spiritual support and psychological well-being: Older adults' perceptions of the religion and health connection. *Alternative Therapies in Health and Medicine, 6*(6), 37–45.

Mako, C., Galek, K., & Poppito, S. R. (2006). Spiritual pain among patients with advanced cancer in palliative care. *Journal of Palliative Medicine, 9*(5), 1106–1113. doi:10.1089/jpm.2006.9.1106

Maslach, C., & Jackson, S. E. (1979). The measurement of experienced burnout (Unpublished manuscript). Department of Psychology, University of California, Berkeley.

Matthews, D. (1999, March). *The faith factor: Is religion good for your health?* Paper presented at the Harvard University Spirituality and Healing Conference, Denver, CO.

McDavis, R., Parker, W., & Parker, W. (1995). Counseling African Americans. In N. Vace, S. DeVaney, & J. Wittmer (Eds.), *Experiencing and counseling multicultural and diverse populations* (pp. 217–248). Bristol, PA: Accelerated Development.

McGann, J. (1997). *Comfort my people: Finding peace as life ends.* Rockville Center, NY: Long Island Catholic.

McGrath, P., Vun, M., & McLeod, L. (2001). Needs and experiences of non-English-speaking hospice patients and families in an English-speaking country. *American Journal of Hospice and Palliative Care, 18*(5), 305–312. doi:10.1177/104990910101800505

Meagher, D., & Bell, C. (1993). Perspectives on death in the African American community. In K. Doka & J. D. Morgan (Eds.), *Death and spirituality* (pp. 113–130). Amityville, NY: Baywood.

Meraviglia, M. G. (2004). The effects of spirituality on well-being of people with lung cancer. *Oncology Nursing Forum, 31*(1), 89–94. doi:10.1188/04.ONF.89-94

Miller, E. (1993). A Roman Catholic view of death. In K. Doka & J. D. Morgan (Eds.), *Death and spirituality* (pp. 33–49). Amityville, NY: Baywood.

Millspaugh, C. D. (2005a). Assessment and response to spiritual pain: Part I. *Journal of Palliative Medicine, 8*(5), 919–923. doi:10.1089/jpm.2005.8.919

Millspaugh, C. D. (2005b). Assessment and response to spiritual pain: Part II. *Journal of Palliative Medicine, 8*(6), 1110–1117. doi:10.1089/jpm.2005.8.1110

Mitchell, D. R. (1997). The "good" death: Three promises to make at the bedside. *Geriatrics, 52*(8), 91–92.

Moore, T. (1992). *Care of the soul: A guide for cultivating depth and sacredness in everyday life.* New York, NY: Harper Collins.

Musgrave, C. F., & McFarlane, E. A. (2004). Israeli oncology nurses' religiosity, spiritual well-being, and attitudes toward spiritual care: A path analysis. *Oncology Nursing Forum, 31*(2), 321–327. doi:10.1188/04.ONF.321-327

Nathan Cummings Foundation and the Fetzer Institute. (1997). Spiritual beliefs and the dying process: A report on a national survey. Conducted by the George H. Gallup International Institute.

National Consensus Project. (2013). National consensus guidelines for quality palliative care. Retrieved from www.nationalconsensusproject.org

O'Connor, P. (1993). A clinical paradigm for exploring spiritual concerns. In K. Doka & J. D. Morgan (Eds.), *Death and spirituality* (pp. 133–150). Amityville, NY: Baywood.

O'Mara, S. K., & Zborovskaya, Y. (2016). End-of-life care in the Hispanic community. *Journal of Hospice and Palliative Nursing, 18*(1), 53–59. doi:10.1097/NJH.0000000000000210

Orion, P. (1993). Spiritual issues in death and dying for those who do not have conventional religious beliefs. In K. Doka & J. D. Morgan (Eds.), *Death and spirituality* (pp. 93–112). Amityville, NY: Baywood.

Parker-Oliver, D. (2002). Redefining hope for the terminally ill. *American Journal of Hospice and Palliative Care, 19*(2), 115–120. doi:10.1177/104990910201900210

Paloutzian, R. F., & Ellison, C. W. (1982). Loneliness, spiritual well-being and quality of life. In Peplau, L. A., & Perlman, D. (Eds.), *Loneliness: A sourcebook of current theory, research and therapy.* New York: Wiley Interscience.

Peterman, A. H., Fitchett, G., Brady, M. J., Hernandez, L., & Cella, D. (2002). Measuring spiritual well-being in people with cancer: The functional assessment of chronic illness therapy–Spiritual Well-Being Scale (FACIT-Sp). *Annals of Behavioral Medicine, 24*(1), 49–58. doi:10.1207/S15324796ABM2401_06

Prince-Paul, M. (2008). Relationships among communicative acts, social well-being, and spiritual well-being on the quality of life at the end of life in patients with cancer enrolled in hospice. *Journal of Palliative Medicine, 11*(1), 20–25. doi:10.1089/jpm.2007.0119

Puchalski, C. M. (1998a). Facing death with dignity. *The World and I, 3*, 34–39.

Puchalski, C. M. (1998b). *FICA: A spiritual assessment.* Unpublished manuscript.

Puchalski, C. M. (2001). Spirituality and health: The art of compassionate medicine. *Hospital Physician, 37*(3), 30–36.

Puchalski, C. M. (2002). Spirituality and end-of-life care: A time for listening and caring. *Journal of Palliative Medicine, 5*(2), 289–294. doi:10.1089/109662102753641287

Puchalski, C. M., & Ferrell, B. (2010). *Making health care whole: Integrating spirituality into patient care.* West Conshohocken, PA: Templeton Press.

Puchalski, C. M., Ferrell, B., Virani, R., Otis-Green, S., Baird, P., Bull, J., . . . Sulmasy, D. (2009). Improving the quality of spiritual care as a dimension of palliative care: The report of the Consensus Conference. *Journal of Palliative Medicine, 12*(10), 885–904. doi:10.1089/jpm.2009.0142

Puchalski, C. M., & Larson, D. B. (1998). Developing curricula in spirituality and medicine. *Journal of the Association of American Medical Colleges, 73*(9), 970–974.

Puchalski, C. M., & Romer, A. L. (2000). Taking a spiritual history allows clinicians to understand patients more fully. *Journal of Palliative Medicine, 3*(1), 129–137. doi:10.1089/jpm.2000.3.129

Purdy, W. A. (2002). Spiritual discernment in palliative care. *Journal of Palliative Medicine, 5*(1), 139–141. doi:10.1089/10966210252785105

Rawdin, B., Evans, C., & Rabow, M. W. (2013). The relationships among hope, pain, psychological distress, and spiritual well-being in oncology outpatients. *Journal of Palliative Medicine, 16*(2), 167–172. doi:10.1089/jpm.2012.0223

Rome, R. B., Luminais, H. H., Bourgeois, D. A., & Blais, C. M. (2011). The role of palliative care at the end of life. *Ochsner Journal, 11*(4), 348–352.

Ryan, D. (1993). Death: Eastern perspectives. In K. Doka & J. D. Morgan (Eds.), *Death and spirituality* (pp. 75–92). Amityville, NY: Baywood.

Ryan, S. (1997). Chaplains are more than what chaplains do. *Visions, 7*(3), 8–9.

Saguil, A., & Phelps, K. (2012). The spiritual assessment. *American Family Physician, 86*(6), 546–550.

Satterly, L. (2001). Guilt, shame, and religious and spiritual pain. *Holistic Nursing Practice, 15*(2), 30–39.

Schroepfer, T. A. (2007). Critical events in the dying process: The potential for physical and psychosocial suffering. *Journal of Palliative Medicine, 10*(1), 136–147. doi:10.1089/jpm.2006.0157

Selsky, C., Kreling, B., Luta, G., Makgoeng, S. B., Gomez-Duarte, J., Barbo, A. G., & Mandelblatt, J. S.; Latin American Cancer Research Coalition. (2012). Hospice knowledge and intentions among Latinos using safety-net clinics. *Journal of Palliative Medicine, 15*(9), 984–990. doi:10.1089/jpm.2011.0517

Sherman, D. W. (1998). Reciprocal suffering: The need to improve family caregivers' quality of life through palliative care. *Journal of Palliative Medicine, 1*(4), 357–366. doi:10.1089/jpm.1998.1.357

Sherman, D. W. (2001). Spiritual and cultural competence in palliative care. In M. Matzo & D. W. Sherman (Eds.), *Palliative care nursing: Quality care to the end of life* (pp. 3–47). New York, NY: Springer.

Sherman, D. W. (2004a). Cultural and spiritual backgrounds of older adults: Considerations for quality palliative care. In M. L. Matzo & D. W. Sherman (Eds.), *Gerontological palliative care nursing* (pp. 3–30). St. Louis, MO: Mosby.

Sherman, D. W. (2004b). Nurses' stress & burnout: How to care for yourself when caring for patients and their families experiencing life-threatening illness. *American Journal of Nursing, 104*(5), 48–56; quiz 57.

Sherman, D. W., McGuire, D., Free, D. C., & Cheon, J. (2013). A pilot study of the experience of family caregivers of patients with advanced pancreatic cancer: A mixed method study. *Journal of Pain and Symptom Management, 48*(3), 385–399.e2. doi: 10.1016/j.jpainsymman.2013.09.006

Sinclair, S., Pereira, J., & Raffin, S. (2006). A thematic review of the spirituality literature within palliative care. *Journal of Palliative Medicine, 9*(2), 464–479. doi:10.1089/jpm.2006.9.464

Smith, R. (1996). Theological perspectives. In B. R. Ferrell (Ed.), *Suffering* (pp. 159–171). Sudbury, MA: Jones & Bartlett.

Smith-Stoner, M. (2006, Summer). Caring for Buddhists at end of life. *American Academy of Hospice and Palliative Medicine Bulletin,* 6–7.

Smith-Stoner, M. (2007). End-of-life preferences for atheists. *Journal of Palliative Medicine, 10*(4), 923–928. doi:10.1089/jpm.2006.0197

Spector, P. E. (1985). Measurement of human service staff satisfaction: Development of the Job Satisfaction Survey. *American Journal of Community Psychology, 13*(6), 693–713. doi:10.1007/bf00929796

Spross, J. (1996). Coaching and suffering: The role of the nurse in helping people face illness. In B. R. Ferrell (Ed.), *Suffering* (pp. 173–208). Sudbury, MA: Jones & Bartlett.

Sullivan, M. (2001). Lost in translation: How Latinos view end of life care. Retrieved from http://www.lastacts.org

Sulmasy, D. (1997). *The healer's calling: A spirituality for physicians and other healthcare professionals.* New York, NY: Paulist Press.

Taxis, J. (2005). Attitudes, values, and questions of African Americans regarding participation in hospice programs. *Journal of Hospice and Palliative Nursing, 8*(2), 77–85. doi:10.1097/00129191-200603000-00011

Taylor, E. J. (2003). Nurses caring for the spirit: Patients with cancer and family caregiver expectations. *Oncology Nursing Forum, 30*(4), 585–590. doi:10.1188/03.ONF.585-590

Taylor, E. J., & Outlaw, F. H. (2002). Use of prayer among persons with cancer. *Holistic Nursing Practice, 16*(3), 46–60.

Taylor, E. J., Outlaw, F. H., Bernardo, T. R., & Roy, A. (1999). Spiritual conflicts associated with praying about cancer. *Psycho-Oncology, 8*(5), 386–394. doi:10.1002/(SICI)1099-1611(199909/10)8:5<386::AID-PON407>3.0.CO;2-C

Theris, T. (2001). Nurturing hope and spirituality in the nursing home. *Holistic Nursing Practice, 15*(4), 45–56. doi:10.1097/00004650-200107000-00008

Thomas, J., & Retsas, A. (1999). Transacting self-preservation: A grounded theory of the spiritual dimensions of people with terminal cancer. *International Journal of Nursing Studies, 36*(3), 191–201. doi:10.1016/S0020-7489(99)00012-7

Tiew, L. H., Kwee, J. H., Creedy, D. K., & Chan, M. F. (2013). Hospice nurses' perspectives of spirituality. *Journal of Clinical Nursing, 22*(19–20), 2923–2933. doi:10.1111/jocn.12358

Timmins, F., & Caldeira, S. (2017). Assessing the spiritual needs of patients. *Nursing Standard, 31*(29), 47–53. doi:10.7748/ns.2017.e10312

Vachon, M., & Huggard, J. (2010). The nurse: Prevention of compassion fatigue. Retrieved from http://txnmhospice.org/docs/2016ELNEChandouts/Module%207%20section%20III.ppt

Vallurupalli, M., Lauderdale, K., Balboni, M. J., Phelps, A. C., Block, S. D., Ng, A. K., . . . Balboni, T. A. (2012). The role of spirituality and religious coping in the quality of life of patients with advanced cancer receiving palliative radiation therapy. *Journal of Supportive Oncology, 10*(2), 81–87. doi:10.1016/j.suponc.2011.09.003

Watson, J. (1986). Suffering and the quest for meaning. In R. DeBellis, E. Marcus, A. Kutscher, C. Smith Torres, V. Barrett, & M. Siegel (Eds.), *Suffering: Psychological and social aspects in loss, grief, and care* (pp. 175–187). New York, NY: Haworth Press.

Wayman, L., & Gaydos, H. (2005). Self-transcending through suffering. *Journal of Hospice and Palliative Nursing, 7*(5), 263–270.

Weaver, A. J., Flannelly, L. T., & Flannelly, K. J. (2001). A review of research on religious and spiritual variables in two primary gerontological nursing journals: 1991 to 1997. *Journal of Gerontological Nursing, 27*(9), 47–54.

Wilson, D. R. (2012). The Editor's Perspective. Spirituality and culture are intertwined. *International Journal of Childbirth Education, 27*(1), 4–5.

Wink, P. (1999). Addressing end of life issues: Spirituality and inner life. *Generations, 23*(1), 75–80.

Yancu, C. N., Farmer, D. F., Graves, M. J., Rhinehardt, A., & Leahman, D. (2015). Accepting transitions: African Americans discuss end of life. *American Journal of Hospice and Palliative Medicine, 32*(4), 380–387. doi:10.1177/1049909114528567

Yoshiko Yamashita, C., & Brown, G. M. (2014). American Indians' experiences of life-threatening illness and end of life. *Journal of Hospice and Palliative Nursing, 16*(7), 404–413. doi:10.1097/NJH.0000000000000086

Yu, J., Chang, L., Jun-Ying, L., Mei-Juan, H., Wen-Xiu, Y., Ru, Z., & Yu-Quan, W. (2007). Different attitudes of Chinese patients and their families toward truth telling of different stages of cancer. *Psycho-Oncology, 16*(10), 928–936. doi:10.1002/pon.1156

Yun, Y. H., Kwon, Y. C., Lee, M. K., Lee, W. J., Jung, K. H., Do, Y. R., . . . Park, S. Y. (2010). Experiences and attitudes of patients with terminal cancer and their family caregivers toward the disclosure of terminal illness. *Journal of Clinical Oncology, 28*(11), 1950–1957. doi:10.1200/JCO.2009.22.9658

Zafiral-Shahri, M., & Al-Khenaizan, A. (2005). Palliative care for Muslim patients. *Journal of Supportive Oncology, 3*(6), 432–436.

Marianne Matzo

Intimacy and Sexual Health

CHAPTER

7

KEY POINTS

- Sexual health concerns exist throughout the trajectory of illness, including late-stage disease.
- Sexual health concerns for seriously ill patients are extremely diverse.
- Illness involving sexual organs increases the likelihood of retraumatization for those who have experienced previous sexual trauma.
- Patients have expectations of assessment and interventions from their practitioner in sexual health concerns.
- There is very little documentation concerning patients with serious illness wishes and expectations regarding their sexual health throughout the course of their illness trajectory.

CASE STUDY

Alice Warton, a 65-year-old retired English teacher, arrived at my outpatient supportive care clinic in a wheelchair wearing pajamas and accompanied by her 28-year-old daughter. Two months ago, Alice was diagnosed with a large vulvar malignancy extending from the clitoris to the anus and involving the lower vagina and urethra (Stage IV squamous cell carcinoma of the vulva). The tumor was unresectable, and she was starting on chemotherapy (six cycles of Cisplatin) and vaginal radiation therapy.

When I talked to Alice, all she did was cry; she was highly anxious and rated her pain as 10/10 in her pudendum. Her daughter reported that she would not get out of bed and expected her to bring her meals on a tray. She would not bathe or change her clothes. She scored 14 out of 27 on the PHQ-9, placing her in the moderate, clinically significant range for depression. Her score on the GAD-7 was 15 out of 21, placing her in the severe, clinically significant range for anxiety. She states she was given Alprazolam to manage her anxiety, but she felt worse ("more agitated and anxious") when taking it. She was taking Effexor 37.5 mg at bedtime for depression. During my assessment, I asked if this was new behavior since the cancer diagnosis, and they both said yes, that she had never had acted this way before.

The focus of my treatment plan for Ms. Warton was pain, mood, and anxiety management. Given that she became more anxious on Alprazolam, I changed her medication to Haldol 0.5 mg every 4 to 6 hours prn for anxiety. The Effexor was changed to duloxetine to help manage both her symptoms of depression and chemotherapy-induced peripheral neuropathy. Her vitamin D_3 level came back at 26.2 when I checked it, so I started her on 50,000 units of cholecalciferol weekly for 10 weeks. Her oxycontin was increased to 40 mg every 12 hours with oxycodone 10 mg every 6 hours prn for breakthrough pain. Yet, I couldn't help but wonder if it was the cancer diagnosis and the effects of treatment alone that resulted in Alice's mood and function devolving.

Quality of life (QOL) issues are very important considerations in the delivery of palliative care. Assessment of an individual's ability to complete activities of daily living and basic needs are an integral part of palliative care. Sexual intimacy is not typically discussed openly, if at all. Sexual health within the context of palliative care may be directly impacted by the disease on anatomical structures. However, direct anatomical effect is not the only concern; changes in a person's sexual interest or desire may also be affected by direct or indirect consequences of medical treatment or in association with being terminally ill.

For many people, when one talks about sexuality, the immediate reference is to intercourse. Different approaches can be taken to the study of sexuality and intimacy, but the focus of this chapter is on *sexual health*, which encompasses both concepts. One definition of sexual health is the integration of somatic, intellectual, and social aspects of being sexual (Epstein & Mamo, 2017). The somatic aspect includes the physical ability to be intimate with a partner, that is, be sexually functional (i.e., to have desire, become aroused, and obtain sexual fulfillment). The intellectual aspect is the ability to communicate about sexual needs and desires, to act intentionally and responsibly, and to set appropriate sexual boundaries. Sexual health affirms sexuality as a positive force that can enhance other aspects of a person's life. Social aspects include the ability to be intimate with a partner, sexual desire, self-acceptance and respect, and the feeling of belonging to and involvement in one's culture (Robinson, Bockting, Simon-Rosser, Miner, & Coleman, 2002).

The sexual healthcare needs of the seriously ill patient facing the end of his or her life has received some recognition in the professional literature, but there are limited research studies to support the assertions made in these publications. There is public health awareness of sexuality related to health, well-being, and QOL and a corresponding need to gather patient data to inform a sexual health plan of care. The World Health Organization (WHO) Department of Reproductive Health and Research recognizes sexual health as a separate dimension of QOL warranting clinical investigation (World Health Organization [WHO], 2004).

An Institute of Medicine (IOM, 2007) report addressed the importance of holistic care for cancer patients. It concluded that in order to ensure appropriate psychosocial health, healthcare practitioners (HCPs) should facilitate effective communication between patients and care providers. In a study by Young (2007),

28% of the patients indicate that their physicians do not pay attention to anything other than their medical needs (Young, 2007). Sexuality assessment is frequently overlooked by palliative care providers when healthcare needs are being assessed. Healthcare professionals may avoid discussion of sexuality for several reasons: (a) embarrassment, (b) assumption that the sex life is over due to the disease, (c) lack of knowledge, and (d) lack of time. Patient-reported barriers can include (a) embarrassment, (b) privacy, and (c) environmental issues (Blagbrough, 2010). Additionally, patients report that psychological distress during diagnosis and treatment of malignancy can impair a healthy sexual response cycle (Krychman, Pereira, Carter, & Amsterdam, 2006).

The Sexual Health Model (Robinson et al., 2002; also see Figure 7.1) is a theoretical framework well suited for palliative care. The model reflects the complexity of human sexuality by identifying 10 broad components posited to be essential aspects of healthy human sexuality:

1. Talking about sex: This is a cornerstone of the model and includes the ability to talk comfortably and explicitly about sexuality, especially one's own sexual values, preferences, attractions, history, and behaviors.
2. Culture and sexual identity: Culture influences one's sexuality and sense of sexual self; understanding how one's cultural heritage impacts sexual identities, attitudes, and behaviors will influence sexual health.
3. Sexual anatomy and functioning: Sexual health assumes a basic knowledge, understanding, and acceptance of one's sexual anatomy, sexual response, and sexual functioning, as well as freedom from sexual dysfunction and other sexual problems.
4. Sexual healthcare: This encompasses knowing one's body, obtaining regular exams for sexually transmitted diseases and cancer, and responding to physical changes with appropriate medical intervention.
5. Overcoming challenges to sexual health: Challenges to sexual health such as sexual abuse, substance abuse, compulsive sexual behavior, sex work, harassment, and discrimination are critical in any discussion of sexual health.
6. Body image: Body image is an important aspect of sexual health; challenging the notion of one's narrow standard of beauty and encouraging self-acceptance is relevant to all populations.
7. Masturbation/fantasy: This includes a realistic appreciation of the important role of masturbation and fantasy. Encouraging masturbation as a normal

adjunct to partnered sex can decrease the pressures on women to engage in penetrative sex with their partners more frequently than they desire.

8. Positive sexuality: This includes a developmental approach to sexual health over the life span, recognizing the reality that all human beings need to explore their sexuality in order to develop and nurture who they are. The importance of exploring and celebrating sexuality from a positive and self-affirming perspective is an essential feature of this model, the assumption being that when people are comfortable with their sexuality they will know and be able to ask for what is sexually pleasurable for them.

9. Intimacy and relationships: Intimacy is a universal need that people try to meet through their relationships.

10. Spirituality and values: The assumption of congruence between one's ethical, spiritual, and moral beliefs and one's sexual behaviors and values. In this context, spirituality may or may not include identification with formal religions, but the need to address moral and ethical concerns (Robinson et al., 2002). Several components of the model will be addressed in this chapter.

■ TALKING ABOUT SEX

HCPs frequently avoid talking about sexuality with cancer patients (Matzo, Whalen, & Pope, 2013). Many studies regarding sexual health document themes related to communication about sexuality and intimacy between patients and their HCPs. These tend to fall into two categories: needs and communication. Regarding needs, patients have questions and concerns about their sexual health that they would like to discuss with their HCPs. A survey of HCPs (N = 1,946; Bachmann, 2006) documented that 60% of the respondents estimated at least three fourths of their patients had sexual dysfunction, but 58% indicated they initiated assessment of sexual health concerns in less than one quarter of their patients. Second, concerning communication, patients indicated they do not initiate these conversations because they think HCPs are too busy, they don't want to "bother" them, they think that they should just be "grateful to be alive," they think that it is a "private matter," or they think if something could be done about the situation, the HCP would raise the issue.

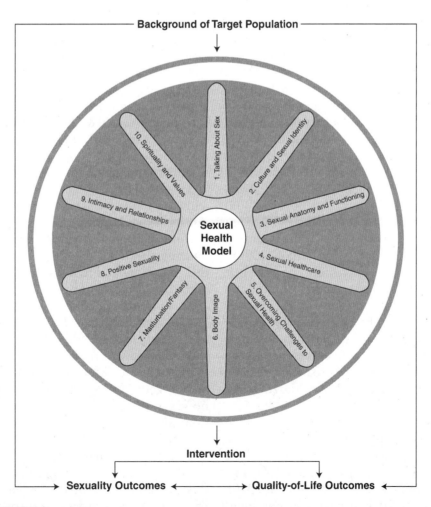

FIGURE 7.1 Sexual Health Model.

Source: Robinson, B. E., Bockting, W. O., Simon-Rosser, B. R., Miner, M., & Coleman, E. (2002). The Sexual Health Model: Application of a sexological approach to HIV prevention. *Health Education Research, 17*(1), 43–57. doi:10.1093/her/17.1.43. With permission from Oxford University Press.

HCPs' barriers to discussing sexuality include embarrassment, misinformed beliefs and assumptions, lack of knowledge, inadequate communication skills, and time constraints. For example, sexual health is not routinely assessed due to the belief that the patient will bring up the topic if it is a concern; the perception that people are "too sick" to be sexual (Caruso-Herman, 1989); lack of their own comfort with the topic (Caruso-Herman, 1989; Dunn, 2004; Epstein & Street, 2007; Grigg, 2002; Wilmoth, 2006); preconceived ideas, attitudes, and values regarding sexuality (Grigg, 2002; Wilmoth, 2006); perceived lack of time for this conversation (Dunn, 2004); and the feeling that there are "more important" issues to be addressed (Ananth, Jones, King, & Tookman, 2003; Smith, 1989). Additionally, lack of communication about sexual health may be the result of the lack of evidence to support raising the issue (Stead, 2004). Sexual health is also not emphasized in HCP professional education (Caruso-Herman, 1989; Dunn, 2004; Grigg, 2002; IOM, 2007; Penson et al., 2000), which can result in this lack of communication, a conspiracy of silence, and a dominant communication pattern of evasiveness (Grigg, 2002).

Communication between the patient and the HCP is an important factor in facilitating the assessment of the patient's sexual health needs. There is disagreement as to who should initiate discussion regarding sexuality between the patient and the caregiver (Levett, 2011). Some literature suggests that health professionals should initiate the discussion regarding changes in sexuality and sexual function that may be occurring related to effects of treatments or secondary to the disease process itself. Patients may not ask these questions themselves because they assume healthcare professionals will initiate the discussion with them (Matzo & Hijjazi, 2009; Rice, 2000). Park, Norris, and Bober (2009) reported that oncology practitioners acknowledge not discussing sexual health issues with patients during the course of treatment; Matzo and Hijjazi (2009) reported that most hospice nurses do not ask their patients about issues related to sexuality or intimacy. Patients, in turn, want the opportunity to discuss their sexual needs with their healthcare provider (Matzo & Hijjazi, 2009). Assessing the patient's needs by obtaining a sexual history and asking pertinent sexual health questions are important components to identify sexual health needs (Matzo & Hijjazi, 2009; Matzo et al., 2013; Rice, 2000).

The most effective communication is that which addresses the needs of the patient at each stage of the illness. The initial assessment should begin when the diagnosis is made and continue throughout the disease process (Mercadante, Vitrano, & Catania, 2010). Communication with cancer patients is a dichotomous situation in that the disease is both life threatening and potentially treatable or curable, which creates much uncertainty and stress on the patient.

■ ADOLESCENTS

Adolescents in palliative care share the same developmental tasks as other adolescents. Cognitive thinking is required to link consequences to behavior; however, in early adolescence, thinking is predominantly concrete (e.g., only the here and now are relevant) and long-term consequences are not considered. Abstract thinking begins in middle adolescence; at this point, consequences of behavior begin to be considered. However, under times of stress, the middle adolescent often reverts to concrete thinking (Wisnieski & Matzo, 2013). Late adolescence is a time when abstract thinking begins to mature and the consequences of behavior are considered. These adolescents strive for autonomy and peer support. Issues of romance, sexuality, and reproduction are normal developmental tasks and should be given attention by healthcare providers. Life-threatening illness may also compromise the development of body image and self-esteem (Knapp, Quinn, Murphy, Brown, & Madden, 2010).

■ SEXUAL ANATOMY AND FUNCTIONING

The complexities of human sexuality are broad, especially for people coping with life-threatening illness (Matzo, 2010). Healthy sexual expression can affirm love, relieve stress and anxiety, foster hope, accentuate spirituality (Matzo, 2015a), and can distract one from the emotional and physical sequelae of chronic illness (Matzo, 2015b). Maintaining sexual health along the trajectory of cancer treatment can be difficult given the physical, emotional, psychological, and communication complexities surrounding this topic (Matzo, Troup, Hijjazi, & Ferrell, 2015). Any aspect of a terminal/life-threatening disease (either from the disease itself or from the treatment) can impact sexual health.

Women diagnosed with breast/gynecological cancers undergo physical and emotional challenges throughout their treatment and recovery, and up to 90% of women with these cancers have sexual dysfunction as a side effect of treatment (Carter, Stabile, Gunn, & Sonoda, 2013; Lutgendorf et al., 2017). The alterations in sexual health include decreased libido, pain with intercourse, trouble reaching orgasm, and vaginal dryness (Matzo et al., 2013). Treatments such as radiation, chemotherapy, and surgery improve prognosis (Salani et al., 2011); however, these treatments result in estrogen depletion, which negatively impacts vaginal health (Matzo, 2015a; Matzo et al., 2013; Mercadante et al., 2010). The resulting vaginal atrophy is manifested by vaginal dryness, discomfort, burning, itching, and dyspareunia; this is a significant problem for female cancer survivors who cannot use estrogen as a treatment intervention because even low-dose estrogen can have effects on tissue outside of the vagina and can present cancer-related health risks (Le et al., 2011). Regardless of interest in sexual activity, vaginal health maintenance is vital for all women; vaginal dryness and/or pain can increase anxiety about gynecological appointments, make exams painful, and potentially result in noncompliance with follow-up care (Carter et al., 2013). Persistent vaginal dryness has been correlated with depression and decreased QOL (Le et al., 2011; Matzo et al., 2015; Tan, Bradshaw, & Carr, 2012) and increased distress (Carter et al., 2013).

Gynecologic cancer therapies exacerbate and accelerate processes seen in normal vaginal aging and are associated with sexual dysfunction. Hormonal therapies such as selective estrogen receptor modulators and aromatase inhibitors decrease vaginal pH and lubrication and increase vasomotor symptoms and dyspareunia. Surgery is also associated with sexual dysfunction, vaginal atrophy, and dyspareunia. Psychological distress that the patient or her partner experiences during diagnosis and treatment of malignancy can also impair a healthy female sexual response cycle. Patients undergoing radiation therapy report more sexual dysfunction than surgical patients and more vaginal atrophy and post-coital bleeding than surgical patients. Radiation therapy decreases blood flow to the vaginal mucosa, which leads to chronic pelvic fibrosis that may persist for up to 2 years after treatment (Matzo, 2015a; Salani et al., 2011).

The vaginal microenvironment directs flora, pH (Linhares, Summers, Larsen, Giraldo, & Witkin, 2011; Oakley, Fiedler, Marrazzo, & Fredricks, 2008), hormonal health (Derzko, Elliott, & Lam, 2007; Moalli, Debes, Meyn, Howden, & Abramowitch, 2008), as well as sexual health (Linhares et al., 2011). Dyspareunia in women with vaginal atrophy is primarily attributed to the lack of vaginal lubrication (Harmanli & Jones, 2010). Lack of vaginal lubrication is also associated with decreased antimicrobial activity. Vaginal dryness, vaginal atrophy, lack of elasticity, dyspareunia, and sexual dysfunction can be improved with the use of vaginal lubricants. Counseling women in the use of vaginal lubricant is one of the most effective methods shown to offset the negative effects of cancer treatments (Le et al., 2011; Linhares et al., 2011; Schover et al., 2011; Table 7.1).

Risk factors for poorer sexual functioning after being diagnosed with gynecological cancer are age, treatment, time since treatment, poor self-esteem/body image, physical symptoms, poor performance status, depression, and anxiety (Pereira & Schattman, 2017). Ovarian cancer is usually treated with a hysterectomy, oophorectomy, and chemotherapy, which can all affect sexual functioning through a decrease in estrogen production (resulting in vaginal atrophy, loss of vaginal lubrication, and hot flashes) and loss of sexual interest resulting from changes in body, fatigue, and nausea (American Cancer Society [ACS], 2017).

Women with advanced ovarian cancer (OVCA) over the age of 55 have reported distress over the loss of reproductive potential (Stewart, Wong, & Duff, 2001). In one study, over 50% of the women with ovarian cancer reported moderate to severely worsened sexual function (Stewart et al., 2001). Carmack Taylor, Basen-Engquist, Shinn, and Bodurka (2004) compared the sexual health of women with breast cancer, ovarian cancer, and postmenopausal women and concluded that low desire, vaginal dryness, and dyspareunia are more common and severe in women with ovarian cancer (Carmack Taylor et al., 2004). Another study documented that for women with ovarian cancer, their satisfaction with care for sexual problems was lower than with their overall cancer care (Lindau et al., 2007).

Treatments for cervical cancer result in numerous issues that can impact sexual health. Surgery shortens the proximal vagina by one third and radiation therapy causes stenosis, drying, and dyspareunia, which typically results in the need for the use of dilator and estrogen creams in order to help prevent vaginal atrophy (Matzo et al., 2015). Hormonal changes result from surgical removal of the ovary or irradiation. Psychological issues related to the diagnosis that can have a negative impact on sexual health are fear of the disease and metastasis, vaginal odor, and the perception of some women that they "deserve" the disease because of their previous sexual behavior (Matzo et al., 2015).

Hughes and De La Garza (2017) studied the sexual health of women diagnosed with breast cancer versus non–breast cancer patients, noting that issues of sexual dysfunction are primarily documented in colorectal or gynecological cancer. However, their study found that regardless of demographic variables, women diagnosed with breast cancer were statistically more likely to report sexual problems (on the NCCN Distress Thermometer checklist). Women living with breast cancer typically experience body image issues, permanent menopause resulting from cancer treatments, and aromatase inhibitors, which negatively affect sexual expression (Hughes & De La Garza, 2017).

Alterations in sexual health for men primarily focus on erectile function. Cancer treatments can interfere with erection by damaging a man's pelvic nerves, pelvic blood vessels, or hormone balance. Prostate, bladder, and colon cancer are often treated with radiation to the pelvis. The higher the total dose of radiation and the wider the section of the pelvis irradiated, the greater the chance of an erection problem later (ACS, 2017). Erectile dysfunction (ED) is a common complication of diabetes (secondary to autonomic neuropathy, vascular insufficiency, or psychological factors) in at least half of men over age 50. ED can also occur as a result of cardiovascular disease, hypertension, hypercholesterolemia, smoking, and the abuse of drugs including alcohol.

Prostate cancer is the most common non–skin cancer in men and sexual dysfunction is the most frequently reported long-term side effect of prostate cancer surgery or radiation (Albaugh, Sufrin, Lapin, Petkewicz, & Tenfelde, 2017). After standard radical prostatectomy, between 65% and 90% of men will become impotent, depending on their age. If the surgeon does not remove

TABLE 7.1   Products to Maintain Vaginal Hydration

Vaginal moisturizers versus vaginal lubricants:

■ **Vaginal moisturizer:** Nonhormonal, over-the-counter, and usually water-based products intended to be used several times a week routinely for overall vaginal health or comfort, regardless of sexual activity. The goal of a vaginal moisturizer is to moisturize the vaginal mucosa for overall comfort. Sometimes a vaginal moisturizer is sufficient for vaginal comfort in regular daily life and for sexual intercourse. Moisturizers restore fluid into the cells of the vagina and vaginal pH. Some female cancer survivors need vaginal moisturizers up to three to five times per week. Most of these moisturizers are gels administered with a tampon-like applicator or as a vaginal suppository. Regular usage is the key to moisturizing performance.

■ **Vaginal lubricant:** Usually a liquid or gel (water-based), but may also be oil- or silicone-based. A vaginal lubricant is meant to be applied around the clitoris and labia minora and inside the vaginal entrance to minimize dryness and pain during sexual activity. Optimally, the lubricant should be applied to both partners' genitals prior to vaginal penetration, to minimize friction and irritation.

Base Types	Brands	Pros	Cons
Water-Based			
Vaginal moisturizers	Replens Lubrin Luvena	Vaginal moisturizers are applied two to five times per week (ideally every 3–4 days) and need not be applied directly prior to sexual activity.	It is possible that a moisturizer alone is insufficient to reduce frictional pain, so during sexual activity a vaginal lubricant may also be needed.
Vaginal lubricants Thin lubricants	K-Y Liquid Astroglide	All water-based vaginal moisturizers and lubricants share the following advantages: ■ Reactivate with a few drops of water ■ Latex compatible ■ Clear and nonstaining ■ Clean up easily with soap and water ■ Absorb into skin and evaporate ■ Water-based lubricants are typically recommended by doctors and healthcare workers, and they are the kind usually made available for free at sexual health clinics	All water-based vaginal moisturizers and lubricants share the following disadvantages: ■ Not compatible with sex acts in water ■ May contain glycerin, an ingredient that turns into sugar in the vagina; thus, it may contribute to yeast infection in persons who are susceptible ■ Tend to dry out ■ May leave sticky residue (especially if high glycerin) ■ Can be dispersed in water (not good for bathtub sex, etc.).
Medium/thick lubricants (thick lubricants are especially helpful when a higher level of lubrication is needed, such as when pain is still experienced while using regular lubricants)	Slippery Stuff Liquid Silk (glycerin-free) ID Lube Astrogel Maximus Probe (paraben-free)		
Other	Maximus (glycerin-free) Sliquid H20 (glycerin-free) Hathor (parabens-free) Aphrodeisia (parabens-free) BioGlide (contains carrageen, which has been shown to protect against HPV and other viruses) K-Y Slide + E, K-Y Liquibeads		
Oil-Based			
Vaginal lubricants	Élégance (only FDA-approved for vaginal application) Vitamin E (puncture caplet and use as suppository) MenoMoist Mineral oil Coconut or olive oil Vegetable shortening	Durable Decreased vaginal bacteria/yeast in testing	Should not be used with condoms (breaks down latex)

(continued)

TABLE 7.1 Products to Maintain Vaginal Hydration (*continued*)			
Silicone-Based			
Vaginal lubricants	Eros Lubricant Liquid Silver Wet Platinum Lubricant I-E Velvet Lubricating Liquid	Always slippery and never tacky feeling A little goes a long way More durable Does not dry up as quickly as other formulations Not absorbed by the skin Good for water use ("water play") Does not change the pH of the vagina (no yeast concerns) Washes away with soap and water Great for full body massage	May leave oily residue on sheets, but will wash out Not recommended with silicone-based toys Usually a little more expensive
Ingredients to consider staying away from include the following: Glycerin or sorbitol may contribute to yeast infections in those susceptible. Petroleum-based lubricants may increase the risk of vaginal infection and also tend to have an unpleasant odor and may damage latex condoms (possible pregnancy or sexually transmitted diseases). Perfume, spermicide, or other additives that may be irritating.			

FDA, Food and Drug Administration.

Source: Carter, J., Goldfrank, D., & Schover, L. R. (2011). Simple strategies for vaginal health promotion in cancer survivors. *Journal of Sexual Medicine, 8*(2), 549–559. doi:10.1111/j.1743-6109.2010.01988.x

or damage the nerves on either side of the prostate, the impotence rate drops to between 25% and 30% for men under 60. The impotence rate is higher for men over 70, even if nerves on both sides are not damaged or removed (Zippe & Pahlajani, 2008). After surgery, there is no ejaculation of semen although, even with a dry orgasm, the sensation should still be pleasurable (ACS, 2017).

Androgen deprivation therapy (ADT) is a common treatment intervention. Most men on ADT for prostate cancer will never return to baseline levels of sexual function (Donovan et al., 2018). Some men diagnosed with cancer report that they were not as sexually active as before diagnosis, experienced reduced potency and diminished pleasure in ejaculation, felt their "manhood" was restricted, and had difficulty discussing sexual problems. A recent systematic review of the impact of prostate treatment on QOL documented that men treated with surgery reported mainly urinary and sexual problems for up to 6 years following treatment (Lardas et al., 2017). Men will sometimes report pain in the genitals during sex, or if the prostate gland or urethra has been irritated from cancer treatment, ejaculation may be painful (ACS, 2017).

Sexual health can be impacted by almost any life-threatening illness and should be assessed in every patient. Assessing a patient's functionality and desire for sexual activity is a necessary skill for HCPs. Asking if there are concerns regarding sexual health may be a good first question in determining how a person's diagnosis,

subsequent treatment, or current health has affected them. Not all patients will report concern regarding their sexual health function; in these cases, no further intervention is needed except to encourage the patient to let the HCP know if their situation changes. Not asking about sexual health may be more comfortable to the HCP, but does not improve the sexual healthcare of the patient (Matzo et al., 2013).

Information to help patients with these concerns primarily focuses on preventing pain (genital and nongenital) during sex and interventions to help men get and keep an erection. In 1998, the Food and Drug Administration (FDA) approved sildenafil citrate (Viagra) to treat impotence. Oral phosphodiesterase-5 inhibitors (PDE-5) help achieve an erection by increasing blood flow to the penis. About half of men with impotence due to medical (rather than psychological) problems are helped to some extent by these drugs (ACS, 2017). Nerve damage from prostate cancer treatment may not respond as well to these drugs as some other physical causes of impotence.

Other treatments for ED include intracavernosal injection therapy and surgically implanted penile prostheses. Noninvasive drug-free solutions such as vacuum erection devices (VED) remain popular despite the availability of PDE-5 inhibitors. The VED is easy to use and a man can produce an erection in 2 to 3 minutes (which can increase spontaneity and patient compliance). Vacuum therapy is a tube, or cylinder, that is placed over the penis. A vacuum is then applied to increase penile blood flow (due to negative pressure). The use of the VED has expanded and can be used in combination with PDE-5 inhibitors in penile rehabilitation following radical prostatectomy and radiation therapy.

Pain during intercourse is one of the most common sexual problems for women (genital or nongenital) and can interfere with the feeling of pleasure during sex (Table 7.2). Nongenital pain may be secondary to soreness in one arm after a radical mastectomy or tingling and numbness in the hands and feet after chemotherapy. The ACS (2017) makes the following recommendations for patients regarding overcoming nongenital pain. First, plan sexual activity for the time of day they feel the least pain. If using pain medicine, take it an hour before planned sexual activity so it will be in full effect during sex. Second, find a position for touching or intercourse that puts as little pressure as possible on the sore areas, support the sore areas, and limit their movement with pillows. If a certain motion is painful, they can choose a position that does not require it or ask their partner to take over the hip movements during intercourse. Encourage patients to talk to their partners regarding what brings the most pleasure. Third, encourage patients to focus on their feelings of pleasure and excitement; with this focus, the pain may fade into the background (ACS, 2017).

Genital-related pain results from a loss of vaginal lubrication and vaginal muscle scarring and shortening. Cancer treatments, aromatase inhibitors, menopause, and hysterectomy or mastectomy decrease the amount of vagina lubrication. Some lubricants include herbal extracts (such as aloe or lavender) that can cause irritation or allergic reactions, and warming gels can cause a burning sensation. Replens and K-Y Liquibeads are vaginal moisturizers that can be used 2 or 3 times a week to help keep the vagina moist and at a more normal acid balance (pH). The effects of these products last longer than those of lubricants, and these products can be purchased without a prescription. Lubrin and Astroglide Silken Secret are other moisturizers that are marketed as longer lasting than typical lubricants (ACS, 2017). Luvena, a prebiotic vaginal moisturizer and lubricant, was the first paraben- and glycerin-free product that utilizes bioactive enzymes naturally found in the vagina (www.luvenacare.com/index.html). Table 7.1 offers the pros and cons of each form of lubricant.

Vaginal dilators are often used after radiation to the pelvis, cervix, or vagina. It is recommended that vaginal dilators are given to patients undergoing radical radiotherapy to the pelvis as part of their cancer treatment, together with support and education. A vaginal dilator is a tube of plastic or rubber used to dilate the vagina and to help women learn to relax the vaginal muscles (ACS, 2017). Regular intercourse and/or the use of vaginal dilators may minimize stenosis. Vaginal changes develop over time, even up to 5 years post treatment, and may impact sexual function and sexual health and well-being in addition to considerable distress for a woman and her partner (Sears, Robinson, & Walker, 2017). Dilators work best when used early after radiation or surgery to prevent vaginal shrinkage prior to the vagina tightening (Matzo et al., 2015). If a woman goes for many months without a sexual relationship, it is very important that the dilator be used to keep the vagina in shape (ACS, 2017). Instructions for use are found in Table 7.3.

Research has shown that up to 50% of women treated for cervix cancers have sexual dysfunction as they recover and become cancer survivors (Shankar et al., 2017).

CASE STUDY Continued

I stopped and went back to my assessment and noticed that Alice had listed in her chart a history of posttraumatic stress disorder (PTSD) and fibromyalgia. When I investigated the origin of her PTSD, she started to sob even harder and said that her father and his friends had sexually abused her, starting at the age of 5. She said she had "dealt with this" in therapy in her 20s, and it was not anything that she thinks about now. It has been my clinical observation that for some women who had experienced sexual assault in their past, gynecological or breast cancer can result in retraumatization. Alice and I talked about this and she agreed to talk with our psychologist.

I was puzzled by Alice's catastrophic reaction to her diagnosis. I suspected that she was having a paradoxical reaction to her prescribed benzodiazepine (Kirkpatrick et al., 2016), but it seemed as though there was something else contributing to her symptoms. She mentioned that she had a history of PTSD, and when I inquired further, she said she had been repeatedly raped starting at the age of 5 by her father and his friends, but it was not something that she had really thought about in a very long time.

TABLE 7.2   BE-FEMM: A Straightforward Approach to Maintaining Sexual Health
Ways to Help Yourself

There is a lot you can do to take back and maintain your sexual health, even while undergoing active treatment. The biggest thing to remember is to be proactive—prevention is much easier than treatment down the road. Although you may not feel up to activities now, you want to keep your body primed for the future!

Just remember BE-FEMM!
- **B**lood Flow
- **E**njoyment
- **F**lora
- **E**lasticity
- **M**oisture
- **M**uscle Tone

Blood Flow

All over your body, healthy tissue needs good blood flow. When your body has had medical or surgical interventions, this becomes even more important. Menopause, whether it occurs naturally over time, or surgically, comes with its own challenges. As estrogen declines, your vagina will begin to atrophy. (Yes, the fun of being a woman goes on and on!) This atrophy can cause thinning of the tissues, shrinkage, and decreased lubrication of the vaginal walls. As if cancer is not enough fun all in itself, chemotherapy is the gift that keeps on giving because it can also directly affect your vaginal health. Not only will all this lead to painful intercourse, but it will also make you more vulnerable to yeast infections. All of these things can be improved with one simple idea—keeping the blood flowing to this area.

Now, the good news. There are some easy (and even fun) things you can do to help improve your blood flow. Stimulation is a great way to accomplish this. You can use vibrators, or even a willing partner if you have one "handy" (no pun intended). You may want to explore a product called an Eros therapy device. This little gem was created to treat female sexual dysfunction. It is a gentle vacuum that will help to restore blood flow to the clitoris and genitalia. (Not a Hoover—I said a gentle vacuum!) The by-product of increased blood flow in this area can be increased orgasms, improved vaginal lubrication, and overall sexual satisfaction. (Let's hear it for overall sexual satisfaction—yeah!) The Eros therapy device is available by prescription only (for more information, visit www.eros-therapy.com).

Enjoyment

Now, with all that increased blood flow, you will be ready to move on to the best advice anyone can give: Please enjoy your sexual relations! Wait, finish reading first! That is better. Unfortunately, some women suffered from unsatisfying sexual relations before they ever got cancer. If you have been suffering in silence all these years, you just got your get-out-of-jail-free card. Look at cancer treatment as an opportunity to make some changes that will make the rest of your life richer, happier, and more rewarding— especially in the orgasm department (which is a very nice department).

If you have been shy about telling your partner what you need or have been afraid of bruising a delicate ego by saying that you have been less than satisfied, this gives you an excuse to open a new dialogue, and try some new techniques. Sometimes, since women can participate in sex without actually feeling any desire for sex, lazy partners can forget to give you adequate stimulation for the encounter to be enjoyable for you. If you are using an Eros therapy device or a vibrator, you may find yourself already stimulated, and take that opportunity to seek out your partner and initiate things yourself. Some guys need that little blue pill to get in the mood—why should not we have some help if we need it? Do not miss the opportunity to tell your partner what you need in the way of stimulation, where your pleasure spots are, and what makes you feel good.

Arousal is very important. We all know it is the key to proper lubrication, but did you know that there are also physical changes to your vagina when you are aroused? It actually causes your vagina to widen and elongate, which will greatly decrease any discomfort you may experience. An interesting note: In most women, the vagina elongates toward the back, but after hysterectomy, it will tend to elongate up more toward your stomach. This may change the angle that feels comfortable to you. The good old missionary position may become uncomfortable. Do not give up on intimacy, just roll over. You may prefer the angle from the back or even the side. Be adventurous. There is nobody there to see you but your partner, and believe me, he or she will want to work to make it better for you. You may also want to try a position where you can control the depth and the angle, such as from the top.

Flora

Now, a word from our sponsor, *Lactobacillus acidophilus*. Kidding. That is the name of the bacteria in "live-culture" yogurt. Did you know that it also plays a starring role in your vagina? That is the busy little bacterium that keeps yeast infections at bay. It occurs naturally in a healthy vagina, and keeps the environment acidic so that harmful bacteria are not happy there. Those little lactobacilli need estrogen too, so menopause can affect the balance of flora in your vagina, which can lead to an increase in urinary tract and yeast infections. You can help maintain the acidic environment in your vagina by using a product such as Luvena.

(continued)

TABLE 7.2 BE-FEMM: A Straightforward Approach to Maintaining Sexual Health (*continued*)

Elasticity

This is a fancy word that means keeping your tissues elastic or stretchy. Remember, "use it or lose it" should be your mantra for elasticity. Tissue atrophy due to reduced estrogen can be minimized by maintaining good blood flow and by stretching the tissues. It is much easier to keep your vagina healthy than it is to return it to good health. It is not that easy with cancer treatments, surgical recovery, and what not to keep a good handle on your vaginal elasticity. (You do not get up every day and say, "Another day, another chance to keep my vagina elastic!") But it is important. If you have not been using these tissues in a while, you may need to start small. Literally. A vaginal dilator can be helpful, and is available online (through online retailers). You can ask your doctor for a prescription if you prefer. A dilator is just a plastic device with tips of various sizes. Used in combination with moisturizers and lubrication, your vaginal opening can gradually be expanded by their use. This can restore natural elasticity and improve comfort in sexual activities (a place where you really want some comfort).

If you experienced sexual pain before your cancer diagnosis, your body may have developed a pain response that can include spasms of the muscles near your vaginal opening, which you should discuss with your doctor.

Moisture

Of all the difficulties you face with the decline of estrogen, the loss of natural lubrication is one of the most heartbreaking. The good news is that with diligent treatment, you can easily improve the symptoms. Once again, your recovery and sexual health are completely in your control. The first component in treatment is a moisturizer. This is a product that you apply at least weekly. It is best to choose a product free of fragrances, dyes, or paraben, and one that is pH-balanced. Replens is available through your doctor; a new product called Luvena has recently become available that is not only moistening, but has a prebiotic formulation that will help you to keep your new commitment to balanced flora!

The second component goes hand-in-hand with moisture, and that is lubrication. You would add lubrication anytime you use dilators, vibrators, or share that magic moment with your partner. You can choose K-Y Jelly, Astroglide, or other lubricating products. See Table 7.1 for pros and cons of each form of lubricant. Each person's preference is different. Fortunately, trying out different lubricants is a really fun way to spend time with that special someone, so have fun, experiment, and decide what is best for you. The important thing to remember is that your lack of natural moisture should not be interpreted as a lack of desire for your partner, or as any kind of hindrance to wonderful love making!

Muscle Tone

The last key to maintaining good sexual health is muscle tone. Perhaps you tried Kegel exercises when you were pregnant? If not, you are about to gain an important tool in keeping both your vagina and your urinary tract healthy. Kegel exercises strengthen the muscles of your pelvic floor (the muscles that support your bladder, bowels, and the walls of your vagina). These muscles are vitally important for maintaining bladder and bowel continence as well as your ability to enjoy sexual relations for the rest of your life. Good. Now that I have your attention, let us try to isolate those pelvic floor muscles.

- Try to tighten the muscles you use to stop urinating, without moving the muscles of your abdomen, legs, or buttocks. If you have trouble isolating them, practice stopping and starting your urine flow (while on the toilet). Once you have found the correct muscles, go on to the next step.
- Squeeze these muscles for about 3 seconds. Then relax them for 3 seconds.
- Do 10–15 repetitions at a time, at least 3 times a day. If you have trouble remembering to do them, associate them with something you do several times a day anyway. Before you start breakfast, lunch, and dinner, try a set of Kegel exercises. If you are doing them right, nobody can tell you are doing them (unless you giggle).

There is a lovely side benefit to doing Kegel exercises. They may actually increase your sexual pleasure. Many women find that they have stronger orgasms after training these muscles, due to increased blood flow and stronger muscle contractions. The increased blood flow to your vaginal area not only speeds healing but also increases sensitivity, and that has got to be a good thing. Your partner will also enjoy the increased muscle tone in your vagina, and if you want to really blow his mind, try doing your Kegel exercises during sex. He will love it.

Getting Help: Finally, cancer does not occur in a vacuum. We are all balancing other concerns in our lives, and cancer is just one more challenge added to your particular mix. Sexual health can be impacted by treatments, by other medical conditions, past abuse or trauma, situational or emotional stress, and relationship issues (or by the absence of a relationship). Instead of letting these concerns cripple this important area of your life, use your cancer as a catalyst to make positive changes in your physical and emotional health! In other words, "Feel positive about your sexuality."

TABLE 7.3 Using a Vaginal Dilator
Minimum use is 3 times weekly for an indefinite time period. Dilators can be used in conjunction with sexual intercourse to achieve a combined frequency of vaginal dilation.
Find a private and comfortable place where you can relax and use the dilator. Dilators can be used in the shower or bath if this provides privacy and/or allows you to relax your pelvic floor muscles. If you wish, your significant other can also be encouraged to be involved.
A water-soluble lubricant should be placed on the dilator and around the entrance to the vagina prior to insertion. Some doctors will prescribe Premarin cream to be used for this purpose.
There are various positions in which to use the dilator: You can either lie down on your back with knees slightly apart and bent, or stand with a leg raised on the side of the bed or bath to insert the dilator.
Inserting the dilator into the vagina requires a firm, gentle pressure. Insert it as deeply as is comfortable, without forcing the dilator. Do pelvic floor exercises during insertion.
Once the dilator is inside the vagina, it should be moved in a forward and backward motion, then a left-to-right motion. If possible, gently rotate the dilator using the handle.
Your doctor will fit you for the dilator. It is usual to start with the smallest size and progress to the largest (size 4) in the days/weeks following treatment, as it is comfortable.
When the dilator is in as far as possible, leave it in your vagina for about 15 minutes. You can pass the time by reading, watching TV, listening to music, or even talking on the phone. If the dilator slips out, gently push it more deeply into your vagina.
The dilator should be removed slowly rotating in clockwise/anticlockwise movements.
Vibrators may also be used in conjunction with the use of dilators.
Slight vaginal loss and blood staining is not uncommon when using dilators. If you experience heavy vaginal bleeding or pain, contact your doctor.
When you remove it, wash it with a mild soap and water. Be sure to rinse all the soap off so no film is left to irritate your vagina the next time you use it.

Source: National Forum of Gynaecological Oncology Nurses. (Ed.). (2005). *Best practice guidelines on the use of vaginal dilators in women receiving pelvic radiotherapy*. Edgbaston, UK: Birmingham Women's Hospital.

■ SEXUAL TRAUMA

Sexual abuse is experienced by approximately 20% of women worldwide (Maseroli et al., 2017). A study by Maseroli et al. documented that women who have been sexually abused had greater anxiety, body image concerns, and sexual distress compared to women who had not. They also reported that sexual abuse had a more negative impact on orgasm and sexual functioning if the abuse occurred in adolescence rather than childhood (Maseroli et al., 2017).

Posttraumatic stress symptoms (PTSS) can be exemplified by reexperiencing the trauma, avoidance of trauma-related stimuli, and negative alterations of cognition, mood, arousal, and reactivity following exposure to a stressor (American Psychiatric Association, 2013). Different longitudinal PTSS trajectories can be found among adult survivors of childhood sexual abuse, typically related to the type of abuse. Abusive experiences considered to be of a high severity level are those of penetrative abuse where the perpetrator was a biological parent or someone the victim trusted. Published literature links childhood sexual abuse to altered neurobiology and stress physiology, increased stress sensitivity later in life, lifelong increased risk of multiple mental and somatic disorders and health problems, and suicide (Steine et al., 2017).

Childhood sexual abuse (CSA) has negative physical and psychological long-term effects. For example, there are published studies documenting that childbirth may retraumatize women who were sexually abused in childhood due to the women's association of the delivery with their earlier maltreatment. For the previously sexually abused woman, the exposure to the medical treatment and medical staff who help handle intimate organs that are associated with sex might also be traumatizing (Daphna-Tekoah, Lev-Wiesel, & Ben-Zion, 2016). Women with a history of CSA may develop symptoms of distress, such as PTSS, depression, and dissociation secondary to a cancer diagnosis involving female sexual organs and breast cancer.

■ OVERCOMING CHALLENGES TO SEXUAL HEALTH AND BODY IMAGE

Some colorectal surgery patients will require either temporary or permanent stomas, as urostomy, colostomy, or ileostomy presents challenges to maintaining sexual health (Albaugh, Tenfelde, & Hayden, 2017). Patients should be reminded to empty the bag and check the seal to reduce the risk of the bag leaking during intercourse. A small-sized ostomy pouch could be worn during sexual activity, or if a two-piece system is used, the pouch can be turned around on the faceplate so that the emptying valve is to the side. If an elastic support belt is worn on the faceplate, it can be tucked into the belt during sex or the bag can be taped to the individual's body. Some people may be more comfortable wearing a T-shirt to cover the appliance. To reduce rubbing against the appliance, encourage patients to choose positions that will keep their partner's weight off the ostomy. If the patient prefers to be on the bottom during intercourse, he or she can put a small pillow above the ostomy faceplate so that the partner can lie on the pillow rather than on the appliance. Those with a colostomy may be able to plan sexual activity for a time of day when the colostomy is not usually active. The colostomy can be irrigated and a stoma cover or a small safety pouch can be used during sex (ACS, 2017).

Some cancers of the head and neck are treated by surgery to remove part of the bone structure of the face. These are public scars that can be devastating to self-image. Surgery on the jaw, palate, or tongue can also change the way people are able to talk. Advances in facial replacement devices and plastic surgery include ears and noses made out of plastic, tinted to match the skin, and attached to the face (ACS, 2017). These interventions can have a tremendous impact on body image and self-esteem.

Treatment for primary tumors of the bone typically includes amputation of the limb, which can result in the need to make some changes during intercourse. Wearing a prosthesis during sex may help with positioning and ease of movement, but the straps that attach it can get in the way. Without a prosthesis, the partner with an amputation may have trouble staying level during intercourse; pillows can be used to support the body. Phantom limb pain can interfere with sexual desire and distract a person during sex; the patient should be encouraged to take pain medications prior to sex.

One quantitative study focused on sexuality in patients with advanced cancer ($n = 65$) assessed their feelings and attitudes regarding sexuality after diagnosis (Vitrano, Catania, & Mercadante, 2011). Over half of the patients still felt attractive despite their diagnosis, and almost half felt that sexuality was important for their psychological well-being; however, only 7.6% were still sexually active. Most patients expressed the importance of communicating their sexual needs with experienced professionals (Vitrano et al., 2011).

■ MASTURBATION

Another component of the Sexual Health Model is masturbation. A stratified probability sample survey of the British general population, aged 16 to 44 years, was conducted from 1999 to 2001 ($N = 11,161$) using face-to-face interviewing and computer-assisted self-interviewing (Gerressu et al., 2008). While a relatively old study, there has not been repeated study related to masturbation. These data were used to estimate the population prevalence of masturbation and to identify sociodemographic, sexual behavioral, and attitudinal factors associated with reporting this behavior. Seventy-three percent of men and 36.8% of women reported masturbating in the 4 weeks prior to interview. Among both men and women, reporting masturbation increased with higher levels of education and social class and was more common among those reporting sexual function problems (Gerressu et al., 2008).

For women, masturbation was more likely among those who reported more frequent vaginal sex in the last 4 weeks, a greater repertoire of sexual activity (such as reporting oral and anal sex), and more sexual partners in the last year. In contrast, the prevalence of masturbation was lower among men reporting more frequent vaginal sex. Both men and women reporting same-sex partner(s) were significantly more likely to report masturbation (Gerressu et al., 2008). Terminally ill people are likely no different than the general population regarding their masturbation habits. Palliative care practitioners should routinely ask their patients if anything interferes in their ability to masturbate and then work with the patient to correct the problem if it is identified.

■ SEXUALITY, INTIMACY, AND RELATIONSHIPS

Sexuality can be seen as the process of giving and receiving sexual pleasure and is associated with a sense of belonging or being accepted by another. Healthcare professionals may focus more on whether a patient is capable of having sex and on the impact of illness on menopause, erectile, or fertility status. This perspective offers a medicalized approach to sexuality, which may be different than the patient's goals. Lemieux, Kaiser, Pereira, and Meadows (2004) conducted a qualitative study that assessed patient perspectives regarding sexuality in palliative care. Overall, it was found that emotional connections took precedence over the physical expressions of love, although sexuality was considered to be very important even during the final stages of life. Barriers to sexual expression included lack of privacy, shared rooms, staff interruptions, and single beds. The patients generally agreed that holistic palliative care should include the impact of illness on sexuality, and these patients would prefer to be asked about these issues in a sensitive manner (Lemieux et al., 2004).

Cort, Monroe, and Oliviere (2004) discussed that sexuality is an integral aspect of palliative care, and couples often seek assistance and support in their relationship. Often, palliative care patients will feel a decreased self-control and a decreased sense of self (Cort et al., 2004). Despite age or physical health, people remain sexual beings, and sexual health needs do not end when a person is diagnosed with a terminal illness (Farrell & Belza, 2012). With respect to relationships, partners often fear causing pain to their significant other. In addition, other problems can occur, such as concerns about body image, altered sexual function, relationship issues, feelings of loss and grief, and bereaved partners (Cort et al., 2004).

Issues related to lesbian, gay, bisexual, transgender, queer (LGBTQ) individuals at the end of life were explored by Rawlings (2012), who reported that there were experienced barriers to sexual health secondary to negative social attitudes. Some subjects reported that they felt pressure to disclose their sexual orientation, while others indicated that they have specifically sought out "gay friendly" practitioners (Rawlings, 2012).

Healthcare professionals may make assumptions based on culture, gender, and sexual orientation, a significant factor highlighted in a review by Harding (Harding, Epiphaniou, & Chidgey-Clark, 2012), who reviewed needs, experiences, and preferences of sexual minorities for end-of-life (EOL) care. Fear of discrimination may prevent disclosure of sexual identity of healthcare professionals. Healthcare professionals should provide services in a nonjudgmental manner, allowing the patient to address sexual needs at the end of life (Matzo et al., 2013; Sears et al., 2017).

Physical barriers to sexual health were reported for hospice patients and included fatigue, pain, and issues of incontinence (Park et al., 2009). A documented environmental barrier was the use of hospital beds for hospice patients (Bowden & Bliss, 2009). Hospital beds facilitate personal care and comfort, but they can interfere with intimacy and sexual expression.

Fertility preservation should be discussed with patients who still want to have children following treatment. Fertility preservation strategies are individualized to the cancer diagnosis, time interval until initiation of treatments, prognosis, pubertal status, and maturity level of patient (Pereira & Schattman, 2017). With the increasing trend for people to defer childbirth to later in life, provision of fertility-related information, access to fertility preservation, and fertility-related psychosocial support should be offered to patients of a reproductive age before they begin cancer treatment (Gerstl et al., 2017).

■ INTIMACY AND LATE-STAGE DISEASE

Vitrano et al. (2011) conducted a study with 65 men and women with advanced cancer to assess their feelings and attitudes on sexuality after diagnosis. Results of the study concluded that over half of the patients still felt attractive despite their diagnosis, and almost half felt that sexuality was important for their psychological well-being. However, only 7.6% were still sexually active for various reasons. Most patients expressed the importance of communicating their sexual needs with experienced professionals (Matzo et al., 2013).

De Vocht, Notter, and de Wiel (2010) interviewed cancer patients and their partners as well as healthcare professionals working in oncology and palliative care. Several themes arose from the interviews, including the need for closeness or intimacy with the partner, changes in sexual expression, and increase in QOL through sexual expression. Interviews highlighted barriers to sexual expression for hospice patients, such as hospital beds that prevent partners from sleeping together, and institutionalized care, which can eliminate privacy and interfere with sexual expression. Interviews with practitioners have documented their self-reported difficulty asking patients questions about sexual health even though they acknowledge that asking would facilitate patients' ability to express their needs. Professionals that addressed patients' sexual concerns reported that patients were not offended by this discussion (de Vocht et al., 2010; Matzo et al., 2013).

■ CONCLUSION

There is a significant lack of literature addressing issues of sexuality in palliative care that can guide evidence-based practice. Sexual health is a broad concept made up of multiple facets such as sexual desire, self as a sexual being, sexual orientation, sexual lifestyles, and relationships (Fogal, 2012). Intimacy, closeness, communication, and emotional support affect all facets of sexuality. Qualitative data obtained from patients reveals that they would prefer to be asked about these topics and given the opportunity to discuss them if so desired (Matzo & Hijjazi, 2009).

However, it appears that practitioners in palliative care settings often feel uncomfortable or unqualified to discuss these issues with their patients. Some suggestions provided for these practitioners to assist in overcoming their discomfort include role-playing, increasing their knowledge base regarding these issues, and ignoring their discomfort and opening the discussion to better meet the patients' needs. If practitioners will pursue sexual assessment with patients, they will quickly experience the gratitude patients express for having the chance to discuss their concerns, and soon their discomfort with the topic will disappear. The practitioner can include general sexual health questions (e.g., "Many patients have concerns about their sexual health and relationships, do you have any concerns about your sexual health?") and proceed to more specific questions about opportunities for physical intimacy, touching, kissing, holding hands, "snuggling," massage, oral sex, and masturbation (e.g., "Are you able to pleasure yourself sexually?" or "Are you able to stimulate yourself to release sexual tension?") as examples of physical intimacy that promotes feelings of love and connectedness. In this way, palliative care clinicians can further enhance the QOL for their patients throughout the trajectory of their illness. Evidence-Based Practice

---

CASE STUDY *Conclusion*

Ms. Warton returned for her 6-week follow-up visit, and I did not recognize her when I walked into the room. She was showered, with her hair done, neatly dressed, wearing make-up, and smiling. Although her daughter was present, she spoke for herself at this visit and no tears were observed. Her affect was bright and she was very engaged in participating in her plan of care. She reports that she is doing extremely well and attributes it to the medication changes. She had been to an appointment with the psychologist, who focused on increasing the number of pleasant events Alice has exposure to and explaining the relationship between mood and behavior. Education also was provided regarding the role of emotions as signals to continue doing something or do something differently.

Alice has purchased an adult coloring journal where she can write about what she is feeling, which helps manage her anxiety with the flow state induced by the adult coloring. She states that she is engaging in pleasant events on a regular basis and is no longer withdrawing from family by staying in her room. She appears to have benefited from a combined approach of medication and behavioral activation to improve her depressive symptoms.

CASE STUDY

AN INTERPROFESSIONAL PERSPECTIVE

Harold B. Bob, MD, CMD, HMDC
Regional Medical Director for Communicare

Mrs. Warton's situation is very compelling and raises complex issues not uncommonly faced by healthcare professionals in the care of patients with issues involving sexuality challenges as a result of their illness and treatment process. In addition to the barriers noted, healthcare providers may not often discuss this, but they are not well trained in providing patients "boundaries" (which are both morally and legally necessary in discussions about sexuality) without building "barriers" to human communication, which may be a large part of what we can offer patients in EOL situations.

Reiki (and other complementary modalities) can be helpful in palliative care since they often focus on presence and breathing and, by the nature of the discipline, seek to combat a sense of loneliness and hopelessness. While at times prescribed pharmacologic products can be helpful in combating pain and anxiety, these products can also have side effects of sedation, constipation, and diminished libido, as well as reduction in normal body fluids and increasing dryness, all of which can make sexuality more difficult. In some cases, verbal discussion of complex past traumas can be healing, but also, in some cases, "opening the scar" of complex suppressed traumas in therapy can be painful, but may well be warranted.

A benefit of Reiki and other mindfulness techniques is a spiritual peace that redirects the physical self to a calmer state. Some studies suggest Reiki impacts the parasympathetic nervous system and reduces "fight or flight response." Finding an intervention pathway where health professionals can honor the concerns of their patients, so that whether or not they can be "cured" they can feel cared about, is crucial. Often, medically ineffective and wasteful processes are carried out, when what some patients need is presence and a sense of being cared about. We certainly need to be aware of how vulnerable our patients are and how important professional boundaries are. Complementary techniques such as Reiki may assist us in maintaining proper boundaries without building barriers that prevent us from providing what is needed the most.

Evidence-Based Practice

Lemke, E. A., Madsen, L. T., & Dains, J. E. (2017). Vaginal testosterone for management of aromatase inhibitor-related sexual dysfunction: An integrative review. *Oncology Nursing Forum, 44*(3), 296–301. doi:10.1188/17.ONF.296-301

Problem Identification
Women taking aromatase inhibitors (AIs) as part of the management of hormone receptor-positive breast cancer experience more symptoms of sexual dysfunction, including vaginal atrophy, as opposed to postmenopausal women and women treated with tamoxifen (Nolvadex). Vaginal testosterone could be an alternative to estrogen, which is contraindicated in this population.

Literature Search
A systematic review was completed by searching PubMed and Scopus databases.

Data Evaluation
Sixty-four search results were reduced to a final sample of three articles after applying inclusion and exclusion criteria.

Synthesis
Published results suggest that vaginally applied testosterone doses of 150 and 300 mcg improve symptoms of sexual dysfunction in women taking AIs. Minimal side effects are observed, and estradiol levels are not affected by vaginally applied testosterone. Additional research is needed to evaluate vaginal testosterone in women taking AIs.

Conclusions
Vaginal testosterone shows preliminary promise as an option to manage sexual side effects of AI therapy in postmenopausal cancer survivors; however, available data are too limited to draw practice-changing conclusions.

Implications for Research
Large-scale randomized, controlled trials need to be completed to evaluate the efficacy and safety of vaginal testosterone in women taking AIs.

■ REFERENCES

Albaugh, J. A., Sufrin, N., Lapin, B. R., Petkewicz, J., & Tenfelde, S. (2017). Life after prostate cancer treatment: A mixed methods study of the experiences of men with sexual dysfunction and their partners. *BMC Urology, 17*(1), 45. doi:10.1186/s12894-017-0231-5

Albaugh, J. A., Tenfelde, S., & Hayden, D. M. (2017). Sexual dysfunction and intimacy for ostomates. *Clinics in Colon and Rectal Surgery, 30*(3), 201–206. doi:10.1055/s-0037-1598161

American Cancer Society. (2017). Ways of dealing with sexual problems. Retrieved from http://www.cancer.org/treatment/treatmentsandsideeffects/physicalsideeffects/sexualsideeffectsinmen/index

American Psychiatric Association. (2013). *Diagnostic and statistical manual of mental disorders* (5th ed.). Arlington, VA: American Psychiatric Publishing.

Ananth, H., Jones, L., King, M., & Tookman, A. (2003). The impact of cancer on sexual function: A controlled study. *Palliative Medicine, 17*, 202–205. doi:10.1191/0269216303pm759oa

Bachmann, G. (2006). Female sexuality and sexual dysfunction: Are we stuck on the learning curve? *Journal of Sexual Medicine, 3*(4), 639–645. doi:10.1111/j.1743-6109.2006.00265.x

Blagbrough, J. (2010). Importance of sexual needs assessment in palliative care. *Nursing Standard, 24*(52), 35–39. doi:10.7748/ns2010.09.24.52.35.c7954

Bowden, G., & Bliss, J. (2009). Does a hospital bed impact on sexuality expression in palliative care? *British Journal of Community Nursing, 14*(3), 122, 124–126. doi:10.12968/bjcn.2009.14.3.40095

Carmack Taylor, C. L., Basen-Engquist, K., Shinn, E. H., & Bodurka, D. C. (2004). Predictors of sexual functioning in ovarian cancer patients. *Journal of Clinical Oncology, 22*(5), 881–889. doi:10.1200/JCO.2004.08.150

Carter, J., Stabile, C., Gunn, A., & Sonoda, Y. (2013). The physical consequences of gynecologic cancer surgery and their impact on sexual, emotional, and quality of life issues. *Journal of Sex Medicine, 10*(Suppl 1), 21–34. doi:10.1111/jsm.12002

Caruso-Herman, D. (1989). Concern for the dying patient and family. *Seminars in Oncology Nursing, 5*(2), 120–123. doi:10.1016/0749-2081(89)90071-5

Cort, E., Monroe, B., & Oliviere, D. (2004). Couples in palliative care. *Sexual and Relationship Therapy, 19*(3), 337–354. doi:10.1080/14681990410001715454

Daphna-Tekoah, S., Lev-Wiesel, R., & Ben-Zion, I. (2016). *Childbirth as retraumitization of childhood's sexual abuse*. In C. Martin, V. Preedy, & V. Patel (Eds.), *Comprehensive guide to post-traumatic stress disorders* (pp. 391–407). New York, NY: Springer.

de Vocht, H., Notter, J., & de Wiel, H. (2010). Sexuality and intimacy in palliative care in the Netherlands. *Palliative Medicine, 24*(2), 215.

Derzko, C., Elliott, S., & Lam, W. (2007). Management of sexual dysfunction in postmenopausal breast cancer patients taking adjuvant aromatase inhibitor therapy. *Current Oncology, 14*(Suppl. 1), S20–S40. doi:10.3747/co.v14i0.178

Donovan, K. A., Gonzalez, B. D., Nelson, A. M., Fishman, M. N., Zachariah, B., & Jacobsen, P. B. (2018). Effect of androgen deprivation therapy on sexual function and bother in men with prostate cancer: A controlled comparison. *Psycho-Oncology, 27*(1), 316–324. doi:10.1002/pon.4463

Dunn, M. E. (2004). Restoration of couple's intimacy and relationship vital to reestablishing erectile function. *Journal of the American Osteopathic Association, 104*(3 Suppl.), S6–S10.

Epstein, R. M., & Street, R. L. (2007). *Patient-centered communication in cancer care: Promoting healing and reducing suffering*. Bethesda, MD: National Cancer Institute.

Epstein, S., & Mamo, L. (2017). The proliferation of sexual health: Diverse social problems and the legitimation of sexuality. *Social Science and Medicine, 188*, 176–190. doi:10.1016/j.socscimed.2017.06.033

Farrell, J., & Belza, B. (2012). Are older patients comfortable discussing sexual health with nurses? *Nursing Research, 61*(1), 51–57. doi:10.1097/NNR.0b013e31823a8600

Fogal, C. I. (2012). Sexuality. In K. D. Schuiling & F. E. Likis (Eds.), *Women's gynecologic health* (2nd ed., pp. 209–226). Burlington, NJ: Jones & Bartlett.

Gerressu, M., Mercer, C. H., Graham, C. A., Wellings, K., Johnson, A. M., Gerressu, M., ... Johnson, A. M. (2008). Prevalence of masturbation and associated factors in a British national probability survey. *Archives of Sexual Behavior, 37*(2), 266–278. doi:10.1007/s10508-006-9123-6

Gerstl, B., Sullivan, E., Ives, A., Saunders, C., Wand, H., & Anazodo, A. (2017). Pregnancy outcomes after a breast cancer diagnosis: A systematic review and meta-analysis. *Clinical Breast Cancer, 18*, e79–e88. doi:10.1016/j.clbc.2017.06.016

Grigg, E. (2002). The issues of sexuality and intimacy in palliative care. In J. Penson & R.A. Fisher, (Eds), *Palliative care for people with cancer* (pp. 202–218). London, UK: Arnold.

Harding, R., Epiphaniou, E., & Chidgey-Clark, J. (2012). Needs, experiences, and preferences of sexual minorities for end-of-life care and palliative care: A systematic review. *Journal of Palliative Medicine, 15*(5), 602–611. doi:10.1089/jpm.2011.0279

Harmanli, O., & Jones, K. A. (2010). Using lubricant for speculum insertion. *Obstetrics and Gynecology, 116* (2 Pt. 1), 415–417. doi:10.1097/AOG.0b013e3181e750f1

Hughes, M., & De La Garza, R. (2017). 040 Self-reported sexual problems are higher in breast cancer vs. non breast cancer patients. *Journal of Sexual Medicine, 14*(6), e365. doi:10.1016/j.jsxm.2017.04.044

Institute of Medicine. (2007). *Cancer care for the whole patient: Meeting psychosocial health needs*. Washington, DC: Author.

Kirkpatrick, D., Smith, T., Kerfeld, M., Ramsdell, T., Sadiq, H., & Sharma, A. (2016). Paradoxical reaction to alprazolam in an elderly woman with a history of anxiety, mood disorders, and hypothyroidism. *Case Reports in Psychiatry, 2016*, 6748947. doi:10.1155/2016/6748947

Knapp, C., Quinn, G. P., Murphy, D., Brown, R., & Madden, V. (2010). Adolescents with life-threatening illnesses. *American Journal of Hospice and Palliative Medicine, 27*(2), 139–144. doi:10.1177/1049909109358310

Krychman, M. L., Pereira, L., Carter, J., & Amsterdam, A. (2006). Sexual oncology: Sexual health issues in women with cancer. *Oncology, 71*(1–2), 18–25. doi:10.1159/000100521

Lardas, M., Liew, M., van den Bergh, R. C., De Santis, M., Bellmunt, J., Van den Broeck, T., … Bourke, L. (2017). Quality of life outcomes after primary treatment for clinically localised prostate cancer: A systematic review. *European Urology, 72*, 869–885. doi:10.1016/j.eururo.2017.06.035

Le, Y.K., Chung, H. H., Kim, J. W., Park, N.H., Song, Y.S., & Kang, S.B. (2011). Vaginal pH-balanced gel for the control of atrophic vaginitis among breast cancer survivors: A randomized controlled trial. *Obstetrics and Gynecology, 117*(4), 922–927. doi:10.1097/AOG.0b013e3182118790

Lemieux, L., Kaiser, S., Pereira, J., & Meadows, L. M. (2004). Sexuality in palliative care: Patient perspectives. *Palliative Medicine, 18*(7), 630–637. doi:10.1191/0269216304pm941oa

Lemke, E. A., Madsen, L. T., & Dains, J. E. (2017). Vaginal testosterone for management of aromatase inhibitor-related sexual dysfunction: An integrative review. *Oncology Nursing Forum, 44*(3), 296–301. doi:10.1188/17.onf.296-301

Levett, T. (2011). How to tackle impaired sexuality in oncology and palliative care patients. *European Journal of Palliative Care, 18*(1), 34–38.

Lindau, S. T., Schumm, L. P., Laumann, E. O., Levinson, W., O'Muircheartaigh, C. A., & Waite, L. J. (2007). A study of sexuality and health among older adults in the United States. *New England Journal of Medicine, 357*, 762–774. doi:10.1056/NEJMoa067423

Linhares, I. M., Summers, P. R., Larsen, B., Giraldo, P. C., & Witkin, S. S. (2011). Contemporary perspectives on vaginal pH and lactobacilli. *American Journal of Obstetrics and Gynecology, 204*(2), 120.e121–125. doi:10.1016/j.ajog.2010.07.010

Lutgendorf, S. K., Shinn, E., Carter, J., Leighton, S., Baggerly, K., Guindani, M., … Sood, A. K. (2017). Quality of life among long-term survivors of advanced stage ovarian cancer: A cross-sectional approach. *Gynecologic Oncology, 146*(1), 101–108. doi:10.1016/j.ygyno.2017.05.008

Maseroli, E., Scavello, I., Fanni, E., Fambrini, M., Maggi, M., & Vignozzi, L. (2017). P-02-009 Psychological and sexual correlates of sexual abuse in women with sexual dysfunction. *Journal of Sexual Medicine, 14*(4), e185. doi:10.1016/j.jsxm.2017.03.210

Matzo, M. (2010). Sexuality. In B. R. Ferrell & N. Coyle (Eds.), *Oxford textbook of palliative nursing* (3rd ed., pp. 477–486). New York, NY: Oxford University Press.

Matzo, M. (2015a). Sexual health and intimacy. In M. Matzo & D. W. Sherman (Eds.), *Palliative care nursing: Quality care to the end of life* (4th ed., pp. 129–146). New York, NY: Springer Publishing.

Matzo, M. (2015b). Sexuality. In B. R. Ferrell, N. Coyle, & J. Paice (Eds.), *Oxford textbook of palliative nursing* (4th ed., pp. 410–421). New York, NY: Oxford University Press.

Matzo, M., & Hijjazi, K. (2009). If you don't ask me … don't expect me to tell: A pilot study of the sexual health of hospice patients. *Journal of Hospice and Palliative Nursing, 11*(5), 271–283. doi:10.1097/NJH.0b013e3181b57b59

Matzo, M., Troup, S., Hijjazi, K., & Ferrell, B. (2015). Evaluating a sexual health patient education resource. *Journal of the Advanced Practitioner in Oncology, 6*(3), 242–248. doi:10.6004/jadpro.2015.6.3.6

Matzo, M., Whalen, J., & Pope, L. (2013). An integrative review of sexual health issues at the end of life. *Journal of Palliative Medicine, 16*(6), 668–691. doi:10.1089/jpm.2012.0416

Mercadante, S., Vitrano, V., & Catania, V. (2010). Sexual issues in early and late stage cancer: A review. *Supportive Care in Cancer, 18*(6), 659–665. doi:10.1007/s00520-010-0814-0

Moalli, P. A., Debes, K. M., Meyn, L. A., Howden, N. S., & Abramowitch, S. D. (2008). Hormones restore biomechanical properties of the vagina and supportive tissues after surgical menopause in young rats. *American Journal of Obstetrics and Gynecology, 199*(2), 161.e1–161.e8. doi:10.1016/j.ajog.2008.01.042

National Forum of Gynaecological Oncology Nurses. (Ed.). (2005). *Best practice guidelines on the use of vaginal dilators in women receiving pelvic radiotherapy*. Edgbaston, UK: Birmingham Women's Hospital.

Oakley, B. B., Fiedler, T. L., Marrazzo, J. M., & Fredricks, D. N. (2008). Diversity of human vaginal bacterial communities and associations with clinically defined bacterial vaginosis. *Applied and Environmental Microbiology, 74*(15), 4898–4909. doi:10.1128/AEM.02884-07

Park, E. R., Norris, R. L., & Bober, S. L. (2009). Sexual health communication during cancer care: Barriers and recommendations. *Cancer Journal, 15*(1), 74–77. doi:10.1097/PPO.0b013e31819587dc

Penson, R. T., Gallagher, J., Gioiella, M. E., Wallace, M., Borden, K., Duska, L. A., … Lynch, T. J. (2000). Sexuality and cancer: Conversation comfort zone. *The Oncologist, 5*, 336–344. doi:10.1634/theoncologist.5-4-336

Pereira, N., & Schattman, G. L. (2017). Fertility preservation and sexual health after cancer therapy. *Journal of Oncology Practice, 13*(10), 643–651. doi:10.1200/jop.2017.023705

Rawlings, D. (2012). End-of-life care considerations for gay, lesbian, bisexual, and transgender individuals. *International Journal of Palliative Nursing, 18*(1), 29–34. doi:10.12968/ijpn.2012.18.1.29

Rice, A. (2000). Sexuality in cancer and palliative care 2: Exploring the issues. *International Journal of Palliative Nursing, 6*(9), 448–453. doi:10.12968/ijpn.2000.6.9.9057

Robinson, B. E., Bockting, W. O., Simon-Rosser, B. R., Miner, M., & Coleman, E. (2002). The Sexual Health Model: Application of a sexological approach to HIV prevention. *Health Education Research, 17*(1), 43–57. doi:10.1093/her/17.1.43

Salani, R., Backes, F. J., Fung, M. F., Holschneider, C. H., Parker, L. P., Bristow, R. E., & Goff, B. A. (2011). Posttreatment surveillance and diagnosis of recurrence in women with gynecologic malignancies: Society of Gynecologic Oncologists recommendations. *American Journal of Obstetrics and Gynecology, 204*(6), 466–478. doi:10.1016/j.ajog.2011.03.008

Schover, L. R., Rhodes, M. M., Baum, G., Adams, J. H., Jenkins, R., Lewis, P., & Jackson, K. E. (2011). Sisters Peer Counseling in Reproductive Issues After Treatment (SPIRIT): A peer counseling program to improve reproductive health among African American breast cancer survivors. *Cancer, 117*(21), 4983–4992. doi:10.1002/cncr.26139

Sears, C. S., Robinson, J. W., & Walker, L. M. (2017). A comprehensive review of sexual health concerns after cancer treatment and the biopsychosocial treatment options available to female patients. *European Journal of Cancer Care (Engl), 7*(2), e12738. doi:10.1111/ecc.12738

Shankar, A., Prasad, N., Roy, S., Chakraborty, A., Biswas, A., Patil, J., & Rath, G. K. (2017). Sexual dysfunction in females after cancer treatment: An unresolved issue. *Asian Pacific Organization for Cancer Prevention, 18*(5), 1177–1182. doi:10.22034/apjcp.2017.18.5.1177

Smith, D. B. (1989). Sexual rehabilitation of the cancer patient. *Cancer Nursing, 12*(1), 10–15.

Stead, M. L. (2004). Sexual function after treatment for gynecological malignancy. *Current Opinion in Oncology, 16*, 492–495.

Steine, I. M., Winje, D., Skogen, J. C., Krystal, J. H., Milde, A. M., Bjorvatn, B., … Pallesen, S. (2017). Posttraumatic symptom profiles among adult survivors of childhood sexual abuse: A longitudinal study. *Child Abuse and Neglect, 67*, 280–293. doi:10.1016/j.chiabu.2017.03.002

Stewart, D. E., Wong, F., & Duff, S. (2001). What doesn't kill you makes you stronger: An ovarian cancer survivor survey. *Gynecologic Oncology, 83*, 537–542. doi:10.1006/gyno.2001.6437

Tan, O., Bradshaw, K., & Carr, B. R. (2012). Management of vulvovaginal atrophy-related sexual dysfunction in postmenopausal women: An up-to-date review. *Menopause, 19*(1), 109–117. doi:10.1097/gme.0b013e31821f92df

Vitrano, V., Catania, V., & Mercadante, S. (2011). Sexuality in patients with advanced cancer: A prospective study in a population admitted to an acute pain relief and palliative care unit. *American Journal of Hospice and Palliative Medicine, 28*(3), 198–202. doi:10.1177/1049909110386044

Wilmoth, M. C. (2006). Life after cancer: What *does* sexuality have to do with it? *Oncology Nursing Forum, 33*(5), 905–910. doi:10.1188/06.ONF.905-910

Wisnieski, D., & Matzo, M. (2013). Promoting healthy sexual behavior in adolescents. *American Journal of Nursing, 113*(6), 67–70. doi:10.1097/01.NAJ.0000431279.98524.f8

World Health Organization. (2004). Sexual health-a new focus for WHO. *Progress in Reproductive Health Research*. Retrieved from http://www.who.int/reproductive-health/hrp/progress/67.pdf

Young, P. (2007). Caring for the whole patient: The Institute of Medicine proposes a new standard of care. *Community Oncology, 4*(12), 748–751.

Zippe, C. D., & Pahlajani, G. (2008). Vacuum erection devices to treat erectile dysfunction and early penile rehabilitation following radical prostatectomy. *Current Urology Reports, 9*(6), 506–513. doi:10.1007/s11934-008-0086-0

Deborah Witt Sherman

Family Caregivers

CHAPTER

8

KEY POINTS

- Families are now defined as two or more people who have come together for a defined purpose, extending the definition of family beyond families of origin or blood relationships.
- Family definitions can be discussed in terms of structure, function, and symbolism and family is whoever the patient says it is.
- The number of family caregivers is staggering and research indicates that they are an at-risk and vulnerable population whose needs and well-being need to be considered as well as those of the patients.
- Although many studies indicate many negative health outcomes related to family caregiving, there are also benefits to the caregiving role.
- Theoretical frameworks related to family caregiving can guide questions for family assessment and the development of family caregiver interventions.
- Caregiver assessment is a systematic process of gathering information specific to the needs, problems, strengths, and resources of the family, and the caregivers' ability to care for the needs of the care recipient.
- Family caregiver interventions include setting realistic goals, having difficult conversations, finding help, and negotiating expectations.
- The needs and concerns of family caregivers should be addressed by all members of the interprofessional palliative or hospice care team.

CASE STUDY

S.M. is a 40-year-old, previously healthy woman who had a seizure while at work. Diagnostic studies indicate that S.M. has had an inoperable brain tumor. S.M. is a single mother of two girls, ages 12 and 14. She now has memory loss, generalized weakness, and increased risk of seizures and therefore cannot be left alone. S.M.'s younger brother, R.C., has taken on the responsibility of being her caregiver and guardian of his nieces. He has brought his sister, nieces, and their two dogs to live with him and his wife. They are expecting their first child and his wife is in the second trimester of a twin pregnancy. In the past year, R.C. and S.M.'s father died because of a heart attack, while 3 years ago their mother died from metastatic ovarian cancer. His wife also lost her father in an accident within the last year. R.C. and his wife have full-time demanding jobs as a respiratory therapist and a registered nurse, respectively. In trying to maintain a sense of normalcy for his nieces, R.C. brings the children to their old school, which is a 45-minute drive from his home. He is also managing his sister's finances, with many medical bills. His wife helps by taking S.M. to her doctor's appointments, managing her healthcare, running her errands, and helping to raise her nieces. Together, they have a complicated set of responsibilities that take up most of their time, while trying to be happy and prepare for their own twin babies. R.C. and his wife are coping not only with their grief associated with the death of their parents, but are experiencing the stress of watching S.M.'s health decline and the realization that they will soon be parents to four children. R.C.'s wife has been experiencing occasional preterm contractions and R.C. has been experiencing physical and emotional exhaustion, leaving him vulnerable to illness himself.

Family is a cultural, legal, sociological, and individually defined concept. Traditional definitions of family include what we refer to as a nuclear family—father, mother, and one or more children—or the extended family which adds grandparents, aunts, uncles, and cousins. In the past, people grew up and lived in the same community for a lifetime in close contact with extended family. Family members counted on each other for help, and there was usually one or more family members available to help with the care of children or older family members. This was usually a wife, mother, or grandmother. After World War II, more and more women moved into the workforce and a new childcare industry emerged. Social forces, such as job mobility, air travel, increased divorce rate, and an increase in cohabitation accelerated during the 1960s and 1970s. This affected the definition of family, as well as the availability of family members to help each other. Simultaneously, advances in healthcare extended the longevity of life, and also increased the number of people living with chronic illness. Today, blended families, those with parents who are on their second or more marriages with children from previous marriages, as well as single-parent families, same-sex families, and families who are childless by choice, are more common. Extended families are either smaller or in other locations and often have limited contact with each other. Legal and illegal immigration has led to communities of immigrants who often live in fear, do not speak English, and delay healthcare because of limited resources or fear of deportation. Homelessness and the increase of people with mental illness, who live on the street, without support or family connections, have created another community with family-like qualities and characteristics. These forces, along with the aging of the population and the incidence of chronic illness, have increased the need for family caregivers and have changed the way we look at family and its involvement in the care of individuals (Marriage and Family Encyclopedia, 2013a).

What, then, is a family? There are several definitions of family in the literature, which describe the structure, function, interactions, and symbolism of family (Carlson & Dermer, 2017). First, structural definitions describe families based on membership and relationships between family members. An example of a structural definition is "a single mother and her children" or "first-degree relatives including step- and half-siblings which would include a father a mother and all their collective children."

A second category for defining families is functional. If the function of families is to procreate and then nurture children, then the evaluation of family function is based on the number of children born within the family. A third category of definitions of family is based on interactions within the family group. It looks at the role of family members, the power dynamics within the family, and how family members relate to each other. This broad category would allow for work groups or societies to be defined as family, as well as a group of friends who view themselves as a family. Finally, the last category of family definitions is a symbolic representation and is defined by the individual family using stories or symbols to define membership. For example, the family may be defined through its generational ownership of a home in which many family members have been born and died. The symbolic representation of a family may be also related to a piece of land on which the family has lived or worked for decades and which represents the experience and livelihood of the whole family.

Most definitions are a combination of these categories. Merely naming the members of a family related by blood or legal arrangements such as adoption or guardianship is the most common, but it defines only a portion of groups who define themselves as families based on their purpose and relationship. Friends and domestic partners, with or without legal sanctions, often depend on each other and have the expectations of loyalty, love, and help that one usually associates with blood relatives and of nuclear families. Even though they are in decline, the nuclear and, to some extent, the extended family are considered the norm legally in medicine when a patient's families are included in the plan of care.

Beyond the definitions of families, there are many different types of family groups based on the structure: (a) couples without dependent children (married and unmarried); (b) single-parent families (never-married, separated, divorced, and widowed); (c) two-parent family household (not married, first marriage, and second/third marriage); (d) foster families; (e) adoptive families; (f) "estranged" families; (g) nuclear, extended, or multigenerational households; (h) none/one/two or multiple wage earners; and (i) "living apart together" families (Policy Institute for Family Impact Seminars, 2013).

Furthermore, the type of family groups varies by socioeconomic characteristics, such as education and income levels. Family groups also vary by the ethnic/racial/cultural background, religion, informal social network (friends and neighbors), relationships to community, and the area where they live (rural/suburban/urban).

Myths about the family may influence the health professionals' assumptions, beliefs, and expectations related to families and their interactions within the healthcare system. The first is that family members have the best interests of the patient at heart. This assumption persists in the face of reports of domestic violence, elder and child abuse, neglect, and abandonment. The second is the belief that children, especially female children, have an obligation to care for chronically ill or impaired family members, especially elders. This expectation is shared by family, medical providers, and cultural norms, irrespective of the burden this places on the individuals, without recognition of their additional family and work responsibilities.

Definitions of Family and Family Caregivers

The 2010 U.S. Census Bureau defines family as two or more people who have come together for a self-defined purpose. That purpose may be procreation or it may be simple companionship, but the persons involved view themselves as family with the bonds and responsibilities one expects from a family of origin or blood relationship.

A family caregiver is a member of this family who has chosen or who has been designated as the caregiver for one or more family members who cannot manage normal activities of daily living without help. There are several definitions of family caregivers, such as the following:

■ Family (Informal) caregiver is an unpaid individual responsible for attending to the daily needs of another person. He or she is responsible for the physical, emotional, and often financial support of another person who is unable to care for himself or herself due to illness, injury, or disability (Family Caregiver Alliance, 2016). The family caregiver may be a spouse, partner, family member, friend, or neighbor.
■ Formal caregivers are paid care providers providing care in one's home or in a care setting (day care, residential facility, long-term care facility; Family Caregiver Alliance, 2013c).

Statistics Related to Family Caregiving

The statistics related to family (informal) caregivers are staggering. The National Alliance for Caregiving in Collaboration with AARP (2015) reported that approximately 43.5 million caregivers have provided unpaid care to an adult or child in the last 12 months. About 34.2 million Americans have provided unpaid care to an adult aged 50 or older in the last 12 months. Most caregivers (82%) care for one other adult, whereas 15% care for two adults, and 3% care for three or more adults. Approximately 39.8 million caregivers provide care to adults (aged 18+ years) with a disability or illness, or 16.6% of Americans. About 15.7 million adult family caregivers care for someone who has dementia. Sixty-five percent of care recipients are female, with an average age of 69.4 years. The younger the care recipient, the more likely the recipient is to be male, whereas 33% of recipients aged 50 or higher are male. More than 75% of all caregivers are female, and may spend as much as 50% more time providing care than males. Female caregivers are more likely than male caregivers to provide personal care. Forty percent of male caregivers use paid assistance for a loved one's personal care. Family caregiver's age increases with the age of the care recipient. The number of hours dedicated to caregiving increases with the age of the caregiver. Higher-hour caregivers are, on average, 51.8 years of age. Lower-hour caregivers are on average 48 years of age.

According to the Family Caregiver Alliance (2013b), it has been estimated that 70 million people will be over 65 years of age in 2030. Therefore, family caregivers increasingly provide care for aging adults, most of whom have one or more chronic conditions and who wish to remain in their own homes and communities. Other family caregivers belong to the "sandwich generation," which describes the caregivers sandwiched between caring for elder parents or grandparents and spouse and/or children. These caregivers are pulled in both directions and often have jobs as well as these dual responsibilities (DeRigne & Ferrante, 2012). They are typically middle-aged women who are overwhelmed with responsibility, act out of duty, and neglect themselves because there are competing demands for their time.

The Burdens and Benefits of Family Caregiving

Family caregivers provide extraordinary uncompensated care, which is physically, emotionally, socially, and financially demanding. The caregiving role begins immediately at the point of diagnosis and continues over the illness trajectory (Given, Given, & Sherwood, 2012) with needs for information about care and the patient's disease (Stajduhar et al., 2010) that vary at the different stages of the patient's illness (Williams & McCorkle, 2011). Caregivers are a conduit for information between patient and provider and between provider and extended family (Given et al., 2012). Family caregivers experience the physical strain associated with caregiving, and also fear, confusion, powerlessness, and a sense of vulnerability, despite their attempts to maintain normalcy (Funk et al., 2010). They often suffer from symptoms of anger, depression, and anxiety and may become demoralized and exhausted (Zarit, 2006). Caregivers, themselves, may experience increased physical illness, exacerbation of comorbid conditions, and a greater risk of mortality

(Family Caregiver Alliance, 2006a). Burdens associated with caregiving include time and logistics, and lost wages or leaving the workforce entirely, which have severe economic implications and personal, social, and institutional impact (Hudson, 2004; Papastavrou, Charalambous, & Tsangari, 2009; Rabow, Hauser, & Adams, 2004; Sherwood et al., 2008; Wong, Liu, Szeto, Sham, & Chan, 2004). Sources of anxiety for caregivers include residual effects of disease and treatment on the patient, altered household and family roles, and altered communication patterns (Given, Sherwood, & Given, 2011). Because caregivers abandon leisure, religious, and social activities, there is heightened marital and family stress, with long-term consequences for the health and the stability of the family (Dumont, Dumont, & Mongeau, 2008).

Changes experienced across the cancer trajectory require caregivers to adapt to a new set of patient needs, creating increased distress, yet caregivers are reluctant to identify themselves as individuals who need support (Funk et al., 2010). This reflects the concept of "legitimacy of needs" or "caregiver ambivalence" because they do not want to "bother" professionals, or shift attention away from the patient (Funk et al., 2010). According to Clukey (2007), some caregivers hide their feelings of loss and grief from the patient, which is termed "bridled grief" (Houldin, 2007; Wells, Cagle, Bradley, & Barnes, 2008). This may lead to increased caregiver isolation, depression, and overwhelming misery when caregivers finally allow themselves to grieve (Moules, Simonson, Prins, Angus, & Bell, 2004; Wells et al., 2008).

The level of stress/strain varies by disease. Previous studies reported that caregivers of dementia patients have higher levels of burden than other caregivers owing to long care hours and physically demanding caregiving (Alzheimer's Association, 2017; Brodaty & Donkin, 2009). A study by Kim and Schulz (2008) compared the strains of family caregivers of cancer patients to the strain of caregivers of frail elders, dementia, and diabetes patients. The results showed that the level of strain of caregivers of cancer patients is greater than the strain on caregivers of elderly or diabetes patients, but cancer caregiver strain is comparable to that of caregivers of dementia patients. Cancer and dementia caregivers reported higher levels of physical strain, emotional stress, and financial hardship because of providing care. The crucial difference between cancer and dementia caregivers was that cancer caregivers were distressed by various acute medical conditions experienced by the patient, such as surgery, chemotherapy, or radiation therapy (e.g., catheter care, or managing patients' emesis or fatigue symptoms), whereas caregivers of dementia patients were distressed by the significant cognitive and functional decline and behavioral changes that progress over time. Alzheimer's takes a devastating toll on caregivers. Compared with caregivers of people without dementia, twice as many dementia caregivers indicate substantial emotional, financial, and physical difficulties (Alzheimer's Association, 2017).

Beyond the burden of family caregiving, the strengths of the family should also be considered. The strengths of individuals and families provide a means of dealing with any problems that exist (Marriage and Family Encyclopedia, 2013b). The goal should be to identify strong families and provide means of developing the strengths of families. Table 8.1 describes the qualities that reflect strength in families. The focus on family strengths does not deny the presence of stressors or perceived burden; rather, it offers a focus on the resources any family can develop and use in reducing the stressors or negative effects associated with caregiving.

Given the strengths of the family, the caregiving experience may also have possible benefits, yet these outcomes have received little attention. Health professionals should not miss the opportunity to identify the rewards and satisfaction that come from caregiving. Studies indicate that family caregivers describe feelings

TABLE 8.1 Qualities of Strong Families	
Categories	**Qualities**
Appreciation and affection	■ Caring for each other ■ Friendship ■ Respect for individuality ■ Playfulness ■ Humor
Positive communication	■ Sharing feelings ■ Giving compliments ■ Avoiding blame ■ Being able to compromise ■ Agreeing to disagree
Spiritual well-being	■ Hope ■ Faith ■ Compassion ■ Shared ethical values ■ Oneness with humankind
Commitment	■ Trust ■ Honesty ■ Dependability ■ Faithfulness ■ Sharing
Time together	■ Quality time in great quantity ■ Good things take time ■ Enjoying each other's company ■ Simple good times ■ Sharing fun times
Ability to cope with stress and crisis	■ Adaptability ■ Seeing crises as challenges and opportunities ■ Growing through crises together ■ Openness to change ■ Resilience

Source: International Encyclopedia of Marriage and Family (2nd ed.). (2003). Reproduced with permission from Cengage. Retrieved from https://www.encyclopedia.com/reference/encyclopedias-almanacs-transcripts-and-maps/family-strengths

of satisfaction for a job well done, particularly when the patient appreciates and acknowledges their care and support, and when caregivers feel a sense of giving back for the care and nurturing they, themselves, received (Narayan, Lewis, Tornatore, Hepburn, & Corcoran-Perry, 2001; Neff, Dy, Frick, & Kasper, 2007; Schumacher, Beck, & Marren, 2006). The positive aspects associated with the caregiving experience may act as a buffer against overwhelming burden and traumatic grief (Gaugler et al., 2005; Hudson, 2004; Salmon, Kwak, Acquaviva, Brandt, & Egan, 2005; Steel, Gamblin, & Carr, 2008). Caregivers with a positive approach to life are better able to cope with caregiving demands (Stajduhar, Martin, Barwich, & Fyles, 2008) and are motivated to maintain their caregiving role (Higginson & Gao, 2008). Based on a comprehensive review of quantitative studies, Stajduhar et al. (2010) reported posttraumatic growth of bereaved caregivers. Funk et al. (2010) reported a sense of existential meaning associated with the caregiver role, including a sense of pride, esteem, mastery, and accomplishment. Using the Stress Process Model, Haley, LaMonde, Han, Burton, and Schonwetter (2003) examined spousal caregiver depression and life satisfaction in the hospice setting, learning that caregivers found meaning and benefits of caregiving, and suggesting the need to identify caregivers at high risk and protective factors that could be incorporated into interventions.

■ THEORETICAL FRAMEWORKS RELATED TO FAMILY CAREGIVING

How then does one begin to assess and intervene in ways that support both the patient and the caregiver? A number of theoretical frameworks has been proposed to evaluate the burdens, benefits, transitions, and associated factors related to family caregiving (Bahr & Bahr, 2001; Fletcher, Miaskowski, Given, & Schumacher, 2012; Grey, Knafl, & McCorkle, 2006; Meleis, Sawyer, Im, Messias, & Schumacher, 2000; Pearlin, Mullan, Semple, & Skaff, 1990; Tsai, 2003).

Traditional family theories are useful for examining family structure and dynamics. From a family theorist perspective, Bahr and Bahr (2001) have explored the concept of self-sacrifice and its meaning in the family. They take this stance in opposition to the theories that stress individual choice and the primacy of the individual over the good of the whole. They assert that self-sacrifice in the interest of the family is viewed as a virtue. Bahr and colleagues go on to say that love is the motivation for this sacrifice manifested as selfless generosity and contrasts with the ethic of personal gain that characterizes social relationships outside the family.

It is understood that serious, acute, chronic, or life-threatening illnesses are disruptive to not only the patient but also his or her family. Illness creates change with respect to daily adjustments and associated transitional events (Schumacher & Meleis, 1994). Caregiver transitions encompass the patient's phases of illness

(Northouse, Katapodi, Schafenacker, & Weiss, 2012), and the caregiver's response to associated deficits, physical/emotional needs, and symptoms (Steinhauser, 2005). Transition is a concept of interest to nurse researchers, theorists, and healthcare providers (Schumacher & Meleis, 1994). Meleis et al. (2000) have developed a middle-range theory of transition, which asserts that clients in transition tend to be more vulnerable to risks that may in turn affect their health. Uncovering these risks may be enhanced by understanding the transition process (Meleis et al., 2000, p. 12). Major concepts of this transition theory (Figure 8.1) include the following: the nature of transitions, including the types, patterns, and properties of transitions; transition conditions (facilitators and inhibitors) within the context of person, community, and society; patterns of response in terms of process and outcome indicators; and nursing therapeutics. More specifically, the types of transitions include developmental, situational, health/illness, and organizational. The pattern of transitions can be single, multiple, sequential, simultaneous, or related/unrelated. The properties of transition experiences include awareness, engagement, change and difference, transition time span, and critical points and events. Meleis et al. (2000) also identify the transition conditions, particularly the importance of personal meaning, cultural beliefs and attitudes, as well as the families' socioeconomic status and their preparation and knowledge of the illness trajectory. For families, they contend that the patterns of response are measured by the process indicators of feeling connected, interacting, location and being situated, developing confidence, and coping. Furthermore, the outcome indicators are measured as mastery and having fluid integrative identities.

The Pearlin Stress Process Model (Pearlin et al., 1990) and a number of stress and coping measures are helpful for researchers studying stress in caregivers. The Pearlin Stress Process Model addresses the experience of caregiving including caregiving transitions and transitional events that occur from one phase of the illness trajectory to another and one stage of caregiving to another. Pearlin's model (as cited in Bastawrous, 2013) suggests that stressors and resources exist that affect an individual's well-being. According to Pearlin et al. (1990), the five major components in caregivers' experience are the following:

1. **Caregiving context,** which includes sociodemographic characteristics of the caregiver and patient, history of illness, history of caregiving, and caregiver living arrangements.
2. **Primary stressors,** which arise directly from the patient's illness and may include the patient's symptoms or impairment, ability to perform activities of daily living, cognitive deficits, and behavioral problems, as well as stressors such as caregiver burden, including the subjective assessment of the degree to which the caregiver perceives each event, including possible role overload (time and energy), role captivity (trapped in

the caregiving role), and the loss of relationship (lost intimacy and social exchanges).

3. **Secondary stressors,** which include tension and conflict in maintaining other roles in one's life such as employment and family relationships; interruptions in other areas of the caregiver's life; and intrapsychic strains that erode a person's self-concept such as sense of caregiver mastery and competence.

4. **Resources,** which include social, financial, and internal resources that increase the ability to manage stressful experiences. Resources include social support, which involves information, material, or financial support, as well as instrumental and emotional support. With resources, caregivers have perceived gains from the caregiving experience.

5. **Outcomes,** which include positive and negative health outcomes related to caregiver, such as self-efficacy or caregiver burden. To summarize Pearlin's model (as cited in Bastawrous, 2013), primary stressors, secondary stressors, and mediators interact in a way that ultimately affects the individuals' well-being outcomes.

As another theory, Tsai (2003) has developed a middle-range theory of caregiver stress. This theory reflects the philosophy and framework of the Roy Adaptation Model. The model and subsequent theory is an input/process/output type model (Figure 8.2) that makes the four following assumptions:

1. Caregivers receive environmental stimuli as input.
2. Caregivers' perceptions determine how they respond to stimuli.
3. Caregivers' adaptation is a function of their environmental stimuli and adaptation level.
4. Caregivers' effector, for example physical function, self-esteem/mastery, role enjoyment, and marital satisfaction, are results of chronic caregiving (Tsai, 2003, p. 139).

Caregivers' adaptation has four adaptive modes: physical function, self-concept mastery and esteem, role function (interdependence), and marital satisfaction.

Fletcher et al. (2012) also developed a theoretical model of cancer family caregiving experience. They reviewed the cancer family caregiving literature, analyzed the concepts and variables used in previous studies, and synthesized the concepts and variables into a conceptual model. Major elements of this model include the following (Figure 8.3):

1. The stress process: primary stressors, secondary stressors, cognitive appraisal, cognitive and behavioral responses, and outcomes of health and well-being
2. Contextual factors: personal, sociocultural, economic, healthcare
3. Cancer diagnosis/Initial treatment →
   a. Remission → surveillance → cancer-free survivorship
   b. Recurrence or second cancer → end-of-life care → bereavement

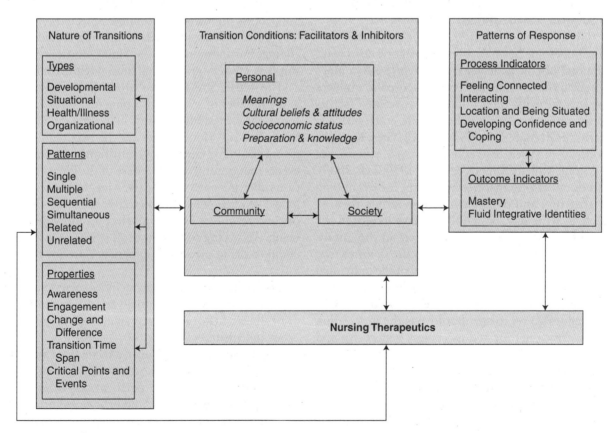

FIGURE 8.1 Transitions: A middle-range theory.

Source: Reprinted from Meleis, A. I., Sawyer, L. M., Im, E. O., Messias, D. K. H., & Schumacher, K. (2000). Experiencing transitions: an emerging middle-range theory. *Advances in Nursing Science, 23*(1), 12–28, with permission from Lippincott Williams & Wilkins.

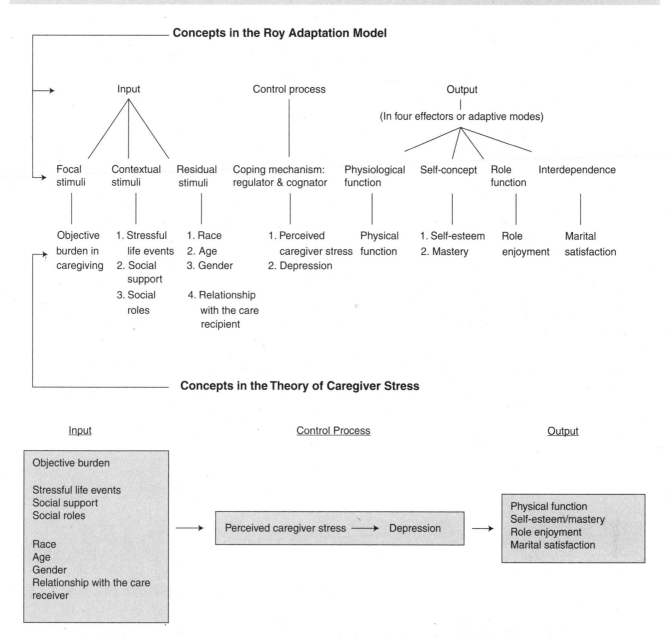

FIGURE 8.2 A middle-range theory of caregiver stress.

Source: Reprinted from Tsai, P. F. (2003). A middle-range theory of caregiver stress. *Nursing Science Quarterly, 16*(2), 137–145, with permission from Elsevier.

Finally, to guide the impact of individual caregiver responses such as compassion fatigue and burden, the Resiliency Model of Family Stress, Adjustment, and Adaptation (RMFSAA), proposed by McCubbin and McCubbin, provides a theoretical framework for studying family caregiving (Lynch, 2013). The resiliency model emphasizes family adaptation and focuses on illness as a stressor affecting family life. Family adaptation rather than adjustment is emphasized, because it is often the most needed response to illness. The resiliency model focuses on a stressor, the family's efforts to use resistance resources, the family's appraisal of the situation, and the family's coping patterns and problem-solving abilities to maintain function while dealing with a stressor. This model explains why some

families are able to overcome crisis and others are not. The level of family appraisal is a force that can facilitate family coping and adaptation by producing optimal problem solving for managing an illness situation (Yeh & Bull, 2012).

These models need to be tested to determine their usefulness in studying caregivers and caregiving behaviors and stresses. Family caregiving is a complex experience, because it involves many dynamics and processes, including the dynamics of family relationships in interaction with the community and healthcare professionals. The family history, social evolution, legal challenges, and medical advancement make decision making a challenge. How then should we view the commitment of family caregivers? Are the activities and responsibilities of caregiving a

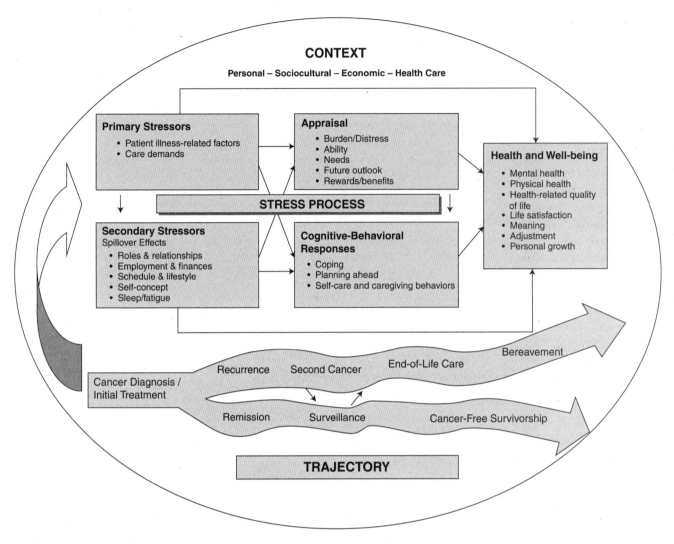

FIGURE 8.3 The cancer family caregiving experience.

Source: Reprinted from Fletcher, B. S., Miaskowski, C., Given, B., & Schumacher, K. (2012). The cancer family caregiving experience: an updated and expanded conceptual model. *European Journal of Oncology Nursing*, 16(4), 387–398. doi:10.1016/j.ejon.2011.09.001 (2012), with permission from Elsevier.

reflection of duty and obligation derived from social and cultural definitions of family? Or are the activities and responsibilities acts of love and self-sacrifice manifesting generosity? Are these family activities and responsibilities merely the reflection of social, political, economic, and medical realities of the time and environment in which we live? Given current economic conditions, is there an ethical or legal obligation of society to care for people in our communities who have progressive, serious, or chronic illnesses or disabilities? If so, how should the limited resources be distributed to support family caregivers?

■ **THE IMPORTANCE OF PATIENT AND FAMILY ASSESSMENT**

The Family Caregiver Alliance sponsors the National Center on Caregiving. The National Center on Caregiving aims to advance the development of high quality, cost-effective policies and programs for caregivers and serves

as a central resource on caregiving and long-term care issues (Gibson, Kelly, & Kaplan, 2012). Speaking at the National Consensus Development Conference for Caregiver Assessment (Family Caregiver Alliance, 2006b), Levine (2006) spoke poignantly about her experience as a caregiver and was very descriptive of the world in which caregivers must navigate. Ahern (2006) commented on how quickly a person's life can change forever and how critical it is to have the support of family and of professionals in the care of loved ones; but ultimately it is an act of love to care for them. Levine's (2006) experience was different in many ways and she vividly described the cruel and insensitive approach of the nurses and therapists at the rehabilitation facility where her brain-injured husband was living. She felt there was no assessment of her commitment, resources, or willingness to be a part of her husband's care although she was doing all she was able. She experienced only judgment, which was rigid and subjective as providers sought a "one-size-fits-all" approach to family caregiving. Her experience is validated in many ways by Thomas

(2006), whose young husband was also brain injured and changed both their lives forever.

One thing is clear: A "one-size-fits-all" approach to caregivers is at best not helpful and at worst destructive. How then does one begin to take a more helpful path in working out the partnership that will lead to successful caregiving for both the caregivers and the care recipients? That path begins with a caregiver assessment. A complete caregiver assessment begins by asking the caregiver about his or her health and well-being, feelings, and stress level to help determine the information, support, and training needed to benefit the caregiver and the person receiving the care (Feinberg & Levine, 2015).

Being a family caregiver can be considered gratifying and meaningful, but the effects on the caregiver can be mostly negative. These negative outcomes include depression, financial disadvantages, social isolation, burden, and decline in physical and mental health (Kim et al., 2017). Caregiver well-being is closely linked with patient well-being (Kutner & Kilbourn, 2009; Porter, Keefe, Garst, McBride, & Baucom, 2008). As a patient's performance status and quality of life declines over time, the caregiver's health often also declines (Northouse et al., 2012; Velanovich & Wollner, 2011). Conversely, without family caregivers, patients' survival rates are lower, societal costs for end-of-life care are greater (Zarit, 2004), and as patients are placed in more costly hospital or nursing home settings (Funk et al., 2010), they may also be at risk for poor care or neglect (Bee, Barnes, & Luker, 2009; Maslow, Levine, & Reinhard, 2006). Steinhauser (2005) wrote, "Characterizing the progression of multiple dimensions of patients' and caregivers' experience from serious illness through death of the patient by appropriate assessment and design is crucial to evidence based understanding of improving end of life care and to capturing transitions and end of life trajectories" (p. 40).

Providing care that is patient- and family-centered is a core priority of the National Quality Forum (Feinberg & Levine, 2015). Despite the National Consensus Guidelines for Quality Palliative Care (National Consensus Project, 2013), which emphasizes that both patient and family should be viewed as the unit of care, health professionals do not always intervene in ways that take caregiver well-being into account. Recent research has found that merely 32% of family caregivers reported that a healthcare provider had asked them if something was needed to care for their family member, and only 16% of family caregivers were asked what was needed for them to care for themselves (Feinberg & Levine, 2015). Inaccessible and unaffordable support puts family caregivers at great risk for burnout, financial disadvantage, and physical and mental health problems (Feinberg & Levine, 2015). The psychosocial needs of family caregivers are usually considered second to that of the patients or disregarded, and there is no standardization or systemic methodology to evaluate their needs (Hudson & Aranda, 2014).

Many caregivers exhibit impaired cognitive functioning (McGuire, Grant, & Park, 2012) and either meet *DSM-IV* criteria for or are being treated for psychiatric problems (Vanderwerker, Laff, Kadan-Lottick, McColl, & Prigerson, 2005). With physical and emotional stress, including sense of burden, depression, and a sense of abandonment by professionals, a comprehensive family assessment and targeted interventions are critical to promoting the health and well-being of individuals of a family, as well as the family as a unit (Given et al., 2004).

Caregiver assessment is "a systematic process of gathering information about a caregiving situation to identify the specific problems, needs, strengths, and resources of the family caregiver, as well as the ability of the caregiver to contribute to the needs of the care recipient" (Feinberg & Hauser, 2012, AARP Fact Sheet, p. 1). A systematic approach to assess caregiver needs and strengths is crucial to develop a dyadic intervention that can improve the outcomes for both caregivers and care recipients (Feinberg & Hauser, 2012). "Caregiver assessments in healthcare have to go beyond burden, stress, and support from family and friends. They have to look at the tasks family caregivers perform, whether the caregiver is physically and emotionally able to do them and the consequences" (Feinberg & Levine, 2015, p. 16). The United Hospital Fund has a self-assessment tool for family caregivers, entitled *Next Step in Care Guide, What Do I Need as a Family Caregiver?*, which allows caregivers to explain their proficiency to complete several common tasks and includes a list of general concerns (Feinberg & Levine, 2015). This tool helps direct appropriate interventions for the caregiver. It is also helpful to understand the ability of the family caregiver to communicate with the healthcare team.

As another dimension of the family caregiver's assessment, it is helpful to understand the family caregiver's communication pattern. The Family Communication Framework proposes that the dimension of family caregiving communication includes conversation and conformity. The pattern of conformity reveals the family caregiver's beliefs and values and their alignment with that of other family members. From the framework has emerged four communication patterns of family caregivers: The manager, who has high conformity and high conversation; the carrier, who has high conformity and low conversation; the partner, who has low conformity and high conversation; and the lone, who has low conformity and low conversation. The manager is the family medical expert whose role usurps other patient or family members' preferences, whereas the carrier relies heavily on the patient to determine care decisions and his or her role depends largely on a sense of family obligation to provide care. In the partner communication pattern, the patient is very involved in his or her own care decisions but is not an actor in the decision-making process. With the lone communication pattern, there is great focus on hope of the efficacy of treatments and the lone caregiver attempts to seek treatments for the patient's condition (Wittenberg, Kravits, Goldsmith, Ferrell, & Jujinami, 2017).

Guberman (2006) discusses the nature of caregiver assessment from a clinical, not research, perspective. Caregiver assessment can be used to determine eligibility for services, identifying unrecognized or subtle problems that might not be obvious although they have great impact on successful caregiving. The assessment process also allows for the development of a strong, trusting, therapeutic relationship between the clinician and the caregivers. Guberman goes on to describe several tools that can be used to perform the assessment, although little consensus exists as to the best strategy. Guberman proposes that the best assessments include all family caregivers and the care recipient. Both the patient and family should be assessed by the same provider in the caregivers' home or another place where they both feel safe to discuss all aspects of the situation.

The advantages of assessment as a basis for accessing services and support are many, but Zarit (2006) outlines some specific benefits. The first is the identification of actual or potential problems in the caregiving context including but not limited to interpersonal, relational, situational, or financial problems. The second advantage is the clarification of roles and responsibilities for family members, as well as a clear estimate of the resources available versus those that will be needed to provide the required care. The assessment can also reveal stresses that can be intervened with before they reach overwhelming and incapacitating anxiety and depression leading to despair. The structured and systematic nature of a good caregiver assessment assures that important aspects are not missed and that a comprehensive approach is implemented.

The Family Caregiver Alliance website is a treasure of resources for caregivers and providers alike. A section on caregiver assessment provides the domains of family caregiver assessment, the constructs, and related assessment questions (Table 8.2).

The Family Caregiver website also provides a list of helpful family assessment tools (see Exhibit 8.1)

Aoun et al. (2015) provide evidence of the value of the Carer Support Needs Assessment Tool (CSNAT), which assesses the physical, psychological, social, practical, financial, and spiritual needs of family caregivers, and has been used in home-based care. Based on the feedback of 233 family caregivers who were administered the tool, most appreciated an opportunity to express their needs, priorities, and focus on solutions. The tool facilitated discussions of health team members with family caregivers and led to timely assessment of needs and early interventions. The CSNAT also helped family caregivers accept the need for assistance and allowed the tailoring of interventions.

Often caregivers are unaware of resources available to them or simply lack the energy to seek them out. Repeatedly family caregivers report that information given to care

for their loved one is insufficient. Caregivers want to feel a sense of readiness and confidence in their role as caregivers. When a caregiver is not prepared, he or she risks suffering from depression, anxiety, guilt, and grief (Hudson & Aranda, 2014). "Preparedness for caregiving is defined as the perceived readiness of caregivers for multiple domains of caregiving role, such as emotional and practical support and managing the stressors of caregiving" (Holm et al., 2016, p. 795). What is not clear is why so many family caregivers fail to have access to these supports and services. What is clear is that caregivers need support and care just as patients do. When caregivers are prepared for their role, there is higher self-perceived hope and rewards for caregiving and lower levels of anxiety (Holm et al., 2016).

■ INTERVENTIONS FOR FAMILY CAREGIVERS

Caring for the Caregiver

Family caregivers must be recognized as "care recipients" in their own right. There is agreement that many times caregivers simply burn out over the course of caregiving. Physical, emotional, and compassion fatigue sets in, AND the caregivers have no reserve to care for the care recipients, much less themselves. This leads to neglect of their own needs and health and the development of depression and other emotional complications as well as physical illness (Family Caregiver Alliance, 2006a).

Family members experience role changes and transitions, stress, and ultimately bereavement as their loved one traverses life's continuum (Dumont et al., 2008; Hebert, Schulz, Copeland, & Arnold, 2009; Hudson et al., 2008). It is important that healthcare professionals recognize physical, emotional, social, spiritual, and financial changes and transitions at the end of life and into bereavement. The transitions and associated needs of family caregivers have not been addressed by the healthcare system. Studies have indicated the existence of issues, such as a lack of continuity of care with multiple care providers and locations of care (Holtslander, 2008; Waldrop, Kramer, Skretny, Milch, & Finn, 2005).

Family caregivers have a right to their own support and assessment of their needs, with their experience evaluated "not as a proxy response for patients but as an outcome itself" (Steinhauser, 2005). Their resources and capabilities are influenced by multiple factors, such as gender, age, ethnicity, education, socioeconomic status, and geographic location (Bernard & Guarnaccia, 2003; Stajduhar et al., 2010). Caregivers' existing psychosocial resources and relationship with patients may indicate vulnerability to challenges of caregiving and may inform interventions that reduce stress and increase caregiver mastery in the role (Kim, Kashy, & Evans, 2007). With a holistic understanding of the caregiver's view, including needs as care recipients, and desired outcomes, limited resources can be appropriately allocated and interventions

TABLE 8.2 Family Caregiver Assessment Domains, Constructs, and Questions

Domain	Constructs	Questions
Context	■ Caregiver relationship to care recipient ■ Physical environment (home, facility) ■ Household status (number in home, etc.) ■ Financial status ■ Quality of family relationships ■ Duration of caregiving ■ Employment status (work/home/volunteer)	■ What is the caregiver's relationship to the care recipient? ■ How long has he/she been in the caregiving role? ■ Does the care recipient live in the same household with the caregiver? ■ Is the caregiver married? Have children? ■ How many people live in the caregiver's household? ■ Are other family members or friends involved in the care? ■ Is the caregiver currently employed? Full-time or part-time? ■ What is the caregiver's household income? ■ How would the caregiver rate his/her quality of family relationships?
Caregiver's perception of health and functional status of care recipient	■ Activities of daily living (ADLs; bathing, dressing) and need for supervision ■ Instrumental activities of daily living (IADLs; managing finances, using the telephone) ■ Psychosocial needs ■ Cognitive impairment ■ Behavioral problems ■ Medical tests and procedures	■ Can the care recipient carry out ADLs without assistance (bathing, dressing, etc.)? ■ Can the care recipient carry out IADLs without assistance (managing finances, shopping)? ■ Can the care recipient administer his/her medications correctly? ■ Does the care recipient have any mental health diagnoses or emotional problems? ■ Does the care recipient have any memory loss or cognitive impairment? ■ Does the care recipient have any behavioral problems? How frequently do they occur and how much do they bother or upset the caregiver when they happen? ■ What medical tests and procedures have been done or are needed?
Caregiver values and preferences	■ Caregiver's/care recipient's willingness to assume/accept care ■ Perceived family obligation to provide care ■ Culture-based norms ■ Preferences for scheduling and delivery of care and services	■ Is the caregiver willing to assume the caregiver role? Is the care recipient willing to accept care? ■ Does the caregiver feel he/she is obligated to provide care? ■ What types of care arrangements are considered culturally acceptable for this family? ■ What are the caregiver's (and the care recipient's) preferences for the scheduling and delivery of care and services?
Well-being of the caregiver	■ Self-rated health ■ Health conditions and symptoms ■ Depression or other emotional distress (e.g., anxiety) ■ Life satisfaction/quality of life	■ How does the caregiver rate his/her own health? Does the caregiver rate his/her health better, about the same, or worse than it was 6 months ago? ■ Does the caregiver have any health conditions or symptoms? ■ How often in the past 6 months has the caregiver had a medical examination or received treatment for physical health problems from a healthcare practitioner? ■ Depression Scale (See Selected Measures in Appendix III) ■ How often does the caregiver feel anxious or angry when he/she is around the care recipient? ■ How often does the caregiver get a full night's sleep? ■ How does the caregiver rate his/her life satisfaction and/or quality of life?

Consequences of caregiving	■ Perceived challenges
	■ Social isolation
	■ Work strain
	■ Emotional and physical health strain
	■ Financial strain
	■ Family relationship strain
		■ Perceived challenges
		  – Does the caregiver have a social support network or is he/she isolated?
		  – Does the caregiver suffer any work-related difficulties due to the caregiving role?
		  – Does the caregiver suffer from any emotional and/or physical health problems as a result of caregiving?
		  – How much does the caregiver's health stand in the way of doing things he/she wants to do?
		  – What has been the financial strain, if any, on the caregiver due to his/her caregiving role?
		  – How much disagreement has the caregiver experienced with other family members over particular care issues?

(continued)

TABLE 8.2   Family Caregiver Assessment Domains, Constructs, and Questions (*continued*)

Domain	Constructs	Questions

	■ Perceived benefits
	■ Satisfaction of helping family member
	■ Developing new skills and competencies
	■ Improved family relationships
		■ Perceived benefits
		  – Does the caregiver feel satisfaction in helping a family member?
		  – Does the caregiver feel he/she has developed new skills and knowledge because of caregiving?
		  – Has there been an improvement in family relationships (general closeness, communication, similarity of views, degree of getting along) as a result of the caregiving situation?

Skills/abilities/ knowledge to provide care recipient with needed care	■ Caregiving confidence and competencies ■ Appropriate knowledge of medical care tasks (wound care, etc.)	■ How knowledgeable does the caregiver feel about the care recipient's condition? ■ What are the skills and abilities needed to provide care for the care recipient? ■ How would the caregiver rate his/her confidence and competence in these areas? ■ Does the caregiver have the appropriate knowledge of medical care tasks (wound care, ability to administer medications correctly, etc.) and transfer techniques (moving from bed to chair, etc.)
Potential resources that caregiver could choose to use	■ Existing or potential strengths (e.g., what is presently going well) ■ Coping strategies ■ Financial resources (healthcare and service benefits, entitlements such as the VA, Medicare) ■ Community resources and services (caregiver support programs, religious organizations, volunteer agencies) ■ Formal and informal helping network and perceived quality of social support	■ Can the caregiver rely on his/her social support network for help (i.e., respite)? ■ What are the caregiver's coping strategies? Are these healthy/constructive? ■ Has the caregiver accessed all financial benefits and entitlements he/she or care recipient is eligible for (e.g., VA)? ■ What other community resources/services is the caregiver utilizing or aware of (e.g., caregiver support groups, religious organizations)?

VA, U. S. Department of Veterans Affairs.

Source: Used with permission from the Family Caregiver Alliance. (2013b, July 25). An online toolkit to help practitioners assess the needs of family caregivers. Retrieved from https://www.caregiver.org/caregivers-count-too-toolkit

Exhibit 8.1
Assessment Tools

www.caregiver.org/caregivers-count-too-toolkit
caregiver.org/caregiver/jsp/content/pdfs/SelCGAssmtMeas_ResInv_FINAL_12.10.12.pdf
myfaf.org
humanservices.ucdavis.edu/Resource/index.aspx
nextstepincare.org/Caregiver_Home/Becoming_a_Family_Caregiver

Assessment Tools by State
www.caregiver.org/caregivers-count-too-s4-fca-assessment-resources

Annotated Bibliography of Assessment References
www.caregiver.org/caregivers-count-too-s4-annotated-bibliography

developed that have a positive impact for caregivers and, in turn, for patients (Guberman, 2006). The family caregiving theoretical frameworks described earlier are not only extremely valuable in identifying important aspects of caregiver assessment, but also can inform health professionals in developing and implementing needed family caregiver interventions.

After one has completed careful family assessment, identification of the family strengths and weaknesses that will have an impact on the caregiver and/or the care recipient and their relationship should be identified, clustered, and organized in a way that they reflect the priorities and function of the dyad. Generally, strategies can be successful by addressing four general areas:

1. Setting realistic goals.
2. Having difficult discussions.
3. Finding help.
4. Negotiating expectations.

■ **Setting Realistic Goals.** Setting realistic goals involves the identification of key tasks and responsibilities, and then priorities for what must and can be accomplished in an hour, a day, or a week (Demiris et al., 2012; Sunnerhagen, Olver, & Francisco, 2013; Wittenberg-Lyles, Goldsmith, Demiris, Oliver, & Stone, 2012). It means looking honestly at the chronic disease or disability that is the focus of palliative care and estimating the level of functioning and participation the caregiver can expect from the care recipient. In the care of patients with various illnesses, clinicians may ask, "Will the husband with the stroke regain any ability to swallow?" "Will the mother with progressive, accelerated memory loss maintain the ability to dress herself?" The answers to these questions may be different from the perspective of clinicians versus family members. The objective observer sees only the reality of permanent dysfunction. If the caregiver can see the situation realistically, then goal setting is easier, but more commonly, the caregivers exhaust themselves trying to reach unrealistic goals and the expectation that they will be able to handle all the care required. It is just as important to be there for the caregiver when they reach the time when they can no longer cope with the enormity of the caregiver experience and admit the need for help and support.

■ **Having Difficult Discussions.** Difficult discussions often involve end-of-life discussions, and there are many areas of life that are difficult to discuss for reasons of history, family dynamics, cognitive dysfunction, or embarrassment (Cherlin et al., 2005; Wright et al., 2008). Chances are that the more difficult the discussion, the more important it is to have that discussion. The imminence of dying often breaks down years of barriers to open, honest communication leading to a restoration of family relationships (Branum, 2002). There is always the possibility that fissures in family structures will become vast crevices, but the potential for healing makes some discussions worth having. Financial discussions may be just as difficult as healing and end-of-life discussions. When a parent or sibling lacks the cognitive ability or judgment to handle his or her own finances, the rational thing to do is manage those components for him/her (Family Caregiver Alliance, 2013a; Marson et al., 2009). However, the care recipients may not see the rationality of that action, particularly if they are paranoid or psychotic.

Difficult discussions require extensive planning and careful selection of place and time. It is best to be very direct with short, simple sentences (Ngo-Metzger, Srinivasan, Solomon, & Meyskens, 2008). It is good not to try to accomplish too much in any one meeting, taking time to work through issues with as little defensiveness and blame as can be accomplished.

■ **Finding Help.** There are two categories of finding help. First, and possibly most straight forward, is help that is available through social programs, support groups, and organizations (National Alliance for Caregiving, 2013; Family Caregiver Alliance, 2013d). There are specific criteria for Medicare, Medicaid, food stamps, even meals-on-wheels. It may be difficult for caregivers to navigate the endless maze of programs and program rules, but help from a case manager or social worker can facilitate this process. Support groups exist for both caregivers and for caregivers and recipients related to diagnosis, disabilities, and specific causes and charities associated with chronic disease and disabilities. For caregivers, simply entering the term "Family Caregivers" into Google returned 2,990,000 results on March 25, 2017. Most notable of those results and in the first 10 returned were the Family Caregiver Alliance, the National Family Caregivers Association, and the Family Caregivers in Cancer (PDQ®) National Cancer Institute. Exhibit 8.2 is a sampling of organizations that exist to support family and informal caregivers.

The second and more difficult task of finding help may be exacting the cooperation and contribution of other family members in the care of the recipient (Barbosa, Figueiredo, Sousa, & Demain, 2011; Family Caregiver Alliance, 2013c; National Alliance for Caregiving in Collaboration with AARP, 2015). Family history and dynamics may make this impossible even with difficult discussions directed at resolving conflicts that fester with anger and resentment and/or blame for past experiences. It may be impossible and inappropriate to request some family members to overcome past abuse that they have finally resolved in order to provide care for the source of their abuse.

■ **Negotiating Expectations.** The most difficult of the four categories of intervention may be negotiating expectations. It depends so much on the other three and time to deal with the realities of caregiving and the development of a trusting relationship with the case manager or palliative care nurse. Caregivers often take on more than one person can honestly accomplish (Stajduhar & Davies, 2005). Whether out of love, duty, or self-interest, the tasks of caring for someone who is physically and/or psychologically dependent may not appear overwhelming until the caregiver tries to get them all accomplished alone in the course of 1 day (Penson et al., 2007). Even if the caregiving activities are not accomplished in addition to a 40+ hours a week job and nuclear family responsibilities, it can be exhausting and mind numbing. Some caregivers persist in spite of pleading from family and friends to get help or give up some of the tasks. Release from the responsibilities comes only after the death of the care recipient. Even placement in a long-term care facility may not release the caregiver from self-imposed responsibilities.

For others, the reality of the responsibilities sinks in quickly and they seek help from family, professional

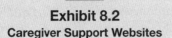

Exhibit 8.2
Caregiver Support Websites

• AARP	www.aarp.org/home-family/caregiving
• Administration on Aging	www.acl.gov/about-acl/administration-aging
• Agingcare.com	www.agingcare.com
• Aging Life Care	www.aginglifecare.org
• American Red Cross	www.redcross.org/prepare/location/home-family
• APA's Family Caregiver Briefcase for Psychologists	www.apa.org/pi/about/publications/caregivers/index.aspx
• ARCH National Respite Network	archrespite.org
• Caregiving.com	www.caregiving.com
• Care Partner	www.carepartner.com
• Caring.com	www.caring.com
• Family Caregiver Alliance	www.caregiver.org
• Family Caregiver Handbook	web.mit.edu/workplacecenter/hndbk
• Family Caregivers Support Network	www.caregiversupportnetwork.org
• Family Caregiver Web	www.familycaregiverweb.com
• Guide to Long Term Care for Veterans	www.va.gov/GERIATRICS/Guide/LongTermCare/index.asp
• Johnson & Johnson Strength for Caring	www.jnj.com/caring/initiatives
• Lotsa Helping Hands	www.lotsahelpinghands.com
• National Alliance for Caregiving	www.caregiving.org
• National Caregivers of Veterans Support Hotline	www.caregiver.va.gov
• National Family Caregivers Association	www.caregiveraction.org
• National Institute on Aging	www.nia.nih.gov
• National Transitions of Care Coalition	www.NTOCC.org
• Next Step in Care	www.nextstepincare.org
• Rosalyn Carter Institute for Caregiving	rci.gsw.edu

This is not an exhaustive list and there are state-specific programs available.

agencies, or through placement in a long-term care facility. There is always some degree of guilt associated with this decision but some deal with their guilt in healthy ways; some do not (Brodaty & Donkin, 2009; Buhr, Kuchibhatla, & Clipp, 2006).

For some family caregivers, the despair and hopelessness that come from being overwhelmed with work and responsibilities, as well as the lack of support and acknowledgement, can manifest in abuse (Funk et al., 2010; Moules et al., 2004; Wells et al., 2008; Zarit, 2006). It would be naive to say there are no mean and naturally abusive people who become caregivers for whatever reason. What then could cause a kind, well-meaning caregiver, who has made a commitment to the care of a family member, go on to starve, slap, pinch, demean, or threaten an elder or disabled family member? Some instances can be explained by despair and hopelessness that lead to acting out on the perceived source of the despair; anger that becomes resentment and develops into rage; and too few resources to meet the demands of the caregiving. A few may have mental illness themselves that manifests in stressful situations such as extreme caregiving (Brodaty & Donkin, 2009). These are potential explanations, not excuses. Consequently, the palliative care nurse or case manager must be vigilant for signs of abuse even in situations where everything seems to be going well. Abuse may be a call for help; it must be identified and stopped. It may take all the negotiating skill of the nurse to protect the care recipient while also getting help for the abuser.

Evidence-Based Family Caregiver Interventions

A recently convened NINR Summit Conference on End of Life and Palliative Care made numerous recommendations for research related to identifying caregiver needs and developing interventions for them as care recipients (McGuire et al., 2012). Systematic reviews of caregiver interventions in terminal illness (Candy, Jones, Drake, Leurent, & King, 2011) and in cancer caregiver populations (Applebaum & Breitbart, 2013; Northouse et al., 2012; Northouse, Katapodi, Song, Zhang, & Mood, 2010) have evaluated the effectiveness of various caregiver interventions (e.g., psychoeducation, problem solving/skills building, supportive therapy, family/couples therapy, interpersonal therapy, complementary therapies) with evidence of short- or long-term benefit to adjustment. Based on a randomized controlled trial conducted by Holm et al. (2016), a psychoeducational intervention was offered to 119 family caregivers enrolled in a palliative care home program to increase their preparation for the caregiving role. The intervention included three sessions with a physician, nurse, and social worker or priest. The results indicated higher levels of caregiver preparedness in both short- and long-term follow-up with increased sense of competence in the short term compared to the control group. However, the intervention did not effect a sense of reward in caregiving or reduce caregiver burden, depression, or anxiety. These results were explained by low to moderate baseline scores on these variables with little room for improvement.

Hudson and Aranda (2014) provide an overview of the development, evaluation, and outcomes arising from a program of research—Melbourne Family Support Program (FSP)—focused on reducing caregiver burden. The transactional model of coping guided the interventions and studies in the program. The program was designed to increase family caregivers' readiness for their role, encourage and support their positive emotions, decrease needs that have been unmet, and reduce their stress. Four psychoeducational interventions, incorporating one-to-one and group format delivery, conducted at the home and inpatient hospital/hospice were evaluated. Statistically significant outcomes included improvements in family caregivers' preparedness, competence, positive emotions, more favorable levels of psychological well-being, and a reduction in unmet needs. The interventions and resources from the Melbourne FSP provide several evidence-based and clinically relevant approaches that focus on reducing the psychosocial burden of the caregiving role (Holm et al., 2016).

Based on a systematic review, Kaltenbaugh et al. (2015) evaluated the effectiveness of web-based interventions to support family caregivers of patients with cancer. Web-based interventions used the Internet for delivery, such as caregiver forums, online support groups, virtual communities, smartphone applications, or online programs offering caregiver information. A total of 795 articles were identified during the extensive search of the literature, with only six studies meeting the inclusion criteria. Two of the studies used the CHESS intervention, which consists of communication, information, and coaching. One study used the virtual portal, HutchWorld, which is an intervention composed of social interaction, diversional activities, and information. One study included was a secondary analysis of data from a randomized trial, whereas another described feasibility testing data, and the sixth reported focused group testing with quantitative results. The results indicated that web-based interventions may positively influence a cancer caregiver's psychological and social health; however, more studies are needed. Given the time constraints faced by family caregivers with multiple roles, Kaltenbaugh et al. (2015) suggest that online education and Internet-based support groups provide an alternative method to offer caregivers support.

■ CONCLUSION

The research clearly indicates the negative outcomes of family caregiving and the need for multimethod interventions to address the physical, emotional, social, spiritual, and practical needs of family caregivers. This is critically important to the well-being of the patient given that caregiver burnout places patients at risk for abuse and neglect. In palliative care, it is recognized that the unit of care is both the patient and family. At many points across the illness continuum, health professionals should conduct a family caregiver assessment to determine the well-being of family caregivers and the functioning of the entire family. Beyond words of encouragement and support, which validate the importance of caregiver roles, it is important for members of the interprofessional team to be consulted to offer their expert advice, advocate for the well-being of caregivers, and assist them in accessing valuable community resources. At the end of life, both the palliative care team and hospice can provide a lifeline to family caregivers, because their health may be at risk and they become second-order patients.

CASE STUDY *Conclusion*

S.M.'s condition continued to decline. Her cognitive and muscular dysfunction and inability to care for her daughters has led to depression. Although she had the help and support of her family, she could not help but feel distressed and had a difficult time accepting her prognosis. S.M.'s ex-husband and father to the two girls became proactive in his daughters' lives, and, in S.M.'s case, restored a friendly relationship. This enabled S.M. to have some peace of mind. Soon thereafter, S.M.'s condition deteriorated and she now needed total care because she was confined to bed. R.C. and K.C. were trying their best, but they felt underprepared and overwhelmed by the experience. The Palliative Care Nurse Practitioner who offered support to S.M. and her family in the hospital's outpatient clinic discussed the value of enrolling in hospice care. She emphasized that hospice would provide assistance in addressing S.M.'s daily physical care needs, management of symptoms, and emotional support to not only S.M., but also her brother, sister-in-law, and her daughters. It was clear to R.C. and his wife, who were both health professionals, that even with healthcare experience they needed support as caregivers.

CASE STUDY

THE INTERPROFESSIONAL PERSPECTIVE OF A SOCIAL WORKER

Mark E. Ritchie, LCSW, Seasons Hospice and Palliative Care, Miami, Florida

The case study of R.C. reveals such a beautiful example of family striving to live by familial values during a time of crisis and upheaval. R.C. models "family taking care of family" behavior and values to S.M.'s children, but encounters how this can readily overwhelm a nuclear family, going through its own losses and stressors.

I'd also like to explore further what the children's understanding is of their mother's health and their own future living with their uncle and aunt. Often families try to "protect" children from information regarding death, dying, and serious illness. With R.C.'s permission, I'd want to talk to the children alone to assess their coping and understanding, also assessing R.C.'s and his wife's current understanding of talking to children about death and dying. How do their recent losses affect their ability to talk to the children about death, dying, and serious illness?

I'd want to offer plenty of validation of the efforts R.C. and his wife are making to keep family together, and how exhausting this must be both emotionally and physically. I would have a discussion of "taking care of the caregiver" with exploration of possible available resources for them. A discussion of family medical leave availability (FMLA), as well as an exploration of other family support and community resources that might be able to help with S.M.'s care, such as hospice/home health, would be important. I would explore whether S.M. qualifies for Medicaid, which might be able to pay for medical bills or for home services.

Caregiving for a seriously ill person is more than a full-time job of its own, and one usually can't sleep well when caregiving due to hypervigilance. R.C. and his wife seem to have come up with a division of associated tasks, but maybe one can take FMLA to care for S.M. while the other can take maternity/paternity leave when their own babies are born. It is a great gesture to drive the children to their former school, but for how long are they going to do that? This family seems to be pacing themselves for a sprint rather than a marathon, and there are already physical consequences occurring suggesting that they may need to find ways to cut themselves some slack and reprioritize.

Evidence-Based Practice

Holm, M., Arestedt, K., Carlander, I., Furst, C., Wengstrom, Y., Ohlen, J., & Alvariza, A. (2016). Short-term and long-term effects of a psychoeducational group intervention for family caregivers in palliative home care—Results from a randomized control trial. *Psycho-Oncology, 25,* 795–802. doi:10.1002/pon.4004

Background

Family caregivers in cancer and palliative care often have tremendous responsibilities and feel inadequately prepared for their roles. This study evaluates the short-term and long-term effects of a psychoeducational group intervention aimed to increase preparedness for family caregiving in specialized palliative home care.

Methods

The study design was a randomized controlled trial where family caregivers were assigned to either an intervention or control group. The intervention was delivered as a program including three sessions by health professionals (physician, nurse, and social worker/priest). Family caregivers from 10 specialized palliative home care settings were included. Questionnaires with validated instruments at baseline, upon completion, and 2 months following the intervention were used to measure effects of the intervention. The primary outcome was preparedness of family caregivers for their role.

Results

In total, 21 intervention programs were delivered, and 119 family caregivers completed all three measurements. The intervention group had a significantly increased sense of preparation for caregiving in both the short-term and long-term follow-up compared with the control group. There were reported effects of the intervention on rewards for caregiving, caregiver burden, health, anxiety, or depression.

Conclusion

The psychoeducational intervention has the potential to be used by health professionals to improve preparedness for caregiving among family caregivers in palliative care both in short and long terms.

■ REFERENCES

Ahern, D. (2006). Holding a mirror to caregiving. In Family Caregiver Alliance (Ed.), *Caregiver assessment: Voices and views from the field: Report from a national consensus development conference* (vol. II; pp. 2–6). San Francisco, CA: Family Caregiver Alliance.

Alzheimer's Association. (2017). *Alzheimer's disease facts and figures.* Chicago, IL: Alzheimer's Association. Retrieved from http://www.caregiver.org/caregiver/jsp/content/pdfs/v2_consensus.pdf

Aoun, S., Deas, K., Toye, C., Weing, G., Grande, G., & Stajduhar, K. (2015). Supporting family caregivers to identify their own needs in end-of-life care: Qualitative findings from a stepped wedge cluster trial. *Palliative Medicine, 29*(6), 508–517. doi:10.1177/0269216314566061

Applebaum, A. J., & Breitbart, W. (2013). Care for the cancer caregiver: A systematic review. *Palliative and Supportive Care, 11*(3), 231–252. doi:10.1017/S1478951512000594

Bahr, H. M., & Bahr, K. S. (2001). Families and self-sacrifice: Alternative models and meanings for family theory. *Social Force, 79*(4), 1231–1258. doi:10.1353/sof.2001.0030

Barbosa, A., Figueiredo, D., Sousa, L., & Demain, S. (2011). Coping with the caregiving role: Differences between primary and secondary caregivers of dependent elderly people. *Aging and Mental Health, 15*(4), 490–499. doi:10.1080/13607863.2010.543660

Bastawrous, M. (2013). Caregiver burden—A critical discussion. *International Journal of Nursing Studies, 50*(3), 431–441. doi:10.1016/j.ijnurstu.2012.10.005

Bee, P. E., Barnes, P., & Luker, K. A. (2009). A systematic review of informal caregivers' needs in providing home-based end-of-life care to people with cancer. *Journal of Clinical Nursing, 18*(10), 1379–1393. doi:10.1111/j.1365-2702.2008.02405.x

Bernard, L. L., & Guarnaccia, C. A. (2003). Two models of caregiver strain and bereavement adjustment: A comparison of husband and daughter caregivers of breast cancer hospice patients. *The Gerontologist, 43*(6), 808–816. doi:10.1093/geront/43.6.808

Branum, K. (2002). Healing in the context of terminal illness. In P. B. Kritek (Ed.), *Reflections on healing: A central nursing construct.* Sudbury, MA: Jones & Bartlett.

Brodaty, H., & Donkin, M. (2009). Family caregivers of people with dementia. *Dialogues in Clinical Neuroscience, 11*(2), 217–228.

Buhr, G. T., Kuchibhatla, M., & Clipp, E. C. (2006). Caregivers' reasons for nursing home placement: Clues for improving discussions with families prior to the transition. *Gerontologist, 46*(1), 52–61. doi:10.1093/geront/46.1.52

Candy, B., Jones, L., Drake, R., Leurent, B., & King, M. (2011). Interventions for supporting informal caregivers of patients in the terminal phase of a disease. *Cochrane Database of Systematic Reviews (Online),* (6), CD007617. doi:10.1002/14651858.CD007617.pub2

Carlson, J., & Dermer, S. B. (2017). *The SAGE encyclopedia of marriage, family, and couples counseling.* Thousand Oaks, CA: SAGE.

Cherlin, E., Fried, T., Prigerson, H. G., Schulman-Green, D., Johnson-Hurzeler, R., & Bradley, E. H. (2005). Communication between physicians and family caregivers about care at the end of life: When do discussions occur and what is said? *Journal of Palliative Medicine, 8*(6), 1176–1185. doi:10.1089/jpm.2005.8.1176

Clukey, L. (2007). "Just be there": Hospice caregivers' anticipatory mourning experience. *Journal of Hospice and Palliative Nursing, 9*(3), 150–158. doi:10.1097/01.NJH.0000269992.13625.00

Demiris, G., Parker Oliver, D., Wittenberg-Lyles, E., Washington, K., Doorenbos, A., Rue, T., & Berry, D. (2012). A noninferiority trial of a problem-solving intervention for hospice caregivers: In person versus videophone. *Journal of Palliative Medicine, 15*(6), 653–660. doi:10.1089/jpm.2011.0488

DeRigne, L., & Ferrante, S. (2012). The sandwich generation: A review of the literature. *Florida Public Health Review, 9,* 95–104.

Dumont, I., Dumont, S., & Mongeau, S. (2008). End-of-life care and the grieving process: Family caregivers who have experienced the loss of a terminal-phase cancer patient. *Qualitative Health Research, 18*(8), 1049–1061. doi:10.1177/1049732308320110

Family Caregiver Alliance. (2006a). *Caregiver assessment: Principles, guidelines and strategies for change: Report from a national consensus development conference* (vol. I). San Francisco, CA: Author. Retrieved from http://www.caregiver.org/caregiver/jsp/content/pdfs/v1_consensus.pdf

Family Caregiver Alliance. (2006b). *Caregiver assessment: Voices and views from the field: Report from a national consensus development conference* (vol. II). San Francisco, CA: Author. Retrieved from http://www.caregiver.org/caregiver/jsp/content/pdfs/v2_consensus.pdf

Family Caregiver Alliance. (2013a, July 31). Alzheimer's disease and caregiving. Retrieved from http://www.caregiver.org/caregiver/jsp/content_node.jsp?nodeid=567

Family Caregiver Alliance. (2013b, July 31). Caregiving. Retrieved from http://caregiver.org/caregiver/jsp/content_node.jsp?nodeid=2313

Family Caregiver Alliance. (2013c, July 31). Definition. Retrieved from http://www.caregiver.org/caregiver/jsp/content_node.jsp?nodeid=1703

Family Caregiver Alliance. (2013d, July 31). Services for family caregivers. Retrieved from https://www.caregiver.org/caregivers-count-too-toolkit

Family Caregiver Alliance. (2016). Caregiver Statistics: Health, Technology, and Caregiving Resources. Retrieved from https://www.caregiver.org/caregiver-statistics-health-technology-and-caregiving-resources

Feinberg, L., & Hauser, A. (2012). *Assessing family caregiver needs: Policy and practice considerations.* Washington, DC: AARP Public Policy Institute. Retrieved from http://www.caregiving.org/wp-content/uploads/2010/11/AARP-caregiver-fact-sheet.pdf

Feinberg, L. F., & Levine, C. (2015). Family caregiving: Looking to the future. *Generations: Journal of the American Society on Aging, 39*(4). Retrieved from http://www.asaging.org/blog/family-caregiving-looking-future

Fletcher, B. S., Miaskowski, C., Given, B., & Schumacher, K. (2012). The cancer family caregiving experience: An updated and expanded conceptual model. *European Journal of Oncology Nursing, 16*(4), 387–398. doi:10.1016/j.ejon.2011.09.001

Funk, L., Stajduhar, K., Toye, C., Aoun, S., Grande, G., & Todd, C. (2010). Part 2: Home-based family caregiving at the end of life: A comprehensive review of published qualitative research (1998–2008). *Palliative Medicine, 24*(6), 594–607. doi:10.1177/0269216310371411

Gaugler, J. E., Hanna, N., Linder, J., Given, C. W., Tolbert, V., Kataria, R., & Regine, W. F. (2005). Cancer caregiving and subjective stress: A multi-site, multi-dimensional analysis. *Psycho-Oncology, 14*(9), 771–785. doi:10.1002/pon.916

Gibson, M. J., Kelly, K. A., & Kaplan, A. K. (2012). Family caregiving and transitional care: A critical review. Family Caregiver Alliance. Retrieved from http://caregiver.org/caregiver/jsp/content/pdfs/FamCGing_TransCare_CritRvw_FINAL10.31.2012.pdf

Given, B. A., Given, C. W., & Sherwood, P. R. (2012). Family and caregiver needs over the course of the cancer trajectory. *Journal of Supportive Oncology, 10*(2), 57–64. doi:10.1016/j.suponc.2011.10.003

Given, B. A., Sherwood, P., & Given, C. W. (2011). Support for caregivers of cancer patients: Transition after active treatment. *Cancer Epidemiology, Biomarkers and Prevention, 20*(10), 2015–2021. doi:10.1158/1055-9965.EPI-11-0611

Given, B. A., Wyatt, G., Given, C., Sherwood, P., Gift, A., DeVoss, D., & Rahbar, M. (2004). Burden and depression among caregivers of patients with cancer at the end of life. *Oncology Nursing Forum, 31*(6), 1105–1117. doi:10.1188/04.ONF.1105-1117

Grey, M., Knafl, K., & McCorkle, R. (2006). A framework for the study of self and family management of chronic conditions. *Nursing Outlook, 54*(5), 278–286. doi:10.1016/j.outlook.2006.06.004

Guberman, N. (2006). Assessment of family caregivers: A practice perspective. In Family Caregiver Alliance (Ed.), *Caregiver assessment: Voices and views from the field report from a national consensus development conference* (vol. II; pp. 38–57). San Francisco, CA: Family Caregiver Alliance.

Haley, W. E., LaMonde, L. A., Han, B., Burton, A. M., & Schonwetter, R. (2003). Predictors of depression and life satisfaction among spousal caregivers in hospice: Application of a stress process model. *Journal of Palliative Medicine, 6*(2), 215–224. doi:10.1089/109662103764978461

Hebert, R. S., Schulz, R., Copeland, V. C., & Arnold, R. M. (2009). Preparing family caregivers for death and bereavement. Insights from caregivers of terminally ill patients. *Journal of Pain and Symptom Management, 37*(1), 3–12. doi:10.1016/j.jpainsymman.2007.12.010

Higginson, I. J., & Gao, W. (2008). Caregiver assessment of patients with advanced cancer: Concordance with patients, effect of burden and positivity. *Health and Quality of Life Outcomes, 6*, 42. doi:10.1186/1477-7525-6-42

Holm, M., Arestedt, K., Carlander, I., Furst, C., Wengstrom, Y., Ohlen, J., & Alvariza, A. (2016). Short-term and long-term effects of a psycho-educational group intervention for family caregivers in palliative home care—Results from a randomized control trial. *Psycho-Oncology, 25*, 795–802. doi:10.1002/pon.4004

Holtslander, L. F. (2008). Caring for bereaved family caregivers: Analyzing the context of care. *Clinical Journal of Oncology Nursing, 12*(3), 501–506. doi:10.1188/08.CJON.501-506

Houldin, A. D. (2007). A qualitative study of caregivers' experiences with newly diagnosed advanced colorectal cancer. *Oncology Nursing Forum, 34*(2), 323–330. doi:10.1188/07.ONF.323-330

Hudson, P. (2004). Positive aspects and challenges associated with caring for a dying relative at home. *International Journal of Palliative Nursing, 10*(2), 58–65. doi:10.12968/ijpn.2004.10.2.12454

Hudson, P., & Aranda, S. (2014). The Melbourne family support program: Evidence-based strategies that prepare family caregivers for supporting palliative care patients. *BMJ Supportive and Palliative Care, 4*(3), 1–7. doi:10.1136/bmjspcare-2013-000500

Hudson, P., Quinn, K., Kristjanson, L., Thomas, T., Braithwaite, M., Fisher, J., & Cockayne, M. (2008). Evaluation of a psycho-educational group programme for family caregivers in home-based palliative care. *Palliative Medicine, 22*(3), 270–280. doi:10.1177/0269216307088187

Kaltenbaugh, D. J., Klem, M. L., Hu, L., Turi, E., Haines, A. J., & Hagerty Lingler, J. (2015). Using web-based interventions to support caregivers of patients with cancer: A systematic review. *Oncology Nursing Forum, 42*(2), 156–164. doi:10.1188/15.ONF.156-164

Kim, S. K., Park, M., Lee, Y., Choi, S. H., Moon, S. Y., Seo, S. W., ... Moon, Y. (2017). Influence of personality on depression, burden, and health-related quality of life in family caregivers of persons with dementia. *International Psychogeriatrics, 29*(2), 227–237. doi:10.1017/S1041610216001770

Kim, Y., Kashy, D. A., & Evans, T. V. (2007). Age and attachment style impact stress and depressive symptoms among caregivers: A prospective investigation. *Journal of Cancer Survivorship: Research and Practice, 1*(1), 35–43. doi:10.1007/s11764-007-0011-4

Kim, Y., & Schulz, R. (2008). Family caregivers' strains: Comparative analysis of cancer caregiving with dementia, diabetes, and frail elderly caregiving. *Journal of Aging and Health, 20*(5), 483–503. doi:10.1177/0898264308317533

Kutner, J. S., & Kilbourn, K. M. (2009). Bereavement: Addressing challenges faced by advanced cancer patients, their caregivers, and their physicians. *Primary Care, 36*(4), 825–844. doi:10.1016/j.pop.2009.07.004

Levine, C. (2006). Notes from the edge of the abyss. In Family Caregiver Alliance (Ed.), *Caregiver assessment: Voices and views from the field: Report from a national consensus development conference* (vol. II; pp. 7–10). San Francisco, CA: Family Caregiver Alliance.

Lynch, S. (2013). Impact of caregiving on family functioning: A theoretical framework. *Communicating Nursing Research, 46*, 567.

Marriage and Family Encyclopedia. (2013a, July 31). Retrieved from http://family.jrank.org

Marriage and Family Encyclopedia. (2013b, July 31). Family strengths—The family strengths perspective. Retrieved from http://family.jrank.org/pages/593/Family-Strengths-Family-Strengths-Perspective.html

Marson, D. C., Martin, R. C., Wadley, V., Griffith, H. R., Snyder, S., Goode, P. S., ... Harrell, L. E. (2009). Clinical interview assessment of financial capacity in older adults with mild cognitive impairment and Alzheimer's disease. *Journal of the American Geriatrics Society, 57*(5), 806–814. doi:10.1111/j.1532-5415.2009.02202.x

Maslow, K., Levine, C., & Reinhard, S. (2006). Assessment of family caregivers: A public policy perspective. *In voices and views from the field* (vol. II; pp. 58–80). San Francisco, CA: Family Caregiver Alliance.

McGuire, D. B., Grant, M., & Park, J. (2012). Palliative care and end of life: The caregiver. *Nursing Outlook, 60*(6), 351–356.e20. doi:10.1016/j.outlook.2012.08.003

Meleis, A. I., Sawyer, L. M., Im, E. O., Messias, D., & Schumacher, K. (2000). Experiencing transitions: An emerging middle range theory. *Advances in Nursing Science, 23*(1), 12–28. doi:10.1097/00012272-200009000-00006

Moules, N. J., Simonson, K., Prins, M., Angus, P., & Bell, J. M. (2004). Making room for grief: Walking backwards and living forward. *Nursing Inquiry, 11*(2), 99–107. doi:10.1111/j.1440-1800.2004.00204.x

Narayan, S., Lewis, M., Tornatore, J., Hepburn, K., & Corcoran-Perry, S. (2001). Subjective responses to caregiving for a spouse with dementia. *Journal of Gerontological Nursing, 27*(3), 19–28. doi:10.3928/0098-9134-20010301-05

National Alliance for Caregiving. (2013). Care for the family caregiver: A place to start. Retrieved from http://www.caregiving.org/data/Emblem_CfC10_Final2.pdf

National Alliance for Caregiving in Collaboration with AARP. (2015). Caregiving in the U.S. Retrieved from http://www.caregiver.org/caregiver-statistics-demographics

National Consensus Project. (2013). *Clinical practice guidelines for quality palliative care* (3rd ed.). Pittsburgh, PA: National Consensus Project for Quality Palliative Care. Retrieved from https://www.nationalcoalitionhpc.org/ncp-guidelines-2013/

Neff, J. L., Dy, S. M., Frick, K. D., & Kasper, J. D. (2007). End-of-life care: Findings from a national survey of informal caregivers. *Archives of Internal Medicine, 167*, 40–46. doi:10.1001/archinte.167.1.40

Ngo-Metzger, Q., Srinivasan, M., Solomon, L., & Meyskens, F. L. (2008). End-of-life care: Guidelines for patient-centered communication. *American Family Physician, 77*(2), 167–174.

Northouse, L. L., Katapodi, M. C., Schafenacker, A. M., & Weiss, D. (2012). The impact of caregiving on the psychological well-being of family caregivers and cancer patients. *Seminars in Oncology Nursing, 28*(4), 236–245. doi:10.1016/j.soncn.2012.09.006

Northouse, L. L., Katapodi, M. C., Song, L., Zhang, L., & Mood, D. W. (2010). Interventions with family caregivers of cancer patients: Meta-analysis of randomized trials. *CA: A Cancer Journal for Clinicians, 60*(5), 317–339. doi:10.3322/caac.20081

Papastavrou, E., Charalambous, A., & Tsangari, H. (2009). Exploring the other side of cancer care: The informal caregiver. *European Journal of Oncology Nursing, 13*(2), 128–136. doi:10.1016/j.ejon.2009.02.003

Pearlin, L. I., Mullan, J. T., Semple, S. J., & Skaff, M. M. (1990). Caregiving and the stress process: An overview of concepts and their measures. *The Gerontologist, 30*(5), 583–594. doi:10.1093/geront/30.5.583

Penson, R. T., Gu, F., Haris, S., Thiel, M. M., Lawton, N., Fuler, A. F., & Lynch, T. J. (2007). Hope. *The Oncologist, 12*(9), 1105–1113. doi:10.1634/theoncologist.12-9-1105

Policy Institute for Family Impact Seminars. (2013, July 31). Key Tool #5: Family diversity and contexts. Retrieved from https://www.purdue.edu/hhs/hdfs/fii/wp-content/uploads/2015/06/fi_toolkit_fdc.pdf

Porter, L. S., Keefe, F. J., Garst, J., McBride, C. M., & Baucom, D. (2008). Self-efficacy for managing pain, symptoms, and function in patients with lung cancer and their informal caregivers: Associations with symptoms and distress. *Pain, 137*(2), 306–315. doi:10.1016/j.pain.2007.09.010

Rabow, M. W., Hauser, J. M., & Adams, J. (2004). Supporting family caregivers at the end of life: "They don't know what they don't know." *Journal of the American Medical Association, 291*(4), 483–491. doi:10.1001/jama.291.4.483

Salmon, J. R., Kwak, J., Acquaviva, K. D., Brandt, K., & Egan, K. A. (2005). Transformative aspects of caregiving at life's end. *Journal of Pain and Symptom Management, 29*(2), 121–129. doi:10.1016/j.jpainsymman.2004.12.008

Schumacher, K. L., Beck, C. A., & Marren, J. M. (2006). Family caregivers: Caring for older adults, working with their families. *American Journal of Nursing, 106*(8), 40–50.

Schumacher, K. L., & Meleis, A. I. (1994). Transitions: A central concept in nursing. *Image—The Journal of Nursing Scholarship, 26*(2), 119–127. doi:10.1111/j.1547-5069.1994.tb00929.x

Sherwood, P. R., Donovan, H. S., Given, C. W., Lu, X., Given, B. A., Hricik, A., & Bradley, S. (2008). Predictors of employment and lost hours from work in cancer caregivers. *Psycho-Oncology, 17*(6), 598–605. doi:10.1002/pon.1287

Stajduhar, K. I., & Davies, B. (2005). Variations in and factors influencing family members' decisions for palliative home care. *Palliative Medicine, 19*(1), 21–32. doi:10.1191/0269216305pm963oa

Stajduhar, K. I., Funk, L., Toye, C., Grande, G., Aoun, S., & Todd, C. (2010). Part 1: Home-based family caregiving at the end of life: A comprehensive review of published quantitative research (1998–2008). *Palliative Medicine, 24*(6), 573–593. doi:10.1177/0269216310371412

Stajduhar, K. I., Martin, W. L., Barwich, D., & Fyles, G. (2008). Factors influencing family caregivers' ability to cope with providing end-of-life cancer care at home. *Cancer Nursing, 31*(1), 77–85. doi:10.1097/01.NCC.0000305686.36637.b5

Steel, J. L., Gamblin, T. C., & Carr, B. I. (2008). Measuring post-traumatic growth in people diagnosed with hepatobiliary cancer: Directions for future research. *Oncology Nursing Forum, 35*(4), 643–650. doi:10.1188/08.ONF.643-650

Steinhauser, K. E. (2005). Measuring end-of-life care outcomes prospectively. *Journal of Palliative Medicine, 8* (Suppl. 1), S30–S41. doi:10.1089/jpm.2005.8.s-30

Sunnerhagen, K. S., Olver, J., & Francisco, G. E. (2013). Assessing and treating functional impairment in poststroke spasticity. *Neurology, 80*(3 Suppl 2), S35–S44. doi:10.1212/WNL.0b013e3182764aa2

Thomas, A. (2006). *A three dog life.* New York, NY: Houghton Mifflin.

Tsai, P. F. (2003). A middle-range theory of caregiver stress. *Nursing Science Quarterly, 16*(2), 137–145. doi:10.1177/0894318403251789

Vanderwerker, L. C., Laff, R. E., Kadan-Lottick, N. S., McColl, S., & Prigerson, H. G. (2005). Psychiatric disorders and mental health service use among caregivers of advanced cancer patients. *Journal of Clinical Oncology, 23*(28), 6899–6907. doi:10.1200/JCO.2005.01.370

Velanovich, V., & Wollner, I. (2011). Quality of life and performance status in patients with pancreatic and periampullary tumors. *International Journal of Clinical Oncology, 16*(4), 401–407. doi:10.1007/s10147-011-0200-z

Waldrop, D. P., Kramer, B. J., Skretny, J. A., Milch, R. A., & Finn, W. (2005). Final transitions: Family caregiving at the end of life. *Journal of Palliative Medicine, 8*(3), 623–638. doi:10.1089/jpm.2005.8.623

Wells, J. N., Cagle, C. S., Bradley, P., & Barnes, D. M. (2008). Voices of Mexican American caregivers for family members with cancer: On becoming stronger. *Journal of Transcultural Nursing, 19*(3), 223–233. doi:10.1177/1043659608317096

Williams, A. L., & McCorkle, R. (2011). Cancer family caregivers during the palliative, hospice, and bereavement phases: A review of the descriptive psychosocial literature. *Palliative and Supportive Care, 9*(3), 315–325. doi:10.1017/S1478951511000265

Wittenberg, E., Kravits, K., Goldsmith, J., Ferrell, B., & Jujinami, R. (2017). Validation of a model of family caregiver communication types and related caregiver outcomes. *Palliative and Supportive Care, 15*, 3–11. doi:10.1017/S1478951516000109

Wittenberg-Lyles, E., Goldsmith, J., Demiris, G., Oliver, D. P., & Stone, J. (2012). The impact of family communication patterns on hospice family caregivers: A new typology. *Journal of Hospice and Palliative Nursing, 14*(1), 25–33. doi:10.1097/NJH.0b013e318233114b

Wong, F. K., Liu, C. F., Szeto, Y., Sham, M., & Chan, T. (2004). Health problems encountered by dying patients receiving palliative home care until death. *Cancer Nursing, 27*(3), 244–251.

Wright, A. A., Zhang, B., Ray, A., Mack, J. W., Trice, E., Balboni, T., ... Prigerson, H. G. (2008). Associations between end-of-life discussions, patient mental health, medical care near death, and caregiver bereavement adjustment. *Journal of the American Medical Association, 300*(14), 1665–1673. doi:10.1001/jama.300.14.1665

Yeh, P., & Bull, M. (2012). Use of the resiliency model of family stress, adjustment and adaptation in the analysis of family caregiver reaction among families of older people with congestive heart failure. *International Journal of Older People Nursing, 7*(2), 117–126. doi:10.1111/j.1748-3743.2011.00275.x

Zarit, S. H. (2004). Family care and burden at the end of life. *Canadian Medical Association Journal, 170*(12), 1811–1812. doi:10.1503/cmaj.1040196

Zarit, S. H. (2006). Assessment of family caregivers: A research perspective. In Family Caregiver Alliance (Ed.), *Caregiver assessment: Voices and views from the field: Report from a national consensus development conference* (vol. II; pp. 12–37). San Francisco, CA: Family Caregiver Alliance.

Kathleen O. Perrin

Communicating With Seriously Ill and Dying Patients, Their Families, and Their Healthcare Practitioners

CHAPTER 9

KEY POINTS

- Conveying or discussing "bad news" requires preparation—locating a private place for the conversation, asking the patient or family to have a significant other present, having as much information available as possible, and practicing what will be said.
- Patients and their families may respond to "bad news" with disbelief, anger, or denial. Nurses and nursing students should practice their reactions to these defense mechanisms.
- Nurses may inappropriately block patient or family communication by ignoring what the patient or family member has to say, offering elaborate explanations or inappropriate advice, and providing their opinions without being asked.
- Nurses may assist patients and their families to decide what is important to them while the patient is dying by asking the patient, "What would be left undone if you died sooner rather than later?"
- Byock believes that it is essential that patients, their families, and significant others find time before the patient dies to say to each other, "Please forgive me; I forgive you; thank you; and I love you."
- It is imperative that nurses demonstrate to patients and their families by their words and deeds that healthcare providers will not abandon the patient after a decision has been made about end-of-life care.

CASE STUDY

Gloria Richards, an 82-year-old woman with severe chronic obstructive lung disease, consented to surgery for an intestinal obstruction. Following the surgery, she required reintubation in the postanesthesia care unit (PACU) and was transported to the ICU for postoperative care. Although she was being ventilated with low tidal volumes, shortly after her arrival in the ICU, several blebs burst in her lungs; she developed crepitus from her chin to her waist and required multiple chest tubes. This marked the beginning of a difficult postoperative course. Three weeks after surgery, her chest tubes could finally be removed. However, she remained intubated, and every effort to wean her from the ventilator resulted in her becoming hypoxic and unresponsive.

After her first week in the ICU, Gloria was awake and responsive during the day. She was able to mouth words to the staff and was involved in developing her plan of care. Although Gloria was able to communicate her wishes clearly, communicating with her was very time consuming. During the second week, Gloria announced that she "was fed up." She believed she was not improving and said she either wanted to get better or have the ventilator removed. Gloria had been living with her brother, who had died 6 months before her hospitalization, so there was concern among members of the healthcare team that she was depressed. During interprofessional rounds, a trial of an antidepressant was proposed, and Gloria and her niece, her next of kin, agreed to the plan. However, as time progressed, Gloria indicated that she was "tired of all this and did not want it anymore." She wanted to know what was happening to her and whether she was likely to get better.

Like Gloria in the case study, seriously ill or dying patients and their families want their healthcare providers to communicate prognoses and treatment options with honesty (Furukawa, 1996; Parker et al., 2007) and care (Czerwiec, 1996; London & Lundstedt, 2007). In 1995, the Study to Understand Prognoses and Preferences for Outcomes and Risks of Treatment (SUPPORT) demonstrated that this discussion does not occur as often as families and hospitalized patients would prefer. Despite years of effort to improve end-of-life (EOL) communication, the SUPPORT finding was reaffirmed in 2007, when a study by Sullivan et al. (2007) found that only 33% of physicians reported that anyone on the healthcare team had spoken with hospitalized patients identified as likely to die about the possibility of dying. However, in the same study, the majority of physicians did report that a few days before the patient's death, someone had spoken about the likelihood of death with the patient's family. Regrettably, the problems with communication continue. In 2011, Curtis et al. reported that a multifaceted, interprofessional intervention intended to improve communication and care at the end of life had not been associated with any improvement in the communication or the quality of dying in critical care units of American hospitals.

Most Americans die in hospitals, so the absence or poor quality of such discussions is a major shortfall in the care of dying Americans. Moreover, even for patients who are cared for at home and referred to hospice, discussion and preparation for death are often avoided until hospice referral. Because most patients are not referred to hospice until the last weeks of their lives, this means that discussion of EOL care is often postponed, as in Gloria's situation, until it is unavoidable.

According to Servaty, Krejci, and Hayslip (1996), healthcare providers with less anxiety about death are more likely to talk meaningfully with dying patients. In their study, nursing students were less anxious and more willing than other college students and beginning medical students to communicate with dying people. Thus, they reasoned, nursing students may be responsive to educational endeavors to promote honest, caring communication with patients and families at the end of life. This chapter explores ways to encourage both nursing students and graduate nurses to facilitate communication with dying patients, their families, and their healthcare providers.

In addition to patients and their families benefiting from communication with nurses at the end of life, the nurses may also benefit. Stiles (1990) described seven types of personal growth that nurses dealing with dying patients felt they experienced as "gifts" from their patients. These gifts are learning to confront their own mortality, learning about self, developing a faith in self and in a higher being, transcending their limitations, learning realistic expectations, and clarifying personal responsibility. Although experienced nurses perceived these opportunities for personal growth as gifts from their patients, undergraduate nursing students may be more distressed by them. Ways in which nursing faculty members might assist undergraduate nursing students to enrich themselves by working with dying patients will also be explored in this chapter.

This chapter is organized according to the phases of the therapeutic relationship because in many ways the phases of the therapeutic relationship—introductory, working, and termination—parallel the dying trajectory. When appropriate in the phases, distinctions are made between the roles and educational needs of the undergraduate nursing student, the nurse with an undergraduate degree, and the nurse with an advanced practice degree.

■ INTRODUCTORY PHASE

During the introductory phase of the therapeutic relationship, the nurse and patient open the relationship, begin to clarify and define the problem that has brought the patient in contact with the nurse, and begin to define their relationship.

Opening the Relationship

The components of this phase include conveying respect for the dying patient and his or her family as well as establishing a trusting relationship. These constituents are no different from their establishment in any therapeutic relationship. The nurse should introduce herself or himself to the patient and identify how the nurse will be involved in the patient's care. If a student nurse is involved, the nursing faculty member ought to note if the student caring for a dying patient seems unusually reluctant to engage in care of that patient. If the student appears hesitant, the faculty member might demonstrate, by introducing himself or herself to the patient, that this portion of the relationship is no different merely because the patient is dying. At this very early stage in the relationship, the healthcare provider probably ought to avoid discussing the subject of death and dying unless the patient brings up the topic (Byock, 1997).

Unfortunately, sometimes, it may be the responsibility of the advanced practice nurse or physician, during one of their initial meetings, to explain to a patient that the patient is severely ill and may be dying. It would always be preferable that the healthcare provider and patient have had an opportunity to establish a trusting relationship before the provider is required to deliver such bad news to the patient. However, in today's fast-paced healthcare environment, especially in emergency departments and critical care units, that is not always possible.

Conveying bad news requires thought and preparation. When preparing for the discussion, Buckman, Lipkin, Sourkes, and Tolle (1997) recommend that the healthcare provider locate a private place for the discussion, ask the patient to have a family member or friend present, have all information available to explain to the patient, and practice what she or he is planning to say. Buckman et al. (1997) suggest that after introductions are made to the patient and family, the patient be asked if it would be permissible to tape the interview. They state that taping the interview and providing the tape to the patient when the interview is finished enhances the patient's long-term adjustment. The steps recommended by Buckman (1992) for breaking bad news are listed in Table 9.1. Although these steps have been advocated and circulated for years, there is little consistent, good-quality evidence to support any interventions to convey "bad news," and they are recommended either on the basis of limited-quality patient-oriented evidence (B level) or consensus and expert opinion (C level; Barclay, Blackhall, & Tulsky, 2007; Ngo-Metzger, August, Srinivasan, Liao, & Meyskens, 2008).

Buckman et al. (1997), Barclay et al. (2007), and Arnold et al. (2010) recommend starting the interview by finding out what the patient knows or suspects. Often the patient has a preconception of the problem, and it may be necessary not only to convey bad news but also to counter the patient's and family's misconceptions of the situation. In numerous studies, families have indicated that prognosis should be conveyed in an honest, caring manner, but that they need to be prepared for a poor prognosis and it should be tempered with hope rather than delivered bluntly (Barclay et al., 2007).

Not all patients want to know the extent of their illness. Therefore, Ngo-Metzger et al. (2008) recommend that patients be asked directly and at the start of the interview how much information they want to know about their prognosis. Kagawa-Singer and Blackhall (2001) note that people from other cultures may not emphasize autonomy as much as Americans do. In some cultures, it is the members of the family and not the individual who learn the prognosis and agree to a plan of care. To uncover the desires of such patients and families, Kagawa-Singer and Blackhall suggest utilizing the following question: "Some patients want to know everything about their condition; others prefer that we talk with their families. How would you like to get information?" (p. 2995).

Before actually stating the problem, Buckman et al. (1997) and Arnold et al. (2010) suggest foreshadowing the news in simple language, such as "I'm sorry, I have some bad news for you." Because patients react immediately to the words "bad news," some physicians suggest substituting the words "serious" or "difficult" for bad (Chesanow, 2016). After the foreshadowing,

TABLE 9.1   Breaking "Bad News"
■ Be sure to get the context right
■ Find out what the patient and family already know
■ Find out how much information the patient or family really wants to know
■ Share the information: start from the viewpoint of the patient and family, and step-by-step bring their understanding closer to the medical facts
■ Respond to their reactions with empathy
■ Explain the treatment plan and prognosis, summarize, and make a contract

Source: Adapted from Buckman, R. (1992). How to break bad news: A guide for health professionals. Baltimore, MD: Johns Hopkins Press.

the situation should be explained in simple terms that are understandable to the patient. Patients and families consistently identify the use of medical jargon as a major deterrent to their understanding of the prognosis. After conveying the information in understandable terms, both Buckman and Arnold and their colleagues recommend something that can be very difficult for the beginning practitioner—at least 10 to 15 seconds of silence. During the period of silence, the patient will have an opportunity to absorb the information, react, and ask questions.

After the information is conveyed to the patient and the patient has had a chance to react, Buckman et al. (1997) and Arnold et al. (2010) suggest an empathetic approach. This implies that the person conveying the bad news should first identify the emotion that the patient or family is experiencing and identify the origins of the emotion. Then, the nurse should respond in a way that tells the person that the nurse understands what the person is experiencing. This means the nurse should "reflect, name, and legitimize the person's feelings" (Buckman et al., 1997, p. 63). For example, the nurse might say, "I can see that this has really upset you. Was that something that you weren't expecting?" (Radziewicz & Baile, 2001, p. 952). Arnold et al. (2010) suggest using the evidence-based mnemonic NURSE to uncover and respond to the patient's or family's emotions. The mnemonic followed by sample statements for the nurse to use is as follows:

- **Name the emotion:** You seem (insert appropriate emotion—e.g., worried).
- **Understand the emotion:** I can see that this is difficult for you.
- **Respect:** I can see that you are trying to _____.
- **Support the participants:** I (or we) will help you to _____.
- **Explore possibilities:** Tell me what options you can envision.

The final step in breaking bad news is providing an initial explanation of potential treatments and prognoses. Later in the therapeutic relationship, the nurse may become involved in empowering the patient to be an active participant in the decision-making process about treatment and developing an agreement about care. At this stage, the possibilities for treatment are usually just described, to provide the patient and family with an opportunity to begin thinking about goals of treatment. Before the interview is complete, the nurse or other member of the healthcare team should summarize the discussion for the patient.

Gordon, Buchman, and Buchman (2007) suggest using the SPIKES mnemonic as a tool to remember the steps for delivering bad news to patients and families. This mnemonic summarizes the steps previously described and serves as a way to remember the steps. The steps of the mnemonic with an explanation of what occurs in each step are as follows:

- **Set up:** Set up an interview with the patient and family.
- **Perception:** Find out what the patient and/or family understands about the prognosis.
- **Invitation:** Ask who should be provided with the prognosis.
- **Knowledge:** Convey the bad news to the appropriate person in an understandable way.
- **Emotions:** Empathize with the person's emotions.
- **Summary and Strategy:** Summarize the discussion and start to think about a plan of care.

Because conveying "bad" news is so difficult, Tulsky, Chesney, and Lo (1996) recommend that a new practitioner be observed several times and offered feedback before being allowed to discuss bad news without supervision. Emanuel (1998) suggests the new practitioner be provided with talking points so that all of the appropriate information is covered. Blackhall, Erickson, Brashers, Owen, and Thomas (2014) have integrated the steps for discussing bad news at the end of life into a "Collaborative Behaviors Objective Assessment Tool for End-of-Life Communication" that identifies specific roles for each member of the multidisciplinary team. The tool has been used to prepare medical and nursing students to collaborate and convey difficult news. Latimer (1998) describes criteria for ethical communication of information that might be used to evaluate the communication skills of a beginning practitioner. To be ethical, according to Latimer, the communication should be timely and desired by the patient. The information must be accurate. The words should be understandable to the patient and family and the information must be conveyed in a gentle, respectful, and compassionate manner.

There is developing awareness that an individual healthcare provider should not confront a patient and family with bad news without informing other members of the healthcare team of the details of the discussion (Davis, Kristjanson, & Blight, 2003; Fallowfield & Jenkins, 2004; Larson & Tobin, 2000; Pattison, 2004). Unfortunately, more than 80% of physicians in a study by Ptacek, Ptacek, and Ellison (2001) did not have another healthcare provider accompany them when they delivered bad news. When individual providers provide bad news to patients and families without informing the other members of the healthcare team, the lack of communication can be a significant barrier to quality EOL care (Yabroff, Mandelblatt, & Ingham, 2004). Patients and families who are anxious often do not hear or understand bad news the first time they hear it. Nurses describe feeling caught "in the middle" or "going in blind" when they don't know what a patient has been told and the patient or family is requesting further information or explanations (Davis et al., 2003). To improve communication and develop an alliance among healthcare providers, patient, and family, Pattison (2004) suggests a policy change requiring that a senior or primary nurse be present when such discussions are initiated in the hospital.

Evidence suggests that family meetings with the multidisciplinary or palliative care (PC) team results in better patient and family understanding of the patient's illness and a more appropriate and coordinated plan of care. Boyle, Miller, and Forbes-Thompson (2005) and Arnold et al. (2010) recommend an initial meeting of the multidisciplinary team, patient (if possible), and family within 48 hours of a patient's ICU admission if the patient is at risk for death. Members of the healthcare team should prepare for the meeting by reviewing any issues, arranging a private location, and coordinating the timing so that the important members of the team can be present. The review of issues should include nurses' perspectives on the difficult or distressing daily patient care decisions that they are already making (Coombs & Long, 2008). Identifying nurses' concerns is of specific importance because nurses raising concerns about family/patient issues has been termed a "red flag" suggesting the presence of obstacles to good quality of EOL care (Ramos et al., 2016). Therefore, it is particularly important to arrange that the patient's nurse not be kept away from the meeting due to patient care concerns or staffing shortages (Brooks, Manias, & Nicholson, 2017).

During the meeting, what family members understand about the illness should be assessed, medical facts and treatment options should be reviewed, the patient's and family's values and goals should be discussed, a plan of care devised, and criteria established to judge whether the plan is succeeding or not developed. Some clinicians use the previously described SPIKES mnemonic as a guide to facilitate family meetings.

Additional meetings may be held to judge the success or failure of the plan and to determine the goals of patient care. To avoid potential conflict, Boyle et al. (2005) also recommend using a screening tool to identify patients and families who are at high risk for conflict. These families are further evaluated by a social worker and recommended for additional interventions, such as regular family meetings or an ethics consult, if appropriate.

The skills and process tasks a nurse needs for this initial, establishment phase of a relationship with a dying patient have been summarized by Coyle et al. (2015) in a communication skills module for oncology nurses. The skills are endorsing question asking, checking for patient and family understanding, and inviting the patient and family to share agenda items. The process tasks are ensuring privacy and comfort and making partnership statements.

Clarifying the Problem

There are several components to the phase of clarifying the problem. They include facilitating the patient's expression of emotions, identifying what the patient and family believe are problems, and identifying and responding to the patient's and family's concerns about care. Nurses should be expert in assisting patients to clarify what they believe are their significant healthcare-related concerns.

When the healthcare provider delivering the bad news has not informed the other members of the healthcare team about the discussion, it is often difficult for a nurse to identify if a patient has received bad news or when the patient is prepared to discuss such news. May (1995) suggests that if the nurse was present at the interview when the bad news was delivered, the patient will feel free to initiate a conversation when the patient is ready. If the nurse was not present during the interview, but suspects such an interview has occurred, the nurse might say to the patient, "I noticed the physician was speaking with you. What did she have to say?" Larson and Tobin (2000) suggest asking a more general question, such as "How is this hospitalization going for you and your family?" or "What has been the most difficult thing about this illness for you?" (p. 1574). May (1995) emphasizes that the nurse should not initiate such a discussion unless the nurse is able to sit down and actively listen to the patient.

Shannon, Long-Sutehall, and Coombs (2011) suggest a structured format for obtaining information about what the patient or family understands: the ASK–TELL–ASK format. Arnold et al. (2010) believe that the ASK–TELL–ASK model is an essential communication skill that all healthcare providers should utilize.

Beginning with the first ASK, the nurse might say, "I was not available during multidisciplinary rounds this morning, would you please tell me about the discussion?" This allows the patient or family to explain what they heard and understood from the meeting. Or, if the nurse was present but wants to learn what the patient or family believes is important, the nurse might ask, "What do you believe is the most important issue for us to talk about after the meeting today?"

The second phase is described by Arnold as the TELL phase when the physician explains to the family what is occurring. However, Shannon notes that it is also the TELL ME MORE phase during which the nurse clarifies that the patient or family understood what was said. For example, the nurse might say, "You mentioned that the team said your wife was holding her own, would you tell me what you understood when they said that?"

Finally, the nurse might summarize and ASK a second time.

> We talked about how your wife is not improving despite having been on a ventilator for some time and the health care team is concerned that although she is stable, she might not improve. Does it make sense to you why the team is concerned? Do you have any questions for me? (Shannon et al., 2011, p. 125)

If the nurse wants to explore the patient's or family's emotional responses, questions may have to be phrased differently.

May (1995) warns that when a nurse asks a patient how the patient feels, the patient usually responds by describing her or his physical condition. Thus, if a nurse wants information about the person's psychological concerns, the question will have to be phrased somewhat differently. Byock (1997) began using the phrase, "How are you feeling within yourself?" after he had noticed that hospice workers in England successfully cut though defenses and learned how the patient was feeling when they were asked that question. He suggests it as a way of getting immediately to the heart of the patient's concerns. Emanuel (1998) recommends several questions including: "During the last few weeks, how often have you felt downhearted or blue?" "What do you believe is bothering you?" "Who are you able to confide in?" (p. 1124).

Wilkinson (1991) examined factors that influenced how nurses communicated with cancer patients. She concluded that in general, nurses had difficulty employing facilitative communication with patients with cancer. She noted that nurses frequently used blocking techniques when dealing with patients who had had a recurrence of their cancer. Because these blocking techniques prevented the nurses from identifying patient concerns, the nurses obtained only a superficial nursing assessment and planned nursing care based on assumptions rather than on actual patient concerns.

Wilkinson (1991) identified three groups of nurses who used different methods to block patient communication. These were ignorers, informers, and mixed responders. *Ignorers* ignored patient cues to talk about specific problems or issues throughout the interview. These nurses changed the subject, engaged in conversation with the patient's relative, or began social chitchat to avoid emotionally laden conversations. *Informers* were nurses who gave elaborate explanations of procedures, offered inappropriate advice, or stated their opinions without being asked. These nurses indicated that providing such detailed, unasked-for information allowed them to maintain control of the situation and avoid difficult or emotionally laden conversations (Wilkinson, 1991). *Mixed responders* were the largest group of nurses in Wilkinson's study. They utilized both facilitative and blocking responses, attempted to understand patient problems, and were more aware of their blocking behaviors when questioned about them.

Although they had been taught facilitative communication, most of the practicing nurses in Wilkinson's 1991 study were unaware that they were blocking their patients' attempts to communicate important needs and concerns until they listened to an audiotape and discussed their responses. In 1996, Heaven and Maguire noted that demonstration with audiotaping and feedback improved the facilitative communication skills of registered nurses. However, since the improvement was not to a statistically significant extent, further study of this approach was recommended. An additional constraint on utilizing audiotaping to improve nursing communication is that there may be issues surrounding patient consent and privacy issues with audiotaping.

Boyd, Merkh, Rutledge, and Randall (2011) found that nurses missed opportunities for important conversations with patients and families about dying and hospice care even though the nurses reported that they were not afraid to engage in such conversations. Searching for low-risk ways to assist nurses to initiate communication with patients about dying, Boyd et al. (2011) recommended role modeling by experienced, effective nurses and providing support and positive reinforcement to nurses when they utilize therapeutic communication skills. Having experienced nurses or encouragement available can prove especially beneficial for nurses who lack confidence in their ability to initiate sensitive conversations (Thompson-Hill, Hookey, Salt, & O'Neill, 2009).

Practice and encouragement in therapeutic communication is important; less than a quarter of the nurses in Wilkinson's 1991 study used primarily facilitative communication techniques when interviewing cancer patients. Nurses who used these techniques were able to do so no matter how ill the patient was or how emotionally laden the material to be divulged. By employing such standard facilitative communication techniques as active listening, use of open-ended questions, reflection or clarification of patient concerns, and empathy, they were able to obtain a more in-depth understanding of their patients' problems and concerns. In "An Interview With Dr. Stuart Farber," Farber states that patients and families most welcomed and remembered interactions with nursing staff that were personalized to the needs of the individual patient and family.

Yabroff et al. (2004) emphasize that it is not only healthcare providers who may establish barriers to good communication and optimal patient care. Patients and families may also establish such barriers by their inability to confront death and their utilization of defense mechanisms like disbelief, anger, and denial. Radziewicz and Baile (2001) describe ways that the nurses might recognize and respond therapeutically to each of these behaviors. They define disbelief as "the patient or family's attempt to make sense of what they have heard" (p. 952). They recommend the nurse respond to the patient's disbelief by saying something like "Accepting such a serious illness must be hard because you have taken such good care of yourself" (p. 952). They believe that anger can be one of the most difficult emotions for an inexperienced nurse to deal with, especially as it may be targeted at healthcare providers. Radziewicz and Baile recommend that the nurse realize the anger often masks another strong emotion such as fear or disappointment. So, the nurse might respond to the angry patient or family member by saying, "I can see how frightening this is for you. Do you want to tell me more about it?" (p. 952).

Radziewicz and Baile (2001) define denial as the patient's refusal to believe bad news, saying that the news is a mistake and not real. Block (2001) notes that denial is a natural response that may help the patient to deal with the illness and should be respected. Radziewicz and Baile (2001) believe the nurse should not argue with the patient or family expressing the denial; should acknowledge the difficulty in accepting the truth; and suggest a possible reason for the difficulty, but avoid continuing any blaming or feeling of mistake (p. 953). For example, a family member might say, "The doctors don't know what they're talking about. My father is going to be fine! He's going to walk again. I don't want anyone to tell me otherwise." The nurse might respond, "It must be difficult believing something so unimaginable could be happening when everything was fine a few days ago." Block (2001) agrees with this approach unless the patient is one of the 10% of patients who are in severe denial and the denial is likely to cause problems. In such a circumstance, Block recommends challenging the patient's denial to achieve a greater good. The nurse might say, "I know that making a decision about this is extremely painful, yet if we don't make plans now, we may lose that chance" (Block, 2001, p. 953).

Rosenbaum and Kreiter (2002), Farrell, Ryan, and Langrick (2001), and Ambuel (2003) have demonstrated that healthcare providers can learn to respond to such patient and family behaviors by role-playing case studies. Some authors suggest scripted case studies; others establish a general style of patient/family behavior and allow the healthcare participants to practice a variety of responses. In either instance, after role-playing, healthcare providers indicate more confidence in their abilities and greater willingness to communicate with patients who have received bad news. It is also important to realize that just because the topic is dying and the problems are serious, the talk does not always have to be solemn. Langley-Evans and Payne (1997) noted that lighthearted talk about illness, symptoms, bereavement, and personal mortality was quite valuable to outpatients in a palliative day care center. What was important was the nursing staff created an atmosphere that facilitated rather than blocked patients' disclosure of their concerns. Nursing administrators can do a great deal to encourage nurses to communicate with dying patients. Studies by Wilkinson (1991) and Booth, Maguire, Butterworth, and Hillier (1996) found that the major predictor of nursing staff's use of facilitative communication with patients with cancer or in hospice was the supportiveness of the nurses' supervisor. In the study by Wilkinson, the ward sisters (unit managers) who took assignments, cared for patients, and demonstrated facilitative communication with patients to their staff were more likely to

communicate therapeutically with their patients. These same ward sisters also encouraged their nurses to work autonomously and make decisions about nursing care. They had negotiated with the physicians who admitted patients to their units to obtain permission for the nurses to talk truthfully with any patient who requested information about her or his prognosis or treatment.

Coyle et al. (2015) summarize the overall strategy of the nurse during this clarifying phase of a relationship as developing an accurate shared understanding of the patient's situation, including disease features, prognosis, and psychosocial needs and concerns. The skills a nurse needs during this phase are checking patient and family understanding, clarifying, and checking for patient preferences. The process tasks are discussing expectations and correcting misunderstandings.

Structuring and Formulating the Care Agreement

There are several components to this phase of the therapeutic relationship. In any therapeutic relationship, the nurse and patient should continue to develop trust during this phase, come to an agreement about the frequency of meetings, and develop goals for care and the relationship. At this point in a dying patient's care, the healthcare team will initiate a discussion of the patient's treatment goals. Murphy and Price (1995) emphasize that the nurse should avoid using any phrase that resembles "There is nothing more that we can do." Ngo-Metzger et al. (2008) place "There is nothing more we can do" foremost in the commonly misconstrued phrases used in EOL discussions with patients. Although the phrase may be intended by the healthcare provider to convey that the patient's disease will progress and the patient will eventually die, it often implies to the patient and family that the healthcare team will abandon the patient.

Instead of focusing on what will not be done, the patient, family, and members of the healthcare team should begin to identify goals for patient care. Patients and families recall feeling supported by healthcare providers when they were told something like "We promise we will work with you to manage your symptoms and we will stay with you as your disease progresses. We can set goals for this portion of your life together."

Farber (1999) identified a number of possible goals that a dying patient might choose. These included living to the last possible second, living until the burden becomes too great, living at home with family, avoiding medical interventions, living as comfortably as possible until death, and avoiding medical treatments unless they will have meaningful outcomes. Once a goal has been identified, the healthcare team, patient, and family can begin to identify interventions that will achieve that goal.

To determine which aspects of physician communication have effects on quality of care at the end of patients' lives, Ramos et al. (2016) had ICU nurses evaluate physician communication with families and patients. Specific aspects of physician communication were associated with an enhanced quality of dying. When physicians were seen answering families' questions about illness, listening to what families had to say, asking about what treatments the patient would want, and helping the family decide what treatment the patient would want, patients experienced an enhanced quality of dying.

In 1993, Cotton noted that many physicians avoid initiating discussions about EOL treatment with their patients for fear the patients will become depressed or distrustful of the physicians' willingness to care for them. Unfortunately, there has been only limited improvement since then. In 2012, Aslakson et al. studied what surgical ICU nurses believed were the most prominent barriers to communication of prognosis and planning for EOL care. One of the four major barriers they identified was inadequate skill and training in communication. Included in this barrier were concerns such as discussions about prognosis being so rushed that patients and families had little time for questions; the use of jargon during conversations so that the patient/family could not understand what was being said; and, sadly, the patients/families not even being able to schedule a meeting with appropriate staff to obtain information or develop plans. In summary, the authors noted that surgical ICU nurses often found that the communication of prognostic information and discussion of goals of care at the end of life was "done quickly, inadequately, and ineffectively" by surgeons (p. 914). To rectify this shortcoming, surgical residency programs are attempting to prepare future surgeons to discuss EOL care. However, the training varies greatly by its length and depth, discipline, institutional culture, and setting (Lamba, Tyrie, Bryczkowski, & Nagurka, 2015). Often physicians of dying patients will delay the conversation until the patient is unresponsive and the family must be consulted (Shmerling, Bedell, Lilienfeld, & Delbanco, 1988; Sullivan et al., 2007). In fact, patients, especially elders, want to identify goals and interventions for EOL care and are relieved when the subject is broached. Most Americans do not have an advance directive, yet as long as they have the capacity to make healthcare decisions, it is their right to have the deciding voice in the type of healthcare they receive. When the members of the healthcare team avoid discussing the goals of EOL care until the patient is unresponsive, the patient is deprived of the right to determine appropriate EOL care.

Multiethnic and multilingual patients experience even more difficulty having effective EOL conversations with physicians (Periyakoil, Neri, & Kraemer, 2016).

Barriers that patients identify include doctor behaviors such as lacking empathy or being too busy to listen. Physicians are often not sensitive to their patients' cultural norms. For example, they may not recognize that there is a superstition about discussing death in some cultures or a cultural bias toward staying alive despite pain. Multiethnic patients describe a "communication chasm between doctors and patients" (p. 376). Patients state physicians communicated as if they do not realize that patients from other cultures might lack knowledge of EOL options, have difficulty understanding medical terms, or might not be able to comprehend significant portions of a conversation.

The role of the nurse is usually to interpret the medical information into terms the patient can understand and repeatedly explain the EOL treatment options to the patient. Even English-speaking patients and families often indicate that listening to the healthcare provider's explanation of a patient's prognosis and possibilities for treatment is like trying to understand a foreign language. In addition, most patients and their families experience stress when they receive bad news. Thus, they are unable to hear or retain much of what has been said to them. Being able to repeatedly replay the taped information is one of the reasons a tape recording of the initial interview may be beneficial for some patients and their families (Buckman et al., 1997). However, most of the time, it is the responsibility of the nurse to translate medical jargon into "lay terms" that the patient can comprehend and to reinforce the information regularly. The nurse might try a variety of teaching strategies, such as diagrams or written explanations, to help the patient and family understand the information. Treece (2007) recommends acknowledging that the information is complex to prevent the patient and family from feeling inadequate, and asking them to explain what they understand.

Coyle et al. (2015) summarize the nursing strategy for this goal-setting phase of the relationship as supporting patients and families following the physician's discussion of death and dying and EOL goals. The skills they have identified as needed during this phase are taking stock, asking open-ended questions, checking patient understanding, endorsing question asking, clarifying, and restating. The process tasks are tailoring information to the patient's level of detail, asking if a discussion of the dying process would be helpful, describing the natural dying process, avoiding jargon and euphemisms, and addressing cultural and religious needs.

During this phase, it is essential that the nurse determine not only what treatment the patient believes she wants but also what the patient believes will happen if she has the treatment that she wants, as shown in the following portion of the case study.

CASE STUDY *Continued*

By the end of the third week, Gloria Richards was more adamant that she wanted the ventilator and endotracheal tube removed. Gloria's niece was scheduled to arrive for a discussion with the interprofessional team after she finished work one Tuesday. That morning a student nurse and a new graduate were caring for her. While giving Gloria her morning bath, the nurse said to her, "Gloria, we'll be meeting this afternoon to talk about your plan of care; would you tell me again what you would like to have done?"

"I want this tube out now," she mouthed.

"Would you please tell me what you believe will happen if we take out the tube?" the nurse asked.

"It will be harder for me to breathe and I probably will die but I have had it," replied Gloria.

Shortly after, Gloria's primary care physician arrived. He asked what she wished to have done and informed her that she would most likely die if the healthcare team followed her wishes. Gloria reaffirmed that she wanted to be extubated.

■ WORKING PHASE

During the working phase of the therapeutic relationship, the nurse explores and understands the patient's feelings and expectations, elaborates on the goals of treatment developed in the previous phase, and facilitates or takes actions that the patient desires. In this case, the feelings and expectations explored relate to the dying process and the goals include defining what the patient believes constitutes dying well.

Exploring and Understanding Patients' Feelings and Expectations About Death and Dying

Nurses should be able to assist a patient to define what she or he believes constitutes dying well or represents a good and timely death. Quill (2000) recognizes that healthcare providers often do not agree about appropriate indications to begin a discussion with patients and families about EOL care. Although he believes the discussion should begin sooner, he states it is urgent to have such a discussion with patients who are facing imminent death, are talking about wanting to die, are inquiring about hospice, have been hospitalized for a severe progressive illness, or are suffering out of proportion to the prognosis. Quill suggests beginning the conversation with a question such as "What would be undone if you were to die sooner rather than later?" (p. 2504). Quill believes this question subtly conveys the message that time may be short and plans ought to be made now. Griffie, Nelson-Marten, and Muchka (2004) suggest a different question that conveys a similar message: "Now that we've discussed the uncertainty of your situation, what's most important to you?" (p. 51).

Nurses should be involved in helping to identify with the patient which issues would be most important

to address so the patient might die well. Some of the issues that may be important to patients at the end of life include participating in those EOL rituals that provide meaning to the patient and family, completing unfinished business, resolving relationship concerns with family and friends, and carrying out a life review. Once the issues are identified, members of the healthcare team may assist in addressing them.

The nurse will need to inquire of the patient and family about any EOL customs or rituals that provide meaning to them. Because a range of responses occurs within cultural and religious groups (Kagawa-Singer & Blackhall, 2001; Mazanec & Tyler, 2004), it is imperative that the nurse not assume that specific rituals will be of significance to a patient and family simply because they are members of a particular ethnic or religious group. The nurse might want to inquire, "What is your faith or belief? Is there a religious or ethnic community that is a source of support for you? Would you like me to notify the community or arrange for something for you?" Once these customs or rituals have been identified, Mazanec and Tyler (2004) state, they should be integrated into the plan of care for the dying patient.

If it is necessary to use an interpreter to have a discussion with a patient about EOL care, the use of a professional interpreter is supported by Grade A evidence. A meeting with the interpreter prior to the discussion is recommended to plan the approach for the discussion, to identify cues for stopping points, and to decide how much should be disclosed before stopping. During the discussion, the healthcare provider needs to continue to respond to the nonverbal cues that the patient and family display and convey empathy. Following the discussion, it is recommended that the healthcare team meet with the interpreter to clarify any misunderstandings (Barclay et al., 2007).

Patients may have a wide variety of unfinished business. Often these issues are related to the patient's age and developmental level. For example, a teenager might want to graduate from high school or an older adult might want to witness the arrival of a first grandchild. To identify what business, if any, the patient would like to complete, the nurse might ask, "If you were to die soon, what would be left undone?" or "Is there some event that would add a great deal of meaning to your life? What do we have to do so that event can take place?" Once the issue has been identified, rules might have to be bent (e.g., a child be allowed to participate in graduation ceremonies without completing required coursework, a grandchild or pet allowed into an ICU), resources expended, or help mobilized to permit the event to happen.

Patients may need both time and assistance to resolve relationship problems with their family and friends. Byock (2004) advocates that patients and their families make every effort to say four things to each other as they prepare to say farewell: "Please forgive me; I forgive you; thank you; and I love you" (p. 5). He believes that saying these four things "offers essential wisdom for completing a lifelong relationship before a final parting." When dying people "can reach out to express love, gratitude, and forgiveness . . . they consistently find that they, and everyone involved, are transformed for the rest of their lives, whether those lives last for decades or just days" (p. 7). Exline, Prince-Paul, Root, Peereboom, and Worthington (2012) demonstrated that unfortunately the opposite is also true. When family members believe that communicating forgiveness at the end of life is important and it does not occur, patients and family members have been shown to become depressed. Emanuel (1998) notes that some patients seem to be able to postpone dying so that they can complete their family business. Often, deaths occur after important events such as birthdays or holidays. One woman who was dying from respiratory failure asked to have her life prolonged by whatever means necessary until her estranged daughter, whom she had not seen in 10 years, arrived from across the country. After the daughter's arrival, arrangements were made for counseling sessions for the mother and daughter. Two days later, the mother died with the daughter present, holding her mother's hand.

Life review is another important part of both the aging process and the dying process. According to Butler, Burt, Foley, Morris, and Morrison (1996), life review is a normal developmental task of the later years characterized by the return of memories and past conflicts. In some cases, this can contribute to psychological growth, including the resolution of past conflicts, reconciliation with significant others, atonement for past wrongdoing, personality integration, and serenity (p. 42).

Mazanec and Tyler (2004) encourage nurses to participate in patients' life reviews. They believe that when patients are encouraged to tell their life stories, the patients are often able to recognize meaning and purpose in their lives. Being present with the patient while the patient begins a life review means a commitment on the part of the nurse to listen actively and devote time to the patient. This is a skill that all nurses ought to have, although it does not require the presence of a nurse or even a professional for the patient to conduct a life review. Life review can provide the patient with a powerful way to work out family relationships and gain a sense of inner peace.

Talking With Patients Across the Life Span and Their Families About Death

A nurse caring for a dying child must establish a trusting relationship with the child and his or her parents. Novice nurses should be especially aware of their emotions and, though empathizing with the family, should avoid burdening them with the nurses' own emotions (Buckman et al., 1997). Children want to know varying amounts of information about their illness. However, most children want to have an appreciation of how the illness will affect the way they will be able to live their lives. Like adults, however, children vary in how much information they are able to understand and absorb even when it is presented at an appropriate level. Young children's verbalization about their potential death can vary across a continuum and may be fluid over time (Buckman et al., 1997). At one end of the continuum, children will state that they are very sick or have a bad disease but will not mention death. Often, children younger than 7 or 8 years of age view death as temporary and reversible, happening only to others and perhaps caused by previous thoughts and actions (Freyer, 2004). Other children may mention an uncertainty about living but will not allude to dying. At the far end of the continuum, usually when the child is older than 7 or 8 years, the child may understand the central aspects of death and may state that she or he could die from this illness. Freyer believes that children today are more insulated from death than in the past and are more likely to learn about death from television and video games than from real-life occurrences. In order to understand children's concerns, the nurse might utilize play therapy or drawing with various colors to help children express their emotions, fears, and realizations about death. Ewing (2009) states that in their drawings, children who are very ill may reveal an edited version of their internal life. If they feel they are different from other children, isolated, and in pain, they may wish to be in a faraway place meeting someone special or possessing a special item. These wishes are often depicted in the children's drawings.

Adolescents, especially ones who have been chronically ill, usually have an accurate understanding of death and are able to verbalize its personal significance as well as its effect on others. Freyer (2004) notes that adolescents "who are medically experienced often demonstrate remarkable insight into their illnesses, prospects for survival, and preferences for how they wish to spend their remaining time" (p. 383). Due to this insight, "adolescents older than 14 are usually assumed to have functional competency to make binding medical decisions for themselves, including decisions relating to the discontinuance of life-sustaining therapy and EOL issues" (Freyer, 2004, p. 383). Freyer emphasizes it is essential that a truthful, honest relationship be established with the adolescent from the very beginning. He believes this can be accomplished if healthcare providers establish an agreement with the adolescent to share all relevant information with the adolescent as soon as it is available and the adolescent agrees to ask all questions, no matter how trivial. To ensure that the adolescent feels free to ask all his or her questions, the nurse will want to ensure that the nurse has time to spend speaking with the adolescent alone, without either parent present. Freyer (2004) notes that because most adolescents really do not believe they can ever die, they may talk about death and plan for their eventual death in ways that seem contradictory. At one moment they may be making plans for termination of chemotherapy and a few moments later they may be talking about attending an event that is years in the future. The nurse may want to help the adolescent arrange to attend important life events (e.g., school prom or graduation) in the near future while helping the adolescent recognize and accept his or her deteriorating condition.

Because there was not sufficient evidence to guide communication with parents of dying children, in 2003 the Institute of Medicine (IOM) put out an urgent call for descriptive research on the process (Hendricks-Ferguson, 2007). Snaman et al. (2016) studied parents' perceptions of the communication patterns of healthcare providers while their children were dying. Overwhelmingly, the most commonly described positive communication strategy healthcare providers utilized was "having a connection with the family and patient, not just treating them as a record number or statistic" (p. 329). Families identified the next two most important communication strategies as providers keeping the family up to date about the steps in the treatment plan and acknowledging the child by interacting and/or playing with him/her. Gilmer, Foster, Bell, Mulder, and Carter (2013) reported on a first multimethod approach to communicating with children at the end of life and their parents. The researchers indicated that although parents were pleased overall with their communication with nurses and involvement in family conferences, they wished they had been offered more assistance and involvement in decision making about EOL care for their children.

Decision making can be very difficult for the parents of seriously ill, possibly dying children. The parents may have difficulty making sense of what is being said or experienced (Anderson & Hall, 1995). They may feel unable to make decisions, especially if they believe that both minor and major decisions are needed simultaneously. At times, according to Anderson and Hall (1995), the parents may feel they cannot differentiate between decisions that merely involve personal preference and ones that have grave implications. They may need help from nurses in untangling these concrete issues, but also in dealing with more philosophical ones such as how to determine the line between what is best or right for their child and what is best or right for them.

Nurses can help these families by reminding them that "forced or hasty decision making may cause them to abrogate responsibility because they have not had an opportunity to understand the issues, their feelings or their roles" (Anderson & Hall, 1995, p. 16). Experienced nurses can assist the parents to understand the issues, express their feelings, and delineate their roles so that the parents can be actively involved in the decision-making process for their children. Crozier and Hancock (2012) emphasize that the importance of silence as a communication tool cannot be underestimated and it should be used at this time both with children with life-threatening illnesses and with their parents.

Most importantly, nurses should ensure that EOL discussions with parents are sensitive and caring. Statements made by a nurse such as "You're young. You can always have another child" makes the family feel the nurse does not value this one, unique child (Mullen, Reynolds, & Larson, 2015). In a descriptive study by Hendricks-Ferguson in 2007, 50% of parents believed that healthcare providers conveyed a recommendation that their child be referred to hospice in an uncaring or insensitive manner. This happened when a healthcare provider said something like the following: "We can treat your child but it will convey no benefit." In contrast, the 17% of parents who felt the recommendation to hospice was conveyed in a caring manner were told, "We have a wonderful hospice team and we will be sure that your child is at peace." Multiple studies of family members of both dying adults and children have indicated that at least as important as the content that is provided is the sensitivity with which the content is conveyed.

Young or middle-aged adults who are dying may feel they have a great deal of unfinished business or many unresolved relationships. The dying patient may need professional assistance in dealing with anger at leaving so much undone. A parent who is dying and leaving young children behind may need assistance from a nurse to find ways to leave mementos or lasting words of wisdom for the children. Some dying parents pick out special Christmas mementos in July for their children. One mother made 12 audiotapes with words of love and encouragement for her only child, one for each year until he would reach age 21.

Older adults are often perceived by healthcare providers as having lived a full life and being prepared to die. Yet, according to Cavendish (1999), nurses should assess all elders' quality of life (QOL) prior to the illness and realize that many have the potential for additional healthy, happy years. Farber (1999) states that adults older than 70 years usually do not believe they have a choice in healthcare treatment. When asked how they had made decisions, they answered, "What do you mean? The doctor told us what to do and we did it." Elders in a study by Schroepfer (2007) on sources of suffering at the end of life indicated that being excluded from discussions and decisions about pain management or withdrawal of treatment resulted in their experiencing unnecessary pain and suffering. Nurses need to assist elders in participating in their treatment decisions whenever they appear to desire a decision-making role. Finally, life review is particularly important for the dying elder (Butler et al., 1996), so time and a compassionate listener should be allotted to this important activity. A nurse might be this compassionate listener, or the nurse might delegate another individual for this task.

Coyle et al. (2015) summarize the strategy for this working phase in the relationship as responding emphatically to a patient's emotional response. They identify the skills needed at this time as asking open-ended questions, encouraging expressions of feelings, then acknowledging, validating, and normalizing the feelings as well as praising patient efforts. The process tasks identified as appropriate to this phase are allowing time for silence, offering tissues, and providing touch when appropriate.

Facilitating and Taking Action

There are several components of this phase. The first part is determining that the patient will die soon. The nurse may be involved with other healthcare providers in deciding when the patient is entering the active dying phase. According to Stein (1999), nurses are the people who guide patients along the path to a peaceful death by recognizing when the patient is suffering needlessly because of inappropriate aggressive treatment. The physician, in some settings, may be the last to realize that the patient is dying. Therefore, it becomes incumbent on nurses to relay their impressions to the physician and possibly to the family. The SUPPORT Principal Investigators' (1995) study indicated that there were problems in the way such information was communicated in hospital settings, and Curtis et al. (2011) indicate that those problems are still ongoing.

Griffie et al. (2004) note that it may be necessary for nurses to act as go-betweens among patients and physicians when there is disagreement about whether a patient is dying and what type of EOL care should be provided. They argue that initiating a discussion of EOL care should be part of standard nursing practice. Crucial elements for nurses to establish effective communication with physicians during disagreement about EOL care include:

- Assessing the patient by learning the details of the situation and identifying any questions that the nurse or patient has prior to contacting the physician
- Focusing on the patient's and family's desires and concerns while identifying their readiness for additional information
- Identifying medications or interventions that the nurse and/or patient believes might be effective, recommending them to the physician, and providing a rationale for their use
- Respectfully questioning interventions chosen by the physician with which the nurse, patient, or family does not agree

An example of a student nurse communicating with a physician about her patient's wishes is shown in the continuation of the case study.

CASE STUDY *Continued*

By midmorning, when multidisciplinary rounds were in progress, Gloria Richards's nurse had another patient who needed to be prepared for emergency surgery and there were several other events occurring in the ICU. The student nurse represented the nursing team at multidisciplinary rounds. The intensivist was hurrying due to the multiple events in the unit and did not have time to have a discussion with the patient. He announced he was concerned that no one was present who had assessed and could voice Gloria's wishes about EOL care, so he wanted to postpone the family meeting planned for the afternoon. He was deeply concerned that Gloria might not understand the repercussions of her decision. The student responded:

> Both Gloria's primary nurse and primary physician spoke with her this morning about her desires. She told each of them separately that she wanted the endotracheal tube and ventilator removed and that she understood that she would probably die when they were discontinued. Repeatedly this morning she has said she has had enough and asked when the meeting and removal would occur.

The intensivist agreed to hold the meeting later in the afternoon.

Determining and agreeing that the patient is dying is extremely important, because most deaths in the United States occur in hospitals and all patients in hospitals must receive CPR unless the physician or advanced practice nurse has written a do-not-resuscitate (DNR) order. Once there is a determination that the patient is dying, the physician or advanced practice nurse should discuss a DNR order with the patient, family, and other healthcare providers.

Inexperienced practitioners commonly make two mistakes when discussing a DNR order. The first is to ask: "Do you want everything done?" Most laypersons do not assume that "everything" means compressing the chest of a person who has already died. They assume it means comfort, care, and support. So, they often answer yes when they really would not want CPR. The second mistake is to use the words: "There is nothing more we can do." Although the patient is dying and medical interventions will not prevent the death, there is much that healthcare providers can do to help the patient die well. The role of the advanced practice nurse is to initiate this discussion using Latimer's (1998) criteria for ethical communication described earlier and listed in Table 9.2. However, Tulsky et al. (1996) stress that new practitioners, such as residents and advanced practice nursing students, should be evaluated by skilled professionals before being allowed to attempt such a discussion on their own.

The nurse is usually the staff member to whom the patient and family turn to discuss exactly what a DNR order is and what the ramifications are likely to be for the patient (Peel, 2003). If that nurse was not present for the discussion, he or she might use the question, "I noticed the physician was speaking with you. What did she say?" The nurse might follow that with, "Many people have questions about what this means for them. What questions do you have?" Most people want reassurance that they are not foregoing an intervention that is likely to offer them benefit. Because only about 12% of all patients survive from CPR to hospital discharge, this reassurance is easy to provide.

As noted previously, the nurse is often the guide on the path to a peaceful death (Stein, 1999). This role is important because the decision to forego CPR is merely the first of many decisions the patient and family may need to make about EOL care. After deciding to forego CPR, the patient and family might choose to forego any further curative therapy, or might opt to have only comfort measures provided for the patient. PC decisions may have to be made regarding the amount of pain medication the patient desires and whether the patient wishes to receive medical interventions for hydration and nutrition or even to continue eating and drinking. Nurses who are caring for a dying patient should be able to describe the benefits and burdens of each of these therapies to the patient. They should also be able to facilitate patient and family decision making about these choices through effective communication.

The nurse may be responsible for advocating for the patient's wishes for EOL care and communicating them to the family and other healthcare providers. This is easier if the patient has verbally expressed a preference to the nurse and is willing to state that preference to the physician and family. It may be more difficult when the nurse, physician, and family are trying to interpret an advance directive that does not fit the patient's situation precisely, when the person who has the durable power of attorney for healthcare purposes is not clear about the patient's wishes, or when there is no advance directive. Harlow, in "Family Letter Writing" (1999), recommends that the family or proxy consider the following:

1. What type of person was the patient?
2. Did the patient ever comment on another person's situation when he or she was incapacitated or on life support?
3. Did the patient relate those experiences to his or her own personal views for himself or herself?
4. What vignettes can you recall from the patient's life that illustrate her or his values and beliefs?

In "Family Letter Writing" (1999), Harlow then asks the family to write a letter incorporating the answers to these questions. He believes that the process is almost a spiritual one for the family that often brings members closer together. It helps them to review and clarify the person's life and understand what was meaningful to the person. Harlow notes that family letter writing may be "experienced by the family as a last act of commitment and caring toward their loved one." The nurse may be the person who encourages the family to begin such an activity.

A more detailed exercise called facilitated values history is suggested by Scheunemann, Arnold, and White (2012).

TABLE 9.2 Criteria for Ethical Communication of Information
■ Ensure that the communication is timely and that the patient desires the information
■ Ensure that the information is accurate
■ Use words that are understandable to the patient and the family
■ Convey the information in a gentle and compassionate manner

Source: Adapted from Latimer, E. J. (1998). Ethical care at the end of life. *Canadian Medical Association Journal, 158*(13), 1741–1747.

They believe that families have difficulty identifying the most important values to utilize when making decisions for patients, especially if they have simply been asked, "What do you think the patient would choose?" They suggest a series of questions that will help the family identify what the patient values about being alive and what he or she is willing to endure for an acceptable QOL. The questions cover eight different domains. Examples include the following: What would your loved one think about living if he or she were unable to speak, unable to interact with people, or unable to think clearly or dress himself or herself?

Either in conjunction with family letter writing, a facilitated values history, or alone, family conferences are often convened to help the patient, family, and healthcare team reach a decision about EOL care. According to Griffie et al. (2004), it is essential to identify the purpose of the conference beforehand. It is also necessary to determine where the meeting should be held. If the patient is able to participate, it may have to be in the patient's room. Some healthcare providers argue that the meeting should always be in the patient's room because it makes everyone consider the patient in the decision. Others believe that if the patient cannot participate, the meeting should be held in a comfortable, private setting away from the patient. If the patient is incapacitated, whoever is the patient's legal decision maker should be present, as well as the people whom the patient considers to be family.

After the purpose of the meeting has been identified and participants have been introduced, Randall Curtis (2008) suggests that healthcare providers focus on specific behaviors that can enhance family satisfaction during a conference. These behaviors include:

- Assuring the family that the patient will not be abandoned by the healthcare team
- Assuring the family that the patient will not suffer
- Providing support for the family's decision whatever the family decides

Furthermore, Randall Curtis recommends that healthcare providers use the mnemonic VALUE to guide their communications with families during the conference. The behaviors described in the VALUE mnemonic have been shown to improve communication between healthcare providers and the families of intensive care patients. The mnemonic stands for

V—Value family statements
A—Acknowledge family emotions
L—Listen to the family
U—Understand the patient as a person
E—Elicit family questions

Once a decision is made to limit further aggressive, curative treatment, the nurse may be involved in establishing a PC understanding with the patient and family.

This is an understanding of what the healthcare team will do for and with the patient and family. Byock (1997) offers the following version of a commitment between the healthcare team and a dying patient:

We will keep you warm and we will keep you dry. We will keep you clean. We will help you with elimination, and your bowels and your bladder function. We will always offer you food and fluid. We will be with you. We will bear witness to your pain and your sorrows, your disappointments and your triumphs; we will listen to the stories of your life and remember the story of your passing. (p. 247)

Although the physician may be the person who establishes this PC understanding, it is the nurse who is responsible for ensuring that it is carried out. It is imperative that the nurse demonstrate, by words and deeds, that the healthcare providers will not abandon the patient after EOL choices are made; that, instead, nurses and other healthcare workers will provide the care the patient needs or will teach and assist family members or friends to provide the care and support the patient requires while dying.

■ TERMINATION PHASE

During this phase in the therapeutic relationship, the nurse, family, and patient prepare for the end of the relationship, accept the feelings of loss, and review or evaluate what has occurred. As a patient is dying, this phase may entail withdrawing medical interventions, preparing the patient and family for the physical signs of impending death, smoothing the passage, consoling the bereaved family, exploring personal reactions, and evaluating nursing responses.

Withdrawing Medical Interventions

During the termination phase, medical interventions, such as ventilators, intravenous (IV) fluids and nutrition, or dialysis, may be withdrawn. The nurse reassures the family that withdrawing such aggressive medical interventions from the dying patient is acceptable to most of the major religious and ethical traditions. The nurse demonstrates that despite the withdrawal of curative measures, the healthcare team will remain present and will provide aggressive comfort measures and respect the patient's individuality.

Preparing the Patient and Family for Physical Signs of Impending Death

The nurse will need to be able to explain the final stages of the dying process to the patient and family. A family that does not understand the dying process may become anxious and feel unable to cope with the patient's care. The nurse may initiate the discussion by stating:

> There are some common signs and symptoms that identify when a person's life is coming to an end. Not all of the signs occur in every person nor do they happen in the same sequence in each person. But it might be helpful if we talk about what may be occurring soon and what you may need or want to do.

Smoothing the Passage

As death approaches, patients may display a variety of typical behaviors. Nurses should be able to explain these behaviors to family members and assist families and dying patients to communicate with each other during the patient's last days and hours. According to Callanan (1994), when a patient is approaching death, she or he may begin to speak in symbolic language. The patient might say, "Oh, here are my mother and brother-in-law, they've come to get me. We have to catch the train." Or, "It's a beautiful place that I'm going to now." Callanan cautions that the family may fear the patient is "losing his mind" or believe she or he is reliving the past. In actuality, it is believed that the patient is preparing to detach from this life. Callanan suggests that nurses should help the family listen to the patient's statements and respond with gentle, open-ended questions such as, "When does the train leave?" The family should be discouraged from trying to reorient the patient ("Your mother died years ago") or contradicting the patient ("You're not going anywhere!"), as these deathbed visions have been shown to calm the patient and ready him or her for death (Fenwick & Brayne, 2011).

Close to the moment of death, the patient may appear more withdrawn, almost detached from the surroundings. The nurse should inform the family that although the patient may appear unresponsive, they should still communicate verbally with the patient because the patient can probably still hear what people in the room are saying. The family may want to say good-bye or one of the four things that Byock (2004) believes matters most—"Please forgive me; I forgive you; thank you; and I love you" (p. 5)—if they have not done so already. This might be a time for the family to recount some favorite memories that illustrate what the dying person meant to them. A member of the family might say, "We will miss you, but we will always love you and we understand that it is time for you to go." Or a family member or close friend might simply be present with the dying person, sitting nearby, holding the person's hand, or lying next to the person and embracing him or her. At the end of life when talking is difficult, nonverbal communication may be an important or even the only way for patients and families to demonstrate caring, or share emotional expressions such as love and convey how they feel about each other (Manusov & Keeley, 2015).

It is the role of the nurse to help the patient and families find an appropriate way to express their feelings and to smooth the patient's passage from this life. Individuals take their own time dying, and each death occurs at its own pace. The nurse may need to help the patient's family understand how idiosyncratically and sometimes how slowly the final moments may pass.

Consoling the Bereaved Family

Nurses need to be able to console families through the bereavement process. If the family was not present during the death, the nurse will want to prepare the body and attempt to create a peaceful environment for the family to view the deceased. Because the nurse is often the professional present at the death or the one who views the body with the family, the nurse will need to demonstrate an acceptance of death and display respect for the deceased. If the family was not present for the death, the members may want a description of the patient's last moments. The nurse should respond both tactfully and truthfully. If it is true, saying to the family, "She was not alone" or "He seemed to be at peace" may be a great source of comfort to the family.

Although students and recent graduates often are worried about what they ought to say to the family at this time, bereaved families usually are more in need of someone to listen to them. Thus, one of the major roles of the nurse at this time is active, compassionate listening. Short statements like "I'm sorry" and "I'll keep you in my thoughts or prayers" may be helpful, but the nurse usually does not need to say much. Trivializing statements such as "She is better off now" or "I know just how you feel" are inappropriate. Depending on the nurse's relationship with the family, a hug might be helpful to both the family and the nurse. The nurse's expression of emotion through tears is not unprofessional when it is an expression of the attachment between the nurse and the patient.

When the death is sudden and unexpected, it is often more difficult for both the healthcare providers and the family to understand. It is usually the physician or the advanced practice nurse who conveys the fact of the death to the family. Buckman et al. (1997) recommend a simple unequivocal statement that the patient (her or his name should be used) has died and state the cause of death. Then the healthcare provider should remain silent and allow an opportunity for the family to respond and ask further questions. A truthful statement that the nurse is sorry helps some families. Though some people prefer a human touch at this point, others may withdraw in grief. When the initial response has subsided, Buckman recommends focusing on the needs of the family, determining whether they need to phone anyone or whether they would like an opportunity to view the body. If there is a possibility of organ donation, the advanced practice nurse would broach the subject at this time.

Coyle et al. (2015) summarize the skills needed during this closing phase of the relationship as taking stock, summarizing, and making partnership statements. The process skills identified during this phase include emphasizing the quality of symptom control and goals of care—a peaceful, natural death and affirming courage.

Review of the Relationship, Exploration of Personal Feelings, and Evaluation of Nursing Responses

Although not a specific step in the therapeutic relationship, it is always wise, following the termination of a relationship, for the nurse to review the process to explore her or his feelings and evaluate her or his behavior. A nursing student encountering his or her first experience with death may need to explore it with the faculty member or preceptor after the patient and family have been cared for. Ambuel (2003) suggests that a faculty member or preceptor who is debriefing a student should include questions such as the following: What went well? What was difficult? What did you learn from this experience that will influence your work with patients and families in the future? In most circumstances, it is helpful for the student to be involved in preparing the body and talking with the family. For the first experience with death, it is helpful if a nursing faculty member or an experienced nurse prepares the body with the student. While preparing the body, most nursing students find it helpful if the faculty member provides simple factual statements of how the body changes after death. Many students will remark how different the deceased seems once the suffering is over and life has departed.

Novice nurses often state that listening to the family helps them to find some meaning in the dying experience. If the death has been anticipated, the family will frequently discuss how the patient felt in the last few days and weeks and will often convey a sense of relief that the patient is no longer struggling. The family may review the person's life and help the student to realize that it had reached its natural end.

When the death is sudden and unexpected, nursing students often are distraught. This is especially true if the patient was close to their own or their parents' ages. A review of what happened to the patient with an emphasis on how the healthcare team responded may at least help the student realize there was no way in which the healthcare team could have prevented the death. Later, many nursing students and nurses question why the person had to die at this time in his or her life. Active listening by the nursing faculty member or perhaps the hospital chaplain is most likely to assist the student to come to some understanding of the death.

Novice nurses may idealize death; they may want each experience to be mystical and transcendent. However, death, like birth, is messy and difficult as well as beautiful and transcendent. Learning to live and care within the realm of what is possible for people at the end of their lives is often difficult for the nursing student and the new graduate. Nursing faculty should help the student recognize the realities that shaped the way in which this particular patient died and identify factors that the student would want to modify when caring for future patients.

■ CONCLUSION

When nurses communicate with their dying patients and the patients' families, they have a clearer understanding of their patients' needs and goals at the end of life. Once these goals are established, the nurse may assist the patient in dying well. That death might include limited technology, symptom relief, life review with resolution of past uncompleted business, and the presence of loving family and friends. Or it might involve fighting for the last breath, remaining alive until the last possible second, using the latest medical technology. However, without thoughtful communication with the patient and family, the nurse cannot be sure which course to take to help the patient die well.

CASE STUDY *Conclusion*

By early afternoon, Gloria announced she was tired of waiting and disconnected the ventilator from her endotracheal tube. Her nurse explained that her niece would be arriving soon for a short discussion so that the niece would understand Gloria's wishes and so she could say good-bye. Gloria wanted to know the precise time. An hour later, Gloria attempted to disconnect the ventilator again and said, "It's time." The nurse explained it was only 3 o'clock and her niece wasn't coming until after 4 and turned Gloria so she could see the clock in the room. The niece arrived promptly at 4 and a conference including the patient, her niece, the nurse, the intensivist, and a social worker took place at the patient's bedside. The nurse asked the patient again if she wanted the tube and ventilator removed. Her niece asked if she was certain, and the patient nodded emphatically yes. An hour later, a morphine drip had been started, Gloria was extubated, and her niece was sitting at her bedside with the lights in the room dimmed, holding her hand. Within an hour Gloria was unresponsive and she died peacefully later that evening.

CASE STUDY *Commentary*

James McGhee, PhD
Professor Emeritus Saint Anselm College
Member of ethics committees of several New Hampshire hospitals and hospices

The detailed medical evaluation of Gloria Richards's physical condition and the description of her eventual death leads to the basic question in bioethics: "When is it justified to withdraw life support from a person who is dying?" Traditionally, the reply would involve distinguishing between extraordinary means of life support and ordinary measures to sustain life. According to this model, one is obliged to take ordinary means that would, for example, be beneficial to one but not extraordinary ones, which would offer no benefit of hope or improvement. In Gloria's case, the lengthy procedures did not seem to offer any hope of benefit, and indeed they proved to be a considerable burden to her and to those around her. Her request to remove the ventilator was thus legitimate, and the cooperation of her family and the hospital personnel was equally sound. As was her right, she died peacefully and with dignity. This approach with its emphasis on PC reflects a hospice mentality and is to be commended.

Two further issues might be raised in Gloria's case. Although compassion is expressed by some of the healthcare practitioners in their effort to comply with her wishes to end treatment quickly, others postponed consideration of her request until they could fit it into their busy schedules. With some planning, such a delay perhaps could have been avoided. More importantly, a holistic approach to the sick would include consideration of their spiritual as well as physical well-being; if desired, they have a right to the consolation of their religion, especially when dying, and caretakers have an obligation to see that this happens where possible. Such a discussion was missing in the presentation of Gloria's EOL story.

Evidence-Based Practice

ASSESSING FAMILY MEMBERS' SATISFACTION WITH INFORMATION SHARING AND COMMUNICATION DURING HOSPITAL CARE AT THE END OF LIFE

Brazil, K., Cupido, C., Tanigushi, A., Howard, M., Akhtar-Danesh, N., & Frolic, A. (2013). Assessing family members satisfaction with information sharing and communication during hospital care at the end of life. *Journal of Palliative Medicine, 16*(1), 82–86. doi:10.1089/jpm.2012.0362
Q: What communication strategies enhance family member satisfaction when a hospitalized patient approaches the end of life?

Methods
Data sources: This was a cross-sectional survey that was performed to determine the relationship among patient variables and satisfaction on the Information Sharing and Communications Scale (ISC).
Study selection and assessment: All of the next of kin of patients who had died during hospitalization at one hospital were contacted by mail 2 weeks after the patient's death

and notified they were eligible to participate in this study. Two weeks later, a consent form and the ISC were mailed if the next of kin had not indicated s/he would not participate. Five hundred and twenty-three surveys were returned, a 43% response rate.

Main Results

The initial scale sent to the next of kin had 23 items developed from two different scales. After factor analysis, one factor (the ISC) with seven items explained 77% of the variance and had high internal consistency (Cronbach's alpha 0.95). Overall, family members who responded were satisfied with communication with healthcare providers. Family members of patients who died following critical care reported the highest satisfaction while family members of male patients and patients who had been hospitalized for long periods of time were less satisfied.

Conclusion

"The ISC scale demonstrated good validity and reliability. It offers acute care facilities a means to assess the quality of information sharing and communication that occurs between health care providers and families with patients at the end of life" (p. 86).

Commentary

■ Many healthcare providers have difficulty initiating conversations about goals of care with families of patients at the end of life. However, having such conversations is critical to developing the plan of care for the dying patient and helping the family prepare for bereavement. This study identified seven healthcare provider behaviors (the ISC scale) that were associated with patient and family satisfaction with the way that the dying process unfolded. The items were:
1. Information provided about the patient's prognosis
2. Information given about how to manage the patient's symptoms
3. When the team initiated EOL discussions (providing enough time for the family to plan)
4. The healthcare team's knowledge of the patient's wishes for EOL care
5. How the healthcare team answered the families' questions
6. The quality of the discussion with the healthcare team about the use of life-sustaining technologies
7. The ability of the family member to talk comfortably with the patient about his/her illness, dying, and death.

The ISC can be used in several ways. It can be available for healthcare providers to view serving as a reminder of how important it is to include all of these items when planning for a patient's EOL care. The scale could be used to review whether or not healthcare providers had utilized appropriate communication strategies when meeting with a family or conducting a family meeting. Or it could be used by a healthcare organization (as in this study) to determine if the organization as a whole is promoting good communication at the end of life.

■ REFERENCES

Ambuel, B. (2003). Delivering bad news and precepting student/resident learners. *Journal of Palliative Medicine, 6*, 265–266. doi:10.1089/109662103764978524

Anderson, B., & Hall, B. (1995). Parents' perceptions of decision making for children. *The Journal of Law, Medicine & Ethics, 23*(1), 15–19. doi:10.1111/j.1748-720X.1995.tb01325.x

Arnold, R., Nelson, J., Prendergast, T., Emlet, L., Weinstein, E., Barnato, A., & Back, A. (2010). Educational modules for the critical care communication course: A communication skills program for intensive care fellows. Retrieved from https://www.uclahealth.org/palliative-care/Workfiles/Educational-Modules-Critical-Care-Communication.pdf

Aslakson, R., Wyskiel, R., Thornton, I., Copley, C., Shaffer, D., Ayra, M., . . . Pronovost, P. (2012). Nurse-perceived barriers to effective communication regarding prognosis and optimal end-of-life care for surgical ICU patients: A qualitative exploration. *Journal of Palliative Medicine, 15*(8), 910–915. doi:10.1089/jpm.2011.0481

Barclay, J. S., Blackhall, L. J., & Tulsky, J. A. (2007). Communication strategies and cultural issues in the delivery of bad news. *Journal of Palliative Medicine, 10*(4), 958–977. doi:10.1089/jpm.2007.9929

Blackhall, L., Erickson, J., Brashers, V., Owen, J., & Thomas, S. (2014). Development and validation of a collaborative behaviours objective assessment tool for end-of-life communication. *Journal of Palliative Medicine, 17*(1), 68–74. doi:10.1089/jpm.2013.0262

Block, S. D. (2001). Perspectives on care at the close of life. Psychological considerations, growth, and transcendence at the end of life: The art of the possible. *The Journal of the American Medical Association, 285*(22), 2898–2905. doi:10.1001/jama.285.22.2898

Booth, K., Maguire, P. M., Butterworth, T., & Hillier, V. F. (1996). Perceived professional support and the use of blocking behaviours by hospice nurses. *Journal of Advanced Nursing, 24*(3), 522–527. doi:10.1046/j.1365-2648.1996.22012.x

Boyd, D., Merkh, K., Rutledge, D. N., & Randall, V. (2011). Nurses' perceptions and experiences with end-of-life communication and care. *Oncology Nursing Forum, 38*(3), E229–E239. doi:10.1188/11.ONF.E229-E239

Boyle, D. K., Miller, P. A., & Forbes-Thompson, S. A. (2005). Communication and end-of-life care in the intensive care unit: Patient, family, and clinician outcomes. *Critical Care Nursing Quarterly, 28*(4), 302–316.

Brazil, K., Cupido, C., Taniguishi, A., Howard, M., Akhtar-Danesh, N., & Frolic, A. (2013). Assessing family members satisfaction with information sharing and communication during hospital care at the end of life. *Journal of Palliatve Medicine, 16*(1), 82–86. doi:10.1089/jpm.2012.0362

Brooks, L., Manias, E., & Nicholson, P. (2017). Communication and decisioin making about end-of-life care in the intensive care unit. *American Journal of Critical Care, 26*(4), 336–341. doi:10.4037/ajcc2017774

Buckman, R. (1992). *How to break bad news: A guide for health professionals.* Baltimore, MD: Johns Hopkins Press.

Buckman, R., Lipkin, M., Sourkes, B., & Tolle, S. (1997, June 15). Strategies and skills for breaking bad news. *Patient Care, 6*, 61–66.

Butler, R. N., Burt, R., Foley, K. M., Morris, J., & Morrison, R. S. (1996). A peaceful death: How to manage pain and provide quality care. A Roundtable Discussion: Part 2. *Geriatrics, 51*(6), 32–42.

Byock, I. (1997). *Dying well: Peace and possibilities at the end of life.* New York, NY: Riverhead Books.

Byock, I. (2004). *The four things that matter most: A book about living.* New York, NY: Free Press.

Callanan, M. (1994). Farewell messages. *American Journal of Nursing, 94*(5), 19–20.

Cavendish, R. (1999). Improving care for the elderly. *American Journal of Nursing, 99*(5), 88.

Chesanow, N. (2016). Delivering "bad" versus "serious" news to patients. *Medscape Critical Care.* Retrieved from https://www.medscape.com/viewarticle/856955_2

Coombs, M., & Long, T. (2008). Managing a good death in critical care: Can health policy help? *Nursing in Critical Care, 13*(4), 208–214. doi:10.1111/j.1478-5153.2008.00280.x

Cotton, P. (1993). Talk to people about dying: They can handle it, say geriatricians and patients. *Journal of the American Medical Association, 269*(3), 321–322. doi:10.1001/jama.1993.03500030013002

Coyle, N., Manna, R., Shen, M., Banerjee, S., Penn, S., Pehrson, C., ... Bylund, C. (2015). Discussing death, dying, and end-of-life goals: A communication skills training module for oncology nurses. *Clinical Journal of Oncology Nursing, 19*(6), 697–702. doi:10.1188/15.CJON.697-702

Crozier, F., & Hancock, L. E. (2012). Pediatric palliative care: Beyond the end of life. *Pediatric Nursing, 38*(4), 198–203, 227; quiz 204.

Curtis, J. R. (2008). Caring for patients with critical illness and their families: The value of the integrated clinical team. *Respiratory Care, 53*, 480–487.

Curtis, J. R., Nielson, E., Treece, R., Downey, L., Dotolo, D., Shannon, S., ..., Engelberg, R. (2011). Effect of a quality improvement intervention on end-of-life care in the intensive care unit: A randomized intervention. *American Journal of Respiratory Critical Care Medicine, 183*, 343–355. doi:10.1164/rccm.201006-1004OC

Czerwiec, M. (1996). When a loved one is dying: Families talk about nursing care. *American Journal of Nursing, 96*(5), 32–36.

Davis, S., Kristjanson, L. J., & Blight, J. (2003). Communicating with families of patients in an acute hospital with advanced cancer: Problems and strategies identified by nurses. *Cancer Nursing, 26*(5), 337–345.

Emanuel, E. J. (1998). The promise of a good death. *The Lancet, 351*(9114, Suppl.), S1121–1126. doi:10.1016/S0140-6736(98)90329-4

Ewing, B. (2009). Wish fulfillment: Palliative care and end-of-life intervention. *Pediatric Nursing, 35*(2), 81–85.

Exline, J. J., Prince-Paul, M., Root, B. L., Peereboom, K. S., & Worthington, E. L. (2012). Forgiveness, depressive symptoms, and communication at the end of life: A study with family members of hospice patients. *Journal of Palliative Medicine, 15*(10), 1113–1119. doi:10.1089/jpm.2012.0138

Fallowfield, L., & Jenkins, V. (2004). Communicating sad, bad, and difficult news in medicine. *The Lancet, 363*(9405), 312–319. doi:10.1016/S0140-6736(03)15392-5

Family Letter Writing. (1999). An interview with Nathan Harlow. *Innovations in End-of-Life Care: An International Journal of Leaders in End-of-Life Care.*

Farrell, M., Ryan, S., & Langrick, B. (2001). "Breaking bad news" within a paediatric setting: An evaluation report of a collaborative education workshop to support health professionals. *Journal of Advanced Nursing, 36*(6), 765–775. doi:10.1046/j.1365-2648.2001.02042.x

Fenwick, P., & Brayne, S. (2011). End-of-life experiences: Reaching out for compassion, communication, and connection-meaning of deathbed visions and coincidences. *American Journal of Hospice and Palliative Care, 28*(1), 7–15. doi:10.1177/1049909110374301

Freyer, D. R. (2004). Care of the dying adolescent: Special considerations. *Pediatrics, 113*(2), 381–388. doi:10.1542/peds.113.2.381

Furukawa, M. M. (1996). Meeting the needs of the dying patient's family. *Critical Care Nurse, 16*(1), 51–57.

Gilmer, M. J., Foster, T. L., Bell, C. J., Mulder, J., & Carter, B. S. (2013). Parental perceptions of care of children at end of life. *American Journal of Hospice and Palliative Care, 30*(1), 53–58. doi:10.1177/1049909112440836

Gordon, M., Buchman, D., & Buchman, S. (2007). "Bad news" communication in palliative care: A challenge and a key to success. *Annals of Long-Term Care, 15*(4), 32–38.

Griffie, J., Nelson-Marten, P., & Muchka, S. (2004). Acknowledging the "elephant": Communication in palliative care. *American Journal of Nursing, 104*(1), 48–57; quiz 58.

Heaven, C. M., & Maguire, P. (1996). Training hospice nurses to elicit patient concerns. *Journal of Advanced Nursing, 23*(2), 280–286. doi:10.1111/j.1365-2648.1996.tb02668.x

Hendricks-Ferguson, B. (2007). Parental perspectives of initial end-of-life care communication. *International Journal of Palliative Nursing, 13*, 522–531. doi:10.12968/ijpn.2007.13.11.27587

Kagawa-Singer, M., & Blackhall, L. J. (2001). Negotiating cross-cultural issues at the end of life: "You got to go where he lives." *Journal of the American Medical Association, 286*(23), 2993–3001. doi:10.1001/jama.286.23.2993

Lamba, S., Tyrie, L., Bryczkowski, S., & Nagurka, R. (2015). Teaching surgery residents the skills to communicate difficult news to patient and family members: A literature review. *Journal of Palliative Medicine, 19*(1), 101–107. doi:10.1089/jpm.2015.0292

Langley-Evans, A., & Payne, S. (1997). Light-hearted death talk in a palliative day care context. *Journal of Advanced Nursing, 26*(6), 1091–1097. doi:10.1046/j.1365-2648.1997.00422.x

Larson, D. G., & Tobin, D. R. (2000). End-of-life conversations: Evolving practice and theory. *Journal of the American Medical Association, 284*(12), 1573–1578. doi:10.1001/jama.284.12.1573

Latimer, E. J. (1998). Ethical care at the end of life. *Canadian Medical Association Journal, 158*(13), 1741–1747.

London, M. R., & Lundstedt, J. (2007). Families speak about inpatient end-of-life care. *Journal of Nursing Care Quality, 22*(2), 152–158. doi:10.1097/01.NCQ.0000263105.08096.b1

Manusov, V., & Keeley, M. (2015). When family talk is difficult: Making sense of nonverbal communication at the end-of-life. *Journal of Family Communication, 15*(4), 387–409. doi:10.1080/15267431.2015.1076424

May, C. (1995). "To call it work somehow demeans it": The social construction of talk in the care of terminally ill patients. *Journal of Advanced Nursing, 22*(3), 556–561. doi:10.1046/j.1365-2648.1995.22030556.x

Mazanec, P., & Tyler, M. K. (2004). Cultural considerations in end-of-life care: How ethnicity, age, and spirituality affect decisions when death is imminent. *Home Healthcare Now, 22*, 317–324.

Mullen, J., Reynolds, M., & Larson, J. (2015). Caring for pediatric patients' families at the child's end of life. *Critical Care Nurse, 35*(6), 46–56. doi:10.4037/ccn2015614

Murphy, P. A., & Price, D. M. (1995). "ACT": Taking a positive approach to end-of-life care. *American Journal of Nursing, 95*(3), 42–43.

Ngo-Metzger, Q., August, K. J., Srinivasan, M., Liao, S., & Meyskens, F. L. (2008). End-of-life care: Guidelines for patient-centered communication. *American Family Physician, 77*(2), 167–174.

Parker, S. M., Clayton, J. M., Hancock, K., Walder, S., Butow, P. N., Carrick, S., … Tattersall, M. H. (2007). A systematic review of prognostic/end-of-life communication with adults in the advanced stages of a life-limiting illness: Patient/caregiver preferences for the content, style, and timing of information. *Journal of Pain and Symptom Management, 34*(1), 81–93. doi:10.1016/j.jpainsymman.2006.09.035

Pattison, N. (2004). Integration of critical care and palliative care at end of life. *British Journal of Nursing, 13*(3), 132–136, 138. doi:10.12968/bjon.2004.13.3.12109

Peel, N. (2003). The role of the critical care nurse in the delivery of bad news. *British Journal of Nursing, 12*(16), 966–971. doi:10.12968/bjon.2003.12.16.11443

Periyakoil, V., Neri, E., & Kraemer, H. (2016). Patient-reported barriers to high-quality, end-of-life: A multiethnic, multilingual, mixed methods study. *Journal of Palliative Medicine, 19*(4), 373–379. doi:10.1089/jpm.2015.0403

Ptacek, J. T., Ptacek, J. J., & Ellison, N. M. (2001). "I'm sorry to tell you." Physicians' reports of breaking bad news. *Journal of Behavioral Medicine, 24*(2), 205–217. doi:10.1023/A:1010766732373

Quill, T. E. (2000). Perspectives on care at the close of life. Initiating end-of-life discussions with seriously ill patients: Addressing the "elephant in the room." *Journal of the American Medical Association, 284*(19), 2502–2507. doi:10.1001/jama.284.19.2502

Radziewicz, R., & Baile, W. F. (2001). Communication skills: Breaking bad news in the clinical setting. *Oncology Nursing Forum, 28*(6), 951–953.

Ramos, K. J., Downey, L., Nielsen, E. L., Treece, P. D., Shannon, S. E., Curtis, J. R., & Engelberg, R. A. (2016). Using nurse ratings of physician communication in the ICU to identify potential targets for intervention to improve end of life care. *Journal of Palliative Medicine, 19*(3), 292–299. doi:10.1089/jpm.2015.0155

Rosenbaum, M. E., & Kreiter, C. (2002). Teaching delivery of bad news using experiential sessions with standardized patients. *Teaching and Learning in Medicine, 14*(3), 144–149. doi:10.1207/S15328015TLM1403_2

Scheunemann, L., Arnold, R., & White, D. (2012). The facilitated values history: Helping surrogates make authentic decisions for incapacitated patients with advanced illness. *American Journal of Respiratory and Critical Care Medicine, 186*(6), 480–486. doi:10.1164/rccm.201204-0710CP

Schroepfer, T. A. (2007). Critical events in the dying process: The potential for physical and psychosocial suffering. *Journal of Palliative Medicine, 10*(1), 136–147. doi:10.1089/jpm.2006.0157

Servaty, H. L., Krejci, M. J., & Hayslip, B. (1996). Relationships among death anxiety, communication apprehension with the dying, and empathy in those seeking occupations as nurses and physicians. *Death Studies, 20*(2), 149–161. doi:10.1080/07481189608252747

Shannon, S. E., Long-Sutehall, T., & Coombs, M. (2011). Conversations in end-of-life care: Communication tools for critical care practitioners. *Nursing in Critical Care, 16*(3), 124–130. doi:10.1111/j.1478-5153.2011.00456.x

Shmerling, R. H., Bedell, S. E., Lilienfeld, A., & Delbanco, T. L. (1988). Discussing cardiopulmonary resuscitation: A study of elderly outpatients. *Journal of General Internal Medicine, 3*(4), 317–321. doi:10.1007/BF02595786

Snaman, J., Torres, C., Duffy, B., Levine, D., Gibson, D., & Baker J. (2016). Parental perspectives of communication at the end of life at a pediatric oncology institution. *Journal of Palliative Medicine, 19*(3), 326–332. doi:10.1089/jpm.2015.0253

Stein, C. (1999). Ending a life. *Boston Globe Magazine, 13*, 24, 30–34, 39–42.

Stiles, M. K. (1990). The shining stranger: Nurse-family spiritual relationship. *Cancer Nursing, 13*(4), 235–245.

Sullivan, A. M., Lakoma, M. D., Matsuyama, R. K., Rosenblatt, L., Arnold, R. M., & Block, S. D. (2007). Diagnosing and discussing imminent death in the hospital: A secondary analysis of physician interviews. *Journal of Palliative Medicine, 10*(4), 882–893. doi:10.1089/jpm.2007.0189

SUPPORT Principal Investigators. (1995). A controlled trial to improve care for seriously ill, hospitalized patients: The Study to Understand Prognoses and Preferences for Outcomes and Risks of Treatments (SUPPORT). *Journal of the American Medical Association, 274*, 1591–1598. doi:10.1001/jama.1995.03530200027032

Thompson-Hill, J., Hookey, C., Salt, E., & O'Neill, T. (2009). The supportive care plan: A tool to improve communication in end-of-life care. *International Journal of Palliative Nursing, 15*(5), 250–255. doi:10.12968/ijpn.2009.15.5.47391

Treece, P. D. (2007). Communication in the intensive care unit about the end of life. *AACN Advanced Critical Care, 18*(4), 406–414. doi:10.4037/15597768-2007-4009

Tulsky, J. A., Chesney, M. A., & Lo, B. (1996). See one, do one, teach one? House staff experience discussing do-not-resuscitate orders. *Archives of Internal Medicine, 156*(12), 1285–1289. doi:10.1001/archinte.1996.00440110047007

Wilkinson, S. (1991). Factors which influence how nurses communicate with cancer patients. *Journal of Advanced Nursing, 16*(6), 677–688. doi:10.1111/j.1365-2648.1991.tb01726.x

Yabroff, K. R., Mandelblatt, J. S., & Ingham, J. (2004). The quality of medical care at the end-of-life in the USA: Existing barriers and examples of process and outcome measures. *Palliative Medicine, 18*(3), 202–216. doi:10.1191/0269216304pm880oa

John P. Rosenberg & Kathrine Hammill

Health Promotion and Rehabilitation in Palliative Care

KEY POINTS

- The provision of palliative and end-of-life (EOL) care does not preclude interventions that optimize health, well-being, and functional status even in the presence of incurable illness.
- The application of the principles and practices of health promotion to palliative and EOL care enhances the health and well-being of individuals, families, and communities.
- Rehabilitation is a valid intervention in advanced disease, promoting optimal function and mitigating deficits in activities of daily living, well-being, and quality of life (QOL).
- The role of the nurse in rehabilitation is vital in responding to the complex needs of those with advanced disease.

CASE STUDY

Jack is a 55-year-old man with a diagnosis of lung cancer. On admission to the palliative care (PC) service, he is still receiving chemotherapy. He is moderately breathless at rest and needs home oxygen. Jack reports pain and fatigue on mobilizing, is unable to walk more than 5 m on flat ground, and is also unable to climb more than three stairs without needing to sit down. He needs minimal assistance with getting to the toilet and moderate assistance with showering. When seated or in bed, Jack needs to be sat upright to be comfortable.

Jack lives with his wife, Mandy, and has two stepchildren who visit them on weekends. He worked as a maintenance worker at a local school and has been a heavy smoker in the past. He and Mandy have always struggled financially and would often forfeit purchasing medication so they could afford food. Jack and Mandy are functionally illiterate and are supported by Mandy's ex-partner to complete paperwork.

Jack and Mandy live in a two-story public housing building, with about 20 steps between levels. Jack sleeps on a mattress on the floor in the upstairs bedroom where there is an adjacent bathroom. The toilet, laundry, kitchen, and living areas are all downstairs.

■ OPTIMIZING HEALTH AT THE END OF LIFE

At first glance, thinking about health and well-being at the end of life might seem contradictory. But there is a growing sense that when we talk about holistic palliative care (PC) and optimal comfort, we are actually talking about health and well-being. Even in the presence of advanced, life-limiting illness, people can—and do—report feeling "as well as possible" in all the levels that holistic care addresses. These include physical, psychological (or emotional), spiritual, and social domains of wellness. Promoting wellness also has the potential to restore some functional deficits that come with advanced disease. It's in this sense that we discuss palliative rehabilitation and the promotion of optimal health as key issues for nursing practice in PC.

Understanding Health-Promoting Palliative Care

Health-promoting palliative care (HPPC) emerged in the 1990s as a concept that proposes that even in the event of advancing disease, a person can maintain a sense of health and wellness. The notion of integrating health promotion and PC is not a new one in the global PC world. Australian sociologist Allan Kellehear (1999) provided the first substantive consideration of this in his groundbreaking book *Health-Promoting Palliative Care*. In this book, Kellehear proposes that the principles of health promotion, as articulated in the World Health Organization's (WHO) *Ottawa Charter for Health Promotion* (WHO, 1987), could not only enhance the care and support of seriously ill and dying people but also address some of the emerging deficits in contemporary models of PC. Kellehear's premise was that "if health is everyone's responsibility then it is also the responsibility of those living with a life-threatening or terminal illness as well as those who care for them" (p. 31). He applies the five action statements of the *Ottawa Charter* to PC, identifying five core concerns of HPPC:

■ Provide education and information for health, dying, and death
■ Provide social support at both personal and community levels
■ Encourage interpersonal reorientation
■ Encourage reorientation of PC services
■ Combat death-denying health policies and attitudes (Kellehear, 1999, pp. 19–20)

Kellehear's *Health-Promoting Palliative Care* is a social model of care based on a perspective that promotes optimal health even in the presence of incurable disease. In *Compassionate Cities* (Kellehear, 2005), he again observed the transference of responsibility for dying from the community to the healthcare professions across the 20th century, with much of the care provision determined by clinical services rather than by consumers of those services. He suggested that the PC profession continues to focus upon individualized responses to need rather than to social change, as this quote illustrates:

> Dying, death and loss are defined as personal problems rather than targets of social change in community attitudes, values and behaviour. This reinforces the view that clinical rather than community skills should take priority in palliative care education and training. (Kellehear, 2005, p. 9)

It should be clear, then, that HPPC addresses not only the ways in which clinicians support the seriously ill and dying, but also how communities can be more effectively engaged in the care and support of their dying members; this speaks to the nature of the relationship between health services and the communities they serve. In North America, you can find examples of these in the end-of-life (EOL) coalitions found in many states and provinces.

■ Utilizing the Ottawa Charter to Change Practice.

To better understand the implications of HPPC for PC nursing practice, it's important to be familiar with its foundational concepts. HPPC sits within the public health paradigm, to which health promotion belongs, and PC is understood at a global level to be a public health concern (Stjernswärd, 2007). In Table 10.1, the five core components of the *Ottawa Charter for Health Promotion* (WHO, 1987) are mapped against PC (Rosenberg, 2012). Each component that promotes health has application to the provision of PC, which, in turn, has implications for nursing practice.

Although the key action areas of the *Ottawa Charter* were described discretely, their interrelatedness was acknowledged by its authors; each represents an area of strategic action to promote the physical, social, and personal aspects of health and well-being. Significantly, the *Ottawa Charter* explicitly asserted that responsibility for health promotion rests not simply with the health sector and its clinicians but also with governments, social and economic sectors, industry and the media, and communities themselves. Health promotion, therefore, was proposed not as just another health program but as an entire approach to the health and well-being of people.

Take note that the foundations upon which HPPC has been built are evident in a number of places in the *Ottawa Charter*. In the key action area of *developing personal skills*, for example, it explicitly mentions lifelong learning for people preparing themselves for *all of life's stages* (author's emphasis). Although dying was not mentioned in the *Ottawa Charter*, or for many years thereafter in the health promotion literature, it is interesting to note this phrasing in such a key document in light of the later development of HPPC.

In the United States, a critique of these approaches to EOL care was offered by D'Onofrio and Ryndes

TABLE 10.1   Translating the Ottawa Charter to Palliative Care

Key Action Areas to Support Health	Health Promotion Description	Application to Palliative Care
Build public policies that support health	Health is on the agenda of all policy makers who consider the health consequences of policy decisions.	Participation of organizations in the development and uptake of public policy relating to palliative care.
Create supportive environments	Health cannot be separated from other societal goals. The links between people and their environment are embraced.	Contributions from palliative care organizations to enhance well-being for consumers and employees.
Strengthen community action	Communities set their own health priorities, make decisions, and plan and implement strategies to promote their empowerment. Community development enhances participation in health matters.	Palliative care organizations engage with the community beyond the provision of clinical services to promote communication toward improved support of the seriously ill and dying.
Develop personal skills	Enhanced life skills are attained through personal and social development that promotes people exercising control of their health throughout life.	Participation of palliative care organizations in the development of personal skills to deal with issues of illness, dying, death, grief, and loss.
Reorient health services	Health services move beyond clinical and curative services to support individuals and communities for a healthier life. Strategies include research, professional education, and training.	Palliative care organizations reorient their members from a conventional to a health-promoting approach, focusing particularly on holistic needs of patients and organizational attitudes.

(2003). In considering WHO's definition of health, consumer stakeholders identified the *preservation of social relationships* at the end of life as a priority; this clearly sits within the psychological and social domains of holistic care. Yet, do our approaches to PC support this? D'Onofrio and Ryndes (2003) identified that EOL care is currently considered a lower priority in the allocation of scarce health resources and noted that this represents a structural barrier within the health system that disadvantages the seriously ill and dying. However, they also suggested that public health approaches could bring about improvement to care at the end of life through its whole-population perspective and policy development. To achieve this, public health systems would need to acknowledge death as the outcome of chronic disease and aging, find new means to measure quality of dying, and consider a reevaluation of resource allocation policies.

■ **Wholeness and Health at the End of Life.** Wholeness and health have close conceptual associations—early definitions of health were built upon pre–World War II assumptions about the relationship between health and disease, where to be healthy was to be without disease (DeSpelder & Strickland, 2002). WHO's definition, in acknowledging the multifaceted and interrelated nature of health and well-being, instead asserted the place of a whole-person approach (WHO, 1978). The concept of wholeness for people at the end of life presents few philosophical hurdles to commentators

on health promotion in PC. Suffering is regarded as a complex, subjective experience, the amelioration of which produces an optimal state in a person even in the presence of incurable illness (Woodruff, 2004). The founder of the modern hospice movement, Dame Cicely Saunders (1987), described good PC in terms now commonly ascribed to holism: namely, indicating the care begins at the time of diagnosis with serious, progressive, or chronic illness and addresses the physical, psychological, social, and spiritual dimensions of a person's experience, through the expertise of an interprofessional healthcare team. She is joined by others who describe a *whole-person response* to the *whole-person experience* (Woodruff, 2004), moving beyond a philosophical position to providing guidelines for the provision of care.

Significantly, public health has explored in detail the relationship between human health and well-being with social and environmental factors (Talbot & Verrinder, 2005). Contemporary understandings of health recognize the impact of disease, illness, and health-related issues upon all aspects of human existence (McMurray, 2003) and the participation of individuals, communities, and societies in determining their own health outcomes. Recipients of care and their family caregivers are recognized as the unit of care, with sympathetic stakeholders in the wider public who are engaged in the kind of local activism that has brought many hospice and PC services into existence (Small, 2003). A central tenet in the support of the seriously ill and dying is the relief of suffering for the whole person—a state often described as a *good death*. Indeed, the hospice pioneers' work shows that to die well was to die with ease of distress across the range of domains of human existence: physical, psychological, social, and spiritual.

Byock, Norris, Curtis, and Patrick (2001) also undertook substantial work toward facilitating a transition from EOL care that focused upon individuals to care that focused on the community, which is a *social* approach. Their justification for this links strongly to the principles of social models of PC:

> The experiences of serious illness, dying, caregiving, grieving and death cannot be completely understood within a medical framework alone. These events are personal, but also fundamentally communal. Medical care and health services constitute essential components of a community's response, but not its entirety. (Byock et al., 2001, p. 760)

These authors saw the community's engagement in EOL issues as having a reciprocal effect: The community members' perspectives of death and dying inform their engagement while their engagement reshapes their perspectives.

■ **Health Promotion in PC.** In North America, Rao and colleagues (Rao, Anderson, & Smith, 2002; Rao et al., 2005) have been asserting the need for the concrete inclusion of a public health foundation in PC service planning for a number of years. They have argued that connecting health to the community by providing information and establishing partnerships will raise awareness of palliative and EOL care and empower the community to contribute to the debate of issues related to quality of life (QOL) at the end of life. Indeed, in their study of public health priorities for EOL initiatives, Rao et al. (2005) identified nine clusters of public health activity that were directly relevant to the provision of PC. Of these, five were identified as most feasible:

■ Public education
■ Patient and family caregiver education
■ Research, epidemiology, and evaluation
■ Professional education
■ Policy and planning

Importantly, each of these clusters was accompanied by a set of recommendations for action that can inform practice. For example, in the public education cluster, Rao et al. (2005) advised the use of strategies to raise public awareness of PC, increase the use of advance health directives, integrate palliative and EOL issues into chronic disease educational materials, and operate some form of information clearinghouse for EOL issues. One can see ways in which PC nursing, as a specialty, can and does contribute in these clusters.

It's also possible to see ways in which PC nursing, as a discrete component of healthcare, can and does contribute in these clusters. You might be able to immediately identify some of the ways this already takes place with your service. With reflection, you may also be able to identify some gaps in your model of care relating to HPPC. So, where do you start?

The framework that follows is one approach to understanding the integration of HPPC in your practice, in your workplace, and the community it serves, as well as in the health systems that govern your clinical practice. It's the *macro–meso–micro* framework, perhaps already familiar to some of you in other contexts.

■ **Macro-Systems Level.** In considering the possibilities for HPPC at the *macro* level, you are examining systems of palliative and EOL care. Do systems that are in place

■ Support changing knowledge, attitudes, and behaviors around illness, dying, and death, and aim to encourage a greater willingness to discuss death and bereavement issues?
■ Promote political and policy action?
■ Incorporate research into the HPPC approach?

It might be unfamiliar territory to consider advocating for a systemic approach to wholeness across the illness-dying trajectory as part of the scope of practice for PC nurses. But nurses, of course, are well positioned to understand and represent the needs of the people who receive their clinical care. Whether individually or collectively, PC nurses have an important knowledge base that may be very valuable in public education programs addressing issues of death and dying.

■ **Meso-Organizational Level.** In thinking about HPPC at the *meso* level, consider the activities regarding PC and EOL care at the service level. Does the organization

■ Include life-and-death education activities for the wider community?
■ Support professional development of its staff toward HPPC approaches?
■ Create partnerships for media engagement, research, and community engagement (e.g., through schools, clubs, church groups, etc.)?
■ Promote organizational HPPC (after the WHO *Ottawa Charter*)?

Once again, you can see how, in a supportive organization, PC nurses can contribute to an approach that promotes optimal health and well-being along the illness-dying continuum. Nurse educators in particular can include these strategies in their role.

■ **Micro-Individual Level.** This is perhaps the most familiar level for most PC nurses. When considering how, at the individual level, you can promote whole-person care, ask yourself the following questions:

■ How do you promote the normalization of illness, and dying, and engage the community in your clinical practice?
■ Do you have an understanding of demographics of the community in order to tailor an appropriate, individualized, or community response?
■ Do you provide a follow-up program for patient, family, and caregiver education?
■ Do you lead support groups for carers/bereaved?
■ Do you assist in creating supportive environments for your colleagues?

These approaches are well within the scope of practice of the PC nurse. As you can see, much of it is attitudinal; it relates to how you understand your role. These are just some ideas regarding an HPPC approach—but in the spirit of community development, there is no one way, no recipe that spells it all out for you. Each organization, community, and practitioner must be assessed so that the strategies developed in response are relevant, focused, and "owned" by all the key stakeholders.

Implementing HPPC Into Organizations

For PC organizations committed to the implementation of HPPC, it's essential to utilize existing, effective quality improvement approaches. It is most effective to take a comprehensive approach, including obtaining strategic buy-in from the executive management, as it cannot rest in the hands of a few champions. It is important to build within the organization a critical mass of health professionals with knowledge and vision. With a realistic plan for service development that includes a sustainable approach to robust evaluation, then HPPC becomes a realistic goal.

CASE STUDY Continued

The registered nurse looking after Jack requested permission from him and Mandy to provide face-to-face learning about his condition and its impact. His stepchildren were invited and the teaching activities were action oriented, rather than provided as written information. A support group of carers was found nearby for Mandy. With her children's help, she was able to attend weekly meetings. She was aware that they also provide support to bereaved carers.

The nurses and other staff of the PC service were concerned about Jack and Mandy's living conditions. A referral was made to the occupational therapist to assist with equipment prescription and environmental modifications to improve his QOL and enable Jack to continue to complete his meaningful activities of daily living in his home. With the support of their organization's CEO, the interprofessional team began to lobby local housing authorities about the impact of the design of public housing on people living with advanced disease, seeking a review of housing allocation practices.

Mandy's new friends within the support group raised public awareness of the challenges facing families in their predicament. They approached the local community newspaper to feature this story. With the PC organization's help, the group ran life-and-death education activities for their community.

The nurses caring for Jack and Mandy identified the need for more robust community evaluation processes that promote appropriate care for the communities they serve. They have entered into a mentoring partnership with a nearby university with expertise in community development, to develop, test, and evaluate a community assessment tool for ongoing use in their service's model of care.

■ REHABILITATION IN PALLIATIVE CARE

As the illness progresses, a patient often experiences increasing deterioration in his or her ability to complete his or her everyday activities. This functional decline often results in a person being unable to participate in life as he or she once did. Patients' functional limitations often result from the progression of advanced disease, extended bed rest, chemotherapy or radiotherapy, surgery, or other treatments. These factors typically present symptomatically as pain, dyspnea, depression, generalized weakness, fatigue, nausea, and vomiting (Lorenz et al., 2008; Santiago-Palma & Payne, 2001). Although the journey at the end of life is different for each person, most want to maintain as much independence as possible for as long as possible and aim to remain symptom free (Belchamber, 2004). However, functional decline that results in an increasing dependency on others negatively affects a person's overall QOL.

Typically, if a patient presents with functional limitations and an inability to complete his or her day-to-day activities, he or she would be offered rehabilitation. Rehabilitation centers on restoring a person's functional ability by addressing any physical, social, psychological, vocational, or spiritual problems that arise due to illness or disability (Barawid, Covarrubias, Tribuzio, & Liao, 2015; Jones & Bunnell, 2011; Santiago-Palma & Payne, 2001). These are familiar terms from our earlier discussion about wholeness. However, in PC, patients present with fluctuating health statuses that will ultimately result in a loss of function rather than restoration of previous functional abilities.

Palliative rehabilitation focuses on maintaining a person's independence and increasing his or her QOL by supporting and enabling him or her to live as normal a life as possible despite the stage of illness or age (Barawid et al., 2015; Cooper & Glaetzer, 2004; Namasivayam & Barnett, 2016). This phenomenon has previously been defined as "rehabilitation in reverse" (Pizzi & Briggs, 2004, p. 123), as it is at odds with the traditional rehabilitation approach that encourages skill development and increased independence to enable a person to reach his or her previous functional ability. This creates a paradox of practice approaches and requires health professionals to reconceptualize their practice to focus on assisting the person to adjust to his or her current and future health and functioning status, while still valuing his or her remaining life (Bye, 1998; Pizzi & Briggs, 2004).

While at present the effectiveness of palliative rehabilitation has not been supported with high-level evidence, it's known that palliative rehabilitation can help with symptom control, improving QOL, providing hope, and assisting people to continue to live until they die (Barawid et al., 2015; Belchamber, Gousy, & Ellis-Hill, 2013; Cramp & Byron-Daniel, 2012; M. Mills et al., 2013; Okamura, 2011; Rueda, Sola, Pascual, & Casacuberta, 2004;

Salakari, Surakka, Nurminen, & Pylkkänen, 2015). This is achieved by enabling people to use aids and equipment, modifying their daily activities, implementing emotional support and coping strategies, remediating their symptoms, and conserving energy (Hammill, Bye, & Cook, 2014; Tester, 2008a). To assist a patient to maintain as much independence as possible, health professionals need to view each person and his or her situation individually and acknowledge that the person's abilities will fluctuate and deteriorate over time (Tester, 2008b).

Palliative rehabilitation is appropriate to start from the time of diagnosis through to the terminal phase of illness (Okamura, 2011), and can occur in the home, hospital, and hospice settings. Before commencing interventions with patients with advanced illnesses, it is important to have an understanding of the person's needs and his or her expected illness trajectory. The most accepted classification system to determine a person's needs that is used in palliative rehabilitation was initially designed for use in cancer care; it classifies people based on their physical and psychosocial needs (Dietz, 1981). Because it classifies people on a needs basis rather than a diagnosis basis, this classification system has strong relevance for any advanced illness, regardless of diagnosis (Okamura, 2011; Tookman, Hopkins, & Scharpen-von-Heussen, 2004). Although Dietz's classification (Table 10.2) system dates back to 1981, it remains helpful for identifying different rehabilitation goals and planning interventions dependent on the current phase of a person's illness (Bray & Cooper, 2004; Okamura, 2011; Tookman et al., 2004).

The Role of the Interprofessional Team in PC Rehabilitation

Interprofessional teams are critical to the success of palliative rehabilitation (Chasen, Feldstain, Gravelle, MacDonald, & Pereira, 2013; Silver et al., 2015). Interprofessional

TABLE 10.2 Rehabilitation Phases in Palliative Care	
Phases of Rehabilitation	**Goal**
Preventive rehabilitation	Should commence at the time of diagnosis to reduce the impact and severity of disease impairment. Can be performed pre- or postoperatively or posttreatment and without functional impairment being present. Typically occurs in inpatient settings and focuses on education and information provision.
Restorative rehabilitation	Commences when functional impairments are present. Aims to restore a person to his or her pre-illness level of functional ability. May occur in inpatient, outpatient, or home settings.
Supportive rehabilitation	Commences when impairments cause functioning to continue to decline and disease advances. Goal is to maintain functional ability through adaptation of the person and the environment, rather than restoration. Compensatory methods such as task modification, energy conservation, equipment, and environmental modifications may be prescribed. Working with families and caregivers is vital.
Palliative rehabilitation	Commences in the terminal stages of illness. Aim is to reduce the impact of advanced disease by increasing a person's quality of life through symptom control. Treatment is client centered and targets symptoms such as pain, dyspnea, edema, and contractures through positioning, breathing assistance, relaxation, and assistive devices. Ongoing support of families and caregivers continues.

teams involve the coordination of care from a variety of specialized health professionals who work together to assist a patient and his or her family to adapt and cope with the impact of the illness or disability (Hearn & Higginson, 1997; Silver et al., 2015; Waldron et al., 2011). Interprofessional teams may include general practitioners, PC specialists, surgeons, oncologists, nurses, social workers, occupational therapists, physiotherapists, speech and language therapists, dietitians, psychologists, chaplains, and pharmacists (Palliative Care Australia, 2008). Most PC services should also have access to alternative therapies to complement mainstream care (Palliative Care Australia, 2008). Working as part of the interprofessional team is critical in palliative rehabilitation, as it enables the patient to be viewed holistically and receive planned, effective, integrated interventions (Hearn & Higginson, 1997; Gopalraj, Grooms, Setters, Kaundar, & Furman, 2012; Silver et al., 2015; Tookman et al., 2004).

The Role of Nurses in Palliative Rehabilitation

Nurses are essential in interprofessional care teams in palliative rehabilitation. An early systematic review identified that PC interprofessional teams have been found to be more effective in improving patient and family satisfaction levels and meeting patient and family needs when compared to conventional care (Hearn & Higginson, 1997). Studies have also found that nurses have the role of communicating care plans, updating health professionals on patients' current symptoms and the progression of illness, and providing practical, hands-on assistance both physically and emotionally to health professionals, patients, and their families (Chapple, Ziebland, & McPherson, 2006; Dunne, Sullivan, & Kernohan, 2005; Skilbeck & Payne, 2003).

■ **Goal Setting.** Goal setting is an integral part of the rehabilitation process. However, establishing meaningful and achievable goals in the PC setting can be challenging (Chen & Bradley, 2010). Challenges exist due to a patient's fluctuating functional ability, rate of disease progression, acceptance of diagnosis, and hopes and expectations for the future (Cheville, Khemka, & O'Mahony, 2007; Namasivayam & Barnett, 2016). While the central goal of PC is to support, enhance, and preserve a person's function in order to achieve his or her best QOL (Santiago-Palma & Payne, 2001), setting goals in PC can be problematic if the person and family are not viewed holistically. Goals should therefore be tailored individually to each person, and their family, and take into account his or her disease trajectory, current medical status, functional limitations, presenting symptoms, and psychosocial status (Chen & Bradley, 2010; Jones & Bunnell, 2011).

In order for goals to be achievable with this patient group, it is preferable to set short-term goals due to patients' fluctuating functional performance levels and the uncertainty of time. Short-term goals should relate to the completion of activities that are meaningful to the patient and enable a person to live as normal a life as possible during this period (Jones & Bunnell, 2011). Regardless of the type of goal set, each goal should be continually reassessed. Frequent reassessment ensures that goals remain realistic regardless of disease progression or increased functional limitations. If it becomes evident during reassessment that goals are no longer realistic, discussion must occur with the patient or family member on how to best change or modify the goal to enhance its achievability (Cheville, 2001; Jones & Bunnell, 2011).

It is also important to acknowledge that while goals may be initially set with the patient, the goals and wishes of the family members and caregivers are also relevant and have to be addressed. A meta-analysis of randomized trials found that involving the patient's family resulted in enhanced treatment outcomes for both the patient and the caregiver (Northouse, Katapodi, Song, Zhang, & Mood, 2010). Furthermore, involving family and caregivers has been shown to facilitate the achievement of goals, improve QOL, and enhance effective discharge planning (Harding & Higginson, 2003; Northouse et al., 2010).

■ **Interventions.** Patients with palliative diagnoses will present with varying levels of physical limitations and differing symptoms. Each patient will have his or her own needs, hopes, desires, fears, and goals that he or she needs to face prior to death. There may also be differing support systems and anticipated life expectancy, and thus each person will require his or her own tailored rehabilitation intervention plan (Chang et al., 2007; Tester, 2008b). Planning interventions in palliative rehabilitation should always occur with involvement of the patient and his or her family, with each patient being considered as an individual.

Nursing interventions in palliative rehabilitation that have been demonstrated to be effective in increasing a patient's independence predominantly revolve around symptom control and provision of psychosocial support to both the patient and his or her family. The most common nursing rehabilitation interventions in PC nursing are related to managing a patient's symptoms of pain, fatigue, and breathlessness (Qaseem et al., 2008; Rueda et al., 2004).

■ **Symptom Control.** Pain is a common symptom experienced by people with a palliative illness. It is estimated that up to 70% of all people with a palliative illness experience some form of pain regardless of their diagnosis (Chang et al., 2007; Dy, 2010). Pain has been found to have acute and chronic origins in people with cancer (Foley, 2004). Acute pain can be related to diagnostic or therapeutic interventions, anticancer treatments, and infections or complications, whereas chronic pain occurs from tumor infiltration into the nervous system or internal organs and from bony metastases (Dy, 2010). Functionally, pain can affect a person's ability to mobilize, transfer, or participate in meaningful activities of daily living and engage in relationships (Chang et al., 2007; Foley, 2004).

A systematic review that looked at effective treatment strategies for pain found strong evidence to support the use of nonsteroidal anti-inflammatory drugs (NSAIDs), opioids, radionuclides, and radiotherapy to treat cancer pain, and weak evidence to support the prescription of opioids for noncancer pain in patients with a palliative illness (Lorenz et al., 2008). Nonpharmacological rehabilitative interventions found to be effective for pain relief include cognitive behavioral therapy, pain education, and exercise (Dy, 2010).

Nurses are essential for delivering pain education and evaluating its effectiveness for patients. Numerous studies have demonstrated the effectiveness of nurse-led pain management education in the reduction of pain levels and should include the use of verbal and written information (Ferrell, Rhiner, & Ferrell, 1993; Oliver, Kravitz, Kaplan, & Meyers, 2001). Pain education should address misconceptions and fears about pain treatments, explanation of the WHO pain control ladder, and identification of pain management goals, which in turn include discussing pain with the treating physician and developing strategies to meet these goals (Oliver et al., 2001). Written information should be given to complement the verbal information received and should contain information on pain management, pain treatments, guidelines for discussing pain with the physician, free space to write down any questions or goals, and a pain scale to document changes in pain intensity with daily activities of daily living (Oliver et al., 2001). However, research suggests that nurses do not always feel confident with administering pain medications for patients with palliative care needs (Burns & McIlfatrick, 2015; Namasivayam & Barnett, 2016; Thomas & Barclay, 2015). Thus, it is recommended that nurses receive ongoing education in the identification of pain in PC patients (Burns & McIlfatrick, 2015; Namasivayam & Barnett, 2016), and the principles of pharmacological management (Nunn, 2014), including the use of syringe drivers (Thomas & Barclay, 2015), from experienced colleagues.

Fatigue is a multidimensional symptom that is widely prevalent in people with a palliative illness; it has been linked with anxiety, depression, pain, dyspnea, insomnia, anorexia, nausea, and drowsiness (Belchamber, 2004; Eyigor, 2010). These symptoms have a direct impact on a person's ability to engage with his or her daily life, often resulting in a reduced QOL (Belchamber, 2004; Eyigor, 2010). While there has been no formal consensus on a definition of fatigue, it is characterized by a prolonged lack of energy and a feeling of exhaustion that does not resolve with rest (Anderson, Dean, & Piech, 2010; Tester, 2008a). However, unlike typical fatigue, in PC

and hospice patients, fatigue is not proportional to activity expenditure, and consists of physical, emotional, and cognitive elements (Saarik & Hartley, 2010). Interventions for fatigue are varied and can involve fatigue management strategies, psychological interventions, and exercise (Anderson et al., 2010; Belchamber, 2004; Tester, 2008b). The goal of fatigue management in palliative rehabilitation is to assist the patient to reduce the effects of fatigue and to maximize the person's existing energy levels (Borneman, 2013).

General fatigue management strategies are often completed in conjunction with other members of the interprofessional team such as occupational therapists, dietitians, and physiotherapists. Occupational therapy strategies to manage fatigue include energy conservation education, task modification, and pacing to ensure a balance of activity and rest, and distraction therapy (Kealey & McIntyre, 2005; Lowrie, 2006; Vockins, 2004). Dietitians focus on optimizing a person's nutritional intake and prevention of weight loss in order to reduce feelings of fatigue (Borneman, 2013; Lowrie, 2006; Saarik & Hartley, 2010). Exercise has been demonstrated to be the most beneficial intervention for patients with cancer-related fatigue, regardless of their stage of disease (Kumar & Jim, 2010; Saarik & Hartley, 2010). Physiotherapists will tailor an exercise program to meet the patient's needs and stage of disease (Kumar & Jim, 2010). Exercise programs may include walking, resistive exercises, or a combination of exercises (Saarik & Hartley, 2010). Two meta-analyses have been conducted to look at the effect of exercise interventions on cancer-related fatigue (E. M. McMillan & Newhouse, 2011; Puetz & Herring, 2012). E. M. McMillan and Newhouse (2011) found that aerobic exercise has the most significant effect when compared to aerobic, resistance, and mixed training exercises in patients with breast or prostate cancer. Puetz and Herring (2012) found that exercise not only improved fatigue, but also increased a person's QOL and decreased depression and anxiety both during and after treatment.

Nurses can assist in the palliative rehabilitation process through thorough assessment of a patient's fatigue levels (Borneman, 2013). Assessment should include the use of a visual pain scale as well as discussion surrounding the impact of the fatigue on the patient's QOL and his or her ability to complete activities of daily living. Nurses play a role in empowering the patient and the family by educating them on fatigue management, pain control, proper nutrition and hydration, the importance of exercise, and energy conservation (Borneman, 2013).

Breathing difficulties are an issue for many patients with PC illnesses and tend to become more frequent as the person nears the end of life (Bausewein, Booth, Gysels, & Higginson, 2008). Breathing difficulties are most commonly present in patients with diagnoses such as lung cancer (including lung metastases to the chest region or obstruction of the airways or mediastinum) and other end-stage respiratory diseases, end-stage cardiac disease, and neuromuscular diseases (Barton, English, Nabb, Rigby, & Johnson, 2010). Common symptoms of breathlessness include dyspnea, hemoptysis, obstruction, cough, and respiratory secretions (Bausewein et al., 2008; K. S. Chan, Sham, Tse, & Thorsen, 2005).

Remediating breathlessness is important because they affect a person's well-being on physical, emotional, social, and functional levels (Bredin et al., 1999). For example, breathlessness can raise a person's fatigue levels, resulting in poor concentration, decreased appetite, pain, and memory loss (K. S. Chan et al., 2005). Emotionally, breathlessness can cause anxiety and fear, as patients panic because of their uncomfortable awareness of breathing (Belchamber, 2004). Functionally, breathlessness may limit a person's ability to complete his or her activities of daily living, resulting in the person moving less, or dependency while completing simple tasks such as showering and dressing. Breathlessness can also affect how frequently a person interacts with others and the type of activities that he or she continues to pursue (Belchamber, 2004; Fialka-Moser, Crevenna, Korpan, & Quittan, 2003). The goal of palliative rehabilitation is to decrease breathlessness and improve a patient's functioning (Fialka-Moser et al., 2003).

Both pharmacological and nonpharmacological interventions have been effective for breathlessness (Bausewein et al., 2008; K. S. Chan et al., 2005; Lorenz et al., 2008; Rueda et al., 2004). The strongest evidence for pharmacological interventions for breathlessness is opioid use for people with chronic obstructive pulmonary disease (COPD). However, a nursing-led nonpharmacological intervention that was found to be effective in reducing breathlessness, regardless of the stage of illness, was education on symptom control (Rueda et al., 2004).

A pilot study looked at the effectiveness of providing breathlessness interventions over one or three sessions (Barton et al., 2010). Twenty-two participants were randomized to receive either a single session or three sessions of education on activity pacing, anxiety management and relaxation, and diaphragmatic breathing. Education was given in person by either a physical therapist or a trained nurse; however, each participant also received a DVD and written material, as well as a telephone call from a research nurse at the conclusion of his or her final session. This study showed a reduction in perceived breathlessness, an increase in coping abilities, and satisfaction in care in the group who received three intervention sessions as opposed to the group who received a single session. While no statistical significance was found, due to the small number of participants and the high attrition rate, this study showed benefits to administering breathlessness interventions over three sessions rather than one session (Barton et al., 2010).

Exercise, diaphragmatic and pursed-lips breathing, and walking and stair-climbing exercises prescribed by physiotherapists have also been shown to be effective in the reduction of breathlessness symptoms (LeGrand, 2002; Lorenz et al., 2008; Syrett & Taylor, 2003).

Occupational therapy interventions of task modification, positioning, home modification, and the prescription of bathroom and bedroom equipment have also been found to reduce symptoms of breathlessness for patients (Cooper, 2006; Fialka-Moser et al., 2003). While these types of interventions are typically prescribed by other health professionals, nurses play a role in encouraging patients to remain engaged in activities of daily living and complete the intervention programs that have been recommended by members of the interprofessional team.

▪ **Psychosocial Support for Patients and Families.** Psychological distress is common in patients with advanced illness, and has links to fatigue, pain, nausea, and breathlessness (Belchamber, 2004). At present, there is limited evidence to support the role of nurses in the provision of psychosocial support interventions with patients who have palliative illnesses (Rueda et al., 2004). However, one randomized controlled study by C. W. Chan, Richardson, and Richardson (2011) assessed the feasibility of running two 40-minute educational sessions combined with progressive muscle relaxation exercises for patients with advanced lung cancer who were receiving palliative radiotherapy, when compared to standard care. Each education session was given by a registered nurse; participants were invited to discuss their related symptoms and self-care management and were given written information. Results showed statistically significant changes in the reduction of anxiety, breathlessness, and fatigue in the psychoeducational intervention group as compared with the control group who received standard care (C. W. Chan et al., 2011).

Nurses' role in rehabilitation includes having conversations with the family (Long, Kneafsey, Ryan, & Berry, 2002). Through communication and rapport building with the family, the palliative rehabilitation nurse is able to provide information, give emotional support, and coordinate care for the family's loved one, thus enhancing a patient's rehabilitation process (Long et al., 2002). Studies have shown that health professionals, including nurses, should routinely assess a patient's family or caregivers' emotional, practical, and supportive needs while caring for a patient with a palliative illness (Qaseem et al., 2008).

However, the exact needs of the family and caregivers of people with a palliative illness have received little research attention. Few interventions have been directly aimed at caregivers, with most focused on patient outcomes (Northouse et al., 2010). Caregivers' needs must be addressed for them to maintain optimal health and provide the best possible care to the patient. A meta-analysis of caregiver studies found that nursing interventions developed for caregivers were found to reduce caregiver burden, improve coping abilities, increase confidence as caregivers, reduce anxiety, and improve marital and family relationships (Northouse et al., 2010).

Nurses can reduce caregiver burden and improve coping abilities by providing education on the nature of the disease and treatment options for the patient; identifying caregivers' physical, emotional, and supportive needs; and problem solving and evaluating any negative reactions to caregiving (Given et al., 2006). A randomized controlled trial by S. C. McMillan et al. (2006) provided coping skills education to caregivers of people with cancer over three 1-hour sessions. Nurses taught a problem-solving method that assisted the caregiver to assess and manage patient symptoms by focusing on creativity, optimism, and respite care resources. Findings from this study showed an increase in caregiver QOL scores and a reduction in caregiver burden related to the patients' symptoms and caregiving tasks (S. C. McMillan et al., 2006).

Improving caregiving skills was seen to be an effective way to increase caregivers' confidence in caring for their loved ones (Mokuau, Braun, Wong, Higuchi, & Gotay, 2008). Given et al. (2006) completed a randomized controlled trial with the aim of lowering caregivers' reactions to chemotherapy symptoms and increasing caregivers' involvement in the symptom management of patients with cancer. This 10-week cognitive behavioral intervention was administered by registered nurses with oncology experience to both the patients and their caregivers. Results showed that caregivers who were given education strategies on symptom management, such as monitoring the effectiveness of pain relief medications for pain control, had significantly lower reactions to assisting patients with symptoms and also assisted with significantly fewer symptoms as the patients had improved in their symptom severity (Given et al., 2006).

A randomized controlled trial found that caregiver anxiety can be managed through the provision of telephone counseling and low-impact exercise (Badger, Segrin, Dorros, Meek, & Lopez, 2007). This intervention focused on both the patient with a cancer diagnosis and the patient's partner, and was delivered by a psychiatric registered nurse with oncology expertise. The patient received a weekly telephone call for 6 weeks and was given cancer education and interpersonal counseling. While the patient was receiving his or her intervention, his or her partner received a biweekly phone call to discuss his or her own emotional well-being and relationship issues. Counseling for the partner addressed cancer education, social support, identification and management of depression and anxiety, and role transitions. A second group was given a self-directed 6-week exercise protocol, which focused on regular, low-impact exercise such as walking. These patients received a weekly phone call to monitor their progress and encourage them to exercise, while their partners received a biweekly call to encourage exercise and monitor their progress. At the conclusion of the 6 weeks, both the patient and his or her partner's anxiety symptoms had decreased significantly in both the interpersonal counseling and the exercise groups (Badger et al., 2007).

Additionally, nurses have been found to play a role in maintaining marital satisfaction, providing family support, and improving couple communication in patients with cancer (Northouse et al., 2010). A secondary analysis of data collected from a previous randomized controlled trial looked at a standardized nursing intervention protocol aimed at improving the QOL for people who had a prostatectomy and their partners (McCorkle, Siefert, Dowd, Robinson, & Pickett, 2007). In the original study, each participant received a home visit biweekly, and a weekly telephone call during the alternate week, for a total of 16 weeks. Interventions focused on educating the patient and his or her spouse on symptoms, symptom management, and caregiver-related skills, communication techniques, and intimacy expectations. Results showed that spouses reported significantly higher levels of depressive symptoms and distress relating to marital interactions than the patients. Patients reported significantly higher distress levels relating to sexual function than their spouses. Findings suggest that standardized nursing interventions focusing on symptom management and communication techniques may help patients and their spouses to develop realistic expectations and perceptions of their sexual functioning, as well as increasing their ability to discuss their expectations of each other (McCorkle et al., 2007).

■ **Outcome Measurement.** Health professionals are continually being asked to employ outcome measures to determine if they are providing effective interventions and relevant services for their client group (Bausewein, Daveson, Benalia, Simon, & Higginson, 2011). Outcome measures provide quantifiable evidence of the effectiveness of an intervention by determining if there have been positive or negative health-related changes (which can be attributed to their healthcare) in a person's health status over time (Bausewein et al., 2011; Hearn & Higginson, 1997).

Measuring outcomes in PC is often difficult, as clients will continue to decline in their function or they may die before a reassessment of their abilities has been performed, confounding the observable effectiveness of the intervention (Pearson, Todd, & Futcher, 2007). Gail (2006) suggested that outcome measurement in PC should focus on reflecting the values and goals of PC, which are to improve QOL before death, enhance symptom control, and provide support to the family, rather than on measuring functional gains or losses. Therefore, it is more appropriate to select an outcome measure that will reflect a meaningful outcome for the patient who is dying (Gail, 2006).

A review of the literature was unable to provide a consensus on which standardized outcome measures should be used in practice to measure changes in PC (Stiel et al., 2012). This was due to the wide scope of PC outcome measures currently being utilized in clinical practice and research (Table 10.3; Stiel et al.,

TABLE 10.3 Examples of Outcome Measures for Use in Palliative Rehabilitation	
Multidimensional outcome measures	Distress Thermometer European Organization for Research and Treatment of Cancer Quality of Life Questionnaire (EORTC QLQ-C30) Palliative Care Assessment Tool (PACA) Palliative Care Outcome Scale (POS) Phase (Stable–Unstable–Deteriorating–Terminal) Support Team Assessment Schedule (STAS)
Quality-of-life measures	Functional Assessment of Cancer Therapy: General (FACT-G) McGill Quality of Life Questionnaire (MGQOL) McMaster Quality of Life Scale (MQLS) Palliative Care Problem Severity Score (PCPSS) Quality of Life at the End of Life Measure (QUAL-E) Quality of Life Index WHO Quality of Life Assessment Instrument (WHOQOL)
Symptom assessments	6 Minute Walk Test Edmonton Symptom Assessment Scale (ESAS) Memorial Symptom Assessment Scale (MSAS) POS-S Symptom List Problem Severity Scale Symptom Assessment Scale (SAS) Symptom Distress Scale (SDS)
Functional status assessments	Australian Modified Karnofsky Scale (AKPS) Eastern Cooperative Oncology Group (ECOG) Hospice Care Performance Inventory (HCPI) Karnofsky Performance Scale (KPS) RUG-ADL
Caregiver assessments	Caregiver Quality of Life Index (CQOL-C) Carer Coping Scale Carer Distress Thermometer Family Satisfaction With Advanced Cancer Care for the Evaluation of Families' Satisfaction and Perception of Care (FamCare)

2012). Findings suggested that outcome measures in PC were selected based on the need to measure a certain dimension or domain of care (Bausewein et al., 2011). Dimensions of care involve physical, social, psychological, or spiritual elements, which provide the health professional with more in-depth knowledge of the problem. For example, a dimension of care may rate the patient's perception of the severity of fatigue as it relates to his or her activities of daily living. Domains may involve the patient, family, and caregiver or multiple physical or psychosocial elements (Bausewein et al., 2011).

When selecting an outcome measure for use, one should assess the dimensions of the domains that are appropriate for the client. For example, their need may relate to individual symptoms, their functional status, QOL, or their caregiver, or they may need an outcome measure that is multidimensional (Bausewein et al., 2011).

Regardless of which outcome measure is chosen, nurses should ensure that the measure has adequate validity and reliability and is responsive to change in the palliative population. Thought should also go into the timing of the measurements taking place (e.g., at the commencement of treatment), and the frequency of measurement, to ensure that each measurement point is long enough to elicit change.

■ CONCLUSION

A core concept in understanding the issue of QOL in PC is that the experience of incurable illness and dying, taking on a caregiver's role, grieving, and death itself cannot be fully understood solely within a medical context (Byock et al., 2001; Howarth, 2007). The perspective of PC services is deeply founded upon notions of holistic care. Health promotion and rehabilitation are critical to maximizing an individual's function and well-being even in the face of life-threatening illness. Nurses play a key role in promoting the health of the patient and his or her family caregivers across the illness trajectory.

CASE STUDY *Conclusion*

Jack was assessed as needing education about his illness, medications, and positioning; psychological support; a social worker to sort out finances and offer support to his family; an occupational therapist for home modification (hospital bed installed downstairs, bathroom changed to downstairs); equipment prescription (hospital bed, pressure care mattress, over-toilet seat, shower chair); task modification/energy conservation education; and a physiotherapist for the prescription of a mobility aid and breathing exercises.

The goals of Jack's rehabilitation are:

■ Increased independence in mobility, toileting, and self-care tasks
■ Decreased caregiver burden
■ Increased emotional support
■ Education regarding the disease trajectory, symptoms, breathlessness, and so forth
■ Assistance regarding financial concerns
■ Increased feelings of control

CASE STUDY

AN INTERPROFESSIONAL PERSPECTIVE: THOUGHTS OF AN OCCUPATIONAL THERAPIST

Part A of Case Study

The first flag I have identified in this case study is Jack's age—55 years. He is in an age bracket more likely to be associated with a specific set of issues that, for example, an 85-year-old man may not have. Specific issues for men of Jack's age may include loss of income, possible social issues around family/age of children/grandchildren, difficulty accessing services at home as he is under 65 years, and relationship/marriage/intimacy issues.

The next issue to consider is that Jack is still receiving chemotherapy and we should consider whether his symptom management is associated with chemotherapy side effects or actual disease progression. The PC team may also need to have a discussion around the actual goal of chemotherapy and whether ceasing it might be appropriate. A key question in this conversation is this: Is the chemotherapy a continuation of active treatment or for palliative symptom management?

Psychosocial impacts of chemotherapy might also impact Jack and his family, including costs of treatment, transport, and parking involved with his appointments; time spent at appointments may detract from quality time to spend with his family and friends. When I read about Jack being on home oxygen, a few other things come to mind for consideration. Costs of the oxygen, electricity to run the concentrator, issues with tubing, and mobilizing around the home space are just a few areas that might need attention.

The case study also talks about his social situation. It mentions he has stepchildren and his wife's ex-partner assists with paperwork. This may impact on Jack regarding his emotional and relationship issues, and family dynamics—all of these factors may require psychosocial support to navigate.

Jack has had a working role as a maintenance worker. We should consider the loss of role identity as a worker and loss of income. It might be worth conducting an interest/leisure checklist to try and engage Jack in some sort of meaningful activity as he can't go to work and a referral to a social worker regarding his financial situation like income protection, access to superannuation, and carer allowances for his wife.[1]

---

[1] These are Australia social support payments.

The case study mentions Jack and his wife are functionally illiterate and are supported by Mandy's ex-partner to complete paperwork. This flags questions about whether an enduring power of attorney has been appointed; has Jack completed an advance health directive and a will so that information about his prognosis, treatment, medications, and services can be conveyed?

The next part of the case study talks about his home environment. As they live in public housing, modifications in the home may be difficult and support may be required to ensure their rent is being paid if Jack can no longer work. Jack is sleeping on a mattress on the floor, so an occupational therapy assessment can look at a hospital bed and pressure care issues; a physiotherapy review can assess how Jack could transfer from the floor, and then of course look at the financial issues about the supply of equipment and appropriate bedding.

Part B of Case Study

This part of the case study talks about a support group for Jack's wife; however, other things to consider include arranging in-home respite support for him while Mandy attends the support group. Does Jack want to talk to others in his situation? Do the stepchildren have enough support?

The case study then continues on to discuss how the service began life-and-death education activities for the community. These activities could include death cafes, focus groups, movie/social events, education forums, advance care planning drop-in clinics, case studies, and open days of the local hospice or PC service.

The case study then looks at partnerships with a nearby university in regard to developing a community assessment tool. What sort of assessment tool could this be? What other types of partnerships could be used in addition to the local university? The case study talks about the service's model of care—what model of care could best meet the needs of its community-based clients?

Part C of Case Study

The final part of the case study looks at the involvement of other members of Allied Health in caring for Jack. Apart from the occupational therapist, social worker, and physiotherapist mentioned, there could be a role for a dietitian, psychologist, and recreation therapist. There might also be a need for a family meeting to discuss Jack's goals of care and interprofessional team meetings to coordinate interdisciplinary care.

Several goals of rehabilitation are listed for Jack. There are a number of goal-setting tools that could be used as well as outcome measures to determine the success of Jack's rehabilitation.

The final goal talks about Jack's increasing feelings of control; how could the team assist in the achievement of this goal? This may include interventions to improve QOL, promote meaningful activity, identify community access goals, undertake dignity therapy, and so on.

Evidence-Based Practice

Mills, J., Rosenberg, J., & McInerney, F. (2015). Building community capacity for end of life: An investigation of community capacity and its implications for health-promoting palliative care in the Australian Capital Territory. *Critical Public Health*, 25(2), 218–230. doi:10.1080/09581596.2014.945396

Background
Community-based activities around death, dying, and EOL care that reflect the philosophy of health-promoting palliative care are of interest beyond an orientation toward service provision.

Purpose
This study identified and examined community-based activities in health-promoting palliative care.

Method
A qualitative interpretative approach was used to engage eight local community groups. Ten representatives were recruited using purposive sampling. Data were collected using a semi-structured interview guide. Nine of the 10 participants were women, reflecting the female role in community caring. The community groups represented included those associated with dementia, cancer, caregivers of patients with life-limiting illness, respite care, motor neuron disease, and muscular dystrophy.

Results
The themes that emerged were: practical support, respect and responsiveness, and connection and empowerment, which reflect community activities initiated in response to life-threatening illness.

Discussion and Implications
Health-promoting palliative care is provided by both community groups and healthcare providers. It is important to build community capacity in providing EOL care to restore community agency while developing collaborative partnerships with healthcare professionals. Promoting community capacity in the care of the seriously ill and dying can be demonstrated by activities that promote socialization, peer support, and normalization of the experience of dying and death.

■ REFERENCES

Anderson, P. R., Dean, G. E., & Piech, M. A. (2010). Fatigue. In B. R. Ferrell & N. Coyle (Eds.), *Oxford textbook of palliative medicine* (3rd ed., pp. 187–211). New York, NY: Oxford University Press.

Badger, T., Segrin, C., Dorros, S. M., Meek, P., & Lopez, A. M. (2007). Depression and anxiety in women with breast cancer and their partners. *Nursing Research, 56*(1), 44–53. doi:10.1097/00006199-200701000-00006

Barawid, E., Covarrubias, N., Tribuzio, B., & Liao, S. (2015). The benefits of rehabilitation for palliative care patients. *American Journal of Hospice and Palliative Medicine, 32*(1), 34–43. doi:10.1177/1049909113514474

Barton, R., English, A., Nabb, S., Rigby, A. S., & Johnson, M. J. (2010). A randomised trial of high vs low intensity training in breathing techniques for breathless patients with malignant lung disease: A feasibility study. *Lung Cancer, 70*(3), 313–319. doi:10.1016/j.lungcan.2010.03.007

Bausewein, C., Booth, S., Gysels, M., & Higginson, I. J. (2008). Non-pharmacological interventions for breathlessness in advanced stages of malignant and non-malignant diseases (Review). *Cochrane Database of Systematic Reviews,* (2), CD005623. doi:10.1002/14651858.CD005623.pub2

Bausewein, C., Daveson, B., Benalia, H., Simon, S. T., & Higginson, I. J. (2011). Outcome measurement in palliative care: The essentials. Retrieved from http://www.csi.kcl.ac.uk/files/Guidance_on_Outcome_Measurement_in_Palliative_Care.pdf

Belchamber, C. A. (2004). Rehabilitative care in a specialist palliative day care centre: A study of patients' perspectives. *International Journal of Therapy and Rehabilitation, 11*(9), 425–434. doi:10.12968/ijtr.2004.11.9.19590

Belchamber, C. A., Gousy, M. H., & Ellis-Hill, C. (2013). Fostering hope through palliative rehabilitation. *European Journal of Palliative Care, 20*(3), 136–139.

Borneman, T. (2013). Assessment and management of cancer-related fatigue. *Journal of Hospice and Palliative Nursing, 15*(2), 77–86. doi:10.1097/NJH.0b013e318286dc19

Bray, J., & Cooper, J. (2004). The contribution of occupational therapy to palliative medicine. In D. Doyle, G. Hanks, & K. Calman (Eds.), *Oxford textbook of palliative medicine* (3rd ed., pp. 1036–1041). New York, NY: Oxford University Press.

Bredin, M., Corner, J., Krishnasamy, M., Plant, H., Bailey, C., & A'Hern, R. (1999). Multicentre randomised controlled trial of nursing intervention for breathlessness in patients with lung cancer. *British Medical Journal, 318*(7188), 901. doi:10.1136/bmj.318.7188.901

Burns, M., & McIlfatrick, S. (2015). Palliative care in dementia: Literature review of nurses' knowledge and attitudes towards pain assessment. *International Journal of Palliative Nursing, 21*(8), 400–407. doi:10.12968/ijpn.2015.21.8.400

Bye, R. (1998). When clients are dying: Occupational therapists' perspectives. *Occupational Therapy Journal of Research, 18*(1), 3–24. doi:10.1177/153944929801800101

Byock, I., Norris, K., Curtis, J. R., & Patrick, D. L. (2001). Improving end-of-life experience and care in the community: A conceptual framework. *Journal of Pain and Symptom Management, 22*(3), 759–772. doi:10.1016/S0885-3924(01)00332-3

Chan, C. W., Richardson, A., & Richardson, J. (2011). Managing symptoms in patients with advanced lung cancer during radiotherapy: Results of a psychoeducational randomized controlled trial. *Journal of Pain and Symptom Management, 41*(2), 347–357. doi:10.1016/j.jpainsymman.2010.04.024

Chan, K. S., Sham, M. M. K., Tse, D. M. V., & Thorsen, A. B. (2005). Palliative medicine in malignant respiratory diseases. In H. G. Doyle, N. I. Cherny, & K. Calman (Eds.), *Oxford textbook of palliative medicine* (3rd ed., pp. 587–618). New York, NY: Oxford University Press.

Chang, V. T., Sorger, B., Rosenfeld, K. E., Lorenz, K. A., Bailey, A. F., Bui, T., … Montagnini, M. (2007). Pain and palliative medicine. *Journal of Rehabilitation Research and Development, 44*(2), 279–294. doi:10.1682/JRRD.2006.06.0067

Chapple, A., Ziebland, S., & McPherson, A. (2006). The specialist palliative care nurse: A qualitative study of the patients' perspective. *International Journal of Nursing Studies, 43*(8), 1011–1022. doi:10.1016/j.ijnurstu.2005.11.007

Chasen, M. R., Feldstain, A., Gravelle, D., MacDonald, N., & Pereira, J. (2013). Results from a structured interprofessional palliative care rehabilitation program in oncology. *Current Oncology, 20*(6), 301–309. doi:10.3747/co.20.1607

Chen, L., & Bradley, S. L. (2010). Rehabilitation goal-setting for a terminally ill patient: A case study. *Journal of the Australasian Rehabilitation Nurses Association, 13*(4), 7–9.

Cheville, A. (2001). Rehabilitation of patients with advanced cancer. *Cancer, 92*(4 Suppl.), 1039–1048. doi:10.1002/1097-0142(20010815)92:4+<1039::AID-CNCR1417>3.0.CO;2-L

Cheville, A., Khemka, V., & O'Mahony, S. (2007). The role of cancer rehabilitation in the maintenance of functional integrity and quality of life. In A. E. Blank, S. O'Mahoney, & A. Selwyn (Eds.), *Choices in palliative care: Issues in care delivery* (pp. 62–83). New York, NY: Springer.

Cooper, J. (2006). Occupational therapy in the management of breathlessness. In J. Cooper (Ed.), *Occupational therapy in oncology and palliative care* (2nd ed., pp. 51–60). West Sussex, UK: John Wiley & Sons.

Cooper, J., & Glaetzer, K. (2004). Recognising the need for palliative care in aged care. *Australasian Journal on Ageing, 23*(4), 162–166. doi:10.1111/j.1741-6612.2004.00043.x

Cramp, F., & Byron-Daniel, J. (2012). Exercise for the management of cancer-related fatigue in adults. *Cochrane Database Systematic Reviews,* (11), CD006145. doi:10.1002/14651858.CD006145.pub2

D'Onofrio, C., & Ryndes, T. (2003). The relevance of public health in improving access to end of life care. In B. Jennings, T. Ryndes, C. D'Onofrio, & M. A. Baily (Eds.), *Access to hospice care: Expanding boundaries, overcoming barriers* (Supplement ed.; pp. S30–S32). New York, NY: The Hastings Center.

DeSpelder, L. A., & Strickland, A. L. (2002). *The last dance: Encountering death and dying* (6th ed.). Boston, MA: McGraw-Hill.

Dietz, J. H. (1981). *Rehabilitation oncology.* New York, NY: Wiley.

Dunne, K., Sullivan, K., & Kernohan, G. (2005). Palliative care for patients with cancer: District nurses' experiences. *Journal of Advanced Nursing, 50*(4), 372–380. doi:10.1111/j.1365-2648.2005.03402.x

Dy, S. M. (2010). Evidence-based approaches to pain in advanced cancer. *Cancer Journal, 16*(5), 500–506. doi:10.1097/PPO.0b013e3181f45853

Eyigor, S. (2010). Physical activity and rehabilitation programs should be recommended on palliative care for patients with cancer. *Journal of Palliative Medicine, 13*(10), 1183–1184. doi:10.1089/jpm.2010.0064

Ferrell, B. R., Rhiner, M., & Ferrell, B. A. (1993). Development and implementation of a pain education program. *Cancer, 72*(Suppl. 11), 3426–3432. doi:10.1002/1097-0142(19931201)72:11+<3426::AID-CNCR2820721608>3.0.CO;2-D

Fialka-Moser, V., Crevenna, R., Korpan, M., & Quittan, M. (2003). Cancer rehabilitation: Particularly with aspects on physical impairments. *Journal of Rehabilitation Medicine, 35*(4), 153–162. doi:10.1080/16501970310000511

Foley, K. (2004). Acute and chronic cancer pain syndromes. In H. G. Doyle, N. I. Cherny, & K. Calman (Eds.), *Oxford textbook of palliative medicine* (pp. 298–315). New York, NY: Oxford University Press.

Gail, E. (2006). Measuring occupational therapy outcomes in cancer and palliative care. In J. Cooper (Ed.), *Occupational therapy in oncology and palliative care* (2nd ed., pp. 189–200). West Sussex, UK: John Wiley & Sons.

Given, B., Given, C. W., Sikorskii, A., Jeon, S., Sherwood, P., & Rahbar, M. (2006). The impact of providing symptom management assistance on caregiver reaction: Results of a randomized trial. *Journal of Pain and Symptom Management, 32*(5), 433–443. doi:10.1016/j.jpainsymman.2006.05.019

Gopalraj, R. K., Grooms, L. J., Setters, B. K., Kaundar, A., & Furman, C. D. (2012). Decision-making in older adults with serious illness: Barriers to the goals of care discussion. *Aging Health, 8*(4), 367–376. doi:10.2217/ahe.12.41

Hammill, K., Bye, R., & Cook, C. (2014). Occupational therapy for people living with a life-limiting illness: A thematic review. *British Journal of Occupational Therapy, 77*(11), 582–589. doi:10.4276/030802214X14151078348594

Harding, R., & Higginson, I. J. (2003). What is the best way to help caregivers in cancer and palliative care? A systematic literature review of interventions and their effectiveness. *Palliative Medicine, 17*(1), 63–74. doi:10.1191/0269216303pm667oa

Hearn, J., & Higginson, I. J. (1997). Outcome measures in palliative care for advanced cancer patients: A review. *Journal of Public Health Medicine, 19*(2), 193–199.

Howarth, G. (2007). *Death and dying: A sociological introduction.* Cambridge, UK: Polity.

Jones, C., & Bunnell, A. (2011). Rehabilitation in palliative care. In M. A. Baldwin & J. Woodhouse (Eds.), *Key concepts in palliative care* (1st ed., pp. 170–175). London, UK: Sage.

Kealey, P., & McIntyre, I. (2005). An evaluation of the domiciliary occupational therapy service in palliative cancer care in a community trust: A patient and carers perspective. *European Journal of Cancer Care, 14*(3), 232–243. doi:10.1111/j.1365-2354.2005.00559.x

Kellehear, A. (1999). *Health-promoting palliative care*. Oxford, UK: Oxford University Press.

Kellehear, A. (2005). *Compassionate cities: Public health and end-of-life care*. London, UK: Routledge.

Kumar, S. P., & Jim, A. (2010). Physical therapy in palliative care: From symptom control to quality of life: A critical review. *Indian Journal of Palliative Care, 16*(3), 138–146. doi:10.4103/0973-1075.73670

LeGrand, S. B. (2002). Dyspnea: The continuing challenge of palliative management. *Current Opinion in Oncology, 14*(4), 394–398. doi:10.1097/01.CCO.0000018317.59235.5F

Long, A. F., Kneafsey, R., Ryan, J., & Berry, J. (2002). The role of the nurse within the multi-professional rehabilitation team. *Journal of Advanced Nursing, 37*(1), 70–78. doi:10.1046/j.1365-2648.2002.02059.x

Lorenz, K. A., Lynn, J., Dy, S. M., Shugarman, L. R., Wilkinson, A., Mularski, R. A., …Shekelle, P. G. (2008). Evidence for improving palliative care at the end of life: A systematic review. *Annals of Internal Medicine, 148*(2), 147–159. doi:10.7326/0003-4819-148-2-200801150-00010

Lowrie, D. (2006). Occupational therapy and cancer related fatigue. In J. Cooper (Ed.), *Occupational therapy in oncology and palliative care* (2nd ed., pp. 61–82). West Sussex, UK: John Wiley & Sons.

McCorkle, R., Siefert, M. L., Dowd, M. F., Robinson, J. P., & Pickett, M. (2007). Effects of advanced practice nursing on patient and spouse depressive symptoms, sexual function, and marital interaction after radical prostatectomy. *Urologic Nursing, 27*(1), 65–77; discussion 78.

McMillan, E. M., & Newhouse, I. J. (2011). Exercise is an effective treatment modality for reducing cancer-related fatigue and improving physical capacity in cancer patients and survivors: A meta-analysis. *Applied Physiology, Nutrition, and Metabolism, 36*(6), 892–903. doi:10.1139/h11-082

McMillan, S. C., Small, B. J., Weitzner, M., Schonwetter, R., Tittle, M., Moody, L., & Haley, W. E. (2006). Impact of coping skills intervention with family caregivers of hospice patients with cancer: A randomized clinical trial. *Cancer, 106*(1), 214–222. doi:10.1002/cncr.21567

McMurray, A. (2003). *Community health and wellness: A socioecological approach* (2nd ed.). Marrickville, Australia: Elsevier.

Mills, J., Rosenberg, J., & McInerney, F. (2015). Building community capacity for end of life: An investigation of community capacity and its implications for health-promoting palliative care in the Australian Capital Territory. *Critical Public Health, 25*(2), 218–230. doi:10.1080/09581596.2014.945396

Mills, M., Black, A., Campbell, A., Cardwell, C. R., Galway, K., & Donnelly, M. (2013, May 21). Multidimensional rehabilitation programmes for adult cancer survivors. *Cochrane Database of Systematic Reviews*, (3), CD007730. Retrieved from http://onlinelibrary.wiley.com/doi/10.1002/14651858.CD007730.pub2/pdf/standard

Mokuau, N., Braun, K. L., Wong, L. K., Higuchi, P., & Gotay, C. C. (2008). Development of a family intervention for Native Hawaiian women with cancer: A pilot study. *Social Work, 53*(1), 9–19. doi:10.1093/sw/53.1.9

Namasivayam, P., & Barnett, T. (2016). Providing palliative care in a rehabilitation setting: A staff needs assessment. *Journal of the Australasian Rehabilitation Nurses' Association, 19*(2), 8–14.

Northouse, L. L., Katapodi, M. C., Song, L., Zhang, L., & Mood, D. W. (2010). Interventions with family caregivers of cancer patients: Meta-analysis of randomized trials. *CA: A Cancer Journal for Clinicians, 60*(5), 317–339. doi:10.3322/caac.20081

Nunn, C. (2014). It's not just about pain: Symptom management in palliative care. *Nurse Prescribing, 12*(7), 338–344. doi:10.12968/npre.2014.12.7.338

Okamura, H. (2011). Importance of rehabilitation in cancer treatment and palliative medicine. *Japanese Journal of Clinical Oncology, 41*(6), 733–738. doi:10.1093/jjco/hyr061

Oliver, J. W., Kravitz, R. L., Kaplan, S. H., & Meyers, F. J. (2001). Individualized patient education and coaching to improve pain control among cancer outpatients. *Journal of Clinical Oncology, 19*(8), 2206–2212. doi:10.1200/JCO.2001.19.8.2206

Palliative Care Australia. (2008). *Palliative and end of life care: Glossary of terms*. Deakin, Australia: Author.

Pearson, E. J., Todd, J. G., & Futcher, J. M. (2007). How can occupational therapists measure outcomes in palliative care? *Palliative Medicine, 21*(6), 477–485. doi:10.1177/0269216307081941

Pizzi, M. A., & Briggs, R. (2004). Occupational and physical therapy in hospice: The facilitation of meaning, quality of life, and well-being. *Topics in Geriatric Rehabilitation, 20*(2), 120–130. doi:10.1097/00013614-200404000-00007

Puetz, T. W., & Herring, M. P. (2012). Differential effects of exercise on cancer-related fatigue during and following treatment: A meta-analysis. *American Journal of Preventive Medicine, 43*(2), e1–e24. doi:10.1016/j.amepre.2012.04.027

Qaseem, A., Snow, V., Shekelle, P., Casey, D. E., Cross, J. T., & Owens, D. K. (2008). Evidence-based interventions to improve the palliative care of pain, dyspnea, and depression at the end of life: A clinical practice guideline from the American College of Physicians. *Annals of Internal Medicine, 148*(2), 141–146. doi:10.7326/0003-4819-148-2-200801150-00009

Rao, J. K., Alongi, J., Anderson, L. A., Jenkins, L., Stokes, G. A., & Kane, M. (2005). Development of public health priorities for end-of-life initiatives. *American Journal of Preventive Medicine, 29*(5), 453–460. doi:10.1016/j.amepre.2005.08.014

Rao, J. K., Anderson, L. A., & Smith, S. M. (2002). End of life is a public health issue. *American Journal of Preventive Medicine, 23*(3), 215–220. doi:10.1016/S0749-3797(02)00500-7

Rosenberg, J. P. (2012). "But we're already doing it!" Examining conceptual blurring between health promotion and palliative care. In L. Sallnow, S. Kumar, & A. Kellehear (Eds.), *International perspectives on public health and palliative care* (pp. 13–29). London, UK: Routledge.

Rueda, J. R., Sola, I., Pascual, A., & Casacuberta, M. S. (2004). Non-invasive interventions for improving well-being and quality of life in patients with lung cancer. *Cochrane Database of Systematic Reviews*, (10), CD004282. doi:10.1002/14651858.CD004282.pub3

Saarik, J., & Hartley, J. (2010). Living with cancer-related fatigue: Developing an effective management programme. *International Journal of Palliative Nursing, 16*(1), 6, 8–12. doi:10.12968/ijpn.2010.16.1.46178

Salakari, M. R. J., Surakka, T., Nurminen, R., & Pylkkänen, L. (2015). Effects of rehabilitation among patients with advanced cancer: A systematic review. *Acta Oncologica, 54*(5), 618–628. doi:10.3109/0284186X.2014.996661

Santiago-Palma, J., & Payne, R. (2001). Palliative care and rehabilitation. *Cancer, 92*(4 Suppl.), 1049–1052. doi:10.1002/1097-0142(20010815)92:4+<1049::AID-CNCR1418>3.0.CO;2-H

Saunders, C. (1987). What's in a name? *Palliative Medicine, 1,* 57–61. doi:10.1177/026921638700100108

Silver, J. K., Raj, V. S., Fu, J. B., Wisotzky, E. M., Smith, S. R., & Kirch, R. A. (2015). Cancer rehabilitation and palliative care: Critical components in the delivery of high-quality oncology services. *Supportive Care in Cancer, 23*(12), 3633–3643. doi:10.1007/s00520-015-2916-1

Skilbeck, J., & Payne, S. (2003). Emotional support and the role of clinical nurse specialists in palliative care. *Journal of Advanced Nursing, 43*(5), 521–530. doi:10.1046/j.1365-2648.2003.02749.x

Small, N. (2003). The changing National Health Service, user involvement and palliative care. In B. Monroe & D. Oliviere (Eds.), *Patient participation in palliative care: A voice for the voiceless* (pp. 8–22). Oxford, UK: Oxford University Press.

Stiel, S., Pastrana, T., Balzer, C., Elsner, F., Ostgathe, C., & Radbruch, L. (2012). Outcome assessment instruments in palliative and hospice care: A review of the literature. *Supportive Care in Cancer, 20*(11), 2879–2893. doi:10.1007/s00520-012-1415-x

Stjernswärd, J. (2007). Palliative care: The public health strategy. *Journal of Public Health Policy, 28*(1), 42–55. doi:10.1057/palgrave.jphp.3200115

Syrett, E., & Taylor, J. (2003). Non-pharmacological management of breathlessness: A collaborative nurse–physiotherapist approach. *International Journal of Palliative Nursing, 9*(4), 150–156. doi:10.12968/ijpn.2003.9.4.11499

Talbot, L., & Verrinder, G. (2005). *Promoting health: The primary health care approach* (3rd ed.). Sydney, Australia: Churchill Livingstone.

Tester, C. Y. (2008a). Impact. In K. M. Boog & C. Y. Tester (Eds.), *Palliative care: A practical guide for the health professional. Finding meaning and purpose in life and death.* (pp. 17–30). Edinburgh, UK: Churchill Livingstone Elsevier.

Tester, C. Y. (2008b). Palliative rehabilitation. In K. M. Boog & C. Y. Tester (Eds.), *Palliative care: A practical guide for the health professional. Finding meaning and purpose in life and death* (pp. 45–62). Philadelphia, PA: Elsevier.

Thomas, T., & Barclay, S. (2015). Continuous subcutaneous infusion in palliative care: A review of current practice. *International Journal of Palliative Nursing, 21*(2), 60–64. doi:10.12968/ijpn.2015.21.2.60

Tookman, A., Hopkins, C., & Scharpen-von-Heussen, K. (2004). Rehabilitation in palliative medicine. In H. G. Doyle, N. I. Cherny, & K. Calman (Eds.), *Textbook of palliative medicine* (3rd ed., pp. 1021–1032). New York, NY: Oxford University Press.

Vockins, H. (2004). Occupational therapy intervention with patients with breast cancer: A survey. *European Journal of Cancer Care, 13*(1), 45–52. doi:10.1111/j.1365-2354.2004.00443.x

Waldron, M., Kernohan, W. G., Hasson, F., Foster, S., Cochrane, B., & Payne, C. (2011). Allied health professionals' views on palliative care for people with advanced Parkinson's disease. *International Journal of Therapy and Rehabilitation, 18*(1), 48–58.

Woodruff, R. (2004). *Palliative medicine: Evidence-based symptomatic and supportive care for patients with advanced cancer.* New York, NY: Oxford University Press.

World Health Organization. (1978). *The declaration of Alma-Ata.* Geneva, Switzerland: Author.

World Health Organization. (1987). *The Ottawa charter for health promotion.* Geneva, Switzerland: Author.

Mertie L. Potter & Brendan P. Wynne

Loss, Grief, and Bereavement

KEY POINTS

- Loss and suffering are universal experiences that occur across the life span.
- Traditional grieving theories view the process in stages with closure or resolution; more contemporary theories view the process as nonstaged, individual, and ongoing.
- Although culture and ethnicity may influence an individual's views on living with and dying from life-threatening illness, individuals must be recognized as unique and encouraged to grieve as is most appropriate for them.
- Nurses are on their own journeys along with patients, families, and significant others as patients face living with and dying from life-threatening illness.
- Nursing presence is an important aspect that can enhance healing in others who are grieving.

CASE STUDY

Ms. Lopez, a 54-year-old divorced female, is hospitalized in the medical–surgical unit. She always has said she "doesn't like doctors" and rarely seeks out medical care. Three months ago she presented to the emergency room for pelvic pain and vaginal bleeding. The workup at that time showed that she had advanced endometrial cancer with metastasis to the stomach and lungs. At that time she had a central venous catheter in place and was started on chemotherapy. Last week it was discovered Ms. Lopez developed septicemia and her chemotherapy treatments were placed on hold. Several days ago, the hospitalist caring for her suggested a palliative care (PC) consult. At the suggestion, Ms. Lopez became angry and demanded to leave the hospital against medical advice (AMA), stating she was going to get "a second opinion." She was discharged AMA and returned home with visiting nurse services. Within 24 hours the visiting nurse determined that Ms. Lopez was unsafe to care for herself alone and she was readmitted to the hospital. Since her readmission, Ms. Lopez has been angry and only partially cooperative with her care. She frequently asks to be left alone.

Ms. Lopez has two adult children: Martin, a single 29-year-old who lives in the next state, and Camila, a 30-year-old mother of 7-year-old Victoria. Prior to her illness, Ms. Lopez would care for Victoria 3 days a week while Camila was at work. Camila and Victoria have been visiting Ms. Lopez every evening, and Victoria is somewhat frightened by all the equipment in the room. She asks many questions to both her mother and grandmother about what is happening, why Lita (Spanish nickname for "grandmother") is so sick, and when will she get better.

LOSS AND SUFFERING

Like 7-year-old Victoria, I was very moved by two deaths in my early childhood: my grandmother's and a little bird's. I was 6 years old. My sister and I were doing our nightly routine. My mother came into our room and sat down on my bed. Mom was crying. She had just received a phone call from "way far away" (my 6-year-old mind's concept of distance) informing us my grandmother had died. Although I had seen my grandmother only a few times in my young life, I felt very connected to her. I loved her very much, because I felt cherished by her. I also knew my mom and dad loved her greatly, and that Grammie had been sick for a long time. Mom answered our questions and prayed with my sister and me. After my mom and big sister left the room, I remember that I "talked to" Grammie from my bedroom window. I said, "I don't know if you can hear me, but I love you a lot and will miss you." I felt sad and cried. I waited, half expecting to hear an answer from her; it was okay when I did not. It was our little good-bye with one another. I felt secure that she was in Heaven and that Heaven seemed like a good place for her to be if she were dead and no longer on earth. I felt at peace.

The other striking memory related to death occurred at the same period of time. My sister and I were playing in one of our favorite pine-needle-laden spots on our farm. We came upon a dead robin. We were horror struck to see this beautiful creature lifeless on the ground. We ran and got a dustpan and gently scooted the bird onto it with a little pine branch. We dug a hole, wrapped the bird in a paper towel, respectfully placed it in a shoebox, and laid the bird to rest in its grave. We read Scripture, sang a hymn, and prayed for the bird. I was very grateful I had an older sister who knew how to conduct a proper funeral service for this dear little creature. We were both sad and cried. That also was the first time I remember questioning if animals have souls and where they go when they die.

Loss and suffering are major experiences along life's journey. How one learns to accept, adapt to, and advance through these experiences determines how the individual will move through life itself. Are loss and suffering perceived as natural, functional, growth-promoting, and normal dimensions in and transitions through life, or are they perceived as unnatural, dysfunctional, harmful, and abnormal circumstances to be avoided?

CASE STUDY *Continued*

On Day 5 Martin arrives. His sister has been keeping him updated on their mother's condition, and he has taken time off from work as Camila has informed him that "things are getting more serious." Ms. Lopez is in pain, has a fever, and has had difficulty breathing. Last night she was started on oxygen. Martin is upset by both Ms. Lopez's angry account of how "they aren't doing anything for me, they just want me to die" and how frail his mother looks. On separate occasions both Camila and Martin speak to Kate, Ms. Lopez's primary nurse, outside of her room. Martin says that he wants everything possible done for his mother and wants to know what else can be done to "beat this thing." Camila, on the other hand, wants her mother kept as comfortable as possible and wants to know more about the PC consult.

■ LIVING WITH AND DYING FROM LIFE-THREATENING ILLNESS

"Losing, leaving, and letting go" are normal processes that help individuals grow (Viorst, 1987, p. 3). However, contemporary grief theorists suggest that grief may be an ongoing experience in which one connects with the lost relationship via memories, heritage, or spirit, rather than sever the relationship (Moules, Simonson, Fleiszer, Prins, & Glasgow, 2007; Moules, Simonson, Prins, Angus, & Bell, 2004). Loss and suffering are inescapable dimensions of life. How an individual transitions through loss and suffering is what remains variable. When planning the patient's care, it is important for the nurse to note how the patient with a life-threatening illness and his or her significant others view loss, suffering, and living with

TABLE 11.1	ACCESS Method of Transcultural Nursing
Assessment	Focus on cultural aspects of clients' lifestyle, health beliefs, and health practices
Communication	Be aware of variations in verbal and nonverbal responses
Cultural negotiation and compromise	Become more aware of aspects of other people's culture as well as understanding
Establishing respect and rapport	Establish a therapeutic relation that portrays genuine respect for clients' cultural beliefs and values
Sensitivity	Deliver diverse culturally sensitive care to culturally diverse groups
Safety	Enable clients to derive a sense of cultural safety

Source: From Narayanasamy, A. (2006). The impact of empirical studies of spirituality and culture on nurse education. *Journal of Clinical Nursing, 15*(7), 840–851. doi:10.1111/j.1365-2702.2006.01616.x

and dying from such an illness. It also is important for nurses to examine their own beliefs related to these life experiences. Developing awareness of and attending to each person's perspective is key in formulating successful interventions.

Provision of nursing care takes place within a person's cultural context. Having an awareness of a patient's cultural background, as well as his or her usual cultural interventions, is both helpful and important. Variations within specific cultures exist, so it is important to discern with a patient and significant others what specific customs and rituals around death and grief are important and preferred (Choi & Lee, 2007; Clements et al., 2003; Mystakidou, Tsilika, Parpa, Katsouda, & Vlahos, 2003). Holloway (2006) considers death to be a leveler in the context of culture; death causes individuals to face the common humanity of mankind. However, nurses must explore the individual's specific view of dying and death while considering the individual's view of self within a given culture or ethnicity. Narayanasamy (2006, p. 841)

details an "ACCESS" model of transcultural nursing (see Table 11.1).

The living–dying interval often is a time of great uncertainty and questioning. Patients may question, Why? Why me? Why now? Patients often seek answers to questions related to the meaning of life, the meaning of suffering, the meaning of death, and the meaning of loss. This may be a time of opportunity for the patient to grow and sense a greater wholeness than ever before in spite of an acute awareness of loss, suffering, and grief. Helping patients living with and dying from a life-threatening illness focus on what they are able to do rather than on what they cannot do is an important nursing intervention.

Grief is considered by clinicians in both traditional and contemporary views as work. Grief work involves cognitive and emotional realms. At the heart of grief is "excruciating sorrow," and at the core of grief work is "spiritual comfort" and "spiritual healing" (Moules et al., 2007, p. 127).

CASE STUDY *Continued*

Kate has been Ms. Lopez's primary nurse for most of the time she has been hospitalized. Kate is upset by Ms. Lopez's anger, her frequent refusal of care, and her rejection of Kate's efforts to connect with her. She is frustrated that Ms. Lopez does not seem to recognize that she is at the end stage of her disease and blames Kate and the rest of the team for being unable to treat her cancer. On several occasions, Kate has driven home from her shift in tears. Kate lost her own mother 3 years ago and identifies with what Camila and Martin are going through; she sets up an appointment to meet with her supervisor to process her feelings.

The Nurse's Role

Nurses meet individuals across the life span and often at the crossroads of their suffering and loss. Regardless of the setting, nurses are in a unique position to help individuals and their significant others who may be in physical, emotional, social, and spiritual pain related

to suffering and loss. The nurse has a broad-based background in providing competent nursing care to individuals across the health–illness continuum. The breadth and depth of each nurse's skills in the specific area of giving care to those living with and dying from terminal illness will be dependent on numerous factors. Some of these include the nurse's personal beliefs and values, life experiences (professional/nonprofessional), level of comfort with death and dying, educational level, licensure, and interest in this area.

Every nurse must be committed to providing patients, either directly or indirectly, quality care at the end of life. Critical to helping the nurse fulfill this obligation is a degree of comfort in dealing with death and dying. Student nurses need experience and support coping with dying and deceased patients. One student nurse shared how traumatic it was for her during her senior preceptorship to be left alone while providing her first postmortem care; the staff member assisting her had to step out of the room temporarily. The student nurse expressed frustration with herself that she felt "frozen" and "scared" until the staff member returned. Processing this experience with her faculty member helped her.

Knowledge of the process of dying and the degree of comfort in dealing with others who are experiencing death and dying are two important areas in which the advanced practitioner's education, experience, and expertise will provide more depth in discerning the special needs of the patient. Furthermore, the advanced practice nurse's skill level is more appropriate for dealing with high-risk and complicated situations.

A number of endeavors have been supported to enhance end-of-life (EOL) care and further education around death, grief, and bereavement. One project is the End of Life Nursing Education Consortium (ELNEC) funded by the Robert Wood Johnson Foundation. Nurses involved with the ELNEC project developed a curriculum to improve EOL nursing care. Nurses are taught interventions that assist patients and families experiencing loss, grief, death, and bereavement, particularly in relation to effective and supportive communication strategies (Matzo et al., 2003; Matzo & Sherman, 2006). To date, ELNEC has trained over 21,000 nurses across the United States. Its curriculum has been adapted for critical care, geriatrics, veterans, pediatrics, oncology, and public hospitals—and has specialty courses for advanced practice registered nurses (APRNs) and graduate nurses. The curriculum has been translated into many languages and is being taught in places such as Japan and Africa (American Association of Colleges of Nursing [AACN], 2016). With a growing body of evidence supporting its efficacy, ELNEC arguably is becoming the gold standard in EOL education for nurses.

Communication may be impaired or even unintelligible in the dying patient. In such circumstances, the nurse needs to inform the patient that the nurse is attempting to understand. It also is important for the nurse to convey an understanding of how difficult it must be for the patient to be unable to communicate and that the nurse will make every effort to meet the patient's needs.

Living with and dying from a life-threatening illness can thrust a patient into a sense of uncertainty. Each patient must be allowed to live and die in his or her own way. The nurse may assist patients to express what this

way is and help them regain some semblance of control (Ferrell & Coyle, 2008). Nurses must be educated to promote holistic care, recognizing that quality-of-life (QOL) issues that are important to dying patients include finding peace of mind, having a voice and being heard, finding meaning, experiencing comfort, and seeking spiritual understanding (Ferrell & Coyle, 2008).

Fostering patterns that are health promoting and positive for individuals is the ideal in nursing care. Unhealthy patterns need to be identified and interventions provided to promote health and healing even as death approaches.

■ EXPERIENCE OF LOSS AND SUFFERING ACROSS THE LIFE SPAN

At birth, an infant is thrust or pulled into a new environment through expulsion and separation from the mother's womb. The infant has no control over this experience. A fairly traumatic transition takes place; one no longer is in the safe and warm environment that provided nourishment and protection during this critical developmental stage. The infant now has to adjust to a new home. This new environment includes the experiences of suffering and loss.

Nearing the sixth month, the infant usually develops an acute awareness of separation from the mother or mother figure. This state is referred to as separation anxiety. This keen awareness of loss may initiate a rudimentary development of death awareness (Backer, Hannon, & Gregg, 1994). This hypothesis is based on Bowlby's (1980) model of attachment between mother and infant and the infant's experience of separation from the mother. As the individual continues to develop, suffering and loss continue to occur. Generally, this occurrence causes the individual to move from a dependent state to an interdependent state and then to an independent state. In some cases, usually due to more loss and suffering, the individual may return to a dependent or interdependent state prior to death. Thus, life often involves a rhythm of change, interfacing with suffering and loss, from the time an individual is born.

Children under the age of 2 years usually have a sense of separation but little understanding of the concept of death. For children between 2 and 5 years of age, death is seen as a transient state but not a permanent event.

Between 6 and 10 years of age, children begin to grasp the reality of death (McIntier, 1995). Adolescents conceptualize death in a way similar to adults; namely, they are mortal and will eventually die. As the adolescent comes to terms with his or her individuality and increasing independence, there is an increasing awareness of one's own mortality. Although death is considered a future event to adolescents and young adults, death anxiety is more evident than at earlier ages. Middle-aged adults and older adults are more aware and accepting of death.

TABLE 11.2 Developmental Views of Death

Age (Years)	Stage of Development	Task/Area of Resolution
Birth to <2	Infancy	Sense of separation; no concept of death
2–5	Early childhood	Death is transient; is not a permanent state
6–10	Late childhood	Beginning awareness of the reality of death
11–25	Adolescence–young adulthood	Similar to adult view—realization of mortality and eventual death; death anxiety more evident; death perceived as a future event
26–65	Middle-aged and older adults	More aware and accepting of death

Sources: Adapted from McIntier, T. M. (1995). Nursing the family when a child dies. *RN, 58*(2), 50–54, quiz 55. doi:10.1016/j.ejon.2013.11.004; Rando, T. A. (1984). *Grief, dying, and death*. Champaign, IL: Research Press.

However, no assumptions can be made concerning any age group, and the previous remarks are generalizations. Each individual's response to death is unique (Rando, 1984; see Table 11.2 for developmental views of death).

■ THEORETICAL UNDERPINNINGS AND THEORIES ON DEATH AND DYING

Stage theory of grief, although widely accepted, has been empirically tested only recently (Maciejewski, Zhang, Block, & Prigerson, 2007). This longitudinal study consisted of 233 individuals experiencing grief after the loss of a family member to natural causes. The stages encompassing disbelief, yearning, anger, depression, and acceptance attained peak values in the given sequence when rescaled but not in the expected sequencing when examined for most frequently endorsed at initial checkpoints. An interesting finding was that the first four negative indicators all reached maximum values within a 6-month period (disbelief—1 month; yearning—4 months; anger—5 months; and depression—6 months). Acceptance increased throughout the entire 24-month observation period.

As will be reviewed, Engel (1964), Freud (1957), Glasser and Strauss (1965), Kubler-Ross (1969), and Lindemann (1944) developed classical work related to dying and death. Bowlby (1980), Pattison (1977), Rando (1984), and Worden (1991) broadened knowledge in the field with their work. More recent writings by Buckman (1993), Copp (1997), Corr (1992), Evans (1994), and Mallinson (1999) have challenged, as well as added to, previous theoretical information. New information relevant to theories on death and dying is expanding rapidly. Contemporary research on death and dying views the time frame for grief resolution in a less restrictive way than earlier writings. Although different in some ways, most of the authors demonstrate a similar thread and core knowledge related to grief work that is helpful to both the beginning clinician and the advanced practitioner.

Freud (1957) brought the concept of grief work to the forefront after examining his personal feelings and societal observations following the mass losses brought about by World War I. He saw grief as a necessary process to assist an individual in adapting to loss. He also felt an individual needed to free himself or herself from attachment to the "lost object."

Lindemann (1944) studied bereavement in individuals who were survivors of the Coconut Grove Hotel fire in Boston (as well as their close relatives), patients who lost a relative while in treatment, relatives of members of the service, and relatives of patients who died while in the hospital. He determined that common physical symptoms, affective symptoms, behavioral manifestations, and physiological changes accompanied each grief experience. Lindemann also first alluded to anticipatory grief in relation to women anticipating the potential death of significant males in their lives during World War II.

Engel (1964) cited three stages through which one progresses in uncomplicated bereavement: shock and disbelief, developing awareness, and restitution and recovery. Engel pointed out that denial predominates initially and helps prevent the individual from being totally overwhelmed. During the second stage, the individual may express guilt and cry. Finally, thoughts and memories of the deceased are discussed and behaviors of the deceased may be displayed by the bereaved.

Glasser and Strauss (1965) examined different contexts related to caregivers' and patients' relation to knowledge about a patient's dying. They suggested that there are four states of awareness related to dying: closed awareness, suspicion awareness, mutual pretense awareness, and open awareness. In the first context, closed awareness, caregivers are aware that the patient is dying but keep that information from the patient. In suspicion awareness, the caregivers know that the patient is dying, but the patient only suspects he or she is dying. The patient is ambivalent about wanting to know and not wanting to know that he or she is dying. In the mutual pretense context, both the caregiver and the patient act as though they do not know the patient is dying, but both know that the patient is. Within the context of open awareness, there is a sharing of knowledge, information, and communication about the patient's dying between the caregiver and the patient (Glasser & Strauss, 1965; Rando, 1984).

Kubler-Ross (1969) studied more than 200 patients diagnosed with terminal cancer. Her work was pivotal in theorizing that individuals move through (not necessarily sequentially) five phases when trying to cope with pending death. These five stages are denial and isolation, anger, bargaining, depression, and acceptance. In the denial and isolation phase, an individual experiences shock and disbelief. A comment such as "I don't believe this is happening" may be made. During the anger phase, the individual questions, "Why me?" Anger often is displaced. The individual may try to rationalize during the bargaining phase by pleading or regretting, "Yes, me, but ..."; bargaining is an attempt to postpone death and extend life. It involves self-imposed deadlines. During the depression phase, the individual may express feelings of guilt or sadness, such as "Yes, this is happening to me." There often is an awareness of great loss for the patient. In the acceptance stage, the struggle is over. The individual has come to accept imminent death and is ready to let go and move on. A comment such as "My time is close; it's all right now" may be made.

Pattison (1977) was the first to focus on a model that examined the "living–dying interval." He defined that interval as existing between knowing that death was imminent and the actual point of death. He incorporates three clinical phases within the living–dying interval: the acute crisis phase, the chronic living–dying phase, and the terminal phase. During the acute crisis phase, the patient is confronted with the knowledge that a process beyond the patient's control influences his or her death. The chronic living–dying phase involves an acute awareness of living and dying simultaneously. Finally, the terminal phase commences when the patient starts withdrawing from the outside world. There is an internal awareness that the patient must conserve energies for himself/herself.

Bowlby (1980) described four phases of bereavement: numbness, yearning and searching, disorganization and despair, and reorganization. His theory is based on an attachment model in which the child must separate from the mother. The process includes (a) shock and disbelief related to the loss (numbness); (b) protest involving an attempt to regain the lost object (yearning and searching); (c) an intense sense of despair in which the individual tries to regain the lost object (disorganization and despair); and (d) completion of the mourning when the individual stops searching and develops new relationships (reorganization; Evans, 1994).

Worden (1991) refers to four tasks of mourning: accepting the reality of the loss, experiencing the pain of grief, adjusting to an environment in which the deceased is not there, and emotionally relocating the deceased and

moving on with life. Mourning may become maladaptive if an individual's response is to avoid, distort, amplify, or prolong grief (Kissane & Bloch, 2002).

Rando (1984) cites six processes of mourning or grief work: recognizing the loss, reacting to the separation, recollecting and reexperiencing the deceased and the relationship in a realistic way, relinquishing old attachments to the deceased and the assumptive world, readjusting to move adaptively in the new world without forgetting the old, and reinvesting. Rando (1984) considers that complicated grief may exist if there is compromise, distortion, or failure of one or more of the six "R" processes occurring after consideration of the amount of time since death.

As mentioned, Buckman (1993), Copp (1997), and Corr (1992) developed more contemporary theories. Corr expanded the theoretical premise of task work postulated by Pattison (1977) and Kalish (1979) to include four major areas of task work in coping with dying, specifically physical, psychological, social, and spiritual loss. Addressing physical tasks involves meeting bodily needs satisfactorily and minimizing the individual's physical distress. Working through psychological tasks maximizes the individual's psychological security, autonomy, and richness of living. In order to meet social tasks, interpersonal attachments of significance must be sustained and enhanced; in addition, individuals must be assisted to explore social implications of dying. Likewise, spiritual task work involves determining and affirming sources of spiritual energy that, in turn, stimulate hope.

Buckman (1993) promoted the concept that grief is more characteristic of the individual than of the individual's progression through particular grief stages. The second major point made by Buckman is that an individual's movement during the grieving process is dependent on resolution of various issues related to emotions rather than changing from one emotion to another, as in Kubler-Ross's model. Additionally, Buckman addressed other responses to dying, such as fear of dying, guilt, hope, despair, and humor (Buckman, 1993).

Copp's (1997) work with dying individuals and the nurses caring for them examined two additional dimensions that seem to occur within the dying individual: readiness to die and a body–person split. Copp observed many direct and indirect actions between patients and nurses: protecting and letting go, watching and waiting, and holding on and letting go. Copp further noted a distinct reference by nurses and patients to the body as separate from the self in relation to patients who were nearing death. A dying individual's personal acceptance of imminent death and physical condition determined the individual's readiness to die. The states of readiness included the following: (a) person ready, body not ready; (b) person ready, body ready; (c) person not ready, body ready; and (d) person not ready, body not ready. One major thrust of Copp's (1998) work is that the dying experience impacts everyone who is involved with the dying patient.

Theories are emerging that demonstrate the ongoing process and complexity of reconstructing meaning for individuals who have experienced a loss versus traditional, linear, stage theories (Pilkington, 2008). These theories are supported through qualitative studies, such as those related to parents dealing with loss of an infant through sudden infant death syndrome (SIDS; Krueger, 2006).

Florczak (2008) incorporates Parse's (2007) human becoming theory in her contemporary conceptualization of grief. Florczak's views vary from traditional ones in that she asserts as follows: (a) The loss is maintained, not severed; (b) a changed meaning about the loss occurs; and (c) sorrow persists related to unfamiliar–familiar patterns being woven into one's life related to the loss (Florczak, 2008).

In contemporary grief theory, grief is seen as dynamic, individualized, pervasive, ongoing, and normative (Cowles & Rodgers, 2000). Contemporary theorists address masculine and feminine differences in grieving (Baum, 2003; McCreight, 2004; Thomas, 2004).

As Pilkington (2006) points out, many of the studies done in relation to human becoming theory are qualitative. Thus, they are not generalizable. However, they provide knowledge for nurses to better understand the importance of presence and to better relate to those who are grieving. Although sorrow related to the loss may continue, the meaning attributed to the loss may change as the individual continues to journey through the process of separating–connecting (Florczak, 2008).

In recent years, Bonanno has challenged many assumptions regarding the way in which people react to bereavement and grief. Following subjects over long periods of time and utilizing sophisticated modeling techniques, Bonanno's research suggests that the most common reaction to grief is not prolonged distress or depression but a stable trajectory with minimal disruption of healthy functioning (Bonanno, Westphal, & Mancini, 2011). Termed *resilience*, this method of coping is often predicted by a number of personality traits present prior to the grief experience. Some of these traits include hardiness, self-enhancement, and a tendency toward positive emotions (Bonanno, 2004). Additionally, Bonanno rejects the notion that people grieve in stages or react to grief experiences in similar ways and instead reports that there is wide variability in response to grief.

■ DIMENSIONS OF LOSS, SUFFERING, GRIEF, AND BEREAVEMENT: DEFINITIONS

Loss

Defined as being deprived of something or someone, loss can be actual, potential, physical, or symbolic. Loss related to health, function, roles, relationships, and life itself is the central focus of this book. Losses other than the death of the loved one are referred to as secondary losses (Rando, 1984).

K. R. Mitchell and Anderson (1983) describe six types of loss: materialistic, relational, intrapsychic, functional, role, and systemic. Material loss involves separation from a physical object or surroundings. In relationship loss, an individual no longer has the ability to relate to another individual. Intrapsychic loss impacts an individual's self-image through loss of what might have been changed perceptions, lost emotions (i.e., faith, hope, or courage), or emotions that result when a major task has been completed successfully. Functional loss occurs through bodily decline or deterioration in illness or aging. Role loss results when an individual changes or loses a customary role (e.g., healthy person to terminally ill person) or acquires a new role (e.g., patient). Systemic loss involves the loss of contact with customary behaviors or functions within a system, such as absence from a usual work environment or home environment.

Loss can be primary or secondary. Primary loss refers to the initial loss (whether of health for the patient or possibly loss of the patient through death for the significant others). Secondary losses stem from the initial loss. As a result of being diagnosed with a terminal illness, the patient also may experience secondary losses of roles, job, income, and so forth. Significant others may experience secondary losses of roles, income, their own health, and so forth.

CASE STUDY *Continued*

Until today, Ms. Lopez has been able to ambulate to the bathroom with assistance. Today she is too weak to walk, and Kate asked Martin, Camila, and Victoria to step out of the room while she and a nursing assistant help Ms. Lopez with a bedpan. Ms. Lopez's family members begin to experience "anticipatory grief" as they watch her condition decline. After finishing with the bedpan, Ms. Lopez touches Kate's hand and thanks her.

Suffering

Suffering is defined as the bearing of pain or distress. It impacts a patient's body, mind, and spirit. Cassell (1991) defines suffering as "the state of severe distress associated with events that threaten the intactness of person" (p. 33). He recognizes the importance of human suffering within any of the human dimensions, such as body, mind, and spirit. He also advocates asking individuals about the presence or absence of suffering because suffering is a very individualized experience and may result from treatment as well as from the disease process or a number of other events. Ferrell and Coyle (2008) assert that relieving suffering is the crux of nurses' professional work.

According to Georgesen and Dungan (1996), the presence of pain compounds suffering and results in spiritual distress. Pain is a frequent companion of terminal illness. Suffering can be present with or without the presence of pain. Suffering, however, cannot be treated or managed like pain. Suffering is a personal experience. Framing suffering in a religious, philosophical, or personally meaningful perspective can help patients endure it better (Rando, 1984). Physical pain is associated with psychological, social, and spiritual distress; pain that continues without meaning results in suffering (Ferrell & Coyle, 2008).

Suffering can be acute or chronic. Acute suffering occurs when the patient is in crisis and confronted with an immediate loss. Chronic suffering results from the longer-term realization and impact of a loss that carries a great deal of significance for, and meaning to, the patient. The patient with a terminal illness may experience only one type of suffering, both types at different times, or both simultaneously. Intervention involves trying to understand the patient's suffering and trying to help the patient cope effectively with suffering. Key to helping the suffering patient is attempting to understand the meaning of the suffering and to comfort and sustain the individual through it.

Similar to chronic suffering is the middle-range nursing theory of chronic sorrow introduced by Eakes, Burke, and Hainsworth (1998). Chronic sorrow is viewed as normal in response to the recurrent experience of ongoing, significant loss that may be actual or symbolic or both. Major concepts within this theory relate to the following: losses, disparity between reality and idealism, trigger events or milestones, and an individual's internal and external means of managing recurring grief that accompanies chronic sorrow. One of the key antecedents to chronic sorrow, namely, disparity between the individual's current reality and idealized reality, is what differentiates chronic sorrow from chronic suffering. An individual experiencing chronic suffering does not necessarily face disparity with chronic suffering. Interventions are aimed at helping the patient with chronic sorrow acknowledge and bear his or her pain, with the goal of redefining the overwhelming scope and impact of a loss into more manageable proportions, thereby decreasing the impact of chronic sorrow on daily living (Rossheim & McAdams, 2010).

CASE STUDY *Continued*

On her way out from visiting with her mother, Camila informs Kate that her mother is in more pain. Kate assures her she will do a pain assessment. During her assessment Ms. Lopez tells Kate that she is afraid. She is afraid of being in pain and she is afraid of dying. She asks Kate to stay with her a while as she does not want to be alone. As they sit, Ms. Lopez questions Kate about her knowledge of the "palliative care the doctors are suggesting." Ms. Lopez admits that she feels as if having the consult is a sign she is "giving up." After a long conversation she asks Kate if she would sit with her and her family during the PC consult.

Grief

Grief is defined as deep or intense sorrow or distress, particularly arising from bereavement concerning someone with whom a close bond was formed. Rando (1984) describes grief as a normal reaction to the perception of loss. Grief is generally a transitory, acute state in response to loss with the possibility that the individual's ability to function may be disrupted temporarily. In addition, the individual may be distracted, disoriented, distressed, or all of these (Mallinson, 1999). Feelings that may accompany grief include anger, shame, helplessness, sadness, guilt, despair, relief, peacefulness, calm, and release (McCall, 1999). Charleton (2003) asserts that stages of grieving might include any or all of the following: "distress, shock, denial, anger, feeling 'low in spirits,' depression, resignation, acceptance, resolution" (p. 671).

Common grief responses are listed in Table 11.3. These responses may involve physical, psychological, and spiritual/sociocultural responses. They may have aspects that seem contradictory in nature. The impact of grief can be extensive and pervasive. Anticipatory grief, those feelings of grief experienced prior to an expected loss, generally assists individuals in working through depression related to the upcoming death, rehearsing of the death, adjusting to the consequences of the death, and having an increased concern for the terminally ill (Fulton & Fulton, 1971). Rando (1984)

TABLE 11.3	Grief Responses		
Physical	**Psychological**	**Spiritual/Sociocultural**	**Dichotomous Nature**
■ Shortness of breath ■ Insomnia ■ Loss of appetite ■ Loss of sleep ■ Energy loss ■ Greater susceptibility to illness ■ Sighing ■ Nervousness and restlessness ■ Sensation of something in the throat ■ Feelings of emptiness or heaviness[a] ■ Heart palpitations ■ Crying ■ Psychomotor retardation ■ Decreased libido or hypersexuality ■ Weight loss[b]	■ Depression ■ Anxiety ■ Guilt ■ Anger and hostility ■ Anhedonia ■ Self-reproach ■ Low self-esteem ■ Helplessness and hopelessness ■ Sense of unreality ■ Suspiciousness ■ Interpersonal problems ■ Imitation of the deceased's behaviors ■ Idealization of the deceased ■ Ambivalent feelings about the deceased[c]	■ Spiritual pain and suffering ■ Spiritual loneliness ■ Fear of God, the unknown, and/or the future ■ Feelings of failure and guilt ■ Feelings of unfairness and anger ■ Loss of transcendence ■ Hopelessness[d] ■ Search for meaning ■ A need for love and hope ■ A sense of forgiveness[e] ■ Participation or lack of participation in formal religious groups ■ Views related to use of "extraordinary" life-prolonging measures ■ Beliefs related to afterlife ■ Handling of the body after death ■ Rituals performed after death[f]	■ Universal/individual ■ Benign/malignant ■ Life-giving/life-requiring ■ Active/passive ■ Internal/external ■ State/process ■ Heart/head ■ Inarticulate/poetic ■ Celebration/bereavement[g]

Physical—[a]taken from Lindemann, E. (1944). Symptomatology and management of acute grief. *American Journal of Psychiatry, 101*, 141–148. doi:10.1176/ajp.101.2.141; [b]taken from Rando, T. A. (1984). *Grief, dying, and death*. Champaign, IL: Research Press.
Psychological—[c]taken from Lindemann, E. (1944). Symptomatology and management of acute grief. *American Journal of Psychiatry, 101*, 141–148. doi:10.1176/ajp.101.2.141.
Spiritual/sociocultural—[d]taken from Stuart, G. W., & Sundeen, S. J. (1991). *Principles and practices of psychiatric nursing* (p. 154). Boston, MA: Mosby Year Book; [e]taken from Pritchett, K. T., & Lucas, P. M. (1997). Grief and loss. In B. S. Johnson (Ed.), *Psychiatric-mental health nursing: Adaptation and growth* (4th ed., p. 203). New York, NY: Lippincott; [f]taken from Kazanowski, M. (2013). End-of-life care. In D. D. Ignatavicius & M. L. Workman (Eds.), *Medical-surgical nursing: Patient-centered collaborative care* (7th ed.). St. Louis, MO: Elsevier Saunders.
Dichotomous—[g]taken from Moules, N. J., Simonson, K., Fleiszer, A. R., Prins, M., & Glasgow, R. B. (2007). The soul of sorrow work: Grief and therapeutic interventions with families. *Journal of Family Nursing, 13*(1), 122. doi:10.1177/1074840706297484

views anticipatory grief as also allowing for gradual absorption of the reality of the loss, helping resolve unfinished business, changing assumptions about life and identity, and making future plans.

Evans (1994) challenges the belief that anticipatory grief experienced prior to death is the same process as the conventional grief experienced in the postdeath period. He proposes the use of the label "terminal response" to describe the process that occurs between diagnosis of terminal illness and death. Differences noted between pre- and postdeath grieving include the following: (a) anticipatory grieving ends at the time of death, whereas conventional grieving can go on indefinitely; and (b) anticipatory grieving increases as death draws nearer, but conventional grieving usually diminishes in intensity with time.

CASE STUDY *Continued*

On the day of the PC consult, Kate is there with Ms. Lopez's treatment team. Today, Ms. Lopez's breathing is much worse, and she has a fever of 102.1° F. She has had her pain medication increased. During the meeting, Ms. Lopez is not angry but asks some questions. They discuss with Ms. Lopez, Camila, and Martin treatment options to improve Ms. Lopez's quality of life in the time she has available. During the meeting, Ms. Lopez states her wish to initiate a do-not-resuscitate (DNR) order. This greatly upsets Martin, who begins to cry and excuses himself from the meeting. Afterward Kate offers the family resources that might help them deal with their mother's pending death. Martin decides he would like to talk to the hospital's spiritual care advisor.

Bereavement

Bereavement is defined as the state or act of being deprived of a loved one. McCall (1999) describes bereavement as the "overall reaction to the loss of a close relationship" and sees it as a description of various "patterns, phrases, and/or stages that an individual goes through when grieving" (p. 42). Mallinson (1999) depicts bereavement as the long-term process of the survivor accommodating his or her life without the loved one. Bereavement is a major life event that can result in an individual having impaired health (Charleton, 2003).

Mourning, grief, and *bereavement* often are used interchangeably. Mourning often encompasses a sociocultural dimension and involves customs and rituals that are influenced by sociocultural and religious beliefs and values. Rando (1984) differentiates among the three in the following ways: (a) Grief is the response to the perception of loss and is a transitional phase in the overall process of mourning; (b) mourning is the intrapsychic process initiated by loss; and (c) bereavement is the state of having suffered a loss (pp. 15–16).

CASE STUDY *Continued*

Seeing Martin upset at the meeting reminds Kate of the loss of her own mother 3 years ago. That night she goes through her old photo albums at home and reexperiences the feelings of loss. The next day she schedules some time with her supervisor to discuss her feelings about Ms. Lopez and her family. Kate voices her concerns that her emotions might interfere with the care she is giving.

■ SIGNIFICANCE AND MEANING OF THE RELATIONSHIP TO LOSS AND SUFFERING

The intensity of loss for the dying patient and his or her significant others relates directly to each individual's perceptions of how close the relationship is and how great the loss of this relationship will be. The significance of the relationship impacts how the individual will interpret the loss and the accompanying suffering. The meaning that the patient, significant others, and nurse assign to loss and suffering also will determine how each individual faces the patient's dying and death. The interpretation of loss and suffering is unique to each individual and to each individual's particular circumstances.

Relationships fall into three categories: social, intimate, and therapeutic (Brady, 1997). Social relationships incorporate the everyday contacts individuals have, such as work colleagues and casual friends. Both individuals in this type of relationship are attempting to have their needs met. There is no particular goal within this relationship. Intimate relationships imply commitment by both individuals to each other. Therapeutic relationships involve goal-directed interaction with the purpose of helping one individual obtain an anticipated outcome to meet an identified need and facilitate growth.

The degree of intimacy and involvement within a relationship is not necessarily dependent on the relationship being a long-term one versus a short-term one or a blood relationship versus a nonblood relationship. Many factors determine how an individual will view his or her relationship with another individual. Some of these factors include respect, responsibility, commitment, compatibility, values, biases, beliefs, and time.

The stage of growth and development of the individual with terminal illness influences his or her ability to cope with the loss, suffering, and grief related to terminal illness. The stage of growth and development of significant others and the nurse also determines their ability to cope with the loss, suffering, grief, and bereavement related to the patient with a terminal illness. In addition, the stages of growth and development for all three groups (patient, significant others, and nurse) significantly impact how each will deal with the other.

Two of the most difficult aspects of a terminal illness are the accompanying uncertainty and unpredictability. These two factors may stress the relationships between the patient, the significant others, and the nurse. For some individuals, not knowing what is going to happen to the patient and when it might happen are difficult and unbearable aspects of coping with the patient's terminal illness.

Balancing aspects of "getting through it" and "accepting that it will take time and a lot of hard work" were critical in a study involving 39 families who each had a child diagnosed with cancer (Woodgate & Degner, 2003, p. 117). In addition, support from the family unit was considered most important for helping maintain one's spirit and keeping the family together. Families wanted to share the entire experience of their children's having cancer and not focus on symptomatology.

Some terminal conditions, such as HIV/AIDS, may not be discussed by the patient or significant others who fear stigma or repercussions. In such situations, it is imperative that the nurse understand and be ready to assist the patient and significant others in sharing the pain associated with these conditions.

Often overlooked are the relationships patients have with their pets and the significance these relationships can have in a person's life. Companion animals provide social contact, comfort, and exercise and help their owners feel more relaxed and happy. Companion animals, however, also can add risk to patients' lives. Some patients may delay, avoid, or refuse treatment if they cannot bring their animals or find them proper care. The impact of the loss of a companion animal is poorly recognized and often the grief related to the death of a pet can be as intense as it is for a human. It is important for the nurse to appreciate and assess how patients' relationships with their pets impact their plan of care (Williams, 2016).

Nurses, patients, and caregivers assigned similar meaning to pain in a study of patients with cancer (Ferrell, Taylor, Sattler, Fowler, & Cheyney, 1993). Although both nurses and patients viewed pain as a challenge, nurses saw the challenge to eliminate pain, whereas patients saw the challenge to live with the pain in order to obtain vitality. Caregivers greatly empathized with the patient's pain and experienced personal suffering and grief. Grief was triggered by pain, as it represented death to the caregivers.

Furthermore, an individual's view of change itself will help determine how that individual will accept loss and suffering related to his or her terminal illness. Has the individual's pattern been to welcome and embrace change or resist and fear change? The answer to that question can assist the nurse in implementing care that will help the patient and significant others to grow through the loss and suffering associated with the patient's terminal illness. Knowledge of change theory can help the advanced nurse facilitate acceptance of, and growth through, loss and suffering for the patient, significant others, and the nurse. Knowing the benefits and risks of change, change strategies, and resistance to change can help the nurse maximize the many changes within the patient's life.

■ ASSESSMENT—WHERE AM I (THE NURSE) ON THE JOURNEY?

In order to be an effective caregiver to the dying patient and the significant others, nurses must come to terms with their own mortality and views on dying and death. Death is an inevitable outcome of life for each individual. The death of a patient with a terminal illness forces the nurse to acknowledge that a cure cannot always be achieved. Fear related to death and dying is normal. Likewise, issues related to grief and bereavement during the death and dying process also are normal and even necessary for healthy adaptation to the preceding loss and suffering.

In American culture, individuals generally believe that explanations for dying always should be given. Furthermore, Americans feel that options to deal with the dying process always should be available (Kazanowski, 2013). This widely held belief impacts the nurse, as well

as the patient and significant others, in relation to high expectations of cure, treatment, care, and avoidance of a painful death. This approach is considered by some to be the "medicalization of human mortality"; this approach has limitations, however, because it cannot address psychological and spiritual factors associated with the suffering related to dying (Kissane & Bloch, 2002, pp. 78–79). Furthermore, with an increasing number of states examining physician-assisted suicide or death with dignity laws, the nurse will be called upon to determine further how to participate and assist—or not—in this process.

Nurses are encouraged to maintain their composure when caring for patients. However, professionalism for the nurse within this context does not require that the nurse deny emotional engagement with the patient and significant others during the dying process and bereavement period. It does require, however, that the nurse's needs be subordinate to the needs of the patient and significant others. Constructive self-disclosure of feelings by the nurse may role model to others a healthy process of acknowledging and resolving the suffering of loss. The nurse may or may not actually cry with the patient and significant others. If crying occurs, the nurse needs to be able to direct this situation into a meaningful and positive one for the patient and significant others. Empathy appropriately shared in this manner may well be described as a "therapeutic tear."

Lewis (1998) describes a strategy used to assist nursing students in working with patients and significant others who are experiencing loss and grieving. The learning activity is called Culture and Loss: A Project of Self-Reflection. Student nurses are requested to examine how their culture handles loss, to prepare a creative presentation for a small group of peers on how their culture responds to loss, and to describe to their class the meaning of their project and how it connects to their culture. Goals for implementing this strategy are identifying personal responses to loss, recognizing differing responses to loss and the influence of individual and cultural factors, and learning skills related to supporting individuals who are grieving.

Spencer (1994) examined which strategies were helpful to nurses in dealing with their own grieving. The most significant strategy noted was the nurse's informal network of peer group support. In addition, the nurses recommended formal group support and increased grief resolution training. When a team is involved, it is helpful to provide an opportunity for staff members to have open communication and to sustain and care for one another (Leichtling, 2004). There are numerous other health-promoting strategies to help the nurse cope with caring for dying patients. These include regular exercise, good nutrition, diversional activities, focus on caring rather than curing, emphasizing the positive dimensions of the nurse's role, and recalling positive experiences with families (Pritchett & Lucas, 1997).

Advances in technology have prolonged dying and death in our culture. As a result, advance directives have taken on greater significance in relation to EOL care. Studies have indicated that patients who have prepared advance directives select PC more frequently, are more accepting of death, and have less expensive care and less aggressive treatment (Danis, 1998).

There are incongruences between the ideal and reality in EOL care. First, clinicians are expected to be able to predict the expected time of death for a terminally ill patient; however, this involves a great deal of uncertainty. Goals of care may need to change quickly as the patient's condition changes or therapeutic trials fail. Second, it is expected that the patient's clinicians know the patient's wishes concerning dying and death. In reality, organizational factors may impact the patient's care more than the patient's wishes during the EOL process. Third, it is thought that the patient's care is well coordinated. Often this is not the case because some intensive-care facilities are staffed with their own primary care providers who may not know the patient admitted with a terminal illness. Therefore, it is important for the nurse to work closely with the patient and the significant others concerning the patient's priorities and wishes. Finally, the measurement of goals and outcomes may not be congruent. Measures of care for dying patients usually focus upon frequency of DNR orders and lengths of time a patient spends on life support or in a coma. It may be more important to patients and significant others to examine issues related to pain management and satisfaction with care (Danis, 1998).

Confronting death with a terminal illness is difficult, painful, and complex. Nurses need to be strong advocates for satisfactory pain management. Keeping abreast of the patient's treatment wishes (which may change during the dying process) and coordinating care between facilities and providers also are important. Additionally, nurses may need to coordinate EOL care through use of hospice programs or PC in various settings: hospital, nursing home, or community (Kazanowski, 2013).

Personal Experiences With Death

Personal experiences with dying and death influence how nurses give care to those who are dying and their significant others. For example, examining personal experiences can help nurses understand their own fears and anxieties related to dying and death. Understanding the meaning and significance of relationships helps put the loss in perspective. The nurse's ability to articulate feelings regarding a good or bad death is important when working with individuals who are dying. Exploring individual values and biases can enhance the nurse's competence; this helps the nurse better understand an individual's healthcare attitudes and behaviors (Warren, 1999).

Kazanowski, Perrin, Potter, and Sheehan (2007) developed a course in which student nurses examine their personal losses in a progressive manner, in terms of both the level of difficulty and the level of disclosure. The intent of the course is to assist students in coping with the suffering of patients with whom they are working as well as the suffering they are experiencing themselves in witnessing such suffering. Ideas from the course have broadened to assist nurses in processing the patient's and their own suffering in various settings and points in their professional journey (Perrin, Sheehan, Potter, & Kazanowski, 2012).

Offering one's presence to patients, families, and significant others affects nurses. The impact on a nurse researcher, supervisor, and two transcribers was examined in addition to data obtained from the original sample group of 38 pregnant women in a grounded theory study exploring their experiences after hearing they had a diagnosis of fetal abnormality (Lalor, Begley, & Devane, 2006). The three themes that emerged were as follows: bearing to watch, bearing to listen, and bearing to support. Painful stories cause strong emotional reactions to those interacting with such information (Lalor et al., 2006). Nurses identify sources of suffering for patients and offer their presence to help patients move through the suffering (Ferrell & Coyle, 2008).

Use the following exercises to help you expand your self-understanding in relation to loss and suffering, dying and death, and grief and bereavement.

Self-Reflective Questions

■ What experiences have you had with death? Describe your earliest memory of death. Was anything positive about it? Was anything negative about it? Have you experienced what you would call a "good death"? Have you experienced what you would describe as a "bad death?"
■ Can you picture yourself helping someone who is dying? How? What do you have to offer that is special and unique?
■ Relate what you believe happens when someone dies. What do you fear about death? What do you fear about your own death?
■ Assume you have just received news that you have been diagnosed with a terminal illness. What would be the most difficult things for you to have to give up during this time?
■ How do you feel about cultural attitudes or behaviors that may be different from your own?

■ ASSESSMENT—WHERE IS THE PATIENT ON THE JOURNEY? THE LIFE CYCLE CONTINUUM—ACROSS THE LIFE SPAN ON THE JOURNEY

Living with and dying from a terminal illness can be best understood within the context of a continuum. One generally does not remain on a fixed point along the continuum. Like one's view of health and illness, living with and dying from terminal illness is a dynamic and fluid experience in which the individual moves back and forth across the continuum.

Reactions to dying and death vary across the life span. They also are dependent on physical, psychological, spiritual, and sociocultural factors that impact the individual's sense of wellness. Physiological change can lead to a sequelae of loss: function, body image, self-esteem, sexuality, and role competence. Furthermore, interfacing of the various factors has the potential to result in grief over lost health (Talerico, 2003). The living–dying interval occurs from the time death is acknowledged as imminent to the point of the actual death. A difficult task during this period is continuing to treat the individual as still living, in other words, as a person and not just a patient. Tasks that the individual needs to attend to are arranging his or her affairs, coping with loss (loved ones and self), attending to future care needs, planning remaining time, confronting loss of self and identity, facing one's own death encounter, deciding whether to succumb to or resist the dying process, and struggling with the psychosocial problems of dying. Some of the issues for the individual during this period of time include treatment choices, remissions and exacerbations, expression of sexuality, financial pressures, employment concerns, struggle for control, and suffering (Rando, 1984).

Depending on the level of maturity, the patient may be confronted with the meaning of life, relationship with God and others, and the reality of death (Georgesen & Dungan, 1996). In addition, the patient may face losses related to independence, control, work, physical comfort, a sense of normalcy, sexual activity, and usefulness when living with a life-threatening condition (Ferrell et al., 1993). For example, it may be difficult for older adults who have served as caregivers to receive care from another because of loss of independence. An aid to this transition of caregiving may be to enable older adults to focus on ways they can affirm the individuals now serving as caregivers to them (Talerico, 2003).

Once rapport has been developed, the nurse may suggest that the patient and the patient's significant others consider attending a support group. Support groups have been found to be particularly helpful for significant others facing traumatic (e.g., loss of a child) or stigmatized (e.g., AIDS) deaths, as well as for individuals who themselves are dying (Callanan & Kelley, 1992; Goodkin et al., 1999; McCreight, 2004; Rando, 1984; Vigil & Clements, 2003).

Individual Needs

During the illness/dying trajectory, the nurse needs to assess the patient's immediate and specific needs. Certain simple pleasures may be more important to the patient than a nurse-perceived need for oxygen. For a peaceful death, a patient may need the comfort and joy that a

treat, such as food or music, may represent. Asking the patient (or significant others if the patient is unable to respond) what the immediate and specific needs are may bring insight as to what intervention is needed to help the patient be more comfortable.

Maintaining some control is especially important during this time, as the patient may have had to relinquish control in many areas. Studies have demonstrated that physical and psychological outcomes can be linked to perceptions of control (Volker & Wu, 2011). Moreover, having control over pain is critical. Patients with a terminal illness and their significant others fear lack of pain control during EOL care (Danis, 1998; Ferrell & Coyle, 2008).

Having a sense of order and a sense of closure in personal affairs is an important aspect to address with the patient also. Sharing what one needs to say to others, through direct contact (e.g., in person or phone) or indirect contact (e.g., written communication), may help the patient have a more peaceful death.

Sensitivity to the patient's wishes in this area is critical.

Areas of Assessment

Use the following questions to assess the patient on his or her journey living with and dying from a terminal illness in relation to loss and suffering, dying and death, and grief and bereavement.

■ How do you view your illness?
■ What is the meaning of your illness to you?
■ What fears or concerns do you have regarding your illness?
■ In what ways are you experiencing loss and suffering?
■ Are there any unresolved issues or business matters that need to be resolved?
■ Do you have any specific fears about dying and death in general? About your own dying and death?
■ What concerns do you have for others now and after your death?
■ What helps you maintain a sense of hope during difficult times?
■ What specific needs do you have at this time?
■ In what ways might I be most helpful to you in meeting those needs?

■ ASSESSMENT—WHERE ARE THE SIGNIFICANT OTHERS ON THE JOURNEY?

Healthy spouses of terminally ill cancer patients were studied (Siegel, Karus, Raveis, Christ, & Mesagno, 1996). Males were found to be more at risk for depressive symptoms than females if they were parents of school-aged children. Part of this could be due to their having less of a social network than females in general, and part of this may be due to their having to assume additional parenting responsibilities as the result of their spouse's illness and subsequent death. Overall adjustment was better for well spouses and inversely proportional to the number of children in the household. Work was perceived as both a stressor due to the demands of the job and a stress buffer due to the potential emotional support, sense of control, and predictability it may provide for the significant other. Masculine and feminine differences have been explored more recently as well, indicating that feminine grieving involves more talking, help seeking, and social involvement than masculine styles of grieving that involve solitude, self-medication, and expression of grief through activities (Baum, 2003; McCreight, 2004; Thomas, 2004).

Elderly males have been found to be at an increased risk for suicide after the death of a spouse, especially within the first year (Ajdacic-Gross et al., 2008). In general, older adults face multiple losses for numerous reasons, including declining health with increasing age (Talerico, 2003).

Family often plays a central role in providing support to a patient diagnosed with a terminal illness. Such informal caring may involve considerable physical, psychological, and economic stresses on significant others (Candy, Jones, Drake, Leurent, & King, 2011). As a result, there is reciprocal suffering inherent in being a family member or significant other of a patient diagnosed with a terminal illness. This suffering results from the expectations and responsibilities placed upon the significant other to care for the patient, the mutual experience of intensified needs brought about by the patient's illness, and the often rapidly changing needs of both the patient and the significant other. QOL issues arise for the family members and significant others as well as for the patient (Sherman, 1998). In addition to the needs of the patient, nurses should assess the concerns of caregivers and consider that they may also benefit from additional support (Candy et al., 2011)

Koop and Strang (1997) reviewed a number of studies to determine correlates of greater satisfaction in families of patients with a terminal illness. They found higher satisfaction in families in which there had been psychosocial support from the nurse, fulfillment of basic needs, high frequency of home visits, support at night, connection to other services, visits to the bereaved caregiver, choices in treatments, privacy during hospitalizations, treatment of respiratory symptoms, the presence of professional caregivers (especially if the patient is at home), and participation in a hospice program.

There is interdependence between the patient, the significant others, and the nurse in relation to providing optimal care for the patient with a terminal illness. The nurse can maximize the positive aspects of this interdependence by recognizing and affirming the patient's significant others, incorporating them into the patient's care as desired by the patient, and assisting the significant others in their loss, suffering, and grief related to the patient's dying and

death. Kissane and Bloch (2002) recognized the influence of family in Reiss's (1990) study on renal disease, claiming, "This research highlights the potential influence of the family on both the course of illness and survival" (p. 26). Woodgate and Degner (2003) note in their research of children with cancer, "It is important for those involved in the care to recognize that maintaining the family unit was equally important to families as was beating the child's cancer" (p. 117). In addition, the patient's significant others will experience bereavement issues once the patient dies. Research by Jordan and Neimeyer (2003) demonstrates that "with the help of family and friends, apparently most mourners are able to work through and integrate their losses relatively well" (p. 772).

How does one know when the patient is ready to die? Four types or stages of death occur, usually in the following order: social death, psychological death, biological death, and physiological death (Sudnow, 1967). Social death marks the narrowing of the patient's world, as he or she has known it. This is a highly individualized stage that is dependent on the patient's level of involvement versus detachment in his or her social world. Psychological death is a death of the patient's personality. Relationships change. The patient withdraws and distances himself or herself from others. Terminal illness places demands that result in the patient becoming regressed and dependent. Biological death involves the loss of consciousness and awareness on a self-sustaining basis; the patient may be on life supports at this point. Finally, physiological death occurs. All vital organs cease to function (Rando, 1984). At this point, a nurse or physician (depending on state law) pronounces death. The moment of finality has arrived. Life as the patient and the significant others knew it for the patient has ceased.

Relationships

Support from significant others can aid in decision making and acceptance of death for a patient with a terminal illness. Patients and their significant others may determine together if they want to pursue life-sustaining procedures or to forego them in light of the uncertainty and potential trauma that surround the situation. With the availability of advanced, and potentially life-extending, technology, patients and their significant others often seek the nurse's advice around treatment options at the end of life. The nurse can initiate conversations focused on the patient's expressed goals and values to help guide these decisions. This close communication is essential because as the needs of the patient at the EOL transition, the nurse can utilize these transition points to revisit with the patient and the patient's significant others their prognosis, goals of care, and treatment options. It is especially important to maintain communication because these transition periods can be times of physical, psychological, and existential crisis for patients and significant others (Peereboom & Coyle, 2012).

Significant others who care for a terminally ill patient are faced with increased feelings of powerlessness, anger, and grief when the patient's pain is unrelieved (Ferrell & Coyle, 2008; Ferrell et al., 1993). When patients choose to spend the end of life at home, it is often the significant others who are directly responsible for the patients' care. It is important for the nurse to support, educate, and work collaboratively with the significant other to both control the pain of the patient and reduce the distress that unrelieved pain causes the caregiver. Strategizing a pain management "game plan" with the significant other can help achieve both of these goals.

Areas of Assessment

- Determine with significant others what they perceive as the patient's needs.
- Provide education in pain assessment and pain management strategies.
- Assess how the significant others feel they are doing and what degree of loss and suffering they are currently experiencing.
- What types of secondary losses are being experienced or anticipated as a result of the primary loss (i.e., anticipatory death or actual death of the patient)?
- Determine the level of emotional support needed.
- Ascertain if spiritual support is desired.
- Assure significant others that they are not an imposition to professionals who also are providing care for the patient.
- Identify available resources to help significant others care for the patient.
- Encourage significant others to grieve in whatever ways are best for them.

Normal Grief

Grief is a normal response to loss. Grief may become manifest in feelings, physical sensations, cognition, and behaviors (see Table 11.3). Psychological, sociocultural, and physical factors influence the grief reaction. The nurse needs to assess which factors are influencing the significant others. Rando (1984, pp. 43–57) addresses these influences as follows:
Psychological factors:

- Significance of the loss
- Attachment level
- Family role of the deceased
- Individual coping behaviors, such as avoidance, distraction, preoccupation, impulsivity, rationalization, intellectualization, prayer, and connection with others
- Intelligence and maturity levels
- Previous experience with death and loss
- Conditioned sex roles
- Age of the individual grieving
- Age and characteristics of the deceased

- The death of a parent represents loss of the past
- The death of a spouse represents loss of the present
- The death of a child represents loss of the future and may be the most difficult death to handle
- Unattended business between the griever and the deceased
- Perception of fulfilled life for deceased
- Circumstances related to death including location, type, reason, and preparedness
- Timing of the death (is the death psychologically acceptable?)
- Perception of death's prevention
- Sudden or anticipated death
- Chronic versus acute illness
- Impact of anticipatory grief on the relationship with the dying patient
- Impact of secondary losses
- Additional stresses or crises

Social factors:

- Level, acceptance, timing, and duration of support
- Religious, sociocultural, ethnic, and philosophical backgrounds
- Bereaved's educational, economic, and occupational status
- Positive or negative funeral rituals

Physiological factors:

- Positive and negative impact of medications
- Need for nutrition, sleep and rest, exercise, and physical health

A way to distinguish between grief and depression is to note if the individual in question is able to experience pleasure. Grieving individuals generally can experience pleasure; depressed individuals often have difficulty experiencing pleasure and may lose morale and hope (Kissane & Bloch, 2002). There has been much controversy over the *Diagnostic and Statistical Manual of Mental Disorders, 5th edition* (American Psychiatric Assocation, 2013) inclusion of grief as a psychiatric disorder. What is clear is that bereavement can result in acutely debilitating symptoms; such symptoms usually are temporary but may result in more chronic symptomatology (Shear et al., 2011).

■ CHILD'S EXPERIENCE OF LOSS

The death of a parent impacts a child greatly. Family life and daily routine are disrupted permanently. A child may have a depressed mood, cry, be sad or irritable, withdraw, or have sleep disturbances during the first 4 months after the loss of a parent. Physical, behavioral, and emotional responses occur immediately for young children. Although infants and toddlers are not at a developmental stage to be able to comprehend loss or death, they are distraught that someone important to them is absent (Hames, 2003). A child's reaction may be impacted by individual personality factors, sociocultural factors, the child's age, the child's history, the child's religious beliefs, family dynamics, family's socioeconomic status, sex of the child and the remaining parent, additional stress in the child's life, parental substitutes, nature of the death, and how the child was notified (Geis, Whittlesey, McDonald, Smith, & Pfefferbaum, 1998).

Children who have lost a parent, especially by suicide, are at an increased risk of psychiatric problems. The most common psychiatric complaints in bereaved children are depressive symptoms. Regression may occur temporarily. Having a baseline of a child's behaviors is important when discerning if there is a serious problem. Suicide bereavement is compounded by the stigma and lack of social support oftentimes in such circumstances (Gray, Weller, Fristad, & Weller, 2011; A. M. Mitchell et al., 2007). Melhem, Porta, Shamseddeen, Walker Payne, and Brent (2011) report that

one of the best predictors of a child's well-being after the death of a parent is the well-being of the surviving parent. For example, the risk of the child developing depression increases if the surviving parent is experiencing complicated grief after the death of his or her spouse.

Caregivers must recognize the importance of age in relation to a child's ability to experience loss and grief. Saldinger, Cain, and Porterfield (2003) note that children may have a very difficult experience with anticipatory grief if they are expected to demonstrate levels of "self-sacrifice" that exceed their "levels of maturity" (p. 175). The ELNEC curriculum provides a table of children's ages and expected grief reactions that can be valuable to caregivers (see Table 11.4).

The degree of attachment also impacts how a child will respond to the loss of a parent. Stroebe (2002) found that individuals who had a more secure attachment to the lost figure had a more fluid movement between loss and restoration orientations and experienced less complications with grieving.

CASE STUDY *Continued*

On the weekend Victoria visits with her mother. She has drawn a picture of her Lita in bed with a big band-aid on her. She tries to give her the picture. However, Ms. Lopez opens her eyes only briefly. Victoria cries and asks Camila why Lita won't wake up. Camila tells Victoria that Lita can't wake up because she is very sick. Camila assures Victoria that the nurse said Lita could still hear Victoria if she wants to talk. Victoria tells her she wants Lita to stop being sick so she can come to her house again when mommy is at work.

Children often experience separation anxiety after the death of a parent. Coming to terms with surviving in a world without the presence of the deceased parent can be traumatic for the child. Secondary to that trauma may be the additional stress of observing a surviving parent cope with the loss or the anticipated loss if such were the case (Saldinger et al., 2003). Nurses can help a dying parent communicate with children who will be left behind; this can enhance meaning and comfort to the dying by making a contribution to their child's journey with grief. Likewise, a surviving parent inadvertently becomes a role model for grieving to children left behind by a deceased parent (Hames, 2003).

If a child loses a sibling, other issues, such as guilt, ambivalence, denial, increased vulnerability, and fear for his own well-being, may arise. Parental response to surviving siblings helps determine the child's adjustment. Similar responses may occur for adolescents with possible reframing of the adolescent's self-concept, self-identity, and family role (Geis et al., 1998). Tasks that occur for all siblings of a deceased child, regardless of age, include grieving the deceased sibling, coping with family changes, realigning relationships, and attempting to understand the meaning of the tragedy within the family (Kiser, Ostoja, & Pruitt, 1998). Research related to the loss of a sibling through suicide indicated younger siblings living at home experience a more difficult time than either older siblings or parents; intervention resources frequently are focused upon parents (Dyregrov & Dyregrov, 2005).

Areas of Assessment

■ How is the child functioning socially according to his or her developmental level? What is the child's involvement in relationships, recreation, and routines?
■ Is the child exhibiting any changed behaviors?

■ What is the child's predominant mood (sad, withdrawn, hyperactive, angry)?
■ How does the child express his or her suffering or "pain" related to the loss?
■ What does the child feel might help make the "pain" better (besides the return of the lost loved one)?

TABLE 11.4 Grief and Bereavement in Children

Characteristics of Age	View of Death and Response	What Helps
Birth to 6 Months		
Basic needs must be met; cries if needs aren't met. Needs emotional and physical closeness of a consistent caregiver. Derives identity from caregiver. Views caregiver as a source of comfort and all needs fulfillment	Has no concept of death. Experiences death like any other separation; no sense of "finality." Nonspecific expressions of distress (crying). Reacts to loss of caregiver. Reacts to caregiver's distress	Progressively disengage child from primary caregiver if possible. Introduce a new primary caregiver. Nurture and comfort the child. Anticipate physical and emotional needs and provide them. Maintain routines
6 Months to 2 Years		
Begins to individuate. Remembers face of caregiver when absent. Demonstrates full range of emotions. Identifies caregiver as a source of good feelings and interactions	May see death as reversible. Experiences bona fide grief. Grief response only to the death of a significant person in child's life. Screams, panics, withdraws, becomes disinterested in food, toys, activities. Reacts in concert with distress experienced by caregiver. No control over feelings and responses; anticipates regressive behavior	Needs continual support and comfort. Avoid separation from significant others. Establish close physical and emotional connections by significant others. Maintain daily structure and schedule of routine activities. Support caregiver to reduce distress and maintain a stable environment. Acknowledge sadness that loved one will not return—offer comfort
2 Years to 5 Years		
Egocentric cause–effect not understood. Developing conscience. Developing trust. Attributes life to objects. Feelings expressed mostly by behaviors. Can recall events from past	Sees death like sleep: reversible. Believes in magical causes. Has sense of loss. Curiosity, questioning. Anticipates regression, clinging. Aggressive behavior is common. Worries about who will care for them	Remind that loved one will not return. Give realistic information, answer questions. Involve in "farewell" ceremonies. Encourage questions and expression of feelings. Keep home environment stable, structured. Help put words to feelings; reassure/comfort. Reassure child about who will take care of them; provide ways to remember loved one
5 Years to 9 Years		
Attributes life to things that move; may fear the dark. Begins to develop intellect. Begins to relate cause and effect; understands consequences. Literal, concrete. Decreasing fantasy life, increasing control of feelings	Personifies death as ghosts, "bogeyman." Shows interest in biological aspects of life and death. Begins to see death as irreversible. May see death as punishment; may feel responsible. Problems concentrating on tasks; may deny or hide feelings, vulnerability	Give clear and realistic information. Include child in funeral ceremonies if he or she chooses. Give permission to express feelings and provide opportunities; reduce guilt by providing factual information. Maintain structured schedule, individual and family activities; needs strong parent. Notify school of what is occurring, gentle confirmation, reassurance
Preadolescent Through Teens		
Individuation outside home. Identifies with peer group; needs family attachment. Understands life processes; can verbalize feelings. Physical maturation	Views death as permanent. Sense of own mortality; sense of future. Strong emotional reaction; may regress, revert to fantasy. May somaticize, intellectualize, morbid preoccupation	Unambiguous information. Provide opportunities to express self, feelings; encourage outside relationships with mentors. Provide tangible means to remember loved one; encourage self-expression, verbal and nonverbal. Dispel fears about physical concerns; educate about maturation; provide outlets for energy and strong feelings (recreation, sports, etc.); needs mentoring and direction

Source: Fine, P. G. (1998). *The hospice companion* (2nd ed). New York, NY: Oxford University Press with permission from Oxford University Press.

■ FAMILY CAREGIVING—PARENTAL EXPERIENCE OF LOSS

Living with dying can tax a patient and his or her significant others economically, as well as physically, spiritually, and psychologically. Often the patient or his or her significant others lose work time due to the patient's care requirements. Additional expenses may arise with treatments, hospitalizations, or other hidden expenses, such as transportation, child care, out-of-home food purchases, lodging, and so forth. Dying patients often experience much stress because of the financial burdens that fall upon the significant others (Rando, 1984). If the nurse feels unprepared to counsel the patient and significant others in this area, it is imperative to refer them to someone who can.

The loss of a child often is devastating to the parents and to the family. Parents feel responsible for their child's health, well-being, and safety. In the case of a newborn with a serious condition, there is accompanying parental blame and guilt for the infant's condition. Parents must grieve the healthy, "normal" child they lost in addition to the anticipated death of the infant.

Parents usually do not expect their child to die. This is true even in the case of adult children who die before parents. As adults are living longer, it is now less certain that children will outlive their parents (White & Beach, 2012). Older adults may experience "survivor guilt, powerlessness, and loss of religious faith"; the deceased child may be idealized, which can complicate grief resolution (Talerico, 2003, p. 14).

Grief related to the loss of a child is apt to be severe and complicated. Anniversary events and developmental milestones for the deceased child reopen the grief experience throughout the parents' lifetime (Kiser et al., 1998). Acknowledging that their lives have changed forever is part of the grief resolution that takes place for parents; however, recovery from the death of a child is a lifelong process (Geis et al., 1998). For the single parent, aloneness may be magnified (Backer et al., 1994). Controversy exists about parents' viewing prenatally deceased infants and stillborn infants; in general, viewing the body is thought to help with grieving (Haas, 2003). Nurses must be sensitive to family members' readiness and wishes related to viewing the body of their deceased loved one.

Areas of Assessment

■ How has your loved one's illness impacted your life?
■ In what ways will you remember your child who died?
■ What is the most significant type of suffering you are experiencing right now?
■ What are your specific needs at this time and how can I help you meet them?

■ GERONTOLOGIC GRIEF

Parker et al. (2002) have asserted that successful aging involves achieving competency in four distinct areas:

■ Engaging in life actively
■ Maximizing cognitive and physical function
■ Preventing disease and disability
■ Experiencing spirituality in relation to developmental processes

However, what happens when one does become ill, either physically or mentally, or acquires chronic illness and/or disability? Hardiness can assist older adults as they age with diagnoses, such as HIV; hardiness includes factors such as control, commitment, and challenge (Vance, Burrage, Couch, & Raper, 2008). Obstacles may become perceived as opportunities. Although there are conflicting reports, more research is needed to determine if an association exists between hardiness and immunological responsiveness in adults with HIV (Vance et al., 2008).

Recognizing whether an older adult is grieving or depressed is important. Although an older adult may deny feeling sad or depressed, it is important to look for the following additional signs of depression, such as

■ Complaints of unexplained aches and pains
■ Expressions of hopelessness or helplessness
■ Symptoms of anxiety
■ Memory impairment
■ Loss of pleasure
■ Decreased movement
■ Irritability
■ Forgetful of meals, personal hygiene, or taking medications (Segal, Jaffe, Davies, & Smith, 2007)

■ RISK FACTORS FOR COMPLICATED GRIEF

Predicting bereavement outcomes is difficult because the subjects are considered to be a vulnerable study population. A balance between the need for protection and the benefits of participation must be attained. Studies suggest that individual differences such as self-enhancing biases, attachment style, coping styles, belief systems, personal identity, and positive emotions can be predictors of well-being during bereavement. For example, those who tend to display more positive emotions prior to the loss of a loved one have lower levels of distress following the loss (Mancini & Bonanno, 2009). The persistence of what some perceive as negative emotions of grieving— namely, disbelief, yearning, anger, and depression—may be an additional predictor of the need for intervention (Maciejewski et al., 2007).

Although each individual's grieving is unique, the bereavement process may be functional or dysfunctional, adaptive or maladaptive. The length of time for grief resolution varies considerably between cultural groups and from person to person (Zisook & Shear, 2009). The majority of individuals experience uncomplicated grief after a loss; however, approximately 10% to 20% of bereaved individuals will experience the prolonged, debilitating phenomenon known as complicated grief (CG; Claxton & Reynolds, 2012). CG is a condition noted for prolonged and recurrent distressing emotions, avoidance of reminders, and intrusive thoughts about the loss of a loved one (Baker et al., 2016, p. 214). These prolonged reactions range from exaggerated normal reactions to abnormal grief reactions. Furthermore, grief may be unresolved or compounded if a loss or losses occur within a community of individuals where the losses are minimized or ignored; this may result in further complications with subsequent losses (Talerico, 2003).

Backer et al. (1994) describe three basic types of CG reactions: delayed, inhibited, and chronic grief. In delayed grief, the grief is triggered by the loss of someone or something else. There is minimal impact in this situation. For example, someone whose father has recently died may experience delayed grief related to the death of the individual's mother 10 years prior to the father's death. The individual has never experienced full grief for the death of the mother until the death of the father. His death triggers the deeply felt but unexpressed loss of the mother. Inhibited grief occurs when an individual never grieves. It also may occur if the individual feels great distress related to a lost relationship. This type of grief becomes complicated if another condition develops related to the unfelt grief. Last, chronic grief exists when the grieving is unending, and the intense yearning for the lost relationship continues. A cause for this type of grief could be unspeakable deaths, such as those due to AIDS or suicide.

Rando (1984) addresses delayed, inhibited, and chronic grief reactions but also includes absent grief, conflicted grief, unanticipated grief, and abbreviated grief in her list of CG types. Absent grief is characterized by a total lack of grief emotions and processes of mourning. Conflicted grief involves an amplification of the characteristics of normal grief partnered with a suppression of other manifestations of normal grief. Unanticipated grief takes place after an unexpected loss that the individual cannot grasp. Abbreviated grief is normal grief that lasts a short period of time because of swift replacement of the lost individual or lack of attachment to the lost individual. One study (Prigerson et al., 1997) identifies grief involving trauma and separation as traumatic grief and indicates that psychiatric sequelae, such as traumatic grief, puts bereaved individuals at risk for CG.

Families grieve in unique ways. Family members all fill unique roles. A lost family member means the family must reassign the lost role. Likewise, families may distort circumstances through idealization, blame, anger, or despair. Families who do not share their grief may experience poor coping or breakdown (Kissane & Bloch, 2002).

There are a number of individuals at risk for CG after the death of a close one with a terminal illness. Some of the best predictors are excessive dependency and insecure attachment styles, which suggest that the loss of a person who provides emotional stability may lead to an exacerbated grief reaction (Claxton & Reynolds, 2012). Others include those with a history of childhood abuse, insomnia, female gender, marital closeness, parents, those experiencing the loss of loved ones through unspeakable deaths, and those with a psychiatric history (Kristjanson, Lobb, Aoun, & Monterosso, 2006; Lobb et al., 2010).

Work done by Pennebaker, Mayne, and Francis (1997) indicates that language usage can help to impact bereavement outcomes in a positive way. Encouraging individuals to talk about traumatic events forces a disorganized event and emotions to become more organized, coherent, and insightful. Over time, the use of insight and causation words in relation to the event and its accompanying emotions helps cognitively reframe the experience that results in more adaptive outcomes.

Frank, Prigerson, Shear, and Reynolds (1997) postulate that individuals experiencing elongated periods of distress (for several months) and exhibiting criteria for major depressive episodes undergo traumatic grief reactions. They advocate treatment interventions that involve reexperiencing the moment of death, saying good-bye to the deceased while still retaining special memories of the person, and gradually being exposed to situations that the bereaved has avoided since the deceased's death. The outcome of this traumatic grief treatment has been reduced subjective distress. They do not advocate for pathologizing or treating brief periods of bereavement-related distress.

Previous editions of the *DSM* excluded a diagnosis of major depression in the bereaved unless their symptoms lasted longer than 2 months. With the publication of the *DSM-5*, this exclusion criterion was eliminated. Without this criterion, nurses may be uncertain how to distinguish between a patient who is experiencing depressive symptoms within the context of bereavement and a patient who is experiencing non-bereavement-related depression as many of the symptoms overlap (McCabe & Christopher, 2015). McCabe and Christopher (2015) studied differences between these two groups and found that feelings of guilt and worthlessness, difficulty making decisions, weight and appetite loss, and thoughts of suicide were more prevalent in patients experiencing a non-bereavement-related major depressive episode than those experiencing depressive symptoms within the context of bereavement.

A number of factors were examined in a study attempting to predict depressive symptomatology in the postbereavement period (Kurtz, Kurtz, Given, & Given,

1997). Prebereavement depressive symptomatology scores, levels of support from friends, and caregiver optimism were most predictive of postbereavement depressive symptomatology. The link between prebereavement and postbereavement depressive symptomatology scores was anticipated. The role of optimism is important for nurses to capitalize on and strengthen when working with significant others. The connection between high social support in the prebereavement period from friends and postbereavement depressive symptomatology was strong. This phenomenon could be caused by altered or lost relationships due to the dying and death of the spouse. Possibly friends experience a social death before the physical death of the bereaved's spouse.

Poor bereavement recovery is apt to occur if the death is unexpected, untimely, or traumatic for the bereaved, such as with homicide or suicide (Kristjanson et al., 2006). Moreover, maladaptive grieving may occur if the significant other had an ambivalent or dependent relationship with the deceased, perceives his or her social networks as unsupportive, and is experiencing concurrent loss. Family coping styles that negatively impact outcomes are (a) hostile (high conflict, low cohesiveness, and poor expressiveness); (b) sullen (limited but less in comparison with the hostile group); and (c) intermediate (intermediate cohesiveness and low control and achievement orientation). Additional correlates for poor outcome include use of medications or alcohol, concern for self, level of contentment, and not viewing the deceased's body. Positive bereavement outcomes are more apt to occur in families who are supportive (high cohesion) and resolve conflict well (Kissane, McKenzie, & Bloch, 1997).

In more dysfunctional grieving situations, the advanced nurse practitioner must treat symptoms of pathological grief. Three major symptom categories of pathological grief are intrusion, denial, and dysfunctional adaptation (Horowitz, Bonanno, & Holen, 1993). Spending long periods of time idealizing the memory of the deceased is a sign of an intrusive thought process. Living as if the deceased were still alive for more than 6 months is evidence of denial. Minimal dysfunction is evidenced in having difficulty making decisions, whereas major dysfunction is evidenced in more severe impairments. Such severe dysfunctional parameters involve extreme fatigue or somatic symptoms that last more than 1 month; inability to resume work, other interests, routines, and responsibilities after more than 1 month; and reluctance to develop new relationships after 13 months of grieving (Lev & McCorkle, 1998, p. 147).

Use the following exercises to expand your understanding of helping the patient's significant others on their journey with the patient who is living with and dying from a terminal illness in relation to suffering and loss, death and dying, and grief and bereavement:

Exercise I—Discuss how you might feel and what you might do if you were the nurse who walked into a patient's room just as the patient has died and the family or significant others are there.

Exercise II—A family member who has been estranged from the dying patient on your floor is in the room as you come in to check on the patient who is unconscious. The family member says, "He wasn't a very good father. He abused my sister and me. I'll be glad when he's dead." How would you respond to this family member?

Exercise III—You are the advanced practice nurse heading up the first meeting of nursing staff since a patient on your floor died from cancer. What would be your objectives for the meeting?

■ CONTEXT OF CAREGIVING AND RELATED INTERVENTIONS

Working with the patient who is living with and dying from a terminal illness and that person's significant others requires compassion, skill, energy, sensitivity, and patience. Compassion promotes a positive connection among the nurse, the patient, and the significant others. Skill gives the nurse credibility in working with them. Energy, often in the form of providing hope for the moment, moves the patient and significant others forward when they feel like giving up. Sensitivity enhances understanding and rapport in the relationships. Patience allows individuals the time needed to face and plan for an uncertain and unpredictable future.

The nurse attempts to help meet the needs of the patient and the significant others. Addressing immediate needs may take on greater significance with the patient experiencing a terminal illness than addressing either short- or long-term needs. Values, control issues, and goals of both the patient and significant others need to be taken into consideration, addressed directly, and handled tactfully and sensitively.

The nurse has a unique window into the patient's circumstances. Depending on the setting, nurses may provide 24-hour care. Even if nursing coverage is not for 24 direct-care hours, nursing care may be accessible for that period of time. Generally, it is the nurse who gets the most consistent, current, and constant view of what is actually happening with the patient and significant others. With few exceptions, the nurse usually is the most readily available and informed team player to help coordinate the patient's care.

Developing goals with the patient and family provides some stability and security during this time. It can empower the patient and the significant others to take an active role in planning the patient's remaining earthbound journey, uncertain and unpredictable as it may be. Furthermore, it helps set the stage for the continuing connection between the nurse and the patient's family in the bereavement period following the patient's death.

Nurse

Nurses care for themselves by seeking support from colleagues, ensuring time for themselves by maintaining healthy boundaries with the patient and significant others, and tending to their own physical, emotional, sociocultural, and spiritual needs. After a patient's death, nurses may work through their grief by attending the memorial service or funeral of the deceased patient if this is deemed acceptable by the nurse's employing agency policy and the deceased patient's family. Sending a sympathy card to significant others, doing follow-up bereavement work with significant others, and reminiscing about the deceased patient with empathic colleagues usually help nurses in dealing with their own grief.

CASE STUDY *Continued*

The morning after her meeting with her supervisor, Kate felt better. She went into Ms. Lopez's room just as the spiritual care advisor was leaving. Ms. Lopez had been awake and talking that morning. As Kate moved around the bed providing care, Ms. Lopez touched her arm and told her, "I think it is almost my time. It's OK. Thank you, Kate, you have been an angel. You all have." They talked a bit more until Ms. Lopez closed her eyes. She did not wake again for the remainder of Kate's shift. Kate stopped in at the end of her shift to check on Martin and Camila. She asked if there was anything she could do for them before she went home.

Nursing Interventions

Nurses are accustomed to action-oriented, "doing for" interventions. However, when caring for the patient with a terminal illness, the nurse's role may be less action oriented and more presence oriented. Presence is being with a patient in an authentic relationship that promotes mutual respect, honesty, and dignity. Establishing presence requires self-awareness, openness, flexibility, and willingness to embrace another person's situation—even when that situation involves suffering for which we can do nothing other than accompany the patient as he or she experiences it (Anderson & Gaugler, 2007; Lavoie, Blondeau, & De Koninck, 2008).

Dodd, Guerin, Delaney, and Dodd (2017) performed a systematic review exploring CG in relation to attitudes, skills, and training of mental health professionals. They noted that in spite of CG being included in *DSM-5* as a persistent complex bereavement disorder, application of research to practice still takes a lot of time. This is especially true in the area of mental health. They determined there is a need to educate practitioners to treat CG, be aware of attitudinal barriers, and recognize the impact of clinicians' personal grief on their work with patients.

Given that so many American deaths occur in hospitals, the nurse is most apt to be with the patient and significant others at the exact time of death. Becoming comfortable with viewing the dying and death process, touching the deceased's body, talking with significant others about the death and their feelings, and dealing with the patient's death among staff are important aspects with which the nurse will be confronted.

The nurse's relationship with the patient will be critical in determining how she or he handles grief and bereavement in relation to the patient's dying and death. Was it a short-term nurse–patient relationship, or did the nurse have a professional relationship with the patient for an extended period of time? In addition, how comfortable does the nurse feel sharing feelings, and how appropriate is it to share feelings with the patient? Nurses need to answer for themselves what the goal is of sharing their feelings and what the expected outcome is of doing so before proceeding.

Johns (2007) contends that reflection is a helpful practice to respond to a patient's suffering. He suggests that reflection should be structured and guided to maximize benefits and deepen attainment of the kind of healthcare provider one wants to be during a patient's suffering. He also encourages construction of the story that is taking place to discover meaning and insight related to the total experience.

The level of intervention by the nurse will be based on professional skills, theoretical background, and clinical setting. The nurse will develop therapeutic relationships; ensure the patient's physical comfort to maintain function; explore the meaning of physical suffering and loss with the patient and significant others; reframe the patient's limitations to identify areas of value that will enhance the patient's QOL; encourage patient and significant others' attendance at support groups; and identify and maximize prior coping skills of the patient and the significant others. Advanced practice nurses will offer more intensive and extensive interventions for grieving and bereavement needs and be involved in conducting or participating in research studies. For example, the advanced practice nurse may prescribe various medications, offer individual or family counseling, lead a bereavement group, or conduct research on QOL and quality of dying outcomes.

Patient

Each patient who is living with and dying from a terminal illness is unique. His or her experiences living with and dying from terminal illness also are unique. A critical factor in promoting good nursing care of this patient and significant others is affirming this uniqueness. Affirming the individual's growth and wholeness during this difficult living–dying interval is critical (Georgesen & Dungan, 1996; Talerico, 2003). Empowering patients to integrate the living–dying experience and optimize their QOL will affirm the patient further.

For example, the patient is affirmed when the nurse acknowledges the patient's level of acceptance of dying and death. The patient's acceptance or denial may seem selective at times. In reality, varying levels of acceptance or denial may serve an adaptive function in which only specific aspects of dying are tolerable at a given point in time. The patient is aided when the nurse accepts and supports the patient's coping in this way to deal with the extensive and intensive challenges during the living–dying interval (Kastenbaum, 1997).

False reassurances prevent patients from accepting reality; the nurse must be honest and not foster false pretenses (Matzo et al., 2003).

Medical science has limitations, and often patients feel dehumanized during some medical procedures. In addition to addressing comfort needs, patients need assurance that their humanity will be respected and valued. The nursing profession has reawakened to the importance of integrating spiritual care within total patient care. Patients have indicated that their spiritual needs are best met through nurses' listening to, talking with, supporting religious practices of, and being with them (O'Neill & Kenny, 1998). Even in the midst of suffering through the loss of physical well-being, patients may sense spiritual well-being. Buckwalter (2003) refers to "moments of ministry" or "ministry of the moment" as those times when nurses or others assist patients in a "holy moment of connection," especially for someone who may be experiencing profound memory loss (p. 22). If a nurse feels inadequate or uncomfortable assisting dying patients in this area in any way, a pastoral care referral may be indicated. In addition, the patient may desire to have clergy closely involved even if the nurse is comfortable meeting the patient's spiritual needs.

Saying good-bye is painful for the patient with a terminal illness, for his or her significant others, and for the nurse. Discerning when (timing) and how (tone) to say and facilitate others' saying good-bye takes sensitivity (touch, emotional, and physical) and skill (training/technique) on the nurse's part. This intervention can be illustrated as follows:

Discernment of readiness to facilitate
good-byes = Nurse sensitivity (touch) +
Skill (training/technique) + When (timing) +
How (tone)

An important question to ask when caring for the patient who is dying from and living with a terminal illness is "What type of patient has the disease, rather than what type of disease does the patient have?" (Harris, 1991, p. 111). Respecting and affirming the patient as a unique and valuable human being will help promote wholeness during a time of brokenness. As the individual is faced with imminent death, he or she must reorient his or her life to adapt to this realization and the accompanying losses. Minimizing losses due to isolation, rejection, and loss of control can decrease the individual's suffering (Rando, 1984). Optimizing patients' strengths is essential in helping them achieve the QOL they would like to pursue in this living–dying interval.

Chronic sorrow is the distinct grief reaction that occurs when loss is not final but continues to be present in the life of the griever (Rossheim & McAdams, 2010). Chronic sorrow may be triggered if the individual senses a disparity with norms. For example, the individual may feel different from others. Situations such as hospitalization accentuate this discrepancy to the individual. Both patients and significant others may experience chronic sorrow.

Nurses can assist individuals with chronic sorrow by helping with internal and external management methods. Internal management methods consist of individualized coping interventions such as stress-relieving practices like journaling. External management methods are those provided by professionals to aid in effective coping such as professional counseling, pastoral care, or pharmaceutical interventions (Ahmann & Dokken, 2009). The nurse may advocate for a patient with a terminal illness by employing the following interventions: advancing grief work, encouraging health-promoting strategies despite a compromised health state, making referrals, meeting with significant others, utilizing cognitive reframing of negative patterns, and engaging the patient in individual or group therapy to work through unresolved situations. The nurse may be asked to work with support staff and significant others to help them accept, support, and devise strategies to work with a patient or significant other who has a dysfunctional approach to suffering and loss.

However, the most meaningful "intervention" that may be provided to a patient with a terminal illness is the gift of presence. Presence validates one's existence amid the experience of suffering (Lavoie et al., 2008).

Family and/or Significant Others

The term "family" will be used to represent both family and significant others. The family of a patient dying from and living with a terminal illness experiences great turmoil and disequilibrium. Often, the illness becomes the focal point of family activity and organization. If the patient is a child and has siblings, the family struggles at maintaining life within the household as well as preparing for the death of one of its members. The child simultaneously may be growing in many ways while dying in others. Treatment programs and appointments may consume much of the family's energy, possibly for extended periods of time. Helping the family maintain a sense of normalcy and balance throughout this period will be an important task for the nurse. Keeping the family as involved as possible in the patient's care applies to the patient with a terminal illness of any age (Matzo et al., 2003; Rando, 1984).

The question of where the patient and family would like the anticipated death to occur must be answered. With shortened hospital stays, families have been forced to assume extended and at times intensive care responsibilities for the dying patient in addition to their usual role expectations and demands. Helping the patient and family decide where and when care will take place becomes an important goal (Lev & McCorkle, 1998). The patient may wish to die at home, in a hospice setting, in a hospital, or in another setting. Assisting the patient and family to communicate what they each can handle at different stages of the patient's dying will be critical.

A family's response to the patient's death is as unique as the individuals making up the family constellation. Each family has its own management style in responding to the death of a member. Management styles include families that progress, that is, are able to move forward as a family; accommodate, adapt to the loss, and adjust; maintain, where family members are variable in their response; struggle, where the family is in conflict; and flounder, where the family is having difficulty both as individuals and as a unit (Wiegand, 2012). A family may seek or need to be referred for counseling if maladaptive symptoms develop. Family bereavement therapy involves assessing the circumstances related to the family member's death; the role of the deceased in the family before and after death; timing of the death in relation to the family member's stage of growth and development; previous and current levels of family functioning; the context of the death; and the meaning assigned by the family to the death (Kiser et al., 1998, p. 97). There is little scientific evidence related to the impact of formal interventions with those bereaved; one reason for this may be that uncomplicated grieving resolves on its own (Jordan & Neimeyer, 2003). Jordan and Neimeyer further assert there is more evidence to support relational contexts of therapy (i.e., friends and family) over medical interventions (i.e., psychology or psychiatry) for those bereaved because those aspects promote hope and learning new coping skills.

However, the nurse must now focus attention on helping significant others begin the tasks of bereavement: accepting the reality of the loss, experiencing the pain of grief, adjusting to an environment without the deceased, and reinvesting energy into other relationships (Worden, 1991). Backer et al. (1994, p. 165) have identified guidelines for counseling the bereaved as follows:

1. Help actualize the loss by talking about the loss
2. Identify and express feelings related to the loss
3. Help the bereaved in decision making
4. Facilitate emotional withdrawal and development of new relationships
5. Provide time to grieve and be cognizant of holidays and anniversary dates
6. Reassure the bereaved that their behavior is normal and that they are not abnormal because of their feelings
7. Allow for individual differences in the bereavement process
8. Provide support
9. Examine individual defenses and coping styles (be aware of problems with alcohol or other substance abuse)
10. Identify pathological behaviors and refer to treatment

The length of time for intense grief to lessen varies from individual to individual. As long as the bereaved's grieving behavior does not interfere significantly with their physiological or psychosocial functioning, it is not considered abnormal. In general, intense responses to grief generally subside in about 6 to 12 months (Rando, 1984). Grieving, however, continues throughout the bereaved's life. The loss, in some cases, may be replaced but, in all cases, it is never recovered. Grief can inflict a woundedness of spirit, much different than a physical wound, that calls for the nurse to wait patiently versus debride quickly and that allows the body and soul to heal (Moules et al., 2007).

The living–dying interval comes to an end with the death of the patient, yet how does one know when grieving ends—or in a contemporary view, if grieving is moving forward—for the bereaved? Parkes and Weiss (1983) identified 10 major areas for assessment of recovery:

1. Functioning has returned to a level equal to or better than before bereavement.
2. Outstanding problems are being solved.
3. Acceptance of the loss has occurred.
4. Socialization is as effective as before the death.
5. The future is viewed positively and realistically.
6. General health is at prebereavement level.
7. Anxiety or depression levels are appropriate.
8. Guilt or anger levels are appropriate.
9. Self-esteem levels are appropriate.
10. Coping with future loss is feasible.

The process of bereavement differs from individual to individual. Some respond with minimal disruptions, some recover over time, while others experience a state of chronic distress (Bonanno et al., 2011). Some individuals' bereavement may occur in ways unfamiliar to the nurse. Through appropriate interventions, the nurse can help the bereaved adapt to their loss in a way that will foster their growth and wholeness as well. The nurse might determine with the bereaved what trajectory the individual may be on and adapt nursing interventions accordingly.

■ CONCLUSION

Living with and dying from a terminal illness results in many losses—for the patient, for the family, and for the nurse. Terminal illness can occur over an extended period of time or a brief period of time. The nurse functions as both facilitator and participant in this process. The nurse also can add objectivity while the patient and family resolve many feelings, issues, and decisions related to the living–dying experience.

This period of time frequently involves suffering in multiple dimensions. The nurse can utilize technical skills to alleviate certain attributes of the suffering, such as the patient's physical pain. When these technical skills are accompanied by the nurse's sensitivity, compassion, empathy, and presence, the patient and family are better equipped to face the other attributes of suffering as well. Thus, the nurse, as a caring professional, may contribute meaningfully to the health and wholeness of the patient and his or her family through one of life's most challenging and difficult transitions.

CASE STUDY *Conclusion*

Twelve days after her arrival on the unit, Ms. Lopez's respirations became irregular. Martin, Camila, and her husband were in the room at the time, and they held her hands. They each kissed her on the forehead and said a personal good-bye. At 3:30 p.m. Ms. Lopez stopped breathing. As a DNR order was in her chart, no resuscitation was attempted. She was pronounced dead at 3:43 p.m. Her children looked at one another, hugged one another, and cried.

Kate was off duty that day. Her supervisor called her to tell her and to praise her for the care she provided for both the patient and her family. They discussed the appropriateness of her attending Ms. Lopez's funeral. After the call, Kate sat on her couch with her dog and reflected on the care she had given Ms. Lopez and her family.

Camila wrote a letter to the hospital unit. She thanked the staff, and especially Kate, for the care they provided her mother

Victoria selected a favorite toy to place in Lita's casket. She commented to Camila, "Lita doesn't look like Lita, I hope she will be happy in Heaven now."

CASE STUDY *Commentary*

Lori Sipes, PhD (Psychology)

What strikes me about Ms. Lopez's treatment were many of the beneficial approaches Kate took to providing care for Ms. Lopez and her family. First, Kate acknowledged that, as caregivers/providers, our experiences with feelings similar to those experienced by our patients do play a role in the care that we provide for them. Although our first impulse usually is to provide the care that we believe someone needs, taking care of ourselves provides the foundation for the care we provide our patients. Kate did an excellent job of self-care by processing her own feelings related to death and loss and accessed available supports such as meeting with her supervisor to process her feelings.

As a caregiver, Kate was understandably frustrated and upset by Ms. Lopez's anger and refusal of care that was unable to heal her illness. Rather than defending the doctor's decision to recommend PC, Kate allowed Ms. Lopez her anger, which, although it may have seemed to be directed at the doctors for not treating her condition, was an expression of Ms. Lopez's hurt, fear, and anger that her body was failing her and that she could not save herself. Ms. Lopez needed her anger, and Kate allowed her to have it and express it. If time was available, and Ms. Lopez were cooperative, she may have benefited from discussing her prior experiences with people in her life having had significant illnesses. If Ms. Lopez was not cooperative because of her need to have and express her anger, the most compassionate care would be to quietly and matter-of-factly provide Ms. Lopez medical care and little comforts, as Kate did. As Ms. Lopez became more verbal about her fears of giving up, she may benefit from acknowledging her accomplishments and the love she shares with her family members.

Through their anticipatory grieving process, Ms. Lopez and her family may have benefited from sharing treasured memories with one another and letting each other (especially Ms. Lopez) know the "lessons" that they learned from her and will carry with them through life. Death and dying often include a time of evaluating the meaning and significance of life. This family is clearly very connected to one another, and that connection is an important component of Ms. Lopez's significance and purpose in life. Referral to spiritual support was a helpful intervention as well.

Evidence-Based Practice

Nam, I. S. (2016). Effects of psychoeducation on helpful support for complicated grief: A preliminary randomized controlled single-blind study. *Psychological Medicine,* 46, 189–195.

Q: What work can clinicians do in helping significant others support a loved one experiencing complicated grief?

Background

Individuals facing the loss of a loved one may experience a distinct psychological response, namely, complicated grief (CG). Adverse health outcomes may result. It often has been thought social support may be beneficial. However, few studies have explored the beneficial effects of helpful support on CG following bereavement. Nam wanted to address: (1) "Are levels of CG and depressive symptoms diminished by access to appropriately trained supportive individuals?" and (2) "Does perceived helpfulness of supporters mediate the effects of the intervention on the CG and depressive symptoms?"

Method

Forty-two participants ranging in age from 21 to 73 years were recruited from two hospice service centers and one community service center in South Korea. These individuals were known to be seeking bereavement support. A randomized controlled trial was conducted. Bereaved participants and supporters were randomized to: (1) psychoeducation on CG and helpful social support or (2) psychoeducation on CG. Rating instruments used included: (1) The Inventory of Complicated Grief (ICD), a 19-item tool, and (2) The Center for Epidmeiologic Studies Depression Scale (CES-D), a 20-item instrument.

Results

The results showed that intervention provided by psychoeducation with supporters of bereaved individuals had significant beneficial effects, namely, decreased CES-D scores postintervention. Particularly, symptoms of CG were decreased in bereaved individuals with supporters that received psychoeducation. Of note, the experimental group also reported large decreases in CG and depressive symptoms postintervention, whereas the control group did not.

Conclusions

This study was seminal in demonstrating the benefits of psychoeducaton for the bereaved and for educating helpers in the provision of support to the bereaved. It also provided a better understanding of the process by which provision of helpful support for CG and depressive symptoms occurs.

■ REFERENCES

Ahmann, E., & Dokken, D. (2009). An evidence-based approach for supporting parents experiencing chronic sorrow. *Pediatric Nursing, 35*(2), 115–119.

Ajdacic-Gross, V., Ring, M., Gadola, E., Lauber, C., Bopp, M., Gutzwiller, F., & Rössler, W. (2008). Suicide after bereavement: An overlooked problem. *Psychological Medicine, 38*(5), 673–676. doi:10.1017/S0033291708002754

American Association of Colleges of Nursing. (2016). ELNEC fact sheet. Retrieved from http://www.aacnnursing.org/Portals/42/ELNEC/PDF/FactSheet.pdf

Anderson, K. A., & Gaugler, J. E. (2007). The grief experiences of certified nursing assistants: Personal growth and complicated grief. *OMEGA: Journal of Death and Dying, 54*(4), 301–318. doi:10.2190/T14N-W223-7612-0224

Backer, B. A., Hannon, N. R., & Gregg, J. Y. (1994). *To listen, to comfort, to care: Reflections on death and dying.* Albany, NY: Delmar.

Baker, A. W., Goetter, E. M., Bui, E., Shah, R., Charney, M. E., Mauro, C., ... Simon, N. M. (2016). The influence of anxiety sensitivity on a wish to die in complicated grief. *Journal of Nervous and Mental Disorder, 204*(4), 314–316. doi:10.1097/NMD.0000000000000465

Baum, N. (2003). The male way of mourning divorce: When, what, and how. *Clinical Social Work Journal, 31*(1), 37–67. doi:10.1037/0033-2909.111.1.108

Bonanno, G. A. (2004). Loss, trauma, and human resilience: Have we underestimated the human capacity to thrive after extremely aversive events? *American Psychologist, 59*(1), 20–28. doi:10.1037/0003-066X.59.1.20

Bonanno, G. A., Westphal, M., & Mancini, A. D. (2011). Resilience to loss and potential trauma. *Annual Review of Clinical Psychology, 7,* 511–535. doi:10.1146/annurev-clinpsy-032210-104526

Bowlby, J. (1980). *Attachment and loss: Loss, sadness and depression* (Vol. III). New York, NY: Basic Books.

Brady, P. F. (1997). The therapeutic relationship. In B. S. Johnson (Ed.), *Psychiatric-mental health nursing: Adaptation and growth* (4th ed., pp. 49–57). New York, NY: Lippincott.

Buckman, R. (1993). Communication in palliative care: A practical guide. In D. Doyle, G. W. C. Hanks, & N. Macdonald (Eds.), *Oxford textbook of palliative medicine* (pp. 47–61). Oxford, UK: Oxford Medical.

Buckwalter, G. L. (2003). Addressing the spiritual & religious needs of persons with profound memory loss. *Home Healthcare Nurse, 21*(1), 20–24. doi:10.1097/00004045-200301000-00005

Callanan, M., & Kelley, P. (1992). *Final gifts.* New York, NY: Poseidon Press.

Candy, B., Jones, L., Drake, R., Leurent, B., & King, M. (2011). Interventions for supporting informal caregivers of patients in the terminal phase of a disease. *Cochrane Database of Systematic Reviews,* (6), CD007617. doi:10.1002/14651858.CD007617.pub2

Cassell, E. (1991). *The nature of suffering and the goals of medicine.* New York, NY: Oxford University Press.

Charleton, R. (2003). Managing bereavement. *Practitioner, 247,* 667, 671–674.

Choi, Y. J., & Lee, K. J. (2007). Evidence-based nursing: Effects of a structured nursing program for the health promotion of Korean women with Hwa-Byung. *Archives of Psychiatric Nursing, 21*(1), 12–16. doi:10.1016/j.apnu.2006.07.006

Claxton, R., & Reynolds, C. F. (2012). Complicated grief #254. *Journal of Palliative Medicine, 15*(7), 829–830. doi:10.1089/jpm.2012.9577

Clements, P. T., Vigil, G. J., Manno, M. S., Henry, G. C., Wilks, J., Das Sarthak, ... Foster, W. (2003). Cultural perspectives of death, grief, and bereavement. *Journal of Psychosocial Nursing and Mental Health Services, 41*(7), 18–26.

Copp, G. (1997). Patients' and nurses' constructions of death and dying in a hospice setting. *Journal of Cancer Nursing, 1*(1), 2–13. doi:10.1016/S1364-9825(97)80345-8

Copp, G. (1998). A review of current theories of death and dying. *Journal of Advanced Nursing, 28*(2), 382–390. doi:10.1046/j.1365-2648.1998.00794.x

Corr, C. A. (1992). A task-based approach to coping with dying. *Omega, 24*(2), 81–94. doi:10.2190/CNNF-CX1P-BFXU-GGN4

Cowles, K., & Rodgers, B. (2000). The concept of grief: An evolutionary perspective. In B. Rodgers & K. Knafl (Eds.), *Concept development in nursing* (pp. 103–117). Philadelphia, PA: W. B. Saunders.

Danis, M. (1998). Improving end-of-life care in the intensive care unit: What's to be learned from outcomes research? *New Horizons, 6*(1), 110–118.

Dodd, A., Guerin, S., Delaney, S., & Dodd, P. (2017). Complicated grief: Knowledge, attitudes, skills and training of mental health professionals: A systematic review. *Patient Education and Counseling, 100*(8), 1447–1458. doi:10.1016/j.pec.2017.03.010

Dyregrov, K., & Dyregrov, A. (2005). Siblings after suicide—"the forgotten bereaved." *Suicide and Life-Threatening Behavior, 35*(6), 714–724. doi:10.1521/suli.2005.35.6.714

Eakes, G. G., Burke, M. L., & Hainsworth, M. A. (1998). Middle-range theory of chronic sorrow. *Image–The Journal of Nursing Scholarship, 30*(2), 179–184. doi:10.1111/j.1547-5069.1998.tb01276.x

Engel, G. L. (1964). Grief and grieving. *The American Journal of Nursing, 64,* 93–98.

Evans, A. J. (1994). Anticipatory grief: A theoretical challenge. *Palliative Medicine, 8*(2), 159–165. doi:10.1177/026921639400800211

Ferrell, B. R., & Coyle, N. (2008). The nature of suffering and the goals of nursing. *Oncology Nursing Forum, 35*(2), 241–247. doi:10.1188/08.ONF.241-247

Ferrell, B. R., Taylor, E. J., Sattler, G. R., Fowler, M., & Cheyney, B. L. (1993). Searching for the meaning of pain. *Cancer Practice, 1,* 185–194.

Fine, P. (Ed.). (1998). *Processes to optimize care during the last phase of life.* Scottsdale, AZ: Vista Care Hospice.

Florczak, K. L. (2008). The persistent yet ever-changing nature of grieving a loss. *Nursing Science Quarterly, 21*(1), 7–11. doi:10.1177/0894318407311163

Frank, E., Prigerson, H. G., Shear, M. K., & Reynolds, C. F. (1997). Phenomenology and treatment of bereavement-related distress in the elderly. *International Clinical Psychopharmacology, 12*(suppl. 7), S25–S29. doi:10.1097/00004850-199712007-00005

Freud, S. (1957). The disillusionment of the war. In J. Strachey (Ed.), *The complete psychological works of Sigmund Freud, Vol. 14 (1914–1916)*. London, UK: Hogarth Press and the Institute of Psychoanalysis.

Fulton, R., & Fulton, J. A. (1971). A psychosocial aspect of terminal care: Anticipatory grief. *Omega, 2*, 91–99. doi:10.2190/0WEH-QUBG-67VG-YKJK

Geis, H. K., Whittlesey, S. W., McDonald, N. B., Smith, K. L., & Pfefferbaum, B. (1998). Bereavement and loss in childhood. *Child and Adolescent Psychiatric Clinics of North America, 7*(1), 73–85, viii. doi:10.1080/135 76270310001613392

Georgesen, J., & Dungan, J. M. (1996). Managing spiritual distress in patients with advanced cancer pain. *Cancer Nursing, 19*(5), 376–383. doi:10.1111/j.1365-2354.2005.00646.x

Glasser, B. G., & Strauss, A. L. (1965). *Awareness of dying*. Chicago, IL: Aldine.

Goodkin, K., Blaney, N. T., Feaster, D. J., Baldewicz, T., Burkhalter, J. E., & Leeds, B. (1999). A randomized controlled clinical trial of a bereavement support group intervention in human immunodeficiency virus type 1-seropositive and -seronegative homosexual men. *Archives of General Psychiatry, 56*(1), 52–59.

Gray, L. B., Weller, R. A., Fristad, M., & Weller, E. B. (2011). Depression in children and adolescents two months after the death of a parent. *Journal of Affective Disorders, 135*(1–3), 277–283. doi:10.1016/j.jad.2011.08.009

Haas, F. (2003). Bereavement care: Seeing the body. *Nursing Standard, 17*(28), 33–37. doi:10.7748/ns2003.03.17.28.33 .c3364

Hames, C. C. (2003). Helping infants and toddlers when a family member dies. *Journal of Hospice and Palliative Nursing, 5*, 103–112. doi:10.1080/07481181003697613

Harris, J. M. (1991). Death and bereavement. *Problems in Veterinary Medicine, 3*(1), 111–117.

Holloway, M. (2006). Death the great leveller? Towards a transcultural spirituality of dying and bereavement. *Journal of Clinical Nursing, 15*(7), 833–839. doi:10.1111/j.1365-2702.2006.01662.x

Horowitz, M. J., Bonanno, G. A., & Holen, A. (1993). Pathological grief: Diagnosis and explanation. *Psychosomatic Medicine, 55*(3), 260–273. doi:10.1097/00006842-199305000-00004

Johns, C. (2007). Toward easing suffering through reflection. *Journal of Holistic Nursing, 25*(3), 204–210. doi:10.1177/0898010106297234

Jordan, J. R., & Neimeyer, R. A. (2003). Does grief counseling work? *Death Studies, 27*(9), 765–786. doi:10.1080/713842360

Kalish, R. A. (1979). The onset of the dying process. In R. A. Kalish (Ed.), *Death, dying, transcending* (pp. 5–17). New York, NY: Baywood.

Kastenbaum, R. A. (1997). *Death, society, and human experience*. Boston, MA: Allyn & Bacon.

Kazanowski, M. (2013). End-of-life care. In D. D. Ignatavicius & M. L. Workman (Eds.), *Medical-surgical nursing: Patient-centered collaborative care* (7th ed.). St. Louis, MO: Elsevier Saunders.

Kazanowski, M., Perrin, K., Potter, M., & Sheehan, C. (2007). The silence of suffering. *Journal of Holistic Nursing, 25*(3), 195–203. doi:10.1177/0898010107305501

Kiser, L. J., Ostoja, E., & Pruitt, D. B. (1998). Dealing with stress and trauma in families. *Child and Adolescent Psychiatric Clinics of North America, 7*(1), 87–103, viii–ix.

Kissane, D. W., & Bloch, S. (2002). *Family focused grief therapy*. Philadelphia, PA: Open University Press.

Kissane, D. W., McKenzie, D. P., & Bloch, S. (1997). Family coping and bereavement outcome. *Palliative Medicine, 11*(3), 191–201. doi:10.1177/026921639701100303

Koop, P. M., & Strang, V. (1997). Predictors of bereavement outcomes in families of patients with cancer: A literature review. *The Canadian Journal of Nursing Research, 29*(4), 33–50.

Kristjanson, L. J., Lobb, E., Aoun, S., & Monterosso, L.(2006). *A systematic review of the literature on complicated grief*. Perth, Australia: Commonwealth of Australia, Department of Health and Ageing.

Krueger, G. (2006). Meaning-making in the aftermath of sudden infant death syndrome. *Nursing Inquiry, 13*(3), 163–171.

Kubler-Ross, E. (1969). *On death and dying*. New York, NY: Macmillan.

Kurtz, M. E., Kurtz, J. C., Given, C. W., & Given, B. (1997). Predictors of postbereavement depressive symptomatology among family caregivers of cancer patients. *Supportive Care in Cancer, 5*(1), 53–60.

Lalor, J. G., Begley, C. M., & Devane, D. (2006). Exploring painful experiences: Impact of emotional narratives on members of a qualitative research team. *Journal of Advanced Nursing, 56*(6), 607–616. doi:10.1111/j.1365-2648.2006.04039.x

Lavoie, M., Blondeau, D., & De Koninck, T. (2008). The dying person: An existential being until the end of life. *Nursing Philosophy, 9*(2), 89–97. doi:10.1111/j.1466-769X.2008.00347.x

Leichtling, B. (2004). Dealing with dying, death and grief. *Caring: National Association for Home Care Magazine, 23*(1), 38–39.

Lev, E. L., & McCorkle, R. (1998). Loss, grief, and bereavement in family members of cancer patients. *Seminars in Oncology Nursing, 14*(2), 145–151. doi:10.1016/S0749-2081(98)80020-X

Lewis, M. L. (1998). Culture and loss: A project of self-reflection. *The Journal of Nursing Education, 37*(9), 398–400.

Lindemann, E. (1944). Symptomatology and management of acute grief. *American Journal of Psychiatry, 101*, 141–148. doi:10.1176/ajp.101.2.141

Lobb, E. A., Kirstjanson, L. J., Aoun, S. M., Monterosso, L., Halkett, G. K. B., & Davies, A. (2010). Predictors of complicated grief: A systematic review of empirical studies. *Death Studies, 34*, 673–698. doi:10.1080/07 481187.2010.496686

Maciejewski, P. K., Zhang, B., Block, S. D., & Prigerson, H. G. (2007). An empirical examination of the stage theory of grief. *Journal of the American Medical Association, 297*(7), 716–723. doi:10.1001/jama.297.7.716

Mallinson, R. K. (1999). Grief work of HIV positive persons and their survivors. *The Nursing Clinics of North America, 34*(1), 163–177.

Mancini, A. D., & Bonanno, G. A. (2009). Predictors and parameters of resilience to loss: Toward an individual differences model. *Journal of Personality, 77*(6), 1805–1832. doi:10.1111/j.1467-6494.2009.00601.x

Matzo, M. L., & Sherman, D. W. (2006). *Palliative care nursing: Quality care to the end of life* (2nd ed.). New York, NY: Springer Publishing.

Matzo, M. L., Sherman, D. W., Lo, K., Egan, K. A., Grant, M., & Rhome, A. (2003). Strategies for teaching loss, grief, and bereavement. *Nurse Educator, 28*(2), 71–76. doi:10.1097/00006223-200303000-00009

McCabe, P. J., & Christopher, P. P. (2015). Symptoms and functional traits of brief major depressive episodes and discrimination of bereavement. *Depression and Anxiety, 33,* 112–119. doi:10.1002/da.22446

McCall, J. B. (1999). *Grief education for care-givers of the elderly.* New York, NY: Haworth Pastoral Press.

McCreight, B. S. (2004). A grief ignored: Narratives of pregnancy loss from a male perspective. *Sociology of Health and Illness, 26*(3), 326–350. doi:10.1111/j.1467-9566.2004.00393.x

McIntier, T. M. (1995). Nursing the family when a child dies. *RN, 58*(2), 50–54; quiz 55. doi:10.1016/j.ejon.2013.11.004

Melhem, N. M., Porta, G., Shamseddeen, W., Walker Payne, M., & Brent, D. A. (2011). Grief in children and adolescents bereaved by sudden parental death. *Archives of General Psychiatry, 68*(9), 911–919. doi:10.1001/archgenpsychiatry.2011.101

Mitchell, A. M., Wesner, S., Garand, L., Gale, D. D., Havill, A., & Brownson, L. (2007). A support group intervention for children bereaved by parental suicide. *Journal of Child and Adolescent Psychiatric Nursing, 20*(1), 3–13. doi:10.1111/j.1744-6171.2007.00073.x

Mitchell, K. R., & Anderson, H. (1983). *All our losses, all our griefs.* Philadelphia, PA: Westminster Press.

Moules, N. J., Simonson, K., Fleiszer, A. R., Prins, M., & Glasgow, R. B. (2007). The soul of sorrow work: Grief and therapeutic interventions with families. *Journal of Family Nursing, 13*(1), 117–141. doi:10.1177/1074840706297484

Moules, N. J., Simonson, K., Prins, M., Angus, P., & Bell, J. M. (2004). Making room for grief: Walking backwards and living forward. *Nursing Inquiry, 11*(2), 99–107. doi:10.1111/j.1440-1800.2004.00204.x

Mystakidou, K., Tsilika, E., Parpa, E., Katsouda, E., & Vlahos, L. (2003). A Greek perspective on concepts of death and expression of grief, with implications for practice. *International Journal of Palliative Nursing, 9*(12), 534–537. doi:10.12968/ijpn.2003.9.12.11989

Nam, I. S. (2016). Effects of psychoeducation on helpful support for complicated grief: A preliminary randomized controlled single-blind study. *Psychological Medicine, 46,* 189–195. doi:10.1017/S0033291715001658

Narayanasamy, A. (2006). The impact of empirical studies of spirituality and culture on nurse education. *Journal of Clinical Nursing, 15*(7), 840–851. doi:10.1111/j.1365-2702.2006.01616.x

O'Neill, D. P., & Kenny, E. K. (1998). Spirituality and chronic illness. *Image—The Journal of Nursing Scholarship, 30*(3), 275–280. doi:10.1111/j.1547-5069.1998.tb01305.x

Parker, B., Alex, L., Jonsen, E., Gustafson, Y., Norgber, A., & Lundman, B. (2002) Resilience, sense of coherence, purpose in life and self-transcendence in relation to perceived physical and mental health among the oldest old. *Aging and Mental Health, 9,* 342–362. doi:10.1080/1360500114415

Parkes, C. M., & Weiss, R. S. (1983). *Recovery from bereavement.* New York, NY: Basic Books.

Parse, R. R. (2007). The human becoming school of thought in 2050. *Nursing Science Quarterly, 20*(4), 308–311. doi:10.1177/0894318407307160

Pattison, E. M. (1977). *The experience of dying.* New York, NY: Simon & Schuster.

Peereboom, K., & Coyle, N. (2012). Facilitating goals-of-care discussions for patients with life-limiting disease: Communication strategies for nurses. *Journal of Hospice and Palliative Nursing, 14*(4), 251–258. doi:10.1097/NJH.0b013e3182533a7f

Pennebaker, J. W., Mayne, T. J., & Francis, M. E. (1997). Linguistic predictors of adaptive bereavement. *Journal of Personality and Social Psychology, 72*(4), 863–871. doi:10.1037/0022-3514.72.4.863

Perrin, K. O., Sheehan, C. A., Potter, M. L., & Kazanowski, M. K. (2012). *Palliative care nursing: Caring for suffering patients.* Sudbury, MA: Jones & Bartlett.

Pilkington, F. B. (2006). Developing nursing knowledge on grieving: A human becoming perspective. *Nursing Science Quarterly, 19*(4), 299–303. doi:10.1177/0894318406293130

Pilkington, F. B. (2008). Expanding nursing perspectives on loss and grieving. *Nursing Science Quarterly, 21*(1), 6–7. doi:10.1177/0894318407310753

Prigerson, H. G., Bierhals, A. J., Kasl, S. V., Reynolds, C. F., Shear, M. K., Day, N., … Jacobs, S. (1997). Traumatic grief as a risk factor for mental and physical morbidity. *The American Journal of Psychiatry, 154*(5), 616–623. doi:10.1176/ajp.154.5.616

Pritchett, K. T., & Lucas, P. M. (1997). Grief and loss. In B. S. Johnson (Ed.), *Psychiatric-mental health nursing: Adaptation and growth* (4th ed., pp. 199–218). New York, NY: Lippincott.

Rando, T. A. (1984). *Grief, dying, and death.* Champaign, IL: Research Press.

Reiss, D. (1990). Patient, family, and staff responses to end-stage renal disease. *American Journal of Kidney Diseases, 15*(3), 194–200. doi:10.1016/S0272-6386(12)80762-1

Rossheim, B., & McAdams, C. (2010). Addressing the chronic sorrow of long-term spousal caregivers: A primer for counselors. *Journal of Counseling and Development, 88,* 477–482. doi:10.1002/j.1556-6678.2010.tb00048.x

Saldinger, A., Cain, A., & Porterfield, K. (2003). Managing traumatic stress in children anticipating parental death. *Psychiatry, 66*(2), 168–181. doi:10.1521/psyc.66.2.168.20613

Segal, J., Jaffe, J., Davies, P., & Smith, M. (2007). Depression in older adults and the elderly: Recognizing signs and getting help. Retrieved from http://www.helpguide.org/mental/depression_elderly.htm

Shear, M. K., Simon, N., Wall, M., Zisook, S., Neimeyer, R., Duan, N., … Keshaviah, A. (2011). Complicated grief and related bereavement issues for *DSM-5. Depression and Anxiety, 28*(2), 103–117. doi:10.1002/da.20780

Sherman, D. W. (1998). Reciprocal suffering: The need to improve family caregivers' quality of life through palliative care. *Journal of Palliative Medicine, 1*(4), 357–366. doi:10.1089/jpm.1998.1.357

Siegel, K., Karus, D. G., Raveis, V. H., Christ, G. H., & Mesagno, F. P. (1996). Depressive distress among the spouses of terminally ill cancer patients. *Cancer Practice, 4*(1), 25–30.

Spencer, L. (1994). How do nurses deal with their own grief when a patient dies on an intensive care unit, and what help can be given to enable them to overcome their grief effectively? *Journal of Advanced Nursing, 19*(6), 1141–1150.

Stroebe, M. S. (2002). Paving the way: From early attachment theory to contemporary bereavement research. *Mortality, 7*, 127–138. doi:10.1080/13576270220136267

Sudnow, D. (1967). *Passing on: The social organization of dying.* Englewood Cliffs, NJ: Prentice Hall.

Talerico, K. A. (2003). Grief and older adults. *Journal of Psychosocial Nursing, 41*(7), 12–16. doi:10.1037/1089-2680.9.1.48

Thomas, S. P. (2004). Men's health and psychosocial issues affecting men. *The Nursing Clinics of North America, 39*(2), 259–270. doi:10.1016/j.cnur.2004.01.002

Vance, D. E., Burrage, J., Couch, A., & Raper, J. (2008). Promoting successful aging with HIV through hardiness: Implications for nursing practice and research. *Journal of Gerontological Nursing, 34*(6), 22–29; quiz 30. doi:10.3928/00989134-20080601-11

Vigil, G. J., & Clements, P. T. (2003). Child and adolescent homicide survivors: Complicated grief and altered worldviews. *Journal of Psychosocial Nursing, 41*(1), 30–39. doi:10.3928/0279-3695-20030101-11

Viorst, J. (1987). *Necessary losses.* New York, NY: Ballantine Books.

Volker, D. L., & Wu, H. L. (2011). Cancer patients' preferences for control at the end of life. *Qualitative Health Research, 21*(12), 1618–1631. doi:10.1177/1049732311415287

Warren, B. J. (1999). Cultural competence in psychiatric nursing: An interlocking paradigm approach. In N. L. Keltner, L. H. Schwecke, & C. E. Bostrom (Eds.), *Psychiatric nursing* (3rd ed., pp. 98–148). Boston, MA: Mosby.

White, B., & Beach, P. (2012). In the shadows of family-centered care. *Journal of Hospice and Palliative Nursing, 14*(1), 53–60. doi:10.1097/NJH.0b013e3182350f1a

Wiegand, D. L. (2012). Family management after the sudden death of a family member. *Journal of Family Nursing, 18*(1), 146–163. doi:10.1177/1074840711428451

Williams, B. (2016). The impact of animals on patient wellbeing. *Nursing Times, 112*(25), 12–13.

Woodgate, R. L., & Degner, L. F. (2003). A substantive theory of keeping the spirit alive: The spirit within children with cancer and their families. *Journal of Pediatric Oncology Nursing, 20*(3), 103–119. doi:10.1053/jpon.2003.75

Worden, J. W. (1991). *Grief counseling and grief therapy: Handbook for the mental health practitioner.* New York, NY: Springer Publishing.

Zisook, S., & Shear, K. (2009). Grief and bereavement: What psychiatrists need to know. *World Psychiatry, 8*(2), 67–74. doi:10.1002/j.2051-5545.2009.tb00217

Carla Mariano

Holistic Integrative Therapies in Palliative Care

KEY POINTS

- Holism focuses on unity, mutuality, meaning, and the interrelationship of all beings events and things.
- People can grow and learn from illness and dying. Individuals can die healed.
- Holism is the theoretical and philosophical foundation for all complementary integrative healing modalities.
- Holistic integrative therapies can be used by the nurse, client/patient, and family. They are therapies of healing and empowerment.
- Relaxation is the basis for most holistic modalities.
- Imagination and imagery can play a powerful role in healing.
- Although there are many forms of meditation, all attempt to quiet the mind and focus one's attention inward.
- Sense therapies such as music (sound), aromas (smell), and touch (kinesthetics) have very potent natural healing properties that can adjust chemical or other imbalances with the body.
- Reminiscence and life review allow one to reintegrate past issues and experiences in the present to achieve a sense of meaning and ego integrity.
- Journal writing often helps those who cannot express verbally how they feel or what they are experiencing.
- Touch is essential to the quality of one's existence. It needs to be reintroduced as a significant modality in nursing practice.
- Herbs have many healing qualities but should be used knowledgeably.
- Homeopathy is a long-standing method of holistic medicine in which "like cures like" and remedies are tailored to the individual.
- Prayer is unique to each individual both in form and in content.
- There is a consciousness in dying where individuals become aware of their own deaths in phases.
- Self-care for health professionals who care for dying persons is imperative. Self-care areas include spiritual, emotional, physical, mental, and relationships.

CASE STUDY

J. A., a 40-year-old male diagnosed with advanced AIDS, was admitted to the hospital 1 week ago. This was his third hospitalization in 6 months. He was experiencing difficulty breathing, dehydration, extreme weakness, and fatigue. Because J. A. had lost so much weight, he was uncomfortable much of the time with muscle and joint aches. Additionally, J. A. was very anxious and found it difficult to sleep at night or rest during the day, increasing his discomfort and fatigue. He was fearful that any physical treatments or manipulation would exaggerate his pain, and he often became angry when the nurses administered morning and evening care.

J. A. was offered therapeutic touch (TT) treatments to see if it might be helpful in relaxing him. At first he refused, stating that he did not want to be touched. The nurse clarified that TT would not cause him any physical pain and that it did not in fact involve touching his body. She explained that it might be relaxing for him and might also help him to rest and sleep. The nurse suggested that, if J. A. was willing, she would do a 10-minute "trial" session to see if TT helped. After putting a sign on the door "Do not disturb for 15 minutes," the nurse encouraged J. A. to breathe slowly and deeply and close his eyes. She then centered herself, breathing slowly and deeply, and set the intention for the wholeness and well-being of J. A. Working about 7 to 10 inches away from his body, she began to assess J. A.'s energy field to ascertain his energy flow and any blockages. She then passed her hands repeatedly through his field from head to toe to get the energy flowing and balance J. A.'s field. The nurse continued for about 5 minutes, noticing that J. A.'s muscles relaxed, his expression softened, and he became quiet.

This chapter introduces the reader to a variety of holistic modalities that are used in nursing practice today and can be used in palliative care (PC). The modalities are defined and shown where they are most useful. In addition, this chapter includes a section on exercises that can be used readily by nurses and incorporated into their practice. It also includes resources where more information on each of these modalities can be obtained. In the education of nurses, it is particularly important for nursing faculty to incorporate these healing modalities into the curriculum for both undergraduate and graduate-level students.

Holism focuses on unity, mutuality, meaning, and the interrelationship of all beings, events, and things. The words "heal" and "health" come from *haelan*, which means to be or become whole. Holism emphasizes the basic wholeness and integrity of the individual. It views the body, mind, emotion, and spirit as inseparable and interdependent. All behaviors, including health, illness, and dying, are manifestations and natural unfolding of the life process of the whole person (Quinn, 2016).

Holistic nursing care draws on nursing knowledge, theories, expertise, and intuition, as nurses and clients become therapeutic partners in a shared evolving process toward healing. Holistic care:

■ Believes that people can grow and learn from health, illness, and dying
■ Promotes clients' active participation in their own healthcare, wellness, and healing
■ Uses appropriate interventions in the context of the client's total needs
■ Works to alleviate clients' physical signs and symptoms
■ Concentrates on the underlying meanings of symptoms and illness events and changes in the clients' life patterns and perceptions (Mariano, 2016b)

Numerous modalities (Dossey & Keegan, 2016; Fontaine, 2015; Micozzi, 2015) are used in the provision of holistic care. Some of these that are particularly useful in end-of-life (EOL) care are discussed in this chapter. Nurses can practice holistic care in any setting where healing occurs.

■ HEALTHCARE AND USE OF COMPLEMENTARY/INTEGRATIVE HEALTH APPROACHES IN THE UNITED STATES

The American public is increasingly demanding healthcare that is compassionate and respectful, provides options, is economically feasible, and is grounded in holistic ideals. A shift is occurring in healthcare, where people desire to be more actively involved in health decision making. They have expressed their dissatisfaction with conventional (Western allopathic) medicine and are calling for a care system that encompasses health, quality of life (QOL), and relationship with their providers.

The most recent survey, the 2012 National Health Interview Survey (NHIS), indicates that 33.2% of the adult population and 11.6% of children use complementary health approaches (Clarke, Black, Stussman, Barnes, & Nahin, 2015). The five most common complementary health approaches were natural products (herbs, vitamins and minerals, probiotics) 17.7%; deep breathing 10.9%; yoga, tai chi, or qi gong 10.1%; chiropractic or osteopathic manipulation 8.4%; and meditation 8% (Clarke et al., 2015; National Institutes of Health/National Center for Complementary and Integrative Health).

According to the NHIS, Americans spent $30.2 billion out of pocket on complementary health approaches (1.1% of total healthcare expenditures in the United States and 14.7 billion out of pocket on visits to complementary practitioners [or 30% of what they spent out of pocket on services by conventional physicians]). Americans spent 12.8 billion out of pocket on natural product supplements, which is about one-quarter of what they spent out of pocket on prescription drugs (Nahin, Barnes, & Stussman, 2016).

People who use complementary/integrative health approaches (CIHA) seek ways to improve their health and well-being, attempt to relieve symptoms associated with chronic or even terminal illnesses or the side effects of conventional treatments, have a holistic health philosophy or desire a transformational experience that changes their worldview, and want greater control over their health. CIHA provides individualized diagnosis and treatment of individuals; an emphasis on maximizing the body's inherent healing ability; and treatment of the "whole" person by addressing his or her physical, mental, and spiritual attributes.

Western medicine is proving wholly or partially ineffective for a significant proportion of the common chronic diseases. Furthermore, highly technological healthcare is too expensive to be universally affordable. Holistic care that promotes health is more cost effective and culturally acceptable to diverse and disparate populations whose belief systems are more congruent with whole-system and holistic approaches to treatment. The use of alternative methods for economic and cultural reasons by these populations often outweighs their use of conventional treatments (Mariano, 2016a).

In the past 5 to 7 years, many conventional healthcare institutions have developed complementary and integrative health programs, including stress management, energy therapies, healers in the operating rooms, and acupuncture. Programs such as TT or Reiki for chronic pain, support groups using imagery for breast cancer, and groups espousing meditation for health and wellness are commonly advertised across the United States. Similarly, local pharmacies and health food stores are selling an array of supplements, herbs, homeopathic preparations, vitamins, hormones, and various combinations of these that were not considered marketable 5 years ago. The number of books, journals, and websites devoted to complementary, integrative, and holistic healing practices has also dramatically increased.

Barnes, Bloom, and Nahin (2008) found that complementary and alternative medicine (CAM) usage was positively associated with the number of health conditions and number of doctor visits in the past 12 months. When worry about cost delayed the receipt of conventional medical care, adults were more likely to use CAM than when the cost of conventional care was not a worry. When unable to afford conventional medical care, adults were more likely to use CAM.

A survey of consumer use of CIHA by the American Association of Retired Persons (AARP) and the National Center for Complementary and Alternative Medicine (NCCAM) found that people 50 years of age and older tend to be high users of CAM (AARP/NCCAM, 2011). More than one-half (53%) of people 50 years and older reported using CIHA at some point in their lives, and nearly as many (47%) reported using it in the past 12 months. The most common reasons for using CIHA were to prevent illness or for overall wellness (77%), to reduce pain or treat painful conditions (73%), to treat a specific health condition (59%), or to supplement conventional medicine (53%). Three fourths (75%) of the respondents who had used herbal products or dietary supplements reported that they currently take one or more prescription medicines.

It is clear that people aged 50 years and older are likely to be using CAM. It is also clear that this population is frequently using prescription medications. Most users of CIHA do so without the knowledge or guidance of any healthcare professional. Common use of CAM as a complement to conventional medicine—and the high use of multiple prescription drugs—further underscores the need for healthcare providers and clients/patients/families to have an open dialogue to ensure safe and appropriate integrated healthcare. The lack of this dialogue points to a need to educate both consumers and healthcare providers about the importance of discussing the use of CAM, how to begin that dialogue, and the implications of not doing so.

The chronically and terminally ill consume more healthcare resources than the rest of the population. Chronic diseases and conditions—such as heart disease, stroke, cancer, diabetes, obesity, arthritis, hypertension, and depression—are some of the most common causes of death and disability in the United States (Centers for Disease Control and Prevention [CDC], 2015). About half of all adults (117 million people) have one or more chronic health conditions. One in four adults has two or more chronic health conditions. Chronic diseases account for 70% of all deaths in the United States, which is 1.7 million deaths each year. These diseases also cause major limitations in daily living for almost 1 out of 10 Americans, or about 25 million people (CDC, 2014). More than 75% of all healthcare spending in the United States currently is for the treatment of chronic disease, and 25% of Medicare spending is for costs incurred during the last year of life (Kaiser

Family Foundation, 2010). The great interest in CAM practices among the chronically ill, those with life-threatening conditions, and those at the end of their lives suggests that increased access to some services among these groups could have significant implications for the healthcare system.

With the number of older Americans expected to increase dramatically over the next 20 years, alternative strategies for dealing with the elderly population and EOL processes will be increasingly important in public policy. If evaluations show that some uses of CIHA can lessen the need for more expensive conventional care in these populations, the economic implications for Medicare and Medicaid could be significant. If safe and effective CIHA practices become more available to the general population, special and vulnerable populations should also have access to these services, along with conventional healthcare. CIHA would not be a replacement for conventional healthcare, but would be part of the treatment options available. In some cases, CIHA practices may be an equal or superior option. CIHA offers the possibility of a new paradigm of integrated healthcare that could affect the affordability, accessibility, and delivery of healthcare services for millions of Americans (Mariano, 2016a, p. 82).

■ HEALING AND DYING

Healing the dying sounds like an oxymoron.... But to heal is not necessarily to cure.... To heal is to bring various levels of oneself—cellular, physical, intrapersonal, interpersonal, societal, spiritual, perhaps even cosmic—into new relationship with each other. (Olson, 2001, p. 3)

The nurse must assess the relationship of the dying individual with self, others, and a higher power, and provide appropriate interventions to assist in the development or maintenance of new or right relationships.

"Dying healed means that a person has finished the business of life, said goodbyes, and reached life's goals. An individual knows who he is, and has a sense of integration of self and life" (Olson, 2001, p. 3). He or she realizes that one's life was unique and one's death matters to someone. One looks inward and realizes that life's difficulties have created a certain wisdom. Significant others have had time to grieve and plan for changes, and comfort and peace are attained. Control of the dying process is maintained as long as possible by the individual and as much as possible as the person is willing. Dying is seen as a stage of life. It is part of a larger philosophy and perception in which both life and death have meaning.

As mentioned previously, healing the dying necessitates regard for relationships and connectedness. We speak of transcendence when implying a sense of connectedness between self and a greater reality. Self-transcendence integrates self with past and future, giving meaning to the present. It reflects concern for others and/or for meaning (Keegan & Drick, 2016). Many of the integrative modalities described in this chapter facilitate self-transcendence. As noted by Keegan and Drick (2016), positive outcomes for the self-transcendent person, even when nearing death, include less depression, neglect, and hopelessness; a greater sense of well-being and ability to cope with grief and death; and the ability to live and find meaning in the present and connect with a higher power.

This caring relationship emphasizes quality rather than length of life. Healing the dying includes PC and focuses on relationships of all kinds. There is the provision for opportunities and choices where the dying person can live life to its fullest, and at some point comfortably forgive, let go, release, and experience a peaceful death.

The nurse is in a partnership with the dying client, sharing rather than denying the experience. The focus of nursing care is on providing sacred space and the milieu for a calm and peaceful death. The nurse works with the client to foster hope and cultivate an appreciation of the seemingly irrelevant things in life. Learning to appreciate simple occurrences such as a sunset or the joys of life can cultivate a more positive view of life and one's present experience. Enhancing avenues of support, whether professional, social (family and friends), or support groups, can often facilitate grieving and increase a sense of meaning in illness. Developing unrecognized inner strengths and resources is of great importance to the person who is dying or grieving.

The Chinese symbol for crisis indicates that crisis can be a challenge but simultaneously offers an opportunity for growth and a different perspective. The Greek word for crisis (krisis) signifies a "turning point." Grief can serve as a building block for personal growth and healing. Asking the dying person about spiritual needs gives the client an occasion to verbalize unmet needs. All of this requires skill, knowledge, compassion, caring, anticipation, and organization on the part of the nurse as well as a willingness to face one's own impermanence and mortality. It also necessitates caring for oneself.

■ SPECIFIC HOLISTIC HEALING MODALITIES

Holism is the theoretical and philosophical foundation for complementary integrative healing modalities. Numerous kinds of these modalities are used in healthcare today. This chapter will cover only a few of those that are most useful in EOL care or PC. Many of these modalities can be used effectively by the nurse as well as the client/patient, for example, centering, relaxation, imagery, meditation, prayer, herbology, and homeopathy. Others are described in use with clients/patients, such as sense therapies, reminiscence and life review, touch, and Reiki. In addition to their calming influence and physiological benefits, these techniques also may alter the perception of pain. Another valuable aspect of these modalities is that their use can empower clients and families. When clients learn to heal themselves, they are empowered. When they learn these techniques, they can do it themselves, which oftentimes gives them a sense of control (Mariano, 2016b). And when families are taught to use these modalities, they feel as if they are contributing something positive to the care of their loved one.

Centering

Centering is a process by which one quiets the mind and focuses one's thoughts. It calms the mind and allows the practitioner to access innermost resources that are powerful forces in healing. Krieger (1997) notes that

> Being on-center does not mean being still, immobile, rigid.... . In centering, we are quiet and "listen" to another language. Our attention goes to the heart region, where we find our own center of peace and know it as an attribute of our true self. We find that this sense of deep serenity is reminiscent of the truer peace we find in untrammeled nature and, with a thrill of personal discovery, realize that it is through such profound natural experiences that we can be at-one with the universe. (p. 22)

Centering is a shift in consciousness, an integrated sense of being. It is "a calm and focused sense of self-relatedness that can be thought of as a place of inner being, a place of quietude within oneself where one feels integrated and focused" (Jackson & Latini, 2016, p. 299). Bodily movements become quieted, and yet one is in an actively conscious state. One feels a unique stillness and peace. There is a sense of inner equilibrium and well-being. Perception deepens, and one is less aware of the chaos of the moment, the day, and the mind's chatter. Practice in the act of centering (closing eyes, quieting one's mind and activities, focusing on one's center or inner peace) leads to intuition and inner wisdom (Krieger, 2002).

By remaining "on-center," the nurse is able to convey to the client an awareness, a sensitivity, an empathy, and a deep sense of peace and regard that often creates a relaxation response in the client. One must give oneself permission to center, as the environment is always calling us to be present for it rather than for ourselves. But when one is centered and personally present, compassion becomes real, and this state is needed for those who would facilitate healing. One important exercise that the nurse can practice is to center before entering into each client encounter—detaching from any prior encounter—and to approach each client with awareness

and with, as Carl Rogers says, "unconditional positive regard" (Laurant & Shlien, 1984).

Creating Intention

Creating intention affects the mental, emotional, and physical realms. It is a powerful way to establish an optimal milieu for a caring–healing interaction.

> Examine the following intention: "I am here for the greater good of this person. I set aside my own concerns and worries and am fully present to the person here and now." With this intention the nurse is consciously setting aside his or her own concerns and focusing on the patient; s/he has set into motion the dynamic that this interaction will be "for the greater good of this person"; and s/he is making a conscious decision to be fully present. The nurse, through this intention, creates an environment that promotes and sustains a caring–healing interaction. (Thornton & Mariano, 2016, p. 471)

Relaxation

Relaxation is a state in which there is an absence of physical, mental, and emotional tension. A pleasant sensation and the lack of stressful or uncomfortable thoughts also accompany relaxation. It is often referred to as the opposite of the fight-or-flight or freeze response.

Relaxation allows the body/mind to quiet and focus inward. One can retreat mentally from one's surroundings, still thoughts, relax muscles, and maintain a state of relaxation, attaining the benefits of decreased tension, anxiety, and pain. Regardless of the approach (use of meditation, yoga, muscle and breathing exercises, hypnosis, prayer, and other forms of stress management), the end result of the relaxation response is a movement of the person toward calmness, balance, and healing. The guidelines for relaxation are found in Exhibit 12.1.

Relaxation techniques are the basis of many holistic modalities. Relaxation has three aims: (a) as a prevention to protect body organs from unnecessary stress and wear; (b) as a treatment to alleviate stress in numerous conditions, for example, hypertension, tension headache, insomnia, asthma, immune deficiency, panic, and pain; and (c) as a coping skill to calm the mind and to help thinking to become clearer and more effective (Micozzi & Jawer, 2015; Pestka, Bee, & Evans, 2014). Positive information in memory also becomes more accessible when a person is relaxed.

There are numerous benefits to the relaxed state, including lowered blood pressure, decreased heart rate, increased body temperature, decreased anxiety associated with painful situations, easing of muscle tension pain such as in contractures, a general sense of intense calm, decreased symptoms of depression and stress, and decreasing fatigue. Other benefits include helping the client to sleep, increasing the effects of medications, improvements in side effects of

Exhibit 12.1
Guidelines for Relaxation

- Be familiar with the relaxation exercise before introducing it to the client.
- Encourage use of familiar relaxation techniques that the client knows.
- Assess the client's level of tension, level of readiness to learn to relax, pain, anxiety, fear, and perception of reality or history of depersonalization.
- Ask the client what it means for him or her to be relaxed.
- Assess the client's ability to remain comfortably in one position for 10 to 20 minutes.
- Decrease as much environmental stimuli as possible.
- Assist the client to develop a positive expectation of what is to occur.
- Describe the potential benefits of relaxation and enlist cooperation.
- Reduce the opportunity for self-blame if the session does not go as expected.
- Have the client close his or her eyes.
- Use a tone of voice that is quiet and calm, conversational at first, and decreasing in volume as the session goes on.
- Use either tapes or a live voice. Music can provide background if desired.
- Guide the client through a basic breathing exercise (see "Exercises" section).
- Phrase all suggestions in a positive form, for example, "*Let go* of your tension," "Feel the tightness *melting* away," "*Loosen and soften* your muscles," "Allow the tension to *drift* away."
- Clients may experience a release of emotion as they relax, such as tears, vomiting, or faster and more shallow breathing. Gently ask if the client can put words to those feelings. Allow time for expression before continuing.
- At the completion of the session, bring the client gradually back to reality by having the client take deep breaths, move the hands and feet, and stretch if able.
- Have the client evaluate the experience.
- Engage the client's cooperation in continuing practice until the next session.

cancer therapy (decreased nausea, vomiting, and anxiety) and AIDS therapy, assisting in preparation for surgery or other treatments, and helping to dissociate from pain (Anselmo, 2016; Eliopoulos, 2018; Freeman, 2009; Payne & Donaghy, 2010). In addition to the therapeutic benefits, relaxation techniques also give clients a sense of control by enabling them to bring about certain psychological and mental responses by themselves.

Anselmo (2016); Davis, Eshelman, and McKay (2008); and Payne and Donaghy (2010) provide excellent guidelines for the nurse in preparing the client for relaxation and actual scripts to guide one through various relaxation exercises. Exhibit 12.1 includes guidelines or key points for relaxation.

A basic breathing exercise and relaxation exercise that can be used with the client or by the nurse are found in the "Exercises" section at the end of this chapter.

Imagery

Imagining is a powerful technique of focusing and directing the imagination. One uses all the senses—vision, sound, smell, taste, movement, position, and touch. Imagery influences an individual's attitudes, feelings, behaviors, and anxiety, which can either lead to a sense of hopelessness or promote a perception of well-being that assists in changing opinions about the disease, treatment, and healing potential. "Imagery [is the] internal experience of memories, dreams, fantasies, and visions—sometimes involving one, several, or all the senses that serve as the bridge for connecting body, mind, and spirit" (Schaub & Burt, 2016, p. 269). Imagery can affect people physically, emotionally, mentally, and biochemically, and the body and mind respond as if the event is actually occurring.

Guided imagery and interactive guided imagery (having the client directly interact with the image) are techniques to access the imagination through a guide. There are numerous types of imagery:

- Receptive imagery (inner knowing or "bubble-up" images)
- Active imagery (a focus on the conscious formation of an image)
- Correct biological imagery (recognizing the impact of negative images on physiology and creating positive correct biological images)
- Symbolic imagery (images emerging from both the unconscious and the conscious that shape attitudes, belief systems, and cultural experiences, often mythic symbols)
- Process imagery (a step-by-step rehearsal of any procedure, treatment, surgery, or other event prior to its occurrence)
- End-state imagery (rehearsal of an image of being in a final, healed state)
- General healing imagery (images that have a personal healing significance such as a wise person, an animal, the sun, etc.)
- Packaged imagery (another person's images such as commercial tapes)
- Customized imagery (images specific to an individual)

Guided imagery has many applications in EOL care or PC, including relaxation, stress reduction, pain relief, symptom management, grief work, and assisting clients to comprehend meaning in their illness experience (Fitzgerald & Langevin, 2014; Fontaine, 2015). It is useful not only in mobilizing latent, innate healing abilities of the client by intensifying the impact of healing messages that the autonomic nervous system sends to the immune system and other bodily functions, but also in the self-care of the nurse. It has been found helpful in relieving chronic pain and headaches, stimulating healing, tolerating medical procedures, exploring emotions that may have caused illness, understanding symptoms, solving difficult problems, enhancing self-esteem and self-confidence, envisioning and planning for the future, and listening to one's inner advisor.

It is usually helpful for the nurse to have training in the use of interactive guided imagery because of possibly overwhelming effects with this type of imagery. Otherwise, as Schaub and Burt (2016) note, imagery scripts are more effective when one learns the speaking skills of voice modulation, specific word emphasis, and the use of pauses. Guidelines for the nurse to use in teaching the client the imagery process are presented in Exhibit 12.2.

Basic imagery exercises that nurses can use with clients are listed under the "Exercises" section at the end of this chapter.

Meditation

Meditation is a quiet turning inward. It is the practice of focusing one's attention internally to achieve clearer consciousness and inner stillness. There are numerous methods and schools of meditation, all having an individual interpretation of the practice. However, all methods believe in emptying the mind and letting go of the mind's chatter that preoccupies us.

Meditation, which originated in the Eastern tradition and is integral to Hinduism, Taoism, and Buddhism, is both a state of mind and a method. The state is one where the mind is quiet and listening to itself. The practitioner is relaxed but alert. The method involves the focusing of attention on something such as the breath, an image, a word, or an action such as tai chi or qigong. There is a sustained concentration, but it should be effortless.

The objective of meditation is to detach from external events as well as one's own mental activity. Rather than examining thoughts that may enter the mind, the person puts them aside and allows them to drift away. There is no criticism or judgment, but an attitude of a beginner's mind: a mind that is open and receptive, clear of attachment to any thoughts. The body is relaxed and the mind is emptied of all thoughts except the awareness of the image, word, or breath. "Passive concentration" keeps the meditator in a state of awareness and alertness rather than drowsiness and intently focused on the present moment. There should be no blame, guilt, or recrimination if the meditator loses focus or if the mind wanders; one is instructed simply to return the mind to its original focus. Reentry into the normal waking state should be gentle and relaxed. Meditation requires practice on a regular schedule, usually once or twice daily to achieve maximal results.

There are various reasons for practicing meditation: to find peace, achieve awareness and enlightenment, find oneself, experience true reality, and enhance a sense of well-being. Research has demonstrated that relaxed forms of meditation decrease heart rate and blood pressure, increase breathing volume while decreasing the number of breaths per minute, increase peripheral blood flow, improve immune function, decrease anxiety, decrease insomnia, and decrease skeletal muscle tension, epinephrine level, gastric acidity, motility, anxiety, depression, traumatic stress, and alcohol and drug consumption (Anselmo, 2016; Fontaine, 2015; Freeman, 2009; Gauding, 2017; Gross, Christopher, & Reilly-Spong, 2014). It is believed that meditation activates the right cerebral hemisphere and the parasympathetic nervous system, thereby quieting the nerves and allowing intuitive, wordless thinking to occur. In addition to physiological benefits, the advantages of meditation cited by Payne and Donaghy (2010) are listed in Exhibit 12.3.

A simple meditation that can be practiced by the nurse or with a client is discussed in the "Exercises" section at the end of this chapter.

Exhibit 12.2
Guidelines to Imagery

- Have the client relax. Help the client to identify the problem or goal of imagery.
- Develop a basic understanding of the physiology involved in the healing process. Begin with a few minutes of relaxation, meditation, or paying attention to the breath exercise.
- Assist the client to develop images of
  - The problem
  - Inner healing resources (beliefs, coping strategies, etc.)
  - External healing resources (medications, treatments, family, etc.)
  - End with images of the desired state of well-being

Exhibit 12.3
Advantages of Meditation

- A better understanding of the self and increased receptivity to insights arising from one's deeper being; practicing meditation can bring the experience of self for the dying, where the individual may attain calm and often a sense of purpose
- A new sense of relaxation and inner peace
- A clearer mind and improved concentration
- More harmony with and within the self
- As a result of the detachment, an acceptance that many unpleasant emotional responses are short-lived sensations created by one's thoughts
- An emphasis on living in the present and valuing the here and now

Sense Therapies

Sense therapies use the senses to treat physical and psychological problems and to adjust chemical or other imbalances within the body. These can include behavioral vision therapy, eye movement, desensitization, flower remedies, hydrotherapy, and light therapy. Three therapies will be explored under sense therapies: music therapy, music thanatology, and aromatherapy.

■ **Music Therapy.** Morris (2009) defines music therapy as the "behavioral science concerned with the systematic application of music to produce relaxation and desired changes in emotions, behavior, and physiology" (p. 327). The elements of music, sound, rhythm, hearing, melody, harmony, and movement are part of people's primary experiences. Listening to, creating, or moving to music assists people in improving, changing, or better integrating aspects of themselves. Music has a power that cannot be expressed in verbal language.

There are references to the therapeutic powers of music in philosophy, art, and literature throughout the ages (Ingersoll & Schaper, 2013). Music is used in healing ceremonies throughout the world. Our own experiences demonstrate the psychological effect that music has on us. Despite varying musical tastes, certain types of music create specific moods: for example, a march, ominous music, lively music at sports events, quiet and relaxing music in waiting rooms, or a mother's singing and rocking her baby in times of distress.

Music therapy can reduce biopsychological stress, pain, anxiety, and isolation. It assists clients in reaching a deep state of relaxation, developing self-awareness and creativity, improving learning, clarifying personal values, and coping with a variety of psychophysiological problems. It also provides clients with integrated body/mind episodes and encourages them to become active participants in their own healing. Appropriate music produces the relaxation response, often removing a client's inner restlessness and quieting ceaseless thinking. It is used as a healing technique to quiet the mind and bring about inner relaxation (Morris, 2009). Research has demonstrated that music reduces acute and chronic pain, is beneficial in treating or managing dementia symptoms, provides distraction, reduces agitated behaviors in elderly individuals, decreases the intensity of depression, reduces pain and nausea, and increases QOL and spiritual well-being (Fontaine, 2015; Ingersoll & Schaper, 2013).

Because music therapy focuses on process and not on outcome, one need not have any musical skills or talents to derive benefits. Clients can be induced to a relaxed state through breathing, suggestive imagery, or a relaxation exercise. Music selected by the client or the nurse is played, and the client is invited to explore images, sensations, emotions, memories, and visions brought on by the music. No one type of music works

Exhibit 12.4
Assessment of Music Therapy

- The client's music history and music preferences
- The client's identification of music that make the client happy, excited, sad, or relaxed
- The client's identification of music that is distasteful and that makes the client tense
- Assessment of the importance of music in the client's life
- The frequency of music playing in the client's life
- Previous participation in relaxation/imagery techniques combined with music
- The client's mood—this will determine the type of music to be played

well for all individuals in all situations. A variety of soothing selections (popular, new age, classical, country, opera, folk, jazz, choral hymns, etc.) should be available because one cannot always predict a client's particular preference or response to the music. Often the client experiences an altered state of consciousness, which is usually very relaxing. After the listening, the client is brought back to reality to discuss the experience. In some instances, the client chooses the music and moves to the music. The nurse should assess the factors described in Exhibit 12.4 in preparing to use music therapy (Chlan & Heiderscheit, 2014).

Music has the greatest effect when the client is appropriately prepared. Find a quiet environment and have the client assume a comfortable position. Suggest that the client maintain a passive attitude, neither forcing nor resisting the experience, and remind the client to focus all concentration on the music.

■ **Music Thanatology.** Music thanatology, developed by Schroeder-Sheker (1994, 2005) and Hollis (2010), is a field that addresses the needs of the dying by assisting the client in completing the transition between life and death. Specially trained therapists, using harp, voice, and chanting, assist the client in leave-taking during the last hours of life by reinforcing peace, acceptance, and a calm anticipation of death. Schroeder-Sheker (1994) describes music thanatology as a

palliative medical modality employing prescriptive music to tend the complex physical and spiritual needs of the dying ... music thanatology is concerned with the possibility of a blessed death and the gift that conscious dying can bring to the fullness of life. (p. 83)

This music is live (not taped), dynamic, and prescriptive. It is individual to each patient and each death, much like childbirth. According to Schroeder-Sheker

(2005), music thanatology has been found to be most effective in deaths from cancer, AIDS, burns, and slowly degenerative diseases.

Schroeder-Sheker (1994) identifies six foundational assumptions of music thanatology:

1. It recognizes dying as a spiritual process and as an opportunity for growth.
2. The musical deathbed vigil, often called "musical-sacramental-midwifery," is a contemplative practice requiring serious inner work and integration of the physical, emotional, mental, and spiritual aspects of the caregiver.
3. Death is not an enemy and it is not a failure; it is a critical chapter of human biography.
4. The way in which each person dies is equally important as the way in which that person lived. Beauty, reverence, dignity, and intimacy are central to life and especially so for death. The infirmary music can bring things to the surface in a nonthreatening way or serve the role of meditation. Music is a flow, weaving the body, soul, and spirit together.
5. This work is a vocation, not merely a career. It requires clear intention and attention at each deathbed vigil.
6. Death and dying should be returned to the human, personal realm rather than denying or ignoring loss and leave-taking and thus reducing them to legal or corporate medical matters.

Music thanatology focuses on music for the dying versus music for the living. The dying person should not spend energy, only receive energy.

The entire surface of the skin can become an extension of the ear, thus enabling the patient to absorb infirmary music, creating the possibility for even deeper emotional, mental, and spiritual reception.... . The sole focus is to help the person move toward completion and to unbind from anything that prevents, impedes, or clouds a tranquil passage. (Schroeder-Sheker, 1994, pp. 93–94)

■ **Aromatherapy.** Aromatherapy is an offshoot of herbal medicine, in which aromatic plant extracts are inhaled or applied to the skin as a means of treating illness and promoting physical, psychological, and spiritual benefits as well as positive changes in mood and outlook (Buckle, 2016). Though aromatherapy and herbal medicine use many of the same plants, in aromatherapy the plants are distilled into oils of exceptional potency (Halcon, 2014).

The advantage of these oils comes from their influence on the limbic system, which coordinates mind and body activity. This system is very sensitive to odors and encodes them into associations and memories, which when awakened alter basic physical functions such as heart rate, blood pressure, breathing, and hormone level. When these oils are rubbed into the skin or inhaled, they set off a reaction leading to rapid and significant alterations in memory, heart rate, and other bodily mechanisms. Some boost energy, some promote relaxation, and others have pharmaceutical effects. However, no treatment should ever involve more than a few drops of oil.

Hundreds of plants are used for aromatherapy (Buckle, 2016; Davis, 2011; Fontaine, 2015; Lewis, 2015; Price & Price, 2011). Some of the more common ones that are useful in the care of the dying include chamomile, which is used to overcome anxiety, anger, tension, stress, and insomnia; lavender, for exhaustion, depression, and stress; marjoram, for those who are physically debilitated; neroli, for countering depression, anxiety, nervous tension, and fearfulness; peppermint and rosewood, for treating nausea; and chamomile, camphor, fennel, lavender, peppermint, and rose, for relieving vomiting. Aromatherapy also is used in the relief of pain (lavender, capsicum, bergamot, chamomile, rose, ginger, rosemary, lemongrass, sage, and camphor). It is most useful in the enhancement of mood, increasing vitality, and relaxation. These plants and oils can be found in natural or health food stores.

Reminiscence and Life Review

Life review or reminiscence therapy is the remembering of significant past events that enables one to reintegrate past issues and experiences in the present for the purpose of achieving a sense of meaning and ego integrity. The concept has been most frequently used with elderly individuals but is just as effective with those nearing the end of life. Reminiscence is a natural phenomenon. It is the process of recounting past events to someone else, or it can be a more complex process of transpersonal focusing and inward reflection. The level of complexity depends on the wish of the client and the training of the nurse. Life review can be oral, including audio and video recordings, or written. Journal and letter writing can also be useful techniques in life review. Photographs and personal items often provide the opportunity for reminiscence and give information about the client that assists the nurse in providing personal and meaningful care.

Life review is a process of unfolding and emerging and therefore cannot be hurried. A life review can be one or many sessions. Keegan and Drick (2016) and Haight and Haight (2007) provide a guide for a structured life review that usually includes six to eight sessions:

■ Use open-ended questions. Ask about childhood and earliest memories and be sure to be supportive if the client recalls sad events.
■ Again using open-ended questions, proceed through the client's life history by asking about adolescence, family and home, adulthood, and later life.
■ Have a summary session inquiring about the following: "Generally, what kind of life do you think you have had? What would you do over again?"

To promote the process, the nurse should encourage the client to express himself or herself, involve significant others, assure confidentiality of the information, be sure the client has sufficient physical strength and a desire for sharing, listen carefully, use touch as appropriate, and allow the client periods of silence to reflect. Life review provides integration, a feeling that this life was individual and unique. The client may verbalize sadness as well as achievement, but the objective is to allow a person to see the meaning in his or her life.

Journal Writing

Keeping a log or journal is a very effective healing technique to use for individuals who are experiencing life-threatening illness and during the grieving process. It allows the person to express his or her innermost feelings and thoughts without fear of criticism. It is often helpful for those who are uncomfortable or unable to articulate how they feel or what they are going through. Writing can also assist the person to make new connections and reframe past experiences. The healing emanates from the actual writing and expression, and not from an analysis of the content of the journal. The writing may be totally private or shared with others. Many clients do not think of this technique, and the nurse may suggest it. Levin and Reich (2013) and Snyder (2014) offer some suggested topics for journal writing:

- Special thoughts of the dying person or about the deceased
- Feelings that were never expressed
- Saying good-bye
- Ways that grief or dying has helped one grow
- Lessons learned from life that one wants to share
- Positive aspects of the past, present, and future
- Transitions
- Fears about treatment/outcomes

There are numerous topics for journal writing, or the client can just write thoughts and feelings as they occur. The individual may find comfort in writing when difficult times occur, for example, unanticipated news about a diagnosis or prognosis, dealing with family members, or writing to God, a loved one, or one's disease. Often the journal becomes one's own record of grieving. It often serves as a chronicle of personal growth, insights, and wisdom gleaned from the experience of dying or loss.

Touch

In the later stages of life, individuals are often deprived of tender and nurturing physical contact such as being touched in a way that is healing, nourishing, relaxing, and pleasurable. Touch is essential to one's quality of existence. It provides comfort, warmth, and renewed vitality—a sense of security and assurance that we are not alone. Reasons for the lack of touch of the dying include fear, discomfort, stereotypes about dying people, and a sense of one's own vulnerability. However, the benefits of touch on individuals are many. There is an increase of circulation and mobility (e.g., range of motion or hand grasp), a decrease in pain, increase in vitality, increase in physical functioning, the experience of being nurtured and cared for, a boost in self-esteem, increased motivation to receive and give attention to self and others, energy and emotional release, a sense memory triggering a relaxation response, relief from loneliness and isolation, decreased feelings of abandonment and deprivation, verbal interaction, and calming reassurance and support (Goldschmidt & van Meines, 2012; Rose, 2009). It often induces much-needed sleep. In this day of technological care, touch may be the one caring tool to help a client feel better.

There are many forms of touch considered to be holistic/integrative modalities (DeLany, 2015; Fontaine, 2015; Jackson & Latini, 2016; Lindquist, Snyder, & Tracy, 2014; Micozzi, 2015). These include, but are not limited to, the following:

- **Acupressure**—The application of pressure, using fingers, thumbs, palms, or elbows, to specific sites along the body's energy meridians to stimulate, disperse, and regulate the body's healing energy for the purpose of relieving tension and reestablishing the flow of energy along the meridian lines.
- **Body therapy**—A general term used for approaches (e.g., Alexander technique, chiropractice, Rolfing, shiatsu, Feldenkrais) that use hands-on techniques to manipulate and balance the musculoskeletal system to facilitate healing, increase energy, relieve pain, and promote relaxation and well-being.
- **Reflexology**—The application of pressure to specific reflex areas on the feet or hands that correspond to other parts of the body in order to locate and correct problems in the body.
- **Massage**—The practice of kneading or otherwise manipulating a person's muscles and other soft tissue with the intent of inducing physical and psychological relaxation, improving circulation, relieving pain and sore muscles, and improving the individual's well-being. Procedural massage is done to diagnose, monitor, or treat the illness itself, focusing on the end result of curing the illness or preventing further complications. In the past, massage has been one of nurses' most important interventions for pain reduction, comfort, tension release, prevention of atrophy of muscles and stiffness of joints, and inducing sleep. A back massage has left many a patient refreshed and feeling cared for. It would behoove us in nursing to reintroduce massage into our practice armamentarium.

Therapeutic Touch was developed by Dolores Krieger and Dora Kunz. This is a specific modality of centering intention while the practitioner moves the hands through the client's energy field for the purpose of assessment and treatment. It is based on the philosophy that universal life energy flows through and around us, and any interruption in this free flow of energy leads to illness. The goal is to balance and repattern the body's energy so that it flows most efficiently to promote health and prevent disease. The TT practitioner scans the client's energy flow, replenishing it where necessary, releasing congestion, removing obstructions, and restoring order and balance in the ill system. This approach is also an effective complementary care approach for facilitation of the body's natural restorative processes, thereby accelerating healing, promoting relaxation, reducing pain and anxiety, and treating chronic conditions.

According to Macrae (2013), a well-known TT practitioner,

> Since therapeutic touch is an interaction, it has the potential to heal the practitioner as well as the patient. ... You can also use the principles of TT to assist in healing yourself ... the use of mental imagery can facilitate both the energy transfer and the rebalancing of the [practitioner's] field. If you have pain or discomfort somewhere: (1) Sit quietly and center yourself; (2) visualize the healing energy (as light, if you wish) coming down from above and flowing through you; (3) visualize the energy clearing away the pain or discomfort (as light shines through a dark area). (pp. 79–80)

Compassionate touch, developed by Nelson (1994, 2006) specifically for hands-on care given to those who are elderly, ill, or dying, is described as

> a gentle, sensitive, and nonintrusive program of massage, attentive touch, and supportive comfort care for those individuals who are temporarily or permanently less active.... . It also includes individuals of any age who are actively beginning the mysterious life transition that we call death. (p. 1)

Compassionate touch is a hands-on technique stemming not from the hands but from the heart. It combines massage and attentive touch with active listening, reflective communication, relaxation, imagery, and breathing awareness exercises. It focuses not only on the physical condition of the client but also on the psychosocial, emotional, and spiritual needs.

According to Nelson (1994),

> Compassion for another implies a feeling of unconditional regard for that other; it also implies a genuine, sincere interest in that person's well-being. The compassionate heart shares in, and is affected by the suffering of another.... . The compassionate individual is able to put aside his or her own concerns for a time in order to give attention to someone else. Some say compassion is love in action. (p. 1)

Compassionate touch is not something we give; it is a way of being. It is a way of providing contact, reassurance, relief, and comfort for those who may be frightened, depressed, out of control, abandoned, overwhelmed, confused, or in despair. It is a means of relating to others rather than a prescribed set of techniques to be practiced on others. It is a spontaneous event of relationship that unfolds moment to moment. Compassionate touch can be administered by anyone who feels inspired to reach out to a fellow human being in need.

Reiki is based on Buddhist teachings, using hands-on touch to support and intensify energy in the physical, emotional, intellectual, and spiritual areas. Universal and personal energy are aligned and balanced by applying gentle hands-on touch to energy pathways of the body. Those who use Reiki attribute it with reducing stress and stress-related illnesses, including acute and chronic conditions; helping in debilitating disease because it bolsters the immune system by increasing energy; and contributing to an overall sense of well-being in the client (Jackson & Latini, 2016; Ringdahl, 2014).

The philosophy of Reiki contends that a person is vitalized by an essential energy that comes from the universal life force. Everyone has access to this life force, and one becomes ill when the energy flow is interrupted or stopped. Opening pathways for energy flow is the prime objective of Reiki. Learners of Reiki must themselves receive an attunement by an expert Reiki master in an initiation ceremony so that they are attuned to the energy transfer process.

Reiki bodywork is not massage. The touch is gentle and aims not to manipulate tissue, but rather to transmit universal life force to the client. The practitioner uses both hands, palms down, fingers held together, and proceeds in a pattern over the client's body. Each positioning of the hands is maintained for 3 to 5 minutes without any movement of the fingers or change in the initial gentle touch. During these hand placements, the universal life force flows through the practitioner to the client to balance the client's energy where necessary (Ringdahl, 2014).

Reiki bodywork is very individualized, and the client's perception of the energy transfer is unique to each person. Most find it rejuvenating and relaxing. The effects may be felt immediately or several days later. Following attunement/initiation of the caregiver, Reiki can be used as a method of self-healing as well as caring for others. As can be seen, numerous holistic healing modalities can be used during EOL care.

Herbology

Herbology is also known as *phytotherapy* or *phytomedicine*. Herbal remedies have been used in various cultures for centuries and are increasingly popular in the United States as health products and medicines. In fact, herbal use is the fastest growing category of alternative/complementary therapy in the United States.

Micozzi and Meserole (2015) define herbs as plants or plant parts (bark, fruit, flower, leaves, stem, root, or seed) that are used in fresh, dried, or extracted form for food, medicine, or promoting, maintaining, or restoring health. Herbs are prepared in many forms: tinctures, extracts, capsules, tablets, lozenges, teas, juices, vapor treatments, poultices, compresses, salves, liniments, and bath products (Springhouse Corporation, 2005).

Herbs are classified based on their effects as follows (Braun & Cohen, 2015; Gladstar, 2012; Helming, 2016; Pursell, 2016; Skidmore-Roth, 2009):

- Adaptogenic herbs (which increase the body's resistance to illness)
- Anti-inflammatory herbs
- Antimicrobial herbs
- Antispasmodic herbs
- Astringent herbs (which are applied externally)
- Bitter herbs to increase the secretion of digestive juices, stimulate appetite, and promote liver detoxification
- Carminative herbs (aromatic oils) to soothe the lining of the gastrointestinal (GI) tract and reduce gas, inflammation, and pain
- Demulcent herbs to soothe and protect inflamed and irritated tissue and mucous membranes
- Diuretic herbs
- Expectorant herbs
- Hepatic herbs to tone the liver and increase the production of hepatocytes
- Hypotensive herbs
- Laxative herbs
- Nervine herbs to strengthen and restore, ease anxiety and tension, and stimulate nerve activity
- Stimulating herbs to stimulate physiologic and metabolic activities
- Tonic herbs, which enliven and invigorate by promoting the "vital force," which is key to health and longevity
- Pain-relieving herbs

Although herbs are natural substances and their overall risk seems to be low, they cannot be used indiscriminately. Herbs are medicinal and may have serious side effects and interactions with prescription drugs. Additionally, there is a lack of regulation of commercial herbal products in the United States and lack of standardized dosage ranges and preparations. Yet, so many Americans choose to take herbal remedies because they are much less costly than prescription drugs, their access is virtually unlimited and unrestricted, they are effective, and many people are becoming disenchanted with traditional healthcare. However, before taking any herbal remedy, one must know what it does, how to use it, and the possible adverse effects.

Many clients may hesitate to inform their healthcare provider that they are using herbs. It is therefore important for the nurse to assess clients' use of herbs and advise them accordingly. Several researchers offer the following guidelines regarding herbal therapy (Fontaine, 2015; Micozzi & Meserole, 2015; Plontikoff, 2014; Skidmore-Roth, 2009):

1. Encourage the client to disclose use of herbal treatments and obtain a history of herb use as complete as possible, including all products taken, amounts, and brand names. If the client is seeing a herbalist, report any prescription drugs.
2. Determine if the client is using herbal remedies instead of, or as an adjunct to, conventional treatment. Is the herb being used to treat a specific condition or for general health?
3. Inform the client of various benefits, risks, and side effects of the herbal remedy, and any potentially serious adverse reactions that may occur when herbs are used with other drugs or substances the client is using. Labels on the products should contain information about product ingredients and use. Recommend standardized herbs.
4. Warn elderly clients, pregnant women, children, and those with known adverse drug reactions, allergies, chronic skin rashes, or preexisting liver disease that they have an increased risk of adverse effects from herbal medicines.
5. Advise the client to notice any unusual symptoms and to report these to the healthcare provider immediately.
6. Advise the client not to take herbal products for serious medical conditions unless they are used under the care of a well-trained healthcare provider. Urge clients to take only the recommended dosages of herbal remedies.
7. Advise the client to be informed of reputable herbal companies and be careful about products sold through magazines, brochures, and the Internet.
8. Tell the client to see a healthcare provider well trained in herbology when using herbal remedies. Health food store clerks are salespersons, not trained practitioners.
9. Keep a referral list of knowledgeable herbologists.

The field of herbology is expanding at an enormous rate, and many books are now available for the nurse to refer to in the care of clients. It is important that the nurse become informed about herbs because increasingly our clients will be coming to us while concurrently using herbal remedies.

Homeopathy

"Homeopathy" comes from the Greek words *homeo*, which means similar, and *pathos*, which means disease or suffering (Boiron Group, 2009). It is based on the law of similars, or like cures like, where stimulating the natural healing properties in the body cures a disease or alleviates a symptom (Freeman, 2009). In other words, when a substance identical to what would produce the symptoms of the disease is introduced into the body in very small or minute doses, it stimulates the person's healing energy. This is very different from what Hahnemann (the father of homeopathy) called allopathy, from the Greek words *allos*, meaning different, and *pathein* or *pathos*, meaning disease or suffering (Weiner, 1998).

The philosophy of homeopathy strongly contends that health and disease are holistic phenomena and the individual must be considered from a body, mind, and spirit perspective; that there is an inherent capacity in all living things to respond to illness in a self-curative way; that there is an "unknowability" about certain disease processes; and that rather than focusing on the disease, treatment may begin with the symptom, but the client is treated as a whole and as an individual rather than as a diagnosis with common symptoms. Treatment is individualized and tailored to the uniqueness of each person.

Homeopathic remedies are prepared from natural substances—plant, animal, and mineral. The use of micro-doses, that is, highly diluted doses, ensures the minimization of toxicity and side effects. Homeopathic medicines are available in various dosage forms: pellets, tablets, liquids, suppositories, and ointments. The U.S. Food and Drug Administration (FDA) recognizes homeopathic remedies as official drugs and regulates the manufacturing, labeling, and dispensing of homeopathic remedies. Simple homeopathic medications of low potencies are available over the counter; however, dilutions for more complicated and chronic conditions are available only from a homeopathic practitioner. Homeopathic remedies are safe, economical, simple to administer, and mild in action, and have very few serious or prolonged adverse effects (Carlston, 2011).

Homeopathic remedies are valuable for a number of symptoms: arnica (marked muscle soreness and acute pain); hypericum (nerve pain, shooting pain); bryonia (trauma, pain on movement); bellis perennis (muscle injury from surgery); ipecacuanha (nausea and vomiting); aconite (fear and shock); calendula (bleeding, preventing infection, increasing granulation); chamomilla (irritability, sensitivity); belladonna (fever); and nux vomica (insomnia; Cummings & Ullman, 2010; Fontaine, 2015; Wauters, 2007).

Prayer

Whatever holistic/complementary therapy we use may not be as important as how we use it. Providing safe space where healing can occur is what is most important—and that means using ourselves as an instrument of healing. Clients with life-threatening illness often question "Why?" and may need support in their desire to connect with something larger and outside of themselves. Focusing on them as spiritual beings allows them to explore the meaning and purpose of their illness and can bring comfort, often alleviating pain (Dossey, 1996, 1998;

Wright, 2005). Burkhardt and Nagai-Jacobson (2016) and Eliopoulos (2018) offer a number of useful guides and instruments to facilitate spiritual assessment.

As O'Brien (2017) notes, prayer is as unique as the individual who is praying. Whether it is of petition, adoration, reparation, or thanksgiving, both the form and the content may vary greatly. Prayer is a simple act of turning our attention to the sacred. Depending on one's beliefs, this can be the God of whatever religion or culture, a higher power, or the ultimate reality. Prayer can be active or passive, involve words, or be wordless. It can involve asking something for oneself or another, expressing repentance for wrongdoing and asking for forgiveness, giving praise and honor, summoning the presence of the Almighty, or offering gratitude (O'Brien, 2003; Snyder & Lathrop, 2014). Many forms of prayer are meditative in nature and have the benefits of meditation previously discussed in the section on meditation. Others are intercessory, an active form of prayer that seeks an outcome through intentionality where we ask for healing for others or ourselves. This also can be done at a distance, which is referred to as nonlocal healing (Dossey, 1998). Clients also can benefit from prayerful listening to sacred music or sounds, writing or art, or expressing their intent toward the sacred through some body movement or posture (Taylor, 2003).

Prayer is often an important solace to clients who are ill; however, illness may create a barrier to prayer. In those instances, nurses' prayers for and with the client can be a meaningful spiritual intervention as long as permission is obtained when possible. The nurse should assess the client to ascertain if prayer is desired and then follow the client's expressed wish. Fontaine (2015) and Taylor (2003) suggest some assessment questions that the nurse can use:

- "How important or helpful is prayer to you?"
- "Would praying together now be comforting?"
- "What type of prayer would be helpful or comforting to you now?"
- "What helps or hinders you as you pray?"
- "How has your illness affected the way you pray or think about prayer?"
- "Have your prayers changed since you became sick?"
- "Do you find it harder to pray sometimes? How do you deal with that?"
- "Have your beliefs about prayer been challenged or changed by illness?"
- "At times like this, some start thinking about if and how their prayers 'get answered.' Have you thought about this?"

A few minutes spent on assessing and possibly praying with a client can often lower a client's anxiety or assist the nurse's understanding of how prayer facilitates the client's coping.

■ THE HEALING JOURNEY AT THE END OF LIFE

Individuals become aware of their own deaths in phases, and this awareness can lead to consciousness in dying. Keegan and Drick (2016) and Olson (1997) identify some tasks for dying consciously, specifically,

1. *Live fully* until death comes. Direct or participate in treatment decisions, determinations about the kinds of care, and other decisions until you are comfortable with accepting the assistance of others.
2. *Plan* to say good-bye to family and friends, finish things you wanted to do, and make final decisions regarding the last will and testament, the estate, organ donation, and so forth. Consider what an ideal death would be like. Who do you want with you, or do you want to be alone? Who are the important people in your life and have you told them? Are there certain rituals you want at your death, for example, a memorial service or cremation? What kind of ceremony do you want? Are there certain treasures that you want particular people to have? Are there particular prayers, poems, or music you want read or played?
3. *Participate* in emotional and spiritual tasks such as forgiving yourself and others, feeling that life mattered and the world is different because you were here, and knowing and accepting love as one changes. Forgiving yourself and others necessitates recognizing that we are responsible for what we are holding onto; confessing one's story to self and others, looking for the good points in ourselves and others; making amends where possible; looking to a higher power for help; and considering what we have learned. Forgiving others and ourselves helps us recognize unconditional love and connect more with the source of our joy instead of focusing on loss, sadness, and pain. Unconditional love helps release one from fear and anxiety.
4. *Rehearse* the dying process. Through an awareness of dying, learn to diminish the fear of death and to "let go of this life" when it is time to do so. Imagery, relaxation, meditation, and prayer scripts on learning forgiveness, becoming peaceful, letting go, opening the heart, forgiving self and others, releasing pain and grief, conscious dying, moving into the light, and closure can facilitate the detachment from pain and grief, the establishment of comfort and peace, and the achievement of closure. Keegan and Drick (2016) is an excellent source for some of these scripts. However, the nurse should have some practice experience prior to their use with clients.

■ BENEFITS OF HOLISTIC INTEGRATIVE THERAPIES

Nurses can make a critical difference in ensuring that clients receiving PC obtain the maximum benefit at a minimum risk when they integrate complementary/alternative modalities and conventional therapies. Clients benefit because of the following:

- Holistic therapies build on the body's capabilities and are aimed toward strengthening the body's own defenses and healing abilities so that the body can heal itself. Strengthened and healthy defenses offer relief that exceeds symptom management.
- Holistic integrative therapies view people holistically, realizing that they are complex combinations of unique bodies, minds, emotion, and spirits. CIHA consider this interconnectedness, as they assess and address the physical, mental, emotional, environmental, and spiritual aspects of the person. Healing practices are tailored to the individual. This is especially important for PC, where each person is experiencing a unique dying process. As a result, questions, emotional problems, socioeconomic concerns, and spiritual issues that affect health can be shared. Learning about the total person facilitates addressing needs holistically. Whole-person practices offer attentive and customized healing measures.
- Holistic therapies empower clients and families. People are taught about self-care practices, guided in using them, and assisted in exploring obstacles that could stand in the way of doing so. Also, family members and caregivers can be taught simple holistic techniques to use with their loved ones and themselves, thereby empowering the caregivers/family to participate in their loved one's care and reduce their own stress.
- Most holistic therapies are safer and gentler than conventional therapies. A variety of physical and mental changes, combined with the high volume and nature of medications used in terminal phases of illness, carry many risks for dying clients. Although there are conditions for which drugs and invasive procedures provide remarkable benefit, there are other conditions that can be managed and improved through lower risk CIHA.

With the many benefits that can be derived from using complementary/integrative therapies and a holistic approach, nurses can best assist those in the dying process by integrating CIHA with conventional therapies. This requires that nurses understand the intended and safe use of various CIHA therapies, educate clients/families in appropriate CIHA use, and prepare themselves to offer selected CIHA therapies as part of their practice.

■ SELF-CARE FOR THE HEALER

Working with the dying and their families can create much stress for the nurse. It is sometimes referred to as "death overload." Olson (1997) notes that caregivers of dying persons often reexamine their own belief systems and may suffer an existential crisis of faith. Health professionals grieve the loss of their clients, and when the losses come too quickly, they may not complete the grieving process before the next death. This may lead to feelings of guilt, anger, irritability, frustration, helplessness, inadequacy, sleeplessness, and depression. Problems may arise in interaction with clients, family members, and other staff. Olson (1997) further notes the consequences when staff are not dealing well with the deaths of clients (p. 207):

■ Avoiding patients/families
■ Poor clinical judgment
■ Unrealistic expectations
■ Staff absences
■ Outbursts of anger
■ Lack of anticipatory planning
■ Staff conflict
■ Scapegoating
■ Interprofessional power struggles
■ Staff fatigue
■ Ambivalence toward patients/families

These problems can affect an individual or an entire team. Therefore, it is imperative that healthcare professionals learn self-care techniques. In discussing bereavement care and the role of nurse healers, Roach and Nieto (1997) identify five self-care areas and questions that need to be explored when working with the dying and their families:

1. Spiritual self-care—Is spirituality important in my life? What is my relationship with God or a higher power? Why am I here and what is my purpose? What is my relationship to the universe?
2. Emotional self-care—Can I identify my emotions? How do I deal with them? Am I usually in control? Can I discuss my emotions? Am I open to others and do I respect the feelings of others or do I jump to conclusions? When do my emotions get out of control?
3. Physical self-care—What areas of my lifestyle are unhealthy, or do I have a healthy lifestyle? What can I do to improve my lifestyle?
4. Mental self-care—Am I knowledgeable, and do I continually increase my knowledge? Am I satisfied with the status quo, or am I open to new ideas? What am I doing to stimulate my mind?
5. Relationship self-care—Am I open and honest with myself and others? Do I have satisfying relationships with others? Am I willing to accept the thoughts and feelings of others even though they are different from my own, or am I judgmental? Must I have all the control, or can I share it? Do I have a balance among work, home, and leisure? (pp. 171–175)

Worden (2009) identified four tasks of mourning that are equally applicable to staff. Accepting the reality of

the loss, although painful, is necessary for healing to occur. It may sometimes feel as if the nurse in EOL care is in chronic grieving because of the number of dying clients. But denying the emotional pain, especially of a favored patient, only slows or inhibits the healing process from occurring.

Although more obvious in the significant others, experiencing the pain of the loss also occurs in the staff, including anger, depression, and guilt. Healing support of each other involves encouraging the expression of feelings and emotions such as sadness, anger, guilt, resentment, and pain. Validating the normalcy of the feelings and emotions is also important. One should identify coping strategies that might work or are not working, forgive oneself and others, and remember shared experiences with the deceased client.

Rediscovering meaning is a period of yearning, searching, and discovery. One yearns for the lost person(s) or assumed state of ordinariness, searches for some type of normalcy to reenter the everyday living or working situation, and then discovers the meaning of the loss or losses. Meaning to each of us is individual, unique, and personal. But if one can find meaning, one seems to adjust more easily. Some find meaning in religion, some in support or supportive groups, and some in going inward. Some may never find the answer to the questions "Why did they have to die?" or "Why am I surrounded by so much death?" However, even if these questions are not answered, one may find a new meaning to life—to the present and to the future.

Reinvesting in life or work is somewhat like hope (Roach & Nieto, 1997). One realizes that there is a purpose to this type of work, that the future can be full and good. There is a letting go of remorse and fear of the future, a sense of empowerment, and a sense of one's place in the world. With letting go, the nurse is free to remember the meaningful times with clients and the lessons learned. Although many techniques described in the previous text help in reinvesting in work, they are also useful for one to engage in an area of interest outside of work: enroll in a class, take a trip, do special things for oneself, or review one's job goals and setting. Reinvesting in work does not necessarily mean that everything is solved; however, it can be the motivation for growth. This growth can be expressed as feeling more intensely, empathizing more completely, caring more fully, and developing more sensitivity to and compassion for others.

As noted earlier, those who care for the terminally ill are at risk for stress associated with many losses. There is also opportunity for a career leading to joy, a sense of personal and professional proficiency, and a capability of living life to the fullest. Olson (1997) identifies three aspects of developing growth when working with the dying. Identifying one's motivation for practicing EOL care is important. Is it unresolved personal issues; a professional challenge beyond the physical that involves a search for meaning and peace; a desire to witness the growth of each individual as one comes to terms with mortality and the nature of life; a spiritual calling; a joy in physical care that involves a variety of techniques including complementary modalities such as breathing, TT, and relaxation? Whatever the motivation, exploring this question leads the nurse in EOL care to a certain insight and wisdom.

Coping techniques include those strategies used to change the negative effects of stress (Mariano, 2007). It can be forgiving self and others, and maintaining health through good nutrition, weight control, regular exercise, adequate sleep, and sufficient resources to maintain oneself in a healthy state. Other kinds of physical activities include massage, diaphragmatic breathing, and distraction. Time needs to be scheduled so that the staff can focus on themselves. An example of diaphragmatic breathing is found in the "Exercises" section of this chapter. Those who use this technique regularly can do so on cue, even at the bedside of a dying patient. Distraction includes humor, a massage break, having lunch out, or a day off. One needs these distractions to rest and refresh one's spirit. Scheduling things that are not reminders of patients, death, or dying is an important aspect in addition to grieving and remembering.

Hill (2011) and Eliopoulos (2018) offer many tools and techniques for transforming oneself and impacting one's practice through the art of self-care or replenishing one's body, mind, and spirit.

> The road you take to self-care creates an endless journey to learning and self-awareness. Self-awareness ... allows us to see ourselves and the world differently. This is what allows us to live and nurse from the highest point of our consciousness. (Hill, 2011, p. xvi)

Developing the spiritual self includes knowing that one's life has meaning and confronting one's mortality. These are key aspects in caring for the dying and their significant others. "*Healing the dying* means healing oneself by forming connections with the Universe and all that it is. It means a path one can count on, a way one travels with confidence" (Olson, 2001, p. 252). Searching for meaning necessitates learning to listen, quieting the mind's chatter, hearing the whisper of the inner self, and connecting to one's spirituality. A sense of connection with meaningfulness and purpose can be with an organized religion, with a group, or on the path of an inner process. There are many ways to develop an ability to listen to the inner self: meditation, creating an environment that supports peace, for example, nature or sound; reading literature about the development of a spiritual path; setting a regular time to practice; keeping a journal; sharing one's spiritual journey with like-minded people; and enjoying life. Whatever the technique, there is a growing sense of unity and purpose in being. One belongs here; one has a mission and a purpose.

■ A COMMENTARY ON EVIDENCE-BASED PRACTICE RESEARCH AND HOLISTIC INTEGRATIVE THERAPIES

There is a great need for an evidence base to establish the effectiveness and efficacy of holistic/integrative therapies, and research in this area will become increasingly important in the future. However, according to Hyman (2006), there are two fundamental problems with using randomized controlled clinical trials (RCT) to study holistic healing modalities. The first is that holistic healing modalities are often part of a system, a philosophical approach that is centered on facilitating and promoting balance and health in the body, rather than ameliorating a particular symptom. In an RCT, the holistic/healing modality often is examined out of context, and, consequently, the results often do not indicate the accurate effectiveness of these treatments. Second, most outcome measures used in the scientific community today are based on tangible physical/mental or disease symptomatology. One of the formidable tasks for nurses will be to identify and describe outcomes of holistic/integrative therapies such as healing, well-being, and harmony to develop instruments to measure these outcomes. In addition, methodologies need to be expanded to capture the wholeness of the individual's experience because the philosophy of these therapies rests on a paradigm of wholeness.

There is presently much discussion about what method is most appropriate for the study of holistic phenomena. Evidence-based medicine (EBM) often falls short in the clinical context of patients with chronic complex illnesses. EBM tends to concentrate on research methodology and reduces clinical practice to the technical implementation of research findings. Clinical practice most often employs multiple interventions that do not add up to an evidence-based approach focused on a single intervention. Clinical research fails to focus on the combined outcome of multiple interventions because of the complexity, cost, and absence of effective tools for studying such approaches.

Researchers are being challenged to look at alternative philosophies of science and research methods that are compatible with investigations of humanistic and holistic occurrences. We need to study phenomena by exploring the context in which they occur and the meaning of patterns that evolve. Also needed are approaches to intervention studies, which are more holistic, taking into consideration the interactive nature of the body–mind–emotion–spirit–environment. Rather than isolating the effects of one part of an intervention, we need more comprehensive interventions and more sensitive instruments that measure the interactive nature of each client's biological, psychological, emotional, spiritual, sociological, and environmental patterns. Researchers must begin to look at whole practices and whole systems, which typify whole-person treatment. Comprehensive comparative outcome studies are needed to ascertain the usefulness, indications, and contraindications of integrative therapies. And researchers must also evaluate these interventions for their usefulness in promoting wellness as well as preventing illness (Mariano, 2008).

The Institute of Medicine (IOM, 2005) report, titled *Complementary and Alternative Medicine in the United States*, and participants at the "IOM Summit on Integrative Medicine and the Health of the Public" strongly emphasized that investigations of CAM (holistic/healing) practices entail a moral commitment of openness to diverse interpretations of health and healing, a commitment to finding innovative ways of obtaining evidence, and an expansion of the knowledge base relevant and appropriate to practice. One way to honor social pluralism is in the recognition of medical pluralism, meaning the broad differences in preferences and values expressed through the public's prevalent use of CAM modalities. The proper attitude is one of skepticism about any claim that conventional biomedical research and practice exhaustively account for the human experiences of health and healing.

The nature of many holistic phenomena presents a challenge to their "scientific" exploration and understanding. Because of the nonempirical effects of some healing therapies, how do we ascertain the effectiveness of some therapies when we presently can only measure the physical, emotional, or psychological parameters? How do we know something is useful to the client when there is no biophysical change and yet the client reports positive evaluations of these interventions? How do we know something works? How do we measure existential peace, or well-being, or openheartedness, or spiritual truth and connection, or psychic power? How do we measure transcendence or the universal life force? Do we need to measure their things? Are practice, theory, and research partly based on faith and mystery? Answers to these questions are beyond the scope of this discussion; however, other ways of knowing such as intuition, esthetic and personal knowing, and unknowing as a way of knowing must be given credibility in the research world focusing on healing and holistic/integrative therapies (Mariano, 2008).

■ CONCLUSION

This chapter has presented some of the more common alternative/complementary/integrative healing modalities that are and can be used by nurses and by students of nursing. It should be noted that centering, relaxation, imagery, meditation, reminiscence and life review, and journal writing are basic and can be practiced by nurses and students with little or no experience. The sense therapies, touch therapies, and Reiki bodywork necessitate further study, which are offered through a few master's degree programs and workshops. Whenever one learns these therapies, it is imperative that nurses practicing in palliative and hospice care be familiar with healing modalities and their beneficial effects for patients and families during the illness experience.

CASE STUDY

AN INTERPROFESSIONAL PERSPECTIVE

Andrew Fantin, Minister of Music

This chapter describes the value of many complementary therapies that provide comfort and support to patients with serious or life-threatening illness. J.A., although reluctant to touch therapy, was willing to have a "trial" of TT, which appeared to provide a sense of relaxation and comfort. A second complementary modality often of value is the use of music. Throughout a person's life time, people are exposed to music, from the sounds of a mother's soft bedtime lullaby to music that is a reflection of a person's culture or a period in his or her personal life history. Music reflects a range of emotions from feelings of joy, exaltation, anger, sorrow, or despair, often mirroring a person's inner life.

Music therapy can be used by all practitioners who care for patients with acute, chronic, progressive, or life-threatening illness to alleviate the emotional pain of loneliness, depression, and anxiety, or the physical pain associated with illness or its treatment. In conversation with patients, practitioners can ask about the importance or value of music in a patient's life. Do they play an instrument? Do they like to sing? Do they listen to music daily, and if so, what is their favorite music, favorite artists, or favorite songs? Listening to music with patients and talking about the meaning of a song or the associated memories gives practitioners a glimpse into a person's spirit and perhaps an understanding of how to heal or make whole.

What is important is that you need not be a music therapist to use music to offer comfort. It is important to find music that the patient prefers rather than the music you, as practitioner, prefer. Through a mutual process of understanding, practitioners can suggest music that hopefully results in the desired health outcome. If a patient is anxious and having trouble sleeping, as in the case of J.A., quiet classical or new age music may help calm him or her, and create a sense of peace and serenity. In order to encourage activity or alert brain function, choosing music that the patient is familiar with and is associated with good memories from their past can be played. Care should be taken to avoid music that upsets the patient or brings back painful memories as the intent is to comfort and support.

As a minister of music, I come to realize that music simulates the brain and enhances learning. Listening to music stimulates the whole brain through diverse neural circuitry that stimulates better brain metabolism and blood flow. Listening to enjoyable music improves brain function and releases endogenous opioids, promoting a general sense of well-being. Classical or easy listening music can help to calm and relax a person, even lowering his or her blood pressure.

As a man in his forties, J.A. spoke about music as boosting his creative energy. He explained that he enjoyed the most music with words, as this type of music stimulated his emotions and visual senses, and inspired his own self-expression. In thinking about types of music, someone who has a left-brain-focused job, such as an accountant, may experience an increased level of peace and stability when he or she listens to classical music or other right-brain-style music. Someone who uses predominantly his or her right brain (such as an artist) may do well with rock-n-roll or other lyric-based music to charge up the left brain. This is all relative to the unique personality and tendencies of an individual, but research suggests that music balances and stabilizes the brain hemispheres.

The important message is there are many ways of showing love, care, and empathy and of promoting physical, emotional, and spiritual well-being—one of which may be through the use of music. Families may bring in headsets or CD players, or even cell phones can play a huge array of songs; the sounds of music can be close at hand even in institutional settings. At the bedside of a seriously ill or dying person, your own sweet voice can be the instrument of connection—a therapeutic use of self—when a sense of human connection is so desperately needed and so deeply valued.

EXERCISES

■ PASSIVE RELAXATION[1]

Procedure for participants who are lying down:

■ With your eyes closed, let your attention focus on your breathing ... notice how gentle, slow, and regular it is becoming ... imagine each breath out carrying your tensions away, leaving you more relaxed than you were before ... if you want to, take one deep breath ... then allow your breathing to settle into its own rhythm ... easy, calm, and even ... and forget about it.

■ I'm going to ask you to take a trip around the body, checking that all the muscle groups are as relaxed as possible and letting go any tension that might still remain. If outside thoughts creep in, hold them in a bubble and let them flow away. I'll begin with the feet.

■ Bring your attention to your toes ... are they lying still? If they are curled or stretched out in some way not entirely comfortable, wiggle them gently. As they come to rest, feel all the tension leaving them ... feel them sinking down, heavy and motionless.

■ Let your feet roll out at the ankles. This is the most relaxed position for them. Let all the tension flow out of them ... enjoy the sensation of just letting them go.

---

[1] From Payne (2005). Reprinted with permission.

- Moving on to the lower legs: Feel the tension leaving the calf muscles and the shins. As the tension goes, they feel heavier ... they feel warm and pleasantly tingling.
- The thighs next: To be fully relaxed they need to be slightly rolling outwards ... feel the relaxing effect of this position ... make sure you have released all tension, and feel your thighs resting heavily on the surface you are resting on.
- Focus for a moment on the sensation of sagging heaviness throughout your legs ... let the muscles shed their last remaining hint of tension and settle into a deep relaxation. And now, think of your hips. Let them settle into the surface you are lying on ... recognize any tension that lingers in the muscles ... then relax it away ... let it go on relaxing a bit further than you thought possible.
- Settle your spine into the rug or mattress ... become aware of how it is resting on a surface. Let it sink down, making contact whenever it wants to ... all tension draining out of it.
- Let your abdominal muscles lose their tension. Let them go soft and loose. Feel them spreading as they give their last vestige of tension ... notice how your relaxed abdomen rises and falls with your breathing ... rises as the air is drawn in and falls as the air is expelled ... abdominal breathing is relaxed breathing.
- Move up to your chest and shoulders, to muscles that are prone to carry tension ... feel them letting go ... feel them spreading ... feel them easing into the surface, limp and heavy ... feel them drooping down toward your feet ... imagine them shedding their burdens ... and as the space between your shoulders and your neck opens out, imagine your neck a bit longer than it was before.
- Now, direct your thoughts to the muscles of your left arm. Check that it lies limply on a surface. Notice the feeling of relaxation and allow this feeling to sweep down to your wrist and hand. Think of the fingers, are they curved and still? ... neither drawn up nor stretched out ... neither opened nor closed, but gently resting ... totally relaxed. As you breathe out, let the arm relax a little bit more ... let it lie heavy and loose ... so heavy and loose that if someone were to pick it up, then let it go, it would flop down again like the arm of a rag doll.
- Repeat the last paragraph with the muscles of the right arm.
- Your neck muscles have no need to work with your head supported, so let them go ... enjoy the feeling of letting go in muscles that work so hard the rest of the time to keep your head upright. If you find any tension in the neck, release it and let this process of releasing continue, even below the surface ... feel how pleasant it is when you let go the tension in these muscles.
- Bring your attention now to your face, to the many small muscles whose job it is to manage your expressions. At the moment there's no need to have any expression at all on your face, so allow your muscles to feel relaxed ... imagine how your face is when you are asleep ... calm and motionless.
- Now, think about the jaw ... and as you do, allow it to drop slightly so that your teeth are separated ... feel it relaxing with your lips gently touching. Check that your tongue is still, and lying in the middle of your mouth, soft and shapeless. Relax your throat so that all tension leaves it and the muscles feel smooth and resting.
- With no expression on your face, your cheeks are relaxed and soft. If you think of your nose, it is just to register the passage of cool air traveling up your nostrils while the warmer air passes down ... breathe tension out with the warm air ... breathe stillness in with cool air.
- Check that your forehead is smooth ... not furrowed in any direction ... and as you release its remaining tension, imagine it being a little higher and a little wider than it was before ... continue this feeling into your scalp and behind your ears ... feel a sense of calm as you do this.
- Let your thoughts focus on your eyes as they lie behind gently closed lids. Think of them resting in their sockets, floating, rather than fixed ... and as they come to rest, so do your thoughts.
- Spend a few minutes continuing to relax, deepening the effect of the previous sequences ...
- You now have relaxed all the major muscle groups in your body. Think about them now as a whole ... a totally relaxed whole ... soothed by your gentle breathing rhythm, feel the peacefulness of this idea ....
- Images may drift in and out of your mind ... see them as thoughts passing through. Feel yourself letting go of them. Say to yourself, "I am feeling calm, I am feeling peaceful." Let your mind conjure up a sense of contentment.

■ IMAGERY

The instructor picks one of the following: a sunny beach, a river bank, or a scented garden. If trainees suffer from hay fever, the first item is the best choice. Imagery is best used after a short relaxation exercise.

A Sunny Beach

■ See yourself lying on the hot sand of a sunny beach within an enclosed bay. It is sheltered from storms and protected from ocean currents. It is safe. You watch the light dancing on the water; you smell the sea air as it fills your nostrils; you hear the gulls calling above the sound of waves; you feel the warm sun on your skin. The grains of dry sand run through your fingers, forming little bumps and hollows beneath your hand.

A River Bank

■ Imagine you are lying in the soft, juicy long grass of early summer. You are in a green meadow that rolls down to the river. Scents rise up from the wildflowers, sweeping over you in waves. The sun is warm, but a gentle breeze softens its intensity. Closing your eyes, you become aware of the sound of water flowing, of birds calling, and of leaves rustling.

A Scented Garden

■ Picture yourself lying on a newly mown lawn with the sun beating down on the moist cuttings, drawing out their fragrance. Reach out and feel the coolness of the damp grass. Through your half-closed eyelids you can see the tops of the trees swaying against the sky. Light breezes carry the scent of honeysuckle.

Following one of these short passages of visualization, trainees can relax for a few minutes, before the session is brought to an end.

■ RELAXATION[2]

I would like you to be as comfortable as you possibly can. Take a couple of deep breaths. Inhale deeply. Exhale very slowly and very completely. Focus on your breathing. Again, inhale very deeply and exhale very slowly. Become aware of your ability to relax your muscles. Allow every muscle in your body to be as relaxed as possible, starting with the feet. Allow the feet to become very, very comfortable. Relax the feet completely. As the muscles relax, you may notice a tingling sensation in the soles and toes of the feet. This simply indicates that the muscles are relaxing.

Be aware as this sensation of relaxation begins to move upward from the feet to the ankles. This sensation of relaxation flows from the ankles to the calves of the legs. The muscles of the calves release the tension and relax. The calves become very comfortable as the tension is released.

This comfortable, relaxed sensation moves from the calves to the upper legs and thighs. These muscles also relax and become very comfortable. Feel the muscles on the sides of the legs, the outside of the legs, the inner legs, and the top of the legs as they become very comfortable and relaxed.

The sensation of relaxation moves up toward the buttocks and toward the pelvic area. Occasionally you may feel a muscle twitch. This is just another sign that relaxation is occurring.

---

[2] From Roach & Nieto (1997).

The tension of the muscles of the buttocks, pelvic area, and the lower abdomen is released. The internal organs relax and the muscles that surround them feel completely tension free.

The sensation of relaxation moves up the body to the upper abdomen and to the chest and from the lower back toward the upper back. The muscles are relaxing from the chest and the upper back to the shoulders.

This relaxation extends to the neck and the throat. Feel the tension draining from the back of the neck. Tension is draining away from the back of the neck and the back of the head. As tension drains away, a sense of relaxation settles in. These feelings are so comfortable and so pleasant. Feel the muscles of the throat, the jaw, and across the bridge of the nose relaxing.

The tension in the arms is released, and these muscles feel relaxed. Relaxation spreads to the hands and the fingers as the tension is released.

From the feet, to the head, to the arms, to the fingertips, the whole body is completely and totally relaxed. Take a few moments to savor this comfortable state of total relaxation of body and mind.

■ **Closure.** Allow time for the client to appreciate this restful state of complete relaxation. After a few minutes, instruct the client to bring his or her attention back to the present. At times, the nurse may want to count slowly from 1 to 10 as the client progressively returns to a more wakeful state.

■ MEDITATION[3]

Using a Mantra

1. Select a word to focus on. It can be a neutral word, such as "one," or a Sanskrit mantra such as "Om Shanti," "Sri Ram," "So-Hum." It could also be a word or phrase that has some special significance within your personal belief system. In his recent book, *Beyond the Relaxation Response*, Benson describes how a word or phrase of special personal significance (such as "I am at peace" or "Let go, let God") deepens the effects of meditation.
2. Repeat this word or phrase, ideally on each exhalation.
3. As any thoughts come to mind, just let them pass over and through you, and gently bring your attention back to the repetitive word or phrase.

Counting Breaths

1. As you sit quietly, focus on the inflow and outflow of your breath. Each time you breathe out, count the breath. You can count up to 10 and start over again, or keep counting as high as you like, or you can use Benson's method of repeating "one" on each exhalation.
2. Each time your focus wanders, bring it back to your breathing and counting. If you get caught in an internal monologue or fantasy, don't worry about it or judge yourself. Just relax and return to the count again.
3. If you lose track of the count, start over at 1 or at a round number like 50 or 100.
4. After practicing breath-counting meditation for a while, you may want to let go of the counting and just focus on the inflow and outflow of your breathing.

Whichever form of meditation you try, you might want to start out with short periods of 5 to 10 minutes and gradually lengthen them to 20 to 30 minutes over a period of 2 to 3 weeks. Most people find that it takes persistent and disciplined effort over a period of several months to become proficient at meditating. Even though meditation is the most demanding of relaxation techniques to learn, it is for many people the most rewarding. Research has found that among all relaxation techniques, meditation is the one that people are most likely to persist in doing regularly.

---

[3] From Bourne (1995). All rights reserved.

If you are truly interested in establishing a meditation practice, you may want to find a class, group, or teacher to study with. This will make it easier for you to continue your practice.

■ SCRIPT FOR BREATHING FOR RELAXATION AND HEALTH[4]

- Close your eyes.... Focus your mind on your breath.... Just follow the air as it goes in ... and as it goes out.
- Feel it as it comes in ... and as it goes out. ... If your mind begins to wander, just bring it back to your breath.
- Feel your stomach rise ... your ribs expand ... and your collarbone rise. ... Breathe in naturally and slowly.
- On your next exhalation, release all the air from your lungs without straining. ... Let it all go. ... Let it all out. ... Prepare your lungs to receive fresh oxygen.
- Now take in a full, deep breath and let the air go to the bottom of your lungs. ... Feel your stomach rise ... your chest expand, and the collarbone area fill.
- Now empty your lungs from top to bottom. ... Let all the air out. ... Compress your stomach to squeeze out all the stale air and carbon dioxide. Squeeze out every bit of air. ... Let it all go.
- Take in another deep breath.... As you breathe in, your diaphragm expands and massages all the internal organs in the abdominal region ... aiding your digestion.
- Breathe out. ... Relax. ... Feel the knots in your stomach untie. ... Let go.
- Breathe in.... Your diaphragm is stimulating your vagus nerve, slowing down the beating of your heart ... relaxing you.
- Breathe out.... Let it all go.... Relax.... Relax more and more.... Breathing heals you ... calms you ... soothes you.
- Breathe in again, fully and completely. Oxygen is entering your bloodstream, nourishing all your organs and cells ... protecting you.
- Breathe out. ... Release all the poisons and toxins with your breath. ... Your breathing is cleansing you ... healing you.
- Breathe in.
- Now imagine exhaling confusion ... and inhaling clarity.
- Imagine exhaling darkness ... and inhaling light.
- Imagine exhaling hatred ... and inhaling love.
- Exhaling anxiety ... and inhaling peace.
- Exhaling selfishness ... and inhaling generosity.
- Exhaling guilt ... and inhaling forgiveness.
- Exhaling weakness ... and inhaling courage.
- Breathe in through your nose and sigh out through your mouth. Let the air stay out of your lungs as long as it is comfortable, and then take another breath.
- Let your breath return to its normal and natural pace. Continue to breathe in slowly, smoothly, and deeply. ... Your breathing is steady, easy, silent.
- Each time you exhale ... allow yourself to feel peaceful ... calm ... and completely relaxed. ... If your mind wanders, bring your attention back to your breath.
- Stretch and open your eyes, feeling refreshed and rejuvenated, alert, and fully alive.

Repeat the previous instructions until everyone is alert.

---

[4] From Lusk (1992, Vol. 1). Copyright 1992 by Julie T. Lusk. Vols. 1 and 2 are available from Whole Persons Associates, 210 W. Michigan, Duluth, Minnesota 55802, 800-247-6789. Julie T. Lusk is also the author of *Refreshing Journeys,* a relaxation audiotape available from Whole Persons Associates, and *Desktop Yoga,* available from Perigee Books, 800-631-8751.

■ GENERAL GUIDED IMAGERY TECHNIQUE[5]

1. Achieving a relaxed state
   A. Find a comfortable sitting or reclining position (not lying down).
   B. Uncross any extremities.
   C. Close your eyes or focus on one spot or object in the room.
   D. Focus on breathing with abdominal muscles—being aware of the breath as it enters through your nose and leaves through your mouth. With your next breath let the exhalation be longer and notice how the inhalation that follows is deeper. And as you notice that, let your body become even more relaxed. Continue to breathe deeply, gradually letting the exhalation become twice as long as the inhalation.
   E. Bring your mind back to thinking of your breathing and your relaxed body if your thoughts roam.
2. Specific suggestions for imagery
   A. Picture a place you enjoy and where you feel good.
   B. Notice what you see, hear, taste, smell, and feel.
   C. Let yourself enjoy being in this place.
   D. Imagine yourself the way you want to be (describe the desired goal specifically).
   E. Imagine what steps you will need to take to be the way you want to be.
   F. Practice these steps now—in this place where you feel good.
   G. What is the first thing you are doing to help you be the way you want to be?
   H. What will you do next?
   I. When you reach your goal of the way you want to be, notice how you feel.
3. Summarize process and reinforce practice
   A. Remember that you can return to this place, this feeling, and this way of being anytime you want.
   B. You can feel this way again by focusing on your breathing, relaxing, and imagining yourself in your special place.
   C. Come back to this place and envision yourself the way you want to be every day.
4. Return to present
   A. Be aware again of the favorite place.
   B. Bring your focus back to your breathing.
   C. Become aware of the room you are in (drawing attention to the temperature, sounds, or lights).
   D. You will feel relaxed and refreshed and be ready to resume your activities.
   E. You may open your eyes when you are ready.

Imagery: Finding One's Special Place[6]

Begin by placing your body in a comfortable position, arms and legs uncrossed, your back well supported. Now take three deep breaths, and during each breath relax even more. Let the exhalation be a letting go kind of breath, letting go of tension. With each breath, take in what you need, and with each exhalation, release anything you don't need. Bring your attention to the top of your head. Feel your scalp relax and let your brow soften and smooth out. Allow the muscles around your eyes to relax. And let any tension flow out through your cheeks as you exhale. Suggest that your jaw relax. Imagine a wave of relaxation flowing down your shoulders, into your arms, elbows, and forearms, all the way into your hands and fingers. Now focus on your chest; releasing any tension around your heart or lungs, relax the muscles around your ribs. Wrap that relaxation around your back and let a wave of relaxation travel down the spine. Allow the muscles along the spine to lengthen and release. Soften and relax the buttocks and pelvis. Let the belly be very soft so that the

---

[5] From Lindquist, Snyder, and Tracy (2014).
[6] From Shames (1996).

breath moves easily down into the abdomen. Invite the legs to join in the relaxation now, as it moves through the thighs, knees, calves, ankles, and feet. Let any last bit of tension or tightness drain out through your feet or toes. When you feel relaxed and comfortable, let me know with a nod of your head. As your body remains relaxed and comfortable, imagine yourself in a very special place, somewhere that is full of natural beauty, safety, and peace. It may be a place you have been to before or it may be a place you want to create in your imagination. Take some time and let yourself be drawn to one place that is just right for you today. Let me know when you are present there (wait for response). Describe what it is like there. What do you see? Are there any smells? Are there any sounds? What is the temperature like? Where are you in this special place? How do you feel here? Take some time to do whatever you would like to do here, to relax or do some activity. Feel free to do whatever you want. This is your place (pause 3 to 4 minutes).

In a few moments, it will be time to come back into a waking state. Know that you can return to this place again anytime you want. Now gently bring yourself back, letting the images fade but keeping with you this relaxed and peaceful feeling. Remember what has been important about this experience. Become aware of the current time and place. Begin to move your body, take a deep breath, open your eyes, and feel relaxed and awake.

At this point, the guide can take a few minutes to allow the person to share his or her experience.

Imagery in Oncology[7]

Many people live their lives in dread and fear of cancer and its treatment. Many nurses find it beneficial to work with the client's negative images and beliefs.

Some nurses have reported making tapes (there are also some available commercially) in which the client is encouraged to imagine chemotherapy or radiation therapy as something positive. Some clients prefer to view it as beams of energy or light.

The practitioner might ask, "How do you imagine the chemotherapy?" Despite the response, the nurse can be helpful in supporting the transformation of the images into something beneficial and positive. "Imagine the medicine going into exactly the cells that most need it. The side effects will be minimal." There are a great variety of techniques and applications that enhance the healing journey through the experience of cancer.

■ QUICK USES OF IMAGERY IN THE CLINICAL SETTING

- ■ **Intravenous Therapy.** When a patient is receiving IV fluids, he or she can envision fluid flowing to every part of the body, removing toxins and flushing them out. The patient can see nutrients providing nourishment to every cell.
- ■ **Pain Medications.** Similarly, the patient can enhance the benefits of pain medication by envisioning its soothing effects as it travels through the bloodstream, sedating any irritated areas and bringing a deep sense of relief throughout. It is suggested that relaxation be used at the first sign of discomfort; focus the patient on the breath. Imagine the body releasing its natural medicine to all areas that are tense or uncomfortable. If pain begins to interfere with activity or rest, ask for medication before becoming so uncomfortable that it would be difficult to work with relaxation and the following imagery:

Imagine the pain medication to be exactly the strength it needs to be. See, feel, or sense the muscles around the painful area softening and relaxing as you breathe into the discomfort. See or feel the pain medication moving to that area, numbing the pain as if it had deposited a layer of frost.

---

[7] Ibid.

Imagine a dial registering a number from 1 to 10 that represents your pain now. See the number come down to your tolerance level. Allow an image to form of a special, quiet, restful place and allow yourself to be there as you rest.

- **Antibiotics.** Some patients like to imagine their antibiotic medication in the bloodstream as hunters stalking their prey. They can envision that the medication stays where the most protection is needed, particularly around burns or incisions, ready to pounce. If more medication is needed, there is an endless supply in the imagination.
- **Anticoagulants.** Likewise, clients using anticoagulants can envision their blood becoming thinner, flowing to exactly the right places to prevent clotting. They can see the medication as extraordinarily efficient and relish watching as it does its magic.
- **Oxygen.** As you take a deep breath, send nourishing healing oxygen into every cell of your lungs, expanding each cell like a balloon. As you exhale, imagine letting the balloons completely deflate and blow any tension or toxins that remain in the body out into the air. Continue doing this slowly for a few minutes, watching the balloons expand and contract.
- **Healing Image.** Imagine little workers repairing the muscles and bones while they are resting, allowing the healing process to begin. See the bone rich in calcium, and see little bone cells growing like coral, increasing in number and density.
- **Ideal Images.** Many clients continue to envision their healing process long after the crises have passed. One way to do this is to imagine themselves in 3 or 6 months. They can imagine themselves exactly as they would wish to be. They can observe how they look, how they walk, and their facial expressions. They might imagine themselves running or swimming, looking healthy and happy.

It is also a good practice for nurses to see themselves as they want to be. Focus on the image; how does it feel to be whole? Many nurses find that using imagery supports their patients totally and empowers them in their work. According to one nurse, after incorporating imagery frequently, "I finally felt as if I were making a difference."

■ DIAPHRAGMATIC BREATHING

Diaphragmatic breathing is a useful technique for relaxing and beginning the centering process. Consciously realizing the path each inhalation takes through the respiratory passages, and inhaling so that the abdomen and lungs expand, allowing each breath to move to the bottom of the respiratory tree by moving the diaphragm downward and outward moves the whole person toward feeling more relaxed. As the slow, long exhalation occurs, a person feels shoulders moving downward and tensions slowly leaving the body. To help with stress at work, a nurse should practice diaphragmatic breathing at home, in either a supine or a sitting position. Putting one's hand on the abdomen is an easy way to know if the abdomen is involved in the breath, or if shallow, tense breaths are a pattern. Once a pattern of abdominal breathing is the norm, the nurse can think of phrases such as, "I can feel this way whenever I take a deep breath and cross my fingers." Connecting the relaxed feeling to the physical act of crossing fingers (or another physical cue) helps the body remember how it feels to relax. A nurse who regularly practices this technique will have the ability to break the cycle of stress and muscle tension in just a few seconds, even at the bedside of a patient. The pattern is as follows:

- Recognize the feeling of tension;
- Take an abdominal breath—on inhalation the stomach expands; and
- On exhalation the stomach contracts—allow the shoulders to sag and experience the relaxation during the exhalation.

This technique, or pattern, is useful by itself to help relax for a few minutes or to lead to more profound states of relaxation.

■ RESOURCES

Academy for Guided Imagery
10780 Santa Monica Blvd., Suite 290, Los Angeles, CA 90025
(800) 726–2070
www.academyforguidedimagery.com

American Herbalist Guild
PO Box 3076
Asheville, NC 28802
617-520-4372
office@americanherbalistguild.com

American Holistic Nurses Association
2900 SW Plass Ct, Topeka, KA 66611
(800) 278–2462
www.ahna.org

American Institute of Homeopathy
801 N. Fairfax Street, Suite 306, Alexandria, VA 22314
(888) 445–9988
www.homeopathyusa.org

American Massage Therapy Association
500 Davis Street, Suite 900, Evanston, IL 60201
(877) 905–2700
www.amtamassage.org

American Meditation Institute
60 Garner Road, Averill Park, New York, NY 12018
(518) 674–8714
www.americanmeditation.org

American Music Therapy Association
8455 Colesville Road, Suite 1000, Silver Spring, MD 20910
(301) 589–3300
www.musictherapy.org

American Psychological Association
750 First Street NE, Washington, DC 20002-4242
(800) 374–2721
www.apa.org

Association for Applied Psychophysiology and Biofeedback
Biofeedback Certification Institute of America
10200 W. 44th Avenue, Suite 304, Wheat Ridge, CO 80003
(303) 422–8436
www.aapb.org
www.bcia.org

Center for Mindfulness in Medicine, Health Care and Society
University of Massachusetts Medical Center
419 Belmond Avenue, Worcester, MA 01604
www.mindfulnesstapes.com

Compassionate Touch
20 Swan Court, Walnut Creek, CA 94596
(510) 935–3906
Info@ageucate.com

Contemplative Outreach, Ltd. [centering prayer]
P.O. Box 737, 10 Park Place, Suite 2B, Butler, NJ 07405
(973) 838–3384
Email: office@coutreach.org
www.centeringprayer.com

Healing Touch International
445 Union Blvd., Lakewood, CO 80228
(303) 989–7982
www.healingtouch.net

International Center for Reiki Training
21421 Hilltop Street, Suite 28, Southfield, MI 48034
(800) 332–8112
www.rekiindia.org

Maharishi Foundation USA
1100 N., 4th Street, Suite 128, Fairfield, IA 52556

Maharishi Vedic School [TM program]
636 Michigan Avenue, Chicago, IL 60605
(312) 431–0110
www.maharishi.org
www.maharishi-medical.com

National Association for Holistic Aromatherapy
3327 W. Indian Trail Road, Spokane, WA 99208
(509) 325–3419
www.naha.org

National Association of Music Therapy (NAMT)
8455 Colesville Road, Suite 930, Silver Spring, MD 20910
(301) 589–3300
www.musictherapy.org

National Association of Nurse Massage Therapists
28 Lowry Drive, P.O. Box 232, West Milton, OH 45383
(800) 262–4017
www.nanmt.org

National Center for Complementary and Integrative Health (NCCIH)
P.O. Box 7923, Gaithersburg, MD 20898
(888) 644–6226
http://nccih.nih.gov

National Certification Commission for Acupuncture and Oriental Medicine (NCCAOM)
11 Canal Center Plaza, Suite 300, Alexandria, VA 22314
(703) 548–9004
www.nccaom.org

Nurse Healers—Professional Associates International [Therapeutic Touch]
P.O. Box 419, Craryville, NY 12521
(877) 326–4724
www.therapeutic-touch.org

Transcendental Meditation
Transcendental Meditation Program (888)LEARN TM
(888) 532–7686
www.tm.org

Evidence-Based Practice

Goldberg, D., Wardell, D., & Kilgarrif, N. (2016). An initial study using healing touch for women undergoing a breast biopsy. *Journal of Holistic Nursing, 34*(2), 123–124.

Purpose

To determine if a noninvasive complementary therapy, healing touch, would benefit women undergoing diagnostic procedures for the determination of breast cancer. Women often experience high levels of fear and anxiety during this diagnostic period.

Design

A randomized controlled pilot study.

Method

An outpatient clinic specializing in breast cancer management was used. Seventy-three women aged 18 to 85 years old participated, with 31 in the control group of standard care and 42 in the intervention group receiving healing touch. A specific technique, magnetic clearing, was provided by a practitioner for 15 minutes prior to the biopsy procedure. Both the State-Trait Anxiety Inventory and the Coping Resources Inventory were administered prior to the procedure and the following day to assess changes.

Results

A mixed analysis of variance indicated that State Anxiety for the Healing Touch group showed a statistically significant reduction in anxiety that was sustained into the following day $F(2, 142) = 10.94, p < .001$. For Trait Anxiety, there was a significant change pre- and postintervention to the day after, $F(2, 142) = 5.15, p < .007$. The Coping Resources Inventory had significant changes in two subcategories, Emotional, $F(2, 142) = 6.10, p > .003$, and Spiritual/Philosophical, $F(2, 142) = 6.10, p < .001$, in the Healing Touch group.

Conclusion

Healing touch may have benefits in reducing anxiety from diagnostic breast procedures.

■ REFERENCES

American Association for Retired Persons/National Center for Complementary and Alternative Medicine. (2011). *Complementary and alternative medicine: What people aged 50 and older discuss with their health care providers.* Washington, DC: U.S. Department of Health and Human Services.

Anselmo, J. (2016). Relaxation. In B. Dossey & L. Keegan (Eds.), *Holistic nursing: A handbook for practice* (7th ed., pp. 239–267). Burlington, MA: Jones & Bartlett.

Barnes, P. M., Bloom, B., & Nahin, R. L. (2008). Complementary and alternative medicine use among adults and children: United States, 2007. *National Health Statistics Reports*, (12), 1–23.

Boiron Group. (2009). *The smart guide to homeopathy.* Newtown Square, PA: Author.

Bourne, E. J. (1995). *The anxiety and phobia workbook* (2nd ed.). Oakland, CA: New Harbinger Publications.

Braun, L., & Cohen, M. (2015). *Herbs and natural substances 2 volume set: Evidence based guide* (4th ed.). London, UK: Churchill Livingston.

Buckle, J. (2016). Aromatherapy. In B. Dossey & L. Keegan (Eds.), *Holistic nursing: A handbook for practice* (7th ed., pp. 345–363). Burlington, MA: Jones & Bartlett.

Burkhardt, M., & Nagai-Jacobson, M. (2016). Spirituality and health. In B. Dossey & L. Keegan (Eds.), *Holistic nursing: A handbook for practice* (7th ed., pp. 135–163). Burlington, MA: Jones & Bartlett.

Carlston, M. (2011). Homeopathy. In M. Marcozzi (Ed.), *Fundamentals of complementary and alternative medicine* (4th ed., pp. 343–354). St. Louis, MO: Saunders Elsevier.

Centers for Disease Control and Prevention. (2014, January 17). *National prevention strategy: America's plan for better health and wellness*. Retrieved from http://www.cdc.gov/Features/PreventionStrategy

Centers for Disease Control and Prevention. (2015). Chronic disease overview. Retrieved from https://www.cdc.gov/chronicdisease/overview/index.htm

Chlan, L., & Heiderscheit, A. (2014). Music intervention. In R. Lindquist, M. Snyder, & M. Tracy (Eds.), *Complementary and alternative therapies in nursing* (7th ed., pp. 99–116). New York, NY: Springer Publishing.

Clarke, T., Black, L., Stussman, B., Barnes, P., & Nahin, R. (2015). Trends in the use of complementary health approaches among adults United States, 2002–2012. *National Health Statistics Report*, (79), 1–16.

Cummings, S., & Ullman, D. (2010). *Everybody's guide to homeopathic medicines* (3rd ed.). Los Angeles, CA: Penguin.

Davis, M., Eshelman, E., & McKay, M. (2008). *The relaxation and stress reduction workbook* (6th ed.). Oakland, CA: New Harbinger Publications.

Davis, P. (2011). *Aromatherapy: An a–z: The most comprehensive guide to aromatherapy ever published* (revised ed.). London, UK: Random House.

DeLany, J. (2015). Massage, bodywork, and touch therapies. In M. Marcozzi (Ed.), *Fundamentals of complementary and alternative medicine* (5th ed., pp. 247–274). St. Louis, MO: Saunders Elsevier.

Dossey, B., & Keegan, L. (2016). *Holistic nursing: A handbook for practice* (7th ed.). Burlington, MA: Jones & Bartlett.

Dossey, L. (1996). *Prayer is good medicine*. San Francisco, CA: HarperCollins.

Dossey, L. (1998). *Reinventing medicine: Beyond mind-body to a new era of healing*. San Francisco, CA: HarperCollins.

Eliopoulos, C. (2018). *Invitation to holistic health: A guide to living a balanced life* (4th ed.). Burlington, MA: Jones & Bartlett.

Fitzgerald, M., & Langevin, M. (2014). Imagery. In R. Lindquist, M. Snyder, & M. Tracy (Eds.), *Complementary and alternative therapies in nursing* (7th ed., pp. 73–98). New York, NY: Springer Publishing.

Fontaine, K. (2015). *Complementary & alternative therapies for nursing practice* (4th ed.). Upper Saddle River, NJ: Pearson.

Freeman, L. (2009). *Mosby's complementary and alternative medicine: A research-based approach* (3rd ed.). St. Louis, MO: Mosby Elsevier.

Gauding, M. (2017). *The meditation bible: The definitive guide to meditations for every purpose*. New York, NY: Sterling.

Gladstar, R. (2012). *Medicinal herbs*. North Adams, MA: Storey.

Goldschmidt, B., & van Meines, N. (2012). *Comforting touch in dementia and end of life care*. Philadelphia, PA: Singing Dragon.

Gross, C., Christopher, M., & Reilly-Spong, M. (2014). Meditation. In R. Lindquist, M. Snyder, & M. Tracy (Eds.), *Complementary and alternative therapies in nursing* (7th ed., pp. 167–190). New York, NY: Springer Publishing.

Haight, B. K., & Haight, B. S. (2007). *The handbook for the structured life review*. Baltimore, MD: Health Professions Press.

Halcon, L. (2014). Aromatherapy. In R. Lindquist, M. Snyder, & M. Tracy (Eds.), *Complementary and alternative therapies in nursing* (7th ed., pp. 323–343). New York, NY: Springer Publishing.

Helming, M. (2016). Herbs and dietary supplements. In B. Dossey & L. Keegan (Eds.), *Holistic nursing: A handbook for practice* (7th ed., pp. 365–413). Burlington, MA: Jones & Bartlett.

Hill, R. (2011). *Nursing from the inside-out: Living and nursing from the highest point of your consciousness*. Sudbury, MA: Jones & Bartlett.

Hollis, J. (2010). *Music at the end of life: Easing the pain and preparing the passage*. Santa Barbara, CA: Praeger.

Hyman, M. (2006). The evolution of research: Meeting the needs of systems medicine, part 1. *Alternative Therapies in Health and Medicine*, 12(3), 10–13.

Ingersoll, S., & Schaper, A. (2013). Music: A caring healing modality. In B. Dossey & L. Keegan (Eds.), *Holistic nursing: A handbook for practice* (6th ed., pp. 397–415). Burlington, MA: Jones & Bartlett.

Institute of Medicine. (2005). *Complementary and alternative medicine in the United States*. Washington, DC: National Academies Press.

Jackson, C., & Latini, C. (2016). Touch and hand-mediated therapies. In B. Dossey & L. Keegan (Eds.), *Holistic nursing: A handbook for practice* (7th ed., pp. 299–319). Burlington, MA: Jones & Bartlett.

Kaiser Family Foundation. (2010). U.S. health care costs: Background brief. Retrieved from http://www.kaiseredu.org/Issue-Modules/US-Health-Care-Costs

Keegan, L., & Drick, C. (2016). Dying in peace. In B. Dossey & L. Keegan (Eds.), *Holistic nursing, a handbook for practice* (7th ed., pp. 415–435). Burlington, MA: Jones & Bartlett.

Krieger, D. (1997). *Therapeutic touch inner workbook*. Santa Fe, NM: Bear.

Krieger, D. (2002). *Therapeutic touch: A transpersonal healing*. New York, NY: Lantern Books.

Laurant, R., & Shlien, J. (1984). *Client centered therapy and the person centered approach*. New York, NY: Praeger.

Levin, J., & Reich, J. (2013). Self-reflection. In B. Dossey & L. Keegan (Eds.), *Holistic nursing: A handbook for practice* (6th ed., pp. 247–260). Burlington, MA: Jones & Bartlett.

Lewis, R. (2015). Aromatherapy. In M. Marcozzi (Ed.), *Fundamentals of complementary and alternative medicine* (5th ed., pp. 411–426). St. Louis, MO: Saunders Elsevier.

Lindquist, R., Snyder, M., & Tracy, M. (2014). *Complementary and alternative therapies in nursing* (7th ed.). New York, NY: Springer Publishing.

Lusk, J. T. (1992). *Scripts for relaxation, imagery and inner healing*. Duluth, MN: Whole Person Associates.

Macrae, J. (2013). *Therapeutic touch: A practical guide*. New York, NY: Knopf.

Mariano, C. (2007). The nursing shortage: Is stress management the answer? *Beginnings*, 27(1), 3.

Mariano, C. (2008). Contributions to holism through critique of theory development and research. *Beginnings*, 28(2), 12–13.

Mariano, C. (2016a). Current trends and issues in holistic nursing. In B. Dossey & L. Keegan (Eds.), *Holistic nursing: A handbook for practice* (7th ed., pp. 77–100). Burlington, MA: Jones & Bartlett.

Mariano, C. (2016b). Holistic nursing: Scope and standards of practice. In B. Dossey & L. Keegan (Eds.), *Holistic nursing: A handbook for practice* (7th ed., pp. 53–76). Burlington, MA: Jones & Bartlett.

Micozzi, M. (2015). *Fundamentals of complementary and alternative medicine* (5th ed.). St. Louis, MO: Saunders Elsevier.

Micozzi, M., & Jawer, M. (2015). Mind-body therapies, stress, and psychometrics. In M. Marcozzi (Ed.), *Fundamentals of complementary and alternative medicine* (5th ed., pp. 114–140). St. Louis, MO: Saunders Elsevier.

Micozzi, M., & Meserole, L. (2015). Ethnobotany and western herbalism. In M. Marcozzi (Ed.), *Fundamentals of complementary and alternative medicine* (5th ed., pp. 387–410). St. Louis, MO: Saunders Elsevier.

Morris, D. (2009). Music therapy. In B. Dossey & L. Keegan (Eds.), *Holistic nursing: A handbook for practice* (5th ed., pp. 327–346). Sudbury, MA: Jones & Bartlett.

Nahin, R., Barnes, P., & Stussman, B. (2016). Expenditures on complementary health approaches: United States, 2012. *National Health Statistics Report*, (95), 1–11.

Nelson, D. (1994). *Compassionate touch: Hands-on care giving for the elderly, the ill and the dying*. Barrytown, NY: Station Hill Press.

Nelson, D. (2006). *From the heart through the hands: The power of touch in caregiving*. Forres, UK: Findhorn Press.

O'Brien, M. (2003). *Prayer in nursing: The spirituality of compassionate caregiving*. Sudbury, MA: Jones & Bartlett.

O'Brien, M. (2017). *Spirituality in nursing: Standing on holy ground* (6th ed.). Sudbury, MA: Jones & Bartlett.

Olson, M. (1997). Death and grief. In B. Dossey (Ed.), *Core curriculum for holistic nursing* (pp. 126–133). Gaithersburg, MD: Aspen.

Olson, M. (2001). *Healing the dying* (2nd ed.). New York, NY: Delmar Thompson.

Payne, R. (2005). *Relaxation techniques: A practical handbook for the health care professional* (3rd ed.). Edinburgh, UK: Elsevier.

Payne, R., & Donaghy, M. (2010). *Relaxation techniques: A practical handbook for the health care professional* (4th ed.). Edinburgh, UK: Elsevier.

Pestka, E., Bee, S., & Evans, M. (2014). Relaxation therapies. In R. Lindquist, M. Snyder, & M. Tracy (Eds.), *Complementary and alternative therapies in nursing* (7th ed., pp. 283–297). New York, NY: Springer Publishing.

Plontikoff, M. (2014). Herbal medicines. In R. Lindquist, M. Snyder, & M. Tracy (Eds.), *Complementary and alternative therapies in nursing* (7th ed., pp. 345–364). New York, NY: Springer Publishing.

Price, L., & Price, S. (2011). *Aromatherapy for health professionals* (4th ed.). New York, NY: Churchill Livingston.

Pursell, J. (2016). *The herbal apothecary*. Portland, OR: Timber Press.

Quinn, J. (2016). Transpersonal human caring and healing. In B. Dossey & L. Keegan (Eds.), *Holistic nursing: A handbook for practice* (7th ed., pp. 101–110). Burlington, MA: Jones & Bartlett.

Ringdahl, D. (2014). Reiki. In R. Lindquist, M. Snyder, & M. Tracy (Eds.), *Complementary and alternative therapies in nursing* (7th ed., pp. 419–439). New York, NY: Springer Publishing.

Roach, S., & Nieto, B. (1997). *Healing and the grief process*. New York, NY: Delmar.

Rose, M. (2009). *Comfort touch: Massage for the elderly and the ill*. Philadelphia, PA: Lippincott Williams & Wilkins.

Schaub, B., & Burt, M. (2016). Imagery. In B. Dossey & L. Keegan (Eds.), *Holistic nursing: A handbook for practice* (7th ed., pp. 269–299). Burlington, MA: Jones & Bartlett.

Schroeder-Sheker, T. (1994). Music for the dying. *Journal of Holistic Nursing, 12*(1), 83–99. doi:10.1177/089801019401200113

Schroeder-Sheker, T. (2005). Prescriptive music: Sounding our transitions. *Explore: The Journal of Science and Healing, 1*(1), 57–58. doi:10.1016/j.explore.2004.10.009

Shames, K. (1996). *Creative imagery in nursing*. Clifton Park, NY: Delmare.

Skidmore-Roth, L. (2009). *Mosby's handbook of herbs and natural supplements* (4th ed.). St. Louis, MO: Mosby.

Snyder, M. (2014). Journaling. In R. Lindquist, M. Snyder, & M. Tracy (Eds.), *Complementary and alternative therapies in nursing* (7th ed., pp. 205–217). New York, NY: Springer Publishing.

Snyder, M., & Lathrop, L. (2014). Prayer. In R. Lindquist, M. Snyder, & M. Tracy (Eds.), *Complementary and alternative therapies in nursing* (7th ed., pp. 191–203). New York, NY: Springer Publishing.

Springhouse Corporation. (2005). *Nursing herbal medicine handbook* (3rd ed.). Springhouse, PA: Author.

Taylor, E. J. (2003). Prayer's clinical issues and implications. *Holistic Nursing Practice, 17*(4), 179–188.

Thornton, L., & Mariano, C. (2016). Evolving from therapeutic to holistic communication. In B. Dossey & L. Keegan (Eds.), *Holistic nursing: A handbook for practice* (7th ed., pp. 465–478). Burlington, MA: Jones & Bartlett.

Wauters, A. (2007). *The homeopathic bible: The definitive guide to remedies*. New York, NY: Sterling.

Weiner, M. (1998). *The complete book of homeopathy*. Arden City Park, NY: Avery.

Worden, J. (2009). *Grief counseling and grief therapy: A handbook for the mental health practitioner* (4th ed.). New York, NY: Springer Publishing.

Wright, L. (2005). *Spirituality, suffering, and illness: Ideas for healing*. Philadelphia, PA: F. A. Davis.

Physical Health: Life-Threatening Diseases

III

Maritza C. Alencar

Cancer

KEY POINTS

- Cancer affects all ages.
- The overall incidence and prevalence of cancer has increased with individuals living with cancer as a chronic illness.
- Treatment options have improved survival rates, decreased toxicity, and provided palliation.
- Symptoms associated with the disease and the toxicities of treatment require a commitment to an interprofessional model of care across healthcare settings.
- Palliative care (PC) focuses on the physical, psychosocial, and spiritual needs of the cancer patient and family as well as bereavement needs of families.

CASE STUDY

Mr. T., a 60-year-old white male, presents to his primary care provider (PCP) with complaints of persistent dry cough and right-sided chest pain over the past 3 months. He also reports unintentional weight loss of 10 pounds during this time. Mr. T. is married, has two teenage children, ages 15 and 17, and recently retired from his job as a police officer. His past medical–surgical criteria were unremarkable, although pertinent history includes smoking a pack of cigarettes per day for 45 years.

His PCP orders a chest x-ray that shows a 6 cm mass in the right lower lobe. A computed tomography (CT) scan of the chest is consequently requested, which shows a 6.5 cm spiculated mass in the right lower lobe with several ipsilateral and contralateral mediastinal lymph nodes. His PCP has a high suspicion for lung carcinoma and refers the patient to the pulmonologist for evaluation and possible biopsy. Based on the biopsy results, Mr. T's diagnosis was Stage IV T2 N3 M1b non–small cell lung adenocarcinoma. His tumor was tested and found to have PD-L1 expression. Brain MRI and PET scan showed no metastases. He was started on systemic immune checkpoint inhibitor therapy with nivolumab after undergoing a video-assisted thoracic surgery (VATS). Current medications include oxycodone 5 mg p.o. every 4 hours as needed for pain.

Mr. T. is receiving care at the Comprehensive Cancer Center. Physical examination at the time of chemotherapy initiation revealed a slightly overweight white male in no acute distress. Vital signs: afebrile, pulse 76 beats/min, with a regular rate and rhythm, respirations 16 breaths per minute and blood pressure of 126/82. Cardiac exam, S1, S2, no S3 or S4, no murmurs, no edema, pulses 2+ throughout, no bruits. Lungs clear to auscultation, well-healed surgical scar. Abdominal examination revealed soft, nontender abdomen; bowel sounds present in all four quadrants; no organomegaly; no palpable masses; or lymphade-nopathy. The musculoskeletal examination was unremarkable. The neurological system was grossly intact. He was determined to have an Eastern Cooperative Oncology Group (ECOG) performance status of 1.

Although Mrs. T. has a strong religious practice in the Roman Catholic faith, Mr. T. is struggling with his spirituality and has no religious affiliation.

Questions that the nurse should consider are as follows:

1. What is the best palliative care (PC) practice model for Mr. T.'s plan of care?
2. What are the benefits and burdens of continued chemotherapy treatment for Mr. T.?
3. What support is needed to help Mr. T. and his family cope with his diagnosis, treatment, disease progression, and loss, grief, and bereavement?
4. How can the nurse support Mr. T. during his spiritual crisis?

Cancer is a devastating diagnosis that many individuals still associate with death. Upon initial diagnosis, individuals embark on a treatment journey that is overwhelming with medical jargon, new healthcare providers, unknown outcomes, and fluctuations of hope amid the distressing effects of the disease and its treatment. Although people are living longer with cancer, and some cancers can be considered chronic in nature, living with cancer can provoke anxiety and a loss of control for the patient and family. Individuals living with cancer rely on family or chosen support people to assist them for physician office visits and treatment, help to decipher and absorb disease and treatment information, and provide physical and emotional support for treatment and possibly end-of-life (EOL) care. Oncology healthcare providers work with a heterogeneous patient population attempting to provide the patient and family with clear communication, the most effective treatment options, and a healthy balance of hope for the future.

Despite continuous improvement in treatment efficacy and survival outcomes, cancer remains the second leading cause of death for both genders and throughout the life span. Adult cancer is second to heart disease, while pediatric cancer is second to accidental death in most age groups through adolescence (Aldridge & Roesch, 2007; Djulbegovic et al., 2008; Wolfe, Friebert, & Hilden, 2002). The American Cancer Society (ACS) estimated 1.6 million new cases of all cancer sites and an estimated 600,000 new cases of cancer in the United States in 2017 (Siegel, Miller, & Jemal, 2017). However, a new cancer diagnosis is no longer synonymous with a limited life expectancy, and could possibly mean a future navigating the healthcare system over the extended survival period. Historically, PC for cancer patients was mainly contained within hospice care. Now, cancer specialists are incorporating the precepts of PC and an interprofessional approach to patient care. Due to medical and nursing certifying boards regulating the specialty of palliative medicine and PC, the increasing number of healthcare professionals certified in PC offers more options for the supportive care of cancer patients actively involved

in curative treatment, receiving expensive physiological supportive treatment, and eventually facing imminent death (Gelfman, Meier, & Morrison, 2008; Griffin, Koch, Nelson, Cooley, & American College of Chest Physicians, 2007; Kuebler, Lynn, & Von Rohen, 2005).

For the majority of the 20th century, cancer was more frequently diagnosed in a later stage. According to the National Cancer Institute (NCI, 2018b), worldwide cancer cases are expected to increase from 14 million to 21 million and cancer deaths from 8 million to 13 million from 2012 to 2030. Cancer care has evolved in the last 20 years not only as a result of changes in treatment efficacy but also due to the interprofessional model of support currently offered. Healthcare consumers prefer honest and more complete information pertaining to diagnosis, prognosis, symptom burden, and survival benefits related to treatment. As a result, healthcare professionals are learning more compassionate communication skills and recognizing the importance of shared decision making with the patient, family, and designated caregivers (Kuebler et al., 2005; Surbone, 2008).

Throughout the various stages of cancer, the needs of the patient and family are complex, requiring special attention to physical, psychological, social, and spiritual distress. Arrangements for an appropriate care setting and adequate caregiving support throughout treatment and at the end of life requires knowledge of specialized treatment providers, available alternatives, and an experience-based understanding of how best to match the needs of the patient and family living with cancer (Griffin et al., 2007).

Although many cancer specialists are experienced in EOL care and consider it relevant to their practice, PC is emerging as an interprofessional specialty with strong support for patient, family, and the clinicians involved in cancer management. Evidence suggests that PC teams assisting in cancer care improve patient care and reduce costs to the family and healthcare system by cultivating an equal exchange of information matching the goals of the patient with treatments offered (Gelfman et al., 2008). In addition, PC teams support the clinicians working so closely with a patient population living with a life-threatening disease by providing emotional and educational support. Where multiple clinicians representing different specialties are involved, PC teams provide the hub of communication and specialized spiritual and bereavement support to patients, families, and clinicians that cancer care requires. PC should be integrated into every cancer patient's treatment, including those pursuing curative or life-prolonging therapies, and whether or not PC specialist teams are available, cancer treatment teams should receive education in the essentials of PC (Griffin et al., 2007).

Future implications for cancer care will include supporting patients through complex treatments offered in a variety of treatment locations and supporting late effects of treatment as seen with survivorship. Young and old, it is important to note that the stage of growth and development, familial support, physiological stamina, psychological reserve, and community resources all present significant consideration for the treatment of adults and children living with cancer (Aldridge & Roesch, 2007; Matsuyama, Reddy, & Smith, 2006). The National Collaborating Centre for Cancer (NCC-C, 2015) has issued guidelines standardizing care services for children and young people with cancer in England and Wales that are applicable to this patient population in the United States. Key recommendations include the following: Care for children and young adults up to 19 years of age should be provided in age-appropriate facilities; there is access to treatment-specific clinical expertise and appropriately trained staff; and coordinated care should be accessible across the continuum of disease providing age- and culture-appropriate information.

■ INCIDENCE AND PREVALENCE

Pediatrics and Young Adults

It is estimated that approximately 15,270 children and young adults are diagnosed yearly with some form of cancer in the United States (NCI, 2017b). Even though childhood cancers are rare, representing less than 1% of all new cancer diagnoses, this is an increase in prevalence in the past 20 years. Due to considerable advances in treatment and high rates of clinical trial participation, 80% of children could experience a long-term remission representing a 30% increase in the 5-year survival rate between the 1970s and the late 1990s and 68% decline in mortality from 1969 to 2009 (Aldridge & Roesch, 2007; American Cancer Society [ACS], 2013). The sites of cancers that occur in children contrast greatly from those affecting adults. Leukemias (mainly acute lymphocytic leukemia) account for approximately 31% of all childhood cancers; brain and nervous system cancers make up about 25% of childhood cancers; while neuroblastoma is the most commonly occurring (6% of all childhood

cancer types) solid tumor outside of the central nervous system (ACS, 2013; Aldridge & Roesch, 2007). Despite advances in early detection and treatment, an estimated 2,000 children die of cancer each year in the United States (NCI, 2017a).

Adult

According to the ACS (2018b), the most frequently diagnosed adult cancer types, considering all sites, are female breast, prostate, lung, and colorectal cancer. These four most commonly occurring cancers will be the focus of this chapter. It is estimated that over 234,000 adult Americans will be diagnosed with lung cancer in 2018, and over 150,000 adult Americans will die of the disease within that same year (ACS, 2018a). Estimated incidence rates for new female breast cancer and prostate cases trail lung cancer rates closely, while colorectal cases affecting both genders could affect approximately 140,000 individuals in the United States (ACS, 2018c). The total estimated cancer death rate for 2018, representing all sites, could reach 609,640 individuals in the United States (ACS, 2018a).

Older Adult

The greatest impact of cancer is seen in the middle-aged and older adult populations since 77% of new cancer incidences occur in individuals 55 years and older (ACS, 2013; Terret, Zulian, Naiem, & Albrand, 2007). The relationship between increasing age and the development of cancer is attributed to cancer growth characteristics (age-related cellular mutations) and the biophysical environment (pro-oncogenic changes in the tissue milieu), allowing mutant cells to survive, proliferate, and express their neoplastic phenotype. Cancer cells may take time to proliferate and growth may not be apparent until later stages of life. The physical environment may impact the life cycle of healthy cells and the propagation of cancer cells. As a result, older adults are at an increased risk for cancer (Extermann & Hurria, 2007; Repetto et al., 2003; Terret et al., 2007).

■ PATHOGENESIS

The etiology of cancer is multifactorial, with genetic (nonmodifiable), environmental (modifiable), medical (modifiable), and lifestyle (modifiable) factors interacting to produce a given malignancy. Knowledge of cancer genetics is rapidly improving our understanding of the biologic aspects of cancer, helping to identify at-risk individuals, furthering the ability to characterize malignancies, establishing treatment tailored to the molecular fingerprint of the disease, and leading to the development of new therapeutic modalities. As a consequence, this expanding knowledge base has implications for all aspects of cancer management, including prevention, screening, treatment, and supportive care.

Malignant tumors are produced by a synergy between the accumulation of mutations and tissue changes that support the survival of mutant cells (Terret et al., 2007). Factors that cause or facilitate cancer development include chemical mutagens, radiation, free radicals, genomic instability, inherited cancer susceptibility, telomere shortening, and altered cellular environment. Modifiable risk factors such as smoking, diet, physical activity, and weight control can alter the cellular environment and influence the proliferation of cancer cells. Carcinogenesis works in a stepwise progression in which a normal cell undergoes malignant transformation. Steps include tumor initiation, promotion, malignant conversion, and, finally, tumor progression (Kufe et al., 2003). Occasionally, family members will question the cause of cancer when a loved one is diagnosed; however, further investigation usually reveals an existential concern that a genetic explanation may not satisfy.

■ DISEASE TRAJECTORY

Breast Cancer

According to the ACS, breast cancer is the most frequently occurring female malignancy in the United States, and approximately 266,120 new cases of invasive breast cancer are estimated to be diagnosed in 2018. Roughly 2,550 new cases will be diagnosed in men while 63,960 women will be diagnosed with in situ breast cancer in 2017 (ACS, 2018b). Roughly 83% of those in situ cases will be ductal carcinoma. Approximately 41,400 women in the United States are expected to die of breast cancer in 2018, despite the current decrease in mortality that has occurred since 1989. Breast cancer is second to lung cancer as a cause of cancer death in women. However, incidence and death rates have steadily decreased in the past 10 years due to reductions in the use of menopausal hormone therapy (MHT), early detection, improved treatment, and increased awareness.

Breast cancer is a complicated disease representing a highly heterogeneous patient population. It originates in two separate cell types: ductal and lobular. Ductal cancers are the most common, with invasive ductal cancer representing approximately 80% of all ductal cancer cases. Lobular breast cancer rarely occurs alone, is more hormonally influenced, and occurs predominantly in premenopausal women. Breast cancer can be estrogen receptor (ER) positive or negative (ER+ or ER–) and progesterone receptor (PR) positive or negative (PR+ or PR–). Most breast cancers are hormone sensitive while non–hormone sensitive breast cancers are found to be faster growing. The goal of treatment for women with early-stage breast cancer is curing the disease and preventing metastasis, death, and recurrence while minimizing side effects from treatment. The goal for women diagnosed with late-stage or metastatic breast cancer is to maintain quality of life (QOL), control the disease, prolong survival, and restrict treatment-related toxicities (Hampton, 2008b; Holcomb, 2006; Smith, 2006).

Pathogenesis involves DNA mutation by genetic alterations or environmental agents, probably occurring early in life. Only 5% to 10% of all breast cancers are inherited and carry the breast cancer–specific gene. Growth factors then increase the growth rate of those mutated cells; finally, progressive alteration of specific oncogenes, or the loss of suppressor genes, leads to advanced metastatic disease (Robinson & Huether, 2009). The environment for breast cancer growth in older women is not as favorable as that in younger women because of the decrease in stimulating growth factor specifically for breast cancer and diminishing mononuclear cell reactions. Breast cancer in older women tends to be more differentiated and rich in hormone receptors than in young women. This renders nonmetastatic tumors more receptive to treatment. However, rather than treating cancer based on the patient's age, it is essential to treat each tumor individually, addressing the characteristics of the tumor and the desires of the patient (Extermann, 2005).

■ **Signs/Symptoms/Staging.** Most generally, breast cancer presents as a painless lump that is hard and has uneven edges. Other signs may include palpable axillary nodes, dimpling, nipple pain or turning inward, changes in breast skin, nipple discharge, or bone pain due to metastasis. Breast cancer is evaluated with mammography, percutaneous needle aspiration, biopsy, and hormone receptor assays. Treatment is determined by cell type, stage, growth rate, and hormone receptor status. The tumor/node/metastasis (TNM) classification system evaluates primary tumor size (TX to T4), regional lymph nodes (NX to N3), and distant metastasis (MX to M1), while staging from 0 to IV is used in addition to the TNM determination. Staging levels increase with tumor size and node involvement; only Stage IV represents metastasis. Rate of growth can be determined by S-phase or Ki-67 tests (Holcomb, 2006; Robinson & Huether, 2009).

■ **Disease Management.** Treatment options take into account tumor size, extent of spread, tumor characteristics, and patient preference regarding QOL. Those options include lumpectomy, simple mastectomy with sentinel node biopsy, radical mastectomy, radiation (external and brachytherapy), and systemic therapy (chemotherapy and hormonal therapy). Imaging studies used for staging include PET/CT, bone scan, ultrasound, and CT.

■ **Surgery.** Options available for the surgical management of breast cancer include lumpectomy, removal of axillary lymph nodes, and mastectomy. Treatment is often multimodal and surgery will frequently be combined with other modalities including radiation and/or systemic therapy. In early breast cancer, long-term survival from breast-conserving surgery coupled with radiation is equal to that of mastectomy (ACS, 2018b; 2018c; Holcomb, 2006).

Axillary node involvement is an important prognostic indicator in breast cancer. Biopsy of axillary sentinel lymph node is a fundamental tool for diagnosing lymph node involvement. Treatment for ductal carcinoma in situ (DCIS) includes excision of the tumor, radiation, and/or hormonal therapy with tamoxifen or aromatase inhibitors (for postmenopausal women).

Treatment for Stage III (locally advanced tumors) involves a combination of surgery, chemotherapy, and radiation for local control of the tumor and to decrease the risk of distant recurrence (Thompson & Chochinov, 2009).

■ **Chemotherapy.** Factors to be evaluated when considering chemotherapy include physical well-being, staging, tumor type, comorbidity, patient preference, and drug efficacy (Extermann, 2005). Tumors rich in hormone receptors are less sensitive to chemotherapy than tumors poor in hormone receptors. Chemotherapy significantly increases survival rates even in older women, who may require more frequent dose adjustments for tolerability (Extermann, 2005). The controversy over chemotoxicity in older adults is a result of the heterogeneous population and the underrepresentation of older adults in clinical trial.

■ **Radiation Therapy.** External beam radiation and brachytherapy are current radiotherapies utilized for the treatment of breast cancer. External radiation is the typical radiation therapy given after lumpectomy and is given to the entire breast with an extra dose ("boost") to the site of the tumor from an external source. Treatment courses last between 3 and 7 weeks with daily treatments for patients with early-stage breast cancer. In brachytherapy, radioactive materials, or "seeds," are placed in or near the tumor bed (tumor location prior to surgical excision). Older women assessed with adequate functional reserves tolerate radiation as well as their younger counterparts (Extermann, 2005).

■ **Hormonal Therapy.** ER+ breast cancer is responsive to tamoxifen (a nonsteroidal selective ER modulator), which significantly reduces the long-term risk of recurrence (Litsas, 2008), and was until recently the most prescribed adjuvant endocrine therapy (ACS, 2018b). Third-generation aromatase inhibitors (AIs) have shown superior outcomes in comparison to tamoxifen in disease-free survival rates, time to recurrence, and occurrence of metastases in postmenopausal women. Both tamoxifen and AIs come with distinct side effects that must be considered on an individual basis. Hormonal therapy is considered the standard of care for treatment of hormone receptor positive breast cancer (Aebi & Pagani, 2007; Mackay, 2000). In premenopausal women with early-stage breast cancer, the use of hormonal therapy for 5 years or longer was associated with a 40% drop in recurrence rate and 30% improvement in mortality rate (Kadakia & Henry, 2015). Systemic adjuvant treatment of breast cancer is most useful for women with a life expectancy of 2 or more years (Extermann, 2005; Litsas, 2008). Third-generation AIs have shown statistically significant improvement in survival in patients with advanced breast cancer as compared with tamoxifen or progestogens (Litsas, 2008; Mauri, Pavlidis, Polyzos, & Ioannidis, 2006).

■ **Palliative Care.** Treatment of women with metastatic breast cancer is palliative. The use of combination therapy presents some benefit over single agents as a front-line option. The Eastern Cooperative Group 1,193 trial randomized 700 women between combination therapy with doxorubicin plus paclitaxel and single-agent therapy with either doxorubicin or paclitaxel. Combination therapy presented a higher response rate (47% vs. 36% vs. 34%, respectively) and longer median time to disease progression (8 vs. 6 vs. 6 months, respectively), but no difference in the overall survival (22 vs. 19 vs. 22 months; Sledge et al., 2003). The use of combination therapy is appropriate when response is required at the expense of increased risk of treatment toxicity, such as highly symptomatic patients with impending organ damage. There is limited data demonstrating the superiority of combination therapy beyond second-line therapy, although it may be considered in heavily pretreated patients or those with significant tumor burden. Anthracycline-based combination therapies such as doxorubicin plus cyclophosphamide, epirubicin with cyclophosphamide and fluorouracil, or doxorubicin and docetaxel plus cyclophosphamide offer overall response rate (ORR) between 50% and 70% (Nabholtz et al., 2003; Nabholtz et al., 2001). No single regimen has been identified as the gold standard for disease control or symptom management (Thompson & Chochinov, 2009).

Prostate Cancer

The ACS (2018b) estimated 164,690 newly diagnosed cases in the year 2018 and about 29,430 deaths. Prostate cancer is common in North and South America, Australia, South Africa, Northwestern Europe, and the Caribbean; conversely, it is rare in Asia and Africa (World Health Organization [WHO], 2012). Incidence rates remain highest in African American men and Jamaican men of African descent (70% higher than in whites). Incidence rates have progressively decreased and death rates fell on average 3.4% yearly from 2005 to 2014. Potential risk factors for prostate cancer include age, race, family history, and dietary factors. However, the only well-established risk factor remains increasing age. Approximately 60% of all prostate diagnoses are in men 65 years and older, while 90% occur in men 50 years of age and older (ACS, 2018b; NCI, 2018a).

Over 95% of prostate malignancies are adenocarcinomas, primarily occurring in the periphery of the prostate. Grading systems represent the glandular pattern, degree of differentiation, or a combination of the two (Robinson & Huether, 2009). The cancer cells metastasize via posterior local extension, lymphatic system, and blood vessels to distant lymph nodes, bone, liver, lungs, and adrenal glands. The most common sites of bone infiltration are pelvis, lumbar and thoracic spine, femur, and ribs. The 5-year survival rate for all stages of prostate cancer is 98.6%. The great majority of patients present with localized (79%) or regional (12%) disease. Of these, there is a 100% 5-year survival, while those with metastatic disease at presentation (5% of cases) have a 5-year survival rate of only 29.8% (NCI, 2018a).

■ **Signs/Symptoms/Staging.** Early and localized stages of prostate cancer generally do not present with symptoms. Hallmark symptoms that occur more frequently in locally advanced cancer are usually associated with urinary outlet obstruction: frequent urination, urinary hesitancy, inability to urinate, nocturia, and dysuria. Impotence, painful ejaculation, bloody urine or semen, pain, and stiffness in the lower back, hips, or upper thighs are additional symptoms suggestive of malignancy. Since many of the common symptoms may mimic other conditions, it is common for men to postpone medical consultation. Symptoms of malignant prostate disease usually do not subside, which distinguishes prostate cancer from benign disorders (Darmber & Aus, 2008; Ryan & Small, 2006).

Digital rectal examination and/or prostate-specific antigen blood test are the most commonly used screening methods for prostate cancer. However, the optimal timing and indication for routine screening remain controversial among medical societies. Diagnosis of prostate cancer is confirmed by prostate biopsy guided by transrectal ultrasonography (TRUS). Additional imaging studies may be obtained when there is suspicion for metastatic disease (extremely elevated PSA, bone pain, abnormal laboratory results; ACS, 2018b).

■ **Disease Management.** Treatment depends on age, life expectancy, overall health status, Gleason Score, and stage. The Gleason Score is a grading scale using numbers 1 to 5 that refer to the appearance and activity of the cancer cells. The Gleason Score adds the grades of the two most prevalent patterns of the cells. Scores may range from 2, representing nonaggressive cancer, to 10, signifying the most aggressive cancer with the greatest potential of spread. Treatments have increased cure rates in men with early and localized tumors, while

interventions for those with advanced disease focus on palliation of symptoms and prolonged survival (Darmber & Aus, 2008).

Expectant management is referred to as "active surveillance" and involves watching for new signs or symptoms of disease progression between regular checkups and testing. Therapy is recommended at the onset of symptoms. Advantages of active surveillance include avoidance of side effects from unnecessary treatment of small indolent cancers (National Comprehensive Cancer Network [NCCN], 2017). Total prostatectomy, radiation therapy, and androgen deprivation therapy are the modalities used for treatment of localized disease (Pignon et al., 1997).

■ **Surgery.** Surgery is a treatment option for individuals with early-stage tumors. Hormonal therapy is usually indicated after surgical treatment, particularly for patients with evidence of pelvic lymph node involvement (NCCN, 2017). Since surgical intervention can result in impotence and incontinence, it is important that treatment discussions involve the spouse or significant other in order to enhance emotional coping and physical healing (Merglen et al., 2007; Willert & Semans, 2000).

■ **Radiation.** Radiation therapy is offered as two different therapeutic approaches: (a) external beam—external application and (b) brachytherapy—internal application of radioactive seed implants. Radiotherapy complications include gastrointestinal toxic effects such as diarrhea, urinary incontinence, and erectile dysfunction. Men diagnosed with prostate cancer are usually older, and treatment burden may be overwhelming if the patient's condition is compromised by comorbidity or presence of a geriatric syndrome (Darmber & Aus, 2008). Patients with hypertension, diabetes mellitus, and pelvic inflammatory disease are not considered optimal candidates for radiation therapy secondary to late effects that may occur and affect QOL (Pignon et al., 1997).

■ **Systemic Therapy and Palliative Care.** Androgen deprivation therapy has been the mainstay systemic treatment of prostate cancer since the 1940s. Responses such as improvement in bone pain in patients with metastatic disease are approximately 70% to 80%. Side effects associated with endocrine manipulation are mild compared to cytotoxic therapies. Hormonal therapy delays disease progression at the expense of potential cardiovascular toxic effects (Darmber & Aus, 2008). Cytotoxic chemotherapy is mostly used for the treatment of hormone-refractory prostate cancer. Cytoxic therapy is associated with an improvement in survival but remains mostly a palliative intervention (Armstrong & Carducci, 2005; Darmber & Aus, 2008). Bone targeted therapies such as denosumab and zoledronic acid are used for prevention of skeletal events such as pathological fractures as well as palliation of metastatic disease to reduce bone pain. Long-term use of either agent carries the risk of osteonecrosis of the jaw (ONJ), thus requiring caution in its use (Boquete-Castro et al., 2016; Diel, 2011; Ryan & Small, 2006).

Lung Cancer

Lung cancer remains the leading cause of cancer death in men and women in the United States and the world with an estimated 234,030 new cases and 154,050 deaths projected for 2018 (ACS, 2018d). The incidence has reached a plateau in women and declined in men, reflecting the trends in smoking patterns over the past few decades (Dubey & Powell, 2008). Most individuals diagnosed with lung cancer are former, rather than current, tobacco smokers. Only 10% of lung cancers occur in individuals with no prior smoking history (Dubey & Powell, 2008). The overall 5-year survival rate is 18.6%, reflecting the poor prognosis associated with this disease (NCI, 2017a).

Lung cancer is divided into two main groups, non–small cell lung cancer (NSCLC) and small cell lung cancer (SCLC). NSCLC accounts for more than 80% of all lung cancers and is further characterized by histology as squamous cell carcinoma, large cell carcinoma, and the most prevalent type, adenocarcinoma (ACS, 2018e). SCLC represents approximately 15% of lung cancers. It typically has a very aggressive clinical course with poorer prognosis. Five-year survival varies between 2% and 30% depending on the stage as compared to 80% in NSCLC (ACS, 2018f; 2018g). SCLC is classified as limited or extensive stage. It is usually detected at a more advanced stage, growing rapidly and metastasizing early in the disease trajectory.

The outcomes of lung cancer are closely defined by staging, with earlier stages being potentially curable while advanced stages are being treated palliatively with generally short survival. Outcomes in NSCLC are further defined by specific genetic mutations that may be potentially targeted by new biologic agents. Individuals with locally advanced NSCLC (Stage IIIA) have a median survival of 14.4 and 16.8 (Stage IIIB) months, respectively, when treated with a combination of operation, chemotherapy, and radiation therapy (Cicenas, Zaliene, & Atkocius, 2009). In another study, patients with Stage IV NSCLC had a median survival rate of 14 months after being treated with chemotherapy and radiotherapy (Su et al., 2014). Individuals with limited disease SCLC who are treated have a median survival of 15 to 20 months, and extensive disease remains poor at approximately 10 months (Chen et al., 2010; Miles, Jacimore, & Nelson, 2011).

About one third of surgically resected NSCLC recur in the ipsilateral or contralateral lung and can metastasize to various sites including bone, liver, adrenal glands, or brain. More than 80% of recurrences occur within 2 years and are complicated by distressing symptoms. Individuals with SCLC are at a much higher risk for brain metastases as compared to those with NSCLC (80% vs. 30%) and are considered for prophylactic brain radiation. Therapeutic strategies to manage brain metastases include surgical resection, stereotactic radiosurgery (SRS), and systemic therapy. These may improve the overall survival for a median of approximately 1 year (Lemjabbar-Alaoui, Hassan, Yang, & Buchanan, 2015; Slotman et al., 2007).

■ **Signs/Symptoms/Staging.** Tissue diagnosis and staging workup determines the type and extent of disease. Accurate staging is critical to determine if surgery is appropriate. PET/CT combined with cranial imaging is more accurate in identifying metastatic disease than conventional imaging (CT scan of chest, abdomen, and pelvis; bone scan; and cranial imaging) in NSCLC (Hampton, 2008a). In NSCLC staging, the TNM classification groups patients according to the size and extent of the tumor (T), lymph node involvement (N), and the presence or absence of metastatic disease (M). Seventy-five percent of patients with NSCLC have locally advanced or unresectable Stage IV disease at the time of diagnosis (Walker, 2003). SCLC has its own staging system. Two thirds of SCLC patients have metastatic disease at diagnosis (NCCN, 2008). Once staging is complete, the treatment plan is individualized and based on the stage, lung cancer genomics, and biomarkers, which predict outcomes and treatment responses, in addition to performance status and the ability to tolerate treatment (Dubey & Powell, 2008).

■ **Disease Management.** Because SCLC is considered a systemic disease, surgery is not a treatment option. Chemotherapy alone or with radiation is the usual treatment for SCLC with a high rate of early remission but frequent recurrences. NSCLC has more treatment options such as chemotherapy, radiation, surgery, immunotherapy, targeted therapy, and kinase inhibitors (NCI, 2018c). However, surgical resection remains the only potential curative treatment for patients with NSCLC presenting with surgically resectable disease. Surgery is recommended for all adults with good performance status. There is no difference in the overall survival between younger and older individuals (Yamamoto et al., 2003). Newer surgical techniques, such as the VATS, have provided a minimally invasive approach with similar long-term survival rates as thoracotomy (Molina, Yang, Cassivi, Schild, & Adjei, 2008). Current treatment options will include surgical resection, systemic therapy, radiation, or combinations of these modalities depending on the stage (Albain et al., 2005; NCCN, 2017).

■ **Radiation Therapy.** Radiation therapy is an important treatment modality in lung cancer. It may be used as an alternative for older patients with NSCLC who are not considered surgical candidates due to comorbid disease states or for those who decline surgery. Combined modality treatment with radiation therapy and chemotherapy in patients with nonresectable advanced-stage NSCLC and limited-stage SCLC is the standard of care for physiologically fit individuals. Radiation has a major role in palliation of symptoms, in particular the pain associated with bone metastases, management of dyspnea and hemoptysis from tumor invasion, and control of symptoms associated with brain metastases such as seizures, confusion, nausea, vomiting, and headache (Kvale, Selecky, & Prakash, 2007).

◼ **Chemotherapy.** Chemotherapy, checkpoint inhibitors, and targeted therapies are the mainstay in advanced NSCLC. Systemic therapy presents survival benefit as an adjuvant therapy for high-risk early-stage NSCLC (NCCN, 2017). Standard chemotherapy includes one of a number of chemotherapy doublet combinations given for four cycles. Double therapy including a platinum-based drug is more effective than single agents or best supportive care in first-line therapies (Obasaju et al., 2007). Concurrent chemoradiotherapy is superior to sequential treatment, but has an increased toxicity (Curran et al., 2011). Single-agent chemotherapy is preferred for patients who have a poor performance status and multiple comorbidities. Therapy of lung cancer has been dramatically impacted over the last decade by the advent of targeted agents, which demonstrate in many scenarios superior outcomes compared to cytotoxic therapy. Precision medicine, tailoring therapy to specific genetic alterations, is an exciting new area that holds profound implications for improvement of response and overall survival (Politi & Herbst, 2015; Walker, 2003).

Treatment options for SCLC are usually limited to chemotherapy and/or radiation. Therapeutic regimens for limited-stage disease consist of concurrent chemotherapy and radiation, followed by prophylactic cranial irradiation, which can increase survival by about 5% (Jassem, 2007). Chemoradiation is difficult to tolerate due to side effects associated with the toxic chemotherapeutic agents and the burden of concurrent radiation.

Extensive-stage SCLC is treated with chemotherapy alone (NCCN, 2017). Slotman et al. (2007) demonstrated that prophylactic brain irradiation in patients with extensive SCLC who responded to chemotherapy reduces the incidence of symptomatic brain metastases and prolongs disease-free and overall survival. Studies of eldery patients suggest they also benefit from treatment for SCLC. However, data on this age group is limited as the elderly population remains underrepresented in clinical trials.

Targeted therapies are aimed at specific tumor pathways in NSCLC. The antiepidermal growth factor receptor (EGFR) inhibitor erlotinib reduces proliferation and survival of tumor cells by inhibiting tyrosine kinase. Bevacizumab, a recombinant vascular endothelial growth factor (VEGF) monoclonal antibody, prohibits angiogenesis, the development of the tumor's vascular supply. Blocking angiogenesis limits local and systemic metastases. Targeted therapies are being used in combination with chemotherapies or as front-line therapy according to current NCCN guidelines (2017). As second-line therapy, erlotinib is especially effective in a subpopulation of females, nonsmokers, individuals who are of East Asian descent, and those who have a histology of adenocarcinoma (Besse, Ropert, & Soria, 2007). Recently, bevacizumab has been shown to be effective in combination with platinum-based chemotherapy for nonsquamous cell advanced NSCLC (NCI, 2018c). Additional targeted agents such as cetuximab, an EGFR inhibitor, and sunitinib and sorafenib, anti-VEGF receptor agents, have been investigated (Besse et al., 2007; Walker, 2003).

Colorectal Cancer

New cases of colorectal cancer (CRC) in the United States in 2018 are estimated to reach approximately 97,220 for colon and 43,030 for rectal cancer (ACS, 2018c). The projected combined death rate has declined 4.1% since 2005 for those 50 years of age and older due to improved screening procedures and significant advances in surgery, radiation, and chemotherapy (Wolpin, Meyerhardt, Mamon, & Mayer, 2007). Conversely, the incidence rate for adults under the age of 55 years has increased 1% per year secondary to lack of early screening when symptoms arise and lack of healthy eating habits and leading active lifestyles (ACS, 2018b). CRC ranks fourth among the most common malignancies in the United States and was the second leading cause of cancer death in 2017 at an estimated rate of 50,260. It is a disease of aging, as the median age of individuals with newly diagnosed CRC is 70 years (Rosati & Bilancia, 2008). In minorities, particularly African Americans, cancer-related mortality remains higher than in whites due to social and economic disparities (65% vs. 55%; Wolpin et al., 2007; ACS, 2016).

CRC is difficult to diagnose at an early stage without screening because patients are usually asymptomatic (ACS, 2018b). Screening to detect polyps and cancer is important for all those deemed to be at risk and for those over the age of 50 years. Diagnosis of CRC in the older adult is especially challenging because many of the common symptoms associated with CRC such as constipation, change in bowel patterns, and fatigue may be inaccurately attributed to the aging process.

Approximately 50% of patients present with hepatic metastases or develop them during the course of the disease (Pawlik, Schulick, & Choti, 2008). Because the portal vein drains the blood supply from the colon, the liver is the most common site of metastasis for advanced disease. Isolated lung or liver metastases may be considered for surgical resection (Engstrom et al., 2007a). As the disease progresses, patients may experience bowel obstruction. Widespread metastases to the abdomen (carcinomatosis), lung, and/or liver are often the cause of death.

■ **Signs/Symptoms/Staging.** Most cancers of the bowel are moderately or well-differentiated adenocarcinomas. These cancers usually develop as a result of progressive colonic polyp mutations (Engstrom et al., 2007b). Screening for and removal of potentially malignant or pre-malignant polyps can prevent the development of more advanced cancer. TNM staging has been modified to correspond with the Astler–Coller Dukes system. This staging process evaluates the depth of bowel wall penetration by the tumor, lymph node involvement, and presence of distant metastasis. The accuracy of the staging in high-risk Stages II and III is associated with the number of nodes surgically removed (Engstrom et al., 2007b). Staging ranges from Stage I to Stage IV, with overall survival declining from greater than 90% in Stage I to less than 10% in Stage IV (Meyerhardt & Mayer, 2005).

■ **Disease Management.** A complete staging workup includes a physical examination; colonoscopy with biopsy; pathologic tissue review; baseline CT of the chest, abdomen, and pelvis; complete blood count; chemistry profile; and carcinoembryonic antigen (CEA) determination.

■ **Surgery.** For resectable colon cancer, surgery remains the standard treatment. Tumor location, blood supply, and lymph node patterns in the area of cancer determine the extent of resection. Examination of a minimum of 12 lymph nodes is necessary for accurate staging (Engstrom et al., 2007a). Laparoscopic advances have allowed the use of minimally invasive surgical procedures to resect colon cancers without increasing recurrence rates (Clinical Outcomes of Surgical Therapy Study Group, 2004). Early mobility, return of pulmonary function, and decreased ileus and adhesion formation have made this procedure desirable for many patients, especially those with advancing age and comorbid illnesses (Baker, 2001).

Surgical management of rectal cancer involves resection with preservation of anorectal sphincter function and sexual and urinary function whenever possible (Engstrom et al., 2007a). Preoperative combined modality therapy (chemotherapy and radiation) has resulted in significant reductions in tumor size and decreased rates of local recurrence in rectal cancer. However, it is associated with increased toxicity when compared to surgery alone (Bosset et al., 2006).

■ **Radiation Therapy.** The role of radiation therapy is not well defined for colon cancer Debate over the value of pre- or postsurgical radiation therapy for rectal cancer continues. Although pre- and postoperative radiotherapy has been shown to reduce local recurrence when compared to surgery alone, neither intervention resulted in a statistically significant improvement in overall survival (Kapiteijn et al., 2001). Preoperative chemoradiotherapy doubled the rate of rectal sphincter-sparing operations and lowered the rates of local recurrence, acute toxicity, and long-term toxicity (Sauer et al., 2004).

■ **Chemotherapy.** Current guidelines for adjuvant therapy do not recommend chemotherapy for individuals with Stage II disease. However, patients with advanced CRC do have a survival benefit from newer chemotherapeutic regimens and targeted agents. Current therapy includes bevacizumab, VEGF blocker, plus FOLFOX infusional 5-fluorouracil (5-FU), leucovorin, oxaliplatin, FOLFIRI (infusional 5-FU, leucovorin, and irinotecan), capecitabine, or 5-FU/LV. The two EGFR monoclonal antibodies, cetuximab and panitumumab, have also been shown to be effective. Genotyping of tumors may help to predict which therapy is most beneficial to an individual. For example, patients with advanced CRC who do not have a mutated form of the gene *KRAS* may benefit from cetuximab and chemotherapy (McBride, 2008). Overall survival is improved with single-agent cetuximab when other treatments fail (Jonker et al., 2007). More recently, immunotherapy has shown promising results with the use of immune checkpoint inhibitors like nivolumab and pembrolizumab. They can be beneficial for advanced CRC that has progressed following conventional treatments. A phase II study with heavily pretreated patients with pembrolizumab showed the objective response rate and progression-free survival of 40% and 78%, respectively (Le et al., 2015).

■ CANCER COMORBIDITIES

For many years, lung cancer risk has been associated with chronic obstructive pulmonary disease (COPD; Dubey & Powell, 2008) and tobacco smoke. Smokers are also known to be at risk for coronary artery disease, peripheral vascular disease, and stroke. These comorbidities may affect the performance status of individuals with lung cancer, limiting treatment options and increasing symptom burden.

Individuals with a first-degree family history of CRC and women with a personal history of ovarian, endometrial, or breast cancer are at a high risk for CRC. Familial adenomatous polyposis (FAP) and hereditary nonpolyposis CRC (HNPCC) are two major conditions that carry a genetic predisposition to CRC. Inflammatory bowel diseases including ulcerative colitis and Crohn's disease are often linked to CRC. FAP, HNPCC, and inflammatory bowel diseases constitute about 10% to 15% of CRC cases. Comorbid conditions that have been identified as increasing the risk of CRC include age, obesity, sedentary lifestyle, diet high in fat or red meats, smoking, and alcohol consumption (no more than 2 drinks/d for men and 1 drink/d for women. The variation in alcohol consumption between men and women relates to the smaller body size of women and slower metabolism; ACS, 2018c).

Frailty at any age adds a risk factor to cancer morbidity. Anticancer therapies often decrease the patient's functional level, leading to catabolic syndrome, muscle wasting, and increased risk of infection. Paraneoplastic syndromes are disorders associated with an altered immune system response to a neoplasm. Symptoms may be endocrine, rheumatological, neuromuscular or musculoskeletal, cardiovascular, cutaneous, hematological, gastrointestinal, or renal, between others. Nonspecific syndromes may precede some of the clinical manifestations of a neoplasm. An example is hypertrophic osteoarthropathy, which may be present in patients with lung cancers. Because of the complexity and variety of clinical presentations with paraneoplastic syndromes, all require expert assessment and rapid management.

■ COMMON ASSOCIATED SYMPTOMS OF CANCER

Palliative care is best initiated at the time of a cancer diagnosis, especially for patients with a life-limiting cancer. Many individuals experience symptoms that interfere with QOL at the time of diagnosis as well as other points in time along the disease trajectory. Hoffman, Given, von Eye, Gift, and Given (2007) have identified a symptom cluster of pain, fatigue, and insomnia in patients who are newly diagnosed and undergoing chemotherapy. Pain, dyspnea, fatigue, weight loss, and cough are commonly associated with lung cancer. Pain may occur because of tumor infiltration into lung parenchyma, the brachial plexus, or spinal cord or from bone or brain metastasis. Dyspnea occurs in as many as 55% of lung cancer patients and in up to 80% of patients at the end of life (Becze, 2008). Risk factors associated with dyspnea may be related to disease or treatment such as disease progression, anemia, or lung irradiation. Interventions for dyspnea have been reviewed, critiqued, and summarized by the Oncology Nursing Society's Putting Evidence into Practice (PEP) Dyspnea Intervention Project Team (Irwin & Johnson, 2014). Fatigue has been described as a very distressing symptom of disease and treatment. Potentially treatable causes such as anemia should be identified and addressed.

More than 95% of individuals with lung cancer are symptomatic at the time of diagnosis (Kvale et al., 2007). Common symptoms such as cough, dyspnea, dysphagia, hoarseness, fatigue, and weight loss are frequently attributed to comorbid illnesses and are often ignored. Unfortunately with lung cancer, these common symptoms are usually the result of locally advanced or metastatic disease. Symptoms may be present as a result of primary cancer itself (dyspnea, wheezing, cough, hemoptysis, chest pain), locoregional metastases within the chest (superior vena cava syndrome, pleural effusions, ribs, or pleura), or distant metastases (back pain; metastases to brain, spinal cord, or bone; Kvale et al., 2007).

Depending on the type of treatment received, additional symptoms may be experienced. For example, persons receiving radiation therapy may have new or increased dysphagia if location of the treatment field involves the esophagus. Individuals receiving chemotherapy or undergoing radiation may experience an increase in fatigue beyond initial presentation. Symptoms at the end of life are dependent on the type of cancer and the sites of metastases. NSCLC frequently goes to the bone, often causing excruciating pain. SCLC often progresses to the brain, causing headaches, nausea, and impaired mental status. These symptoms require aggressive PC intervention (Kvale et al., 2007).

Chemotherapy and targeted agents used to treat lung cancer have the potential to cause side effects that negatively influence QOL. Body image, nausea and vomiting, and chemo-induced neuropathies require aggressive supportive care. However, it is important to note that for all individuals with NSCLC or SCLC, chemotherapy has been shown to relieve tumor-related symptoms such as pain, cough, and dyspnea, as well as offering survival benefit, despite the potential side effects (Stinnett, Williams, & Johnson, 2007).

Chemotherapy-related toxicities are common, undertreated, and underreported. In a review of three randomized clinical trials with a total of 1,090 patients (2,482 cycles), underreporting by physicians ranged from 40.7% to 74.4% (Di Maio et al., 2015). The deleterious effects of anticancer treatments can alter the patient's QOL and inhibit further treatments. Common causes of hospitalization due to chemotherapy toxicity include neutropenic fever, severe electrolyte disorders, or volume depletion related to poorly controlled nausea, vomiting, or diarrhea. Other chemotherapy-induced effects include cytopenias, constipation, mucositis, anxiety/depression, neurotoxicity, hand and foot syndrome, and cardiac toxicity (Moore, Johnson, Fortner, & Houts, 2008).

■ MANAGEMENT

Cancer care should be age appropriate and treatment should be easily accessed to ensure successful management of physical, emotional, and spiritual symptoms. The family or designated caregiver should be considered within the unit of care throughout the life span for effective palliative management. From childhood to frail older adult, the responsibility of decision making shifts from parent (or support group) with possible patient input, to patient with support group input, and back to support group with possible patient input (Scullion, 2005). An interprofessional collaborative care model, sometimes referred to as an integrated approach, is the gold standard for cancer care regardless of age, life expectancy, and treatment choices. The complexity of cancer care requires many members of the healthcare team to work simultaneously to accomplish treatment goals and manage optimally the patient affected with cancer.

Pediatric and Young Adult

Cancer in children and the young adult is rare. It is critical to identify any unexplained signs or symptoms that do not improve with standard management. Such cases should be further worked up.

■ **Children.** The life of a child who has been diagnosed with a life-threatening illness is drastically altered with wide-reaching and long-lasting effects on the child and family unit. PC health professionals working in the field of pediatrics have reported the parental need to provide every available therapy to their child in order to feel confident they have given their child the best chance for survival. Often, the attempt to defy death with anticancer treatment eliminated the chance of expert symptom management occurring simultaneously. Parental direction toward measures to defy death is now considered the reality of pediatric cancer care and healthcare professionals. PC specialists can philosophically support parents when they maintain dual goals of hope for comfort and emotional support at the same time as hope for life extension. This is a healthier alternative not only for the patient and family but also for the healthcare team since it is distressing for healthcare professionals when expert symptom management is delayed until all other options have been exhausted (De Graves & Aranda, 2005; Wolfe, Friebert, & Hilden, 2002). Pediatric oncology nurses report moral distress when "good nursing" is impeded as curative needs of the patient overshadow the patient's physical and emotional needs. It is necessary that cure and palliation goals interface in cancer care, allowing an overlap so the palliative needs of the child are not sacrificed for the hope of a cure.

Symptom management, communication, and shared decision making resemble adult care with few exceptions, while spiritual care often presents slightly differently for children. Identification of meaningful activity will change from one development stage to another. Play and relational connection are two identified mainstays for children. School-age children may desire to maintain a school-day schedule to support their need to remain similar to and receive acceptance by their peers. Routine and normalcy are also recognized as important goals for care of children with life-altering illness, and religious ritual, as in routine visits to a church, synagogue, or mosque, maintains the family's meaningful spiritual routine (De Graves & Aranda, 2005; Wolfe, Grier et al., 2000). Location of care and the pediatric patient's preference continue to merit attention. Some suggest that family adjustment after the child's death is better if the child dies at home, yet others have contended that family relationships are enriched if death occurs during hospitalization. Outpatient clinics resembling day care allow the pediatric cancer patient who is receiving chemotherapy to spend nights at home and receive treatment elsewhere. These day care clinics also encourage play that children need for emotional development. Parents frequently identify the decrease in their child's activity level in play as a source of emotional distress. No matter what the location is for anticancer treatment and EOL care, it is worth noting that healthcare professionals specialized in symptom management and bereavement support make a difference in the family's memory of the illness regardless of the outcome (De Graves & Aranda, 2005; Houlston, 2006; Wolfe, Klar et al., 2000).

High-quality care for children living with cancer includes expert pain and symptom management. Healthcare professionals have an opportunity to make a difference in the perceived and actual experience of the parents of dying children. Children dying of cancer experience many symptoms, and parents who witness the child suffering may experience additional suffering during grief long after the child's death (Pritchard et al., 2008). Wolfe, Grier et al. (2000) discovered that discordance between parents and physicians regarding symptom recognition is similar to that of adults and their healthcare providers. There was also a direct correlation between a parent's report of the child's suffering and the level of involvement the physician displayed during the final phase of the child's life. In other words, a parent was more likely to report the child suffering when the parent also reported feeling that the physician was not actively involved in care at the end of the child's life. Wolfe found that earlier discussions about hospice care were associated with a higher likelihood that the parent would report the child as calm and peaceful during the last month of life. These observations support the theory that active involvement by healthcare providers committed to palliation helps to alleviate the suffering of dying children (Pritchard et al., 2008).

■ **Young Adults.** Uncertainty while living with cancer has been identified as a significant aspect of pediatric cancer and a major concern of adolescent and young adult cancer survivors. Long-lasting disease control and long-term survival during and after childhood is now common due to major advances in surgery, chemotherapy, and radiotherapy. However, treatment success can also have serious implications through each phase of the patient's life. Chemotherapy and radiation therapy can harm developing organs, and surgery can alter normal physical functioning or cause disfigurement (see Table 13.1). Previous studies have reported that as many as 69% of survivors of childhood cancer have physical, mental, or emotional limitations resulting from successful anticancer treatment (Decker, Haase, & Bell, 2007). A study of 226 adult survivors of childhood cancer showed that 12% of those interviewed reported some level of suicidal symptoms. Risk factors associated with a higher significance of suicidal symptoms included younger age at diagnosis, a greater time lapse since diagnosis, and radiation treatments to the head. Add those risk factors to feelings of depression and hopelessness, chronic pain, physical dysfunction, and appearance alterations due to treatment, and the data suggest that healthcare professionals should perform a thorough psychosocial assessment upon long-term follow-up of

TABLE 13.1   Organ-Specific Late Effects of Cancer Therapy and Screening Methodology

Organ	Causes	Screening Tests
Musculoskeletal	RT	■ Physical exam, scoliosis exam (annually if growing) ■ X-ray prn
Breast	Mediastinal RT	■ Breast exam ■ Mammography beginning at age 25–30
Central nervous system	Cranial RT	■ Neurocognitive testing (baseline, q3–5 yrs) ■ MRN (baseline)
Neuroendocrine	Hypothalamic-pituitary RT	■ Growth curve every year, bone age (age 9) ■ GH stimulation test ■ TSH, free T4, T3 (baseline q3–5 yrs prn) ■ LH and FSH test (baseline, prn) ■ Prolactin (baseline, prn) ■ 8 a.m. cortisol (baseline, prn)
Cardiac	Anthracyclines	■ ECHO/ECG (baseline for all; q3–5 yrs after anthracycline)
	T-spine RT	■ Holter q5 yrs prn (high-dose anthracycline) ■ Stress test/dobutamine stress ECHO prn (after RT)
Pulmonary	RT, Bleomycin, CCNU/BCNU	■ PFT baseline, q3–5 yrs prn
Ovary	Alkylating agents, RT	■ Menstrual history annually ■ LH, FSH, and estradiol baseline (age > 12) and prn
Testes	Alkylating agents, RT	■ LH, FSH, and testosterone baseline (age > 12) and prn ■ Spermatoanalysis prn
Renal	Cisplatin (carboplatin)	■ Creatinine q1–2 yrs ■ Magnesium q1–2 yrs ■ Serum phosphate ■ Urine glucose ■ Protein
	Ifosfamide	■ Urinalysis ■ Creatinine clearance baseline and q3–5 yrs prn
	RT	■ Urinalysis
Bladder	Cyclophosphamide, Ifosfamide, RT	■ Urinalysis annually for heme
Thyroid	RT to neck and/or mediastinum	■ TSH, free T4, T3 q yr × 10 ■ Scans (U/S) prn
Liver	6-MP, MTX, Act-d, RT	■ Liver function tests q1–3 yr
Gastrointestinal	Intestinal RT	■ Stool guaiac q yr ■ Colonoscopy (according to ACS)

ACS, American Cancer Society; BCNU, carmustine; CCNU, lomustine; ECHO, echocardiogram; FSH, follicular-stimulating hormone; GH, growth hormone; LH, luteinizing hormone; MTX, methotrexate; PFT, pulmonary function test; RT, radiotherapy; TSH, thyroid stimulating hormone.

Source: From Schwartz, C. (1999). Long-term survivors of childhood cancer: The late effects of therapy. *Oncologist, 4,* 45–54.

survivors (Carroll, 2007). Decker et al. (2007) conducted a cross-sectional, secondary analysis study to examine uncertainty in three "time-since-diagnosis" groups of adolescents and young adults. The most recent diagnosed survivors had significantly higher uncertainty for recurring pain, an unpredictable illness course, and self-care concerns. Interestingly, survivors with 5 or more years from diagnosis had higher uncertainty related to knowing what to expect for disease recurrence. All survivor groups exhibited a significantly high uncertainty about multiple meanings of communication from doctors, leading the investigators to conclude that providers should have direct communication with adolescent and young adult patients. Uncertainty should be considered a concern throughout cancer survivorship, and long-term support of the young cancer survivor is warranted.

Adults and Older Adults

Critical assessment of the individual with cancer is important when determining life expectancy, treatment tolerance, and palliation. Physical reserve, psychosocial support, economic support, and comorbidity impact treatment outcomes (Repetto & Comandini, 2000).

The Zubrod or ECOG (Table 13.2) is the most widely used assessment tool in the field of oncology to determine performance status (West & Jin, 2015). The Karnofsky Performance Scale (KPS; Table 13.2) evaluates physical function and draws a close parallel with mortality (Repetto, Comandini, & Mammoliti, 2001). Assessing performance status plays an important role in determining the best treatment plan. Performance status is a fundamental part of provider assessments, eligibility criteria for clinical trials, and guidelines for standard treatment recommendations (West & Jin, 2015).

The Palliative Performance Scale (PPS; Table 13.3) is correlated with the KPS and has been used by PC specialists, most generally hospice professionals, to determine and monitor a patient's eligibility for hospice services. The PPS is a reliable, valid tool that correlates well with

actual and median survival time for cancer patients (Anderson, Downing, Hill, Casorso, & Lerch, 1996).

Age itself is not the most useful factor to determine prognosis and consider treatment options for older adults. However, a standardized nomenclature is required for a large and growing population. The concept of senescence by the passing of biological time is most useful in predicting survival, chemotherapy toxicity, postoperative morbidity, and mortality as opposed to chronological age (Audisio et al., 2004; Extermann & Hurria, 2007). Chronological age can be used as a functional status indicator for older adults because it is assumed that adults living with cancer are more likely to need functional assistance than their same-age peers without cancer. Predicting functional needs of older adults, geriatric terminology categorizes elders as "young old" (70–74 years), "old-old" (75–84 years), and "oldest old" (85 years and older). These age-related categorizations should be considered with a complete functional assessment when developing a treatment plan since aging involves a progression of the decline in organ systems, coexisting physical conditions, cognitive impairment, social isolation, functional dependence, and economic limitations (Audisio et al., 2004; Extermann, 2005). Natural changes

TABLE 13.2 Performance Status Scales

Zubrod/ECOG Scale		Karnofsky Scale		
Rating	Definition	Rating %	Criteria	Definition
0	Normal activity	100	Normal; no complaints; no evidence of disease	Able to carry on normal activity and to work; no special care needed
		90	Able to carry on normal activity; minor signs or symptoms of disease	
1	Symptomatic and ambulatory; cares for self	80	Normal activity with effort; some signs or symptoms of disease	
		70	Cares for self; unable to carry on normal activity or to do active work	Unable to work; able to live at home and care for most personal needs; varying amount of assistance
2	Ambulatory >50% of the time; occasional assistance	60	Requires occasional assistance, but is able to care for most of personal needs	
3	Ambulatory ≤50% of the time; nursing care needed	50	Requires considerable assistance and frequent medical care	
		40	Disabled; requires special care and assistance	Unable to care for self; requires equivalent of institutional or hospital care; disease may be progressing rapidly
		30	Severely disabled; hospital admission is indicated although death is not imminent	
4	Bedridden	20	Very sick; hospital admission necessary; active supportive treatment necessary	
		10	Moribund; fatal processes progressing rapidly	
5	Dead	0	Dead	

ECOG, Eastern Cooperative Oncology Group.

Source: From West, J., & Jin, J. O. (2015). Performance status in patients with cancer: Patient performance status (PS) is an important part of cancer care and treatment. *Journal of American Medical Association: Oncology, 1*(7), 998. doi:10.1001/jamaoncol.2015.3113

TABLE 13.3 Palliative Performance Scale					
PPS Level	Ambulation	Activity and Evidence of Disease	Self-Care	Intake	Conscious Level
100%	Full	Normal activity and work No evidence of disease	Full	Normal	Full
90%	Full	Normal activity and work Some evidence of disease	Full	Normal	Full
80%	Full	Normal activity *with* effort Some evidence of disease	Full	Normal or reduced	Full
70%	Reduced	Unable to do normal job/work Significant disease	Full	Normal or reduced	Full
60%	Reduced	Unable to do hobby/house work Significant disease	Occasional assistance necessary	Normal or reduced	Full or confusion
50%	Mainly sit/lie	Unable to do any work Extensive disease	Considerable assistance required	Normal or reduced	Full or confusion
40%	Mainly sit/lie	Unable to do most activity Extensive disease	Mainly assistance	Normal or reduced	Full or drowsy +/- confusion
30%	Totally bed bound	Unable to do any activity Extensive disease	Total care	Normal or reduced	Full or drowsy +/- confusion
20%	Totally bed bound	Unable to do any activity Extensive disease	Total care	Minimal to sips	Full or drowsy +/- confusion
10%	Totally bed bound	Unable to do any activity Extensive disease	Total care	Mouth care only	Drowsy or coma +/- confusion
0%	Dead	—	—	—	—

Source: From Victoria Hospice Society. (2001). The Palliative Performance Scale version 2 (PPSv2) tool. Retrieved from http://www.npcrc .org/files/content/pps_for_distribution_2015_-_with_watermark_sample.pdf

associated with age often lead to a greater susceptibility to chronic and acute disease, yet a comprehensive evaluation of the older adult's coexisting disease (comorbidities), cognition, functional status, nutritional status, social supports, psychological state, and personal resolve gives a more accurate definition of age in relation to cancer treatment tolerance (Extermann & Hurria, 2007).

Another commonly used geriatric classification of the older adult is the "frail elder." The use of the term "elder" is most generally reserved for patients older than 65 years, and "frail" is a traditional term not well defined. The medical literature often refers to a frail individual as someone with poor physiological reserves and a high prevalence of repeated chronic illness requiring multiple hospital admissions. Additional characteristics of frailty include complex psychosocial problems and limited social support, which increases the risk of treatment-related complications and cancer-specific mortality (Audisio et al., 2004). In addition, the term is associated with more than one geriatric syndrome, a limited life expectancy not much beyond 2 years, the inability to maintain homeostasis in nonstressed conditions, and a greater risk of developing

treatment-related toxicities with the loss of functional independence (Repetto & Comandini, 2000). Geriatric syndromes should also be included in a comprehensive assessment in order to determine accurately the elder's stage of life and functional capabilities. Geriatric syndromes that have been defined and used in treatment planning within the last 10 years include dementia, depression, abuse/neglect, incontinence, osteoporosis, failure to thrive, and risk for falls (Extermann, 2005).

Since the evaluation of the older adult is obviously influenced by many factors, a geriatric assessment tool can equip healthcare providers to manage the complexity of geriatric oncology healthcare needs. The Comprehensive Geriatric Assessment (CGA; Table 13.4) is recommended to determine the medical, psychological, and functional capabilities of elderly cancer patients. The CGA focuses on frail elderly people with complex conditions and a functional status relating to QOL and incorporates an interprofessional team approach to assessment (Repetto et al., 2003). Activities of daily living (ADLs) and instrumental ADLs (IADLs) are useful tools for assessing functional ability and are incorporated into

TABLE 13.4	Elements of a Comprehensive Geriatric Assessment		
Domain	**Assessment**		**Association with Age**
Level of functional activity	Ability to perform activities of daily living (ADL): ■ transfer from bed to chair ■ ability to feed ■ ability to use restroom	Ability to perform instrumental ADLs: ■ self-administer medications ■ prepare meals ■ make telephone calls	Impact on life expectancy and ability to live on his/her own
Comorbidities	Amount and gravity of illnesses		Impacts life expectancy
Disorders associated with aging	Dementia, depression, delirium, fractures, falls, light-headedness, failure to thrive, lack of care, and ill-treatment		Impacts life expectancy and ability to live on his/her own
Nutritional status	Assessment of dietary status		Dietary risks (i.e., malnutrition) and ability to live on his/her own
Medications	Assess for polypharmacy; amount of medications (both prescription and over-the-counter)		Increased risk of drug interactions and comorbidity
Financial resources	Assess the level of income and savings		Risk for financial toxicity and ability to live on his/her own
Caregiver support	Availability of social support such as family, friends, and neighbors. Consideration of the caregiver's health and functional status and accessibility		Safety risks related to residing at home

Source: Adapted From Balducci, L. (2009). Pharmacology of antineoplastic medications in older cancer patients. Physicians Practice. Retrieved from http://www.physicianspractice.com/oncology-journal/pharmacology-antineoplastic-medications-older-cancer-patients

many comprehensive assessment tools (Table 13.2; Repetto et al., 2003). Dependence for ADLs and IADLs closely parallel limited life expectancy and dependence for IADL correlates with treatment intolerance, while comorbidity, a normal process of age, is known to complicate cancer diagnosis, prognosis, and treatment (Extermann, 2005; Lazzaro & Comandini, 2000). Comorbidity is associated with decreased survival rates and merits attention during a comprehensive assessment.

Family Support

In addition to the physical care of a loved one with advanced cancer, comprehensive care requires family support. PC includes physical, emotional, and spiritual comfort of the patient and family. Spouses, adult children, extended relatives, and neighbors account for the 7 million Americans who consider themselves caregivers. Approximately 15% of those Americans care for individuals with serious illness and disability. Spouses represent roughly 62% of those caregivers, with women representing 72% (Derby & O'Mahony, 2006). Often, primary caregivers are spouses with their own healthcare needs that may make them susceptible to depression, fatigue, and frequent acute illness. Other caregiving relationships involve adult children as dual-role caregivers to parents and their own children, or the staff at the elder's nursing facility or assisted-living environment. Kobayashi (2000) identified that both the patient and his or her

family require medical and psychosocial treatment when evaluating the use of home medical/social services by elders in the last 6 months of life. Symptom management is more intense and requires regular evaluation. Illnesses at an advanced stage frequently require more physical symptom monitoring with similar need for psychosocial care. Utilization of the PC team is vital at the end of life (Kobayashi, 2000). The level of burden placed on caregivers of cancer patients exceeds that experienced by those caring for the elderly or patients suffering from dementia. Furthermore, the level of care required by the patient directly influences the caregiver's life and health, leading to caregiver burnout (Bevans & Sternberg, 2012).

EOL decisions place additional burdens on the family. Those decisions include where the final days will be spent, what impact there will be on loved ones, and whether the family can afford the care involved. Family members often take a leave of absence from their jobs to care for a dying loved one. Those who do not have that option may experience feelings of remorse for taking a more peripheral role in the care of the older adult. Many Americans report they would prefer to die in the comforts of their home; however, a majority die in an acute-care or long-term facility. Nurses can support a dying patient by providing a home-like environment and a familiar surrounding with the patient's personal items, aroma, music, and support people (Beardsmore & Fitzmaurice, 2002; Higginson & Sen-Gupta, 2000; Hsieh, Huang, Lai, & Lin, 2007; Tang, 2003).

When patients reach the terminal phase of cancer, conflict may occur among the patient, family members, and healthcare workers. Conflict at the end of life may be influenced by disparities of patient/family expectations with the patient's function and symptom status as well as the patient's attempt to maintain physical, emotional, and existential control. As the disease progresses, symptoms and physical function are in flux. Family members attempt to adjust to the changes; however, the quick changes associated with advanced cancer may provoke conflict.

Family concerns throughout the course of advanced illness are directed toward the physical comfort of the patient, the emotional impact on the family, and the desire for accurate information (Griffin et al., 2007; Kristjanson & White, 2002; Milberg, Olsson, Jakobsson, Olsson, & Friedrichsen, 2008; Tang, 2003; Valdimarsdóttir et al., 2007). It is commonly perceived by family members that once the terminal prognosis is discussed, healthcare professionals do not feel the need to provide additional information. In view of the rapid change in physical and cognitive status, information updates are just as significant as before the discussion of prognosis. Out of 22 terminally ill patients interviewed, Kutner, Steiner, Corbett, Jahnigen, and Barton, (1999) concluded that 98.2% requested information concerning changes in their disease status. It is interesting to note that even though most patients and families request the truth, they still want healthcare providers to be optimistic and maintain a sense of hope (Kutner et al., 1999). It is also worth noting that bereaved family members report higher satisfaction, fewer concerns, and fewer unmet needs pertaining to the care of a loved one when PC and hospice teams provide EOL care (Teno et al., 2004).

Initially, the family's focus of hope is often on cure. It is also the hope and goal of the family to provide comfort and support to their loved one as death becomes imminent. The PC team assists caregivers to develop the physical, emotional, and mental reserves that are required to maintain hope, coupling that with the provision of timely, accurate, and honest information on the impending death. Nurses should respond to patient and family concerns with patience and assurance of non-abandonment and an increase in attention to aggressive symptom management (Borneman, Stahl, Ferrell, & Smith, 2002; Valdimarsdóttir et al., 2007). Physicians often choose to limit or tailor prognostic information with the intention of maintaining a patient's hope. It is important to disclose information in a timely manner and prepare family members for their family member's death. This allows for participation of the patient and loved ones in the EOL process and a sense of control with the experience leading up to death. Advice and assistance that the patient and caregivers receive before death decrease anxiety and facilitate the grieving process (Dumont, Dumont, & Mongeau, 2008). Dumont et al. (2008) described that the principles that most significantly affected positively or negatively family caregivers' experience are (a) characteristics of the family caregiver (attitudes,

religious and spiritual beliefs, personal competence, psychological and emotional burden); (b) patient characteristics (attitudes, relation to death); (c) symptoms of the illness (confusion, major behavior changes, cachexia); (d) the relational context (relationship with the patient and other family members); (e) social and professional support; and (f) circumstances surrounding the death (moment of death, preparedness for death).

Mack et al. (2007) conducted a cross-sectional, questionnaire-based study of parents and physicians of children with cancer. The study evaluated relationships between parental recall of prognostic disclosure from the physician and how that disclosure affected hope, trust, and emotional distress. In this multivariable model, parents frequently reported that "high quality" physician communication (defined by parents as trusting a familiar physician to give honest information) involving more elements of prognostic disclosure made them feel more hopeful. The study found that when the physician has established a compassionate, trusting relationship with the patient, family prognostic disclosure could support hope, even when the prognosis is poor. In fact, no data are available that show hope can be taken from patients and families despite the long-standing fear of clinicians (Harrington & Smith, 2008).

Parents of dying children often have an intellectual knowledge or emotional awareness of the child's impending death. Valdimarsdóttir et al. (2007) discovered that healthcare providers can influence the awareness of parents, encouraging a "preparatory phase" of care that fosters an environment of talking about the child's impending death and making a long-lasting beneficial effect on bereavement. Emotional awareness enables parents to see the patient's weakening condition, obtain more information and assistance from healthcare providers, and discuss important issues on life and death. As the family's focus of hope shifts due to the patient's weakening physical condition, family members may strengthen the connection with their faith system, their relationship to the patient, and others. The connection made with healthcare providers prior to the death of the loved one is considered integral in the grieving process (Griffin et al., 2007; Kristjanson & White, 2002; Milberg et al., 2008; Tang, 2003; Valdimarsdóttir et al., 2007).

Bereavement Support

Saying good-bye to a loved one is important to survivors. Those who lose a loved one unexpectedly often exhibit less resilience and more anger during the bereavement period. Anticipatory grief has not been shown to alter actual grief, but giving family members sufficient warning of an impending death will foster a shift of focus to meaningful discussions with the cancer patient. That meaningful time will have a lasting impact on the survivor, possibly alleviating any guilt the survivor may normally experience as a grieving caregiver. Since mourning is culture based, this is also a good time for the healthcare provider to inquire about and honor cultural and religious practices surrounding death. This display of respect for cultural and spiritual rituals surrounding the dying process and memorial can make the experience of death less traumatic. Data from two small studies (Cohen et al., 1997) of terminally ill cancer patients show that scores of existential well-being correlate with scores of physical well-being. Even in the presence of physical pain, depression and hopelessness are inversely related to spiritual well-being. After the death, a caring call from a familiar healthcare provider allows the survivor to reconnect with someone who shared the death experience and to discuss concerns regarding emotional and physical responses to grief. The bereaved often report the need to talk about the death experience many times. These phone calls can lend an additional listening ear for that purpose (Griffin et al., 2007). Milberg et al. (2008) learned from bereaved family members that half of them requested bereavement follow-up and many wanted to talk about the events occurring in the palliative phase of the decedent's care, their own response to loneliness, and the future. Follow-up contacts were preferred in person and respondents expressed appreciation to be recognized as a person with specific needs for contact.

■ PALLIATIVE CARE ISSUES

Palliative Chemotherapy

When chemotherapy is given with the intention of improving symptoms and quality of life without a curative intent, it is referred to as palliative chemotherapy. Metastatic cancer that has advanced beyond any curative options commonly may be managed with palliative chemotherapy regimens that may extend life.

■ Goals and Use of Chemotherapy Near the End of Life. Since the 1970s, oncological trials have focused on chemotherapy response rates, disease-free intervals, and overall survival endpoints. At the same time, clinicians have observed and recorded the symptom improvement benefits during curative treatment efforts. As a result, the concept of "palliative chemotherapy" for the purpose of symptom improvement became not only an acceptable practice but also a desirable choice for patients whose cancer was impossible to eradicate (Thompson & Chochinov, 2009). Tolerability to chemotherapy continues to dramatically improve, allowing patients with incurable cancer the option of palliative chemotherapy with an acceptable risk of toxicity despite the uncertainty that symptom burden will be relieved or survival will be extended. Patients and families will put their hope in treatments offered with limited scientific evidence of benefit; consequently, chemotherapy use for patients with advanced disease requires sophisticated oncologic assessment, clarity of the patient's goals for care, and balanced shared decision making between the patient and the oncologist. Like other treatment decisions, it requires a complete burden versus benefit analysis. Despite data to support the palliative benefits of chemotherapy, most hospice agencies are not willing to assume the cost of such treatment. Community resources offering interprofessional support not linked to the hospice benefit provide valuable support to individuals receiving palliative chemotherapy. Cancer clinics may be linked to national and local programs, and area hospices may have additional services for individuals ineligible for hospice benefits.

Knowing what patients and families understand from diagnosis, treatment, and prognosis, discussions with their oncologists is paramount. Many studies have described lack of understanding from patients and families that late-stage chemotherapy was not intended to cure. Harrington and Smith (2008) reported that many patients did not recall a discussion regarding prognosis and the goal of palliative treatment. In an effort to support a patient's hope for disease outcome, it has also been reported that many physicians will offer a wide range of outcomes to allow patients to determine for themselves their most favorable option. Supporting a balanced exchange of information and shared decision making between patients and their oncologists remains important. People living face-to-face with death will choose aggressive treatment with major adverse effects and a small chance of benefit. This is largely different from what their physicians and nurses who are not living with illness would choose. Individuals representing many socioeconomic levels and value systems are willing to place their hope in experimental drugs with a 10% mortality rate for one last chance of benefit (Harrington & Smith, 2008). A conversation with a clear understanding and clarification of a patient's interpretation of the discussion regarding goals of care and treatment options is critical for informed decision making.

A discussion of patient preference for quality and quantity of life with or without chemotherapy is a good start to a palliative treatment discussion. Before chemotherapy is recommended, a definable benefit must be identified, and a straightforward discussion can be initiated by asking patients how much they want to know about their current condition and prognosis. Define the words "response" and "cure." Many patients will use these terms interchangeably. Provide printed resources listing the benefits of adverse reactions to chemotherapy, keeping in mind that there must be a definable benefit to chemotherapy before treatment can be medically justified. Ask patients about their goals for treatment, views on undesirable side effects, and plans for the future. Extending survival time for an upcoming special event may be the benefit that could justify treatment in the patient's mind. Also, initiate discussion, with the intent of revisiting the plan when the cancer is resistant to chemotherapy.

Upon evaluation of the palliative treatment, the nurse can facilitate a meeting with the treating and PC team to clearly report on how the cancer is responding to chemotherapy. Working within an interprofessional framework, the physician, nurse specialist, clergy, patient, and family should be involved in this discussion. Continue a straightforward approach to communication by clearly defining the cancer's response to treatment. Provide hope if there is reason to be hopeful; however, avoid offering false hope. It is a good practice to provide patients and caregivers with factual information based on patient assessment, laboratory data, pathological reports, and diagnostic imaging. Many people are able to be hopeful about something even if the cancer is growing, yet some physicians believe that disclosing a poor prognosis will reduce a patient's hope. In a study of 194 parents of children living with cancer, Mack et al. (2007) discovered that clinician communication can foster hope even when the news is bad. In almost half of the parents receiving more prognostic, high-quality information from their child's physician, a greater communication-related hope was reported (Mack et al., 2007). High-quality care was designated by clinician sensitivity and the clinician's active listening skills. Supporting previous research findings, Mack and colleagues suggest that meaningful experiences and relationships can serve as a foundation for hope, as opposed to a hope based on unrealistic expectations for treatment outcome. In fact, there is no data that support the previous belief that hope can be taken away from patients and that patients are harmed by sensitive, compassionate information exchange regarding prognosis (Harrington & Smith, 2008).

Body image changes associated with targeted agents, including facial and upper body rash and hair loss associated with many of the chemotherapeutic agents, can be devastating for patients and families. The pathophysiology of nausea and vomiting is quite complex and requires strong assessment skills to identify appropriate pharmacologic and nonpharmacologic interventions (Coyne, Lyckholm, & Smith, 2006; Thompson & Chochinov, 2009). Neuropathies associated with thoracic surgical resection and with chemotherapeutic agents, especially the platinum drugs and taxotere, can be very burdensome and require aggressive management. Medications for neuropathic pain, such as gabapentin, pregabalin, duloxetine, or the tricyclic antidepressants, may improve QOL (Coyne et al., 2006).

In addition to addressing physical symptoms associated with cancer, the nurse may be involved with PC to help the patient and family with complex decision making during the staging process, at the time of disease progression, and end of life. With the minimally toxic targeted agents now available, many are opting to choose treatment rather than supportive care alone.

Hospice length of stay may decrease as more patients are continuing treatment late into the disease. The current hospice Medicare regulations require patients to choose either hospice care or continued therapy. Until there is a change in the hospice benefit, many will not have access to needed hospice care until the last days of life (Temel et al., 2008; Thompson & Chochinov, 2009). The role of the nurse as an advocate is needed at this stage.

PC can also improve psychological, social, and spiritual concerns that confront patients and families with cancer. Guilt may increase distress in patients throughout the disease trajectory such as patients with lung cancer with a history of smoking or current tobacco use. Counseling may be helpful to address emotions, fears, and concerns. Changes in roles and relationships as a result of disease progression also may require intervention from the counselors and social workers on the PC team. Involving spiritual care is important as individuals face the reality of the end of life and the importance of life closure. Balboni et al. (2013) described that patients who were well supported by religious communities and received spiritual support from the medical team had higher rates of hospice use, fewer aggressive interventions, and fewer ICU deaths. EOL discussions were also associated with less aggressive interventions.

Over half of all patients with CRCs are diagnosed in an advanced stage. Comfort measures to manage metastatic disease and side effects of treatment are essential for QOL. Trimodality therapy is difficult with patients battling fatigue, nausea and vomiting, diarrhea, and pain. In late-stage disease, bowel obstruction, pain, ascites, nausea, and vomiting require aggressive PC. Pharmacologic and nonpharmacologic interventions may relieve pain and symptoms associated with treatment and disease progression (Thompson & Chochinov, 2009).

Along with managing physical symptoms, the nurse must address the psychological, social, and spiritual issues that may be evident across the disease trajectory. Depression, frequently underdiagnosed and undertreated in patients with cancer, should be managed with medication and counseling. Financial burdens associated with months of expensive treatment and inability to work require help from social work. Spiritual care may alleviate the anxiety that comes from the uncertainty of disease progression and the challenges associated with treatment decisions. As hope and goals change from control of the disease to a comfortable death, the PC team in conjunction with the primary nurse can provide support to the patient and family.

CASE STUDY *Conclusion*

Mr. T. experienced the roller-coaster journey of advanced cancer. Throughout his journey, from diagnosis until death, he was supported by his primary treatment nurse and the cancer center's PC team including advanced practice nurses, social workers, counselors, and spiritual care coordinators. The best approach to patients with life-limiting illness is access to PC throughout the disease trajectory.

For approximately 6 months, Mr. T.'s CT scans demonstrated response to treatment or stable disease. During other times of restaging, CT scans or even clinical symptoms demonstrated evidence of progression. Over the course of the first 6 months, he received a variety of combinations of chemotherapy and targeted agents. Pain, nausea and vomiting, anxiety, and depression were managed with pharmacologic and nonpharmacologic interventions. Mr. and Mrs. T. participated in counseling at the cancer center. The spiritual care counselor provided listening and presence during each of his treatment sessions.

In March 2017, Mr. T. had progressive disease with liver and bone metastases. At that time, he was experiencing right upper quadrant pain from liver metastases, nausea and vomiting related to the treatment, lower extremity peripheral neuropathy, cough, and depression. Medications included oxycontin 10 mg p.o. twice a day (BID), oxycodone 5 mg p.o. every 4 hours as needed for pain, dexamethasone 8 mg daily for bone pain, ondansetron 8 mg p.o. every 6 hours as needed for nausea and vomiting, lorazepam 1 mg p.o. every 8 hours as needed for anxiety, benzonatate 100 mg p.o. every 4 hours for cough, gabapentin 300 mg p.o. BID for chemotherapy-induced neuropathy, magnesium oxide 400 mg p.o. BID, and sertraline 150 mg p.o. daily for depression, which had been increased over time.

As pulmonary metastases progressed, managing Mr. T.'s dyspnea and pain became the major challenge. He was hoping to enroll in a second phase I clinical trial but required hospitalization for worsening shortness of breath. Current recommendations for progressive lung cancer suggest chemotherapy may provide benefit in symptom management and increased survival. Since Mr. T.'s goals were quantity and QOL, continuing chemotherapy was deemed appropriate. However, during this admission, it became evident that he was dying from his pulmonary metastasis and would no longer be a candidate for further treatment.

The PC team worked with the nurses to manage his dyspnea with opioids and an increase in IV lorazepam to alleviate anxiety and restlessness. Mrs. T. met with the team in conjunction with the oncologists to review the goals of care. It was determined by Mr. and Mrs. T. that he did not want aggressive interventions initiated if he continued to deteriorate. Hospice service was called in to help care for him at the end of his life. Mrs. T. was very worried about caring for him at home and preferred to stay in the hospital with the staff she had come to know over the 2 years of care. A decision was made to admit him to inpatient hospice care.

Mr. T's children were at his bedside and spent his remaining days with their dad with the support of child-life counselors. All children participated in decorating squares on a premade quilt on Mr. T.'s bed, expressing their love for him. Time was set aside for Mr. T. and his wife to be alone in the room and their privacy was honored by the staff. Mr. T. died peacefully within 5 days of his sudden decline. The PC team, who had been with him throughout the cancer experience, supported Mrs. T. and her family at this difficult time and hospice continued to provide bereavement support and counseling to the family following his death.

CASE STUDY

AN INTERPROFESSIONAL PERSPECTIVE

Krishna V. Komanduri, MD

An old friend of mine, pursuing graduate work in epidemiology while I was studying medicine, reminded me that cumulative mortality in any cohort will eventually reach 100%. While we often appropriately share with patients the numerical results of studies that have primary endpoints like "progression-free survival" or "non-relapse mortality," we tend to underemphasize how therapies will influence QOL. We are even less likely to discuss, at least initially, how our proposed "standards of care" will impact a patient's ability to work, let alone more private and personal consequences, such as their finances or their sexuality. Why we naturally focus on the "mathematics" is complex—in some cases this focus on response and survival may reflect our inherent optimism as clinicians, or insulate us from other realities. As clinical research on these diverse endpoints is inherently more difficult, it has been underemphasized and underfunded. However, it is critical that we embrace all stages of cancer care, from diagnosis to treatment and (unfortunately too often) the transition from a focus on life extension to support of the dying patient and family.

This case illustrates many events in the typical cycle of cancer diagnosis and treatment. A police officer still in the prime of life experiences symptoms that lead to a diagnosis of advanced lung cancer. Fortunately, his care team did not subscribe to the outdated notion that PC should be provided only after conventional attempts to cure or prolong life fail. In contrast, both the patient and the family were engaged as the unit of care from the point of diagnosis. The PC team helped the patient and his loved ones during phases of treatment that included approved immunotherapies and then transitioned to phase I trials. His needs, and those of his wife and two children, were addressed. Critically, this included both medications to limit physical symptoms, but also therapies directed at the psychosocial impacts of cancer. Ultimately, he transitioned gracefully from active therapy to supportive care and ultimately chose to die in an inpatient hospice setting.

The approach illustrated in this case highlights a modern and still underutilized approach to cancer care. It illustrates why PC and oncology care should be performed concurrently with, and not in opposition to, conventional cancer therapies aimed at prolonging life. We now have objective evidence from studies ranging from solid tumor therapy to hematopoietic cell transplantation that suggest that early PC consultation does not just make theoretical sense, but leads to objective, measurable differences in QOL and indexes of mental health. As a community, we should embrace this approach and encourage controlled basic and clinical research that further improves the quality of palliative oncology care. Each of us will some day face our mortality and expect quality healthcare across the illness experience. For members of oncology teams or PC teams, collaboration is essential. We will reap what we sow when we personally need care or care for our family members.

Evidence-Based Practice

Temel, J. S., Greer, J. A., Muzikansky, A., Gallagher, E. R., Admane, S., Jackson, V. A., ... Lynch, T. J. (2010). Early palliative care for patients with metastatic non-small-cell lung cancer. *New England Journal of Medicine, 363*(8), 733–742.

Research Problem
Examine the effect of early introduction of PC on patient-reported outcomes and EOL care among patients with newly diagnosed NSCLC.

Design
Non-blinded, randomized controlled trial of early PC integrated with standard oncologic care as compared to standard oncologic care alone. Patients were randomly assigned and enrolled within 8 weeks after diagnosis to one of two groups in a 1:1 ratio with stratification. Patients assigned to early PC met with members of the PC team within 3 weeks after enrollment and at least monthly thereafter in the outpatient setting until death. Additional PC visits were scheduled at the discretion of the patient, physician, or PC provider.

Sample and Setting
Sample size: 151 patients underwent randomization, of which 27 died by 12 weeks and 107 completed assessments.
Setting: Single tertiary care site

Methods

Eligible patients had pathologically confirmed metastatic NSCLC diagnosed within 8 weeks and an ECOG Performance Status of 0–2. Scales used: Functional Assessment of Cancer Therapy-Lung (FACT-L) scale; assesses various dimensions of QOL (physical, functional, emotional, and social well-being). Also utilized was the Lung Cancer Subscale (LCS) of the FACT-L; this evaluates seven symptoms specific to lung cancer: (1) shortness of breath, (2) weight loss, (3) clearness of thinking, (4) cough, (5) good appetite, (6) chest tightness, and (7) ease of breathing. Primary outcome was change from baseline to 12 weeks in the score on the Trial Outcome Index (TOI; sum of scores on LCS and physical well-being and functional well-being subscales of FACT-L scale). Mood was also assessed using the Hospital Anxiety and Depression Scale (HADS) and the Patient Health Questionnaire 9 (PHQ-9), a nine-item measure evaluating symptoms of major depressive disorder according to the *Diagnostic and Statistical Manual of Mental Disorders (*4th ed.; *DSM-IV)*.

Results

Although there was no significant difference in overall survival between study participants and eligible patients who were not enrolled, study patients assigned to early PC had significantly higher scores than those assigned to standard care. PC patients had a 2.3-point increase in mean TOI score from baseline to 12 weeks, while the standard group had a 2.3-point decrease. Also, the percentage of patients with depression at 12 weeks was significantly lower in the PC group versus the standard care group, with the proportion of patients receiving antidepressants being similar in both groups. By the time EOL analysis was completed, 105 patients had died. Of those assigned to the standard care group, 54% versus 33% had received more aggressive EOL interventions as compared to those in the PC group. The results also indicated that patients in the PC group had significantly longer survival than those in the standard care group (median survival, 11.6 vs. 8.9 months) and differences in the duration of hospice care (median duration, 11 days in PC group vs. 4 days in standard care group).

Conclusion

This study indicates clear benefits to obtaining PC throughout the continuum of advanced lung cancer care. Incorporating PC into the treatment plan early can lead to better QOL, less aggressive interventions at end of life that ultimately translates to healthcare cost savings, and clear treatment goals set by patients such as resuscitation preferences.

Evidence-Based Practice

Hart, S. L., & Charles, S. T. (2013). Age-related pattern in negative affect and appraisals about colorectal cancer over time. *Health Psychology, 32*(23), 302–310.

Research Problem

Application of a theoretical model of strength and vulnerability integration (SAVI) to understand age-related patterns in emotional responses of individuals diagnosed with CRC.

Design
Diagnosed individuals completed surveys at four time points. Multilevel model.

Sample and Setting
Sample size: 139 respondents in the age range of 28 to 89 years completed surveys prior to surgery (baseline), and 6, 12, and 18 months postsurgery.

Methods
Multilevel modeling examined changes in measures of positive and negative affect, depressive symptoms, and appraisals of cancer over the determined period of time. Scales used: The Positive and Negative Affect Scale (PANAS) includes two 10-item scales rating the extent to which the respondent experiences various feelings on a scale of 1 to 5. The Center for Epidemiologic Studies–Depression Scale (CES-D) is a well-known, validated 20-item scale used to measure depressive symptoms. The Stress Appraisal Measure is a validated measure of a patient's understanding of the nature of his or her illness divided into three scales. Linear and nonlinear patterns of change were examined for a period of 18 months.

Results
This examination discovered that emotional distress and age differences are less pronounced at the initial onset of illness and treatment of CRC. During the 18-month examination, age-related strengths came to light and older adults reported less negative affect than younger adults. In addition, it was found that older adults are more likely to use emotional regulation that allows them to adapt to their diagnosis and treatment plan. In other words, older adults are more likely to evaluate their illness as less threatening and a greater challenge than younger adults through the period of time during and after treatment.

Commentary
This study is one of the first to examine colorectal patients immediately after diagnosis and is focused on the correlation between resiliency and age of patient. This study followed colorectal patients during the most critical and difficult parts of their cancer treatment. This study concluded that older adults present with a greater level of resiliency than their younger counterparts, yet more research is needed to examine the relationship with patients' levels of education and geographic locations.

■ **Acknowledgment.** The editors would like to thank Amy E. Guthrie, MSN, APRN, CHPN for her contribution to the previous edition.

■ REFERENCES

Aebi, S., & Pagani, O. (2007). Treatment of premenopausal women with early breast cancer: Old challenges and new opportunities. *Drugs, 67*(10), 1393–1401. doi:10.2165/00003495-200767100-00002

Albain, S., Swann, R., Rusch, V., Turrisi, A., Sheperd, F., Smith, C., & Miller, R. (2005). Phase III study of concurrent chemotherapy and radiotherapy (CT/RT) vs CT/RT followed by surgical resection for Stage IIIA (pN2) nonsmall cell lung cancer (NSCLC): Outcomes update of North American Intergroup 0139 (RTOG 9309) [Abstract 7014]. *Journal of Clinical Oncology, 23*(Suppl. 16), 7014. doi:10.1200/jco.2005.23.16_suppl.7014

Aldridge, A. A., & Roesch, S. C. (2007). Coping and adjustment in children with cancer: A meta-analytic study. *Journal of Behavioral Medicine, 30*(2), 115–129. doi:10.1007/s10865-006-9087-y

American Cancer Society. (2013). *Cancer facts and figures 2013.* Atlanta, GA: Author.

American Cancer Society. (2016). *Cancer Facts and Figures for African Americans 2016–2018*. Atlanta, GA: Author.

American Cancer Society. (2018a). *Cancer facts and figures 2018*. Atlanta, GA: Author. Retrieved from https://www.cancer.org/content/dam/cancer-org/research/cancer-facts-and-statistics/annual-cancer-facts-and-figures/2018/cancer-facts-and-figures-2018.pdf

American Cancer Society. (2018b). What tests can detect prostate cancer early? Retrieved from https://www.cancer.org/cancer/prostate-cancer/early-detection/tests.html

American Cancer Society. (2018c). Key statistics for colorectal cancer. Retrieved from https://www.cancer.org/cancer/colon-rectal-cancer/about/key-statistics.html

American Cancer Society. (2018d). Key statistics for lung cancer. Retrieved from https://www.cancer.org/cancer/non-small-cell-lung-cancer/about/key-statistics.html

American Cancer Society. (2018e). What is non-small cell lung cancer? Retrieved from https://www.cancer.org/cancer/non-small-cell-lung-cancer/about/key-statistics.html

American Cancer Society. (2018f). Small cell lung cancer survival rates, by stage. Retrieved from https://www.cancer.org/cancer/small-cell-lung-cancer/detection-diagnosis-staging/survival-rates.html

American Cancer Society. (2018g). Non-small cell lung cancer survival rates, by stage. Retrieved from https://www.cancer.org/cancer/non-small-cell-lung-cancer/detection-diagnosis-staging/survival-rates.html

Anderson, F., Downing, G. M., Hill, J., Casorso, L., & Lerch, N. (1996). Palliative performance scale (PPS): A new tool. *Journal of Palliative Care, 12*(1), 5–11.

Armstrong, A. J., & Carducci, M. A. (2005). Chemotherapy for advanced prostate cancer: Results of new clinical trials and future studies. *Current Oncology Reports, 7*(3), 186–195. doi:10.1007/s11912-005-0072-3

Audisio, R. A., Bozzetti, F., Gennari, R., Jaklitsch, M. T., Koperna, T., Longo, W. E., … Zbar, A. P. (2004). The surgical management of elderly cancer patients; recommendations of the SIOG surgical task force. *European Journal of Cancer, 40*(7), 926–938. doi:10.1016/j.ejca.2004.01.016

Baker, D. (2001). Current surgical management of colorectal cancer. *Nursing Clinics of North America, 36*(3), 579–592, xi.

Balboni, T. A., Balboni, M., Enzinger, A. C., Gallivan, K., Paulk, M. E., Wright, A., … Prigerson, H. G. (2013). Provision of spiritual support to patients with advanced cancer by religious communities and associations with medical care at the end of life. *Journal of American Medical Association: Internal Medicine, 173*(12), 1109–1117. doi:10.1001/jamainternmed.2013.903

Beardsmore, S., & Fitzmaurice, N. (2002). Palliative care in pediatric oncology. *European Journal of Cancer, 38*(14), 1900–1907; discussion 1908. doi:10.1016/S0959-8049(02)00216-2

Becze, E. (2008). Put evidence into practice to manage dyspnea. *ONS Connect, 23*(8), 18–19.

Besse, B., Ropert, S., & Soria, J. (2007). Targeted therapies in lung cancer. *Annals of Oncology, 18*(Suppl. 9), 135–142. doi:10.1093/annonc/mdm308

Bevans, M. F., & Sternberg, E. M. (2012). Caregiving burden, stress, and health effects among family caregivers of adult cancer patients. *Journal of American Medical Association, 307*(4), 398–403. doi:10.1001/jama.2012.29

Boquete-Castro, A., Gómez-Moreno, G., Calvo-Guirado J. L., Aguilar-Salvatierra, A., & Delgado-Ruiz, R. A. (2016). Denosumab and osteonecrosis of the jaw. A systematic analysis of events reported in clinical trials. *Clincal Oral Implants Research, 27*(3), 367–375. doi:10.1111/clr.12556

Borneman, T., Stahl, C., Ferrell, B., & Smith, D. (2002). The concept of hope in family caregivers of cancer patients at home. *Journal of Hospice and Palliative Nursing, 4*(1), 21–33. doi:10.1097/00129191-200201000-00012

Bosset, J. F., Collette, L., Calais, G., Mineur, L., Maingon, P., Radosevic-Jelic, L., … Ollier, J. C.; EORTC Radiotherapy Group Trial 22921. (2006). Chemotherapy with preoperative radiotherapy in rectal cancer. *New England Journal of Medicine, 355*(11), 1114–1123. doi:10.1056/NEJMoa060829

Carroll, S. (2007). Adult survivors of childhood cancer are at risk for suicide. *Oncology Nursing, 34*(2), 294.

Chen, J., Jiang, R., Garces, Y. I., Jatoi, A. J., Stoddard, S. M., Sun, Z., … Yang, P. (2010). Prognostic factors for limited-stage small cell lung cancer: A study of 284 patients. *Lung Cancer, 67*(2), 221. doi:1016/j.lungcan.2009.04.006

Cicenas, S., Zaliene, A., & Atkocius. (2009). Treatment outcome of locally advanced stage IIIA/B lung cancer. *Medicina, 45*(6), 452–459.

Clinical Outcomes of Surgical Therapy Study Group. (2004). A comparison of laparoscopically assisted and open colectomy for colon cancer. *New England Journal of Medicine, 350*, 2050–2059. doi:10.1056/NEJMoa032651

Cohen, S. R., Mount, B. M., Bruera, E., Provost, M., Rowe, J., & Tong, K. (1997). Validity of the McGill Quality of Life Questionnaire in the palliative care setting: A multi-centre Canadian study demonstrating the importance of the existential domain. *Palliative Medicine, 11*(1), 3–20. doi:10.1177/026921639701100102

Coyne, P., Lyckholm, L., & Smith, T. J. (2006). Clinical interventions, economic outcomes, and palliative care. In B. Ferrell & N. Coyle (Eds.), *Textbook of palliative nursing* (pp. 429–442). New York, NY: Oxford University Press.

Curran, W., Scott, C., Langer, C., Kmaki, R., Lee, J., Hauser, S, … Cox, J. (2011). Sequential vs. concurrent chemoradiation for Stage III non-small lung cancer: Randomized Phase III trial RTOG 9410. *Journal of National Cancer Institute, 103*(19), 1452–1460. doi:10.1093/jnci/djr325

Darmber, J., & Aus, G. (2008). Prostate cancer. *Lancet, 371*, 1710–1721. doi:10.1016/S0140-6736(08)60729-1

De Graves, S., & Aranda, S. (2005). When a child cannot be cured—reflections of health professionals. *European Journal of Cancer Care, 14*(2), 132–140. doi:10.1111/j.1365-2354.2005.00520.x

Decker, C. L., Haase, J. E., & Bell, C. J. (2007). Uncertainty in adolescents and young adults with cancer. *Oncology Nursing Forum, 34*(3), 681–688. doi:10.1188/07.ONF.681-688

Derby, S., & O'Mahony, S. (2006). Elderly patients. In B. Ferrell & N. Coyle (Eds.), *Textbook of palliative nursing* (pp. 635–660). New York, NY: Oxford University Press.

Di Maio, M., Gallo, C., Leighl, N. B., Piccirillo, M. C., Daniele, G., Nuzzo, F., … Perrone, F. (2015). Symptomatic toxicities experience during anticancer treatment: Agreement between patient and physician reporting in three randomized trials. *Journal of Clinical Oncology, (33)*8, 910–915. doi:10.1200/JCO.2014.57.9334

Diel, I. J. (2011). Bisphosphonates and RANKL antibodies in breast carcinoma with bone metastases. In M. Davis, P. Feyer, P. Ortner, & C. Zimmerman (Eds.), *Supportive oncology* (pp. 245–247). Philadelphia, PA: Elsevier.

Djulbegovic, B., Kumar, A., Soares, H. P., Hozo, I., Bepler, G., Clarke, M., & Bennett, C. L. (2008). Treatment success in cancer: New cancer treatment successes identified in phase 3 randomized controlled trials conducted by the National Cancer Institute-sponsored cooperative oncology groups, 1955 to 2006. *Archives of Internal Medicine, 168*(6), 632–642. doi:10.1001/archinte.168.6.632

Dubey, S., & Powell, C. A. (2008). Update in lung cancer 2007. *American Journal of Respiratory and Critical Care Medicine, 177*(9), 941–946. doi:10.1164/rccm.200801-107UP

Dumont, I., Dumont, S., & Mongeau, S. (2008). End-of-life care and the grieving process: Family caregivers who have experienced the loss of a terminal-phase cancer patient. *Qualitative Health Research, 18*(8), 1049–1061. doi:10.1177/1049732308320110

Engstrom, P. F., Arnoletti, J. P., Benson, A. B., Chen, Y. J., Choti, M. A., Cooper, H. S., … Venook, A. P.; Fox Chase Cancer Center Partners. (2007a). Colon cancer. *Journal of the National Comprehensive Cancer Network, 5*(9), 884–925. doi:10.6004/jnccn.2007.0079

Engstrom, P. F., Arnoletti, J. P., Benson, A. B., Chen, Y. J., Choti, M. A., Cooper, H. S., … Venook, A. P.; National Comprehensive Cancer Network. (2007b). Rectal cancer. *Journal of the National Comprehensive Cancer Network, 5*(9), 940–981. doi:10.6004/jnccn.2007.0081

Extermann, M. (2005). Older patients, cognitive impairment, and cancer: An increasingly frequent triad. *Journal of the National Comprehensive Cancer Network, 3*(4), 593–596. doi:10.6004/jnccn.2005.0033

Extermann, M., & Hurria, A. (2007). Comprehensive geriatric assessment for older patients with cancer. *Journal of Clinical Oncology, 25*(14), 1824–1831. doi:10.1200/JCO.2007.10.6559

Gelfman, L. P., Meier, D. E., & Morrison, R. S. (2008). Does palliative care improve quality? A survey of bereaved family members. *Journal of Pain and Symptom Management, 36*(1), 22–28. doi:10.1016/j.jpainsymman.2007.09.008

Griffin, J. P., Koch, K. A., Nelson, J. E., & Cooley, M. E.; American College of Chest Physicians. (2007). Palliative care consultation, quality-of-life measurements, and bereavement for end-of-life care in patients with lung cancer: ACCP evidence-based clinical practice guidelines (2nd Ed.). *Chest, 132*(Suppl. 3), 404S–422S. doi:10.1378/chest.07-1392

Hampton, T. (2008a). New studies target lung cancer prevention, imaging, and treatment. *Journal of the American Medical Association, 300*(3), 267–268. doi:10.1001/jama.2008.49

Hampton, T. (2008b). New treatment strategies provide more options for patients with breast cancer. *Journal of the American Medical Association, 300*(4), 381–382. doi:10.1001/jama.300.4.381

Harrington, S. E., & Smith, T. J. (2008). The role of chemotherapy at the end of life: Healthcare consultant oncology. *Clinical Geriatrics, 6*(3), 2–3, 7–10. doi:10.1001/jama.299.22.2667

Higginson, I. J., & Sen-Gupta, G. J. (2000). Place of care in advanced cancer: A qualitative systematic literature review of patient preferences. *Journal of Palliative Medicine, 3*(3), 287–300. doi:10.1089/jpm.2000.3.287

Hoffman, A. J., Given, B. A., von Eye, A., Gift, A. G., & Given, C. W. (2007). Relationships among pain, fatigue, insomnia, and gender in persons with lung cancer. *Oncology Nursing Forum, 34*(4), 785–792. doi:10.1188/07.ONF.785-792

Holcomb, S. S. (2006). Breast cancer therapy and treatment guidelines. *Nurse Practitioner, 31*(10), 59–63.

Houlston, A. (2006). Hospital for the children. *Nursing Standard, 20*(25), 70–71. doi:10.7748/ns2006.03.20.25.70.c4081

Hsieh, M. C., Huang, M. C., Lai, Y. L., & Lin, C. C. (2007). Grief reactions in family caregivers of advanced cancer patients in Taiwan: Relationship to place of death. *Cancer Nursing, 30*(4), 278–284. doi:10.1097/01.NCC.0000281728.72243.c4

Irwin, M., & Johnson, L. A. (Eds.). (2014). *Putting evidence into practice: A pocket guide to cancer symptom management*. Pittsburgh, PA: Oncology Nursing Society.

Jassem, J. (2007). The role of radiotherapy in lung cancer: Where is the evidence? *Radiotherapy and Oncology, 83*(2), 203–213. doi:10.1016/j.radonc.2007.04.004

Jonker, D. J., O'Callaghan, C. J., Karapetis, C. S., Zalcberg, J. R., Tu, D., Au, H. J., … Moore, M. J. (2007). Cetuximab for the treatment of colorectal cancer. *New England Journal of Medicine, 357*(20), 2040–2048. doi:10.1056/NEJMoa071834

Kadakia, K. C., & Henry, N. L. (2015). Adjuvant endocrine therapy in premenopausal women with breast cancer. *Clinical Advanced Hematology Oncology, 13*(10), 663–672.

Kapiteijn, E., Marijnen, C. A., Nagtegaal, I. D., Putter, H., Steup, W. H., Wiggers, T., … van de Velde, C. J.; Dutch Colorectal Cancer Group. (2001). Preoperative radiotherapy combined with total mesorectal excision for resectable rectal cancer. *New England Journal of Medicine, 345*(9), 638–646. doi:10.1056/NEJMoa010580

Kobayashi, N. (2000). Formal service utilization by the frail elderly at home during the last 6 months of life. *Nursing and Health Sciences, 2*(4), 201. doi:10.1046/j.1442-2018.2000.00057.x

Kristjanson, L. J., & White, K. (2002). Clinical support for families in the palliative care phase of hematologic or oncologic illness. *Hematology/Oncology Clinics of North America, 16*(3), 745–762, xi. doi:10.1016/S0889-8588(02)00023-0

Kuebler, K. K., Lynn, J., & Von Rohen, J. (2005). Perspectives in palliative care. *Seminars in Oncology Nursing, 21*(1), 2–10. doi:10.1053/j.soncn.2004.10.001

Kufe, D. W., Pollock, R. E., Weichselbaum, R. R., Bast, R. C., Gansler, T. S., Holland, J. F., & Frei, E. (2003). *Holland-frei cancer medicine* (6th ed.). Hamilton, ON, Canada: BC Decker.

Kutner, J. S., Steiner, J. F., Corbett, K. K., Jahnigen, D. W., & Barton, P. L. (1999). Information needs in terminal illness. *Social Science and Medicine (1982), 48*(10), 1341–1352. doi:10.1016/S0277-9536(98)00453-5

Kvale, P., Selecky, P., & Prakash, U. (2007). Palliative care in lung cancer: ACCP evidence-based clinical practice guidelines (2nd ed.). *Chest, 132*(Suppl. 3), 368S–403S. doi:10.1378/chest.07-1391

Lazzaro, R., & Comandini, D. (2000). Cancer in the elderly: Assessing patients for fitness. *Critical Reviews in Oncology/Hematology, 35,* 155–160. doi:10.1016/S1040-8428(00)00091-3

Le, D. T., Uran, J. N., Wang, H., Bartlett, B. R., Kemberling, H., Eyring, A. D., … Diaz, L. A. (2015). PD-1 blockade in tumors with mismatch-repair deficiency. *New England Journal of Medicine, 372*(26), 2509–2520. doi:10.1056/NEJMoa1500596

Lemjabbar-Alaoui, H., Hassan, O., Yang, Y., & Buchanan, P. (2015). Lung cancer: Biology and treatment options. *Biochimica et Biophysica Acta, 1856*(2), 189–210. doi:10.1016/j.bbcan.2015.08.002

Litsas, G. (2008). Sequential therapy with tamoxifen and aromatase inhibitors in early-stage postmenopausal breast cancer: A review of the evidence. *Oncology Nursing Forum, 35*(4), 714–721. doi:10.1188/08.ONF.714-721

Mack, J. W., Wolfe, J., Cook, E. F., Grier, H. E., Cleary, P. D., & Weeks, J. C. (2007). Hope and prognostic disclosure. *Journal of Clinical Oncology, 25*(35), 5636–5642. doi:10.1200/JCO.2007.12.6110

Mackay, H. J. (2000). Metastatic and advanced breast cancer in the elderly. *Clinical Geriatrics.* Retrieved from http://www.mmhc.com/cg/articles/CG9912/mackay.html

Matsuyama, R., Reddy, S., & Smith, T. J. (2006). Why do patients choose chemotherapy near the end of life? A review of the perspective of those facing death from cancer. *Journal of Clinical Oncology, 24*(21), 3490–3496. doi:10.1200/JCO.2005.03.6236

Mauri, D., Pavlidis, N., Polyzos, N. P., & Ioannidis, J. P. (2006). Survival with aromatase inhibitors and inactivators versus standard hormonal therapy in advanced breast cancer: Meta-analysis. *Journal of the National Cancer Institute, 98*(18), 1285–1291. doi:10.1093/jnci/djj357

McBride, D. (2008). KRAS status predicts response to cetuximab for metastatic colorectal cancer. *ONS Connect, 8,* 25.

Merglen, A., Schmidlin, F., Fioretta, G., Verkooijen, H. M., Rapiti, E., Zanetti, R., … Bouchardy, C. (2007). Short- and long-term mortality with localized prostate cancer. *Archives of Internal Medicine, 167*(18), 1944–1950. doi:10.1001/archinte.167.18.1944

Meyerhardt, J., & Mayer, R. (2005). Systemic therapy for colorectal cancer. Palliation of gastrointestinal obstructive disorders. *Nursing Clinics of North America, 36*(4), 761–778.

Milberg, A., Olsson, E. C., Jakobsson, M., Olsson, M., & Friedrichsen, M. (2008). Family members' perceived needs for bereavement follow-up. *Journal of Pain and Symptom Management, 35*(1), 58–69. doi:10.1016/j.jpainsymman.2007.02.039

Miles, E. F., Jacimore, L. L., & Nelson, J. W. (2011). Aggressive palliation in extensive stage small cell lung cancer, practice guidelines versus clinical practice: A case report and review of the literature. *Lung Cancer International, 2011,* 659807. doi:10.4061/2011/659807

Molina, J. R., Yang, P., Cassivi, S. D., Schild, S. E., & Adjei, A. A. (2008). Non-small cell lung cancer: Epidemiology, risk factors, treatment, and survivorship. *Mayo Clinic Proceedings, 83*(5), 584–594. doi:10.4065/83.5.584

Moore, K., Johnson, G., Fortner, B. V., & Houts, A. C. (2008). The AIM Higher Initiative: New procedures implemented for assessment, information, and management of chemotherapy toxicities in community oncology clinics. *Clinical Journal of Oncology Nursing, 12*(2), 229–238. doi:10.1188/08.CJON.229-238

Nabholtz, J. M., Falkson, C., Campos, D., Szanto, J., Martin, M., Chan, S., … Pouillart, P. (2003). Abstract: Docetaxel and doxorubicin compared with doxorubicin and cyclophosphamide as first-line chemotherapy for metastatic breast cancer: Results of a randomized, multicenter, phase III trial. *Journal of Clinical Oncology, 21*(6), 968–975. doi:10.1200/JCO.2003.04.040

Nabholtz, J. M., Mackey, J. R., Smylie, M., Paterson, A., Noël, D. R., Al-Tweigeri, T., … Riva, A. (2001). Abstract: Phase II study of docetaxel, doxorubicin, and cyclophosphamide as first-line chemotherapy for metastatic breast cancer. *Journal of Clinical Oncology, 19*(2), 314–321. doi:10.1200/JCO.2001.19.2.314

National Cancer Institute. (2017a). Surveillance, epidemiology, and end results (SEER) cancer statistics review, 1975–2014. Retrieved from https://seer.cancer.gov/statfacts/html/lungb.html

National Cancer Institute. (2017b). Cancer in children and adolescents. Retrieved from https://www.cancer.gov/types/childhood-cancers/child-adolescent-cancers-fact-sheet

National Cancer Institute. (2018a). Cancer stat facts: Prostate cancer. Retrieved from https://seer.cancer.gov/statfacts/html/prost.html

National Cancer Institute. (2018b). Cancer statistics. Retrieved from https://www.cancer.gov/about-cancer/understanding/statistics

National Cancer Institute. (2018c). Non-small cell lung treatment. Retrieved from https://www.cancer.gov/types/lung/patient/non-small-cell-lung-treatment-pdq#section/_164

National Collaborating Centre for Cancer. (2015). http://www.wales.nhs.uk/sites3/page.cfm?orgid=432&pid=12500

National Comprehensive Cancer Network. (2008). Practice guidelines in oncology: *Nonsmall cell lung cancer [v.2.2008].* Retrieved from http://www.nccn.org/profes-sionals/physician_gls/PDF/palliative.pdf

National Comprehensive Cancer Network. (2017). NCCN clinical practice guidelines in oncology: Non-small cell lung cancer [v.8.2017]. Retrieved from https://www.nccn.org/professionals/physician_gls/pdf/nscl.pdf

Obasaju, C., Conkling, P., Richards, D., Fitzgibbons, J., Arce-neau, K., & Boehm, L.… Reynolds, C. (2007). A randomized phase III trial of gemcitabine with or without carboplatin in performance status 2 (PS2) patients (pts) with advanced (stage IIIB with pleural effusion or stage IV) nonsmall cell lung cancer (NSCLC; Abstract 7533; ASCO Annual Meeting Proceedings, Part I). *Journal of Clinical Oncology, 25*(188), 392s. doi:10.1200/jco.2007.25.18_suppl.7533

Pawlik, T. M., Schulick, R. D., & Choti, M. A. (2008). Expanding criteria for resectability of colorectal liver metastases. *Oncologist, 13*(1), 51–64. doi:10.1634/theoncologist.2007-0142

Pignon, T., Horiot, J. C., Bolla, M., van Poppel, H., Bartelink, H., Roelofsen, F., … Scalliet, P. (1997). Age is not a limiting factor for radical radiotherapy in pelvic malignancies. *Radiotherapy and Oncology, 42*(2), 107–120. doi:10.1016/S0167-8140(96)01861-0

Politi, K., & Herbst, R. S. (2015). Lung cancer in the era of precision medicine. *Clinical Cancer Research, 21*(10), 2213–2220. doi:10.1158/1078-0432.CCR-14-2748

Pritchard, M., Burghen, E., Srivastava, D. K., Okuma, J., Anderson, L., Powell, B., ... Hinds, P. S. (2008). Cancer-related symptoms most concerning to parents during the last week and last day of their child's life. *Pediatrics, 121*(5), e1301–e1309. doi:10.1542/peds.2007-2681

Repetto, L., & Comandini, D. (2000). Cancer in the elderly: Assessing patients for fitness. *Critical Reviews in Oncology/Hematology, 35*(3), 155–160. doi:10.1016/S1040-8428(00)00091-3

Repetto, L., Comandini, D., & Mammoliti, S. (2001). Life expectancy, comorbidity and quality of life: The treatment equation in the older cancer patients. *Critical Reviews in Oncology/Hematology, 37*(2), 147–152. doi:10.1016/S1040-8428(00)00104-9

Repetto, L., Venturino, A., Fratino, L., Serraino, D., Troisi, G., Gianni, W., & Pietropaolo, M. (2003). Geriatric oncology: A clinical approach to the older patient with cancer. *European Journal of Cancer, 39*(7), 870–880. doi:10.1016/S0959-8049(03)00062-5

Robinson, K. M., & Huether, S. E (2009). Structure and function of the reproductive systems. In K. L. McCance & S. L. Huether (Eds.), *Pathophysiology: The biologic basis for disease in adults and children* (6th ed., pp. 659–736). St. Louis, MO: Mosby.

Rosati, G., & Bilancia, D. (2008). Role of chemotherapy and novel biological agents in the treatment of elderly patients with colorectal cancer. *World Journal of Gastroenterology, 14*(12), 1812–1822. doi:10.3748/wjg.14.1812

Ryan, C. J., & Small, E. J. (2006). Prostate cancer update: 2005. *Current Opinion in Oncology, 18*(3), 284–288. doi:10.1097/01.cco.0000219259.83585.f3

Sauer, R., Becker, H., Hohenberger, W., Rödel, C., Wittekind, C., Fietkau, R., ... Raab, R.; German Rectal Cancer Study Group. (2004). Preoperative versus postoperative chemoradiotherapy for rectal cancer. *New England Journal of Medicine, 351*(17), 1731–1740. doi:10.1056/NEJMoa040694

Schwartz, C. (1999). Long-term survivors of childhood cancer: The late effects of therapy. *Oncologist, 4*, 45–54.

Scullion, F. (2005). An integrated model of care is needed for children and young people with cancer. *International Journal of Palliative Nursing, 11*(9), 494–495. doi:10.12968/ijpn.2005.11.9.19785

Siegel, R. L., Miller, K. D., & Jemal, A. (2017). Cancer statistics, 2017. *CA: A Cancer Journal for Clinicians. 67*(1), 7–30. doi:10.3322/caac.21387

Sledge, G. W., Neuberg, D., Bernardo, P., Ingle, J. N., Martino, S., Rowinsky, E. K., & Wood, W. C. (2003). Phase III trial of doxorubicin, paclitaxel, and the combination of doxorubicin and paclitaxel as front-line chemotherapy for metastatic breast cancer: An intergroup trial (E1193). *Journal of Clinical Oncology, 21*(4), 588–592. doi:10.1200/JCO.2003.08.013

Slotman, B., Faivre-Finn, C., Kramer, G., Rankin, E., Snee, M., Hatton, M., ... Senan, S.; EORTC Radiation Oncology Group and Lung Cancer Group. (2007). Prophylactic cranial irradiation in extensive small-cell lung cancer. *New England Journal of Medicine, 357*(7), 664–672. doi:10.1056/NEJMoa071780

Smith, I. (2006). Goals of treatment for patients with metastatic breast cancer. *Seminars in Oncology, 33*(2), 2–5. doi:10.1053/j.seminoncol.2005.07.030

Stinnett, S., Williams, L., & Johnson, D. H. (2007). Role of chemotherapy for palliation in the lung cancer patient. *Journal of Supportive Oncology, 5*(1), 19–24.

Su, S., Hu, Y., Ouyang, W., Ma, Z., Lu, B., Li, Q., ... Wang, Y. (2014). The survival outcomes and prognosis of stage IV non-small-cell lung cancer treated with thoracic three dimensional radiotherapy combined with chemotherapy. *Radiation Oncology, 9*, 290. doi:10.1186/s13014-014-0290-7

Surbone, A. (2008). Information to cancer patients: Ready for new challenges? *Supportive Care in Cancer, 16*(8), 865–868. doi:10.1007/s00520-008-0412-6

Tang, S. T. (2003). When death is imminent: Where terminally ill patients with cancer prefer to die and why. *Cancer Nursing, 26*(3), 245–251.

Temel, J. S., McCannon, J., Greer, J. A., Jackson, V. A., Ostler, P., Pirl, W. F., ... Billings, J. A. (2008). Aggressiveness of care in a prospective cohort of patients with advanced NSCLC. *Cancer, 113*(4), 826–833. doi:10.1002/cncr.23620

Teno, J. M., Clarridge, B. R., Casey, V., Welch, L. C., Wetle, T., Shield, R., & Mor, V. (2004). Family perspectives on end-of-life care at the last place of care. *Journal of the American Medical Association, 291*(1), 88–93. doi:10.1001/jama.291.1.88

Terret, C., Zulian, G. B., Naiem, A., & Albrand, G. (2007). Multidisciplinary approach to the geriatric oncology patient. *Journal of Clinical Oncology, 25*(14), 1876–1881. doi:10.1200/JCO.2006.10.3291

Thompson, G. N., & Chochinov, H. M. (2009). Palliative care: Special considerations for older adults with cancer. In A. Hurria & L. Balducci (Eds.), *Geriatric oncology* (pp. 293–324). Dordrecht, The Netherlands: Springer.

Valdimarsdóttir, U., Kreicbergs, U., Hauksdóttir, A., Hunt, H., Onelöv, E., Henter, J. I., & Steineck, G. (2007). Parents' intellectual and emotional awareness of their child's impending death to cancer: A population-based long-term follow-up study. *Lancet Oncology, 8*(8), 706–714. doi:10.1016/S1470-2045(07)70209-7

Victoria Hospice Society. (2001). The Palliative Performance Scale version 2 (PPSv2) tool. Retrieved from http://www.npcrc.org/files/content/pps_for_distribution_2015_-_with_watermark_sample.pdf

Walker, S. (2003). Updates in nonsmall cell lung cancer. *Clinical Journal of Oncology Nursing, 127*(4), 587–596. doi:10.1188/08.CJON

West, J., & Jin, J. O. (2015). Performance status in patients with cancer: Patient performance status (PS) is an important part of cancer care and treatment. *Journal of American Medical Association: Oncology, 1*(7), 998. doi:10.1001/jamaoncol.2015.3113

Willert, A., & Semans, M. (2000). Knowledge and attitudes about later life sexuality: What clinicians need to know about helping the elderly. *Contemporary Family Therapy, 22*(4), 415–435. doi:10.1023/A:1007896817570

Wolfe, J., Friebert, S., & Hilden, J. (2002). Caring for children with advanced cancer integrating palliative care. *Pediatric Clinics of North America, 49*(5), 1043–1062. doi:10.1016/S0031-3955(02)00034-2

Wolfe, J., Grier, H., Klar, N., Levin, S., Ellenbogen, J., Salem-Schatz, S., … Weeks, J. C. (2000). Symptoms and suffering at the end of life in children with cancer. *New England Journal of Medicine, 342,* 326–33. doi:10.1056/NEJM200002033420506

Wolfe, J., Klar, N., Grier, H. E., Duncan, J., Salem-Schatz, S., Emanuel, E. J., & Weeks, J. C. (2000). Understanding of prognosis among parents of children who died of cancer: Impact on treatment goals and integration of palliative care. *Journal of the American Medical Association, 284*(19), 2469–2475. doi:10.1001/jama.284.19.2469

Wolpin, B. M., Meyerhardt, J. A., Mamon, H. J., & Mayer, R. J. (2007). Adjuvant treatment of colorectal cancer. *CA: A Cancer Journal for Clinicians, 57*(3), 168–185. doi:10.3322/canjclin.57.3.168

World Health Organization. (2012). Estimated prostate cancer incidence worldwide in 2012. Retrieved from http://globocan.iarc.fr/old/FactSheets/cancers/prostate-new.asp

Yamamoto, K., Padilla Alarcón, J., Calvo Medina, V., García-Zarza, A., Pastor Guillen, J., Blasco Armengod, E., & París Romeu, F. (2003). Surgical results of Stage I non-small cell lung cancer: Comparison between elderly and younger patients. *European Journal of Cardio-Thoracic Surgery, 23*(1), 21–25. doi:10.1016/S1010-7940(02)00661-9

Lucie B. Dlugasch

CHAPTER 14

End-Stage Heart Disease

KEY POINTS

- Heart failure (HF) is a terminal disease.
- Eight million patients will have HF by 2030.
- Direct/indirect cost in 2012 was $31 billion.
- Large-scale clinical trials give evidence-based guidelines as to the treatment.
- Predicting the illness trajectory is much harder in HF than in cancer.
- Communication of wishes and goals of care continues to be a problem.
- Nursing has a key role in the management and outcomes of patients with HF.
- Patients often turn to nurses for information on their disease, especially in the end stages of the disease.
- A coordinated effort by nursing has been developed as to how to help patients with not only the physical symptoms of HF but also the psychosocial aspects.

CASE STUDY

Mrs. F. is an 80-year-old woman who has been seen by the cardiologist on a weekly basis for the past 6 weeks in order to closely follow her progressive symptoms of heart failure (heart failure with reduced ejection fraction [HFrEF]). She has a history of an acute myocardial infarction (AMI), hypertension, dyslipidemia, and osteoarthritis. At this point, she appears cachexic and now needs a walker, as she gets dyspneic and exhausted even at rest. She has been given maximal medical therapy, including an angiotensin-converting enzyme inhibitor (ACEI) and beta blocker (BB) for the last 5 years. She also takes a diuretic, statin, aspirin, and an omega 3 supplement, and recently started taking Hawthorn. She felt like her arthritis has been worsening in the past few weeks, so she resumed taking a nonsteroidal anti-inflammatory drug (NSAID). She had a pacemaker and defibrillator implanted 2 years ago. She has been hospitalized three times in the last 6 months and wants to know her medical options.

Her son, who has been bringing her into the office, is confused about why his mom has deteriorated so quickly and does not understand why his mother would not want to go back to the hospital since it always helped her improve in the past. She has been living with him since her last discharge and is requiring more and more care.

Mrs. F. recognizes that the weekly visits are tiring and thinks that the frequent changes in her diuretic doses are making her feel weaker. She also feels the frequent hospitalizations are taking away from the time she enjoys with her grandchildren. Today on examination, she can barely speak in full sentences and her resting SaO$_2$ is 88% on room air. She tells her healthcare provider that she is exhausted and does not know where to turn for help.

The nurse practitioner, who is her healthcare provider today, will need to address the following questions:

1. What concerns should be addressed?
2. What are the treatment options in this case?
3. What referrals would be appropriate and why?

HF is considered a terminal disease. In the final phase, patients and their families experience office visits, hospitalizations, and decreased quality of life (QOL) despite optimal therapy. Patients may suffer with intractable dyspnea, pain, profound fatigue, orthopnea, and psychological despair. The disease is difficult to prognosticate, making it challenging to know when end-of-life (EOL) discussions should occur. In addition, healthcare providers may find it difficult and feel they don't have the skills to discuss EOL issues. As professional nurses and nurse practitioners, how can we intervene with these patients who have very little "life" left and help their families cope with this reality? This chapter provides evidence-based strategies to address these questions.

■ END-STAGE HEART DISEASE OVERVIEW

The majority of end-stage heart disease patients have heart failure (HF) as it is the common endpoint for most cardiovascular diseases such as hypertension (HTN), atrial fibrillation, valvular disease, AMI, cardiomyopathies, and coronary artery disease (CAD). HF is not a disease, but rather a complex clinical syndrome evidenced by the ventricular inability to fill or eject blood, generally as a result of structural or functional impairment (Ponikowski et al., 2016; Yancy et al., 2013). Cardiovascular diseases are more common with aging. Recognition, treatment, and survival from many cardiovascular diseases (e.g., AMI, CAD, HTN) have improved. These patients, however, eventually suffer the long-term effects of the heart damage incurred during the acute event or from having a chronic condition such as decreased left ventricular (LV) function resulting from cardiac muscle damage. While many medications and interventional devices can prolong life, these patients can eventually develop HF as they age and medications or devices become less effective or do not improve the QOL. By 2050, one in five Americans is predicted to be over the age of 65; therefore, the incidence of HF is expected to worsen significantly (U.S. Census Bureau, 2012). According to the most recent numbers from the American Heart Association (AHA) (Benjamin et al., 2017; Go et al., 2013), one in five people in the United States is at risk for developing HF, with one in eight death certificates listing HF as the cause of death.

Evidence-based therapies for HF have improved long-term survival, and this has simultaneously led to a heavy symptom burden resulting in a poor QOL (Alpert, Smith, Hummel, & Hummel, 2017). HF Stage D (Table 14.1), in particular, is associated with a poor prognosis, limited therapies, and a short life span

(Fang et al., 2015). While a majority of hospice admissions for cardiovascular disease (heart and stroke) has surpassed admissions for cancer diagnosis, there is still a low referral rate for HF patients (Fang et al., 2015). Referrals to hospice and palliative care tend to occur in the last 2 weeks of life (Fang et al., 2015; Unroe et al., 2011). Because of the low rate of hospice utilization and pattern of late referrals in end-stage heart disease, there is a need for the infusion of palliative care (PC) principles into general care (Alpert et al., 2017; Whellan et al., 2014). In addition to the human cost of HF, there is a high societal cost as well. HF continues to pose heavy economic burden in the United States with a projected total cost increase from $31 billion in 2012 to $70 billion by 2030 (Benjamin et al., 2017). Much of this cost is driven by frequent hospital admissions and readmissions. PC, with its focus on symptom management and decisional support, has the potential to ameliorate some of the burden of HF.

Heart Failure Is a Condition of Aging

An estimated 6.5 million people have HF, and this is expected to increase by 46% from 2012 to 2030, putting the incidence at 8 million people with HF over the age of 18 (Benjamin et al., 2017). The projected increase in HF incidence and prevalence is strongly associated with the aging of the baby boomers. Almost 75% of those diagnosed with HF are older than 65 years (Benjamin et al., 2017).

HF is the number one hospitalization diagnosis for older adults, with the number of hospitalizations increasing 150% over the last 20 years (Yancy et al., 2013). Despite the prevalence of HF in older adults, cardiovascular clinical trials continue to exclude the typical older adult HF patient. In most of these trials, participants are younger

TABLE 14.1   Stages in the Development of Heart Failure

Stage A	Stage B	Stage C	Stage D
High risk for HF but no structural heart disease or symptoms of HF. For example, patients with: ■ Hypertension ■ Atherosclerotic disease ■ Diabetes ■ Obesity ■ Metabolic syndrome ■ Using cardiotoxins ■ With family history of cardiomyopathy	Structural heart disease but no signs or symptoms of HF. For example, patients with: ■ Previous MI ■ LV remodeling including LVH and low EF ■ Asymptomatic valvular disease	Structural heart disease with prior or current symptoms of HF. For example, patients with: ■ Known structural heart disease ■ Shortness of breath and fatigue, reduced exercise tolerance	Refractory HF requiring specialized interventions. For example, patients with: ■ Marked symptoms at rest despite maximal medical therapy (e.g., those who are recurrently hospitalized or cannot be safely discharged without specialized interventions)

EF, ejection fraction; HF, heart failure; LV, left ventricular; LVH, left ventricular hypertrophy; MI, myocardial infarction.

Source: Adapted from Jessup, M., Abraham, W. T., Casey, D. E., Feldman, A. M., Francis, G. S., Ganiats, T. G., … Yancy, C. W. (2009). Focused update: ACCF/AHA guidelines for the diagnosis and management of heart failure in adults. A report of the American College of Cardiology Foundation/American Heart Association Task Force on practice guidelines. *Circulation, 119*(14), 1977–2016. doi:10.1161/CIRCULATIONAHA.109.192064

than average (50–65 years of age vs. older than 75 years) and the samples are skewed toward males and those with fewer comorbidities. The trials target one specific therapy, whereas it is usual for there to be concurrent medications in the general HF population. Because of selection criteria, the participants are generally compliant with low risk of disability (Colvin et al., 2015). Clinical practice is very different from the controlled environment of a clinical trial, yet this type of research forms the basis of HF evidence-based practice. This disconnection between clinical trials and clinical practice makes it challenging to make generalizations to commonly affected HF populations (e.g., non-Caucasian, elderly, frail) and offers sound evidence on which to base everyday practice. These limitations should be kept in mind when reviewing the literature in this chapter as well as on your own.

Classifying and Determining Prognosis in Heart Failure

There are two complementary classification systems to describe HF. The AHA and the American College of Cardiology Foundation (ACCF) collaboratively developed criteria that describe the stages in the development and progression of HF, which is outlined in Table 14.1. The New York Heart Association (NYHA) Functional Classification System (Exhibit 14.1) focuses on a patient's exercise capacity and symptom status. The patient with advanced heart disease is classified as Stage D or NYHA Class III or IV, both of which are associated with significant clinical dysfunction resulting from symptoms and affecting the QOL. Symptoms include dyspnea, fatigue, or angina. The NYHA functional classification scale is very useful for clinicians who treat HF patients. The scale provides a benchmark to determine whether

Exhibit 14.1
The NYHA Functional Classification

Early-Stage Heart Failure
- **NYHA Class I**
  No symptoms at any level of exertion and no limitation in ordinary physical activity.
- **NYHA Class II**
  Mild symptoms and slight limitation during regular activity. Comfortable at rest.

Advanced-Stage Heart Failure
- **NYHA Class III**
  Noticeable limitation due to symptoms, even during minimal activity. Comfortable only at rest.
- **NYHA Class IV**
  Severe limitations. Experience symptoms even while at rest (sitting in a recliner or watching TV).

Source: Compiled from the New York Heart Association classifications. Retrieved from http://www.heartonline.org.au/.../New_York_Heart_Association_(NYHA)_classification.pdf

the condition is improving, staying the same, or getting worse and to easily communicate the severity of the patient's symptoms. The scale is also used in research studies to evaluate the effectiveness of new treatments.

This variability of symptoms is one of the difficulties in predicting the end of life in HF. There are weeks or months when patients seem to favorably respond to the guideline-based therapies, and other times the same treatments are no longer tolerated and the patient requires multiple hospitalizations. Often it's a balancing act, titrating medications to keep the patient stable and out of the hospital without exacerbating another problem when you think the end may be near. Patients will often explain away an increase in symptoms such as breathlessness as "just getting old" or a process of "deconditioning." Patients and families often think of HF as episodic. If the patient is symptomatic, they will say that the patient has HF, but when symptoms abate, the patient and family often believe that the patient is no longer in HF. Rarely do they think of HF as a terminal diagnosis. Yet the same patient may be stable for many months or even a year or two and then die suddenly due to a new cardiac event or a concomitant or new medical problem.

Difficulty predicting prognosis presents barriers to appropriate treatments, such as when to deactivate devices or referral to hospice, for the last stage of HF. Hospice referral in the United States requires a predicted 6-month prognosis, yet many providers are hesitant in making this determination when the course of HF is often unpredictable. This also complicates decision making about what treatment options should be considered and how helpful treatments will be.

The Role of Comorbidities in Heart Failure

Coexisting conditions such as diabetes mellitus (DM), renal disease, anemia, obesity, pulmonary disease, sleep-disordered breathing (SDB), and depression also factor into HF, with 40% of HF patients having five or more comorbidities (Tevendale & Baxter, 2011; Whellan et al., 2014). Comorbidity impacts both decision making related to treatment options and response to treatments. DM is considered a cardiac risk equivalent. This means that a patient with diabetes is treated medically as if he or she has already had a cardiovascular event. Renal insufficiency, often as a consequence of poor renal perfusion, is common in HF. Renal insufficiency causes fluid retention and activation of the renin system, which leads to vasoconstriction and increases myocardial demand. Pulmonary disease also leads to symptoms such as dyspnea or fatigue, so it is important to ascertain whether the heart, the lungs, or both are the cause of the symptoms. SDB, common in HF, contributes to many cardiovascular symptoms such as pulmonary HTN and right-sided HF. When properly identified, SDB can be easily treated, leading to improved symptoms and functional ability.

Depression and anxiety are important as they relate to the pathophysiology of HF. Depression may independently worsen HF and increase the risk of death (Abete et al., 2012; Moraska et al., 2013). Cortisol levels are persistently high in patients with depression, which, over time, leads to HTN caused by increased afterload and an increase in heart rate resulting from decreased ventricular filling time. Proinflammatory cytokines, which are activated in the stress response, reduce the available serotonin, which leads not only to depression but also to increased platelet aggregation and ultimately coronary artery occlusion (Halaris, 2016).

Prognostic Models to Predict End of Life in Heart Failure

Clinicians and researchers have attempted to address HF's prognostic uncertainty by developing prognostic models. Some of the models are used for calculating a risk score for patients with chronic heart failure (e.g., Seattle Heart Failure Model [SHFM]), while others are for patients with acute decompensated HF (e.g., EFFECT, ESCAPE). A listing of the various models is shown in Table 14.2.

The most widely used prognostic model for chronic HF is the SHFM. This model was developed using data from the prospective randomized amlodipine survival evaluation (PRAISE) clinical trial to predict survival of HF patients, unlike mortality used in other models. Its primary purpose is as an aid for decision making and to determine the impact of treatment on survival in transplantation and other advanced therapies. The model can also be used for predicting the risk of death (Whellan et al., 2014). Demographic and clinical characteristics such as age, gender, NYHA class, ischemic etiology, ejection fraction (EF), systolic blood pressure, lab values, and pharmaceutical use are entered into the online tool. An estimate of survival is provided, allowing for comparisons between different types of interventions and procedures. When populated with these data, the model gives survival and mortality rates at 1, 2, and 5 years, as well as data for mean life expectancy (Levy et al., 2006; Levy, 2013). The SHFM, however, has limited application in PC prognostication, as it can overestimate survival. Bakitas et al. (2013) conducted a retrospective chart audit of HF outpatients and found that the SHFM predicted the median survival time at 2.8 years in their sample when the actual median survival time was 21 days. Although changes to the SHFM have been made to allow application to higher risk hospitalized patients, the SHFM needs further evaluation in an advanced HF population, and therefore, it may underestimate the risk in this population (Whellan et al., 2014). This data suggests that the SHFM should be used with caution in PC populations.

Another prognostic model was developed using the organized program to initiate lifesaving treatment in hospitalized patients with heart failure (OPTIMIZE-HF) registry data. O'Connor et al. (2008) identified factors that predicted early posthospital mortality. Their analysis indicates that the following factors were predictive of both posthospital mortality and rehospitalization:

- Age
- Kidney, liver, or pulmonary (both reactive and obstructive) compromise
- Low systolic blood pressure, serum sodium, or admission weight
- Depression

TABLE 14.2 Risk Scores to Predict Outcomes in HF

Risk Score	Reference (from full-text guideline)/Link
Chronic HF	
All patients with chronic HF	
Seattle Heart Failure Model	(204)/http://SeattleHeartFailureModel.org
Heart Failure Survival Score	(200)/www.amga.org/wcm/PI/Collabs/HF/MO/Mtgs/2015111113/pina.pdf
CHARM Risk Score	(207)
CORONA Risk Score	(208)
Specific to chronic HFpEF	
I-PRESERVE Score	(202)
Acutely Decompensated HF	
ADHERE Classification and Regression Tree (CART) Model	(201)
American Heart Association Get With the Guidelines Score	(206) www.heart.org/HEARTORG/HealthcareProfessional/GetWithTheGuidelinesHFStroke/GetWithTheGuidelinesHeartFailureHomePage/Get-With-The-Guidelines-Heart-Failure-Home-%20Page_UCM_306087_SubHomePage.jsp
EFFECT Risk Score	(203) www.ccort.ca/Research/CHFRiskModel.aspx
ESCAPE Risk Model and Discharge Score	(215)
OPTIMIZE HF Risk Prediction Nomogram	(216)

HF, heart failure; HFpEF, heart failure with preserved ejection fraction.

O'Connor et al. (2010) developed the Evaluation Study of Congestive Heart Failure and Pulmonary Artery Catheterization Effectiveness (ESCAPE). The model is used to predict high risk for death in patients discharged after a hospital stay for advanced decompensated HF. The score is broken down into patients at high, medium, or low risk of death at 6 months. The following factors are used in predicting a score:

■ Age
■ Blood urea nitrogen (BUN)
■ Sodium
■ 6-minute walk
■ CPR/mechanical ventilation
■ Diuretic dose
■ No BB at discharge
■ Brain natriuretic peptide

Despite a large number of prognostic models, there continues to be a need for further refinement. An extensive review of 117 models was conducted to evaluate the strongest variables, models, and model characteristics to predict HF outcome. The researchers found that the strongest predictors of outcome were BUN and sodium, and concluded that the prediction of mortality and hospitalization for HF patients remains moderately successful (Ouwerkerk, Voors, & Zwinderman, 2014).

■ PATHOPHYSIOLOGY OF HEART FAILURE

HF generally results from more than one factor. Cardiac overload, injury, genetics, and changes in the neurohormonal, inflammatory, and biochemical profile all interact to impact the heart (Gaggin & Januzzi, 2015). Development of HF results from both structural changes and neurohormonal compensatory mechanisms, which in turn lead to progression of HF in a downward spiral.

Structural Changes in Heart Failure

Structural heart changes that contribute to HF result from cellular and mechanical cardiovascular abnormalities. HF can be classified according to two different types of pathophysiology that lead to similar symptoms. Systolic HF is caused by impaired ventricular contractility and is characterized by a low EF (less than 40%, normal 55%–60%) and thus termed heart failure with reduced ejection fraction. Contrasting with this, diastolic HF has a normal or near-normal EF and impaired ventricular filling because the heart muscle cannot relax during diastole and is termed heart failure with preserved ejection fraction (HFpEF). Both types of HF are associated with poor cardiac output.

A variety of pathophysiologic mechanisms contribute to LV hypertrophy, which is the structural change responsible for diastolic HF. LV hypertrophy is a common consequence of prolonged HTN. Increased afterload in the aorta and high systemic vascular resistance compromise compliance of the ventricles, leading to problems with cardiac relaxation and filling, which is the underlying problem in diastolic HF. Changes in myocyte shape, size, and number, as well as the development of interstitial fibrosis, also contribute to hypertrophy (Yancy et al., 2013). These changes increase LV wall thickness, causing septal hypertrophy and a reduction in diastolic compliance (Abete et al., 2012).

LV dilation and myocardial weakening are structural changes that commonly cause systolic HF. After cardiac injury, such as AMI, the damaged and weakened heart muscle dilates and fills with more blood in an attempt to compensate for its lower cardiac output. This leads to higher volumes and pressures in the heart. The end result of these pressure and volume changes in the LV is known as cardiac remodeling. In cardiac remodeling, the LV becomes more spherical, increasing the hemodynamic stresses on the chamber wall, decreasing mechanical performance, and increasing the likelihood of mitral regurgitation (Yancy et al., 2013). The ventricle takes on a spherical instead of an elliptical shape as a dynamic of the Starling Law. This law maintains that if the myocardial fibers can be stretched by increasing the volume of blood within it, the force of contraction will be greater and the ventricle will more completely empty (Moser & Riegel, 2008). Over time, further remodeling occurs, leading to increased disease progression.

Valvular malfunction can lead to both systolic and diastolic HF. This occurs because of either pressure overload associated with stenosis (valvular narrowing) or volume overload associated with regurgitation (valvular leakage). In stenosis, the heart valves become calcified, leading to narrowing of the valve diameter and increasing the pressure load on the heart chamber behind the valve. Stenosis is most often seen in the aortic valve and slowly progresses in severity. Volume overload, which is present in valvular insufficiency or regurgitation, most often occurs in the mitral and aortic valves. This condition also progresses insidiously, unless there is an associated acute cause, such as endocarditis, papillary muscle or chordae tendineae rupture, or interventricular rupture following a myocardial infarction (Moser & Riegel, 2008).

Neurohormonal Changes in Heart Failure

Poor cardiac output, in both systolic and diastolic HF, triggers acute compensatory neurohormonal mechanisms (McCance & Huether, 2014). These compensatory responses include the innervations of the sympathetic nervous system (increasing heart rate and peripheral vascular resistance), increased inotropy (increasing contractile state in viable myocardium), arteriolar constriction to maintain vital organ perfusion, and activation of the renin–angiotensin–aldosterone system (RAAS) to maintain cardiac output. The RAAS contributes to homeostasis through the activation of angiotensin II, which is synthesized through angiotensin-converting enzyme stimulation. Angiotensin causes systemic vasoconstriction. Aldosterone, which is primarily stimulated by angiotensin II, promotes retention of sodium and water and leads to volume expansion. In the acute phase, these compensatory mechanisms attempt to maintain adequate cardiac output and vital organ perfusion, which would be appropriate in an acute state such as shock. However, when poor cardiac output becomes chronic, each of these mechanisms leads to detrimental consequences for the patient. Chronic neurohormonal activation is another cause of HF symptoms and worsening heart function over time because ventricular remodeling develops in response to these chronic neurohormonal influences. When neurohormonal response and ventricular remodeling occur, the result is myopathy, which is a response to the increased afterload and fluid retention. Ventricular filling pressures (preload) increase further, the myocardial fibers overstretch, the mechanism of Starling Law fails, cardiac output is compromised, and the increased pressure in the left ventricle backs up into the pulmonary vasculature. The heart can no longer meet the metabolic needs of the body for oxygen delivery to the tissues, and systolic hypoperfusion, severe vasoconstriction (increased afterload), and poor pump performance occur.

Inflammation, oxidative stress, and chronic neurohormonal activation are under current investigation as unique stressors to the myocardium potentially contributing to ongoing cardiac damage, even in the absence of new cardiac events (Gaggin & Januzzi, 2015). Brain natriuretic peptide (BNP) and N-terminal fragment proBNP (NT-proBNP), which rise in response to increasing ventricular pressures or volume, are considered essential markers in diagnosis and determining prognosis in HF. Troponin T and I, commonly used to diagnose myocardial infarction, are often elevated in HF. Prolonged activation of the RAAS leads to long-term deleterious effects. Neurohormonal activation includes the effects of norepinephrine, angiotensin II, aldosterone release, arginine vasopressin, and another marker named mid-regional proadrenomedullin (MR-proADM). This hormone has natriuretic, vasodilatory, and hypotensive effects (Peacock, 2014). MR-proADM is elevated in acute and chronic HF and is used as a predictor of hospitalization and mortality. Two markers, soluble ST2 receptor and Galectin 3, are linked to myocardial remodeling and fibrosis that eventually lead to the myocardial dysfunction and HF and may be considered as prognostic markers of HF (Yancy et al., 2017). C-reactive protein, tumor necrosis factor-α (TNF-α), and interleukins 1, 6, 18 are all inflammatory markers that appear to have direct adverse effects on the myocardium through myocyte apoptosis (programmed cell death) and necrosis (traumatic cell death) and are associated with remodeling. These biomarkers are increasingly being used to assess HF patients, and drug therapies are being developed to target many of these mechanisms to slow the progression of HF and decrease symptom burden. The study of biomarkers to identify anticipated patterns of HF progression and prognosis is another rapidly evolving field of precision medicine that may have important implications for PC. The expert clinician will keep up to date on the latest research and clinical practice guidelines.

■ CLINICAL SIGNS AND PRESENTING SYMPTOMS IN HEART FAILURE

Clinical Signs of Heart Failure

HF can be due to either systolic or diastolic dysfunction, but generally most patients will have varying forms of both dysfunctions (Yancy et al., 2013). Systolic dysfunction (HFrEF) is measured by the left ventricular ejection fraction (LVEF). Normal EF is approximately 60%, but in systolic HF, the EF is usually less than 40%. In end-stage systolic HF, the EF can be as low as 15% to 20% or less. Common causes of HFrEF are ischemic and valvular heart disease and cardiomyopathy. Diastolic HF (HFpEF) occurs when the EF is normal, but ventricular relaxation and filling are compromised (Udelson, 2011). This leads to a lower stroke volume (amount of blood pumped to the body with each cardiac contraction), reducing cardiac output, especially with exertion. Because blood cannot move forward through the heart, it backs up into the pulmonary vasculature, which causes dyspnea and edema.

HFpEF accounts for approximately 20% to 50% of all cases of HF and is commonly seen in older adults, and in women who are obese and have HTN and DM (Udelson, 2011; Yancy et al., 2013). It is important to note that in the aging process, the relaxation of the heart in diastole is sometimes delayed, which causes a decrease in the filling time (Westenbrink, Damman, Rienstra, Maass, & van der Meer, 2012). Determining whether a patient has HFrEF or HFpEF based on examination or history of symptoms is usually challenging, and many patients have systolic and diastolic dysfunction regardless of EF (Yancy et al., 2013). The most accurate method of determining the type of HF is echocardiography; some diagnostic clues are identified in Table 14.3.

HF has been historically classified according to the side of the heart that is affected. It is important to understand that the right ventricle and the left ventricle are independent of each other, yet they are connected through the pulmonary vasculature. To function effectively, both ventricles must maintain equal outputs. Unless the patient has a history of chronic lung disease, the left ventricle is usually the first to become dysfunctional as it must generate higher pressures to pump blood to the systemic circulation.

Right ventricular (RV) failure is generally the result of increased pulmonary pressure. This increased pressure can be due to chronic lung disease, pulmonary emboli, or left-sided HF. The clinical signs of RV failure are those associated with increased systemic venous pressure with dependent peripheral edema or engorgement of the liver and mesenteric vasculature. Although HF may initially be either right or left sided, in end-stage HF it is generally biventricular.

TABLE 14.3 Characteristics of Patients With Diastolic HF (HFpEF) Versus Systolic HF (HFrEF)		
Characteristic	**Diastolic HF (HFpEF)**	**Systolic HF (HFrEF)**
Age	Elderly	All ages (50–70 years)
Sex	Frequently female	Often male
Ejection fraction	Normal or elevated	40% or less
Hypertension	Usually present	Often present
Diabetes mellitus	Usually present	Often present
Previous heart attack	Occasionally present	Usually present
Obesity	Usually present	Occasionally present
Chronic lung disease	Often present	Not present
Sleep apnea	Often present	Often present
Chronic renal disease	Often present	Not present
Atrial fibrillation	Occasionally present	Occasionally present

HF, heart failure; HFpEF, heart failure with preserved ejection fraction; HFrEF, heart failure with reduced ejection fraction.

Source: From Jessup, M., & Brozena, S. (2003). Heart failure. *New England Journal of Medicine, 348*(20), 2007–2018. doi:10.1056/NEJMra021498

TABLE 14.4 Signs and Symptoms of Left and Right Ventricular Heart Failure

Left Heart Failure	Right Heart Failure
■ Dyspnea, orthopnea, paroxysmal nocturnal dyspnea ■ Pulmonary edema ■ Dry cough ■ S3, S4 ■ Fine crackles, wheezing ■ Fatigue ■ Hypoxemia	■ Abdominal pain/bloating ■ Jugular vein distention ■ Peripheral edema ■ Hepatojugular reflex ■ Liver engorgement (increased liver function tests) ■ Splenomegaly ■ Significant, recent weight gain of greater than 2 lbs/d

It is important for clinicians to understand and be able to identify the symptoms of both right and left ventricular HF as treatment often differs. A patient may have typical right or left ventricular HF symptoms, but often in patients with end-stage heart disease, combined symptoms occur. In Table 14.4, the symptoms of both RV and LV failure are outlined. The severity and progression of the symptoms are dependent on the extent of the failure and the type of dysfunction.

Presenting Symptoms in Heart Failure

According to the ACC/AHA guidelines (Yancy et al., 2013), patients with HF usually present in three ways:

■ A recent syndrome of decreased exercise tolerance, usually due to dyspnea and/or fatigue; in this case, it is important for the provider to ascertain whether these symptoms represent HF or another condition such as pulmonary disease
■ Fluid retention with complaints of leg edema or abdominal bloating
■ With or without any symptoms of another cardiac or noncardiac disorder, such as DM, abnormal heart sounds, abnormal ECG, arrhythmia, HTN/hypotension, AMI, pulmonary emboli/other systemic thrombosis, or a chest x-ray that has evidence of cardiac enlargement

Dyspnea is the initial manifestation of HF in most patients and occurs from hypoxemia due to low cardiac output. At first, this may be a subtle change, but as the condition progresses, this is the most common presenting symptom, especially in left-sided HF. As the LV fails, blood backs up to the left atrium and the pulmonary veins. As pressure rises in the pulmonary vasculature, blood moves into the alveoli and pulmonary edema occurs. Orthopnea and paroxysmal nocturnal dyspnea increase and often patients have to sleep in upright positions to rest. A dry or nonproductive cough is another common HF symptom, which can often be attributed to another cause (postnasal drip or cough from ACEI medication).

When fulminate pulmonary edema occurs, there is pink frothy expectorant and a feeling of "suffocating" or "drowning."

Fatigue increases as HF progresses. Patients often report the inability to "do what they used to do." Activity tolerance decreases and the smallest of tasks can be overwhelming. Cachexia and malnutrition are also seen and muscle mass diminishes. Patients are often too tired to eat and say that it "takes too much energy" (which it does as eating increases myocardial oxygen demand). These men and women become frail and often have a low albumin level that only adds to their overall peripheral edema. The cardiac output becomes so low that the gut does not get adequate perfusion and becomes hypoxic. An oxygen-deprived gastrointestinal system does not function efficiently, which contributes to anorexia, early satiety, additional cachexia, and weight loss. In HF, blood flow to the kidneys decreases, reducing urinary output and compromising the effectiveness of diuretics. Renal insufficiency and eventually renal failure occur in many cases as the creatinine rises and the patient and family are faced with the decision as to whether renal replacement therapy should be initiated. When oliguria and anuria occur, fluid retention increases, and peripheral edema and pulmonary edema become more pronounced. Eventually, cardiogenic shock occurs with marked hypoperfusion of poorly oxygenated blood to the tissues, which causes metabolic acidosis and death. HF should be ruled out in patients who present with recurrent pulmonary infections, individuals with frequent exacerbations of chronic obstructive pulmonary disease (COPD), and elders who experience acute confusion.

■ CLINICAL ASSESSMENT IN HEART FAILURE

According to the practice guidelines by the ACC/AHA (Yancy et al., 2013), the causal mechanism of the patient's HF should be determined. Some conditions that lead to LV dysfunction are treatable and can be reversed. Measurement of BNP can be helpful in confirming the diagnosis of HF. BNP is a naturally occurring cardiac neurohormone secreted by the ventricular membrane in response to volume expansion and pressure overload. Other BNP functions are to regulate vascular tone and extracellular volume status as well as to counteract the effects of the RAAS. BNP is elevated in the failing heart when ventricular stretching occurs. BNP can be used to help differentiate between HF and chronic fibrotic lung changes, or an exacerbation of COPD, which can present similarly (Yancy et al., 2017). Therefore, BNP levels should be ordered when it is unclear as to the cause of presenting symptoms. A negative value of BNP is under 100 pg/mL, and BNP trends are effective in showing changes in fluid status over time or in response to therapies. The finding of a BNP of less than 50 pg/mL is good evidence of the absence of HF. An alternative lab assay is

NT-proBNP—inactive fragment of BNP, negative value is under 900 pg/mL, and less than 300 pg/mL is normal (Gaggin & Januzzi, 2015). Ranges of NT-proBNP can vary by age, and reference ranges vary in the literature.

The clinical assessment of HF begins with a thorough history and physical, and with the assessment of the following conditions or comorbidities: HTN, DM, dyslipidemia, valvular heart disease, CAD, peripheral vascular disease (PVD), cardiomyopathy, rheumatic fever, SDB, exposure to cardiotoxic medication (chemotherapy regimens; especially anthracyclines, herceptin, cyclophosphamide), current or past alcohol consumption, smoking, collagen vascular disease, thyroid disorder, obesity, pheochromocytoma, and exposure to sexually transmitted diseases. A family history should be taken with a focus on premature CAD in a first-degree relative, sudden cardiac death, conduction system problems, cardiomyopathy, and history of strokes or PVD. Assess the family history for three generations.

The goal of the targeted HF assessment is to determine the type (right, left, and biventricular), severity, and progression of the HF. HF assessment includes cardiac, pulmonary, integumentary, and gastrointestinal systems as well as functional symptoms, self-care, and psychosocial/spiritual status assessments (Table 14.5).

Cardiac Assessment

Assessment of the heart rate and rhythm is essential to determine whether there are any dysrhythmias that are compromising the function of the heart. Arrhythmias are common in advanced HF and may contribute to symptoms such as fatigue. The pulse is usually the initial response to decreased cardiac output. In HF, the pulse is often weak, or pulsus alternans may be present due to the altered function of the left ventricle. Pulsus alternans is exhibited by strong beats, alternating with weak beats with a regular heart rhythm and low-voltage QRS complexes on the EKG.

TABLE 14.5 Heart Failure Assessment		
Assessment Domain	**Assessment Parameters**	**Indicators of HF**
Cardiac assessment	■ Palpate rate and rhythm ■ Auscultate heart sounds ■ Palpate the chest wall ■ Inspect jugular pressure	■ Dysrhythmias ■ S3, murmurs ■ Displaced PMI ■ Increased JVD
Pulmonary assessment	■ Auscultate lung sounds	■ Crackles, pleural effusions
Integumentary assessment	■ Palpate skin	■ Dependent edema ■ Venous stasis ■ Cool, clammy skin
Gastrointestinal assessment	■ Palpate abdomen	■ Liver, spleen enlargement ■ Hepatojugular reflux ■ Ascites

Functional status assessment	■ Interview for
	  – Ambulation
	  – Activity level
	  – Self-care
	  – Intake
	  – Level of consciousness
		■ Reduced to bedbound
		■ Normal with effort to reduced
		■ Assistance needed to total care
		■ Reduced to minimal
		■ Full to confused

Symptom status assessment	■ Interview for
	  – Number of symptoms
	  – Severity of symptoms
	  – Distress caused by symptoms
		■ Fatigue
		■ Dyspnea
		■ Decreased activity levels

Self-care status assessment	■ Interview for
	  – Medication, dietary, daily weight patterns
	  – Symptom response
		■ Decreases in self-care
		■ Increasing symptoms and/or fluid imbalance despite adequate self-care

Psychosocial/spiritual status assessment	■ Interview for
	  – Psychological distress/adjustment
	  – Family resources/needs
	  – Spiritual needs
	  – Advanced care planning
		■ Increasing distress as condition progresses

JVD, jugular vein distention; PMI, point of maximum impulse.

On palpation of the chest wall, the point of maximum impulse (PMI), which normally is at the fifth intercostal space, midclavicular line, will be displaced laterally to the left toward the axilla. This displacement is due to the enlarged hypertrophied left ventricle. In HF patients, a third heart sound (S3) is often the first clinical sign of HF and is highly specific. An S3 occurs in early diastole soon after S2 and occurs in HF when the blood flows from the atrium into an already overloaded ventricle. A fourth heart sound (S4) may also be heard, which may indicate chronic ischemic disease and lack of ventricular compliance. An S4 occurs at the end of diastole just before S1, which is a marker of the beginning of systole. An S4 is caused by a forceful atrium contracting against an abnormally stiff or hypertrophic ventricle. While the S4 may be present in HF, it may also be a normal finding in some older adults. It is also important to be alert for murmurs, which indicate valvular malfunction or septal defects. A systolic murmur may be present in systolic HF with LV dilation and fluid overload, becoming more pronounced when fluid overload increases LV pressures, dilating the mitral valve.

Jugular venous pulses can estimate the central venous pressure and should be examined in the right internal jugular vein while the patient is positioned supine at a 30° to 45° angle. If the jugular vein is distended, it indicates RV failure and fluid overload. The hepatojugular reflex should also be elicited and is done by pressing on the right upper quadrant of the abdomen. With engorgement of the liver in right HF, the compression of the abdomen fills the jugular vein, causing increased jugular vein distention (JVD). Assessing daily weight patterns and changes from the "dry weight" will also provide information about fluid retention related to cardiac dysfunction. The "dry weight" is the patient's stable weight with no signs of fluid overload. These are key findings of HF and usually indicate a need for additional diuretic therapy.

Pulmonary Assessment

When pulmonary pressures are elevated, the hydrostatic pressure within the pulmonary capillaries surrounding the alveoli is elevated. This occurs as the left ventricle fails and causes backward flow. This increased pressure causes transudation of the fluid within the capillary into the alveoli. Dyspnea increases as fluid accumulates in the alveoli (pulmonary edema), oxygen saturation decreases, and the patient feels as if he or she is drowning.

The accumulated fluid can be heard when the patient inspires as "crackles." These crackles do not clear with coughing and are initially heard in the dependent portions of the lung. As pulmonary pressures continue to rise with left HF, these breath sounds can be heard throughout both lung fields. It is important to note that some people with HF do not exhibit pulmonary crackles when

fluid volume is elevated, as their pulmonary lymphatic drainage has increased to compensate for this chronic condition (Leier & Chatterjee, 2007). Pleural effusions may also be present.

Integumentary Assessment

Dependent edema is a hallmark sign of right and biventricular HF. Edema is felt in dependent areas such as in the hips, legs, ankles and feet, or the sacral area for those who are bedridden. It is important to accurately assess the extent of the edema by looking for pitting beginning at the ankle and continuing up to the leg, thigh, and even hip, if necessary, until it is no longer seen. Extensive edema is often accompanied by weeping of the tissue and scrotal edema in men. Extensive edema is also accompanied by decreased mobility, as the weakened patient struggles to lift his or her fluid-filled legs. This edema may lead to stasis dermatitis, hyperpigmentation, and ulceration. The temperature of the skin is also very helpful in assessing cardiac output. Cool, clammy, or diaphoretic skin is an indicator of peripheral vasoconstriction, which is a sign of increased sympathetic nervous system response, a compensation for decreased cardiac output.

Gastrointestinal Assessment

As mentioned in Table 14.4, liver enlargement occurs with right or biventricular HF due to venous congestion. The engorged liver can be felt below the right costal margin of the ribs. In advanced HF, the spleen can also be palpated below the left costal margin. End-stage HF may also result in ascites (peritoneal cavity fluid accumulation) that can contribute to dyspnea, abdominal discomfort, and decreased mobility.

Functional Status

In end-stage heart disease, symptoms of biventricular failure such as dyspnea, weakness, fatigue, and pain are present. Healthcare providers need to evaluate the impact of these symptoms on daily function by doing patient interviews or questionnaires at every visit. The Palliative Performance Scale (PP) developed by Anderson, Downing, Hill, Casorso, and Lerch (1996) is an easy-to-use assessment of functional status. The clinician interviews the patient or caregiver, asking about the patient's ambulation, activity level, self-care practice, oral intake, and level of consciousness. Information from each of the items is recorded and the clinician then assigns a score that has been shown to be predictive of survival (Morita, Tsunoda, Inoue, & Chihara, 1999). The PPS identifies not only changes in condition but also potential care needs.

More information on the PPS is available at palliative. org/NewPC/professionals/tools/pps.html

Another functional status measure is the Duke Activity Status Index (DASI). It is a 12-item questionnaire that can be self-administered. The DASI scale attempts to capture major aspects of physical function: personal hygiene, ambulation, daily routine tasks, recreational/sports, and sexual function. Lower scores are related to poor function and prognosis, and higher scores are indicative of better functioning. The DASI scale has been found to be an independent predictor of mortality in patients with stable HF (Grodin, Hammadah, Fan, Hazen, & Tang, 2015).

Symptom Status

Patients' self-report is the gold standard for symptom assessment. The symptoms of HF are often associated with inflammatory and neurohormonal activation. HF symptoms commonly experienced are fatigue, dyspnea, and decreased activity levels. Older HF patients also commonly have symptoms associated with geriatric syndromes such as osteoarthritic pain. While NYHA status is often used to assess for and track the patient's symptom status, clinician and patient reports do not correlate well. A better instrument is the widely used Edmonton Symptom Assessment Scale (ESAS; Chang, Hwang, & Feuerman, 2000). The ESAS assesses for pain, tiredness, nausea, depression, anxiety, drowsiness, appetite, well-being, and dyspnea using a 0 to 10 visual analog scale. The clinical interview can identify which factors precipitate, worsen, or improve each symptom.

Self-Care Status

Self-care is a key in maintaining the HF patient's status at home and is critical to health promotion and rehabilitation. Self-care involves adhering to the plan of care, monitoring symptom status, and then responding in an appropriate way to symptoms when they occur (Riegel, Lee, & Dickson, 2011). However, many HF patients have difficulty with self-care due to cognitive changes, decreasing activity levels, lack of family support, and the complexity of the self-care regimen itself. The clinical interview should explore such issues as medication use, dietary intake, and daily weight patterns followed by questions assessing for correct responses to changes in weight or increasing shortness of breath. Motivational interviewing techniques would be useful to encourage adherence, provide education, and support successful practices. To validate and improve understanding, a teach-back technique can be used. The teach-back method allows an opportunity for the healthcare provider to confirm that the patient has understood information given and is useful when a lot of information is shared (Xu, 2012).

Psychosocial/Spiritual Status

A hallmark of quality PC is the assessment of the psychological, social, and spiritual/existential aspects of care (National Consensus Project for Quality Palliative Care, 2013). Particular areas for assessment involve taking a psychological history and assessing for reaction to the current condition, indicators of distress, family structure and function, strengths and vulnerabilities, caregiving needs, access to community services and resources, and advanced care planning. It should also include a spiritual assessment, which has been mandated by the Joint Commission since 2001. One spiritual assessment tool is the FICA, developed by Puchalski, Lunsford, Harris, and Miller (2006). Using the acronym *FICA*, the clinician assesses for *f*aith or belief systems, *i*mportant influences in the person's life, community support, and *a*ddressing the issues in the person's healthcare. Other instruments specific to the assessment of individuals with end-stage disease are available at TIME: Toolkit of Instruments to Measure EOL care, available at www.chcr.brown.edu/pcoc/toolkit.htm

In addition to the complete physical examination needed for patients with HF, the following diagnostic studies may be indicated:

1. Complete blood count (CBC), urinalysis
2. Serum electrolytes, glycohemoglobin, lipid profile, BUN, creatinine, liver function tests, magnesium, calcium
3. BNP or NT-proBNP
4. Chest x-ray and 12-lead EKG (should not be used as a primary determinant of cause of HF)
5. Thyroid studies (especially in those with atrial fibrillation and unexplained HF)
6. Transthoracic Doppler—two-dimensional echocardiography (most relevant diagnostic test)
7. Noninvasive stress testing (in patients with a previous history of coronary artery disease/myocardial infarction)
8. Cardiac catheterization in patients with angina or large areas of ischemic myocardium
9. MRI may need to be done to determine myocardial viability and scar tissue

Other diagnostic studies may be indicated depending on clinical evaluation such as fasting transferrin saturation (to rule out hemochromatosis, or the cause of cardiomyopathy) or HIV and so forth.

■ HEART FAILURE MANAGEMENT

Disease Management Guidelines in Heart Failure

The management of patients with various cardiovascular diseases is now widely based on the latest ACC/AHA and other societal guidelines (Table 14.6). These guidelines

TABLE 14.6 Joint Guidelines and Statements	
Title	Year Guideline/ Update Published
2014 AHA/ACC/HRS Guideline for the Management of Patients With Atrial Fibrillation (Compilation of 2006 ACCF/AHA/ESC and 2011 ACCF/AHA/HRS Recommendations)	2014
2012 ACCF/AHA/ACP/AATS/PCNA/SCAI/STS Guideline for the Diagnosis and Management of Patients With Stable Ischemic Heart Disease **WITH** 2014 ACC/AHA/ACP/AATS/PCNA/SCAI/STS Focused Update of the Guideline for the Diagnosis and Management of Patients With Stable Ischemic Heart Disease	2012/2014
2008 ACCF/AHA/HRS Guidelines for Device-Based Therapy of Cardiac Rhythm Abnormalities **WITH** 2012 ACCF/AHA/HRS Focused Update of the 2008 Guidelines for Device-Based Therapy of Cardiac Rhythm Abnormalities	2008/2012
2012 ACCF/AHA Focused Update of the Guideline for the Management of Patients With Unstable Angina/Non-ST–Elevation Myocardial Infarction (Updating the 2007 Guideline and Replacing the 2011 Focused Update)	2012
Management of Patients With Peripheral Artery Disease (Compilation of 2005 and 2011 ACCF/AHA Guideline Recommendations)	2013
2011 ACCF/AHA Focused Update of the Guideline for the Management of Patients With Peripheral Artery Disease (Updating the 2005 Guideline)	2011
ACCF/AHA 2011 Expert Consensus Document on Hypertension in the Elderly	2011
ACCF/AHA/ACP/HFSA/ISHLT 2010 Clinical Competence Statement on Management of Patients With Advanced Heart Failure and Cardiac Transplant	2010
2010 ACCF/AHA/AATS/ACR/ASA/SCA/SCAI/SIR/STS/SVM Guidelines for the Diagnosis and Management of Patients With Thoracic Aortic Disease: Full Text	2010
2013 ACCF/AHA Guidelines for the Diagnosis and Management of Heart Failure in Adults **WITH** 2017 Focused Update of the 2013 ACCF/AHA 2013 Guideline for the Management of Heart Failure	2013/2017
ACC/AHA 2008 Guidelines for the Management of Adults With Congenital Heart Disease: Full Text	2008
2014 AHA/ACC Guideline for the Management of Patients With Valvular Heart Disease **WITH** 2017 AHA/ACC Focused Update of the 2014 AHA/ACC Guideline for the Management of Patients With Valvular Heart Disease	2014/2017
ACC/AHA/ESC 2006 Guidelines for Management of Patients With Ventricular Arrhythmias and the Prevention of Sudden Cardiac Death—Full Text	2006
AHA 2016 Drugs That May Cause or Exacerbate Heart Failure: A Scientific Statement From the American Heart Association	2016
2010 Heart Rhythm Society Expert Consensus Statement on the Management of Cardiovascular Implantable Electronic Devices (CIEDs) in Patients Nearing End of Life or Requesting Withdrawal of Therapy	2010

AATS, American Association for Thoracic Surgery; ACC, American College of Cardiology; ACCF, American College of Cardiology Foundation; ACP, American College of Physicians; ACR, American College of Radiology; AHA, American Heart Association; ASA, American Stroke Association; ESC, European Society of Cardiology; HFSA, Heart Failure Society of America; HRS, Heart Rhythm Society; ISHLT, International Society for Heart and Lung Transplantation; PCNA, Preventive Cardiovascular Nurses Association; SCA, Society of Cardiovascular Anesthesiologists; SCAI, Society for Cardiovascular Angiography and Interventions; SIR, Society of Interventional Radiology; STS, Society of Thoracic Surgeons; SVM, Society for Vascular Medicine.

were developed after reviewing multiple, large-scale studies. Most HF patients have other cardiovascular diseases, so reviewing related guidelines may be helpful in HF management. While there are certainly principles to guide the management of patients with HFpEF, there are no specific guidelines or clear recommendations. So take note that most of the medication and device recommendations described in this chapter are specifically for patients with HFrEF.

■ GENERAL MEDICATION GUIDELINES FOR PATIENTS WITH HEART FAILURE WITH REDUCED EJECTION FRACTION AS PER JOINT GUIDELINES AND STATEMENTS

General medication guidelines for patients with HFrEF in Stages B through D and the landmark trials support the use of the following medications.

All patients with HF, unless contraindicated, should be on an ACEI or angiotensin receptor blocker (ARB) or ARNI and a BB:

1. **ACEIs,** based on the CONSENSUS, SOLVD, and ATLAS trials, are a key component in the treatment of HF antagonizing the RAAS. They have been shown to promote disease regression, symptom improvement, reduced hospitalization, and decreased mortality. *Or*
2. **ARBs** are used when the patient is not able to take an ACEI. The ELITE and CHARM-Alternative trials showed that ARBs reduce endpoint mortality and morbidity and improve clinical signs and symptoms. *Or*
3. **ARBs with Neprilysin Inhibitor (ARNI)**—While ACEIs or ARBs have been mainstays and the first-line therapy for several years, an ARB has been combined with a neprilysin inhibitor (ARNI) to create a new combination medication for HF. In a focused update for AHA/ACC/HFSA guidelines for the management of HF (2017), ARNI is now recommended as a replacement for ACEI or ARB therapy. The recommendations for ARNI as a substitution for ACEIs or ARBs are based on the PARADIGM-HF trials (Yancy et al., 2017). ARNIs reduce HF hospitalizations and mortality (McMurray et al., 2014). Side effects include hypotension, renal insufficiency, and angioedema, with the latter occurring at a lower incidence than ACEIs. *And*
4. **BBs** are a standard of HF care based on the MDC, MERIT-HF, MOCHA, PRECISE, COPERNICUS, COMET, BEST, CIBIS, and CIBIS-II trials. BBs improve mortality and symptoms and prevent hospitalizations in patients with chronic HF. BBs are best initiated when the patient is stable rather than during decompensation, as they may worsen symptoms. The benefit of BBs is long term, and they should be initiated and the dose up-titrated while evaluated for tolerance. The three types of BBs proven to be effective in HF are bisoprolol, carvedilol, or sustained release metopolol succinate. Other types of BBs do not have the same efficacy.

■ ADDITIONAL MEDICATIONS USED IN HEART DISEASE

Other medications such as diuretics, aldosterone antagonists, hydralazine and nitrates, digoxin, and ivabradine are prescribed based on the circumstances described in the following list:

1. **Diuretics** with salt restriction are the mainstay for patients with fluid overload. Loop diuretics or thiazides are most often used.
2. **Aldosterone antagonists,** such as Spironolactone or Eplerenone, were shown in the RALES, EPHESUS, and EMPHASIS-HF trials to decrease mortality though they need to be used in conjunction with potassium monitoring due to the risk of hyperkalemia. This potassium-sparing effect is often beneficial when they are used in combination with potassium-wasting diuretics such as furosemide. These medications are indicated in patients with a NYHA Class II to IV HF with an EF of 35% or less. Glomerular filtration rate needs to be >30/ml/min/1.73 m^2 and potassium levels need to be less than 5.0 mEq/L.
3. **Hydralazine and nitrates,** based on V-HEFT trial, are used when patients cannot be on an ACEI or ARB. The A-HEFT trial demonstrated improved mortality and reduced hospitalization rates in African Americans when added to optimal therapy with ACEI or ARB and BBs.
4. **Ivabradine** is a new class of medication that inhibits current (funny current—I_f) in the sinoatrial node. This effect leads to a reduction in heart rate. Reduction in heart rate, in turn, is associated with a reduction in hospitalizations and mortality similar to principles guiding BB use. Ivabradine is indicated when a patient is in sinus rhythm with a resting heart rate of more than 70 beats per minute despite a maximally tolerated dose of BBs (Yancy et al., 2017). These recommendations were based on the SHIFT and BEAUTIFUL trials (Bohm et al., 2015; Fox et al., 2010). Major side effects include bradycardia, atrial fibrillation, and increased blood pressure.
5. **Digoxin** is a positive inotropic medication that improves pump contractility. While it was widely used in the past, its substantial risk profile and limited benefit to long-term patient outcomes have reduced its use currently to those patients in whom other therapies, noted previously, have not improved symptoms.

Evidence for use of the aforementioned medications in patients with HFpEF have not yielded the same results as in patients with HFrEF. Medication management in HFpEF is geared toward symptomatology, comorbidities, and risk factors leading to cardiovascular disease. Diuretics are recommended for symptoms of fluid overload. One of the key comorbidities in patients with HFpEF is hypertension, and ACEI or ARBs are considered first-line treatment (Yancy et al., 2013). Blood pressure should be reduced to less than 140/90 mmHg.

■ DISCUSSION OF SPECIFIC CATEGORIES OF MEDICATIONS USED IN HEART FAILURE

Angiotensin-Converting Enzyme Inhibitors

ACEIs have been studied extensively over the last 10 years in many large series studies. ACEIs were introduced initially as treatment for HTN. It was felt that since these agents vasodilated the peripheral blood vessels by inhibiting the RAAS, there might be an indication for use in HF. Extensive studies found that not only did these agents decrease afterload and preload as expected, but more importantly they had a significant effect on ventricular remodeling. Through the mechanisms of decreasing aldosterone secretion and response of the sympathetic nervous system, symptoms improved quickly and dramatically. There continues to be concern with hypotension and the use of ACEI, especially in the older adult, and further large-scale studies should be done with patients older than 65 years. Enalapril, one of the earliest ACEIs studied, has been shown to benefit older adults. ACEIs are better tolerated if patients are hydrated and electrolytes are within normal limits. ACEIs should not be used in patients with a history of angioedema or anuria. Also cautious use of ACEIs is warranted in those with high serum creatinine levels (greater than 3 mg/dL), bilateral renal stenosis, high serum potassium levels (greater than 5.5 mmol/L), and low systolic blood pressure who are symptomatic (Yancy et al., 2013). Many patients complain of an irritating dry cough, which is a common side effect. The cough can occur shortly after initiation of therapy to several months later. The mechanism of the cough is generally thought to be caused by inhibition of ACE, which causes accumulation of bradykinin and tachykinins, which are normally metabolized by ACE. The cough can be a major reason for treatment discontinuation. Once discontinued, the cough resolution usually takes from 1 to 4 weeks to resolve but can linger for up to 3 months

Angiotensin Receptor Blockers

These agents block angiotensin II and angiotensin-dependent aldosterone at the receptor level. Hemodynamic effects are the same as with ACEI as far as reducing preload and afterload and increasing cardiac output, but these agents do not increase bradykinin levels, thus diminishing the side effect of cough (Moser & Riegel, 2008). However, there are reports of patients receiving ARBs who complain of cough, thereby proposing that bradykinin is not the only mechanism by which cough is induced (Rodgers & Patterson, 2001). The first of these agents, Losartan, was found to be well tolerated in older patients.

Angiotensin Receptor Blockers With Neprilysin Inhibitor (ARBNIs)

ACEIs and ARBs are very effective in blocking the deleterious effects of prolonged activation of the RAAS system. While both medications have significantly impacted the mortality rate in HF patients, there is still need for improvement as HF patients continue to decline while on treatment. While RAAS activation

becomes pathologic in HF, in contrast, other neurohormonal pathways that are activated in HF exert a protective, beneficial response. The most well known of those pathways is the natriuretic peptide (NP) systems composed of atrial (ANP), brain (BNP), and C-type peptides. These peptides cause vasodilation and natriuresis (sodium excretion in urine) and prevents development of fibrosis. Neprilysin is an enzyme that is the major way in which beneficial peptides are degraded and eliminated. The first attempts at blocking neprilysin to enhance the effects of the NPs did not yield the positive effects intended. The lack of effectiveness was possibly due to neprilysin inhibition leading to the degrading of angiotensin II and increased vasoconstriction (Kirby & Bakhai, 2016). Omapatrilat, which was a combination of an ACEI and a neprilysin inhibitor, was then developed. However, in this combination there was a higher rate of angioedema and hypotension than with an ACEI only. ACE and neprilysin are involved in the bradykinin metabolism, and the inhibition then leads to an accumulation of bradykinins and substance P, which are considered the source of the risk for development of angioedema (McMurray, 2015). ARBs, as opposed to ACEIs, do not affect bradykinin and other angioedema mediators. This led to the pairing of an ARB (valsartan) with a neprilysin inhibitor (sacubitril) and the development of the first medication known as ARNIs. The positive effects of ARNI in HF patients are the inhibition of vasoconstriction and remodeling of angiotensin II and the prevention of the catabolism of NPs, leading to diuresis of sodium and water. In the PARADIGM-HF trials, ARNIs reduced HF hospitalizations and mortality by 21% in comparison to ACEI alone (McMurray et al., 2014). ARNI is recommended as a substitution for ACEI or ARB in patients with HF (Yancy et al., 2017). Side effects include hypotension, cough, and hyperkalemia. The ARNI should be started 36 hours after the discontinuation of the ACEI to reduce the risk of angioedema and a cumulative effect. Neprilysin enzymes have an effect on several systems, and of particular concern is the clearance of amyloid-beta peptides, which are implicated in the development of Alzheimer's. In the PARADIGM-HF and OVERTURE trials, dementia and cognitive changes were not increased, but further research is necessary to continue to evaluate long-term effects of neprilysin inhibition (Gori, Volterrani, Piepoli & Senni, 2017; McMurray, 2015).

Beta-Adrenergic Blocking Agents

BB use in patients with chronic HF has been studied in 20 clinical trials with over 10,000 patients. These trials have shown that these agents reduce the risk of sudden death by 40% to 50% and the need for hospital admission, and improve the overall functional capacity

(Hunt et al., 2009). The beneficial effects of BB in HF result from the blocking of adrenergic stimulation of the heart, specifically norepinephrine, which in HF is related to increased mortality (Maack, Elter, & Bohm, 2007). BBs do have a negative inotropic effect, so for many years they were contraindicated in HF patients. In clinical trials, however, it was shown that this decrease in cardiac output was transient; in fact, BBs were shown to increase LVEF. These benefits were found in patients who were receiving therapeutic responses to diuretics and ACEI. Patients with NYHA Class II to IV HF were studied in multiple trials; one trial was able to show the decrease in mortality of 35% (Goldstein et al., 2001). The studies looking at BB in HF examined three agents: carvedilol, bisoprolol, and metoprolol CR/XL. The CIBIS-I trial found that there was a 34% reduction in hospital admission rates for patients who were on bisoprolol, and many showed improvements in overall QOL (Cardiac Insufficiency Bisoprolol Study [CIBIS], 1994). In the second trial, CIBIS-II, in patients with NYHA Class III and IV HF, there was a 34% reduction in mortality and a 20% reduction in hospital admissions in those treated with bisoprolol (CIBIS-II, 1999). BBs must be used with caution in patients with bronchospastic disease or asymptomatic bradycardia and should be used with caution in those with low systolic blood pressure. BBs generally are added with or after ACEIs have been optimized, and the patient is clinically stable and euvolemic.

Diuretics

Loop diuretics are the preferred class of diuretic, as these high-ceiling diuretics promote sodium and water excretion even when renal function is compromised. Loop diuretics provide immediate relief of symptoms associated with fluid overload but should not be used as the only pharmacologic agent. When used on a chronic basis, diuretics can increase renin, magnifying the activation of the RAAS. Therefore, they should be combined with ACEIs (von Lueder, Atar, & Krum, 2013). Common loop diuretics used in HF are furosemide (Lasix), torsemide (Demadex), and bumetanide (Bumex). Because loop diuretics cause loss of essential electrolytes (hypokalemia, hypomagnesemia, hyponatremia), ongoing assessment of these lab values is recommended. The determination of the proper initial dose and readjustment of doses require an ongoing evaluation of symptoms and careful titration based on daily weight and symptom patterns, especially in the older adult. Absorption of loop diuretics in the engorged, poorly perfused gastrointestinal tract is often compromised in the patient with worsening HF, and increased diuretic dosages may be necessary (von Lueder et al.,2013). In end-stage disease, periodic oral metolazone (Zaroxolyn) dosing may be necessary to promote diuresis, especially in patients with renal insufficiency. Metolazone should be used with extreme caution and careful assessment of the patient response, as it may cause overdiuresis, hypotension, and severe hypokalemia.

Aldosterone Antagonists

Low-dose aldosterone antagonists, such as spironolactone (12.5–25 mg/d) or eplerenone, have been found to be helpful in patients with NYHA Class II to IV HF with an EF of 35% or less. Class II HF patients should also have a history of hospitalization for cardiovascular reasons or elevated BNP. These agents block aldosterone, which then causes diuresis and decreases preload. Patients, however, should have normal serum potassium levels (less than 5.0 mEq/L) and adequate renal function (creatinine less than 2.5 mg/dL for men and less than 2.0 mg/dL for women) when taking these, and potassium should be monitored for hyperkalemia.

Ivabradine

Several studies have revealed that increases in heart rate in patients with HF are associated with an increased risk of hospitalization or death (Komajda, 2014). Ivabradine is a selective funny current (I_f) inhibitor, which slows heart rate without weakening myocardial contraction. In SHIFT trials, ivabradine significantly reduced HF hospitalizations and mortality (Swedberg et al., 2010). Ivabradine can be beneficial for patients with symptomatic but stable HF who are on maximum BB dose but still have a resting heart rate >70 beats per minute. Patients must also be in sinus rhythm.

Digitalis

Digitalis glycosides, positive inotropic agents, have been a part of the medical regime for patients in HF for over 200 years. These agents are still indicated for use in patients with HFrEF and ongoing symptoms of HF despite already being on optimum doses of ACEIs or ARBs and BBs (Yancy et al., 2013). Patients with mild-to-moderate HF on digoxin experienced a decrease in the progression of HF and had decreased hospital admissions (28%), but had no overall decrease in mortality (Yancy et al., 2013). Digoxin is also indicated in patients with HF with atrial fibrillation and uncontrolled ventricular response. However, this drug must be used carefully, monitoring for and preventing digoxin toxicity. Digoxin toxicity may cause arrhythmias, and it is potentiated by low potassium and magnesium levels, common electrolyte abnormalities in patients with HF due to diuretic use.

The suggested dosing of these medications is as shown in Table 14.7. The titration of each medication dose is based on a careful evaluation of the patient's tolerance and response.

TABLE 14.7 Evidence-Based Medications for Heart Failure With Reduced Ejection Fraction

Drug Name	Starting Dose	Target Dose
Vasodilators (ACEI)		
Captopril	6.25 mg 3×/d	50 mg 3×/d
Enalapril	2.5 mg 2×/d	10 mg 2×/d
Lisinopril	2.5–5 mg/d	20 mg/d
Ramipril	1.25–2.5 mg/d	5 mg/d
Fosinopril	2.5 mg 2×/d	20 mg 2×/d
Quinapril	5 mg 2×/d	20 mg 2×/d
Trandolapril	1 mg/d	4 mg/d
Vasodilators (ARB)		
Candesartan	4–8 mg/d	32 mg/d
Valsartan	20–40 mg 2×/d	80 mg 2×/d
Valsartan with Sacubitril (neprilysin inhibitor)	49 mg/51 mg 2×/d	97 mg/103 mg 2×/d
Vasodilators (direct acting, a = arterial, v = venous)		
■ Hydralazine (a)	25 mg 4×/d	–
■ Isosorbide dinitrate (v)	10 mg 3×/d	–
■ Isosorbide mononitrate (v)	30–60 mg/d	–
Beta Blockers		
Carvedilol	3.125→6.25→12.5→25→50 mg	25 mg 2×/d (less than 85 kg)
Carvedilol CR	10→20→40→80 mg	50 mg 2×/d (greater than 85 kg) 80 mg once daily
Metoprolol succinate extended release (CR/XL)	25→50→100→150→200 mg	200 mg/d
Bisoprolol	1.25→2.5→5→10 mg	10 mg/d
Nebivolol	1.25→2.5→5→10 mg	10 mg/d
If Current Inhibitors		
Ivabradine	5 mg 2×/d	Adjust to achieve HR 50–60/min (maximum) 7.5 mg 2×/d
Cardiac Glycoside Therapy		
Digitalis	0.125–0.25 mg/d	0.5 mg/d[a]
Aldosterone Antagonists[b]		
Spironolactone	12.5–25 mg/d (use low dose)	25 mg 2×/d
Eplerenone	25 mg/d × 4 weeks→50 mg/d	50 mg/d
Diuretics (Type)	**Relative Potency**	**Note**
Furosemide (loop)	40 mg/d	
Bumetanide (loop)	1 mg/d	
Ethacrynic acid (loop)	50 mg/d	Take with/before loop diuretic
Torsemide (loop)	20–40 mg/d	Used to treat hypertension
HCTZ (thiazide)	–	
Chlorthalidone (thiazide)	25–100 mg/d	
Metolazone (thiazide-like)	2.5–5 mg/d	Take with/before loop diuretic
Triamterene	–	Does not inhibit aldosterone
Amiloride	–	Does not inhibit aldosterone

[a]Refer to facility formularies for target dosing of digitalis.
[b]Base dosing on eGFR and potassium levels.

ACEI, angiotensin converting enzyme inhibitor; ARB, angiotensin receptor blocker; HCTZ, hydrochlorothiazide.

Source: Albert, N. M., Anderson, D., Besthoff, C. M., Byrne-Barta, D., Cecil, R. Y., Cichocki, M., ... Lucarelli, P. (2013). Care of the chronically ill patient. In C. B. Laughlin (Ed.), *Core curriculum for ambulatory care nursing* (pp. 361–470). Pittman, NJ: American Academy of Ambulatory Care Nursing.

Drugs That Cause or Exacerbate Heart Failure

There are several classes of drugs and medications that need to be evaluated and/or avoided in HF patients. The following is a partial list of common medications. A complete listing along with the level of evidence and effect on HF can be found in the AHA scientific statement (Page et al., 2016).

1. Analgesics: Nonsteroidal anti-inflammatory drugs cause sodium retention and peripheral vasoconstriction, as well as decrease in efficacy and increase in toxicity of diuretics and ACEI. In addition, they increase the risk of bleeding when used with anticoagulants such as warfarin, a drug widely used in this population. Because this important class of analgesics cannot be safely used in HF, pain management can be challenging in this population.
2. Antidiabetics:
   a. Thiazolidinediones, which are antidiabetic agents, can cause or exacerbate HF symptoms and therefore are contraindicated.
   b. Biguanides are not recommended in unstable or hospitalized HF patients, and renal function criteria need to be concomitantly evaluated.
   c. Dipeptyl Peptidase 4-Inhibitors possibly increase in HF hospitalizations although the reason behind this is unknown.
3. Antiarrhythmic agents (Class I, III, and others) may lead to cardiodepression and proarrhythmic effects.
4. Antihypertensives:
   a. Calcium channel blockers have negative inotropic properties and should be used with caution because they may lead to increased risk of cardiovascular events and decreased survival.
   b. Alpha blockers and centrally acting alpha blockers have been associated with worse clinical outcomes and mortality and are not recommended in HF.
5. Other major classifications included in the AHA statement include anesthetics, anticancer, antiinfective, hematologic, pulmonary, rheumatological, urological, ophthalmologic, neurological, and psychiatric medications.

Complementary and Alternative Medicine in Heart Failure

People frequently use holistic modalities in prevention and treatment of disease. Natural treatments, vitamins, herbs, antioxidants, and other nontraditional (at least to Western or allopathic medicine) therapies are used by many patients to complement or even replace drugs and other interventions. Adjuvant healing modalities can be a benefit to allopathic medicine. There are specific complementary and alternative medicine (CAM) therapies that have shown some efficacy in HF. According to the National Health Interview Survey (Centers for Disease Control and Prevention [CDC], 2012), 34% of all U.S. adults used some form of CAM in the prior 12 months. A study of older HF patients from eight medical centers found that 93% used over-the-counter (OTC) drugs, while 11.5% used herbal therapies (Albert et al., 2009). While the literature yields no specific information on the number of HF patients using all CAM modalities, a breakdown by age of CAM use shows that there is a substantive usage in populations known to be at high risk for HF (Barnes, Bloom, & Nahin, 2008), with the highest use being of biologically based (natural product) therapies.

■ **Evidence-Based Complementary and Alternative Medicine.** According to the classification of therapies by the National Center for Complementary and Alternative Medicine (NCCAM; one of the institutes of the National Institutes of Health [NIH]), there is sufficient evidence to warrant considering recommending certain mind–body therapies in HF (Table 14.8).

Spirituality is another mind–body modality used by patients to cope with the uncertainty of HF. Spirituality influences the manner in which a patient adjusts to a chronic illness. Patients with end-stage heart disease often reflect on their past and attempt to nurture hopes for the future. Symptomatic HF patients have been found to have higher depression scores and lower spiritual well-being than patients with advanced cancer, suggesting the need for support in this important area, particularly because of links between spirituality and hope (Bekelman et al., 2009; Davidson, Dracup, Phillips, Daly, & Padilla, 2007). Park et al. (2015) investigated spirituality as a predictor of mortality in HF patients. Spirituality was defined as a sense of inner peace and harmony. The participants were 191 patients with HF who were interviewed at baseline and followed for 5 years. During the study 32% of the participants died. The researchers found that while religion and spirituality were both associated with better health behaviors at baseline, only spirituality was associated with a reduced mortality risk (20%).

Dietary supplements, herbs, and botanicals, as well as traditional medicine formulations, make up the category known as natural products (formerly classified as biologically based). There are varying levels of evidence to support the efficacy of these products in HF (Table 14.9). In addition to studies on these products, there have been numerous recent calls for additional research on the role of micronutrients in HF and for careful nutritional assessment (Agarwal, Phan, Willix, Barber, & Schwarz, 2011; Azizi-Namini, Ahmed, Yan, & Keith, 2012; Kamalov, Bhattacharya, & Weber, 2010; Lee et al., 2011; McKeag, McKinley, Woodside, Harbinson, & McKeown, 2012; Song & Kang, 2017).

TABLE 14.8 Mind–Body Therapies

CAM Modality	Evidence
Exercise and relaxation	■ Two randomized controlled quantitative/qualitative studies (RCT; $n = 95$, $n = 57$) of U.S. veterans with moderately severe HF showed significant improvement in QOL measures/reported emotional improvement after participating in relaxation response interventions (Chang et al., 2004, 2005). ■ Two RCTs of older Chinese HF patients ($n = 121$, $n = 59$) examined effects of relaxation therapy and found significant improvement in psychological well-being compared to the control group (Yu, Lee, Woo, & Hui, 2007; Yu, Lee, & Woo, 2010).
Meditation	■ RCT ($n = 19$) of older patients with HF showed significant improvement in the QOL and improved measurements on cardiopulmonary exercise testing (Curiati et al., 2005). ■ Clinical trial ($n = 23$) of older African American patients with HF found improved QOL and measurements on cardiopulmonary exercise testing (Jayadevappa et al., 2007). ■ Systematic review of relaxation, meditation, and guided imagery strategies for symptom management in HF report that the quality of studies vary and findings are mixed, but data indicates a potential benefit (Kwekkeboom & Bratke, 2016).
Acupuncture	■ RCT ($n = 17$) of stable HF Class II to III patients found no improvement in cardiac ejection fraction or peak oxygen uptake, but significant improvement in the 6-min walk test and postexercise recovery (Kristen et al., 2010).
Yoga	■ RCT ($n = 40$) of predominantly African American HF patients showed significant improvement in flexibility, treadmill time, VO$_2$ peak, and inflammatory biomarkers compared to controls, and in posttest versus pretest scores (Pullen et al., 2010). ■ RCT ($n = 19$) of Class I to II HF patients showed significantly improved exercise tolerance and inflammatory biomarkers, with a trend toward improvement in QOL (Pullen et al., 2008).

Tai chi/qi gong	■ Systematic review of tai chi (TC) exercise effectiveness for individuals with heart disease summarized evidence of effectiveness in heart disease from three studies (Ng et al., 2012).
	  – *Evidence suggests TC exercise may improve perceived symptoms, mood, and QOL*
	  – *Evidence suggests improvement in EF and BNP*
	  – *Mixed results found an effect on exercise capacity and inflammatory biomarker levels*
	  – *One study demonstrated improvement in sleep stability (Yeh, Wayne, & Phillips, 2008)*
	■ RCT ($n = 100$) of NYHA Class I to II HF outpatients found TC patients showed significant improvement in QOL, exercise self-efficacy, and mood. However, there were no differences in 6-min walk distance or peak O$_2$ uptake (Yeh et al., 2011).
	■ Clinical trial ($n = 28$) found TC reduced somatic subscore on a depression scale but did not significantly reduce fatigue (Redwine et al., 2012).

CAM, complementary and alternative medicine; HF, heart failure; NYHA, New York Heart Association; QOL, quality of life; RCT, randomized controlled trial.

■ EXPERIMENTAL TREATMENTS

Cardiovascular Regeneration and Cell-Based Therapies

Regeneration of myocardial cells and activation of myocardial stem cells to replace infarcted myocardial cells has the potential for a positive effect on HF patients but is in the experimental stages (Le, Thavapalachandran, Kizana, & Chong, 2017). Major advancements over the past decade have occurred in investigating the mechanisms of action and the clinical application of cell-based therapy for ischemic heart disease. This field is evolving rapidly and large numbers of studies are testing a variety of cell sources, delivery methods, and patient characteristics. These therapies show incredible promise as a treatment to prevent or reverse myocardial remodeling and to promote cell regeneration in the future (Behfar, Crespo-Diaz, Terzic, & Gersh, 2014).

Xenotransplantation

In the future, this may become a therapeutic option for those people dying each year of heart, kidney, lung, and liver failure. Xenotransplantation involves the transplantation of nonhuman tissues or organs into human recipients. Xenotransplantation between closely related species, such as baboons or pigs and humans, offers an alternative to allotransplantation as a source of human organ replacement, but problems with rejection remain a major concern (Ekser & Cooper, 2008).

TABLE 14.9 Natural Products

CAM Modality	Evidence
Dietary supplements	■ Systematic review of evidence on studies of micronutrients and HF (McKeag et al., 2012): – *Selenium, zinc, and copper*—Evidence that patients with HF have lower levels of circulating selenium and zinc and higher levels of copper. Higher selenium levels were associated with O_2 uptake in bicycle stress test. – *Vitamins A, C, or E*—No conclusive evidence they are related to improved outcomes in HF. – *B vitamins: Thiamine, riboflavin, pyridoxine, B12, and folate*—Inconclusive evidence on the role of these in HF. – *Vitamin D* ■ Evidence that HF patients have lower circulating levels of vitamin D than those without. ■ Observational study evidence of a relationship between vitamin D status and prevalence and incidence of HF; possible relationship between vitamin D and physical function in HF; possible relationship between vitamin D and prognosis in HF. ■ Intervention study evidence that higher level of vitamin D supplementation is associated with significant increase in levels of IL-10. ■ Caution that vitamin D supplementation up to 10k units daily is not associated with toxicity, while hypercalcemia and other toxic effects are commonly associated with doses of 50k units or more daily.
Herbs and botanicals	*Crategus* spp. (common name: Hawthorn) ■ Cochrane systematic review of 10 double-blind RCTs ($n = 855$) using extract of Hawthorn flower or leaf as an adjuvant therapy to treat patients with NYHA Class I to III HF (Pittler, Guo, & Ernst, 2008) found that compared to controls. – Exercise tolerance significantly increased – Maximal workload improved – Decreased cardiac oxygen consumption observed – Symptoms of shortness of breath and fatigue significantly improved – Adverse events were infrequent, mild, and transient and included dizziness, nausea, and cardiac and GI complaints ■ Systematic review of 24 studies ($n = 5,577$) with dosage ranging from 160 to 1,800 mg taken over 3–24 weeks found a total of 166 AEs reported. Most were mild to moderate including dizziness, nausea, headache, migraine, palpitation, and GI complaints. Eight involving use of the extract LI132 were severe: GI hemorrhage (2), circulation failure (2), erythematous rash (2), and fall (2) (Daniele, Mazzanti, Pittler, & Ernst, 2006). ■ Clinical implications of potential interactions: Since clinical trials have shown Hawthorn causes a slight reduction in BP in patients with heart conditions, monitor use in conjunction with antihypertensives. Contains OPCs, which could theoretically reduce absorption of alkaloids and alkaline drugs—take 2 hours away from medication (Mills & Bone, 2005).
Traditional medicine formulations	■ Cochrane systematic review updated in 2012 included nine RCTs ($n = 600$; Chen, Yao, Chen, Kwong, & Chen, 2012). – Seven of the studies compared Shengmai, a traditional Chinese herbal medication, with standard treatment to standard treatment alone; three studies compared Shengmai to placebo (one did both). – The seven trials reported significant improvement in patients taking Shengmai as opposed to those with standard treatment alone using various outcome measures. – Three RCTs likewise reported significant improvement in patients taking Shengmai as opposed to controls using various outcome measures. – Evidence lacks strength due to poor study quality, small sample sizes, and lack of comparability of outcome measures. – Mild AEs were reported in six patients from three of the studies, generally in the higher dosage cohorts (60 mL/d). They included dry mouth and fidgety (2), mild sleep disorder (2), stomach discomfort, and hypoglycemia (2).

AEs, adverse effects; BP, blood pressure; CAM, complementary and alternative medicine; GI, gastrointestinal; HF, heart failure; IL-10, interleukin 10; NYHA, New York Heart Association; OPCs, oligomeric procyanidins; RCT, randomized controlled trial.

Device Therapies in Heart Failure

Because pharmacologic agents alone rarely improved QOL and prognosis, especially in those with chronic ventricular dysfunction, device therapies are options in HF. These therapies include biventricular pacing, implantable cardioverter defibrillators (ICDs), and LV assist devices (LVAD).

Biventricular Pacing or Cardiac Resynchronization Therapy

Since the early 1990s, there have been numerous approaches to improve LV function in patients with HF by means of cardiac pacing. In the last 10 years, the most promising of these approaches has been biventricular pacing, or cardiac resynchronization therapy (CRT).

Normally, electrical impulses arise in the sinoatrial node of the heart, travel down through the atrioventricular node, to the bundle of His, through the left and the right bundle branches to the Purkinje fibers, where simultaneous depolarization of the atrium and the ventricles occurs. This coordinated conduction enables stroke volume to be maximized. If one or more of these conduction pathways (left bundle or right bundle) is damaged or blocked, the impulse will reach one ventricle before the other, causing asynchrony of the ventricular contraction. When this occurs, it is called intraventricular conduction defect (IVCD). This can be seen in the QRS (measurement of time for ventricular depolarization) of the EKG, which becomes prolonged: more than 120 ms. IVCD has been found in 30% to 50% of patients with HF (Saxon et al., 1999). These conduction delays cause inefficient ventricular contraction, with segments of the ventricle contracting at different times. Short diastole occurs with overlapping of systole and diastole and cardiac output decreases. If the patient already has a failing left ventricle, this dyssynchrony with decrease in cardiac output leads to further dysfunction and increased symptoms.

The biventricular pacemaker looks like other pacemakers, but it has three leads instead of two. Electrical leads are threaded to both the left and the right ventricle, as well as the right atrium. This device provides electrical stimulation that is programmed precisely to synchronize and coordinate the right and left ventricular contraction.

Evidence of the use of biventricular pacing with HF patients in large-series clinical trials has been found in the COMPANION, MUSTIC, and REVERSE trials (Daubert et al., 2009), and the efficacy of this treatment has been well documented (Cleland et al., 2005; Young et al., 2003). Most patients in these trials had NYHA Class II to IV HF and prolonged QRS duration (greater than 150 ms) and were on optimum medical therapy (Saxon et al., 1999). Primary endpoints for these trials were 6-minute walk tests, QOL, and O_2 consumption at peak exercise (Cazeau et al., 2002). Consistently, it was found that there was an almost immediate increase in cardiac output, a positive effect on LV remodeling, and an improvement in diastolic function.

Implantable Cardiac Defibrillators and Cardiac Resynchronization Therapy in Combination

Sudden death occurs in 30% to 59% of patients in NYHA Class IV (Cazeau et al., 2002). Because of these alarming statistics, the role of combining implantable cardiac defibrillators (ICDs) and CRT devices in chronic HF patients has been investigated. ICD implantation is a lifesaving option for the patient who has a substrate for sudden cardiac death due to lethal ventricular arrhythmia. In the VENTAK CHF, Insync ICD, and COMPANION MADIT-CRT and MIRACLE ICD trials, both of these devices were investigated (Barsheshet et al., 2011; Dresing & Natale, 2001; Young et al., 2003). The results of these studies in primary reports have indicated an improvement in symptoms, increased QOL, and decreased incidence of sudden death. The efficacy of biventricular pacing and ICDs in patients with HF and IVCDs in the general HF population is now a proven therapy and a lifesaving device in those patients who meet criteria for placement. However, ICDs and/or CRTs are considered of uncertain benefit to patients with advanced frailty, multiple comorbid conditions, and high risk for nonsudden death as are usually seen in PC settings (Yancy et al., 2013).

Left Ventricular Assist Devices

These mechanical devices are percutaneous or implanted into the abdomen or chest of the recipient. LVADs are attached to a weakened heart to assist with pumping. LVADs were first used as a bridge therapy to help keep heart transplant candidates alive while they waited for a donor heart. LVADs are now considered as destination therapy or an alternative to transplantation. Implanted heart pumps can significantly extend and improve the lives of some people with end-stage HF who are not eligible for or able to undergo heart transplantation. There is now evidence that mechanical circulatory support, such as LVADs, is considered reasonable in carefully vetted end-stage HF patients to improve survival, functional capacity, and QOL (Yancy et al., 2013). The Randomized Evaluation of Mechanical Assistance for the Treatment of Congestive Heart Failure (REMATCH) trial evaluated the survival benefit of this implanted left heart pumping device after 2 years and found that there was significantly more improvement in QOL than in those patients who were receiving optimal medical therapy (52% vs. 25%; Stevenson et al., 2004). The REMATCH trial evaluated the LVADs that used older pulsatile technology. There are serious side effects of LVAD device use, which include infection, bleeding, and stroke. Pulsatile LVADs have been replaced by continuous flow technology, either axial or centrifugal flow. Studies of the newer models are being conducted for safety and efficacy in advanced HF patients with a particular focus on the incidence of stroke and death. ENDURANCE and MOMENTUM3 are two large-scale trials conducted to evaluate the two types of continuous flow devices (centrifugal vs. axial) in advanced HF patients. The primary outcome in the ENDURANCE trial was the survival from disabling stroke or device removal for malfunction or failure. The researchers found that the centrifugal device was noninferior to the axial flow device (Rogers et al., 2017). In the MOMENTUM3 study, there were also no differences in death or disabling stroke when comparing the two types of devices, but reoperation for pump malfunction was higher in the axial flow device (Mehra et al., 2017). LVAD implantation is generally not recommended for use in PC, but it is required by CMS that all LVAD recipients be referred to PC for symptom management and decision-making support (Swetz et al., 2011).

Evidence for Heart Failure Management

The evidence in the literature is robust regarding the management of HF patients. There are multiple meta-analyses, considered the strongest evidence, describing effective HF systems of care, treatment recommendations, and communication principles. Included in Table 14.10 is a selection of HF meta-analyses.

In addition to the meta-analyses, there are many evidence-based clinical trials as to the appropriate treatment of end-stage HF: COACH, I-, CHARM, TOPCAT, PARADIGM-HF, PREVENT-HF, OptiLink, DOSE, trials, and OPTIMIZE-HF and ADHERE registries. Information on these clinical trials can be accessed from the Internet by searching for the name of the particular trial. The most recent clinical trials can be accessed on www.clinicaltrials.gov. When reviewing the evidence from these clinical trials, remember to assess the patient sample. Ask whether the clinical trial sample is reflective of the HF population in your practice. While it is important to keep up with the current state of the HF science, there are also structured guidelines that have been developed

and are updated regularly from the strongest clinical trials (Ponikowski et al., 2016). HF care, unlike some other conditions, is guideline driven.

Acute Decompensated Heart Failure Management

Guidelines are lacking for the management of acute decompensated HF (ADHF), so therapy is based on the best available clinical research and expert consensus. When patients develop signs and symptoms of HF, they often need to be hospitalized. Hospitalization is typical when a patient is first diagnosed with HF. However, readmission of patients who already have been diagnosed with HF is extremely common, usually due to fluid overload. Many of these rehospitalizations are preventable through close outpatient follow-up and self-care. Changes in hospital reimbursement guidelines have made this a critical issue. Earlier referral to PC is one solution to the burgeoning problem of repeat HF admissions.

The primary goal for HF-related hospitalization is to relieve symptoms, particularly congestion. Determining the etiology of the HF and EF will help determine what therapies are initiated. Another key goal while in the hospital is to identify and address precipitating factors for

TABLE 14.10 Select Heart Failure Meta-Analyses

Meta-Analysis Topic	Citation	Findings
Palliative care interventions for patients with heart failure	Diop, Rudolph, Zimmerman, Richter, and Skarf (2017)	n = 15 prospective, 10 retrospective studies; home- and team-based palliative interventions for HF patients improve patient-centered outcomes, documentation of preferences, and utilization. Need for better quality studies.
Heart rate and rhythm and benefits of beta blockers	Kotecha et al. (2017)	n = 11 RCTs; beta blockers reduce mortality in HFrEF regardless of pretreatment rate for those in sinus rhythm, but there was no mortality effect for those with atrial fibrillation.
Self-management interventions efficacy in HF	Jonkman et al. (2016)	n = 20 RCTs; self-management interventions had a beneficial effect on all-cause death and HF-related hospitalization and a small increase in HF-related quality of life; increased mortality in depressed patients warrants caution in applying self-management strategies in these patients.
Preventing HF hospital readmission	Benbassat and Taragin (2013)	n = 99 systematic reviews of RCTs; disease management programs significantly reduce hospital readmissions.
Effectiveness of disease management in HF	Takeda et al. (2012)	n = 25 RCTs; case management nurses reduce mortality and readmission rates.
Efficacy of BNP-guided therapy	Li, Luo, and Chen (2013)	n = 11 RCTs; BNP-guided therapy reduces mortality and rehospitalization, particularly in younger or higher BNP patients.
Efficacy of different beta blockers in reduced ejection fraction HF	Chatterjee et al. (2013)	n = 21 RCTs; beta blockers provide mortality benefits as a class effect, no superiority of a single agent over another.

BNP, brain natriuretic peptide; HF, heart failure; HFrEF, heart failure with reduced ejection fraction; RCT, randomized controlled trial.

the decompensation such as poor adherence to medications or diet and fluid recommendations, poor social support or financial resources, lack of self-care education, or inadequate medical regimen prior to admission, as well as medical conditions such as atrial fibrillation, worsening renal function, HTN, or ischemia (Gheorghiade, Vaduganathan, Fonarow, & Bonow, 2013; Ziaeian & Fonarow, 2016).

The majority of patients are admitted due to fluid overload resulting in symptoms such as dyspnea, orthopnea, weight gain, or edema. Initially, these are treated with IV loop diuretics with the goal of getting the patient back to his or her "dry weight." Most patients respond to standard IV diuretics and transition to oral diuretics, but for those patients with chronic HF and cardiorenal syndrome, other therapies may be needed such as ultrafiltration. Ultrafiltration is a mechanical strategy developed to affect diuresis in patients unresponsive to pharmacologic diuresis. It involves the movement of water and solutes across a semipermeable membrane from higher to lower concentration. Ultrafiltration in refractory HF is considered a reasonable alternative; however, a nephrologist should be consulted prior to implementation (Yancy et al., 2013). The efficacy of ultrafiltration in HF with renal impairment, a common comorbidity with HF, has not been established and there may be significant deterioration in renal function and more adverse events (Bart et al., 2012; Raichlin et al., 2013).

Many episodes of ADHF are precipitated by new cardiac events or other medical conditions. Identification and treatment of these events is paramount such as rate and/or rhythm control in atrial fibrillation, controlling HTN, and determining if a patient is ischemic. The number one cause for developing HF is CAD, so if this is the first presentation of HF, ruling out CAD is essential. If the patient has evidence of ischemia, revascularization with percutaneous coronary intervention may improve symptoms, prevent further hospitalizations, and have a survival benefit (Lindenfeld et al., 2010).

If the patient exhibits low perfusion HF, this is a more complicated picture and will require more advanced therapies such as inotropes or mechanical support. However, most patients admitted with HF are perfusing well and may even be hypertensive. Once the newly diagnosed HF patient is euvolemic and decongested, oral evidence-based medications can be started and doses optimized. While in the hospital, the patient should also be evaluated for further advanced therapies such as device therapy—if this is consistent with his or her goals of care.

The discharge process starts early in the hospitalization. To prepare patients and families for HF self-care, the acronym DAMES highlights areas of needed education:

Diet and fluid recommendations
Activity/work recommendations
Medications education
Everyday weights
Symptoms to monitor and how to manage if they occur

Instilling the importance of adherence to the treatment plan and to follow up with a practitioner within 7 to 10 days of discharge is the standard of care. Patients admitted to the hospital with HF are at a high risk for readmission. There are various determinants that influence engagement in patient self-care and caregiver support in HF that must be considered during discharge planning. These determinants include the presence of impaired activity of daily living, comorbid burden, impaired cognition, depression, sleep impairment, and high symptom burden. Other factors that will influence self-care and support are HF duration, QOL, relationship quality and role, and hospitalizations (Bidwell et al., 2015). Consider, where possible, a referral to a formal HF disease management program where much time and effort is spent on preventing readmissions.

Disease Management Programs

Disease management is increasing the use of evidence-based therapies to improve patient education and decrease readmissions. Postdischarge interventions have been identified by multiple studies as being imperative for HF patients. These interventions include clinical follow-up with a nurse practitioner under the supervision of cardiology or a primary care physician, home nursing follow-up, or a telephone follow-up with a nurse practitioner or specialized registered nurses (Takeda et al., 2012). It is suggested that algorithms, tables, development of "pocket cards," HF preprinted discharge sheets, and systematic use of guideline summaries be developed to help nurses to manage HF patients so that the practice is more uniform and effective. The American Association of Heart Failure Nurses (AAHFN) website (www.aahfn .org) is a good resource for this information and tools.

Team-Based Care in Heart Failure

Nurses are active in the planning and management of care of HF patients. Care that is collaborative, often nurse directed, and in many areas multidisciplinary is available in HF clinics. The optimal treatment for patients with HF involves considerably more than prescribing the right medicine. It requires the full support of the patient and family, working with the healthcare team, to manage his or her HF. The main reasons for rehospitalization are the discontinuation of prescribed medications, dietary indiscretions, and the failure to identify early signs of worsening HF.

Care provided by specialists or board-certified HF nurses in outpatient clinics has been shown to improve outcomes for patients, significantly reducing the number of unplanned readmissions (Takeda et al., 2012). As part of the interprofessional integrated team, nurses, dieticians, social workers, pastoral care, physical therapists, occupational therapists, case managers, pharmacists, and physicians must take part in a coordinated approach in counseling and educating patients and families with end-stage heart disease. A consistent plan of care should be maintained across all settings of care.

Palliative Care Guidelines

There is a common misperception that disease management and PC are synonymous types of care (Buck & Zambroski, 2012). Disease management, while evidence based, does not include all of the domains identified in quality care for people with life-limiting conditions such as HF. For example, the psychological and psychiatric, social, spiritual, religious, and existential cultural aspects of care and care of the patient at the end of life are not addressed in the scientific statement from the AHA disease management taxonomy writing group (Krumholz et al., 2006). Disease management is currently defined as a system of care that coordinates medical interventions, including communication, for populations with chronic disease. The focus of disease management is on supporting clinician/patient dyads, practicing evidence-based medicine, empowering patients, and evaluating outcomes (Krumholz et al., 2006). PC is not just a system of care; it is a philosophy of care, which focuses on anticipating, preventing, and alleviating suffering, and improving QOL for patients and families (National Consensus Project for Quality Palliative Care, 2013). For optimal HF management, PC should be offered simultaneously with disease-oriented care.

While disease management and PC are not synonymous, PC and hospice care are also not synonymous. Hospice care is one type of PC that is delivered at the end of life. When it is time for hospice care, criterion from the National Hospice and Palliative Care Organization can help in determining when a patient is appropriate for hospice. In addition to the general hospice referral criteria, there are criteria specific to heart disease patients; these include the following:

- Intractable or recurrent symptoms of HF
- Optimal medical treatment for HF should be in place
- Presence of symptomatic arrhythmias
- History of cardiac arrest and resuscitation or syncope
- Cardiogenic brain embolism
- Co-occurring HIV disease

For those patients covered by the hospice benefit, an advanced practice clinician must manage their care and certify that they are expected to survive 6 months or less. It is hard to predict who is at the end of life in HF because the trajectory of HF is so uncertain and deterioration can be rapid and sudden. Therefore, to deliver high-quality, comprehensive care, the nurse needs to blend aspects from both PC and disease management with all HF patients. Patients should receive evidence-based treatments in a holistic framework that addresses every part of their life—not just their HF (Fahlberg, Donoho, Paire, & Davidson, 2011; Whellan et al., 2014).

The evidence-based management of HF has improved considerably over the last 10 years, but those who will eventually die from this condition are first and foremost in need of respectful and comprehensive PC. Consensus statements and guidelines have addressed the need and can be used as benchmarks for PC of the HF patient (Fang et al., 2015; Whellan et al., 2014; Yancy et al., 2013). The EOL considerations in these documents are as follows:

1. Ongoing patient and family education should include discussion of prognosis
2. Patient and family discussions regarding advanced directives and the role of palliative and hospice care should occur
3. There should be discussion of the option of deactivating implantable assistive devices
4. Continuity of medical care between inpatient and outpatient settings should be ensured
5. Components of hospice care should include opiate use, inotropes, and IV diuretics
6. All professionals should examine current EOL processes and work toward improvement of approaches to PC
7. Aggressive procedures performed in the final days of life are not appropriate

Although hospice and palliative care are recommended options for patients with HF, the use of these services is not optimal. The number of patients who are referred to hospice is relatively small. In a retrospective review of approximately 300,000 Medicare beneficiaries with HF, while overall hospice use increased between 2000 and 2007, the percentage of HF patients with short stays (less than 3 days) remained steady at 19%. Approximately 37% of HF patients had stays of less than 7 days, demonstrating the need for more timely hospice referrals in this population (Unroe et al., 2011). A cross-sectional analysis was conducted to evaluate trends in PC use in patients over 70 years old with severe HF. Data was retrieved from the Veterans Affair Healthcare System over a 7-year period (2007–2013). The researchers found that only 7.6% (338 of 4,474) patients with severe HF were seen by PC. Of those 338 patients, 72.8% (246 of 338) died within 1 year. Additionally, of the total 4,474 with severe HF, more than half (51.2%) died within 1 year of hospitalization (Mandawat, Heidenreich, Mandawat, & Bhatt, 2016). One limitation of this study was the predominance of male population. Robinson, Al-Kindi, and Oliveira (2017) found similar results in PC use in a larger cohort of nonveterans of both sexes. Data was retrieved from Explorys, which is a large clinical registry of 50 million patients from inpatient and outpatient settings at 360 hospitals in the United States. Of the 37,270 patients over 70 with severe HF, only 9.6% (3,590) were seen by PC within 1 year. The findings from these studies indicate the need for increased incorporation of PC into HF care.

There are various gaps in the research pertaining to the delivery of palliative (non-hospice) care for patients with HF. Gelfman, Bakitas, Warner Stevenson, Kirkpatrick, and Goldstein (2017) identified four key areas that are research priorities pertaining to PC in HF: (1) to better understand advanced HF patients' limiting symptoms and focus treatment on their relief; (2) to better characterize and address the needs of caregivers of advanced HF patients' limiting symptoms and focus treatment on their relief; (3) to improve patient and family understanding of the HF disease trajectory and the importance of advance care planning; and (4) to determine the best models of PC, including models for those who want to continue life-prolonging therapies.

Communication

Providers need to be aware that many patients die before Stage D (advanced) HF occurs and HF deterioration can progress suddenly and unpredictably (Whellan et al., 2014). Therefore, discussions about prognosis and care preferences should begin early in the disease process. It is too late to discuss PC and EOL wishes when the patient is near death. As with all patients at this stage of life, ongoing communication is the key in achieving the goal of dying well. Communication skills needed for the discussions necessary are often lacking in healthcare education. Providers who work with HF patients may feel poorly prepared or uncomfortable having these conversations. Care philosophies of providers often impact the decisions they make, determining options offered to patients and families, and whether palliative approaches to care are utilized (Low, Pattenden, Candy, Beattie, & Jones, 2011). Confounding the discussions regarding PC and EOL are the very interventions that relieve symptoms also prolong life (Gelfman et al., 2017; Psotka, McKee, Liu, Elia, & De Marco, 2017). In a descriptive and comparative study conducted in Sweden, researchers evaluated how often and why nurses in outpatient HF clinics discussed prognosis and EOL care. The researchers found that these topics were not routinely discussed. The reasons the nurses gave for not discussing prognosis and EOL topics were clinical routines dictated that these topics were to be discussed only when a patient was in an advanced stage or was deteriorating. Other reasons for not discussing these topics included the patient's situation, which meant that the nurses felt that other matters such as self-care and medications were more important than EOL discussions. Nurses also felt that these topics were not part of their role and were best discussed or initiated by physicians (Hjelmfors et al., 2015).

Most patients are aware they are dying and appreciate the discussion of their death. Many patients are not aware of the choices they have and can make. When patients reach the place where they want and need to discuss their wishes for their end of life, they often depend on their healthcare provider to initiate the conversation. These discussions need to happen before the patients become too ill to participate because these decisions impact not only their own lives but also the lives of their loved ones. Healthcare providers rarely raise these issues for fear of "decreasing hope" or increasing anxiety.

Shared Decision Making

The AHA released a recent scientific statement on shared decision making (Allen et al., 2012). In this important document, high-quality decisions involve medically reasonable care options, which align with the values, goals, and preferences of an informed patient. Decision making is seen as an iterative process that allows for change over time. Over the course of a person's illness, advanced therapies such as a pacemaker, ICD, LVAD, heart transplantation, or transcatheter aortic-valve implantation may be discussed. Surgical or interventional revascularization options may be appropriate when patients experience new cardiac events, if these are in keeping with the patient's goals of care. Shared decision making involving a trusted clinician will help ensure that the patient's goals and wishes match proposed therapies. It is recommended that HF patients and their clinicians have yearly "HF review" conversations to discuss concerns and preferences about therapies, potential adverse events, current symptom burden, changes in functional status, QOL, and caregiver burden.

Symptom Management

Aggressive symptom management is a hallmark of quality PC. The four most prevalent symptoms in HF are dyspnea, pain, depression, and fatigue (Adler, Goldfinger, Kalman, Park, & Meier, 2009). In addition to depression, anxiety may occur. Gastrointestinal symptoms can include nausea, anorexia, and constipation. Other systemic symptoms that can occur are weakness, edema, and sleep disorders. Cough is another symptom in advanced HF (Whellan et al., 2014). The strongest evidence for managing dyspnea supports the use of ACEI, ARBs with or without neprilysin and mineralocorticoid antagonists (spironolactone). Digoxin and intravenous inotropic infusion may provide relief of symptoms when other therapies have been maximized. If edema is present, loop diuretics with or without thiazides, along with dietary salt and fluid restriction, are recommended. The source of cough should be evaluated and managed based on the cause; for example, if ACEI is the source of the cough, switch to an ARB or ARNI. If fluid overload is the source of the cough, then diuresis is warranted. Pain management involves assessing the source of pain and treating according to the source. The strongest evidence is the use of opioids for general pain and bisphosphonates for bone pain as NSAIDs are contraindicated due to their potential to worsen HF and renal failure. Nitrates, BBs, and vasoselective calcium channel blockers such as amlodipine, ranolazine, and coronary revascularization should be used for anginal pain. Depression and anxiety can be managed by selective serotonin reuptake inhibitors (SSRIs), which have the most evidence to support their safety and efficacy in advanced HF. Other alternative agents that have been identified as safe in HF are bupropion, mirtazapine, venlafaxine, and duloxetine (Harris & Heil, 2013). The SSRIs can induce fluid retention and hyponatremia, and therefore, patients should be started on low doses and carefully monitored. At this time, there isn't strong evidence for the treatment of fatigue and weakness, but exercise can be encouraged in those who can. Optimizing the management for other causes of fatigue such as anemia, infection, sleep disorders, and deconditioning is recommended. There is a divergence of opinion on the usefulness of treating fatigue with stimulants, especially if the etiology is ischemia or CAD (Whellan et al., 2014). Management of anorexia and nausea is complex as treatments such as megesterol have significant side effects and appetite supplements are of unproven benefit in HF. A thorough review of potential offending agents should be conducted and a determination of their necessity evaluated (e.g., aspirin). Constipation can be managed with high-fiber diet foods and laxatives. Additional strategies to consider that could relieve multiple symptoms such as dyspnea, pain, fatigue, and depression are physical therapy, mindfulness training, and cognitive behavioral therapy (Psotka et al., 2017). Use of fans and beds that allow head elevation are environmental adaptations that could also alleviate dyspnea.

Deactivation of Devices in Heart Failure

Cardiologists who implant devices rarely discuss EOL issues or device deactivation at the time of implantation (Barclay, Momen, Case-Upton, Kuhn, & Smith, 2011). The American Academy of Hospice and Palliative Medicine recommends that the status of the device (whether activated or deactivated) should be consistent with patient and family goals of care. The ACC has issued guidelines related to deactivation of device-based therapies (Epstein et al., 2008). These deactivation guidelines state the following:

■ Patients or surrogate decision makers should be fully informed of the consequences to deactivation and offered alternatives.
■ An order for a do not resuscitate (DNR) should accompany the deactivation.
■ Psychiatric and ethics consultations should be arranged in the setting of impaired decision making or disagreement.
■ If the clinician has personal beliefs that prohibit deactivation, the patient should be referred to another clinician.
■ Deactivation can occur at the implanting center or a local site at the patient's request.

■ Implanting clinicians should encourage, at the time of the implantation, the completion of advanced directives, which include device management and deactivation at end of life. The Heart Rhythm Society (HRS) in collaboration with five other national and international EOL or cardiology societies issued an expert consensus statement guideline related to the deactivation of device-based therapies for those requesting withdrawal and/or the end of life (Lampert et al., 2010). The HRS consensus statement also discusses the ethical, legal, religious, and procedural issues surrounding the deactivation of cardiac devices in patients nearing the end of life or who were requesting withdrawal of therapy.

Concurrent Care With Disease Management

Concurrent care is a care delivery model where the patient receives standard HF care while also being followed closely by a PC clinician (Maloney et al., 2013). This model is borrowed from oncology, where patients are routinely referred to PC while still in active treatment, particularly if there is need for symptom management and decision-making support. A recent HF chart review assessing the reasons for PC consultations was conducted at a large healthcare system with almost 4,000 PC consultations (inpatient and outpatient) per year. This review of the electronic medical record showed that 80% of palliative consultations were for goals of care conversations, followed by decision making and hospice referral/discussion (Bakitas et al., 2013). These numbers support the idea that there is a need for a concurrent model of care.

In the concurrent care model, HF medications, discussed earlier in this chapter, can continue as they are palliative in scope. But frequent review of medications is important to determine their continued necessity and effects on symptoms and QOL. Medications that can potentially be discontinued as EOL approaches are statins, digoxin (digitoxicity increases as renal function decreases), and anticoagulation and antiplatelet therapy. Furthermore, if the patient has symptomatic hypotension, ACEI, ARBs, and other antihypertensives may need to be stopped. If the patient is in fluid overload, the BB should be tapered. Diuretics are often a key to symptom management in HF requiring careful titration based on daily weights and symptoms/signs of fluid overload, while avoiding dehydration and orthostatic hypotension. Many patients and families find additional "as needed" dosing of furosemide to be useful, allowing the patient more dietary choices during this time when appetite is often limited. Depression is common and normal during this time and should be treated. SSRI are usually well tolerated and improve QOL. The defibrillator function of an ICD may be turned off during this period, but this option should be addressed early in the disease process and agreed upon by the patient, family, and healthcare provider. This needs to be included in advance directives.

PC has now been widely accepted and incorporated in the care of the HF population. Nurses play a key role in the delivery of PC and need to take advantage of the findings of these studies and discuss them with patients. Oncology nurses are a great role model for integrating PC, and their models should be emulated by those who care for HF patients. Nurses' efforts should begin with becoming knowledgeable about PC and remaining current of all the nursing interventions that are evidence based so that they are reflected in standards of care. There is a wealth of information available in resources such as the End-of-Life Nursing Education Consortium (ELNEC) and the National Hospice and Palliative Care Organization.

■ OLDER ADULTS AND HEART FAILURE

There can be many adverse reactions to cardiovascular therapies when used in the older adult population. Physiologically, changes in the metabolism and excretion of drugs occur with age, including a decrease in the glomerular filtration and tubular secretion. Cardiac medications that are dependent on the kidney for excretion should be titrated appropriately; digoxin and ACEI are those that fit into this category. The hepatic metabolism of drugs also decreases with age. The commonly used medications for relief of symptoms in HF can therefore have a delayed absorption that can be variable in the older patient. Careful dosing and titration of these drugs on an individual basis is imperative.

General Pharmacologic Recommendations for Older Adults

The following recommendations should be considered when prescribing cardiac medications for older adults:

1. Start low and go slow. Always begin with the smallest effective dose; titrate up in small increments, keeping in mind the patient's comorbid conditions that could influence the pharmacokinetics of the drug(s).
2. As dose adjustment is made, clinical evaluation should occur.
3. Review each medication the patient is currently taking, even OTC medications and herbal remedies, and be aware of contraindications or adjustments needed.
4. Avoid empiric treatment of symptoms. Have a diagnosis before initiating drug therapy.
5. Keep it simple! Adherence decreases as the number of medications and frequency of dosing increases.
6. Make sure that the patient can read the labels; if not, a family member or home care nurse should set up

a weekly pill dispenser. Patients can also have large print labels on their prescription bottles.
7. Patient education is key. Make sure that each patient understands the adverse reactions to watch for and knows when to call for assistance.

Specific Pharmacologic Recommendations for Older Adults

Health practitioners should be familiar with the cardiovascular recommendations for older adults by the American Geriatrics Society (American Geriatrics Society 2015 Beers Criteria Update Expert Panel, 2015). The following recommendations should be considered when prescribing cardiac medications for older adults:

1. Alpha blockers, such as doxazosin, prazosin, and terazosin, should be avoided as antihypertensives. They create a high risk for orthostatic hypotension.
2. Central alpha agonists, such as clonidine, reserpine (greater than 0.1 mg/d), and methyldopa, should be avoided as antihypertensives. They create a high risk for adverse central nervous system (CNS) effects, bradyarrhythmias, and orthostatic hypotension.
3. Class Ia, Ic, and III antiarrhythmic drugs, such as procainamide and quinidine, should be avoided. They have been associated with multiple toxicities. Rate control is recommended over rhythm control for older adults. Avoid Amiodarone as a first-line treatment for atrial fibrillation (AF) unless there is concomitant HF and if rhythm control is preferred over rate control.
4. Disopyramide is a potent negative inotrope in older adults and should be used with caution as it may induce HF.
5. Dronedarone is to be avoided in patients with HF.
6. Avoid digoxin (greater than 0.125 mg/d). Higher doses increase the risk of toxicity in the presence of slow renal clearance common in older adults.
7. Avoid nifedipine (immediate release). Increases the risk of hypotension or myocardial ischemia
8. Avoid spironolactone greater than 25 mg/d. Risk of hyperkalemia. Avoid in CrCl less than 30 mL/min
9. Antithrombotic dipyridamole (oral short acting) should be avoided due to the risk for orthostatic hypotension. Extended release with aspirin is acceptable.

The AHA scientific statement on drugs that can cause or exacerbate AHA (2016) should also be reviewed when evaluating drug therapy in HF patients regardless of age.

Nonpharmacologic Recommendations

For older adults (as well as those younger than 65), aggressive use of the nonpharmacologic measures is imperative. Drug therapy can often cause unpleasant side effects, which often lead to nonadherence, and are costly now that Medicare D plans are in place. General measures are recommended as follows:

1. Decreasing more or new cardiac injury by risk factor reduction
2. Limiting alcohol use to two glasses/d for men and one glass/d for women
3. Maintaining fluid balance by restricted salt intake (2 g/d)
4. Improving physical conditioning
5. Careful management of comorbid conditions
6. Patient education regarding self-care
7. Smoking cessation when appropriate
8. Influenza vaccination every fall
9. Pneumococcal immunizations: 13 valent pneumococcal conjugate vaccine (PCV13) and 23 valent pneumococcal polysaccharide vaccine (PPSV23). Review latest Centers for Disease Control vaccine administration guidelines.
10. Care of patients with HF across settings and by interprofessional teams
11. Careful monitoring of fluid status

■ CONCLUSION

In caring for the patient with advanced HF, there are clinical, evidence-based therapies that should drive clinical decision making. Hopefully, this chapter has helped the reader to understand the disease of HF: how important disease management is, how nurse-based HF interventions can lead to positive outcomes, and, most importantly, how to communicate with patients and families regarding their treatment options and what is important to them in the final phase of their life.

■ HELPFUL RESOURCES AND WEBSITES REGARDING HEART FAILURE

1. AHA (www.heart.org)
   - Very helpful in assessing data regarding statistics, patient information, risk factor identification, publications/brochures for patient education
2. AAHFN (www.aahfn.org)
   - Provides latest, guideline-directed professional education materials, caregiver resources, and patient education materials
3. National Guideline Clearinghouse
   - Latest evidence-based guidelines on the care of patients with heart disease
4. National Heart, Lung and Blood Institute (www.nhlbi.nih.gov)
   - Health information on cardiac risk factors with guidelines for management
5. Center to Advance Palliative Care (www.capc.org)
   - Publications, resources, conferences on PC
6. Heart Failure Society of America (www.hfsa.org)

CASE STUDY *Conclusion*

Now back to Mrs. F., the 80-year-old patient presented at the beginning of this chapter. She is in her final phase of life and is very ill with Class IV symptoms, associated with Stage D, and is interested in knowing what to do next. Her son is also struggling with the fact that his mom is getting worse and yet she doesn't want the treatment that helped her in the past. In his own mind he thinks that maximal medical care and hospitalization should be planned for his mom, but this may be contradictory to what Mrs. F. wishes at this point. The priority concerns to be addressed today are as follows: address their hopes and worries, determine her goals of care, symptom management, and discussion of care options consistent with her goals.

These conversations take time and thoughtful planning. Research has shown that healthcare practitioners do not feel prepared or confident to have these difficult EOL discussions. Why are we hesitant to talk about the full spectrum of HF? Why can't we share the prognosis of heart disease with our patients? Why can't we make their fears and misunderstandings about how they feel a priority in their care? Is it because we have trouble with the idea of death ourselves? Is it because we are afraid that it would be somehow a failure on our part? There are patient and family barriers to these conversations as well as a lack of understanding of what the disease entails and what to expect, their own fears around death, fear of not wanting to disappoint or question their healthcare provider, or not knowing how to bring up such topics. We know from multiple studies that patients want to talk about these issues and that many patients feel that a frank discussion about their diagnosis and prognosis would be helpful and even welcome.

Preparing Mrs. F. and her son for what was happening at this point in her HF trajectory is important but often overlooked. Shared decision making at each interaction throughout the course of her illness would have prepared her and her son for the future and what to expect. By having advance care planning discussions at each clinical encounter, it normalizes these often hard conversations. The first of these conversations may be suggesting an advance directive and choosing a surrogate decision maker and later bringing up decompensation events and EOL issues. While not every situation can be anticipated, helping the patient and family have these conversations will facilitate the process of developing a preparedness plan. The plan could include explanation that the HF course and prognosis is uncertain at first, the possibility of hospitalizations, suggestions of advanced therapies, decreasing functional status, and even sudden death. As HF progresses, the patient's goals may change. Health practitioners have an obligation to review the goals of care regularly in order to make the appropriate treatment recommendations.

To begin a goals of care conversation, practitioners need to have a sense of Mrs. F.'s prognosis. An ask–tell–ask method of communication would be appropriate. EOL discussions require the use of empathic responses which are demonstrated by the use of "wish" statements, good listening skills, and an understanding of another person's perspective. Given her recent hospitalizations, declining functional status, and progression of symptoms, it is evident that she is nearing the end of her life. Next, it is important to determine her and her son's understanding of her illness and their prognostic awareness so they are able to make the right treatment choices. Building this foundation fosters and guides the rest of the conversation, allows the correction of misconceptions, clarifies concerns/worries, and gently helps patients and families to understand the illness trajectory. Upon determination of what is most important to the patient and what she is hoping for in the context of her illness, clinicians can help to match the patient's goals of care with the appropriate treatment plan. Mrs. F. verbalized that she wanted to be home and spend as much time with her family and to feel as good as possible for whatever time she had left. Being in the hospital or continuing some of her HF therapies would not help meet these goals. Since her goals valued QOL over life-prolonging therapies, the deactivation of her ICD was also discussed. While this therapy was appropriate for her earlier in her disease process, it was no longer the recommended treatment.

The second priority to address is Mrs. F.'s symptoms, their burden on her and her family, and how best to manage them. Again, an understanding of her goals and where she is on her disease trajectory will inform how the symptoms should be managed, given their impact on her QOL. It may actually be time to discontinue some of her medications like ACEI and BBs to allow her blood pressure to increase. This may improve her fatigue and shortness of breath. The ACEI, however, might reduce her afterload reduction, and therefore, it would be reasonable to keep her on an ACEI to help with symptom management. By increasing her diuretics, the swelling and dyspnea may improve. Reinforcing the low-sodium diet and fluid recommendations may also be appropriate. At some point, the burden of the diuretics will also have to be balanced with QOL issues. Home oxygen therapy may improve her energy and can help even when oxygen saturation levels are within normal range. General measures to alleviate breathlessness can be suggested, such as use of a fan, pursed lip breathing, and proper body positioning. Oral morphine prior to exertional activities and with episodes of dyspnea can also be beneficial. Oral morphine can also be helpful in managing her increasing osteoarthritis pain. Her use of NSAIDs may be causing sodium and water retention and may render the diuretics less effective and should be discontinued. Depression and anxiety can make patients more dyspneic, so screening for these symptoms is essential, and appropriate medication may be prescribed. Exploring the role of spirituality is important in our treatment of Mrs. F. because it often brings inner peace and comfort in these end stages.

An evaluation of her other medications for other conditions and use of supplements is warranted. Mrs. F. is taking a statin for her dyslipidemia. Statins and Omega 3 are important in preventing long-term consequences and have no benefit in HF and therefore could be discontinued. Aspirin is used to prevent long-term cardiovascular sequelae and is not necessary for Mrs. F. Hawthorn is probably not effective and can be discontinued.

Since Mrs. F. desires to be at home, discussions about future hospitalizations need to be clarified, as well as EOL care planning, including where she would want to be when she dies. Her symptoms and prognosis qualify her for hospice, and both she and her family would benefit from the support hospice provides. Consideration of other referrals, such as support groups, a social worker, or psychologist, may also meet the patient's and family's needs. It may even be appropriate at this time for referral for physical therapy to help with energy conservation. Mrs. F. and her son agreed that a hospice plan of care would best meet their needs and welcomed the referral. Although this conversation is often difficult and emotional, it is valuable and appreciated to know the resources available. Mrs. F.'s primary care practitioner was notified of the discussion, and with the collaboration of the cardiologist and other members of the healthcare team, including nurses, a coordinated and comprehensive plan of care was provided to promote Mrs. F.'s QOL until its end.

CASE STUDY

AN INTERPROFESSIONAL PERSPECTIVE

Amit Badiye, MD, FACC

HF is a complex, costly disease with multiple comorbidities, and its incidence is increasing with a constantly aging population. Mortality is 50% in 5 years after the first admission for HF. It is imperative that such a deadly disease be tackled from all fronts. It starts from focusing on prevention from Stage A HF to optimizing medical therapy through Stages B to D. Newer medications, CRT devices, and LVADs have revolutionized the care of HF patients. Every clinical visit is thus an opportunity to improve care. Providing patient-centered care with a team-based approach is key. This builds patient and family confidence and also resolves conflicts and confusion as care becomes complex and the patient becomes sicker.

In this patient, for example, there is an opportunity to add spironolactone or eplerenone, which has been shown to reduce hospital readmissions and decrease mortality. Advice to discontinue NSAIDs is well aligned with the recent scientific statement from AHA that addresses drugs that may cause or exacerbate HF. Inability to up-titrate medications, such as ACEIs, ARBs, BBs, and ARNIs, suggests worsening HF and the need for preemptive referral to a cardiologist. In Mrs. F.'s case, advanced age and frailty may preclude her candidacy for many therapies. Diuretics used for decongestion is appropriate when needed. In select patients with advanced disease on optimal medical therapy, continuous home inotrope infusion can also be used for palliation and symptom relief (ACCF/AHA Class IIB indication).

Considering the limited options in Mrs. F.'s case, initiation of palliative therapy consult is most appropriate. It is important to have open-ended focused conversation regarding goals of care and involve the patient and key family members/caregivers in the conversation. Many times having an interdisciplinary meeting with the patient, caregivers, and all the providers (especially inpatient setting) helps enormously in decision making. In fact, there are multiple (missed) opportunities of introduction and application of PC principles while taking care of a patient with HF. The possible opportunities are during HF hospitalizations (e.g., first admission to intensive care unit), worsening of disease process or symptoms (e.g., readmissions), escalation of therapies (e.g., need for dialysis, home O_2 use), evaluation for advanced therapies like transplant/LVAD, intolerance or inability to tolerate up-titration of therapies, de-escalation of therapies (e.g., reduction in doses of BB or ACE inhibitors due to hypotension), and lastly when no other therapies are available. I strongly believe that treatment should not be worse than the disease itself and PC has a special role in patients with advanced HF.

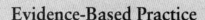

Evidence-Based Practice

Sidebottom, A. C, Jorgenson, A., Richards, H., Kirven, J., & Sillah, A. (2015). Inpatient palliative care for patients with acute heart failure: Outcomes from a randomized trial. *Journal of Palliative Medicine, 18*(2), 134–142.

Background

Models and guidelines for integrating PC into HF management have been proposed, but there is a need for more evidence to determine their impact on patient outcomes. The purpose of this study was to determine if there was an improvement in health status or use of health services for HF patients who had PC incorporated into their inpatient care. Specific research questions included: Is the provision of PC to HF patients in the inpatient setting associated with differences in QOL, symptom management, or depression, or differences in advance care planning (ACP), 30-day readmission, hospice use, or mortality compared with standard care?

Methods

Patients hospitalized with acute HF were randomized to receive a PC consult with follow-up as determined by provider or standard care. Two hundred thirty-two patients (116 intervention/116 control) from a large tertiary-care urban hospital were recruited over a 10-month period. Primary outcomes were symptom burden measured with the ESAS, depressive symptoms measured with the Patient Health Questionnaire-9 (PHQ-9), and QOL measured with the Minnesota Living With Heart Failure Questionnaire. Data were collected at baseline, 1, and 3 months. Secondary outcomes included ACP, inpatient 30-day readmission, hospice use, and death.

Results

Improvements were greater at both 1 and 3 months in the intervention group for the three primary outcome summary measures of symptom burden, depression, and QOL. Particular symptoms on the ESAS that were statistically significant were shortness of breath, anxiety, tiredness, and pain. Of the secondary outcomes, those in the intervention group were more likely to have ACP. There were no differences in 30-day readmission, hospice use, or death.

Conclusions

PC in this acute care inpatient model was associated with improvement in symptom burden, QOL, and depressive symptoms. Discussions with providers also improve ACP.

■ **Acknowledgment.** The editors would like to thank Judith B. Dyne, MS, RN, APRN, BC for her contribution to the previous edition.

■ REFERENCES

Abete, P., Testa, G., Della-Morte, D., Gargiulo, G., Galizia, G., de Santis, D., ... Cacciatore, F. (2012). Treatment for chronic heart failure in the elderly: Current practice and problems. *Heart Failure Reviews, 18*, 529–551. doi:10.1007/s10741-012-9363-6

Adler, E. D., Goldfinger, J. Z., Kalman, J., Park, M. E., & Meier, D. E. (2009). Palliative care in the treatment of advanced heart failure. *Circulation, 120*(25), 2597–2606. doi:10.1161/CIRCULATIONAHA.109.869123

Agarwal, M., Phan, A., Willix, R., Jr., Barber, M., & Schwarz, E. R. (2011). Is vitamin D deficiency associated with heart failure? A review of current evidence. *Journal of Cardiovascular Pharmacology and Therapeutics, 16*(3–4), 354–363. doi:10.1177/1074248410390214

Albert, N. M., Anderson, D., Besthoff, C. M., Byrne-Barta, D., Cecil, R. Y., Cichocki, M., … Lucarelli, P. (2013). Care of the chronically ill patient. In C. B. Laughlin (Ed.), *Core curriculum for ambulatory care nursing* (pp. 361–470). Pittman, NJ: American Academy of Ambulatory Care Nursing.

Albert, N. M., Rathman, L., Ross, D., Walker, D., Bena, J., McIntyre, S., … Zielinski, P. (2009). Predictors of over-the-counter drug and herbal therapies use in elderly patients with heart failure. *Journal of Cardiac Failure, 15*(7), 600–606. doi:10.1016/j.cardfail.2009.02.001

Allen, L. A., Stevenson, L. W., Grady, K. L., Goldstein, N. E., Matlock, D. D., Arnold, R. M., … Spertus, J. A. (2012). Decision making in advanced heart failure: A scientific statement from the American Heart Association. *Circulation, 125*(15), 1928–1952. doi:10.1161/CIR.0b013e31824f2173

Alpert, C. M., Smith, M. A., Hummel, S. L., & Hummel, E. K. (2017). Symptom burden in heart failure: Assessment, impact on outcomes and management. *Heart Failure Reviews, 22*(1), 25–39. doi:10.1007/s10741-016-9581-4

American Geriatrics Society 2015 Beers Criteria Update Expert Panel. (2015). American Geriatrics Society 2015 updated Beers Criteria for potentially inappropriate medication use in older adults. *Journal of the American Geriatrics Society, 63*, 2227–2246. doi:10.1111/jgs.13702

Anderson, F., Downing, G. M., Hill, J., Casorso, L., & Lerch, N. (1996). Palliative performance scale (PPS): A new tool. *Journal of Palliative Care, 12*(1), 5–11.

Azizi-Namini, P., Ahmed, M., Yan, A. T., & Keith, M. (2012). The role of B vitamins in the management of heart failure. *Nutrition in Clinical Practice, 27*(3), 363–374. doi:10.1177/0884533612444539

Bakitas, M., MacMartin, M., Trzepkowski, K., Robert, A., Jackson, L., Brown, J. R., … Kono, A. (2013). Palliative care consultations for heart failure patients: How many, when, and why? *Journal of Cardiac Failure, 19*(3), 193–201. doi:10.1016/j.cardfail.2013.01.011

Barclay, S., Momen, N., Case-Upton, S., Kuhn, I., & Smith, E. (2011). End-of-life care conversations with heart failure patients: A systematic literature review and narrative synthesis. *The British Journal of General Practice, 61*(582), e49–e62. doi:10.3399/bjgp11X549018

Barnes, P. M., Bloom, B., & Nahin, R. L. (2008). Complementary and alternative medicine use among adults and children: United States, 2007. *National Health Statistics Reports*, (12), 1–23.

Barsheshet, A., Wang, P. J., Moss, A. J., Solomon, S. D., Al-Ahmad, A., McNitt, S., … Goldenberg, I. (2011). Reverse remodeling and the risk of ventricular tachyarrhythmias in the MADIT-CRT (Multicenter Automatic Defibrillator Implantation Trial-Cardiac Resynchronization Therapy). *Journal of the American College of Cardiology, 57*, 2416–2423. doi:10.1016/j.hrthm.2014.11.014

Bart, B. A., Goldsmith, S. R., Lee, K. L., Givertz, M. M., O'Connor, C. M., Bull, D. A., … Braunwald, E.; Heart Failure Clinical Research Network. (2012). Ultrafiltration in decompensated heart failure with cardiorenal syndrome. *New England Journal of Medicine, 367*(24), 2296–2304. doi:10.1056/NEJMoa1210357

Behfar, A., Crespo-Diaz, R., Terzic, A., & Gersh, B. J. (2014). Cell therapy for cardiac repair—lessons from clinical trials. *Nature Reviews of Cardiology, 11*, 232–246. doi:10.1038/nrcardio.2014.9

Bekelman, D. B., Rumsfeld, J. S., Havranek, E. P., Yamashita, T. E., Hutt, E., Gottlieb, S. H., … Kutner, J. S. (2009). Symptom burden, depression, and spiritual well-being: A comparison of heart failure and advanced cancer patients. *Journal of General Internal Medicine, 24*(5), 592–598. doi:10.1007/s11606-009-0931-y

Benbassat, J., & Taragin, M. I. (2013). The effect of clinical interventions on hospital readmissions: A meta-review of published meta-analyses. *Israel Journal of Health Policy Research, 2*(1), 1. doi:10.1186/2045-4015-2-1

Benjamin, E. J., Blaha, M. J., Chieve, S. E., Cushman, M., Das, D. R., Deo, R., … Muntner, P. (2017). Heart disease and stroke statistics—2017 update: A report from the American Heart Association. *Circulation, 135*, e146–e603. doi:10.1161/CIR.0000000000000485

Bidwell, J. T., Vellone, E., Lyons, K. S., D'Agostino, F., Riegel, B., Juarez-Vela, R., … Lee, C. S. (2015). Determinants of heart failure self-care maintenance and management in patients and caregivers: A dyadic analysis. *Research in Nursing and Health, 38*, 392–402. doi:10.1002/nur.21675

Bohm, M., Robertson, M., Ford, I., Borer, J. S., Komajda, M., Kindermann, I., … Swedberg, K. (2015). Influence of cardiovascular and noncardiovascular co-morbidities on outcomes and treatment effect of heart rate reduction with ivabradine in stable heart failure (from the SHIFT Trial). *American Journal of Cardiology, 116*(12), 1890–1897. doi:10.1016/j.amjcard.2015.09.029

Buck, H. G., & Zambroski, C. H. (2012). Upstreaming palliative care for patients with heart failure. *The Journal of Cardiovascular Nursing, 27*(2), 147–153. doi:10.1097/JCN.0b013e318239f629

Cardiac Insufficiency Bisoprolol Study. (1994). A randomized trial of beta-blockade in heart failure. CIBIS Investigators and Committees. *Circulation, 90*(4), 1765–1773. doi:10.1161/01.CIR.90.4.1765

Cazeau, S., Leclercq, C., Lavergne, T., Garrigue, S., Bailleul, C., & Daubert, J. C.; Groupe des investigateurs MUSTIC. (2002). [MUSTIC trial]. *Archives Des Maladies du Coeur et des Vaisseaux, 95* (Spec 4; 5 Spec 4), 33–36.

Centers for Disease Control and Prevention. (2012). National Health Interview Survey-2012. Retrieved from http://www.cdc.gov/nchs/nhis/nhis_2012_data_release.htm

Chang, B. H., Hendricks, A., Zhao, Y., Rothendler, J. A., LoCastro, J. S., & Slawsky, M. T. (2005). A relaxation response randomized trial on patients with chronic heart failure. *Journal of Cardiopulmonary Rehabilitation, 25*(3), 149–157.

Chang, B. H., Jones, D., Hendricks, A., Boehmer, U., LoCastro, J. S., & Slawsky, M. (2004). Relaxation response for Veterans Affairs patients with congestive heart failure: Results from a qualitative study within a clinical trial. *Preventive Cardiology, 7*(2), 64–70. doi:10.1111/j.1520-037X.2004.3164.x

Chang, V. T., Hwang, S. S., & Feuerman, M. (2000). Validation of the Edmonton symptom assessment scale. *Cancer, 88*(9), 2164–2171.

Chatterjee, S., Biondi-Zoccai, G., Abbate, A., D'Ascenzo, F., Castagno, D., Van Tassell, B., ... Lichstein, E. (2013). Benefits of ß blockers in patients with heart failure and reduced ejection fraction: Network meta-analysis. *BMJ, 346*, f55. doi:10.1136/bmj.f55

Chen, J., Yao, Y., Chen, H., Kwong, J. S., & Chen, J. (2012). Shengmai (a traditional Chinese herbal medicine) for heart failure. *Cochrane Database of Systematic Reviews, 11*, CD005052. doi:10.1002/14651858

CIBIS-II. (1999). The cardiac insufficiency Bisoprolol study II; A randomized trial. *The Lancet, 353*(9146), 9–13.

Cleland, J. G., Daubert, J. C., Erdmann, E., Freemantle, N., Gras, D., Kappenberger, L., & Tavazzi, L; CardiacResynchronization-Heart Failure (CARE-HF) Study Investigators. (2005). The effect of cardiac resynchronization on morbidity and mortality in heart failure. *New England Journal of Medicine, 352*, 1539–1549. doi:10.1093/eurheartj/ehl099

Colvin, M., Sweitzer, M. K., Albert, N. M., Krishnamani, R., Rich, M. W., Stough, W. G., ... Givertz, M. M. (2015). Heart failure in non-caucasians, women and older adults: A white paper on special populations from the Heart Failure Society of America guideline committee. *Journal of Cardiac Failure, 21*(8), 674–693. doi:10.1016/j.cardfail.2015.05.013

Curiati, J. A., Bocchi, E., Freire, J. O., Arantes, A. C., Braga, M., Garcia, Y., ... Fo, W. J. (2005). Meditation reduces sympathetic activation and improves the quality of life in elderly patients with optimally treated heart failure: A prospective randomized study. *Journal of Alternative and Complementary Medicine, 11*(3), 465–472. doi:10.1089/acm.2005.11.465

Daniele, C., Mazzanti, G., Pittler, M. H., & Ernst, E. (2006). Adverse-event profile of Crataegus spp.: A systematic review. *Drug Safety, 29*(6), 523–535.

Daubert, C., Gold, M. R., Abraham, W. T., Ghio, S., Hassager, C., Goode, G., ... Linde, C; REVERSE Study Group. (2009). Prevention of disease progression by cardiac resynchronization therapy in patients with asymptomatic or mildly symptomatic left ventricular dysfunction: insights from the European cohort of the REVERSE (Resynchronization Reverses Remodeling in Systolic Left Ventricular Dysfunction) trial. *Journal of the American College of Cardiology, 54*, 1837–1846. doi:10.1016/j.jacc.2009.08.011

Davidson, P. M., Dracup, K., Phillips, J., Daly, J., & Padilla, G. (2007). Preparing for the worst while hoping for the best: The relevance of hope in the heart failure illness trajectory. *The Journal of Cardiovascular Nursing, 22*(3), 159–165. doi:10.1097/01.JCN.0000267821.74084.72

Diop, M. S., Rudolph, J. L., Zimmerman, K. M., Richter, M. A., & Skarf, L. M. (2017). Palliative care interventions for patients with heart failure: A systematic review and meta-analysis. *Journal of Palliative Care, 20*(1), 84–92. doi:10.1093/eurheartj/ehl099

Dresing, T. J., & Natale, A. (2001). Congestive heart failure treatment: The pacing approach. *Heart Failure Reviews, 6*(1), 15–25. doi.org/10.1023/A:1009899023118

Ekser, B., & Cooper, D. K. (2008). Update: Cardiac xenotransplantation. *Current Opinion in Organ Transplantation, 13*(5), 531–535. doi:10.1097/MOT.0b013e32830fdf89

Epstein, A. E., DiMarco, J. P., Ellenbogen, K. A., Estes, N. A., Freedman, R. A., Gettes, L. S., ... Sweeney, M. O.. (2008). ACC/AHA/HRS 2008 guidelines for device-based therapy of cardiac rhythm abnormalities: A report of the American College of Cardiology/American Heart Association Task Force on Practice Guidelines (writing committee to revise the *ACC/AHA/NASPE 2002 Guideline Update for Implantation of Cardiac pacemakers and Antiarrhythmia Devices*): Developed in collaboration with the American Association for Thoracic Surgery and Society of Thoracic Surgeons. *Circulation, 117*(21), e350–e408. doi:10.1161/CIRCUALTIONAHA.108.189742

Fahlberg, B., Donoho, E. K., Paire, S., & Davidson, P. M. (2011). Ten principles of integrated palliative and supportive care in heart failure. Retrieved from https://www.aahfn.org/application/views/ce/ce_45/SPC_Article_Overview.pdf

Fang, J. C., Ewald, G. A., Allen, L. A., Butler, J., Westlake-Canary, C. A., Colvin-Adams, M., ... Givertz, M. M. (2015). Advanced (Stage D) heart failure: A statement from the Heart Failure Society of America guidelines committee. *Journal of Cardiac Failure, 21*(6), 519–534. doi:10.1016/j.cardfail.2015.04.013

Fox, K., Komajda, M., Ford, I., Roberston, M., Bohm, M. Borer J., Steg, Pl, Tavazzi, L., & Tendera, M. (2010). Effect of ivabradine in patients with left-ventricular systolic dysfunction: A pooled analysis of individual patient data from the BEAUTIFUL and SHIFT trails. *European Heart Journal, 34*(9), 2263–2270.

Gaggin, H. K., & Januzzi, J. L. (2015, February 10). Cardiac markers and heart failure. Retrieved from http://www.acc.org/latest-in-cardiology/articles/2015/02/09/13/00/cardiac-biomarkers-and-heart-failure

Gelfman, L. P., Bakitas, M., Warner Stevenson, L., Kirkpatrick, J. N., & Goldstein, N. E. (2017). The state of the science on integrating palliative care in heart failure. *Journal of Palliative Medicine, 20*(6), 592–603. doi:10.1089/jpm.2017.0178

Gheorghiade, M., Vaduganathan, M., Fonarow, G. C., & Bonow, R. O. (2013). Rehospitalization for heart failure. *Journal of the American College of Cardiology, 61*(4), 391–403. doi:10.1016/j.jacc.2012.09.038

Go, A. S., Mozaffarian, D., Roger, V. L., Benjamin, E. J., Berry, J. D., Borden, W. B., ... Turner, M. B. (2013). Heart disease and stroke statistics–2013 update: A report from the American Heart Association. *Circulation, 127*(1), e6–e245. doi:10.1161/CIR.0b013e31828124ad

Goldstein, S., Fagerberg, B., Hjalmarson, A., Kjekshus, J., Waagstein, F., Wedel, H., & Wikstrand, J. (2001). Metoprolol controlled release/extended release in patients with severe heart failure: analysis of the experience in the MERIT-HF study. *Journal of the American College of Cardiology, 38*(4), 932–938. doi:10.1016/S0735-1097(01)01516-9

Gori, M., Volterrani, M., Piepoli, M., & Senni, M. (2017). Angiotensin receptor-neprilysin inhibitor (ARNI): Clinical studies on a new class of drugs. *International Journal of Cardiology, 226*, 136–140. doi:10.1016/j.ijcard.2016.06.083

Grodin, J. L., Hammadah, M., Fan, Y., Hazen, S. L., & Tang, W. H. W. (2015). Prognostic value of estimating functional capacity with the use of the Duke activity status index in stable patients with chronic heart failure. *Journal of Cardiac Failure, 21*(1), 44–50. doi:10.1016/j.cardfail.2014.08.013

Halaris, A. (2016). Inflammation associated co-morbidity between depression and cardiovascular disease. *Current Topics in Behavioral Neurosciences, 31,* 45–70. doi:10.1007/7854_2016_28

Harris, J., & Heil, J. S. (2013). Managing depression in patients with advanced heart failure awaiting transplantation. *American Journal of Health-System Pharmacy, 70*(10), 867–873. doi:10.2146/ajhp110738

Hjelmfors, L., van der Wal, M. H. L., Friedrichsen, M. J., Mårtensson, J., Strömberg, A., & Jaarsma, T. (2015). Patient-nurse communication about prognosis and end-of-life care. *Journal of Palliative Medicine, 18*(10), 865–871. doi:10.1089/jpm.2015.0037

Hunt, S. A., Abraham, W. T., Chin, M. H., Feldman, A. M., Francis, G. S., Ganiats, T. G., ... Yancy, C. W. (2009). 2009 focused update incorporated into the *ACC/AHA 2005 Guidelines for the Diagnosis and Management of Heart Failure in Adults*: A report of the American College of Cardiology Foundation/American Heart Association Task Force on Practice Guidelines: Developed in collaboration with the International Society for Heart and Lung Transplantation. *Circulation, 119*(14), e391–e479. doi:10.1161/CIRCULATIONAHA.109.192065

Jayadevappa, R., Johnson, J. C., Bloom, B. S., Nidich, S., Desai, S., Chhatre, S., ... Schneider, R. (2007). Effectiveness of transcendental meditation on functional capacity and quality of life of African Americans with congestive heart failure: A randomized control study. *Ethnicity & Disease, 17*(1), 72–77.

Jessup, M., & Brozena, S. (2003). Heart failure. *New England Journal of Medicine, 348*(20), 2007–2018. doi:10.1056/NEJMra021498

Jessup, M., Abraham, W. T., Casey, D. E., Feldman, A. M., Francis, G. S., Ganiats, T. G., ... Yancy, C. W. (2009). Focused update: ACCF/AHA guidelines for the diagnosis and management of heart failure in adults. A report of the American College of Cardiology Foundation/American Heart Association Task Force on practice guidelines. *Circulation, 119*(14), 1977–2016. doi:10.1161/CIRCULATIONAHA.109.192064

Jonkman, N. H., Westland, H., Groenwold, R. H. H., Ågren, S., Atienza, F., Blue, L., ... Riegel, B. (2016). Do self-management interventions work in patients with heart failure? An individual patient data meta-analysis. *Circulation, 133*(112), 1189–1198. doi:10.1161/CIRCULATIONAHA.115.018006

Kamalov, G., Bhattacharya, S. K., & Weber, K. T. (2010). Congestive heart failure: Where homeostasis begets dyshomeostasis. *Journal of Cardiovascular Pharmacology, 56*(3), 320–328. doi:10.1097/FJC.0b013e3181ed064f

Kirby, M., & Bakhai, A. (2016). Sacubitril/valsartan: The first ARNI. *Primary Care Cardiovascular Journal, 9*(1), S17–S20.

Komajda, M. (2014). Heart rate in chronic heart failure: An overlooked risk factor. *European Heart Journal, 36,* 348–349. doi:10.1093/eurheartj/ehu440

Kotecha, D., Flather, M. D., Altman, D. G., Holmes, J., Rosano, G., Wikstrand, J., ... Cleland, J. G. F.; Beta-Blockers in Heart Failure Collaborative Group. (2017). Heart rate, heart rhythm, and prognostic benefits of beta-blockers in heart failure: Individual patient-data meta-analysis. *Journal of the American College of Cardiology, 69*(24), 2885–2896. doi:10.1016/j.jacc.2017.04.001

Kristen, A. V., Schuhmacher, B., Strych, K., Lossnitzer, D., Friederich, H. C., Hilbel, T., ... Backs, J. (2010). Acupuncture improves exercise tolerance of patients with heart failure: A placebo-controlled pilot study. *Heart, 96*(17), 1396–1400. doi:10.1136/hrt.2009.187930

Krumholz, H. M., Currie, P. M., Riegel, B., Phillips, C. O., Peterson, E. D., Smith, R., ... Faxon, D. P. (2006). A taxonomy for disease management: A scientific statement from the American Heart Association Disease Management Taxonomy Writing Group. *Circulation, 114*(13), 1432–1445. doi:10.1161/CIRCULATIONAHA.106.177322

Kwekkeboom, J., & Bratke, P. (2016). Systematic review of relaxation, meditation, guided imagery strategies for symptom management in HF. *Journal of Cardiovascular nursing, 31*(5), 457–468.

Lampert, R., Hayes, D. L., Annas, G. J., Farley, M. A., Goldstein, N. E., Hamilton, R. M., ... Zellner, R. (2010). HRS expert consensus statement on the management of cardiovascular implantable electronic devices (CIEDs) in patients nearing end of life or requesting withdrawal of therapy. *Heart Rhythm, 7*(7), 1008–1026. doi:10.1016/j.hrthm.2010.04.033

Le, T. Y. L., Thavapalachandran, S., Kizana, E., & Chong, J. J. H. (2017). New developments in cardiac regeneration. *Heart, Lung and Circulation, 26,* 316–322. doi:10.15171/jcvtr.2017.22

Lee, J. H., Jarreau, T., Prasad, A., Lavie, C., O'Keefe, J., & Ventura, H. (2011). Nutritional assessment in heart failure patients. *Congestive Heart Failure, 17*(4), 199–203. doi:10.1111/j.1751-7133.2011.00239.x

Leier, C. V., & Chatterjee, K. (2007). The physical examination in heart failure–Part II. *Congestive Heart Failure, 13*(2), 99–104. doi:10.1111/j.1527-5299.2007.06491.x

Levy, W. C., Mozaffarian, D., Linker, D. T., Sutradhar, S. C., Anker, S. D., Cropp, A. B., ... Packer, M. (2006). The Seattle Heart Failure Model: Prediction of survival in heart failure. *Circulation, 113*(11), 1424–1433. doi:10.1161/CIRCULATIONAHA.105.584102

Levy, W. C. (2013). Seattle heart failure model. *The American Journal of Cardiology, 111* (8)1123–1132.

Li, P., Luo, Y., & Chen, Y. M. (2013). B-type natriuretic peptide-guided chronic heart failure therapy: A meta-analysis of 11 randomized controlled trials. *Heart, Lung & Circulation, 22*(10), 852–860. doi:10.1016/j.hlc.2013.03.077

Lindenfeld, J., Albert, N. M., Boehmer, J. P., Collins, S. P., Ezekowitz, J. A., Givertz, M. M., ... Walsh, M. N. (2010). HFSA 2010 comprehensive heart failure practice guideline. *Journal of Cardiac Failure, 16*(6), e1–e194. doi:10.1016/j.cardfail.2010.04.004

Low, J., Pattenden, J., Candy, B., Beattie, J. M., & Jones, L. (2011). Palliative care in advanced heart failure: An international review of the perspectives of recipients and health professionals on care provision. *Journal of Cardiac Failure, 17*(3), 231–252. doi:10.1016/j.cardfail.2010.10.003

Maack, C., Elter, T., & Bohm, M. (2007). Beta-blocker treatment of chronic heart failure: Comparison of carvedilol and metoprolol. *Congestive Heart Failure, 9*(5), 263–270.

Maloney, C., Lyons, K. D., Li, Z., Hegel, M., Ahles, T. A., & Bakitas, M. (2013). Patient perspectives on participation in the ENABLE II randomized controlled trial of a concurrent oncology palliative care intervention: Benefits and burdens. *Palliative Medicine, 27*(4), 375–383. doi:10.1177/0269216312445188

Mandawat, A., Heidenreich, P. A., Mandawat, A., & Bhatt, D. L. (2016). Trends in palliative care use in veterans with severe heart failure using a large national cohort. *Journal of the American Medical Association, 1*(5), 617–619. doi:10.1001/jamacardio.2016.1687

McCance, K. L., & Huether, S. E. (2014). *Pathophysiology: The biologic basis for disease in adults and children* (7th ed.). St. Louis, MO: Mosby.

McKeag, N. A., McKinley, M. C., Woodside, J. V., Harbinson, M. T., & McKeown, P. P. (2012). The role of micronutrients in heart failure. *Journal of the Academy of Nutrition and Dietetics, 112*(6), 870–886. doi:10.1016/j.jand.2012.01.016

McMurray, J. J. V. (2015). Neprilysin inhibition to treat heart failure: A tale of science, serendipity, and second chances. *European Journal of Heart Failure, 17*, 242–247. doi:10.1002/ejhf.250

McMurray, J. J. V., Packer, M. D., Desai, A. S., Gong, J., Lefkowitz, M. P., Rizkala, A. R., ... Zile, M. R. (2014). Angiotensin-neprilysin inhibition versus enalapril in heart failure. *New England Journal of Medicine 371*(11), 993–1004. doi:10.1056/NEJMoa1409077

Mehra, M. R., Naka, Y., Uriel, N., Goldstein, D. J., Cleveland, J. C., Jr., Colombo, P.C., ... Salerno, C. (2017). A fully magnetically levitated circulatory pump for advanced heart failure. *New England Journal of Medicine, 376*, 440–450. doi:10.1056/NEJMoa1610426

Mills, S., & Bone, K. (2005). *The essential guide to herbal safety*. St. Louis, MO: Churchill Livingston.

Moraska, A. R., Chamberlain, A. M., Sha, N. D., Vickers, K. S., Rummans, T. A., Dunaly, S. M., ... Roger, V. L. (2013). Depression, healthcare utilization, and death in heart failure: A community study. *Circulation: Heart Failure, 6*(3), 387–394. doi:10.1161/CIRCHEARTFAILURE.112.000118

Morita, T., Tsunoda, J., Inoue, S., & Chihara, S. (1999). Validity of the palliative performance scale from a survival perspective. *Journal of Pain and Symptom Management, 18*(1), 2–3.

Moser, D. K., & Riegel, B. (2008). *Cardiac nursing: A companion to Braunwald's heart disease*. St. Louis, MO: Edinburgh.

National Consensus Project for Quality Palliative Care. (2013). *Clinical practice guidelines for quality palliative care* (3rd ed.). Retrieved from http://www.nationalconsensusproject.org

Ng, S. M., Wang, C. W., Ho, R. T., Tin-Hung Ho, R., Ziea, T. C., Tat-Chi Ziea, E., ... Lai-Wan Chan, C. (2012). Tai chi exercise for patients with heart disease: A systematic review of controlled clinical trials. *Alternative Therapies in Health and Medicine, 18*(3), 16–22.

O'Connor, C. M., Abraham, W. T., Albert, N. M., Clare, R., Gattis Stough, W., Gheorghiade, M., ... Fonarow, G. C. (2008). Predictors of mortality after discharge in patients hospitalized with heart failure: An analysis from the Organized Program to Initiate Lifesaving Treatment in Hospitalized Patients with Heart Failure (OPTIMIZE-HF). *American Heart Journal, 156*(4), 662–673. doi:10.1016/j.ahj.2008.04.030

O'Connor, C. M., Hasselblad, V., Mehta, R. H., Tasissa, G., Califf, R. M., Fiuzat, M., ... Stevenson, L.W. (2010). Triage after hospitalization with advanced heart failure: The ESCAPE risk model and discharge score. *Journal of the American College of Cardiology, 55*(9), 872–878. doi:10.1016/j.jacc.2009.08.083

Ouwerkerk, W., Voors, A. A., & Zwinderman, A. H, (2014). Factors influencing the predictive power of models for predicting mortality and/or heart failure hospitalization in patients with heart failure. *Journal of the American College of Cardiology, 2*(5), 429–436. doi:10.1016/j.jchf.2014.04.006

Page, R. L., O'Bryant, C. L., Cheng, D., Dow, T. J., Ky, B., Stein, C. M., ... Lindenfeld, J. (2016). Drugs that may cause or exacerbate heart failure: A scientific statement from the American Heart Association. *Circulation, 34*, e32–e69. doi:10.1161/CIR.0000000000000426

Park, C. L., Aldwin, C. M., Choun, S., George, L., Suresh, D. P., & Bliss, D. (2015). Spiritual peach predicts 5-year mortality in congestive heart failure patients. *Health Psychology, 35*(3), 203–210. doi:10.1037/hea0000271

Peacock, W. F. (2014). Novel biomarkers in acute heart failure: MR-pro-adrnomedullin. *Clinical Chemistry and Laboratory Medicine, 52*(10), 1433–1435. doi:10.1515/cclm-2014-0222

Pittler, M. H., Guo, R., & Ernst, E. (2008). Hawthorn extract for treating chronic heart failure. *Cochrane Database of Systematic Reviews*, (1), CD005312. doi:10.1002/14651858.CD005312.pub2

Ponikowski, P., Voors, A. A., Anker, S. D., Bueno, H., Cleland, J. G. F, Coats, A. J. S, ... ESC Scientific Document Group. (2016). 2016 ESC Guidelines for the diagnosis and treatment of acute and chronic heart failure: The Task Force for the diagnosis and treatment of acute and chronic heart failure of the European Society of Cardiology (ESC) Developed with the special contribution of the Heart Failure Association (HFA) of the ESC. *European Heart Journal. 2016 Jul 14;37*(27):2129–2200. doi:10.1093/eurheartj/ehw128

Psotka, M. A., McKee, K. Y., Liu, A. Y., Elia, G., & De Marco, T. (2017). Palliative care in heart failure: What triggers specialist consultation? *Progress in Cardiovascular Diseases, 60*(2), 215–225. doi:10.1016/j.pcad.2017.05.001

Puchalski, C. M., Lunsford, B., Harris, M. H., & Miller, R. T. (2006). Interdisciplinary spiritual care for seriously ill and dying patients: A collaborative model. *Cancer Journal, 12*(5), 398–416.

Pullen, P. R., Nagamia, S. H., Mehta, P. K., Thompson, W. R., Benardot, D., Hammoud, R., ... Khan, B. V. (2008). Effects of yoga on inflammation and exercise capacity in patients with chronic heart failure. *Journal of Cardiac Failure, 14*(5), 407–413. doi:10.1016/j.cardfail.2007.12.007

Pullen, P.·R., Thompson, W. R., Benardot, D., Brandon, L. J., Mehta, P. K., Rifai, L., ... Khan, B. V. (2010). Benefits of yoga for African American heart failure patients. *Medicine and Science in Sports and Exercise, 42*(4), 651–657. doi:10.1249/MSS.0b013e3181bf24c4

Raichlin, E., Haglund, N. A., Dumitru, I., Lyden, E. R., Johnston, M. D., Mack, J. M., ... Lowes, B. D. (2013). Worsening renal function in patients with acute decompensated heart failure treated with ultrafiltration: Predictors and outcomes. *Journal of Cardiac Failure, 19*(12), 787–794. doi:10.1016/j.cardfail.2013.10.011

Redwine, L. S., Tsuang, M., Rusiewicz, A., Pandzic, I., Cammarata, S., Rutledge, T., ... Mills, P. J. (2012). A pilot study exploring the effects of a 12-week t'ai chi intervention on somatic symptoms of depression in patients with heart failure. *Journal of Alternative and Complementary Medicine, 18*(8), 744–748. doi:10.1089/acm.2011.0314

Riegel, B., Lee, C. S., & Dickson, V. V. (2011). Self care in patients with chronic heart failure. *Nature Reviews. Cardiology, 8*(11), 644–654. doi:10.1038/nrcardio.2011.95

Robinson, M. R., Al-Kindi, S. G., & Oliveira, G. H. (2017). Trends in palliative care use in elderly men and women with severe heart failure in the United States. *Journal of the American Medical Association: Cardiology, 2*(3), 344. doi:10.1001/jamacardio.2016.4517

Rodgers, J. E., & Patterson, J. H. (2001). Angiotensin II-receptor blockers: Clinical relevance and therapeutic role. *American Journal of Health Systems Pharmarcists, 58*, 671–683.

Rogers, J. G., Pagani, F. D., Tatooles, A. J., Bhat, G., Slaughter, M. S., Birks, E. J., ... Milano, C. A. (2017). Intrapericardial left ventricular assist device for advanced heart failure. *New England Journal of Medicine, 376*, 451–460. doi:10.1056/NEJMoa1602954

Saxon, L. A., Boehmer, J. P., Hummel, J., Kacet, S., De Marco, T., Naccarelli, G., & Daoud, E. (1999). Biventricular pacing in patients with congestive heart failure: Two prospective randomized trials. The VIGOR CHF and VENTAK CHF Investigators. *American Journal of Cardiology, 83*(5B), 120D–123D. doi:10.1161/01.CIR.101.8.836

Sidebottom, A. C., Jorgenson, A., Richards, H., Kirven, J., & Sillah, A. (2015). Inpatient palliative care for patients with acute heart failure: Outcomes from a randomized trial. *Journal of Palliative Medicine, 18*(2), 134–142. doi:2010.1089/jpm.2014.0192

Song, E. K., & Kang, S. (2017). Micronutrient deficiency indepntly predicts adverse health outcomes in patients with heart failure. *The Journal of Cardiovascular Nursing, 32*(1), 47–53. doi:10.1097/JCN.0000000000000304

Stevenson, L. W., Miller, L. W., Desvigne-Nickens, P., Ascheim, D. D., Parides, M. K., Renlund, D. G., ... Mancini, D.; REMATCH Investigators. (2004). Left ventricular assist device as destination for patients undergoing intravenous inotropic therapy: A subset analysis from REMATCH (Randomized Evaluation of Mechanical Assistance in Treatment of Chronic Heart Failure). *Circulation, 110*(8), 975–981. doi:10.1161/01.CIR.0000139862.48167.23

Swedberg, K., Komajda, M., Böhm, M., Borer, J., Ford, I., Dubost-Brama, A., ... Tavazzi, L. (2010). Ivabradine and outcomes in chronic heart failure (SHIFT): Arandomised placebo-controlled trial. *Lancet, 376*, 875–885. doi:10.1016/S0140-6736(10)61198-1

Swetz, K. M., Freeman, M. R., AbouEzzeddine, O. F., Carter, K. A., Boilson, B. A., Ottenberg, A. L., ... Mueller, P. S. (2011). Palliative medicine consultation for preparedness planning in patients receiving left ventricular assist devices as destination therapy. *Mayo Clinic Proceedings, 86*(6), 493–500. doi:10.4065/mcp.2010.0747

Takeda, A., Taylor, S. J., Taylor, R. S., Khan, F., Krum, H., & Underwood, M. (2012). Clinical service organisation for heart failure. *Cochrane Database of Systematic Reviews*, (9), CD002752. doi:10.1002/14651858.CD002752.pub3

Tevendale, E., & Baxter, J. (2011). Heart failure comorbidities at the end of life. *Current Opinion in Supportive and Palliative Care, 5*(4), 322–326. doi:10.1097/SPC.0b013e32834d2ee4

Udelson, J. E. (2011). Heart failure with preserved ejection fraction. *Circulation, 124*(21), e540–e543. doi:10.1161/CIRCULATIONAHA.111.071696

Unroe, K. T., Greiner, M. A., Hernandez, A. F., Whellan, D. J., Kaul, P., Schulman, K. A., ... Curtis, L. H. (2011). Resource use in the last 6 months of life among Medicare beneficiaries with heart failure, 2000–2007. *Archives of Internal Medicine, 171*(3), 196–203. doi:10.1001/archinternmed.2010.371

U.S. Census Bureau. (2012). National Population Projections: Summary Tables. Table 2. Projections of the Population by Selected Age Groups and Sex for the United States: 2015 to 2060. Retrieved from https://www.census.gov/library/publications/2011/compendia/statab/131ed.html

von Lueder, T. G., Atar, D., & Krum, H. (2013). Diuretic use in heart failure and outcomes. *Clinical Pharmacology and Therapeutics, 94*(4), 490–498. doi:10.1038/clpt.2013.140

Westenbrink, B. D., Damman, K., Rienstra, M., Maass, A. H., & van der Meer, P. (2012). Heart failure highlights in 2011. *European Journal of Heart Failure, 14*(10), 1090–1096. doi:10.1093/eurjhf/hfs121

Whellan, D. J., Goodlin, S. J., Dickinson, M. J., Heidenrich, P. A., Jaenicke, C., Gattis-Stough, W., & Rich, M. W. (2014). End-of-Life care in patients with heart failure. *Journal of Cardiac Failure, 20*(2), 121–134. doi:10.1016/j.cardfail.2013.12.003

Xu, P. (2012). Using teach back method for patient education and self-management. *American Nurse Today, 7*(3). Retrieved from https://www.americannursetoday.com/using-teach-back-for-patient-education-and-self-management

Yancy, C. W., Jessup, M., Bozkurt, B., Masoudi, F. A., Butler, J., McBride, P. E., ... Wilkoff, B. L. (2013). ACCF/AHA guideline for the management of heart failure: Executive summary: A report of the American College of Cardiology Foundation/American Heart Association Task Force on Practice Guidelines. *Journal of the American College of Cardiology, 62*(16), e147–e239. doi:10.1016/j.jacc.2013.05.019

Yancy, C. W., Jessup, M., Bozkurt, B., Butler, J., Casey, D. E., Jr., Colvin, M. M., Drazner, M. H., ... Westlake C. (2017). 2017 ACC/AHA/HFSA focused update of the *2013 ACCF/AHA Guideline for the Management of Heart Failure*: A report of the American College of Cardiology/American Heart Association Task Force on Clinical Practice Guidelines and the Heart Failure Society of America. *Circulation, 136*(6), e137–e161. doi:10.1161/CIR.0000000000000509

Yeh, G. Y., McCarthy, E. P., Wayne, P. M., Stevenson, L. W., Wood, M. J., Forman, D., ... Phillips, R. S. (2011). Tai chi exercise in patients with chronic heart failure: A randomized clinical trial. *Archives of Internal Medicine, 171*(8), 750–757. doi:10.1001/archinternmed.2011.150

Yeh, G. Y., Wayne, P. M., & Phillips, R. S. (2008). T'ai Chi exercise in patients with chronic heart failure. *Medicine and Sport Science, 52*, 195–208. doi:10.1159/000134300

Young, J. B., Abraham, W. T., Smith, A. L., Leon, A. R., Lieberman, R., Wilkoff, B., ... Wheelan, K; Multicenter InSync ICDRandomized Clinical Evaluation (MIRACLE ICD) Trial Investigators. (2003). Combined cardiac resynchronization and implantable cardioversion defibrillation in advanced chronic heart failure: The MIRACLE ICD Trial. *Journal of the American Medical Association, 289*, 2685–2694. doi:10.1001/jama.289.20.2685

Yu, D. S., Lee, D. T., & Woo, J. (2010). Improving health-related quality of life of patients with chronic heart failure: Effects of relaxation therapy. *Journal of Advanced Nursing, 66*(2), 392–403. doi:10.1111/j.1365-2648.2009.05198.x

Yu, D. S., Lee, D. T., Woo, J., & Hui, E. (2007). Non-pharmacological interventions in older people with heart failure: Effects of exercise training and relaxation therapy. *Gerontology, 53*(2), 74–81. doi:10.1159/000096427

Ziaeian, B., & Fonarow, G. C. (2016). The prevention of hospital readmissions in heart failure. *Progress in Cardiovascular Diseases, 58*, 379–385. doi:10.1016/j.pcad.2015.09.004

Mary M. Brennan

Chronic Lung Disease

KEY POINTS

- What are the pathophysiological changes associated with COPD?
- What are the etiologies involved in the development of COPD?
- How is COPD diagnosed and what are the current medical treatment modalities?
- How are the extrapulmonary manifestations of COPD treated?
- What interventions are effective for smoking cessation?
- Are there alternative/complementary therapies that can assist the older adult with COPD?
- When should conversations regarding prognosis, advance care planning, and end-of-life be initiated?
- What are the goals for patients with COPD and how do they differ according to the severity of the disease?

CASE STUDY

Mrs. S. is a 60-year-old Hispanic female with a 40-pack-year smoking history. Over the past year, she has complained of progressive shortness of breath and dry cough. Pulmonary function tests (PFTs) have revealed Stage II COPD with moderate airflow limitation. Chest x-ray reveals emphysematous changes. Mrs. S. is currently using an albuterol inhaler as necessary when short of breath. Mrs. S. and her family have admitted to a knowledge deficit related to COPD and have asked her physician and nurse to educate them about the disease.

Psychosocial history reveals she has been married for 40 years, has a son and daughter, and retired 5 years ago from a dry-cleaning business. Her physical exam reveals she is a middle-aged, obese female with a dry cough and shortness of breath with exertion. Lung sounds are diminished.

When asked if she was interested in quitting smoking, she replied she had been thinking about quitting recently and wanted to learn more about the nicotine patch. Awareness of the problem of smoking and thinking about quitting indicate she is at the contemplative stage and may be open to receiving information about smoking cessation.

Chronic lung disease, specifically COPD, is the third leading cause of death and is the most common cause of death from respiratory disease in the United States (American Lung Association, 2017). Clients with COPD experience pulmonary complications as well as a spectrum of extrapulmonary complications arising from the disease, including malnutrition, pain, anxiety, and depression (Global Initiative for Chronic Obstructive Lung Disease [GOLD], 2017). As COPD progresses, it is the seventh leading cause of disability and the 12th most common cause of morbidity (American Lung Association, 2017). About 80% to 90% of COPD cases are the result of smoking (American Lung Association, 2017). Eighty percent of patients with COPD die from causes attributable to smoking (Centers for Disease Control and Prevention [CDC], 2017). COPD is progressive, yet variable, and the course of the disease is characterized as a slow decline with intermittent episodes of exacerbations (Curtis, 2008). Due to the progressive nature of COPD, as well as the increased complications and disability, PC should be implemented at the point of diagnosis. According to the National Consensus Project for Quality Palliative Care (2013), the objective of PC is "to prevent and relieve suffering and to support the best possible quality of life (QOL) for patients and families, regardless of the stage of the disease or the need for other therapies" (p. 6). However, due to the variable and often unpredictable course of the disease, fewer patients with COPD receive PC than patients with other chronic diseases (Curtis, 2008; Yohannes, 2007). As part of an interprofessional, team-based approach, integrated PC needs to be initiated at the time of diagnosis and tailored to the individual needs of the patient, the stage of COPD, and his or her symptoms to promote quality of life (QOL) for clients throughout the continuum of the disease. PC is patient centered and family centered. Although the goals of care may be different for each patient, Mrs. S., and her family, require PC, specific to the stage of the disease and to her needs.

■ DEFINITION OF CHRONIC OBSTRUCTIVE PULMONARY DISEASE

COPD is defined as follows:

A common preventable and treatable disease, [it] is characterized by persistent airflow limitation that is progressive and associated with an enhanced chronic inflammatory response in the airways and the lungs to noxious particles or gases. Exacerbations and comorbidities contribute to the overall severity of the disease in individual patients. (GOLD, 2017)

The pulmonary aspect of COPD reflects airflow limitation and includes alterations in the different structures of the lung, including inflammation of the small airways, destruction of the pulmonary alveoli with diminished elastic recoil, and loss of parenchymal tissue (GOLD, 2017). Emphysema, the destruction of alveoli with subsequent dysfunction of gas exchange, is one of the changes that may occur with COPD (GOLD, 2017). Bronchitis, associated with excessive sputum production, may or may not occur with COPD but does not reflect the major airflow obstruction that is characteristic of COPD (GOLD, 2017). The constellation of symptoms including dyspnea on exertion, chronic cough, and chronic sputum production suggests a possible clinical diagnosis of COPD; however, spirometry is required for a definitive diagnosis of COPD.

■ CAUSES

Smoking is a major precursor to the development of COPD. Individuals who have been smoking for 10 years begin to develop pulmonary changes associated with COPD (American Lung Association, 2017). However, only 15% of smokers go on to develop COPD (Mosenifar, 2013). Urban living and air pollution have also been implicated in the development and the exacerbation of COPD (Mosenifar, 2013). Alpha-antitrypsin is a glycoprotein that appears to protect the alveolar walls from destruction; congenital deficiency of alpha-antitrypsin has been implicated in the diagnosis of COPD in persons who are nonsmokers (Mosenifar, 2013). In the 15% of nonsmokers who will develop COPD, a deficiency of alpha-antitrypsin may be suspected (Barnes, 2001).

■ PATHOPHYSIOLOGY

Clients with COPD have a number of pathological changes in the bronchioles, lower airways, lung parenchyma, and pulmonary vessels. Exposure to cigarette smoke, toxic gases, air pollution, and noxious substances induce widespread tissue damage and inflammation. Smokers are thought to have increased levels of inflammatory cells, including neutrophils, macrophages, and T-lymphocytes (GOLD, 2017). These cells damage the airways and stimulate proteases, which destroy connective tissue and overwhelm the number of protective antiproteases. As the pulmonary cells undergo repeated episodes of damage and cell repair, structural changes occur in the normal epithelium of the airways. Fibrosis and inflammation replace normal epithelium, contributing to weakness and narrowing of the airways. The resultant narrowing of the airways causes an obstruction to airflow, particularly expiratory flow. As airways weaken and collapse, air in the airways is unable to be expired and becomes trapped. The residual air causes a breakdown of the alveoli and further damages the structure of the lungs.

Airflow limitation and obstruction of airflow are the hallmark consequences of COPD.

Airflow limitation can be accentuated by three main processes:

1. Loss of elastic recoil of the alveoli
2. Inflammation causing narrowing of the airways
3. Hypertrophy of the mucus-producing goblet cells causing obstruction of the lumen of the airways with thickened mucus. As COPD progresses, there is a decline in lung function that is three to five times more dramatic than in age-related matched groups without COPD (Hardin, Meyers, & Louie, 2008).

■ DIAGNOSIS

The diagnosis of COPD is often considered when a client reports a chronic cough, sputum production, or progressive dyspnea (GOLD, 2017). A comprehensive history should be obtained, including the duration and type of cough, whether dyspnea occurs at rest or with exercise, and the amount of sputum production. The baseline functional status of the client should be established and monitored over the course of the disease. Information regarding smoking history, recent exposure to toxic substances, or exposure to occupational fumes is necessary in establishing a diagnosis.

Once the diagnosis of COPD is considered, PFTs are needed to objectively confirm the diagnosis. PFTs measure the degree of airway obstruction. The stages of COPD are classified according to the degree of airway obstruction and are primarily measured with three spirometric parameters. The first is the forced expiratory volume in 1 second (FEV1). In healthy individuals, 80% of air is forcibly expired in 1 second. In patients with COPD, expiration of the normal volume of air is diminished due to airway limitation with FEV1 measurements less than 80%. The forced vital capacity (FVC) measures the maximum amount of air expired after a maximal inhalation. The FEV1/FVC is the ratio of the forced expiratory volume relative to the FVC and should be greater than 70%. Both the FEV1 and the FEV1/FVC are used to classify the severity of the airflow limitation and, accordingly, the severity of the disease (see severity of airflow limitation in patients with COPD; GOLD, 2017; Table 15.1). For example, if a patient's spirometry reveals FEV1/FVC equal to or less than 70% and if the FEV1 is 60%, the patient is classified as having a moderate degree of airflow obstruction. The different stages of COPD are described as follows: (a) Stage I COPD indicates mild airway obstruction; (b) Stage II COPD indicates moderate airway obstruction; (c) Stage III COPD indicates severe airway obstruction; and (d) Stage IV COPD reveals very severe airway obstruction. Pharmacotherapy and treatments are individualized according to the degree of airway obstruction and symptoms (GOLD, 2017).

TABLE 15.1 Severity of Airflow Classification in COPD	
Patients With FEV1/FVC ≤ 70%	
Classification	Criteria
Mild	FEV1 > 80% predicted
Moderate	50% ≥ FEV1 ≤ 80% predicted
Severe	30% ≥ FEVI ≤ 50% predicted
Very severe	30% < FEVI predicted

Source: Adapted from Global Initiative for Chronic Obstructive Lung Disease. (2017). Global strategy for diagnosis, management and prevention of chronic obstructive pulmonary disease. Retrieved from http://goldcopd.org/gold-2017-global-strategy-diagnosis-management-prevention-copd/

Additional diagnostic tests may be necessary for further investigation, including a chest x-ray, arterial blood gases analysis, and bronchodilator reversibility testing. If a client is diagnosed with COPD before the age of 45, and has a family history, alpha-1 antitrypsin testing may be performed. The chest x-ray examination may demonstrate hyperinflation, flattened diaphragms, and an increased anteroposterior (AP) diameter (Barnes, 2001). The arterial blood gases (ABGs) will remain fairly normal until the later stages of the disease. Use of the modified BORG scale (see Exhibit 15.1) and noninvasive technology, such as pulse oximetry, may also help

Exhibit 15.1
Modified BORG Scale for Perceived Dyspnea

0 = Nothing at all
0.5 = Very, very slight (just noticeable)
1 = Very slight
2 = Slight (light)
3 = Moderate
4 = Somewhat severe
5 = Severe
6-----
7 = Very severe
8-----
9 = Very, very severe (almost maximal)
10 = Worst imaginable

Source: Republished with permission of American Association of Critical-Care Nurses, from Spector, N., & Klein, D. (2001). Chronic critically ill dyspneic patients: Mechanisms and clinical measurement. *AACN Clinical Issues. Advanced Practice in Acute and Critical Care, 12*(2), 220–233; permission conveyed through Copyright Clearance Center, Inc.

to quantify the changes in the respiratory status of the older adult (Duthie, Katz, & Malone, 2007).

Considering that COPD is a disease with myriad physical and psychological consequences, a more comprehensive assessment is required beyond just the spirometry readings. The revised GOLD guidelines (2017) recommend additional assessments to stratify patients. The revised ABCD assessment tool allows providers to consider the patient's spirometry readings in conjunction with the patient's symptoms and history of exacerbations to better tailor treatments to the patient's symptoms. Symptom assessment is conducted using the COPD Assessment Tool (CAT) or the Modified British Medical Research Council (mMRC) Questionnaire. The CAT is an eight-question survey that asks a patient to self-evaluate the frequency of his/her cough and the amount of mucus produced, characterize the severity of chest tightness, describe his/her exercise tolerance, characterize the activities performed at home, assess confidence leaving home, portray his/her sleep quality, and report his/her energy level. The mMRC asks the patient to describe his/her degree of breathlessness, ranging from breathlessness with strenuous exertion only to severe breathlessness preventing the patient from leaving the home.

■ REVIEW OF SYMPTOMS AND PHYSICAL EXAMINATION FINDINGS

The client may complain of dyspnea upon exertion as well as at rest. A decrease in appetite, or a loss of appetite, can occur as dyspneic symptoms worsen. As a result of the increased effort of breathing and decreased food intake, the older adult may report weight loss. Additionally, due to decreased oxygenation, mental status changes may be reported by family members or significant others.

Up to 60% of patients with COPD experience sleep disturbances, yet this symptom is often underassessed by providers or underreported by patients (Jen, Li, Owens, & Malhotra, 2016). Sleep quality is often fragmented, with episodes of dyspnea or coughing interrupting nighttime sleeping. Additionally, COPD patients may also experience sleep apnea, referred to as "overlay syndrome" when sleep apnea is diagnosed with COPD. The coexistence of sleep apnea with COPD is reported to be up to 60% in patients with COPD (Jen et al., 2016).

In the beginning phase of the disease, the patient may not exhibit any visible signs of lung disease. However, as the disease progresses, patients may present with a barrel chest, indicative of the hyperinflation and enlarged volumes that occur with advanced disease. At the advanced stages, patients may demonstrate signs of wasting, with prominence of sternocleidomastoid muscles and bitemporal wasting.

Upon physical examination, auscultation of the lungs may reveal wheezing, rhonchi, or diminished lung sounds. With disease exacerbation, accessory muscle use will become visible—typically involving the sternocleidomastoid and trapezius muscle groups with intercostal muscle retractions as examples. A Hoover's sign may be noticeable, which is a paradoxical inward movement of the lower rib cage that occurs with inspiration, secondary to increased lung volumes and a flattened diaphragm pulling the ribs inward instead of downward. Due to an increased AP diameter, the heart sounds may be distant. If the patient has advanced right-heart failure (RHF) with an enlarged right ventricle, the patient may present with signs of RHF, such as jugular vein distention, an enlarged liver, and edema of the lower extremities.

■ COMPLICATIONS OF CHRONIC OBSTRUCTIVE PULMONARY DISEASE

The systemic and extrapulmonary complications of COPD may include cardiac, pulmonary, and gastrointestinal dysfunction. Some of the complications associated with COPD include pulmonary vascular vasoconstriction, cor pulmonale, atrial arrhythmias, pneumothorax, recurrent respiratory infections (such as pneumonia), respiratory failure, and malnutrition. Pulmonary vascular hypertension develops as the result of hypoxia, which causes vasoconstriction of the pulmonary arterioles. As the vasoconstriction worsens, increased pressure is reflected to the right side of the heart. Cor pulmonale, or enlargement of the right ventricle, occurs in response to increased pulmonary pressures and is a common feature of severe COPD (Sommers & Johnson, 2002). Cor pulmonale accounts for 25% of all types of heart failure and is more common in middle-aged and older males (Sommers & Johnson, 2002). Cor pulmonale is a late sign of COPD and there is a poor response to therapeutic interventions (GOLD, 2017).

A pneumothorax, an accumulation of air within the pleural space, may occur due to rupture of emphysematous bullae. Bullae develop as the result of cell and alveolar damage associated with COPD. Recurrent respiratory infections, commonly viral and bacterial in origin, can cause a transient worsening of COPD symptoms and are the most common cause of acute exacerbations. COPD patients are likely to experience one to two acute exacerbations per year. *Haemophilus* and *Streptococcus* pneumonia infections are the most common bacterial infections. The rhinovirus is responsible for approximately 25% of acute exacerbations (Sethi & Murphy, 2008). Frequent infections are likely to worsen pulmonary function.

The development of malnutrition is multifactorial in the older adult and occurs in up to 25% to 50% of COPD patients (Dine, Williams, & DeLisser, 2009). There is a 20% to 50% increase in metabolic demands associated with COPD as the normal work of breathing becomes more difficult and requires more effort (Dine et al., 2009). Calorie expenditure may increase 10-fold to more than 700 calories/day (Dine et al., 2009). Patients with COPD find it difficult to satisfy the excessive caloric requirements associated with breathing. Early satiety may develop due to the diaphragmatic changes associated with COPD, with the lowering and flattening of the diaphragm resulting in gastric compression. Nutrition is compromised as a result of decreased food intake due to dyspnea and the increased energy expenditure due to the disease process. Fatigue and dyspnea can result in decreased oral intake. Depression due to the chronic illness, progressive changes in lifestyle, and personal losses may decrease the client's interest in eating.

Changes that occur in the lung with normal aging may predispose the patient to COPD or may worsen lung function in patients with COPD. There are changes in lung function that are associated with the aging process. As individuals age, elastic recoil decreases and the chest wall stiffens. As a result of these changes, there is a decrease in compliance of the lungs (GOLD, 2017; Sheahan & Musialowski, 2001). The residual volume, or air remaining in the lungs after a maximal expiration, increases (Duthie et al., 2007). This increase in residual volume contributes to the breakdown in lung elasticity. Airway compression occurs earlier in the expiratory phase of ventilation, resulting in air trapping and altered gas exchange (Sheahan & Musialowski, 2001). Mucociliary clearance in both upper and lower airways may be diminished (Duthie et al., 2007). The alterations in the architecture of the pulmonary parenchyma, airways, and alveoli associated with aging contribute to further compromise of pulmonary function and an increased risk of infection in patients with COPD.

According to Sheahan and Musialowski (2001), exercise capacity can be diminished as a result of decreased muscle mass, decreased cardiac function, and decreased level of conditioning that may occur in some older adults. A decrease in the function of lymphocytes and a decreased humoral response also predispose the older client to viral and bacterial infections (Duthie et al., 2007).

Respiratory failure is a serious complication of COPD and could necessitate hospitalization, intubation, and mechanical ventilation in patients desiring aggressive treatment. Patients with COPD are at an increased risk of developing respiratory failure since the inflammation and damage of the alveoli-capillary membrane are progressive. Respiratory failure is characterized as a failure of either oxygen exchange or carbon dioxide elimination. The clinical criteria of respiratory failure include a PaO_2 of less than 60 mmHg, PCO_2 of greater than 50 mmHg, or respiratory rate of greater than 30 breaths/min (Sharma, 2006). The complication of respiratory failure can be due to an acute insult (such as an infection) or progressive worsening of COPD.

In addition to the physical changes and complications, many patients with COPD experience psychological manifestations, including depression and anxiety. The prevalence of depression increases with the severity of the disease, approaching 80% in individuals with Stage IV obstruction or severe disease (Schneider, Jick, Bothner, & Meier, 2010). Some studies suggest that the development of depression in COPD is related to an increase in inflammatory markers, specifically the levels of interleukin-6 (IL-6; Lu et al., 2013). Although the incidence of depression is greater for patients with COPD than for other chronic illnesses, many clients are not screened for depression and therefore are not treated. Depression is thought to contribute to an increased risk of both hospitalizations and mortality (Yohannes, Willgoss, Baldwin, & Connolly, 2010).

■ TREATMENT

PC is defined as follows:

> Palliative care means patient and family centered care that optimizes quality of life by anticipating, preventing and treating suffering. Palliative care throughout the continuum of illness involves addressing physical, intellectual, emotional, social, and spiritual needs and to facilitate patient autonomy, access to information and choice. (National Consensus Project for Quality Palliative Care, 2013, p. 9)

The National Quality Forum (2012) has approved 14 quality measures designed to address and support the PC needs of patients as well as the end-of-life (EOL) care. The measures encompass diverse concerns of patients with chronic disease including their psychosocial needs, pain management, and care preferences. Specifically, the quality measures address the assessment and screening of dyspnea, pain management, documentation of EOL preferences, and documentation of EOL discussions, important aspects of care to integrate into the treatment plan.

There are numerous barriers to the delivery of PC for patients with COPD. Research suggests that many providers have an inadequate understanding of the nature of PC and often perceive PC as synonymous with EOL care (Spence et al., 2009). The underdiagnosis, undertreatment, and unpredictability of the trajectory of COPD contribute to confusion and uncertainty regarding the diagnosis and prognosis among interdisciplinary providers. In addition, many providers lack the communication skills needed to discuss the trajectory of COPD illness and the needs that patients experience at different stages of the COPD, from managing their illness at diagnosis to discussing their preferences for care at the end of their lives (Spence et al., 2009). Fear of patients' reactions to the diagnosis and treatment may hinder discussions with patients and their families and contributes to a lack of specialized care, including inadequate information regarding prognosis, lack of emotional support, inadequate screening for depression and anxiety, and insufficient assistance with medical decision-making at the end of life (Spence et al., 2009).

Patients with COPD need support managing each stage of the disease, and this specialized care extends beyond the traditional boundaries of medical care. PC, delivered by a specialized group of professionals working within a team, may help to address the medical needs, as well as addressing the physical, emotional, and psychosocial needs and goals of care at each stage of the illness. At the point of diagnosis, a PC team should be engaged.

The goal of PC for patients with COPD is to promote QOL (Hardin et al., 2008). The principles that underlie the provision of PC include effective communication among providers, clients, and their families, as well as maintaining independence and promoting psychosocial, spiritual, and emotional health (Hardin et al., 2008). Patient education is an important component of communication and may help clients adjust to their illness and manage the disease. Providers should educate clients about the causes of COPD as well as the progressive nature of the disease. Effective communication may assist clients with smoking cessation. Discussions about advance directives and EOL care should be carried out throughout the early and late stages of the disease to promote QOL (Bischoff, Sudore, Miao, Boscardin, & Smith, 2013). Additionally, EOL care is a patient safety issue due to the aggressive life-prolonging treatments that some patients receive in the last months of life because other alternative preferences, such as supportive/comfort care, had not been discussed (Joint Commission, 2015). Some studies reveal that patients wish to speak with their providers about EOL care, but fewer than 30% of patients engage in a conversation ("Lake Research Partners and the Coalition for Compassionate Care of California," 2012; The Conversation Project, 2014; Yung, Walling, Min, Wenger, & Ganz, 2010). Education about the nature of COPD, the course of the illness, and advance directives has been shown to allay patients' anxiety (Knauft, Nielsen, Engelberg, Patrick, & Curtis, 2005).

Management of Stable Chronic Obstructive Pulmonary Disease

PC for patients with COPD involves comprehensive care including disease-directed treatment, such as promoting independence and reducing symptoms. The treatment of patients often depends on the stage of their diagnosis and their symptoms. In mild COPD, therapy is targeted toward prolonging life. In contrast, treatment of patients with very severe disease is aimed toward promoting comfort and helping patients and families cope with EOL decisions and issues.

Current treatment modalities for all patients with COPD include smoking cessation, prevention of infection,

maximizing pulmonary function, and education (Barnes, 2001; Hanania, Sharma, & Sharafkhaneh, 2010). After the age of 65, smoking continues to be a major risk factor for death as well as a decreased QOL (Duthie et al., 2007). Cessation of smoking is the most effective intervention to reduce the progression of COPD (GOLD, 2017). Smoking cessation in older adults can improve their QOL, prevent the progression of COPD, and therefore reduce the development of complications due to COPD (Duthie et al., 2007). The risk for the development of influenza and pneumonia decreases as the result of smoking cessation in the older adult.

Counseling has been shown to be a very effective intervention to reduce smoking. The GOLD Guidelines (2013) recommend that clients should receive counseling at every healthcare visit. Counseling can range from a brief, informal episode to longer, more structured interventions; however, both are effective (Fiore et al., 2008a, 2008b). A recommended strategy for healthcare providers is to utilize the five A's approach at every visit (Fiore et al., 2008a, 2008b; GOLD, 2017).

1. *Ask:* Identify all smokers.
2. *Advise:* Advise smokers to quit smoking at every visit.
3. *Assess:* Assess a client's willingness to quit smoking.
4. *Assist:* Assist a client to quit by encouraging the use of counseling and pharmacotherapies.
5. *Arrange:* Arrange for the client to receive follow-up care.

A growing evidence base reveals that several therapies are effective in achieving and sustaining smoking cessation (Fiore et al., 2008a, 2008b; Stead et al., 2012). Guidelines advocate the use of nicotine replacement therapies (NRTs) in the form of nicotine inhalers, lozenges, gum, nasal spray, and patches (Fiore et al., 2008a, 2008b; Stead et al., 2012). The goals of NRT are to reduce the desire to smoke and to decrease the physical, psychological, and physiological signs and symptoms of nicotine withdrawal. In a systematic review (Stead et al., 2012), all of the different NRTs increased the success of smoking cessation by 50% to 70%. The most effective medical therapy to date is Varenicline, a partial agonist of nicotine receptors. Varenicline is thought to increase levels of dopamine in the brain and decrease satisfaction associated with smoking (Cahill, Stead, & Lancaster, 2009). A systematic review found the use of Varenicline was two to three times more effective in achieving smoking cessation when compared with placebo and was superior to Bupropion in achieving abstinence from smoking at 24 and 52 weeks (Cahill et al., 2009). Side effects associated with the use of Varenicline include nausea, insomnia, and bad dreams. Concerns regarding depression and suicide have prompted the Food and Drug Administration (FDA) to issue a black box warning regarding the development of neuropsychiatric syndromes. An assessment of the patient's risk of depression must be conducted prior to prescribing this medication. Bupropion, an antidepressant thought to antagonize nicotinic receptors in the brain, has been found to be effective in increasing smoking cessation; a few studies have shown it to be superior to NRTs (Hughes, Stead, & Lancaster, 2007; Stead, Perrara, Bullen, Mant, & Lancaster, 2008). The addition of NRT to Bupropion is more effective than nicotine replacement alone (Stead et al., 2008). Side effects associated with Bupropion include dry mouth, insomnia, and nausea. Seizures occur in 1 of 1,000 patients treated with this medication and the risk of seizure increases with higher doses. While each of the aforementioned therapies has been successful in achieving outcomes, the combination of counseling and medications greatly increases the rate of cessation (Fiore et al., 2008a, 2008b).

The prevention of infection is an important consideration in the older adult with COPD. Simple interventions, such as handwashing and avoidance of exposure to illness, can reduce the development of respiratory infections. Immunizations, such as the influenza vaccine and the pneumococcal vaccines, are important vaccinations to prevent disease exacerbations (Barnes, 2001). Maximizing pulmonary function includes pharmacologic therapy, pulmonary rehabilitation, breathing retraining, and the prevention of malnutrition. Standard pharmacologic therapies include bronchodilators, steroids, and supplemental oxygen (Exhibit 15.2). If the older client has developed cor pulmonale or atrial arrhythmias, pharmacologic therapy is directed toward reducing the adverse cardiovascular effects that occur.

The importance of good nutrition in patients with COPD cannot be underestimated. A diet high in protein and calories is indicated to counter the possible protein breakdown that may occur with inadequate nutritional intake, particularly as the disease progresses. Small frequent meals with soft, nutrient-dense foods are recommended, such as yogurts, puddings, and omelets (Dine et al., 2009). Oxygen provided with meals may help to treat the shortness of breath while eating. Nutritional supplements in the form of thick shakes may help patients receive their daily amount of vitamins and minerals. Multivitamins should be prescribed for all patients.

Pulmonary rehabilitation is one of the most important recommendations for the treatment of patients with COPD. Pulmonary rehabilitation programs usually include exercise as a key component of the treatment, but many include additional interventions such as counseling, psychological support, and nutrition education. A recent systematic review (SR) and meta-analysis of randomized controlled trials (RCTs) investigated the impact of pulmonary rehabilitation programs with at least 4 weeks of exercise training to usual care on health-related QOL, functional status, and exercise capacity (McCarthy et al., 2015). Sixty-five RCTS with 3,822 participants met the inclusion criteria and were included in the review.

Exhibit 15.2
Pharmacologic Interventions for Chronic Lung Disease

Bronchodilators	Routes
Sympathomimetics	
Epinephrine	Inhaled, oral, parenteral
Isoproterenol	
Beta-2 Agonists	
Short-acting Albuterol	Inhalation—drug of choice in acute exacerbations; oral—duration of action is 4–6 hours
Long-acting Salmeterol	Duration of action is 12 hours
Xanthines	
Theophylline	Oral
Aminophylline	Parenteral
Anticholinergics	
Short-acting Ipratropium	Inhaled
Long-acting Tiotropium, long-acting	Inhaled
Supplemental O₂	
Nasal cannula	Compressed gas, liquid, or concentrate
Steroids[a]	
Corticosteroids	
Prednisone	Oral
Methylprednisolone	Parenteral
Beclomethasone	Inhaled

[a]Not an all-inclusive list of medications.

Overall, the authors found pulmonary rehabilitation to be significantly efficacious for improving QOL and improving exercise and functional capacity, as well as reducing symptoms of COPD such as dyspnea and fatigue. The authors concluded that additional RCTs are not needed; however, researchers should determine the length and duration of pulmonary rehabilitation necessary to improve QOL and determine which components of rehabilitation are the most efficacious.

Exercise is central to the treatment of COPD and helps to improve both the physical symptoms of dyspnea and the psychological symptoms of depression. GOLD Guidelines (2017) recommend that a combination of constant load or continuous exercise and interval exercise training provides the most beneficial outcomes compared to either treatment alone. Constant load exercise training refers to walking or biking at a specific intensity for 30 continuous minutes. Interval training refers to shorter periods of peak intensity, from 30 seconds to 3 minutes, alternating with short periods of rest. As symptoms progress, patients may opt for the shorter training periods due to the increasing breathlessness associated with the advancement of the disease. Although a combination of exercise regimens is preferred, both types of exercise contributed to improved QOL and 6-minute walk tests (Lee & Holland, 2014).

Exercise may also contribute to improved sleep quality in patients with COPD. Additionally, avoiding daytime sleeping and frequent naps may help to promote uninterrupted periods of sleep at night. Melatonin receptor agonists, such as ramelteon, a non-sedative hypnotic, may be used to promote sleep while avoiding the sedative effects that may be problematic for COPD patients.

Respiratory Pharmacologic Therapy of Stable Chronic Obstructive Pulmonary Disease

Pharmacotherapeutic agents are recommended for the treatment of symptoms and prevention of acute exacerbations for clients with COPD. Bronchodilators constitute the foundation of pharmacotherapy for all patients with COPD (GOLD, 2017). Treatment with bronchodilators is associated with a reduction in dyspnea and an improvement in exercise capacity (GOLD, 2017); however, their use is not associated with an improvement in survival. Bronchodilators can be administered via metered-dose inhalers, by nebulizer, or by oral administration. The bronchodilators most often prescribed for patients with COPD include beta-2 agonists and anticholinergic agents. Beta-2 agonists stimulate the beta-receptors in the lung and promote bronchodilation of the proximal airways by relaxing smooth muscle. In mild cases of COPD, the short-acting beta-2 agonist (SABAs), such as albuterol, is prescribed on an as-needed basis to reduce symptoms such as wheezing, shortness of breath, and chest tightness. As COPD increases in severity to moderate and severe forms of the disease, long-acting beta-2 agonists (LABAs) are recommended. LABAs, such as salmeterol, provide sustained bronchodilation with daily or twice daily dosing. Research suggests that LABAs may be associated with improved QOL, reduced symptoms, reduced hospitalizations, and a decrease in the frequency of acute exacerbations (GOLD, 2017). Adverse effects usually occur as a result of beta-2 adrenergic stimulation and contribute to tremors and sinus tachycardia.

Anticholinergic agents promote bronchodilation in patients with COPD and work by activating muscarinic receptors in the airways to decrease bronchoconstriction. Ipratropium, a short-acting antimuscarinic agent (SAMA), and Tiotropium, a long-acting antimuscarinic agent (LAMA), are recommended to improve symptoms.

An SR (Barr, Bourbeau, & Camargo, 2008) compared Ipratropium, administered twice daily as a less-selective agent, with Tiotropium, an agent with greater selectivity. Tiotropium was shown to reduce exacerbations of COPD and decrease the number of hospitalizations (Barr et al., 2008). Patients with moderate to severe COPD, who were managed with Tiotropium, had significant improvements in QOL and reduction in symptom scores when compared with LABAs (Barr et al., 2008). Additionally, when compared with LABAs, treatment with Tiotropium resulted in fewer exacerbations of COPD and a decrease in disease-related hospitalizations (Chong, Karner, & Poole, 2012). The use of Tiotropium in conjunction with a LABA has been shown to improve QOL. The latest recommendations from the GOLD Guidelines (2017) note that both SAMAs and SABAs are Evidence A for maintenance and as-needed treatments in COPD to decrease symptoms and increase the FEV1 scores. Both LABAs and LAMAs are effective in improving lung function and decreasing exacerbations and may be used synergistically if treatment with one or the other is not effective. Combination LABAs and LAMAs constitute an Evidence A recommendation and have been shown to be effective in reducing exacerbations and hospitalizations (GOLD, 2017).

As the severity of COPD increases, and patients are diagnosed with moderate-to-severe forms of the disease, the GOLD Guidelines (2017) recommend as the next step the addition of an inhaled corticosteroid (ICS) to long-acting bronchodilator therapy for all patients diagnosed with moderate-stage COPD, having an FEV1 of less than 50%, with frequent exacerbations of COPD. Inhaled corticosteroids, such as Fluticasone, have been shown to decrease the number and severity of exacerbations (Cayley, 2008; Yang, Fong, Sim, Black, & Lasserson, 2007). Additionally, treatment with inhaled corticosteroids is associated with an improvement in QOL despite the fact that the therapy does not slow the decline of lung function (Yang et al., 2007). Adverse effects associated with inhaled corticosteroids include hoarseness and vocal cord myopathy caused by the topical placement of the steroids on the vocal cords with resultant muscle breakdown. Rinsing after administration of the inhaled steroids helps to reduce the oropharyngeal complications. Some studies suggest an increased risk of pneumonia in patients who use inhaled corticosteroids. At this point, there is insufficient evidence to know whether there is an associated increase in pneumonia as a result of long-term therapy.

As an alternative treatment, theophylline, a methylxanthine, is a bronchodilator with a narrow therapeutic index, requiring frequent monitoring of drug levels and adjustments of the dose. An improvement in pulmonary function may occur with their use; however, most of the beneficial effects occur with doses nearing toxic amounts. Unfavorable side effects including palpitations and tremors are associated with their use and more likely to occur with near-toxic doses, often relegating theophylline to second- or third-line therapy. Changes in cardiac or liver function associated with aging can decrease the clearance of theophylline, contributing to side effects and necessitating dosage adjustments (GOLD, 2017). Cigarette smoking can also negatively influence the metabolism of theophylline, increasing the levels of theophylline and contributing to possible toxicity.

CASE STUDY *Continued*

MRS. S.—2 YEARS LATER

Upon diagnosis, Mrs. S. was educated about COPD, the progressive nature of the disease, and the variable course of illness. At that time, Mrs. S. expressed a need to focus on disease-directed therapy and life-sustaining treatments. The interprofessional team emphasized improvements in QOL. She was started on NRT, yet has not completely stopped smoking. After Mrs. S. complained of shortness of breath with exertion, a LABA was initiated and she reported improvement in the symptoms of shortness of breath. Mrs. S. also visited with her minister twice a month and enjoys their regular discussions. She began a pulmonary rehabilitation program, with noted improvement in her mood over the next several months. The interprofessional team consisting of the pulmonary specialist, nurses, occupational therapists, pulmonary therapists, and their minister continued to work with Mrs. S. to address her emotional, physical, psychosocial, and spiritual needs. At that time, Mrs. S. was interested in aggressive resuscitation efforts including cardiopulmonary resuscitation and intubation in the event her condition deteriorated precipitously. The PC team continued to assess Mrs. S.'s goals of care.

■ MANAGEMENT OF ACUTE EXACERBATIONS

Acute exacerbations may be triggered by both bacterial and viral infections. Infections may exacerbate inflammation and contribute to impairment of cilia and hypersecretion of mucous goblet cells. Oral and intravenous (IV) steroids are administered to patients to treat acute exacerbations of chronic obstructive lung disease. The main advantage to glucocorticoid steroids is their anti-inflammatory effect. Oral and parenteral glucocorticoids are effective in reducing COPD exacerbations (Walters, Gibson, Wood-Baker, Hannay, & Walters, 2009). Glucocorticoids suppress a number of inflammatory mediators and, thus, decrease the inflammation associated with the exacerbation. Evidence revealed that the use of systemic glucocorticoids for acute exacerbations significantly decreased dyspnea, the risk of treatment failure, and appearance of recurrent exacerbations within 30 days (Wood-Baker, Gibson, Hannay, Walters, & Walters, 2008). There was a significant increase in the volume of expired air and an improvement in ABGs within the first 72 hours (Wood-Baker et al., 2008). However, even short-term use is associated with an increased incidence of adverse side effects including increased risk of infection, hyperglycemia, weight gain, and insomnia (Walters et al., 2009). Nonsignificant increases in depression and anxiety have also been noted. Long-term complications include muscle breakdown, suppression of the hypothalamus–pituitary axis, and osteoporosis. Treatment for acute exacerbations is usually short term to avoid complications associated with their use.

Oxygen therapy can decrease the potentially harmful effects of hypoxemia-induced vasoconstriction on the pulmonary vasculature in patients with severe COPD and pulmonary hypertension with severe resting hypoxemia and a resting oxygen saturation of less than 88%. Oxygen is utilized during acute exacerbations (Brashers, 2002) to reduce the dyspnea associated with hypoxemia and the long-term consequences of hypoxemia such as pulmonary hypertension and cor pulmonale (Barnes, 2001). Oxygen therapy is titrated to a PaO_2 of 55 to 60 mmHg in order to avoid "turning off" the hypoxic drive in clients with COPD (Barnes, 2001).

Small breaths and a decreased respiratory rate is a COPD client's response to exercise (Collins, Langbein, Fehr, & Maloney, 2001). As stated previously, the older adult will reduce his or her activity in order to reduce the occurrence of dyspnea. Pulmonary rehabilitation is focused on exercise and muscle reconditioning. Rehabilitation can take place in a community setting as well as in the client's home. By increasing physical activity, muscle atrophy may be reduced and the efficiency of oxygen uptake will be improved (Collins et al., 2001).

Breathing retraining for clients with COPD includes the techniques of pursed-lip breathing and diaphragmatic/abdominal breathing (see Exhibit 15.3). Due to

Exhibit 15.3
Breathing Exercises

Pursed lip:

- Breathe slowly through the nose.
- Hold your breath to a count of 3 seconds.
- Purse lips like you are whistling; breathe out to an inspiration; should drop with expiration; exhale through mouth.
- By exhaling through pursed lips, air is expelled from the lungs and breathing is slowed.

Abdominal/diaphragmatic:

- Sit comfortably with feet on floor.
- Press one hand to the abdomen, rest the other hand on the chest.
- Inhale through the nose slowly; use abdominal muscles.
- Abdominal hand should rise with a count of 3 seconds.
- Hand on chest should stay still.

Source: From Sheahan, S. L., & Musialowski, R. (2001). Clinical implications of respiratory system changes in aging. *Journal of Gerontological Nursing, 27*(5), 26–34.

the pathophysiology of COPD, air becomes trapped in the terminal airways and adequate ventilation decreases. Lung changes associated with aging can result in air trapping without the presence of COPD (Sheahan & Musialowski, 2001). Pursed-lip breathing facilitates the expulsion of air from the lungs by the client controlling and lengthening the expiratory phase of respiration (Collins et al., 2001; Dunn, 2001).

Diaphragmatic/abdominal breathing serves a similar purpose as pursed-lip breathing. The client utilizes the diaphragmatic and abdominal muscles to control both inspiration and expiration. Both techniques assist the client to reduce panic and anxiety associated with dyspneic episodes (Dunn, 2001). The older client can perform both of these exercises while seated comfortably in a chair. A Cochrane Systematic Review investigating the effectiveness of 4 to 12 weeks of breathing retraining/exercises in patients with COPD, including pursed-lip breathing and diaphragmatic breathing, reported an improvement in the patient's functional capacity, but no improvements in dyspnea (Holland, Hill, Jones, & McDonald, 2012).

Malnutrition negatively affects the pulmonary system as well as the immune system in the older adult. Due to the physiologic changes associated with aging, immunity and pulmonary function can already be compromised (Marini & Wheeler, 2010). If an older adult is concurrently on diuretic therapy, losses of phosphorus and potassium can contribute to further muscle weakness (Hanania et al., 2010). Recommendations to improve nutrition include

eating smaller, more frequent meals (Sommers & Johnson, 2002), increasing protein and calories (Berry & Baum, 2001; Collins et al., 2001; Sommers & Johnson, 2002), and limiting carbohydrates to 50% of the total caloric intake (Marini & Wheeler, 2010). In a Cochrane Systematic Review, when nutritional supplementation, defined as oral, enteral, or parenteral caloric substances administered over at least a 2-week period, was compared with usual diet, there were significant improvements in weight gain and the 6-minute walk test (Ferreira, Brooks, White, & Goldstein, 2012). Additional anthropometric parameters revealed a significant increase in fat mass index, lean body mass index, and skinfold thickness (Ferreira et al., 2012).

Administering bronchodilators prior to meals can also facilitate intake by decreasing dyspneic episodes. Oral care prior to meals can improve the eating experience for clients who mouth-breathe or have sputum production. Improving nutritional intake can increase the patient's response to hypoxemia, decrease hypercarbia, and maintain immune function, which is often diminished as a result of the physiologic changes associated with aging as well as the pathophysiologic process of COPD (Barnes, 2001).

Education is incorporated in the care of the older client during each contact. Explanations should be given regarding smoking cessation, medication administration, and potential side effects of these medications. Instructions should be given regarding exercise, retraining, and pulmonary rehabilitation and, if necessary, home oxygen therapy. Because significant others often function as caregivers in the home, they should be included in the education sessions.

Determining Prognosis in End-Stage Pulmonary Disease

Determining prognosis in end-stage lung disease is extremely difficult. There is marked variability in survival. Physician estimates of prognosis vary in accuracy, even in patients who appear end stage. Even at the time of intubation and mechanical ventilation for respiratory failure from acute exacerbation of COPD, 6-month survival cannot be predicted with certainty from simple data easily available to the clinician. Far less information than this is available to most hospice programs at the time of referral.

Although the end stages of various forms of lung disease differ in some respects, most follow a final common pathway leading to progressive hypoxemia, cor pulmonale, and recurrent infections. Once the older adult is diagnosed with COPD, the individual and his or her significant others should be made aware of the predictors of a poor prognosis (see Exhibit 15.4). Although many studies have not been able to link premorbid variables to mortality (Messer, Griffiths, & Baudouin, 2012), the National Institute for Health and Care Excellence Guidelines (2017) have recommended a number of variables as important determinants in decisions regarding intubation, including age, functional status, FEV1, oxygen

Exhibit 15.4
Predictors of Poor Prognosis in Patients With COPD

1. FEV1 less than 30% of predicted
2. Declining performance status, with increasing dependence on others for activities of daily living
3. Uninterrupted walk distance limited to a few steps
4. More than one urgent hospitalization within the past year
5. Left-heart and/or other chronic comorbid disease
6. Depression/anxiety
7. BMI less than 21 kg/m^2
8. Poor QOL per patient
9. Long-term oxygen therapy
10. Intolerable dyspnea
11. BODE Index score greater than 7

Source: From Hardin, K. A., Meyers, F., & Louis, S. (2008). Integrating palliative care in severe chronic obstructive lung disease. *COPD: Journal of Chronic Obstructive Pulmonary Disease, 5,* 207–220.

requirements, and comorbidities. At the present time, it is uncertain what number or combination of these factors might predict 6-month mortality; clinical judgment is required. Patients who fit the following parameters can be expected to have the lowest survival rates:

I. Severity of chronic lung disease documented by:
   A. Disabling dyspnea at rest, poor oxygenation, or unresponsiveness to bronchodilators, resulting in decreased functional activity, for example, bed-to-chair existence, often exacerbated by other debilitating symptoms such as fatigue and cough. FEV1, after bronchodilator, less than 30% of predicted, is helpful supplemental objective evidence, but should not be required if not already available.
   B. Progressive pulmonary disease
      1. Increasing visits to emergency department or hospitalizations for pulmonary infections and/or respiratory failure;
      2. Decrease in FEV1 on serial testing of greater than 40 mL per year is helpful supplemental objective evidence, but should not be required if not already available.
II. Presence of cor pulmonale or RHF
   A. These should be due to advanced pulmonary disease, not primary or secondary to left-heart disease or valvulopathy.
   B. Cor pulmonale may be documented by
      1. Echocardiography
      2. Electrocardiogram (ECG)
      3. Chest x-ray
      4. Physical signs of RHF
III. Hypoxemia at rest on supplemental oxygen
   A. PO$_2$ less than or equal to 55 mmHg on supplemental oxygen
   B. Oxygen saturation less than or equal to 88% on supplemental oxygen
IV. Hypercapnia
   A. PCO$_2$ equal to or greater than 50 mmHg
V. Unintentional progressive weight loss of greater than 10% of body weight over the preceding 6 months
VI. Resting tachycardia greater than 100/min in a patient with known severe COPD (National Hospice Organization, 1996)

The endpoint of the disease is pulmonary hypertension and the development of cor pulmonale (Marini & Wheeler, 2010). All information regarding the diagnosis and prognosis should be delivered honestly to the client and significant others at their level of understanding (Meier, Morrison, & Ahronheim, 1998).

Once the diagnosis of end-stage disease has been made, it is appropriate to begin discussions about advance directives. Discussion regarding advance directives should begin prior to the development of a life-threatening event. If a patient has two or more of the clinical predictors identified in Exhibit 15.4, discussions regarding EOL care are necessary. Even though predicting the exact time of death is difficult, the client and significant others should be offered options in treatment. Information regarding PC can also be included in the treatment plan for clients with COPD.

CASE STUDY *Continued*

MRS. S. PRESENTS 4 YEARS LATER. SHE HAS BEEN FOLLOWED UP IN THE PULMONARY CLINIC.

Mrs. S. is now 66 years old with a 40-pack-year smoking history. She eventually quit smoking 2 years ago. The final driver for Mrs. S. to quit smoking was the diagnosis of a lung nodule on a repeat chest x-ray. Fortunately, after a workup by her pulmonologist, which included a biopsy, the nodule was diagnosed as noncancerous. This significant event coupled with using a nicotine patch created a strong incentive to finally quit smoking. Additionally last year, home oxygen was initiated for an oxygen saturation level of 87% on room air. She has been hospitalized four times in the last year with acute exacerbations of her COPD. Recent PFTs revealed Stage IV COPD/severe airflow limitation.

She has expressed feelings of sadness over the last several weeks and has lost interest in socializing with family and friends. Physical examination reveals an elderly, cachectic woman who looks older than her stated years of age. She wears a nasal cannula that delivers oxygen at 2 L/min and is visibly short of breath. She has a poor appetite, and recently lost 10 lbs. She has lost 60 pounds over the last 5 years. Her examination is also notable for an increased antero-posterior (AP) diameter of her chest. Lung sounds are diminished bilaterally, with extensive wheezing. Intercostal muscle retractions are noted. Mrs. S.'s medication regimen includes an albuterol nebulizer as needed, a combination inhaled corticosteroid and LABA (Symbicort) twice per day, a long-acting muscarinic antagonist (Tiotropium) once per day via nebulizer, Prednisone 5 mgm oral dose once per day, and home oxygen at 2 L/min. Mrs. S. was screened for depression and scored a 16/27 on the Patient Health Questionnaire-9 (PHQ-9), indicating moderate–severe depression. A serotonin reuptake inhibitor was added to her regimen.

Conversations regarding Mrs. S.'s prognosis and end of life were initiated 1 year ago with her provider, family, and minister, prior to the implementation of home oxygen. Although her family was reluctant to discuss these issues, her provider knew that many patients complain that they did not have these important conversations regarding advance care planning.

■ PROGRESSION OF COPD TO END STAGE: SYMPTOM IDENTIFICATION AND TREATMENT

Symptom management is important in the PC of clients with progression of COPD but does not alter the trajectory of the disease or the survival odds. Dyspnea and the resultant development of anxiety are commonly associated with end-stage COPD. Dyspnea may also be associated with cor pulmonale, which is a late sign and poor outcome indicator of COPD (Marini & Wheeler, 2010). However, in the older adult with COPD, dyspnea and complaints of breathlessness may be difficult to ascertain (Duthie et al., 2007). Dyspnea is a subjective symptom of breathlessness, but the older adult may compensate for its development by decreasing his or her level of activity (Duthie et al., 2007).

Once dyspnea has been diagnosed, the underlying cause needs to be identified. In the older adult with COPD, dyspnea can be the result of the disease process itself, the development of cor pulmonale, or a respiratory infection, such as pneumonia. Nonpharmacologic interventions for symptom relief of dyspnea include repositioning the client with his or her head up or to a position of comfort in a chair (Kazanowski, 2001; LaDuke, 2001). A cool environment can decrease the perception of dyspnea (Kazanowski, 2001; Meier et al., 1998). Balancing rest and exercise as tolerated can also assist the client to breathe easier (Kazanowski, 2001; LaDuke, 2001). Frequent reassurance and providing a physical presence can assist in decreasing anxiety and therefore decrease dyspnea.

The pharmacologic interventions chosen to treat dyspnea depend on the underlying etiology. Oxygen can be an initial adjunctive therapy for dyspnea (Kazanowski, 2001; LaDuke, 2001) and can be delivered via nasal cannula, face mask with cool mist, bilevel positive airway pressure (Bi-PAP), or mechanical ventilation. Oxygen is the only therapy associated with increased survival in patients who have chronic respiratory failure and must be administered for a minimum of 15 hours or more (GOLD, 2017). Oxygen therapy should be prescribed for all COPD patients who experience severe hypoxemia while resting and/or who have an oxygen saturation of less than 88% at rest (GOLD, 2017). The administration of oxygen has a number of salient effects, including improvements in pulmonary hemodynamics, functional status, and well-being (GOLD, 2017). Although Bi-PAP is used in the acute care setting to reverse respiratory failure, it may provide some relief from dyspnea. Bi-PAP may also be desirable because it may be chosen as a less invasive alternative to mechanical ventilation. Recent studies have found no mortality benefit with the use of long-term oxygenation in patients who have stable COPD or who experience desaturation to between 89% and 93% while resting or exercising (The Long-Term Oxygen Treatment Trial Research Group, 2016). Additionally, the use of supplemental oxygen in patients with stable COPD did not reduce the risk of hospitalizations, the incidence of COPD exacerbations, or changes in QOL, depression, or functional status.

Since breathlessness is a multidimensional symptom, composed of both uncomfortable physical symptoms and a troubling affective dimension, (Mahler et al., 2010) strongly recommends morphine as the drug of choice to treat breathlessness. Opioids, such as morphine sulfate, can be administered to decrease the perception and sensation of dyspnea and/or breathlessness (Kazanowski, 2001; LaDuke, 2001). Morphine works by primarily activating the mu receptor on certain cells in the central or peripheral nervous system, inhibiting the release of noxious substances, such as Substance P or norepinephrine. Additionally, there is a release of dopamine in the brain, contributing to a feeling of pleasure. Morphine can be administered sublingually,

---

Exhibit 15.5
Pharmacologic Interventions for Dyspnea

Opiates: *Morphine Sulfate*
    Parenteral (1–2 mg IV every 10–15 minutes; 2–5 mg SC initially)
    Orally or sublingually (5–10 mg, repeat as needed every 1 hour prn)
    Rectally (10–20 mg every 4 hours)

Antidepressants: *Selective Serotonin Reuptake Inhibitors*
    Sertraline (Zoloft), oral, treatment initiated at 25 to 50 mg/d. Older adults should start at 25 mg/d.
    Dose may be increased after 4 weeks if symptoms persist.

Anxiolytics: *Benzodiazepines*
    Lorazepam (0.5 mg orally or sublingually every 4 hours)
    Thorazine (25–100 mg orally TID or QID)

Diuretics: *Furosemide*
    Administered orally, SC, IV, or IM for signs/symptoms of fluid volume excess; 20–80 mg orally (per dose)
    20–40 mg IV/IM (per dose)

Source: From Kazanowski, M. K. (2001). Symptom management in palliative care. In M. L. Matzo & D. W. Sherman (Eds.), *Palliative care nursing: Quality care to the end of life* (pp. 327–361). New York, NY: Springer.

---

orally, parenterally, and via nebulizer (see Exhibit 15.5). Studies have revealed that patients with COPD who receive morphine experience improved QOL (Bajwah et al., 2012). Anxiety is also reduced because of the mood-altering effects of morphine (LaDuke, 2001), considered a "double-effect" treatment with morphine. Morphine use and dosing should be tailored to the individual patients. The ethical obligation to treat breathlessness in patients with advanced disease should outweigh providers' concerns regarding addiction or dependence (ATSP, 2010). However, while morphine can reduce breathlessness, there are many associated serious adverse effects, including respiratory depression, somnolence, nausea, vomiting, and confusion. Respiratory depression is one of the most concerning side effects; however, patients develop a tolerance toward respiratory depression. A recent study revealed that almost 75% of patients with COPD are prescribed opioids, but there is twice the risk of death in new patients who begin morphine, thought to be cardiovascular related (Vozoris et al., 2016). The authors advise providers to be careful when initiating opioid use in new patients who have COPD and to be vigilant regarding the development of side effects (Vozoris et al., 2016).

Steroids can be administered to the client with COPD to alleviate the inflammatory effects within the lungs, as well as bronchodilators, to relieve dyspnea (Kazanowski, 2001; LaDuke, 2001). Dyspnea related to cor pulmonale may respond to the administration of diuretics. If the client has tenacious secretions associated with COPD or a respiratory infection, mucolytics may be administered (Kazanowski, 2001). Carbocysteine and *N*-acetylcysteine may help to reduce exacerbations associated with COPD (GOLD, 2017). A SR reveals a reduction in the number of acute exacerbations and a decrease in the number of days of associated disability with mucolytics (Poole & Black, 2010). If a respiratory infection, such as pneumonia, has been identified as the source of dyspnea (fever, congested cough), antibiotic therapy is appropriate (Kazanowski, 2001; LaDuke, 2001). Anxiolytics, such as benzodiazepines, barbiturates, and phenothiazines, may be prescribed to relieve the anxiety and fear associated with the feelings of breathlessness (Kazanowski, 2001; LaDuke, 2001).

Depression and anxiety are common comorbidities in patients with COPD and are associated with an increased morbidity and mortality, dyspnea, declining functional status, and decreased QOL. The prevalence of anxiety ranges from 10% to 96% of individuals (Putman-Casdorph & McCrone, 2009). Some reports indicate that fewer than one-third of patients with COPD receive appropriate care for anxiety and depression, and these untreated comorbidities contribute to increased hospitalization rates and premature deaths when compared to COPD patients without comorbidities (Yohannes & Alexopoulos, 2014). The causes of anxiety and depression arise from multiple biological, psychological, and sociological origins and impair the patient's physical functioning as well as his or her social interactions (Yohannes & Alexopoulos, 2014). Depression is thought to be both a cause and a consequence of COPD, although the exact mechanism explaining how depression causes COPD is not known (Yohannes & Alexopoulos, 2014). Increased anxiety may be associated with difficulty breathing (Putman-Casdorph & McCrone, 2009).

The incidence of depression is higher in clients with COPD than in the general public (Putman-Casdorph & McCrone, 2009). In COPD, depression rates range from 20% to 80% (Putman-Casdorph & McCrone, 2009). Individuals who are African American, elderly, and of lower socioeconomic status experience a disproportionate incidence of depression (Putman-Casdorph & McCrone, 2009). Depression in COPD interferes with the client's ability to participate in activities of daily living, pulmonary rehabilitation, and breathing exercises. Depression may also impede the individual's ability to quit smoking, which is an integral component of care.

Due to the significant morbidity and mortality associated with depression in patients with COPD, it is imperative that clinicians screen patients for depression. Multiple tools have been developed to assess for depression, including the Geriatric Depression Scale, Patient Health Questionnaire-9 (PHQ-9), and the Primary Care Evaluation of Mental Disorders (PRIME-MD).

Although limited, studies to date indicate that antidepressants and psychotherapy may reduce a client's feelings of depression (Putman-Casdorph & McCrone, 2009). Providers should encourage clients to discuss their feelings and proactively encourage communication throughout the continuum of care. Clients should be assessed for depression and offered both antidepressants and/or cognitive/behavioral therapy and psychotherapy.

Norwood and Balkissoon (2005) have developed guidelines for screening and treating COPD patients who satisfy the criteria for major depression. Antidepressant therapy is recommended for all patients with major depression; most commonly, the classes of serotonin reuptake inhibitors (SSRIs) and tricyclic antidepressants (TCA) are prescribed. Although there are limited data to date on antidepressant therapy of COPD patients, most studies suggest that there are fewer adverse effects associated with SSRIs. Studies have recently shown that patients with COPD who are treated with multiple, complex psychological and/or lifestyle interventions such as education, relaxation, counseling, problem solving, and cognitive-behavioral therapy have fewer symptoms of anxiety and depression (Coventry et al., 2013). Additionally, the GOLD Guidelines (2013) suggest that exercise may have beneficial effects in treating depression in patients with chronic illnesses in general.

Many providers are unaware that pain is a common symptom in COPD (Hardin et al., 2008). Often pain occurs as a result of both anxiety and depression, which are prevalent in this population. Due to the lack of knowledge, clients are not routinely assessed for pain, and their pain is often undertreated. Additionally, many providers are concerned that treating pain may depress the patient's respiratory drive or hasten their deaths. Common misperceptions and lack of knowledge may prohibit treatment of both pain and depression.

Mechanical ventilation is an intervention that involves the creation of an artificial airway in order to deliver oxygen. In the setting of end-stage COPD, it is not an option that offers many advantages. There is an increased risk of nosocomial infection in an already compromised host (Hanania et al., 2010). It is difficult to wean a client with COPD from the ventilator because of diaphragmatic muscle weakness and, in the older adult, a decreased physiologic response to hypoxemia and hypercarbia (Phelan, Cooper, & Sangkachand, 2002). Mechanical ventilation also increases the risk of cardiac problems, aspiration, and barotrauma (Hanania et al., 2010). All oxygen delivery options should be offered to the client and family, along with the risks and benefits associated with treatment. In the setting of PC, the least invasive and intrusive therapies will promote comfort (Curtis, 2008).

■ COMPLEMENTARY THERAPIES FOR PATIENTS WITH CHRONIC OBSTRUCTIVE PULMONARY DISEASE

Complementary therapies, when incorporated into the practice of nursing, can increase the repertoire of interventions available to older adult clients (Frisch, 2001). For those clients who are receiving symptom relief at the end of life, complementary therapies can positively enhance what is already being done. Complementary therapies enable the nurse to create care that is client centered and holistic (Frisch, 2001). There is increasing demand by consumers to receive holistic care that takes into account the mind, body, and spirit (Kreitzer & Jensen, 2000). Complementary therapies are already available in the community. The use of complementary therapies can give clients and their families control over their care decisions (Kreitzer & Jensen, 2000); most complementary therapies can be utilized in the home. Examples of complementary therapies include guided imagery, relaxation, massage, and music therapy.

Rest is necessary in order to decrease the intensity of dyspnea; it can also decrease the work of breathing. Promoting rest and sleep can also decrease anxiety. Assessment of the client's sleep habits can be a helpful starting point to the promotion of restful sleep (Tullmann & Dracup, 2000). Assisting the client into a position of comfort can promote sleep (Tullmann & Dracup, 2000), and in the case of the client with COPD, this generally means elevation of the head of the bed, which also facilitates diaphragmatic expansion.

Guided imagery is a technique that can be utilized to promote sleep in the client with COPD (Tusek & Cwynar, 2000). Guided imagery can also assist the client through a stressful experience (Tusek & Cwynar, 2000). The client can practice guided imagery with a partner or via audiotape. Clients focus on the present and then are taken to a safe place in their mind.

Massage can also be explored as an option for sleep promotion (Richards, Gibson, & Overton-McCoy, 2000). Prior to initiating massage, the nurse must first determine that the elder is comfortable with being touched (Richards et al., 2000). In the client at the end stage of COPD, there are no contraindications to massage being utilized for the promotion of rest and sleep.

Music can also be added to the therapeutic plan for the promotion of rest and sleep, and may help to reduce the need for pain medications (Chlan, 2000; O'Kelly & Koffman, 2007; Richards et al., 2000). Music therapy can be helpful in clients with COPD who tire easily; however, music should be selected to their personal preference (Chlan, 2000). Anxiety reduction can also be facilitated through the use of complementary therapies such as massage (Richards et al., 2000), guided imagery (Tusek & Cwynar, 2000), and music therapy (Chlan, 2000). Reducing anxiety can also result in the reduction of dyspnea in the client with COPD.

Clients or their significant others may ask the nurse about the utility of herbal remedies in the treatment of COPD. There are several herbs that are used in the treatment of respiratory ailments. Chaparral, cinnamon, horehound, and pansy have been used in the treatment of bronchitis, although chaparral can cause severe liver damage and cinnamon can precipitate shortness of breath (Skidmore-Roth, 2001). Anise and astragalus have been used in the treatment of COPD. For general respiratory care and cough, lobelia and wild cherry have been used (Skidmore-Roth, 2001). Lobelia is contraindicated in a client who has congestive heart failure or dysrhythmias, and wild cherry is contraindicated in a client who has respiratory or cardiovascular depression (Skidmore-Roth, 2001). If the client is self-medicating with ginseng, tachycardia and hypertension can result if he or she also ingests caffeinated beverages, such as coffee or tea (Kuhn, 2002). St. John's wort taken in combination with theophylline can decrease the serum level of theophylline, making it less effective as a bronchodilator (Kuhn, 2002). Theophylline should not be used concurrently with the herb guarana, as it also contains theophylline (Kuhn, 2002). The benefits of herbal interventions should be weighed against the harmful side effects that could exacerbate COPD or the complications of cor pulmonale and respiratory failure.

More research is needed regarding the benefits of complementary therapies in the treatment plan of end-stage COPD. Spirituality also plays a role in fostering a positive attitude in the client and the maintenance of hope in family members. Complementary therapies can be incorporated with other pharmacologic and nonpharmacologic modalities in the care of the older adult with end-stage COPD.

■ DEATH FROM CHRONIC OBSTRUCTIVE PULMONARY DISEASE

The death of a client with COPD is commonly the result of respiratory failure (Barnes, 2001). Respiratory failure can be due to the development of either hypoxemia or hypercapnia. The client may initially present with dyspnea, disorientation, or confusion. Vague symptoms such as tachypnea, tachycardia, and restlessness can occur. If respiratory failure is due to hypercapnia, the client may become stuporous or lapse into a coma (Barnes, 2001). Cyanosis is a late sign of respiratory failure. Therapeutic interventions are based on the etiology of the respiratory failure. Supplemental oxygen may be delivered either noninvasively or via mechanical ventilation. Dyspneic symptoms are treated with opiates, bronchodilators, and anxiolytics.

Due to the unpredictable and variable trajectory in patients with COPD, few of these patients are offered hospice care at the end of their lives (Curtis, 2008). With greater education for patients and families, EOL discussions and optimal care will be improved. Criteria for admission to hospice have been delineated by the National Hospice and Palliative Care Organization and are listed in Exhibit 15.6.

In order to support the family through the death of their loved one, an honest discussion about the dying process needs to occur. Dyspnea is a symptom that is seen during the dying process of a client with COPD. Family members may panic when these dyspneic episodes occur (Tarzian, 2000). Due to the fact that the patient with COPD has no control over his or her breathlessness (Tarzian, 2000), educating the family and including the family in the

---

Exhibit 15.6
National Hospice and Palliative Care Organization: Criteria for Admission to Hospice in Patients With COPD

Primary
1. Disabling dyspnea at rest
2. Progressive pulmonary disease
3. Increasing emergency department visits or hospitalizations
4. Hypoxemia at rest on supplemental oxygen
   PO_2 less than 55 on O_2
   O_2 sat less than 88 on supplemental
   Or
   Hypercapnia: PCO_2 greater than 50.

Source: Adapted from Weiss, B. D., & Lee, E. (2010). Elder care: A resource for interprofessional care. Hospice eligibility for patients with COPD. Retrieved from https://nursingandhealth.asu.edu/sites/default/files/hospice-care-for-copd.pdf

---

management of dyspneic episodes can decrease his or her sense of panic and increase his or her sense of control.

PC, integrated throughout the continuum of the disease from diagnosis to end of life, may help to provide comprehensive care that improves QOL, reduces symptoms, and eases suffering for both patients experiencing COPD and their family members.

■ CONCLUSION

COPD is the third leading cause of death in the United States and the leading cause of death due to a respiratory condition; development of this disease occurs as the result of cigarette smoking and exposure to environmental pollution. These factors place clients at particular risk for developing COPD because they have been exposed to smoking and pollution for an extended period of time. In addition to this, the normal physiologic changes due to the aging process places individuals at an increased risk for the development of complications, such as cor pulmonale and pneumonia. In order to reduce the risk of developing the complications of COPD, smoking cessation is recommended. Pharmacologic modalities focus on improving ventilation, reducing inflammation, and preventing complications. Nonpharmacologic interventions including exercise, rest, and improved nutrition can be valuable adjunctive therapies in the care of patients with COPD. Patients and families experiencing chronic progressive lung disease benefit from the interprofessional approach offered by a PC team. The physical, emotional, social, and spiritual challenges of lung disease require the expertise of a cadre of health professionals who collaborate effectively across health settings in promoting quality of care across the illness experience.

CASE STUDY *Conclusion*

MRS. S.—5 YEARS LATER

The EOL discussions were initiated approximately 2 years ago when Mrs. S. started on home oxygen. At that time, Mrs. S. determined that she wanted all life-sustaining interventions and refused to sign an advance directive. Mrs. S.'s condition acutely deteriorated, however, when she experienced an episode of hemoptysis. Mrs. S was diagnosed with squamous cell carcinoma of her right bronchus. Given the severe progression of her COPD and low FEV1, Mrs. S. was not considered a surgical candidate because she would not tolerate the pneumonectomy required for treatment. The sudden diagnosis of lung cancer significantly impacted Mrs. S. and her two adult children, and they began to question whether an advance directive was necessary at this time. The PC team called a meeting and invited representatives from pulmonology, anesthesiology, and cardiothoracic surgery. The consultants explained that the risks of surgery were too great and that the prognosis would likely require a hospice admission. Mrs. S. and her family, upon hearing this assessment, signed an advance directive refusing intubation and cardiopulmonary resuscitation, and Mrs. S. was admitted to hospice. Mrs. S., age 71, died at home with her family in attendance 1 month after entering the hospice program.

CASE STUDY

AN INTERPROFESSIONAL PERSPECTIVE

Benjamin M. Sherman, MD, MBA, Cardiothoracic Anesthesiologist

The management of patients with COPD can be challenging for the anesthesiologist. Anesthesiologists must be aware of the sequelae of COPD such as the risks of obstructive sleep apnea, RHF, risks of pneumothorax, and the potential side effects of COPD medications when developing the best anesthetic plans for patients requiring surgery or procedures. It must also be noted that in addition to respiratory compromise, COPD patients may have physical inactivity, anorexia, muscle weakness, and fatigue. Each of these systemic impacts of COPD can lead to the increased frailty of patients. The more frail a patient becomes, the less likely he or she will be able to recover from the stressors of surgery and/or an acute illness. Additionally, given the high morbidity and mortality of COPD patients, anesthesiologists can be thrust into situations where EOL planning must be discussed with patients and/or their families. This conversation can be especially difficult given the acute nature of the situation and the limited time most anesthesiology providers have to build a relationship with the patients and their families.

Historically, the role of the anesthesiologist has been limited in regard to long-term patient optimization, EOL planning, and public health. Anesthesiologists frequently meet their patients on the day of surgery and have limited roles in the early preoperative and postoperative phases of care. COPD patients frequently can benefit from early interventions such as smoking cessation and pulmonary rehabilitation. Fortunately, a new care paradigm has been developed in recent years to help address these issues. The American Society of Anesthesiologists has developed and championed a new model of care called the Perioperative Surgical Home (PSH). The PSH is a system for managing and coordinating care that is patient centered and team based. PSH care extends from the time a decision for surgery is made and until there is a completion of the patient's recovery. The main goals are to improve the patient experience, improve the safety and health outcomes, and reduce the costs.

Specifically for COPD patients, the PSH paradigm helps improve care in several ways. Smoking cessation is very difficult for many tobacco-dependent patients, and it is not uncommon for patients to have several unsuccessful attempts at quitting. The perioperative period has been identified as a powerful teaching moment for smoking cessation, and identification and treatment of tobacco dependence during this period can be particularly effective. Smoking cessation reduces the risks of perioperative complications as well as improves the overall health of the patient in the long term. The PSH has therefore incorporated smoking cessation as one of the goals prior to surgery. Additionally, early identification of COPD patients who display high frailty scores can be enrolled into pulmonary prehabilitation programs and nutrition programs, which help reduce the amount of frailty and respiratory dysfunction prior to undergoing surgery. Lastly, the PSH model can help begin and continue EOL discussions with COPD patients regarding resuscitative wishes if the patient's condition deteriorates postoperatively. The PSH model of care is an extension of PC into the perioperative phase of a patient's life. Through thoughtful consideration and early identification of modifiable risk factors, the patient's perioperative experience can have improved outcomes while reducing patient suffering.

Reflecting specifically about Mrs. S.'s case, her story underscores how the PSH can help many patients like her. In regard to her smoking cessation, only after she was confronted with the possibility of lung cancer (lung nodule) could she find the will to overcome her addiction to tobacco. This underscores the unique opportunity that anesthesiologists have to initiate smoking cessation therapy at a time when it will have a significant impact and the highest opportunity of success. When Mrs. S. was eventually diagnosed with terminal lung cancer, the opportunity for the family to interact with the anesthesiologist in a collaborative manner and in a non-urgent circumstance facilitated their ability to make the difficult choices about EOL planning. The PSH will similarly give patients and families an opportunity to discuss their disease process and implications regarding the risks of anesthesiology and surgery in a nonurgent setting. This will hopefully give patients time to process all the information and make sensible EOL decisions.

Evidence-Based Practice

Horita, N., Gota, A., Shibata, Y., Ota, E., Nakashima, K., Nagai, K., & Kaneko, T. (2017). Which combination of inhaled medications are safe and effective for chronic obstructive pulmonary disease (COPD)? *Cochrane Database of Systematic Reviews*, 2, doi:10.1002/14651858.CD012066.pub2

Research Problem
Patients with COPD experience difficulty breathing along with excessive mucous production and cough. Determining which treatments are best to reduce symptoms of dyspnea and cough is paramount in caring for these patients. Recent guidelines suggest that the combination of a LABA and a LAMA is preferable to the combination of a LABA and ICS.

Design, Setting, Sample, and Methods
The authors conducted a systematic review consisting of 11 RCTs to determine the effectiveness of LAMA and LABA compared with LABA and ICS. Additionally, the benefits and risk associated with each combination were investigated.

Results

The combination of a LABA and a LAMA was more effective than LABA and ICS in reducing symptoms, exacerbations, pneumonia, and QOL. There was no difference in mortality between the two combination therapies.

Implication for Nursing Practice

Helping patients to relieve symptoms of dyspnea and reduce exacerbations of COPD is an important treatment goal for COPD patients. A LABA and LAMA combination treatment can be delivered via one medication device, assisting patients with ease of administration and facilitating compliance.

■ REFERENCES

American Lung Association. (2017). How Serious Is COPD?. Retrieved from http://www.lung.org/lung-health -and-diseases/lung-disease-lookup/copd/learn-about-copd/how-serious-is-copd.html

Bajwah, S., Higginson, I. J., Ross, J. R., Wells, A. U., Birring, S. S., Patel, A., & Riley, J. (2012). Specialist palliative care is more than drugs: A retrospective study of ILD patients. *Lung, 190,* 215–220. doi:10.1007/s00408-011-9355-7

Barnes, P. J. (2001). Modern management of COPD in the elderly. *Annals of Long-Term Care, 9*(5), 51–56.

Barr, R. G., Bourbeau, J., & Camargo, C. A. (2008). Tiotropium for stable chronic obstructive pulmonary disease. *The Cochrane Collaboration, 4,* 1–78. doi:10.1002/14651858.CD002876.pub2

Berry, J. K., & Baum, C. L. (2001). Malnutrition in chronic obstructive pulmonary disease: Adding insult to injury. *AACN Clinical Issues. Advanced Practice in Acute and Critical Care, 12*(2), 210–219. doi:10.1097/00044067-200105000-00005

Bischoff, K. E., Sudore, R., Miao, Y., Boscardin, W. J., & Smith, A. K. (2013). Advance care planning and the quality of end-of-life care among older adults. *Journal of the American Geriatric Society, 61*(2), 209–214. doi:10.1111/jgs.12105

Brashers, V. L. (Ed.). (2002). *Chronic obstructive pulmonary disease. Clinical applications of pathophysiology: Assessment, diagnostic reasoning and management.* St. Louis, MO: Mosby.

Cahill, K., Stead, L. F., & Lancaster, T. (2009). Nicotine receptor partial agonists for smoking cessation. *Cochrane Database of Systematic Reviews, 1,* 1–59. doi:10.1002/14651858.CD006103.pub6.

Cayley, W. E. (2008). Use of inhaled corticosteroids to treat stable COPD. *American Family Physician, 77*(11), 1532–1533.

Centers for Disease Control and Prevention. (2017, May). *Smoking and tobacco use.* Retrieved from https://www .cdc.gov/tobacco/data_statistics/fact_sheets/health_effects/effects_cig_smoking/index.htm

Chlan, L. L. (2000). Music therapy as a nursing intervention for patients supported by mechanical ventilation. *AACN Clinical Issues. Advanced Practice in Acute and Critical Care, 11*(1), 128–138. doi:10.1097/00044067-200002000-00014

Chong, J., Karner, C., & Poole, P. (2012). Tiotropium versus long-acting beta-agonists for stable chronic obstructive pulmonary disease. *Cochrane Database of Systematic Reviews,* (9), CD009157. doi:10.1002/14651858 .CD009157.pub2

Collins, E. G., Langbein, W. E., Fehr, L., & Maloney, C. (2001). Breathing pattern retraining and exercise in persons with chronic obstructive pulmonary disease. *AACN Clinical Issues, 12*(2), 202–209.

Coventry, P. A., Bower, P., Keyworth, C., Kenning, C., Knopp, J., Garrett, C., ... Dickens, C. (2013). The effect of complex interventions on depression and anxiety in chronic obstructive pulmonary disease: Systematic review and meta-analysis. *PLOS ONE, 8*(4), e60532. doi:10.1371/journal.pone.0060532

Curtis, J. R. (2008). Palliative and end-of-life care for patients with severe COPD. *The European Respiratory Journal, 32*(3), 796–803. doi:10.1183/09031936.00126107

Dine, J., Williams, J., & DeLisser, H. (2009). Pulmonary disease. In L. Hark & G. Morrison (Eds.), *Medical nutrition and disease: A case-based approach* (4th ed., pp. 355–373). West Sussex, UK: Wiley-Blackwell.

Dunn, N. A. (2001). Keeping COPD patients out of the ED. *Registered Nurses, 64*(2), 33–38.

Duthie, E., Katz, P., & Malone, M. (2007). *Practice of geriatrics.* Philadelphia, PA: W. B. Saunders.

Ferreira, I. M., Brooks, D., White, J., & Goldstein, R. (2012). Nutritional supplementation for stable chronic obstructive pulmonary disease. *Cochrane Database of Systematic Reviews, 12,* 1–95. doi:10.1002/14651858 .CD000998.pub3

Fiore, M., Jaén, C. R., Baker, T. B., Bailey, W. C., Bennett, G., Benowitz, N. L., ... Williams, C. (2008a). A clinical practice guideline for treating tobacco use and dependence: 2008 update. A U.S. Public Health Service report. *American Journal of Preventive Medicine, 35*(2), 158–176. doi:10.1016/j.amepre.2008.04.009

Fiore, M. C., Jaén, C. R., Baker, T. B., Bailey, W. C., Benowitz, N. L., Curry, S. J., ... Leitzke, C. (2008b). Treating tobacco use and dependence: 2008 update. Clinical practice guideline. Executive Summary. *Respiratory Care, 53*(9), 1217–1222.

Frisch, N. C. (2001). Nursing as a context for alternative/complementary modalities. *Online Journal of Issues in Nursing, 6*(2), 2.

Global Initiative for Chronic Obstructive Lung Disease. (2009, January). Global strategy for the diagnosis, management and prevention of chronic obstructive pulmonary disease. Retrieved from http://www.goldcopd.com

Global Initiative for Chronic Obstructive Lung Disease. (2013). Global strategy for diagnosis, management and prevention of chronic obstructive pulmonary disease. Retrieved from http://www.goldcopd.org

Global Initiative for Chronic Obstructive Lung Disease. (2017). Global strategy for diagnosis, management and prevention of chronic obstructive pulmonary disease. Retrieved from http://goldcopd.org/gold-2017-global -strategy-diagnosis-management-prevention-copd/

Hanania, N., Sharma., G., & Sharafkhaneh, A. (2010). COPD in the elderly patient. *Seminars in Respiratory and Critical Care Medicine, 31*(5), 596–606. doi:10.1055/s-0030-1265900

Hardin, K. A., Meyers, F., & Louie, S. (2008). Integrating palliative care in severe chronic obstructive lung disease. *COPD: Journal of Chronic Obstructive Pulmonary Disease, 5*, 207–220. doi:10.1080/15412550802237366

Holland, A. E., Hill, C. J., Jones, A. Y., & McDonald, C. (2012). Breathing exercises for chronic obstructive pulmonary disease. *Cochrane Dababase of Systematic Review*s, (10), 1–89. doi:10.1002/14651858.CD008250.pub2

Hughes, J. R., Stead, L. F., & Lancaster, T. (2007). Antidepressants for smoking cessation. *Cochrane Database of Systematic Reviews,* (1), 1–106. doi:10.1002/14651858.CD000031.pub3

Jen, R., Li, Y., Owens, R., & Malhotra, Y. (2016). Sleep in chronic obstructive pulmonary disease: Evidence gaps and challenges. *Canadian Respiratory Journal, 2016*, 7947198. doi:10.1155/2016/7947198

Joint Commission. (2015, July). End-of-life care: A patient safety issue. *QuickSafety, 15*, 1–3.

Kazanowski, M. K. (2001). Symptom management in palliative care. In M. L. Matzo & D. W. Sherman (Eds.), *Palliative care nursing: Quality care to the end of life* (pp. 327–361). New York, NY: Springer Publishing.

Knauft, E., Nielsen, E., Engelberg, R., Patrick, D., & Curtis, J. R. (2005). Barriers and facilitators to end-of-life care communication for patients with COPD. *Chest, 127*, 2188–2196. doi:10.1378/chest.127.6.2188

Kreitzer, M. J., & Jensen, D. (2000). Healing practices: Trends, challenges, and opportunities for nurses in acute and critical care. *AACN Clinical Issues. Advanced Practice in Acute and Critical Care, 11*(1), 7–16. doi:10.1097/00044067-200002000-00003

Kuhn, M. A. (2002). Herbal remedies: Drug-herb interactions. *Critical Care Nurse, 22*(2), 22–28, 30.

LaDuke, S. (2001). Terminal dyspnea and palliative care. *American Journal of Nursing, 101*(11), 26–31.

Lake Research Partners and the Coalition for Compassionate Care of California. (2012). Final Chapter: Californians' attitudes and experiences with death and dying. Oakland: California Healthcare Foundation.

Lee, A., & Holland, A. (2014). Time to adapt exercise training regiments in pulmonary rehabilitation—A review of the literature. *International Journal of Chronic Obstructive Disease, 9*(1) 1275–1288. doi:10.2147/COPD .S54925

Lu, Y., Feng, L., Liang, F., Ma Shwe, N., Keng, B. Y., & Tze, P. N. (2013). Systemic inflammation, depression, and obstructive pulmonary function; a population-based study. *Respiratory Research, 14*(53). 1–8. doi:10.1186/1465–9921-14-53

Mahler, D. A. Selecky, P. A., Harrod, C. G., Benditt, J. O., Carrieri-Kohlman, V., Curtis, R., Manning, H. L., ... & Waller, A. (2010). American College of Chest Physicians consensus statement of the management of dyspnea in patients with advanced lung or heart disease. *Chest, 137*(3), 674–688.

Marini, J. J., & Wheeler, A. P. (Eds.). (2010). *Critical care medicine: The essentials.* Baltimore, MD: Williams & Wilkins.

McCarthy, B., Casey, D., Devane, D., Murphy, K., Murphy, E., & Lacasse, Y. (2015). Pulmonary rehabilitation for chronic obstructive pulmonary disease. *Cochrane Database of Systematic Reviews, 2*, 1–208. doi:10.1002/ 14651858.CD003793.pub3

Meier, D. E., Morrison, R. S., & Ahronheim, J. C. (1998). Palliative care. In: E. H. Duthrie & P. R. Katz (Eds.), *Practice of geriatrics* (pp. 99–111). Philadelphia, PA: W. B. Saunders.

Messer, B., Griffiths, J., & Baudouin (2012). The prognostic variables predictive of mortality inpatients with an exacerbation of COPD admitted to the ICU: An integrative review. *The Quality Journal of Medicine, 105*, 115–126. doi:10.1093/qjmed/hcr210

Mosenifar, Z. (2013). Chronic obstructive pulmonary disease. In J. J. Oppenheimer (Ed.), *Medscape.* Retrieved from http://emedicine.medscape.com/article/297664-treatment

National Consensus Project for Quality Palliative Care. (2013). *Clinical practice guidelines for quality palliative care.* Pittsburgh, PA: Author. Retrieved from https://www.nationalcoalitionhpc.org/ncp-guidelines-2013

National Hospice Organization. (1996). *Medical guidelines for determining prognosis in selected non-cancer diseases* (2nd ed.). Arlington, VA: Author.

National Institute for Health and Care Excellence Guidelines. (2017). End of life care for adults. Quality standard. Retrieved from https://www.nice.org.uk/guidance/qs144

National Quality Forum. (2012). National Voluntary Consensus standards: Palliative care and end-of-life—A consensus report. Retrieved from https://www.qualityforum.org/Publications/2012/04/Palliative_Care_and_End -of-Life_Care—A_Consensus_Report.aspx

Norwood, R., & Balkissoon, R. (2005). Current perspectives on the management of co-morbid depression in COPD. *COPD, 2*(1), 185–193. doi:10.1081/COPD-200050740

O'Kelly, J., & Koffman, J. (2007). Multidisciplinary perspectives of music therapy in adult palliative care. *Palliative Medicine, 21*, 235–241. doi:10.1177/0269216307077207

Phelan, B. A., Cooper, D. A., & Sangkachand, P. (2002). Prolonged mechanical ventilation and tracheostomy in the elderly. *AACN Clinical Issues. Advanced Practice in Acute and Critical Care, 13*(1), 84–93. doi:10.1097/00044067-200202000-00009

Poole, P., & Black, P. N. (2010). Mucolytic agents for chronic bronchitis or chronic obstructive pulmonary disease. *Cochrane Database of Systematic Review, 17*(2), 1–79. doi:10.1002/14651858.CD001287.pub2

Putman-Casdorph, H., & McCrone, S. (2009). Chronic obstructive pulmonary disease, anxiety and depression: State of the science. *Heart and Lung, 38*(1), 34–47. doi:10.1016/j.hrtlng.2008.02.005

Richards, K. C., Gibson, R., & Overton-McCoy, A. L. (2000). Effects of massage in acute and critical care. *AACN Clinical Issues. Advanced Practice in Acute and Critical Care, 11*(1), 77–96.

Schneider, C., Jick, S. S., Bothner, U., & Meier, C. (2010). COPD and the risk of depression. *Chest, 137*(2), 341–347. doi:10.1378/chest.09-0614

Sethi, S., & Murphy, T. F. (2008). Infection in the pathogenesis and course of chronic obstructive pulmonary disease. *New England Journal of Medicine, 359*, 2355–2365. doi:10.1056/NEJMra0800353

Sharma, S. (2006). Respiratory failure. E-Medicine. Retrieved from http://emedicine.medscape.com/article/167981-print

Sheahan, S. L., & Musialowski, R. (2001). Clinical implications of respiratory system changes in aging. *Journal of Gerontological Nursing, 27*(5), 26–34. doi:10.3928/0098-9134-20010501-08

Skidmore-Roth, L. (Ed.). (2001). *Handbook of herbs and natural supplements*. St. Louis, MO: Mosby.

Sommers, M. S., & Johnson, S. A. (Eds.). (2002). *Diseases and disorders: A nursing therapeutics manual*. Philadelphia, PA: F. A. Davis.

Spector, N., & Klein, D. (2001). Chronic critically ill dyspneic patients: Mechanisms and clinical measurement. *AACN Clinical Issues. Advanced Practice in Acute and Critical Care, 12*(2), 220–233. doi:10.1097/00044067-200105000-00006

Spence, A., Hasson, F., Waldron, M., Kernohan, W. G., McLaughlin, D., Watson, B., ... Marley, A. M. (2009). Professionals delivering palliative care to people with COPD: Qualitative study. *Palliative Medicine, 23*, 126–131. doi:10.1177/0269216308098804

Stead, L. F., Perera, R., Bullen, C., Mant, D., Hartmann-Boyce, J., Cahill, K., & Lancaster, T. (2012). Nicotine replacement therapy for smoking cessation. *Cochrane Database of Systematic Reviews, 11*, 1–264. doi:10.1002/14651858.CD000146.pub4

Stead, L. F., Perrara, R., Bullen, C., Mant, D., & Lancaster, T. (2008). Nicotine replacement therapy for smoking cessation (Review). *Cochrane Database of Systematic Reviews, 1*, 1–221. doi:10.1002/14651858.CD000146.pub3.

Tarzian, A. J. (2000). Caring for dying patients who have air hunger. *Journal of Nursing Scholarship, 32*(2), 137–143. doi:10.1111/j.1547-5069.2000.00137.x

The Long-Term Oxygen Treatment Trial Research Group. (2016). A randomized trial of long-term oxygen for COPD with moderate saturation. *New England Journal of Medicine, 375*(17), 1617–1627. doi:10.1056/NEJMoa1604344

Tullmann, D. F., & Dracup, K. (2000). Creating a healing environment for elders. *AACN Clinical Issues. Advanced Practice in Acute and Critical Care, 11*(1), 34–50.

Tusek, D. L., & Cwynar, R. E. (2000). Strategies for implementing a guided imagery program to enhance patient experience. *AACN Clinical Issues. Advanced Practice in Acute and Critical Care, 11*(1), 68–76. doi:10.1097/00044067-200002000-00009

Vozoris, N. T., Wang, X., Fischer, H., Bell, C. M., O'Donnell, D. E., Austin, P. C., ... Rochon, P. A. (2016). Incident opioid drug use and adverse respiratory outcomes among older adults with COPD. *European Respiratory Journal, 48*(3), 683–693. doi:10.1183/09031936.00008014

Walters, J. A. E., Gibson, P. G., Wood-Baker, R., Hannay, M., & Walters, E. H. (2009). Systemic corticosteroids for acute exacerbations of chronic obstructive pulmonary disease. *Cochrane Database of Systematic Reviews, 1*(4), 1–57. doi:10.1002/14651858.CD001288.pub3

Weiss, B. D., & Lee, E. (2010). Elder care: A resource for interprofessional care. Hospice eligibility for patients with COPD. Retrieved from https://nursingandhealth.asu.edu/sites/default/files/hospice-care-for-copd.pd

Wood-Baker, R. R., Gibson, P. G., Hannay, M., Walters, E. H., & Walters, J. A. E. (2008). Systemic corticosteroids for acute exacerbations of chronic obstructive pulmonary disease. *Cochrane Database of Systematic Reviews*, (1), 1–63.

Yang, I. A., Fong, K., Sim, E. A., Black, P. N., & Lasserson, T. J. (2007). Inhaled corticosteroids for stable chronic obstructive pulmonary disease. *Cochrane Database of Systematic Review, 2*, 1–19. doi:10.1002/14651858.CD002991.pub2

Yohannes, A. M. (2007). Palliative care provision for patients with chronic obstructive pulmonary disease. *Health and Quality of Life Outcomes, 5*(17), 1–6. Retrieved from http://www.hqlo.com/content/5/1/17

Yohannes, A. M., & Alexopoulos, G. S. (2014). Depression and anxiety in patients with COPD. *European Respiratory Review, 23*(133), 345–349. doi:10.1183/09059180.00007813

Yohannes, A. M., Willgoss, T. G., Baldwin, R. C., & Connolly, M. J. (2010). Depression and anxiety in chronic heart failure and chronic obstructive disease: Prevalence, relevance, clinical implications and management principles. *International Journal of Geriatric Psychiatry, 25*(12), 1209–1221. doi:10.1002/gps.2463

Yung, V. Y., Walling, A. M., Min, L., Wenger, N. S., & Ganz, D. A. (2010). Documentation of advance care planning for community-dwelling elders. *Journal of Palliative Medicine, 13*(7), 861–867. doi:10.1089/jpm.2009.0341

Melody Hope Gallamore

Neurological Disorders

CHAPTER

16

KEY POINTS

- A growing body of evidence supports that symptoms associated with severe stroke and chronic neurological disorders are amenable to palliative treatment and that quality of life is increased from multidisciplinary approaches to care.
- Common problems faced by patients with these disorders include impairments in cognition, communication, sleep, swallowing, breathing, and mobility, as well as pain, fatigue, and depression.
- To improve treatment choices and end-of-life (EOL) decision making, research is needed to disentangle some difficulties with prognostic criteria for receiving hospice benefits and the accuracy of newer technologies in determining irreversible brain death.

CASE STUDY

Mr. M.J. is a 79-year-old male who lives in an assisted living facility. He was found on the bathroom floor and taken to the hospital. Physicians discovered that he had a left middle cerebral artery (MCA) stroke. He has lost movement to his right upper and lower extremity. He has decreased sensation in his right upper extremity and slightly more sensation in his right lower extremity. He is exhibiting the symptoms of expressive aphasia and difficulty swallowing. His medical team is contemplating sending him to a long-term care facility in a few days. Currently, he is resistant to physical and occupational therapy. He yells when his right extremities are moved, as if in pain. He does not seem to have a desire to interact with nurses or support staff.

What methods could the interdisciplinary team employ to attempt to enhance Mr. M.J.'s overall quality of life? What components should be included in Mr. M.J.'s assessment? What interventions would you recommend to treat Mr. M.J.?

This chapter focuses on management of people with stroke, chronic neurological disorders (CNDs), coma, and brain death. Stroke and CNDs, while unique and individualized in many respects, share a cluster of common symptoms and treatment needs. While some people who suffer a stroke recover completely or nearly completely from the event, people with CNDs often exhibit unresponsiveness or only slight or temporary responsiveness to curative treatments. Symptoms associated with severe stroke and CNDs are amenable to palliative treatment, and a growing body of evidence supports that quality of life (QOL) is increased from interdisciplinary palliative care (PC) approaches to symptom management (Bede et al., 2011; Blackhall, 2012; Blacquiere, Gubitz, Dupere, McLeod, & Phillips, 2009; Burton & Payne, 2012; Campbell, Jones, & Merrills, 2010; Higginson et al., 2009; Kuhn & Forrest, 2012; Lökk, 2011; Martin & Sabbagh, 2011; Miller et al., 2009; Miyasaki et al., 2012).

This chapter presents a description of common symptoms experienced from stroke and CNDs, including Alzheimer's disease, Parkinson's disease, multiple sclerosis (MS), and amyotrophic lateral sclerosis (ALS). Comorbid conditions that frequently accompany the latter stages of these illnesses are described as well as interventions aimed to provide symptom management. Due to the unique assessment and management issues that accompany coma and brain death, these problems and their management are presented in separate sections of the chapter. Issues unique to pediatric coma and brain death are also discussed. All disorders discussed in this chapter except MS are more likely to occur in older adulthood; thus, gerontological issues are incorporated throughout the chapter.

■ PREVALENCE, DISEASE TRAJECTORY, AND PATHOGENESIS

Stroke

In the United States, stroke is the fifth leading cause of death and the leading cause of severe long-term disability (C. Davis & Lockhart, 2016), with someone having a stroke every 40 seconds and someone dying of a stroke, on average, every 4 minutes (American Heart Association [AHA], 2017).

It is estimated that each year 795,000 people will experience either a new stroke (77%) or a recurrent stroke (23%). Eighty-seven percent of strokes are ischemic, 10% are hemorrhagic, and 3% are a subarachnoid hemorrhage (AHA, 2017). The prevalence of stroke is higher in older adults, African Americans, American Indians/Alaska Natives, persons with lower levels of education, and persons living in the southeastern United States (Go et al., 2013). Racial and ethnic disparities in stroke care continue to be a major challenge for healthcare providers, with the burden of stroke remaining consistently higher among ethnic minority groups (Qian et al., 2013). Seventeen percent of all strokes occur in people who are older than 85 years (Go et al., 2013). The incidence of stroke is higher in men than in women between the ages of 45 and 84 years. However, this changes after the age of 85 years with women having a higher incidence of strokes than men (Go et al., 2013). While stroke is most common in older adults, it does occur in teenagers, children, infants, and unborn babies. The overall incidence of stroke in children 15 years of age and younger is 6.4/100,000. In contrast to adults, children have as many ischemic as hemorrhagic strokes (Go et al., 2013). Most people

with stroke will survive the initial illness. As a result, there are an estimated 6.8 million stroke survivors in the United States with a projection of an additional 4 million by the year 2030 (Go et al., 2013). Stroke accounts for more than 130,000 deaths in the United States each year, which is 1 in every 20 deaths (AHA, 2017).

There are two types of stroke: ischemic and hemorrhagic. Each type of stroke results in the brain being deprived of oxygen-rich blood leading to tissue hypoxia or death (C. Davis & Lockhart, 2016). An ischemic stroke results in a disruption of blood to a portion of the brain due to an occlusion of the cerebral artery by blood clots (emboli) or plaque and fatty deposits (thrombi). The majority of occlusions occur from the formation of a thrombus. In a thrombotic event, atherosclerotic blood vessels cause complete or partial blockage of blood flow to a local area in the brain. In an embolic event, a clot forms elsewhere in the body, such as in the heart; breaks off; and travels through the arterial system and lodges in a cerebral vessel, blocking blood flow. Atherosclerotic plaques tend to occur at the arterial bifurcations. Common sites for plaque formation include the internal carotid and vertebral arteries, and the junctions of the basilar and vertebral arteries (Book, 2009).

Hemorrhagic stroke occurs when a weakened blood vessel bursts, leaking blood into the brain. A stroke can cause a sudden onset of a focal or global neurological deficit that lasts longer than 24 hours and is caused by disrupted cerebral vascular circulation (Veerbeek et al., 2014). Ruptured intracerebral vessels occur as a result of hypertension, aneurysm, trauma, erosion of vessels by tumors, arteriovenous malformations, blood coagulation disorders, vasculitis, or drugs. The bleeding that occurs within the brain tissue causes increased pressure within the skull, resulting in brain cell death. Hemorrhagic stroke can progress rapidly, resulting in coma and frequently death (Book, 2009).

Signs of impairment may be perceptual, motor, cognitive, or speech related. Risk factors include hypertension, disorders of heart rhythm, high blood cholesterol and other lipids, diabetes mellitus, physical inactivity, family history and genetics, chronic kidney disease, and smoking (AHA, 2017). The effects of an acute stroke are dependent on the site and the extent of the brain damaged. Some of the effects include paralysis, cognitive deficits, speech problems, emotional difficulties, problems with activities of daily living (ADLs), and pain (National Institutes of Health, 2013). Recovery after stroke is complex and varies in terms of outcomes. The greater the initial damage, the longer and more difficult the recovery and residual disability. Neurological function begins to improve within a few days after the onset of a stroke, with the greatest gain occurring within the first 4 to 5 weeks (Kreisel, Hennerici, & Bäzner, 2007). Neurological and functional gains can continue over 3 to 6 months; however, they will do so more slowly, "plateauing" (Langhorne, Bernhardt, &

Kwakkel, 2011). The National Heart, Lung, and Blood Institute's Framingham Heart Study reported that among stroke survivors 65 years of age or older at 6 months after discharge, 50% had some hemiparesis, 35% had depressive symptoms, 30% were unable to walk without assistance, 26% were dependent for ADLs, 26% were institutionalized in a nursing home, and 19% were aphasic (Go et al., 2013). The percentage of people dead at 1 year after stroke ranges from 14% to 19% for 45- to 64-year-olds and 23% to 28% for those older than 65 years of age. The percentage of people who die increases at 5 years, with a range from 26% to 41% for 45- to 64-year-olds and 50% to 57% for those older than 65 years of age (AHA, 2017).

Chronic Neurological Disorders

■ **Alzheimer's Disease.** Alzheimer's disease is the sixth leading cause of death in the United States (Alzheimer's Association, 2017). Approximately 5.4 million people of all ages are living in the United States with Alzheimer's disease and this number is expected to increase as the population ages (Alzheimer's Association, 2017). There are more women than men with Alzheimer's disease because women tend to live longer. The greatest risk factor for Alzheimer's disease is advancing age (Alzheimer's Association, 2017). It is estimated that dementia of the Alzheimer's type affects over 13% of adults older than 65 years or one out of eight people (Alzheimer's Association, 2017). By 2050, the number of people age 65 and older with Alzheimer's disease is projected to almost triple, from 5 million to a projected 16 million (Alzheimer's Association, 2017).

Alzheimer's disease is a chronic, devastating, progressive, incurable neurodegenerative disease and predominant form of dementia (Van Cauwenberghe, Van Broeckhoven, & Sleegers, 2016). It is characterized by severe neuronal and cognitive loss, accumulation of plaques, and formation of neurofibrillary tangles (Van Cauwenberghe et al., 2016). Known risk factors for Alzheimer's disease are increasing age, family history, and genetics; however, biological and lifestyle factors have also been associated with Alzheimer's disease (National Institute on Aging, 2016). The pathophysiological processes that trigger the development and progression of Alzheimer's disease remain unclear and complex. While there is no single event identified to date that explains the development of Alzheimer's disease, several hypotheses are being put forward to explain the disorder (Kumar, Singh, & Ekavali, 2015). The hallmark microscopic features of Alzheimer's disease are the presence of beta-amyloid containing neuritic plaques and neurofibrillary tangles in the brain (Kawczynski Pasch, 2009; Takahashi, Nagao, & Gouras, 2017). Neuritic plaques occur as a result of an abnormal accumulation and clumping of the beta-amyloid protein between the nerve cells early in the disease process. The clumping by the beta-amyloid protein in the brain is thought to be responsible for blocking cell-to-cell signaling at synapses and triggering inflammation leading to neuronal dysfunction and death. Neurofibrillary tangles form an abnormal tau protein conglomerate in a helical fashion inside of abnormal neurons. The neurofibrillary tangle development causes disruption inside the neuron and later neuronal death (Querfurth & LaFerla, 2010). Neuritic plaques and neurofibrillary tangles are found in the hippocampus and other areas of the cerebral cortex. The hippocampus controls information processing, acquisition of new memories, and retrieval of old memories. In contrast, the cerebral cortex is involved in thinking and decision making (Book, 2009). As a result, people with Alzheimer's disease experience progressive memory loss, loss of executive function, language difficulties, and psychiatric and behavioral disturbances, and eventually the disease affects the area of the brain that enables the person to carry out basic bodily functions such as walking or swallowing (Alzheimer's Association, 2017; Burns & Iliffe, 2009).

Alzheimer's disease progression and rate of decline vary from person to person. People with Alzheimer's disease die an average of 4 to 8 years after diagnosis; however, the disease can last for as many as 20 years (Alzheimer's Association, 2017). The underlying pathophysiological process of Alzheimer's disease has been purported to begin years, if not decades, before the clinical symptoms are apparent (Dubois, Padovani, Scheltens, Rossi, & Dell'Agnello, 2016; Sperling et al., 2011). In 2012, the National Institute on Aging and the Alzheimer's Association issued new criteria and guidelines for the diagnosis of Alzheimer's disease. One of the decisions was to consider Alzheimer's disease a disease with two stages—mild cognitive impairment due to Alzheimer's and dementia due to Alzheimer's. Persons with mild cognitive impairment due to Alzheimer's exhibit mild cognitive decline greater than that expected for their age and education level (Alzheimer's Association, 2017), but these changes do not necessarily interfere with normal activities. The second stage, dementia due to Alzheimer's, is characterized by memory, thinking, and behavioral symptoms that impair the person's ability to function in daily activities (Alzheimer's Association, 2017). The new guidelines also propose, for research purposes, a preclinical phase that occurs before symptoms like memory loss develop (Alzheimer's Association, 2017). In this period prior to clinical symptoms, however, changes in the brain, cerebrospinal fluid, and/or blood occur and can be measured (Alzheimer's Association, 2017).

■ **Parkinson's Disease.** Parkinson's disease is the second most common, progressive, neurodegenerative disorder after Alzheimer's disease, affecting approximately 1 million people in the United States, with as many as 60,000 new cases appearing each year (Parkinson's Disease Foundation, 2017). This estimate may be low because diagnosis is uncertain and may take several years to conclude Parkinson's disease. Life expectancy for people with Parkinson's disease is not as good as once thought. One study found the duration between disease onset to death ranged from 7 to 14 years with differences being explained by age at diagnosis and the year the study was performed (MacLeod, Taylor, & Counsell, 2014). The presence of a diagnosis of dementia was found to be an independent predictor of mortality (MacLeod et al., 2014). Parkinson's disease is the 14th leading cause of death in the United States (Kochanek, Murphy, Xu, & Tejada-Vera, 2016). Its symptoms mimic other conditions and there is no biomarker for the disease. These figures are projected to grow as the age of the population increases. The average age of onset of Parkinson's disease is 60 years; however, 5% to 10% are diagnosed younger than the age of 50. Statistics have shown that men are affected more often than women (National Institute of Neurological Disorders and Stroke [NINDS], 2014).

Like Alzheimer's disease, the exact etiology of Parkinson's disease is not known. The only known definitive risk factor for the development of idiopathic Parkinson's disease is aging. Scientists suspect that both genetics and environmental factors play a role in the development of Parkinson's disease; however, they are unsure of the pathogenic role each plays and in what combination and/or dose. Most cases of Parkinson's disease occur without an obvious genetic cause (Parkinson's Disease Foundation, 2017). Possible environmental toxins that have been connected to Parkinson's disease are pesticides/herbicide, exposure to metals, solvents and polychlorinated biphenyls (PCBs), 1-methyl-4-phenyl-1,2,3, 6-tetrahydropyridine (MPTP) found in some synthetic forms of heroin, and viruses (NINDS, 2014). The hallmark features of Parkinson's disease are the loss of dopaminergic neurons in the substantia nigra and the presence of Lewy bodies. Parkinson's disease develops when brain cells in the substantia nigra begin to degenerate and die, resulting in progressive development of motor and nonmotor symptoms (NINDS, 2014). This structure makes and stores the neurotransmitter dopamine; the degenerative process results in the depletion of dopamine, a compound involved in communication between brain cells. Approximately 60% to 80% of dopamine cells are lost before clinical symptoms start to appear. The four primary motor symptoms are bradykinesia (i.e., slowness of movement), rigidity, postural instability or balance problems, and resting tremor (NINDS, 2014). Nonmotor symptoms associated with Parkinson's disease are many; some are minor while others are debilitating, including depression, emotional changes, difficulty with swallowing and chewing, loss of sense of smell, speech changes, urinary problems or constipation, skin problems, sleep problems, dementia, orthostatic hypotension, muscle cramps and dystonia, pain, sexual dysfunction, and fatigue and loss of energy (NINDS, 2014). The progression of Parkinson's disease symptoms manifests differently from person to person. In some people, the disease progresses more quickly and in others it may take 20 years or more (NINDS, 2014). Symptoms usually begin on one side of the body and eventually progress to both sides, causing balance problems and severe disability. In the late stage of Parkinson's disease, people are bedbound and are commonly afflicted by complications such as choking, pneumonia, and falls that can be the contributing factor leading to death (NINDS, 2014). Currently, there are no curative treatments, but early pharmacological treatment can limit the progression of the symptoms associated with Parkinson's disease. Levodopa is considered the first-line treatment for Parkinson's. It is a precursor to dopamine. While levadopa is used because it is able to cross the blood–brain barrier, it is still susceptible to enzymatic breakdown. To minimize the metabolism of levodopa in the body, it is often given in conjunction with carbidopa, which decreases the amount of levodopa breakdown, allowing more levodopa to enter the CNS and be converted to dopamine (Gopalakrishna & Alexander, 2015).

■ **Multiple Sclerosis.** MS occurs when the body's immune system attacks myelin. Myelin is the fatty substance that surrounds and protects the nerve fibers of the central nervous system. MS is thought to be immune mediated (National Multiple Sclerosis Society, 2016). The damaged myelin develops scar tissue (sclerosis), which disrupts or slows the nerve impulses traveling to and from the brain (National Multiple Sclerosis Society, 2016). Many researchers believe that MS is an autoimmune disease (NINDS, 2017b). Approximately 250,000 to 350,000 people in the United States are living with MS, with an estimate of 200 new cases a week (NINDS, 2017b). MS can occur between the ages of 10 and 80 years; however, a majority are diagnosed with their first attack between the ages of 20 and 50 years. Women are two to three times more commonly affected than men. The disease is more common in whites, especially those of Northern European ancestry. There is a strong genetic link, especially for first-degree relatives where there is approximately a 1 in 40 chance of developing MS (National Multiple Sclerosis Society, 2016). Most people with MS have a normal life expectancy. However, a rare form of the illness can be fatal within weeks (National Multiple Sclerosis Society, 2016).

The exact cause of MS is unknown. It is thought to be caused by genetic vulnerabilities combined with environmental factors, which subsequently trigger an autoimmune attack on the myelin, nerve fibers, and neurons in the brain and spinal cord (NINDS, 2017b). Scar tissue forms hard sclerotic plaques in multiple regions of the CNS. Early in the illness, the myelin sheath is affected; however, the nerve fiber does not allow nerve impulses to transmit signals through the nerve. As the damage to nerves progresses, the nerve axons are destroyed and nerve impulses are totally blocked, resulting in permanent loss of function (NINDS, 2017b).

MS is highly unpredictable from person to person. There's no set pattern to nerves affected, thus making it difficult to predict the disease course (NINDS, 2017b). There are four main patterns to the presentation of MS. Relapsing-remitting is the most common form of MS and is characterized by flare-ups that appear for several days to weeks followed by remissions, during which not all symptoms resolve completely. Primary-progressive MS is a less common form in which the disease manifestations gradually worsen over time without periods of remission. The secondary-progressive MS form starts out as a relapsing-remitting course but later progresses to primary-progressive MS. Progressive-relapsing MS is the least common form that is progressive from the beginning, with episodes of acute increased worsening of existing symptoms or new ones (National Multiple Sclerosis Society, 2016). Symptoms of MS are not the same for everyone; it depends on the location and extent of damage to the myelin in the CNS. Symptoms can come and go, range from mild to severe, and differ greatly between one relapse to another (National Multiple Sclerosis Society, 2016). The most common symptoms are fatigue, numbness, walking balance and coordination, bowel and bladder dysfunction, vision problems, dizziness, sexual dysfunction, pain, cognitive dysfunction, emotional changes, depression, and spasticity (National Multiple Sclerosis Society, 2016).

■ **Amyotrophic Lateral Sclerosis.** ALS, or Lou Gehrig disease, is a rare but rapidly progressive neurodegenerative disease that affects both upper and lower motor neurons leading to progressive muscle atrophy of the voluntary muscles in the arms, legs, and trunk (NINDS, 2017c). The incidence of ALS is higher in men than in women and typically strikes people between 40 and 60 years of age (NINDS, 2017c). Roughly, 20,000 to 30,000 Americans are living with ALS at any given time with approximately 5,000 new cases diagnosed each year. ALS is a fatal disease; most die from respiratory failure. The average life expectancy after onset of symptoms is 3 to 5 years; however, approximately 10% will survive 10 or more years (NINDS, 2017c).

The etiology and pathogenesis of ALS remains unclear and multifactorial, possibly involving both genetics and environmental exposures. However, over the years, researchers have identified only a few possible pathogenic processes that occur after symptom onset, such as mitochondrial dysfunction, protein aggregation, generation of free radicals, excitotoxicity, hypermetabolism, inflammation, and apoptosis (Gordon, 2011; van Es et al., 2017). In addition, only 5% to 10% of the cases are of the inherited type, leaving 90% of the cases classified as sporadic or meaning there is no clear cause (NINDS, 2017c). Diagnosis is made primarily on the medical history and the physical and neurological exam showing upper and lower motor neuron damage that cannot be attributed to other diseases (NINDS, 2017c). The sense of sight, touch, hearing, taste, and smell are not affected, while ocular movements, bowel and bladder function, and cognitive abilities are occasionally affected (NINDS, 2017c). ALS onset causes progressive loss of limb strength, dysphagia, dysarthria, and ultimately respiratory failure (Chio, Mora, & Lauria, 2017). Initial symptoms commonly include twitching, cramping, or stiffness of muscles; muscle weakness affecting an arm or a leg; slurred and nasal speech; or difficulty chewing or swallowing. As the disease progresses, muscle weakness and paralysis spread to the muscles of the trunk of the body. Eventually, in the more advanced stage of the disease, muscles that control vital functions are impaired, causing difficulties in speech, swallowing, and breathing. Respiratory failure is the cause of most deaths (NINDS, 2017c).

Treatment of ALS remains focused on symptom management with the goal of maintaining QOL. An interprofessional team is typically established, including a neurologist, nurses, physical therapists, occupational therapists, speech pathologists, psychologists, and many others, to help navigate patient management (Vucic, Rothstein, & Kiernan, 2014). Drug therapy options include riluzole, which was approved in 1995 by the FDA to treat ALS and remains the only approved treatment to date (Poppe, Rue, Robberecht, & Van Den Bosch, 2014). Potential therapeutic approaches focus on causal treatment or modifying treatment. Causal treatment focuses on directly targeting disease-causing genes to prevent their expression, while modifying treatments focus on targeting factors or mechanisms that influence pathological processes related to ALS (Poppe et al., 2014).

■ **Coma.** Coma is the result of injury to the brain and is characterized as a deep state of unconsciousness in which a person cannot be awakened and does not purposefully respond to stimuli (NINDS, 2017a). Those in the deepest coma are not conscious of self or their environment; they show no sleep–wake cycles or auditory or visual responses, and have reflex and postural responses only to external stimuli (Posner, Saper, & Schiff, 2007).

To date, precise estimates of the incidence and prevalence of coma in the United States are not available due to lack of surveillance, incomplete diagnostic codes for stages of recovery, and misdiagnosis in the assessment of disorders of consciousness (McNamee, Howe, Nakase-Richardson, & Peterson, 2012). However, prevalence estimates for vegetative state (now known as unresponsive wakefulness syndrome) and minimally conscious state (MCS) range from 25,000 to 420,000 and 112,000 to 280,000, respectively (Hirschberg & Giacino, 2011). The state of arousal and wakefulness is dependent on functioning cerebral hemispheres and the brainstem's regulatory system called the reticular-activating system (RAS; Posner et al., 2007). The RAS is located at the core of the brainstem. Damage to either the RAS area or both cerebral hemispheres will result in an altered level of consciousness or coma (Posner et al., 2007).

Coma etiology can be classified into one of three main categories: supratentorial lesions, infratentorial lesions, and metabolic encephalopathy. Supratentorial-type coma results from the formation of a mass (i.e., brain tumor, stroke, head trauma with brain swelling, brain abscess) that expands, producing brain herniation through the tentorial opening into the tentorial compartment, causing fatal brainstem hemorrhages and ischemia (L. Davis, King, & Schultz, 2005). Infratentorial-type coma occurs when a tumor or ischemic stroke involving the brainstem or cerebellum damages or compresses reticular formation. Metabolic encephalopathy–type coma results from a variety of sources that affect brain chemistry (i.e., drugs, hypoxia, blood glucose abnormalities, organ diseases, vitamin B deficiencies, poor cerebral perfusion, toxins, etc.). Metabolic coma develops acutely and is often reversible if the underlying disorder is treated (L. Davis et al., 2005). Many comatose patients progress to being brain dead. Diagnosing brain death remains challenging; to date, there is no one specific protocol to determine clinical criteria of brain death (Hills, 2010). Brain death is defined as the irreversible loss of function of the brain, including the brainstem (Posner et al., 2007).

The differential diagnosis for coma includes a structural lesion (stroke, head trauma, tumor), meningeal irritation (infection or bleeding), metabolic encephalopathy (organ failure, drugs), and seizure (Simon, 2000). Getting a history from witnesses or significant others is helpful in making a differential diagnosis. If the coma was preceded by a period of confusion or delirium, this is more consistent with infection or metabolic etiologies, whereas sudden loss of consciousness suggests an intracranial bleed or infarct.

Initial priority in the emergency management of comatose patients is to evaluate and maintain respiratory and circulatory function and then to establish the underlying disease process. Timely diagnosis will improve the likelihood of reversing the coma, when this is possible, and reducing mortality. The Glasgow Coma Scale (GCS) is often used to assess and score the level of consciousness. Eye opening, verbal response, and motor response to stimuli are evaluated. The Consciousness Scale for Palliative Care (CSPC) is designed to assess consciousness in PC patients. It is easy to use and has good psychometrics, with a Cronbach alpha of 0.99, intraclass correlation of 0.99, and correlation with the GCS of 0.82 (Gonçalves, Bento, Alvarenga, Costa, & Costa, 2008).

A pediatric version of the GCS is available (Reilly, Simpson, Sprod, & Thomas, 1988). The CHOP Infant Coma Scale or Infant Face Scale (IFS) may be more useful for children younger than 2 years of age. This scale relies on objective behavioral observations, assesses cortical as well as brainstem function, and is based on infant-appropriate behaviors. It can also be used with intubated patients and has better interrater reliability than the pediatric version of the GCS (Durham et al., 2000).

Some of the causes are treatable and reversible, whereas others are not. The prognosis depends on the cause, the severity of damage, and the site of neurological damage (NINDS, 2017a). Comas vary in their duration from days to weeks, typically lasting no longer than approximately 4 weeks (NINDS, 2017a). The most critical factors involved in determining prognosis is etiology of the coma, the clinical depth of coma, and the length of time the person remains comatose. Other factors include the age of the person, neurological findings, and concurrent medical complications (Posner et al., 2007). Poor prognostic signs are when the coma follows cardiac arrest or if the patient has not regained pupillary function or purposeful movement after 72 hours.

Coma due to traumatic head injury has a worse prognosis in older patients, with patients older than 60 years being three times more likely to die than patients younger than 20 years (Simon, 2000). Most comatose stroke patients do not survive. Medical comorbidities, advanced age, and complications all negatively affect survival. The majority of coma patients will die in the acute care setting, except for those whose coma is persistent. They are transferred to a long-term care facility for supportive nursing care. Similar to stroke, they may die from the initial damage to the brain, which precipitated the coma, or from subsequent complications or comorbid conditions.

After the coma phase, some people gradually recover, some progress into a vegetative state, and others become brain dead. People who do emerge from a coma may have problems with complex thinking, emotional stability, and physical difficulties. The most common cause of death for someone in a persistent vegetative state is infection, such as pneumonia.

The common causes of pediatric coma are injury, shock, metabolic disorders, ingestions, and CNS infections. Altered mental status in children covers a range of behaviors, and irritability, lethargy, changes in feeding or sleeping habits, and other subtle behavioral changes can be indicative of impairments in the child's CNS. History from the caregiver is critical. One recent study suggests that studying reactive encephalographic patterns in comatose children may be useful in prognostication of morbidity and mortality outcomes (Ramachandrannair, Sharma, Weiss, & Cortez, 2005).

■ COMORBIDITIES ASSOCIATED WITH NEUROLOGICAL DISORDERS

Many of the predisposing factors for stroke, Alzheimer's disease, and vascular dementia overlap with cardiovascular disease and include hypertension, diabetes, cigarette smoking, high cholesterol, and African American ethnicity. This can lead to complications with unstable blood pressure, angina, congestive heart failure, myocardial infarction, and arrhythmias (Cechetto, Hachinski, & Whitehead, 2008; Ostwald, Wasserman, & Davis, 2006).

As previously stated, the risk of stroke and most CNDs increases with age and the older patient is also more likely to have coexisting chronic illnesses. People with MS are likely to be younger at age of onset and thus have fewer coexisting chronic problems. Any limitations associated with comorbid conditions can impede functional status and complicate management. Comorbid illnesses have consistently been shown to affect function, mortality, and utilization of services (Studenski, Lai, Duncan, & Rigler, 2004).

People with stroke and CNDs are susceptible to secondary complications, including pressure sores, malnutrition, venous thrombosis, contractures, pneumonia, conjunctivitis, depression, and problems with bowel and bladder function. These complications are frequent enough that they should be anticipated, and nursing care should be aimed at prevention, early recognition, and treatment of problems.

■ COMMON SYMPTOMS AND TREATMENTS

Symptoms vary greatly among people who have had a stroke or neurodegenerative illness, depending on the location(s) and severity of damage or pathology. Specific chapters in this book that cover management of symptoms such as dyspnea, pain, immobility, and gastrointestinal symptoms should be consulted for an overview of treatment options. This section focuses on some of the PC issues and their management for individuals with stroke and chronic neurodegenerative diseases such as cognition and communication, affect and behavior, recognizing and treating pain, eating and swallowing, dyspnea and air hunger, sleep, and infection.

Cognition

There is great heterogeneity in cognitive deficits following a stroke. The person can exhibit a reduced level of consciousness, attention deficits, and an array of perceptual deficits that commonly impact functional ability. For example, some patients develop neglect or a loss of awareness of their affected limbs. It is associated with right hemispheric strokes and, in the extreme, can result in patients being completely unaware of the left side of their body or of stimuli coming from the left side of their environment. Patient safety is compromised as neglect can increase the risk of injury and falls.

Neurodegenerative illnesses are associated with the development of cognitive deficits; symptoms worsen as the illness progresses. Early in Alzheimer's disease, short-term memory, judgment, and visuospatial problems are common. During later stages, the person has severe impairment of all cognitive functions and may no longer recognize family members. Attention, orientation, and short- and long-term memories are impaired. In Parkinson's disease, mild cognitive impairment and dementia are among the most frequent nonmotor symptoms the patient may face (Biundo, Weis, & Antonini, 2016). Cognitive impairments affect a large proportion of people, with MS occurring in 40% to 70% of cases and mainly affecting attention, information-processing speed, and episodic memory (Houtchens et al., 2007; Minden, 2000; Rocca et al., 2015; Bede et al., 2011).

There is evidence that memantine and cholinesterase inhibitors are modestly effective in decreasing the severity of cognitive deficits in Alzheimer's disease and Parkinson's disease. Cholinesterase inhibitors are used in mild-to-moderate dementia, and memantine alone or in combination with cholinesterase inhibitors is used in the late stages of the illness (Buckley & Salpeter, 2015; Lökk & Delbari, 2012). Reality orientation is not recommended for people with Alzheimer's disease, but the use of environmental cues and decreasing visual clutter are recommended. Pleasant music has been found to improve visual attention in patients with unilateral neglect after stroke (M. Chen, Tsai, Huang, & Lin, 2013). Effective treatment often requires an interdisciplinary approach, including nurses, physical therapists, and occupational therapists. Treatment methods include reminding the patient to look toward his or her affected side, continual use of touch on the affected side, and intentionally approaching the patient from the affected side.

Communication

Impairments in communication are common with all disorders discussed in this chapter. Strokes occurring in the left hemisphere, in particular, can impair the ability to communicate. Voice disorders can be grouped into dysarthria and dysphonia. Dysarthria is caused by neurological damage to the motor components of speech. Impairments in neuromuscular function cause dysarthria in people with Parkinson's disease, MS, and ALS. Dysphonia is disordered sound production at the level of the larynx and may have a neurological, structural, or functional etiology (S. M. Cohen, Elackattu, Noordzij, Walsh, & Langmore, 2009).

Cognitive deficits are associated with receptive and expressive aphasia in CNDs. As Alzheimer's disease progresses to late stage, the number of words in the person's vocabulary is usually limited to 20 or less. Those individuals with expressive aphasia may comprehend spoken language but are unable to express themselves verbally to varying degrees. Receptive aphasia is the result of deficits in receiving the message/auditory perception or retaining it. Stroke patients can experience several different forms of aphasia: expressive, receptive, or global aphasia. Due to difficulty expressing their needs or interpreting what is going on around them, aphasic patients may become noncompliant, angry, fearful, or withdrawn.

Difficulty communicating severely reduces QOL. Voice amplifiers may be helpful in the final stages of certain illnesses in which nerve damage or reduced respiratory support for speech contributes to a soft voice. Surgically placing a tracheoesophageal prosthesis and augmenting an atrophic vocal fold with collagen can palliate the dysphonic patient (S. M. Cohen et al., 2009). Another treatment option that has had a promising effect on phonation in patients suffering from dysphagia with dysphonia is laryngopharyngeal neuromuscular electrical stimulation (Ko, Park, Hyun, Seo, & Kim, 2016).

The nurse should develop a plan with the interprofessional team for providing meaningful communication and socialization that considers the wishes of the individual and the accommodations needed because of communication deficits. A consistent caregiver or family member is often able to understand speech that others consider unintelligible. Supporting the remaining demonstrations of attempts to communicate enables the patient to feel connected and accepted; he or she may begin using many more nonverbal cues to communicate needs.

Behaviors listed in Table 16.1 may be used by patients to communicate to the caregiver that there is an unmet need such as pain or hunger, or the need to eliminate or change positions (Kovach et al., 2012).

Anticipating physical needs decreases frustration for the person who is unable to clearly or consistently verbalize needs. Nonverbal communication through touch, massage, and eye contact should be used. Gestures are a three-dimensional language of communication; waving

hello, pointing, beckoning with outstretched hands, and hugging used judiciously by the caregiver may be effective communication tools. The presence of a family member or caregiver conveys to the individual that he or she is not alone and that the individual is respected.

When cognitive impairment is present, the strategies outlined in Table 16.2 may be useful to facilitate communication. A calm, gentle voice communicates safety and security. Listening to the person, even if the message is unclear, communicates respect. Compared to those with mild cognitive impairment, the individual who is severely impaired may require more focused stimulation to elicit a response. Making a compassionate and meaningful connection with a person who has severe dementia will often soothe a troubled anxious state.

Affect and Behavior

The development of depression, apathy, mood disorders, and anxiety associated with stroke and neurodegenerative illnesses is common. Frontal lobe pathology and disturbed neurotransmitter metabolism increase a person's susceptibility to depression. Also, adapting to the loss of physical or cognitive abilities can be overwhelming. The individual's premorbid personality, coping skills, and resources are all factors in making this adaptation. Medications can contribute to depressive and psychotic symptoms. People experiencing CNDs often experience periods of uncontrolled laughing or crying, also known as pseudobulbar affect (PBA). The pathophysiology of PBA appears to be a lack of voluntary control, or disinhibition, but the pathways are yet to be clearly understood (Ahmed & Simmons, 2013). Patients with Parkinson's disease are increasingly seen with impulse control disorders like compulsive gambling or buying and sexual and eating behaviors (Weintraub & Claassen, 2017). These impulse control disorders have been most closely related to the use of dopamine agonists (Weintraub & Claassen, 2017).

People with CNDs are both underdiagnosed and inadequately treated for mood and anxiety disorders (Hallford, McCabe, Mellor, Davison, & Goldhammer, 2012). Depression was exhibited in 31% of stroke survivors at any time from the moment of the stroke to 5 years (Hackett & Pickles, 2014). In people with MS, mental health comorbidities contribute to secondary disability and decrease their QOL (Turner et al., 2016). People with neuromuscular problems may appear less animated at baseline, so flat affect and decreased involvement in activity are not useful cues for depression or mood disorders.

A systematic literature review using Cochrane methodology found a lack of evidence of an association between the severity of Alzheimer's disease and the prevalence of comorbid depressive symptoms or depression (Verkaik, Nuyen, Schellevis, & Francke, 2007). This review suggests that prevention and intervention strategies for depression should be aimed at all people with Alzheimer's disease regardless of their

TABLE 16.1 Behavioral Symptoms of Unmet Needs in People With Impaired Communication and/or Cognition

- Any change in behavior
- Restless movement
- Moaning
- Tense muscles
- Facial grimace
- Agitation
- Combative/angry
- Pulling away
- Changes in mobility
- Rubbing/holding or bracing of a body part
- Crying/tears in eyes
- Change in sleep
- Confusion
- Changes in appetite
- Verbal perseveration
- Withdrawal/quietness
- Increased pulse or respiration

TABLE 16.2   Communication Strategies With the Cognitively Impaired
■ Make sure the person knows you are present before communicating to avoid startling or frightening the person.
■ Touching the person gently may be used to begin the communication. A conventional handshake may be well tolerated. Assess the person's reaction and gradually increase the use of appropriate touch, if tolerated.
■ Keep voice, facial expression, and body movements calm, slow, clear, and positive.
■ Use short, simple, adult sentences.
■ Use the name of the person most familiar to them. Avoid the use of pronouns.
■ Use visual cues to augment verbal message.
■ Limit choices to two options to avoid overwhelming the person's cognitive ability.
■ Avoid "why" questions which may be perceived as threatening.
■ Avoid negative feedback statements such as "Don't. . . . "
■ Avoid working to teach or orient the person. Since short-term memory is severely impaired, this is ineffective.
■ Listen to the person's verbal message attentively and allow enough time for the person to communicate with you.
■ Validate the feelings behind the words. For example, "I hear that you are upset and I am here to help" or "I'm glad you're okay."
■ Tapes of family members may be used to provide simulated presence therapy.
■ End all interactions with positive feedback such as "I appreciate this time with you," or "It was nice to visit with you today."

disease severity. Geropsychiatry consultations are often needed to competently assess and treat those with more complicated symptomatology.

There are few systematic studies of psychotherapy and pharmacotherapy in individuals with CNDs. Evidence supports the use of selective serotonin reuptake inhibitors (SSRIs) as the drugs of choice for depressive disorders because of their safer drug profile, and anxiety disorders may be treated effectively with combined drug and nonpharmacological therapy (Chan, Cordato, & O'Rourke, 2008; Lökk & Delbari, 2012).

Behaviors listed in Table 16.1 are common in people with dementia and may indicate an underlying need such as pain or hunger. People with dementia are very sensitive and reactive to stressful stimuli in the environment, though this behavioral response is somewhat less evident in later stages. The person may have active hands and repetitive movements or vocalizations (i.e., perseverance). Delusions and hallucinations may be present and the person may display agitation, wandering, aggressive outbursts, and spontaneous screaming.

The person who has decreased competence, particularly cognitive competence, is more affected by stressors from the environment and has a decreased threshold for tolerating stressors from the environment (Kovach, 2000). Consideration of this environmental vulnerability creates the need for two foundational interventions:

■ Provide a positive environment with few environmental stressors.
■ Balance sensory stimulating and sensory calming activity throughout the day. (Kovach et al., 2004)

People with dementia have heightened sensitivity to environmental stressors and cues (Chaudhury, Cooke, Cowie, & Razaghi, 2017). High decibel sound is associated with higher levels of agitation in people with dementia (Joosse, 2012). Health professionals should conduct a noise assessment by listening at various times of the day to sources of noxious or extraneous noise. Eliminate echo, background conversations, and television used for background sound. Provide brief periods of music listening with selections that are pleasing to the patient (Padilla, 2011). The visually accessible environment may be quite circumscribed, so it is important that it be pleasant and as stress free as possible. Avoid fluorescent lighting that often creates a glare. Keep some items that are familiar to the person in the immediate area; for example, pictures, afghans, and pillows may convey home and familiarity. Spaces that are too big or too small, as well as cluttered areas, should be avoided. One or two plants or flower arrangements are preferred to an overwhelming clutter of flora. Avoid tactile stressors by keeping the room temperature comfortable. Avoid itchy skin by keeping the skin well lubricated and treating with medicated emollients; flannel sheets and silk pillowcases may provide some comfort.

In addition to decreasing environmental stress, there is a need to balance sensory stimulating and sensory calming activity (Kovach et al., 2004). As the illness progresses, there may be a need for more sensory calming time, and the person will probably tolerate less than 1 hour of activity before needing a decrease in environmental stimulation. Often, only brief visits of 10 minutes or less will be tolerated. The person may need to engage in frequent inner retreat by withdrawing from others.

This need should be explained to the family so they do not feel shunned; if the patient shuns socialization, allow him or her some solitary time and approach again later.

Agitated behaviors are associated with cognitive impairment and increase in frequency as dementia progresses (Y. Chen, Ryden, Feldt, & Savik, 2000; Kales, Gitlin, & Lyketsos, 2015). Physical aggression is a behavioral manifestation for many dementia patients, and it is usually related to identifiable triggers or communication challenges (Wharton & Ford, 2014). Social contact and focused, therapeutic stimulation have been associated with decreases in agitated behavior (Draper et al., 2000; McGonigal-Kenny & Schutte, 2006). Stimulation of multiple senses may enhance engagement in the activity. Friendly visit, hand massage, music listening, and pet therapy are just a few examples of therapeutic activities. Multiple activity therapy books provide suggestions for therapeutic activities that accommodate any level of cognitive or functional deficit and enhance QOL.

Perseverant behavior, defined as repetitive movement or verbalization, may also occur in patients with CNDs. Perseverance may indicate boredom, discomfort, or an unmet need; it may also be a simple tension reduction mechanism. Calm repetitive movements or verbalizations may be a coping mechanism and may not require treatment. It is important to determine if environmental stress needs to be decreased or, alternatively, if stimulating activity should be provided. Health professionals should assess for basic comfort needs: offer a drink, be certain elimination needs have been met, provide a warm blanket or sweater, check for pressure points, and ensure good positioning. If pain is suspected, administer an analgesic.

Aggression and resisting care may also be present. Resisting care may indicate that pain control is inadequate. This behavior is often temporary, so the caregiver should repeat the attempt to provide care following a short break. Paratonia is a primitive reflex that may be present and is often mistaken for resisting care. Paratonia is involuntary resistance of an extremity in response to sudden passive movement. A caregiver who moves a patient's arm may evoke this movement that appears to be resistance to care. Slow and gentle touch decreases the likelihood of inducing paratonia.

Delusions and hallucinations, when present, are a real part of the person's mental life and can be very discomforting. These alterations in perception often respond well to psychotropic drugs. Caregivers should not agree or disagree with the false perception, but there is a need to provide comforting intervention. For example, saying, "I hear that you are afraid and I will keep you safe," validates feelings and provides reassurance. Distraction or provision of a comforting intervention such as a friendly visit will often soothe the person's troubled state. Also, check to be sure the person's glasses and hearing aid are in place and functioning properly. Many suspected delusions are actually mixed messages resulting from impaired hearing.

Eating and Swallowing

Dysphagia and aspiration are problematic in stroke and neurodegenerative illnesses. Swallowing is a complex process that involves precise coordination of the oral cavity and the pharynx (Sasegbon & Hamdy, 2017). Damage to any portion of the complex process of swallowing can lead to dysphagia (Sasegbon & Hamdy, 2017). Dysphagia resulting from stroke is temporary in 90% of cases but is a part of the general progress of the illness for CNDs discussed in this chapter (Broadley et al., 2005). Dysphasia can occur in the oropharyngeal or esophageal phases of swallowing. The oropharyngeal phase is voluntary and depends on motor and sensory pathways triggering a series of movements that move food posteriorly to the oropharynx. Oropharyngeal dysphagia has a neurological cause in 75% of cases (Ertekin & Aydogdu, 2003). Esophageal dysphagia is more likely caused by obstruction or stricture (Navaneethan & Eubanks, 2015; White, O'Rourke, Ong, Cordato, & Chan, 2008). Patients with swallowing disorders are at risk of aspiration pneumonia. Sialorrhoea, or an excessive secretion of saliva, is common for those with Parkinson's disease, ALS, and MS (Andersen et al., 2012; McGeachan & McDermott, 2017). Low food consumption, food pocketing, difficulty manipulating food on the plate and transporting it to the mouth, weight loss, and nutritional impairments are common in Parkinson's disease (Simons, 2017; Westergren, Ohlsson, & Hallberg, 2002).

The swallowing mechanism is quite complex, involving 26 sets of muscles and six nerves, and is dependent on critical timing of several phases and highly coordinated movement (Shapiro & Downe, 2003). Individuals in the late stages of neurodegenerative diseases will have dysphagia and be at risk of aspiration and malnutrition (Altman, Richards, Goldberg, Frucht, & McCabe, 2013; Langmore, Grillone, Elackattu, & Walsh, 2009). Management strategies are important in preventing morbidity. All stroke patients should be evaluated by speech therapy to determine if feeding by mouth is safe and if aspiration precautions are needed. Techniques commonly used to assist individuals with dysphagia to swallow safely will be reviewed. Other options for managing eating problems will be discussed.

Prior to the meal, several interventions may be helpful. For example, oral hygiene is important in maintaining a normal viscosity to the saliva, and aggressive oral care may reduce the risk of pneumonia (Marik & Kaplan, 2003; Sura, Madhavan, Carnaby-Mann, & Crary, 2012). If the person is taking medications that dry the mouth, artificial saliva products should be used. Safe swallowing methods include upright posture, chin-tucking, careful slow swallowing, and specific maneuvers designed to improve swallowing (D. L. Cohen et al., 2016; Marik & Kaplan, 2003). For the person with dementia, providing some cueing that mealtime is coming is helpful. For example, in a long-term setting on units for individuals with late-stage CND, in the late afternoon a tablecloth and a vase of flowers are placed on each table to signal that it is the start of evening mealtime. It is important to reduce distractions during mealtime, so the focus is on eating and swallowing. If the person is in a long-term care facility, the dining room should optimally seat 16 or fewer residents to decrease the potential for overstimulation. Turning up lights, increasing visual contrasts, and improving acoustics have been suggested to enhance mealtimes in group dining rooms (Brush & Calkins, 2008). Be certain the person is comfortable and that the environment is comfortable and free from odors.

Provide verbal cueing to assist the person to eat; for example, say "the food is coming" and "swallow now." Do not rush the person to eat and swallow too quickly, but be aware that excessive time spent at the task may lead to fatigue and decreased eating. Provide positive encouragement during the meal. Plastic utensils should not be used because a biting reflex may occur, especially if the gums or teeth are touched with the utensil. Applying gentle pressure on the jaw and cheek muscles may break the biting reflex. The following feeder behaviors may help to sustain eating behaviors of the patient: talking and reorienting the person to the meal, offering drinks between bites, holding the spoon ready for a bite, and warmly touching the person.

There is a need for research on drugs used to stimulate appetite and promote weight gain in anorexic individuals with neurological illnesses. Dronabinol is a cannabis derivative, which in one study of people with Alzheimer's disease was associated with a 0.5 to 1 kg greater weight gain than with placebo (Chapman, 2007).

The person with dysphagia will require alterations in diet. Dietitians can suggest foods that are easier to swallow. Calorie-dense pureed diets and thickened liquids may be used. One large randomized controlled trial found that honey-thick liquids were more effective than nectar-thick liquids, and chin-tucking was least effective. All three interventions were more effective in people with Parkinson's disease than with Alzheimer's disease (Logemann et al., 2008). Smaller, more frequent meals are used, and the person often takes in more food at meals earlier in the day. For some people, the stimulation of a soft bolus of food, such as mashed potatoes, may provide more stimuli for swallowing than liquids. The person should drink sufficient liquid to produce straw-colored urine. Consuming 20 to 35 g of fiber each day can help to manage constipation (Shagam, 2008).

For patients who have had a stroke, enteral feedings may be seen as a temporary intervention to allow time for rehabilitation and recovery or as a permanent intervention to prolong life. For those with CND, oral feeding may eventually become impossible and a person should never be force fed. The decision to tube feed is complex and controversial; in addition, courts have recognized tube feeding as a medical treatment that can be refused. Prior decision making by the patient

relative to the desire to initiate assisted feeding is helpful. There are no randomized clinical trials examining the outcomes of tube feeding. In the case of ALS, percutaneous endoscopic gastrostomy (PEG) tube placement is common and evidence suggests that nutrition and QOL are improved and survival is prolonged (Andersen et al., 2012; Dorst et al., 2015). There is no evidence that tube feedings reduce the incidence of aspiration pneumonia, prolong life, or improve QOL for people with advanced dementia (Gessert, Mosier, Brown, & Frey, 2000). Other possible problems associated with tube feeding include diarrhea and possible skin breakdown, as well as the need for physical restraints if tubes are pulled and wound infection occurs.

Dyspnea

In people with CND involving motor systems, respiratory insufficiency is common late in the illness. Chronic nocturnal hypoventilation is also common. Weakness of the respiratory muscles produces a restrictive ventilatory defect with resulting atelectasis and a feeling of dyspnea or increased work of breathing. Expiratory weakness is generally more prominent than inspiratory weakness and may contribute to impaired coughing, aspiration, and the development of pneumonia. Thick respiratory secretions may be difficult to manage and uncomfortable. Respiratory insufficiency is particularly severe in ALS and MS.

In people with CND involving motor systems, respiratory insufficiency may cause chronic nocturnal hypoventilation and sleeplessness. Respiratory management of these patients has evolved from no treatment to the use of strategies to avert respiratory failure and to permit the extubation of unweanable patients without a tracheostomy. An international panel, experienced in continuous noninvasive intermittent positive pressure ventilatory support (CNVS), reviewed the strength of evidence for the efficacy of interventions and made recommendations for achieving prolonged survival by CNVS. Controlled studies demonstrated prolongation of survival for several months using nocturnal bilevel positive airway pressure (PAP). Daily air stacking involves the glottis and holding consecutively delivered air volumes from a volume cycled ventilator or a manual resuscitator until no more can be held (maximal insufflation capacity), and is recommended once the vital capacity is lower than 80% of normal. Following air stacking, a cough-timed abdominal thrust was demonstrated to significantly increase cough peak flow. Because bilevel PAP cannot be used for air stacking, expiratory PAP is counterproductive for assisting weak respiratory muscles and, because portable ventilators eventually become necessary for CNVS, the panel recommended that all patients with the ability to air stack use nocturnal noninvasive intermittent positive pressure ventilation rather than bilevel PAP. The panel unanimously recommended tracheotomy only for patients who cannot maintain a SpO_2 of greater than or equal to 95% despite CNVS and mechanically assisted coughing (Bach et al., 2012). Clinicians are challenged to support this strong desire to live while providing appropriate expectations for life after tracheostomy.

Supplemental oxygen therapy for patients with respiratory muscle weakness is not recommended because it has been found to decrease ventilator drive and worsen high CO_2 levels, decrease effectiveness of nocturnal bilevel PAP and NIV, and render oximetry ineffective as a gauge of hypoventilation, airway mucus congestion, atelectasis, and pneumonia (Bach et al., 2012).

People who choose to not receive ventilator support need to be given information regarding the mechanism of terminal hypercapnic coma and the resulting peaceful death, so that fear is decreased. Medications discussed in the chapter on dyspnea need to be administered skillfully to successfully prevent the feeling of "choking to death."

Fatigue, Activity, and Sleep

Fatigue is a subjective feeling of early exhaustion that impacts an individual's ability to interact mentally or physically with his or her environment. It is a commonly reported symptom and can be overwhelmingly debilitating, especially for people with MS (Caminero & Bartolomé, 2011; Mateen, et al., 2017). An understanding of the relationship among fatigue and depression, sleep disturbances, and specific deficits is needed in order to better recognize and treat fatigue.

Sleep disruptions and insomnia are common in people with stroke, dementia, and other neurodegenerative illnesses (Amara, Chahine, & Videnovic, 2017; Brass, Duquette, Proulx-Therrien, & Auerbach, 2010; Subramanian & Surani, 2007). Impaired sleep and alertness affect the majority of patients with Parkinson's disease, negatively impacting safety and QOL (Amara et al., 2017). People with dementia show great alterations in the sleep–wake cycle with increased nighttime awakenings, decreased time spent awake versus time spent in bed, increased daytime napping, and changes in the amount of rapid eye movement and nonrapid eye movement sleep (Ancoli-Israel & Cooke, 2005; Subramanian & Surani, 2007). Sleep-disordered breathing is a common symptom experienced in neurological disorders. Identifying and treating patients experiencing sleep disorders can have a positive effect on their QOL (Deak & Kirsch, 2014). Sleep is greatly impaired by involuntary movements and muscle spasms for those with Parkinson's disease and MS, and dyspnea during the night for those with ALS and MS.

Patients should be carefully evaluated for factors that could be contributing to their fatigue, such as anemia, pain, occult infections, hypothyroidism, medications, malnutrition, and sleep apnea (Oken et al., 2006). Adapting the environment to promote sleep, pacing activities, treating pain, and eliminating or reducing any offending medications should be considered possible interventions for people with CND. Relaxation techniques such as breathing exercises, massage, imagery, or music may also promote sleep and reduce fatigue.

Light and fragmented sleep impairs QOL. Nocturnal hypoventilation is discussed under dyspnea. It is important to keep a consistent schedule so that the diurnal rhythm is encouraged. Most people will need an afternoon nap, but keeping the person engaged in some activities during the daytime might help to improve nighttime sleep.

Sundowning is a term used to describe an increase in a number of behaviors that occur in some patients with dementia in the late afternoon or evening including agitation, aggression, wandering, yelling, and hallucinations (Canevelli et al., 2016; Yevchak, Steis, & Evans, 2012). This often indicates there is a need to improve the balance between sensory stimulating and sensory calming activity earlier in the day (Kovach et al., 2004). Specifically, there may be a need for more physical activity early in the day, followed by an afternoon nap. Then, during the usual sundowning period, the person should be engaged in a quiet one-on-one activity. Also, because of the severe sleep variations experienced by people with CND, try to keep diurnal rhythms intact by keeping lighting low during the night and up during the day. This may require increasing the use of artificial light beginning in the late afternoon.

Movement

Stroke and neurodegenerative disease affect movement. These symptoms can severely impact functional ability and QOL. People who suffer from a stroke may display hemiparesis, aphasia, dysphagia, and a variety of other symptoms, depending on the location and severity of the damage. People with neurodegenerative disease have slowed movement and gait disturbances, which progress so that the person becomes chair- or bedbound. People with late-stage Alzheimer's disease may display primitive reflexes such as hand grasping, sucking reflexes, and paratonia. Paratonia is the involuntary resistance of an arm or leg to movement of the limb by another person. This may be misinterpreted by a caregiver as aggressive behavior, but is actually a reflexive process. Resting tremor occurs when the muscle is relaxed and may be present when the muscle is rigid (Kurlan, Richard, Papka, & Marshall, 2000; NINDS, 2017d; Wilson et al., 2000).

Late in Parkinson's disease, motor problems result from drug therapy and include dyskinesias (involuntary movements), shorter duration of benefit or lack of benefit from medication, and end-of-dose deterioration. Severe muscle rigidity and hypokinesia contribute to the person becoming bed- or chairbound. When movement does occur, the person often needs physical help initiating the movement. Akinesia or freezing of movement becomes debilitating. Giving short-acting levodopa/carbidopa every 3 to 4 hours with catechol-O-methyltransferase

(COMT) inhibitors is recommended to minimize episodes of hypokinesia. This regimen causes the least variation of levodopa in blood levels, with less off-time, more on-time, and better QOL (Lökk & Delbari, 2012).

For people with MS, problems with walking, or gait, can arise from muscle weakness or stiffness, numbness, poor balance, spasticity, lack of ability to coordinate muscle movements, extreme fatigue, or visual disturbances. Depending on the type of MS, symptoms can become progressively worse or recur over time. People with ALS experience weakness, particularly of the upper limbs, and progressive muscle wasting. The person loses muscle strength, muscle mass, and mobility, until becoming completely dependent. Riluzole has antiglutamate properties and has been shown to slow the course of ALS. It is not considered useful in the later stages (Andersen et al., 2012; Poppe et al., 2014).

Physical exercise is a cornerstone of rehabilitation following stroke. However, evidence is inconclusive regarding the benefits of cardiovascular exercises on disability, ADLs, QOL, and death (Meek, Pollock, Potter, & Langhorne, 2003). The goals of treatment of Parkinson's disease are to slow the progression of the illness and to reduce disability without inducing long-term complications. Motor symptoms associated with Parkinson's disease are disabling. While levodopa/carbidopa is the cornerstone of treatment of motor symptoms of Parkinson's disease, optimal response only lasts 5 to 7 years. The classes of drugs approved for the treatment of Parkinson's disease include dopamine agonists, COMT inhibitors, monoamine-oxidase type B (MAO-B) inhibitors, and anticholinergics. These drugs do not prevent neuronal degeneration but decrease motor symptoms (Connolly & Lang, 2014; Lo, Leung, & Shek, 2007). Research is currently focused on developing neuroprotective drugs that will slow or halt the progression of Parkinson's disease. Deep brain stimulation is an option for some patients with Parkinson's disease who are not effectively managed through drug therapy.

Research into exercise for people with Alzheimer's disease and related disorders has shown maintenance of motor skills, decreased falls, reduced rate of cognitive decline, and improved mood (Paillard, Rolland, & de Souto Barreto, 2015; Teri et al., 2003). A systematic review and meta-analysis showed that strengthening and balance exercises in Parkinson's disease provide benefits to physical function, strength, balance, gait speed, and health-related QOL (Goodwin, Richards, Taylor, Taylor, & Campbell, 2008). Rhythmic auditory stimulation, in which rhythms of sounds function as a cue to stabilize and enhance the organization of movement, may be beneficial for improving gait parameters in stroke patients, including gait velocity, cadence, stride length, and gait symmetry (Bradt, Magee, Dileo, Wheeler, & McGilloway, 2010). For people with ALS, exercise can help to maintain the flexibility of muscles but it will not strengthen muscles that have been weakened by ALS. For people with MS, exercise may decrease symptoms but it must be done judiciously as overheating or overstressing the body can actually exacerbate symptoms. Occupational therapy may help patients to maintain independence for longer periods of time as the CNDs progress.

Pain

Spasticity due to increased muscle tone is common, especially post stroke, with MS and Parkinson's disease and presents as resistance to passive range of motion (PROM). Brain lesions can interfere with the descending CNS pathways that regulate muscle tone (Barnes & Campbell, 2010). For people with ALS, spasticity can actually be helpful in maintaining function as the rigidity helps replace normal muscle strength, but it causes jerky, hard-to-control movements.

Shoulder pain after stroke is common, affecting from 16% to 72% of patients (Adey-Wakeling et al., 2016; Walsh, 2001). Both flaccidity and spasticity in the paretic arm can cause subluxation (partial separation), instability of the shoulder joint, pain, and increased risk of subacromial bursitis. Shoulder hand syndrome or reflex sympathetic dystrophy is due to autonomic dysfunction in the affected upper extremity. Paresis in the shoulder and arm can lead to joint instability and trauma that may trigger overstimulation of the sympathetic nervous system. It develops in stages; typically, there is vasoconstriction in the affected arm with complaints of burning pain. If it progresses beyond 3 months, the limb may develop trophic changes with decreased hair, thin shiny skin, increased or decreased sweating, edema, and bone demineralization. Movement and touch usually cause pain, and patients tend to guard the limb, leading to further dysfunction. After 9 months, atrophy and contractures may also occur. Central poststroke pain (CPSP) is described as a neuropathic pain in all or part of the body affected by the stroke that may develop immediately or up to 6 months after the initial stroke (Klit, Finnerup, & Jensen, 2015). It is associated with sensory deficits and tactile allodynia (pain elicited by a normally nonpainful stimulus). This often prompts patients to lie perfectly still in order to avoid discomfort.

Pain in MS occurs as a consequence of both the disease process and the resulting disability. The prevalence of pain in patients with MS is nearly 50%, and approximately 75% of patients report having had pain within 1 month of assessment. The presence of pain in patients with MS is associated with increased age, duration of illness, depression, degree of functional impairment, and fatigue. Pain in MS may originate from trigeminal neuralgia, headache, facial pain, tonic seizures, and limb pain. The pain may indicate an underlying inflammatory process or demyelinating lesion affecting a pain pathway (O'Connor, Schwid, Herrmann, Markman, & Dworkin, 2008).

Dysesthetic extremity pain in people with MS is a result of demyelinating lesions and is described as persistent and burning. The legs and feet are most commonly affected, but the upper extremities and the trunk can also be affected. Pain is often worse at night and after exercise, and may be precipitated by changes in temperature, particularly the use of warm water. Joint pain and back pain are common, resulting from the disease process, steroid-induced osteoporosis, postural changes, immobility, and weakness with improper use of compensatory muscles (Maloni, 2000). Pain in ALS is often undertreated. It can occur at all stages of the disease, can affect QOL, and increase the prevalence of depression (Chio et al., 2017).

Pain experienced by individuals with stroke and neurodegenerative illnesses may also arise from the medical conditions commonly prevalent in the older age group, or as a result of comorbid conditions such as pressure ulcers, urinary retention, constipation, and contractures. Older people more commonly suffer from arthritis, back problems, and other chronic conditions.

The consequences of untreated pain are far reaching, and assessing for pain and treating it early may help to improve psychosocial and functional outcomes. Spasticity is a common problem that can become disabling, affecting ADLs and, ultimately, QOL. While there is a growing interest in the use of cannabinoids for palliation of refractory spasticity and neuropathic pain in CNDs, controversies remain over side effects versus benefits (da Rovare et al., 2017; Peat, 2010). Early and continued ROM exercises done at least twice daily to the affected areas and individualized splinting may reduce the risk of contractures. Given the risk of sedation and mental status changes, particularly in the older adult, the decision to treat pharmacologically must be weighed carefully. Drugs such as baclofen, tizanidine, benzodiazepines, or dantrolene each work slightly differently, but all patients using them must be closely monitored for side effects. Baclofen can also be administered intrathecally for spasticity. Nerve blocks with phenol or botulinum toxin to focal areas of spasticity can be effective for a number of weeks to months but need to be repeated for sustained symptom relief. In order to restore a functional position or facilitate hygiene, surgical tendon release or lengthening can also be an option in extremities with no voluntary movement. Nondrug treatments that may be helpful include the application of heat or cold to areas of spasticity but not if there is reduced sensation given the risk of injury. Gentle massage and relaxation techniques such as imagery or music may also promote comfort (Blatzheim, 2009; Gutgsell et al., 2013).

Establishing the underlying cause of the shoulder pain in patients with stroke is necessary when choosing the appropriate intervention. The effect of electrical stimulation on shoulder pain is inconclusive, but it may offer relief for some patients. Intraarticular steroid injections can be helpful, especially with bursitis. Shoulder pain due to spasticity has also responded to intramuscular botulinum toxin injections. Nonpharmacological treatments such as ice, heat, transcutaneous electrical nerve stimulation (TENS), and ultrasound may also relieve pain in some patients. ROM exercises, proper positioning, and techniques to manage edema should be initiated immediately post stroke in the affected limb.

Treatment options used for neuropathic pain can include anticonvulsants (e.g., gabapentin) and tricyclic antidepressants (e.g., amitriptyline and nortriptyline). The risk versus benefit of a trial of a tricyclic antidepressant in an older adult must be carefully considered given the anticholinergic side effect profile. Opiates play a relatively small role in the management of neuropathic pain. Vestergaard, Andersen, Gottrup, Kristensen, and Jensen (2001) found that the anticonvulsant, lamotrigine, for patients with CPSP reduced pain scores by 30% and, at 200 mg/day, the drug was well tolerated. Another study found gabapentin effective for paroxysmal pain experienced by people with MS (Yetimalar, Gürgör, & Basoglu, 2004). Adapting relaxation techniques to assist patients in coping with neuropathic pain may be helpful.

It may be difficult to recognize pain in people who have dementia and/or communication impairment. While self-report remains the gold standard for assessing pain, for those who do not communicate pain verbally, it is important to be vigilant in assessing for potential causes of pain, to observe for changes in patient behavior that may be indicators of pain, to seek surrogate reports from caregivers, and to attempt an analgesic trial if pain is suspected (Kovach et al., 2012). Refer to Chapter 20 for further discussion of pain management.

■ ADDITIONAL ILLNESS-SPECIFIC SYMPTOMS AND INFECTION

Autonomic nervous system symptoms are most common in MS and Parkinson's disease, and can include postural hypotension, constipation, bowel dysfunction, urine retention, urgency, and incontinence. Bowel dysfunction may result from both a delay in colon transit time and an impaired muscle coordination in the anorectal area (Pfeiffer, 2000). Delayed gastric emptying, caused by reduced parasympathetic activity, can affect the timing of drug response. Damage to the sensory system in MS can cause or contribute to a variety of problems, including loss of sensation and sexual dysfunction. Visual dysfunction is common, including diplopia, vision loss, and nystagmus.

Severe infection, commonly pneumonia and septicemia arising from the urinary tract, may be the cause of death in those with CNDs. Delayed diagnosis of infection may contribute to the severity of infection because of both altered clinical presentations for infection and the inability to clearly report symptoms (Fox et al., 2014; Kovach,

Logan, Simpson, & Reynolds, 2010). Nurses should work to prevent infection through common practices such as good handwashing, skin care, and adequate hydration. As the illness progresses, the question of how vigorously to treat infection or if one should treat infection at all is commonly raised.

■ PALLIATIVE CARE ISSUES

The illness trajectory for patients with CNDs is often long and unpredictable. The prognostic uncertainty is associated with a host of patient, family, caregiving, and reimbursement challenges. Patients with CNDs have heavy physical and emotional care needs. Care in a hospice or long-term care facility may reduce the caregiving required of the family, but may lead to feelings of loss of control as well as feelings of isolation. Deciding on the preferred setting for end-of-life care is complex with many factors to consider; family members may disagree with each other or with the individual himself or herself. The nurse can serve as a nonjudgmental listener, can help to explore options, and can facilitate working through the process of decision making with family members.

Regardless of the setting of care, people with CNDs do not receive enough palliative or hospice care even though the overall QOL is rated highly by family members of decedents. Approximately 12.8% of patients receiving hospice care have a diagnosis of dementia and tend to remain on hospice longer than 6 months (Rothenberg, Doberman, Simon, Gryczynski, & Cordts, 2014). Healthcare providers often do not understand that hospice services are extremely helpful to those with noncancer diseases, nor do they understand the criteria or mechanisms for establishing hospice services in their agencies or homes.

Guidelines established by the National Hospice Organization (NHO) for determining prognosis in selected noncancer diseases, including dementia, stroke, and coma, are designed to predict 6-month mortality so that the person can be entered into Medicare/Medicaid-reimbursed hospice services. The accuracy of these guidelines at predicting mortality is open to debate. Because of the prognostic uncertainty in advanced dementia, the NHO criteria are restrictive, and patients who are clearly terminal may still not qualify. Hospice criteria for dementia include (a) dementia severe enough to have reached Stage 7-C of the Functional Assessment Staging (FAST) scale and (b) the presence of medical comorbid conditions of sufficient severity to warrant medical treatment, whether or not the decision was made to treat the condition. In the chronic phase after stroke, criteria for hospice include either (a) poststroke dementia equivalent to Stage 7-C of the FAST scale; (b) poor functional status, as evidenced by a Karnofsky score of less than 50%; or (c) poor nutritional status as

measured by weight loss and serum albumin. Patients in coma are eligible for hospice if they show any four of the following: (a) abnormal brainstem response; (b) absent verbal response; (c) absent withdrawal response to pain; (d) serum creatinine greater than 1.5 mg/dL; or (e) age older than 70 years (National Hospice Organization [NHO], 1996).

Family members should optimally be a part of a continued process of decision making throughout the illness trajectory. In the case of illnesses that are associated with dementia, early discussions and assignment of trusted family members to decision-making roles when capacity is compromised are essential. With these illnesses, there is a lot of anticipatory grieving that occurs, and family members need to be supported in accepting their feelings. Acknowledging conflicting feelings, particularly both the dread and the desire for the death to occur, as common and natural can be helpful. Early discussions about the typical course of the illness that are honest but sensitive are needed.

Coping with the late stages of chronic neurodegenerative illness is both physically and emotionally demanding. The patient's stress should not be amplified by an awareness of the burden on family or professional caregivers. Discussions about the burdens or problems of caregiving should be held away from the patient. The person should feel cared for and safe.

Brain Death

Improved medical technology capable of sustaining life and organ transplantation protocols has created circumstances in which the individual may have cardiopulmonary functions, but is brain dead. Toward the need to define and determine brain death, the President's Commission (1981) developed the Uniform Determination of Death Act that allowed brain death to be a legal definition of death. Declaring a person dead requires that either his or her heart function has ceased or his or her brain no longer functions due to irreversible damage. There is continued controversy and ongoing research to improve accuracy in determining irreversible brain death, and a variety of confirming tests have been suggested. These include electroencephalography (EEG), computed tomographic angiography, MRI, and testing of cerebrospinal fluid (Owen, Schiff, & Laureys, 2009; Welschehold et al., 2012). Major differences exist in the guidelines used to determine brain death in major neurological hospitals in the United States (Greer et al., 2016; Lessard & Brochu, 2010).

Direct damage to the brainstem (head trauma, intracranial hemorrhage, infarcts, and mass lesions) or diffuse damage to neuronal metabolism (drugs, renal failure, and hypoglycemia) are the mechanisms by which irreversible brain death may occur. Patients who are being evaluated for brain death are most likely being treated in the ICU or ER. Families need significant education and support throughout the diagnostic evaluation and the process of treatment withdrawal. If brain death has occurred as the result of a long illness with multiple organ failure, they may have had time to absorb information and develop realistic expectations about their loved one's survival, as opposed to a sudden unpredictable trauma. It is important to have staff available who are comfortable discussing the implications of brain death, the need for withdrawal of treatment, and how to incorporate any previous wishes of the patient and requests by the family.

Truog et al. (2001) recommend that families be given a very straightforward but compassionate explanation that the patient died when his or her brain died and that treatment is being withdrawn from someone who is already dead. This may relieve feelings of guilt that the withdrawal of treatment contributed to the patient's death. Due to the extent of the brainstem injury, brain-dead patients do not feel pain. Reassurance that they are not suffering and that measures to ensure patient dignity are in place is important as well as incorporating any cultural or spiritual rituals. Nurses can help to establish an environment where the family feels supported and valued.

Before withdrawing life support, families should be offered adequate time to process and cope with the information they have been given and to spend time with the patient if requested. Discussion of any possible organ donation should be separate from the notification of brain death and should be done by those trained to have such discussions.

Pediatric Brain Death

The concept of brain death, particularly in children, remains difficult. Because of the gravity of the outcome of the diagnosis of brain death, the process should never be rushed, requires the expertise of multiple clinicians in pediatric neurocritical care, and should be well documented (Mullen, 2013).

The 1987 Guidelines for the Determination of Brain Death in children (American Academy of Pediatrics Task Force on Brain Death in Children, 1987) were recently updated by an interprofessional team of experts (Nakagawa, Ashwal, Mathur, & Mysore, 2011). The patient's history must provide a proximate cause of the irreversible coma and potentially correctable conditions must be excluded. The guidelines include the need for a diagnosis of coma, absent brainstem function, flaccid tone and absence of spontaneous or induced movements excluding spinal cord reflexes, and meet apnea testing criteria. The period of observation varies by the age of the patient (Mullen, 2013). Waiting periods for establishing brain death, particularly of infants and young children, require further research. Also, it is important to be aware of legal requirements specific to states as well as institutional policies regarding brain death and organ procurement.

Palliative Care Nursing for Comatose and Brain-Dead Patients

Assessing for signs and symptoms of discomfort is difficult due to the lack of response to stimuli from patients who are in a coma. It is possible that some comatose patients may feel painful stimulation, but be unable to respond in any meaningful way depending on the depth of the coma. Physiological responses, such as changes in blood pressure, heart rate, respiratory rate and rhythm, diaphoresis, and decreased oxygen saturation levels, may be possible cues of pain sensation. Monitoring facial electromyography and electroencephalographic tracings have both been used, but they remain invalidated measures. Bispectral analysis using encephalographic signals to assess the level of consciousness and comfort during withdrawal of life support has been attempted (Truog et al., 2001). This technology may assess the level of arousal, but is not able to quantify pain. The use of analgesics to relieve potential pain in unresponsive patients with diagnoses consistent with pain or undergoing painful procedures should be considered.

Although brain-dead patients, by definition, do not feel pain, they should be treated with the intent to maximize their physical integrity and minimize discomfort. Families may be comforted by touching and speaking to them and should be offered privacy to do so. Attention should be focused on the physical and emotional needs of the family members throughout these events.

■ WITHDRAWAL OF LIFE SUPPORT

By the time it is determined that any meaningful recovery is unlikely, healthcare providers may have had the opportunity to process the implications. Families, however, may require additional time and counseling to reconcile with the poor prognosis and the option of treatment withdrawal. It is always a difficult and emotionally charged issue to begin discussing the withdrawal of life support from a patient. Having consistent staff members communicating with families and ongoing opportunities to discuss diagnosis, prognosis, and QOL issues should help to prepare them for potential outcomes.

Information regarding the actual process for withdrawal of treatment can be reviewed to the extent that the family requests; in addition, input from all appropriate disciplines should be encouraged. The actual process of withdrawal needs to incorporate any preferences for timing, those who will be present, and religious and cultural rituals. This promotes the family's ability to infuse personal meaning into the experience. Ideally, this should occur in a calm environment with respect for privacy.

Protocols vary between institutions, and more evidence-based data are needed to determine the optimum management of patients during the withdrawal of life support. Prior to discontinuing mechanical ventilation, all other treatments that do not contribute to the patient's level of comfort and unnecessary electronic monitoring may be discontinued. An intravenous (IV) line may be maintained in order to administer medications. Rubenfeld and Crawford (2001) recommend that, given the uncertainty regarding the potential for pain and suffering in comatose patients, clinicians administer an appropriate level of sedation. However, due to the extent of their neurological injuries, sedation is not required in brain-dead patients. Opioids and benzodiazepines are the primary drugs used for sedation and analgesia in comatose patients before and during the withdrawal of life support (Delaney & Downar, 2016; von Gunten & Weissman, 2001), and these should be titrated up to effect or comfort.

After removing all other life support equipment, ventilator withdrawal in comatose or brain-dead patients can be done by simply removing the endotracheal tube (extubation) or by gradually reducing the ventilator settings (terminal weaning). For unconscious patients unlikely to experience discomfort, Truog et al. (2001) suggest rapidly withdrawing ventilator support by removing the artificial airway or disconnecting the ventilator rather than the process of terminal weaning. For any distress during or after extubation, Pendergast (2002) recommends midazolam (2–5 mg IV every 7–10 minutes) or diazepam (5–10 mg IV every 3–5 minutes) and/or morphine (5–10 mg IV every 10 minutes) or fentanyl (100–250 mcg IV every 3–5 minutes).

Following the withdrawal of supportive measures, the family may need time to share their feelings and have their decisions reaffirmed. Information on grief counseling should be offered to all who were involved in the person's care. Staff members should also have opportunities to debrief after withdrawing a patient from life support. Discussing reactions with coworkers can be therapeutic and can lead to quality improvement initiatives.

■ RESEARCH IMPLICATIONS REGARDING CARE OF COMATOSE AND BRAIN-DEAD PATIENTS

Future research is needed to develop technology that could better assess pain perception in unconscious patients. This same technology might be applied to patients with impairments in cognition or communication as well. Currently, protocols for withdrawal of life support vary within and among institutions. Analysis of staff competencies, perceived patient comfort, and family acceptance to different protocols would support evidence-based clinical guidelines for the care of comatose and brain-dead patients. Putting the available resources of the healthcare system to the most appropriate use takes on added meaning with patients who require advanced technology for life support.

■ CONCLUSION

Patients and their families who are dealing with the consequences of stroke, coma, CNDs, or a diagnosis of brain death face enormous challenges and are ideal candidates for PC. Challenges may occur over a period of hours in the acute care setting with immediate decisions to be made regarding prognosis and life support, or they may be experienced for years and require lifelong coping strategies. Research reveals the importance of having conversations regarding PC earlier in the neurological population, when cognitive and communication abilities are intact (Gofton, Jog, & Schulz, 2009; Liu et al., 2017). From a culturally relevant perspective, nurses in all settings need to combine knowledge of the disease, its trajectory, and related symptoms with appreciation of the values and goals of the patient and his or her family. Comfort and QOL interventions have been found to greatly assist people to cope with an array of debilitating symptoms.

While nursing spends a good deal of time focused on pain management and symptom control, nurses are also responsible for addressing the QOL needs of patients who are at the end of their lives. Family members may need help learning how to avoid just sitting at the bedside in a "death watch" but rather share meaningful moments with their loved one. Family members and caregivers should still engage the person in activities designed to evoke feelings of pleasure, meaningfulness, and being socially connected. Warm conversation, music and pet therapy, massage, and activities designed to share beauty in the world and to maintain social connections should be a part of everyday life for the noncomatose patient. For families whose loved one is in a coma or determined brain dead, PC nursing can provide information and support along the illness trajectory and into the bereavement period. Such support is central in assisting families to cope effectively with illness and to find strength in facing their loss.

Since patients with serious neurological problems are often not able to advocate for themselves, it is the nurses' responsibility to continue to work to improve the care delivered to this population who are nearing the end of their lives. There is a need for the profession of nursing to develop a host of evidence-based interventions to meet the PC needs of people with serious neurological disorders.

CASE STUDY *Conclusion*

Mr. M.J., who was introduced at the beginning of this chapter, is experiencing hemiparesis, dysphagia, and aphasia, which are common outcomes for patients with stroke. He had been living in an assisted living facility and it is unlikely that he will be able to return. He is resistant to nursing care and physical therapy. He is having difficulty adjusting to his new situation and accepting his new deficits.

It was explained to Mr. M.J. that there were certain tasks that had to be completed for his symptoms to improve. Nurses started by explaining that they were going to try to ask him yes/no questions so that he would have an easier time answering. They also explained that they were required to perform frequent neurological assessments and that these were important for him because they allowed the medical team to understand his progress. They also provided him with a communication picture board to help aid him in conveying his feelings. Rather than speaking about him or at him, they spoke to him, and this seemed to help.

Mr. M.J. was also started on acetaminophen 500 mg every 6 hours as needed, because it is known that hemiplegic shoulder pain is a common issue for patients who have experienced a stroke. The nurses also explained the necessity of repositioning him, and that they would be coming in at least every 2 hours to reposition his arm and leg, and to relieve pressure on his coccyx. The acetaminophen seemed to help his pain, allowing for short sessions of ROM exercises.

He was started on a pureed diet with honey-thick liquids. While eating, staff sat at his bedside and patiently coached him through his meals. He began eating more of his meals independently, increasing his feelings of autonomy. It is important to place as much control as possible into the hands of the patient. When they feel they have a say in their care and plan, they feel more control over their lives. This allows the patient to feel more normal and hopefully will increase their participation in interdisciplinary care measures, ultimately improving their QOL.

CASE STUDY

AN INTERDISCIPLINARY FOCUS

Glendora Allen, PT, DPT

As a physiotherapist, my initial assessment for palliative rehabilitation will consist in obtaining a detailed history of pertinent information, reviewing relevant systems, and performing functional evidence-based tests and measurements to document prognostic factors, diagnosis, prognosis, and needed interventions.

I would obtain the medical history from the patient or, if possible, from family members, caregivers, medical records, and other interdisciplinary healthcare team members. The data generated from the patient's history review should include, but not be limited to, demographics, current and past medical conditions, medications, living environment, social status, health status, prior level of function (PLOF), and prior level of care (PLOC).

The systems review and examination should consist of assessment data regarding mental status, cognition level, language, and the physiological and/or anatomical status of the neuromuscular (e.g., pain, sensory loss, vision, coordination, tone/reflexes, balance), musculoskeletal (e.g., ROM, mobility), integumentary (e.g., pressure ulcer, lesions), and cardiopulmonary systems (e.g., resting vitals, activity vitals, activity tolerance). An examination of these systems will help determine which tests and measurements can more specifically determine functional limitations, specific impairments, and disabilities, all of which are important in determining the patient's diagnosis and prognosis, and related therapies.

Mr. M.J. has been diagnosed with a left MCA stroke. He presents with right-sided hemiparesis/paralysis; that is, decreased sensation of the right upper extremity and the lower extremity. He has expressive aphasia and dysphagia. He has poor tolerance to skilled thera-peutic activities secondary to pain. He demonstrates verbal outburst and decreased desire and motivation to participate. As a physiotherapist, I assessed Mr. M.J. for motor systems impairments including muscle weakness, abnormalities of muscle tone, coordination problems, timing problems, involuntary movements, and associated movements. Sensory impairments include somato-sensory deficits, visual deficits, as well as cognitive and perceptual problems.

Palliative rehabilitation focuses on patient-, family-, and caregiver-centered goals and maintaining functional independence within the scope of the patient's disability and limitation until the end of life. The patient has expressive aphasia and increased pain, therefore becoming easily frustrated and refusing to participate in therapy sessions. The family's goal is for the patient to be able to transfer to a wheel chair with only standby assist to allow for increased mobility within the facility and to the bedside commode to decrease urinary incontinence.

Initial goals for Mr. M.J. consisted of pain control using therapeutic and pharmacological interventions. Therapeutic interventions included gentle passive range of motion (PROM), positioning techniques, and therapeutic activities. Pharmacological intervention would be based on the physician or advanced practice nurse's orders and the patient's medical condition.

Within 2 weeks of beginning palliative rehabilitation, Mr. M.J. reported a decrease in pain and was able to increase his tolerance to PROM in order to prevent contractures. He also began to participate in his treatment sessions and tolerated neuromuscular therapeutic activities for initiation of static and dynamic sitting balance. With the support and expertise of the interprofessional healthcare team, Mr. M.J. was soon able to transfer from the bed to a wheelchair, and participate in activities offered on the unit, which were important to his physical and emotional health and sense of well-being.

Evidence-Based Practice

Gilmore-Bykovskyi, A. L., & Bowers, B. J. (2013). Understanding nurses decisions to treat pain in nursing home residents with dementia. *Research in Gerontological Nursing*, 6(2), 127–138. doi:10.3928/19404921-20130110-02

Research Problem
Pain is a common symptom in older adult patients with dementia. Nursing home residents with dementia continue to receive inadequate pain treatment. Nursing home residents with cognitive impairment received significantly fewer analgesics than residents without cognitive impairment. This study seeks to explore how nurses make decisions whether to treat pain pharmacologically in nursing home residents with dementia, to identify the conditions that influence treatment decisions, and to develop a conceptual model to guide further research and practice.

Design
This study employed a qualitative design, Grounded Dimensional Analysis, to explore the understandings that nurses have about pain in persons with dementia, the actions nurses take in relation to the understanding, and how the two are related (Caron & Bowers, 2000). This research also seeks to identify conditions that influence nurses' actions related to pain management.

Sample and Setting
Fifteen in-depth interviews were conducted with 13 nurses from 14 skilled nursing facilities in Wisconsin. The eligibility criterion for the nursing participants was current

licensure (including three licensed practical and 10 registered nurses) with experience caring for nursing home residents with dementia. Researchers worked in collaboration with directors of nursing to recruit participants.

Methods

Data were analyzed following each interview, allowing the researcher to pursue questions in subsequent interviews that are informed by the development of the conceptual model. Analysis progressed through several nonlinear phases: open, axial, and selective coding. Open coding focused on dimensions, axial coding focused on pain management, and selective coding identified a central social process or core category that became the primary goal of analysis. The goal of axial coding was to explore the interactions between different dimensions.

Results

A conceptual model was developed to illustrate the process that nurses engage in while identifying and deciding on whether or not to treat pain in nursing home residents with dementia. Nurses perceived that the level of certainty about the presence of pain was the most significant factor in determining if the patient would be treated pharmacologically or treated at all. Resident characteristics influenced the nurses' level of certainty regarding the presence of pain. Obvious or visible reasons for pain were considered when the patient had a "reason" for pain such as a recent surgery.

The nurses reported the most prominent characteristics were whether the resident was a long-term or short-term stay resident, had dementia, had a history of drug seeking, and was actively dying. The nurses also reported that they engaged in different assessments in response to if they (the nurse) had a high or low level of certainty regarding the presence of pain. This led to two distinct treatment trajectories that the authors labeled Responding to Uncertainty or Responding to Certainty.

The Responding to Uncertainty treatment trajectory led to treatment delays and generally occurred in patients who were long-term residents and/or had dementia, and/or had a history of drug seeking, and/or had no obvious/visible reason for pain. The Responding to Certainty treatment trajectory led to prompt treatment and generally occurred in patients who were short stay and did not have dementia, were actively dying, or had an obvious/visible reason for pain like recent surgery.

Implications for Nursing Practice

As nurses are the gatekeepers to pain medication, especially in long-term care facilities, it is important to examine their decision-making process in relation to treating pain in patients with dementia. This study provides an insight into how the nurses conceptualize pain in nursing home residents with dementia and their decisions to provide a pharmacological treatment. The findings also highlight the reasons for inadequate pain management in dementia patients.

Commentary

This study included a small sample of licensed and registered nurses who worked in a geographically similar area. No demographic information was collected and no participant observation took place. The study was unable to establish with certainty the consistency between reported behavior and action. The study does establish the need for further research in this area. This study highlights the need for clear, specific assessment tools for pain in patients with dementia, as well as the importance of education regarding responding to pain indicators and behavioral symptoms. The study revealed a large degree of inconsistency regarding pain interventions.

■ **Acknowledgments.** The editors would like to thank Christine R. Kovach, PhD, RN and Sheila Reynolds, MS, GCNS, BC for their contributions to the previous edition.

■ REFERENCES

Adey-Wakeling, Z., Liu, E., Crotty, M., Leyden, J., Kleinig, T., Anderson, C. S., & Newbury, J. (2016). Hemiplegic shoulder pain reduces quality of life after acute stroke. *American Journal of Physical Medicine and Rehabilitation, 95*(10), 758–763. doi:10.1097/PHM.0000000000000496

Ahmed, A., & Simmons, Z. (2013). Pseudobulbar affect: Prevalence and management. *Therapeutics and Clinical Risk Management, 9*, 483–489. doi:10.2147/TCRM.S53906

Altman, K. W., Richards, A., Goldberg, L., Frucht, S., & McCabe, D. J. (2013). Dysphagia in stroke, neurogenerative disease, and advanced dementia. *Otolaryngologic Clinics of North America, 46*(6), 1137–1149. doi:10.1016/j.otc.2013.08.005

Alzheimer's Association. (2017). *2017 Alzheimer's disease facts and figures.* Chicago, IL. Retrieved from http://www.alz.org/documents_custom/2017-facts-and-figures.pdf

Amara, A. W., Chahine, L. M., & Videnovic, A. (2017). Treatment of sleep dysfunction in Parkinson's disease. *Current Treatment Options in Neurology, 19*(7), 26. doi:10.1007/s11940-017-0461-6

American Academy of Pediatrics Task Force on Brain Death in Children. (1987). Report of Special Task Force. Guidelines for the determination of brain death in children. *Pediatrics, 80*(2), 298–300.

American Heart Association. (2017). *Heart disease and stroke statistics 2017 Update: A report from the American Heart Association.* Dallas, TX: Author.

Ancoli-Israel, S., & Cooke, J. R. (2005). Prevalence and comorbidity of insomnia and effect on functioning in elderly populations. *Journal of the American Geriatrics Society, 53*(7 Suppl.), S264–S271. doi:10.1111/j.1532-5415.2005.53392.x

Andersen, P. M., Abrahams, S., Borasio, G. D., de Carvalho, M., Chio, A., Van Damme, P., … Weber, M. (2012). EFNS guidelines on the clinical management of amyotrophic lateral sclerosis (MALS)—Revised report of an EFNS task force. *European Journal of Neurology, 19*(3), 360–375. doi:10.1111/j.1468-1331.2011.03501.x

Bach, J. R., Goncalves, M. R., Hon, A. M., Ishikawa, Y. M., De Vito, E. L., Prado, F. M., & Dominguez, M. E. (2012). Changing trends in the management of end-stage neuromuscular respiratory muscle failure: Recommendations of an international consensus. *American Journal of Physical Medicine and Rehabilitation, 92*(3), 267–277. doi:10.1097/PHM.0b013e31826edcf1

Barnes, J., & Campbell, C. (2010). Palliative care in multiple sclerosis and motor neurone disease. *British Journal of Hospital Medicine, 71*(1), 21–25. doi:10.12968/hmed.2010.71.1.45968

Bede, P., Oliver, D., Stodart, J., Simmons, Z., O Brannagáin, D., Borasio, G. D., & Hardiman, O. (2011). Palliative care in amyotrophic lateral sclerosis: A review of current international guidelines and initiatives. *Journal of Neurology, Neurosurgery and Psychiatry, 82*(4), 413–418. doi:10.1136/jnnp.2010.232637

Biundo, R., Weis, L., & Antonini. A. (2016). Cognitive decline in Parkinson's disease: The complex picture. *NPJ Parkinson's Disease, 2*, 16018. doi:10.1038/npjparkd.2016.18

Blackhall, L. J. (2012). Amyotrophic lateral sclerosis and palliative care: Where we are, and the road ahead. *Muscle and Nerve, 45*(3), 311–318. doi:10.1002/mus.22305

Blacquiere, D. P., Gubitz, G. J., Dupere, D., McLeod, D., & Phillips, S. (2009). Evaluating an organized palliative care approach in patients with severe stroke. *Canadian Journal of Neurological Sciences, 36*(6), 731–734. doi:10.1017/S0317167100008349

Blatzheim, K. (2009). Interdisciplinary palliative care, including massage, in treatment of amyotrophic lateral sclerosis. *Journal of Bodywork and Movement Therapies, 13*(4), 328–335. doi:10.1016/j.jbmt.2008.04.040

Book, D. S. (2009). Disorders of brain function. In C. Porth, G. Matfin, & C. Porth (Eds.), *Pathophysiology: Concepts of altered health states* (8th ed., pp. 1299–1337). Philadelphia, PA: Wolters Kluwer Health/Lippincott Williams & Wilkins.

Bradt, J., Magee, W. L., Dileo, C., Wheeler, B. L., & McGilloway, E. (2010). Music therapy for acquired brain injury. *Cochrane Database of Systematic Reviews*, (7), CD006787. doi:10.1002/14651858.CD006787.pub2

Brass, S. D., Duquette, P., Proulx-Therrien, J., & Auerbach, S. (2010). Sleep disorders in patients with multiple sclerosis. *Sleep Medicine Reviews, 14*(2), 121–129. doi:10.1016/j.smrv.2009.07.005

Broadley, S., Cheek, A., Salonikis, S., Whitham, E., Chong, V., Cardone, D., … Thompson, P. (2005). Predicting prolonged dysphagia in acute stroke: The Royal Adelaide Prognostic Index for Dysphagic Stroke (RAPIDS). *Dysphagia, 20*(4), 303–310. doi:10.1007/s00455-005-0032-y

Brush, J. A., & Calkins, M. P. (2008). Environmental interventions and dementia: Enhancing mealtimes in group dining rooms. *ASHA Leader, 13*(8), 24–25. doi:10.1044/leader.FTR4.13082008.24

Buckley, J. S., & Salpeter, S. R. (2015). A risk-benefit assessment of dementia medications: Systematic review of the evidence. *Drugs and Aging, 32*, 453–467. doi:10.1007/s40266-015-0266-9

Burns, A., & Iliffe, S. (2009). Alzheimer's disease. *British Medical Journal, 338*, b158. doi:10.1136/bmj.b158

Burton, C. R., & Payne, S. (2012). Integrating palliative care within acute stroke services: Developing a programme theory of patient and family needs, preferences and staff perspectives. *BMC Palliative Care, 11*, 22. doi:10.1186/1472-684X-11-22

Caminero, A., & Bartolomé, M. (2011). Sleep disturbances in multiple sclerosis. *Journal of the Neurological Sciences, 309*(1–2), 86–91. doi:10.1016/j.jns.2011.07.015

Campbell, C. W., Jones, E. J., & Merrills, J. (2010). Palliative and end-of-life care in advanced Parkinson's disease and multiple sclerosis. *Clinical Medicine, 10*(3), 290–292. doi:10.7861/clinmedicine.10-3-290

Canevelli, M., Valletta, M., Trebbastoni, A., Sarli, G., D'Antonio, F., Tariciotti, L., ... Bruno, G. (2016). Sundowning in dementia: Clinical relevance, pathophysiological determinants, and therapeutic approaches. *Frontiers in Medicine, 3*, 73. doi:10.3389/fmed.2016.00073

Caron C., & Bowers B. (2000). Methods and application of dimensional analysis: A contribution to concept and knowledge development in nursing. In B. Rodgers & K. Knafl (Eds), *Concept development in nursing, foundations, techniques and applications* (pp. 285–319). Philadelphia, PA: W.B. Saunders Co.

Cechetto, D. F., Hachinski, V., & Whitehead, S. N. (2008). Vascular risk factors and Alzheimer's disease. *Expert Review of Neurotherapeutics, 8*(5), 743–750. doi:10.1586/14737175.8.5.743

Chan, D. K., Cordato, D. J., & O'Rourke, F. (2008). Management for motor and non-motor complications in late Parkinson's disease. *Geriatrics, 63*(5), 22–27.

Chapman, I. M. (2007). The anorexia of aging. *Clinics in Geriatric Medicine, 23*(4), 735–756, v. doi:10.1016/j.cger.2007.06.001

Chaudhury, H., Cooke, H. A., Cowie, H., & Razaghi, L. (2017). The influence of the physical environment on residents with dementia in long-term care settings: A review of the empirical literature. *The Gerontologist, 00*, 1–13. doi:10.1093/geront/gnw259

Chen, M. C., Tsai, P. L., Huang, Y. T., & Lin, K. C. (2013). Pleasant music improves visual attention in patients with unilateral neglect after stroke. *Brain Injury, 27*(1), 75–82. doi:10.3109/02699052.2012.722255

Chen, Y., Ryden, M. B., Feldt, K., & Savik, K. (2000). The relationship between social interaction and characteristics of aggressive, cognitive impaired nursing home residents. *American Journal of Alzheimer's Disease and Other Dementias, 15*(1), 10–17. doi:10.1177/153331750001500108

Chio, A., Mora, G., & Lauria, G. (2017). Pain in amyotrophic lateral sclerosis. *Lancet Neurology, 16*, 144–157. doi:10.1016/S1474-4422(16)30358-1

Cohen, D. L., Roffe, C., Beavan, J., Blackett, B., Fairfield, C. A., Hamdy, S., ... Bath, P. M. (2016). Post-stroke dysphagia: A review and design considerations for future trials. *Journal of Stroke, 11*(4), 399–411. doi:10.1177/1747493016639057

Cohen, S. M., Elackattu, A., Noordzij, J. P., Walsh, M. J., & Langmore, S. E. (2009). Palliative treatment of dysphonia and dysarthria. *Otolaryngologic Clinics of North America, 42*(1), 107–121. doi:10.1016/j.otc.2008.09.010

Connolly, B. S., & Lang, A. E. (2014). Pharmacological treatment of Parkinson disease: A review. *Journal of the American Medical Association, 311*(16), 1670–1683. doi:10.1001/jama.2014.3654

da Rovare, V. P., Magalhaes, G. P., Jardini, G. D., Beraldo, M. L., Gameiro, M. O., Agarwal, A., ... El Dib, R. (2017). Cannabinoids for spasticity due to multiple sclerosis or paraplegia: A systematic review and meta-analysis of randomized clinical trials. *Complementary Therapies in Medicine, 34*, 170–184. doi:10.1016/j.ctim.2017.08.010

Davis, C., & Lockhart, L. (2016). Update: Stroke. *Nursing Management, 47*(2), 24–33. doi:10.1097/01.NUMA.0000479442.68020.46

Davis, L. D., King, M. K., & Schultz, J. L. (2005). *Fundamentals of neurologic disease: An introductory text.* New York, NY: Demos Medical Publishing, LLC.

Deak, M. C., & Kirsch, D. B. (2014). Sleep disordered breathing in neurologic conditions. *Clinics in Chest Medicine, 35*(3), 547–556. doi:10.1016/j.ccm.2014.06.009

Delaney, J. W., & Downar, J. (2016). How is life support withdrawn in intensive care units: A narrative review. *Journal of Critical Care, 35*, 12–18. doi:10.1016/j.jcrc.2016.04.006

Dorst, J., Dupuis, L., Petri, S., Kollewe, K., Abdulla, S., Wolf, J., ... Ludolph, A. C. (2015). Percutaneous endoscopic gastronomy in amyotrophic lateral sclerosis: A prospective observational study. *Journal of Neurology, 262*, 849–858. doi:10.1007/s00415-015-7646-2

Draper, B., Snowdon, J., Meares, S., Turner, J., Gonski, P., McMinn, B., ... Luscombe, G. (2000). Case-controlled study of nursing home residents referred for treatment of vocally disruptive behavior. *International Psychogeriatrics/IPA, 12*(3), 333–344. doi:10.1017/s1041610200006438

Dubois, B., Padovani, A., Scheltens, P., Rossi, A., & Dell'Agnello, G. (2016). Timely diagnosis for Alzheimer's disease: A literature review on benefits and challenges. *Journal of Alzheimer's Disease, 14*, 617–631. doi:10.3233/JAD-150692

Durham, S. R., Clancy, R. R., Leuthardt, E., Sun, P., Kamerling, S., Dominguez, T., & Duhaime, A. C. (2000). CHOP Infant Coma Scale ("Infant Face Scale"): A novel coma scale for children less than two years of age. *Journal of Neurotrauma, 17*(9), 729–737. doi:10.1089/neu.2000.17.729

Ertekin, C., & Aydogdu, I. (2003). Neurophysiology of swallowing. *Clinical Neurophysiology, 114*(12), 2226–2244. doi:10.1016/S1388-2457(03)00237-2

Fox, C., Smith, T., Maidment, I., Hebding, J., Madzima, T., Cheater, F., ... Young. J. (2014). The importance of detecting and managing comorbidities in people with dementia? *Age and Ageing, 43*, 741–743. doi:10.1093/ageing/afu101

Gessert, C. E., Mosier, M. C., Brown, E. F., & Frey, B. (2000). Tube feeding in nursing home residents with severe and irreversible cognitive impairment. *Journal of the American Geriatrics Society, 48*(12), 1593–1600. doi:10.1111/j.1532-5415.2000.tb03869.x

Gilmore-Bykovskyi, A. L., & Bowers, B. J. (2013). Understanding nurses' decisions to treat pain in nursing home residents with dementia. *Research in Gerontological Nursing, 6*(2), 127–138. doi:10.3928/19404921-20130110-02

Go, A. S., Mozaffarian, D., Roger, V. L., Benjamin, E. J., Berry, J. D., Borden, W. B., ... Turner, M. B.; American Heart Association Statistics Committee and Stroke Statistics Subcommittee. (2013). Heart disease and stroke statistics—2013 update: A report from the American Heart Association. *Circulation, 127*(1), e6–e245. doi:10.1161/CIR.0b013e31828124ad

Gofton, T. E., Jog, M. S., & Schulz, V. (2009). A palliative approach to neurological care: A literature review. *Canadian Journal of Neurological Sciences, 36*(3), 296–302. doi:10.1017/s0317167100007010

Gonçalves, F., Bento, M. J., Alvarenga, M., Costa, I., & Costa, L. (2008). Validation of a consciousness level scale for palliative care. *Palliative Medicine, 22*(6), 724–729. doi:10.1177/0269216308094104

Goodwin, V. A., Richards, S. H., Taylor, R. S., Taylor, A. H., & Campbell, J. L. (2008). The effectiveness of exercise interventions for people with Parkinson's disease: A systematic review and meta-analysis. *Movement Disorders, 23*(5), 631–640. doi:10.1002/mds.21922

Gopalakrishna, A., & Alexander, S. A. (2015). Understanding Parkinson disease: A complex and multifaceted illness. *Journal of Neuroscience Nursing, 47*(6), 320–326. doi:10.1097/JNN.0000000000000162

Gordon, P. H. (2011). Amyotrophic lateral sclerosis: Pathophysiology, diagnosis and management. *CNS Drugs, 25*(1), 1–15. doi:10.2165/11586000-000000000-00000

Greer, D. M., Wang, H. H., Robinson, J. D., Varelas, P. N., Henderson, G. V., & Wijdicks, E. F. (2016). Variability of brain death policies in the United States. *JAMA Neurology, 73*(2), 213–218. doi:10.1001/*jamaneurol*.2015.3943

Gutgsell, K. J., Schluchter, M., Margevicius, S., DeGolia, P. A., McLaughlin, B., Harris, M., ... Wiencek, C. (2013). Music therapy reduces pain in palliative care patients: A randomized controlled trial. *Journal of Pain and Symptom Management, 45*(5), 822–831. doi:10.1016/j.jpainsymman.2012.05.008

Hackett, M. L., & Pickles, K. (2014). Part 1: Frequency of depression after stroke: An updated systematic review and meta-analysis of observational studies. *International Journal of Stroke, 9*(8), 1017–1025. doi:10.1111/ijs.12357

Hallford, D. J., McCabe, M. P., Mellor, D., Davison, T. E., & Goldhammer, D. L. (2012). Depression in palliative care settings: The need for training for nurses and other health professionals to improve patients' pathways to care. *Nurse Education Today, 32*(5), 556–560. doi:10.1016/j.nedt.2011.07.011

Higginson, I. J., McCrone, P., Hart, S. R., Burman, R., Silber, E., & Edmonds, P. M. (2009). Is short-term palliative care cost-effective in multiple sclerosis? A randomized phase II trial. *Journal of Pain and Symptom Management, 38*(6), 816–826. doi:10.1016/j.jpainsymman.2009.07.002

Hills, T. E. (2010). Determining brain death: A review of evidence-based guidelines. *Nursing, 40*(12), 34–40; quiz 40. doi:10.1097/01.NURSE.0000390667.52579.8e

Hirschberg, R., & Giacino, J. T. (2011). The vegetative and minimally conscious states: Diagnosis, prognosis and treatment. *Neurologic Clinics, 29*(4), 773–786. doi:10.1016/j.ncl.2011.07.009

Houtchens, M. K., Benedict, R. H., Killiany, R., Sharma, J., Jaisani, Z., Singh, B., ... Bakshi, R. (2007). Thalamic atrophy and cognition in multiple sclerosis. *Neurology, 69*(12), 1213–1223. doi:10.1212/01.wnl.0000276992.17011.b5

Joosse, L. L. (2012). Do sound levels and space contribute to agitation in nursing home residents with dementia? *Research in Gerontological Nursing, 5*(3), 174–184. doi:10.3928/19404921-20120605-02

Kales, H. C., Gitlin, L. N., & Lyketsos, C. G. (2015). Assessment and management of behavioral and psychological symptoms of dementia. *British Medical Journal, 350*, h369. doi:10.1136/bmj.h369

Kawczynski Pasch, S. (2009). Disorders of thought, mood, and memory. In C. Porth, G. Matfin, & C. Porth (Eds.), *Pathophysiology: Concepts of altered health states* (8th ed., pp. 1357–1387). Philadelphia, PA: Wolters Kluwer Health/Lippincott Williams & Wilkins.

Klit, H. M., Finnerup, N. B., & Jensen, T. S. (2015). Diagnosis, prevalence, characteristics, and treatment of central poststroke pain. *International Association for the Study of Pain, 23*(3), 1–7.

Ko, K. R., Park, H. J., Hyun, J. K., Seo, I., & Kim, T. U. (2016). Effect of laryngopharyngeal neuromuscular electrical stimulation in dysphagia accompanied in post-stroke and traumatic brain injury patients: A pilot study. *Annals of Rehabilitation Medicine, 40*(4), 600–610. doi:10.5535/arm.2016.40.4.600

Kochanek, M. A., Murphy, S. L., Xu, J., & Tejada-Vera, B. (2016). Deaths: Final data for 2014. *National Vital Statistics Reports, 65*(4), 1–4.

Kovach, C. R. (2000). Sensoristasis and imbalance in persons with dementia. *Journal of Nursing Scholarship, 32*(4), 379–384. doi:10.1111/j.1547-5069.2000.00379.x

Kovach, C. R., Logan, B. R., Simpson, M. R., & Reynolds, S. (2010). Factors associated with time to identify physical problems of nursing home residents with dementia. *American Journal of Alzheimer's Disease and Other Dementias, 25*(4), 317–323. doi:10.1177/1533317510363471

Kovach, C. R., Simpson, M. R., Joosse, L., Logan, B. R., Noonan, P. E., Reynolds, S. A., ... Raff, H. (2012). Comparison of the effectiveness of two protocols for treating nursing home residents with advanced dementia. *Research in Gerontological Nursing, 5*(4), 251–263. doi:10.3928/19404921-20120906-01

Kovach, C. R., Taneli, Y., Dohearty, P., Schlidt, A. M., Cashin, S., & Silva-Smith, A. L. (2004). Effect of the BACE intervention on agitation of people with dementia. *Gerontologist, 44*(6), 797–806. doi:10.1093/geront/44.6.797

Kreisel, S. H., Hennerici, M. G., & Bäzner, H. (2007). Pathophysiology of stroke rehabilitation: The natural course of clinical recovery, use-dependent plasticity and rehabilitative outcome. *Cerebrovascular Diseases, 23*(4), 243–255. doi:10.1159/000098323

Kuhn, D. R., & Forrest, J. M. (2012). Palliative care for advanced dementia: A pilot project in 2 nursing homes. *American Journal of Alzheimer's Disease and Other Dementias, 27*(1), 33–40. doi:10.1177/1533317511432732

Kumar, A., Singh, A., & Ekavali (2015). A review on Alzheimer's disease pathophysiology and its management: An update. *Pharmacological Reports, 67*, 195–203. doi:10.1016/j.pharep.2014.09.004

Kurlan, R., Richard, I. H., Papka, M., & Marshall, F. (2000). Movement disorders in Alzheimer's disease: More rigidity of definitions is needed. *Movement Disorders, 15*(1), 24–29. doi:10.1002/1531-8257(200001)15:1<24::AID-MDS1006>3.0.CO;2-

Langhorne, P., Bernhardt, J., & Kwakkel, G. (2011). Stroke rehabilitation. *Lancet, 377*(9778), 1693–1702. doi:10.1016/S0140-6736(11)60325-5

Langmore, S. E., Grillone, G., Elackattu, A., & Walsh, M. (2009). Disorders of swallowing: Palliative care. *Otolaryngologic Clinics of North America, 42*(1), 87–105, ix. doi:10.1016/j.otc.2008.09.005

Lessard, M. R., & Brochu, J. G. (2010). Challenges in diagnosing brain death. *Canadian Journal of Anaesthesia, 57*(10), 882–887. doi:10.1007/s12630-010-9361-x

Liu, Y., Kline, D., Aerts, S., Youngwerth, J. M., Kutner, J. S., Sillau, S., & Kluger, B. M. (2017). Inpatient palliative care for neurological disorders: Lessons from a large retrospective series. *Journal of Palliative Medicine, 20*(1), 59–64. doi:10.1089/jpm.2016.0240

Lo, K., Leung, K., & Shek, A. (2007). Management of Parkinson disease: Current treatments, recent advances, and future development. *Formulary, 42*, 529–544.

Logemann, J. A., Gensler, G., Robbins, J., Lindblad, A. S., Brandt, D., Hind, J. A., ... Miller Gardner, P. J. (2008). A randomized study of three interventions for aspiration of thin liquids in patients with dementia or Parkinson's disease. *Journal of Speech, Language, and Hearing Research, 51*(1), 173–183. doi:10.1044/1092-4388(2008/013)

Lökk, J. (2011). Parkinson's disease permanent care unit: Managing the chronic-palliative interface. *Journal of Multidisciplinary Healthcare, 4*, 33–38. doi:10.2147/JMDH.S17713

Lökk, J., & Delbari, A. (2012). Clinical aspects of palliative care in advanced Parkinson's disease. *BMC Palliative Care, 11*, 20. doi:10.1186/1472-684X-11-20

MacLeod, A. D., Taylor, K. S., Counsell, C. E. (2014). Mortality in Parkinson's disease: A systematic review and meta-analysis. *Movement Disorders, 29*(13). doi:10.1002/mds.25898

Maloni, H. W. (2000). Pain in multiple sclerosis: An overview of its nature and management. *Journal of Neuroscience Nursing, 32*(3), 139–144, 152. doi:10.1097/01376517-200006000-00004

Marik, P. E., & Kaplan, D. (2003). Aspiration pneumonia and dysphagia in the elderly. *Chest, 124*(1), 328–336. doi:10.1378/chest.124.1.328

Martin, G. A., & Sabbagh, M. N. (2011). *Palliative care for advanced Alzheimer's and dementia: Guidelines and standards for evidence-based care.* New York, NY: Springer.

Mateen, F. J., Manalo, N. C., Grundy S. J., Houghton, M. A., Hotan, G. C., Erickson, H., & Videnovic, A. (2017). Light therapy for multiple sclerosis-associated fatigue. *Medicine, 96*(36), e8037. doi:10.1097/MD.0000000000008037

McGeachan, A. J., & McDermott, C. J. (2017). Management of oral secretions in neurological disease. *Practical Neurology, 17*, 96–103. doi:10.1136/practneurol-2016-001515

McGonigal-Kenny, M. L., & Schutte, D. L. (2006). Nonpharmacologic management of agitated behaviors in persons with Alzheimer disease and other chronic dementing conditions. *Journal of Gerontological Nursing, 32*(2), 9–14.

McNamee, S., Howe, L., Nakase-Richardson, R., & Peterson, M. (2012). Treatment of disorders of consciousness in the Veterans Health Administration polytrauma centers. *Journal of Head Trauma Rehabilitation, 27*(4), 244–252. doi:10.1097/HTR.0b013e31825e12c8

Meek, C., Pollock, A., Potter, J., & Langhorne, P. (2003). A systematic review of exercise trials post stroke. *Clinical Rehabilitation, 17*(1), 6–13. doi:10.1191/0269215503cr579oa

Miller, R. G., Jackson, C. E., Kasarskis, E. J., England, J. D., Forshew, D., Johnston, W., ... Woolley, S. C. (2009). Practice Parameter update: The care of the patient with amyotrophic lateral sclerosis: Multidisciplinary care, symptom management, and cognitive/behavioral impairment (an evidence-based review): Report of the Quality Standards Subcommittee of the American Academy of Neurology. *Neurology, 73*(15), 1227–1233. doi:10.1212/WNL.0b013e3181bc01a4

Minden, S. L. (2000). Mood disorders in multiple sclerosis: Diagnosis and treatment. *Journal of Neurovirology, 6* (Suppl. 2), S160–S167.

Miyasaki, J. M., Long, J., Mancini, D., Moro, E., Fox, S. H., Lang, A. E., ... Hui, J. (2012). Palliative care for advanced Parkinson disease: An interdisciplinary clinic and new scale, the ESAS-PD. *Parkinsonism and Related Disorders, 18*(Suppl. 3), S6–S9. doi:10.1016/j.parkreldis.2012.06.013

Mullen, J. E. (2013). Pediatric brain death: Updated guidelines. *AACN Advanced Critical Care, 24*(1), 33–37. doi:10.1097/NCI.0b013e31827be114

Nakagawa, T. A., Ashwal, S., Mathur, M., & Mysore, M.; Society of Critical Care Medicine, Section on Critical Care and Section on Neurology of American Academy of Pediatrics; Child Neurology Society. (2011). Clinical report—Guidelines for the determination of brain death in infants and children: An update of the 1987 task force recommendations. *Pediatrics, 128*(3), e720–e740. doi:10.1542/peds.2011-1511

National Hospice Organization. (1996). *Medical guidelines for determining prognosis in selected non-cancer diseases* (2nd ed.). Arlington, VA: Author.

National Institute of Neurological Disorders and Stroke. (2014). *Parkinson's disease: Hope through research.* Bethesda, MD National Institutes of Health. Retrieved from https://catalog.ninds.nih.gov/pubstatic//15-139/15-139.pdf

National Institute of Neurological Disorders and Stroke. (2017a). NINDS coma information page. Retrieved from https://www.ninds.nih.gov/Disorders/All-Disorders/Coma-Information-Page

National Institute of Neurological Disorders and Stroke (2017b). *Multiple Sclerosis Information.* Retrieved from https://www.ninds.nih.gov/Disorders/All-Disorders/Multiple-Sclerosis-Information-Page

National Institute of Neurological Disorders and Stroke. (2017c). Amyotrophic lateral sclerosis (ALS) fact sheet. Retrieved from https://www.ninds.nih.gov/Disorders/Patient-Caregiver-Education/Fact-Sheets/Amyotrophic-Lateral-Sclerosis-ALS-Fact-Sheet

National Institute of Neurological Disorders and Stroke. (2017d). Tremor fact sheet. Retrieved from https://www.gov/Disorders/Patient-Caregiver-Education/Fact-Sheets/Tremor-Fact-Sheet

National Institute on Aging. (2016). Alzheimer's disease fact sheet. Retrieved from https://www.nia.nih.gov/health/alzheimers-disease-fact-sheet

National Institutes of Health. (2013). *Stroke: Hope through research (NIH Publication No. 99–2222).* Bethesda, MD: National Institute of Neurological Disorders and Stroke. Retrieved from http://www.ninds.nih.gov/disorders/stroke/detail_stroke.htm

National Multiple Sclerosis Society. (2016). About MS. Retrieved from http://www.nationalmssociety.org

Navaneethan, U., & Eubanks, S. (2015). Approach to patients with esophageal dysphagia. *Surgical Clinics of North America, 95*(3), 483–489. doi:10.1016/j.suc.2015.02.004

O'Connor, A. B., Schwid, S. R., Herrmann, D. N., Markman, J. D., & Dworkin, R. H. (2008). Pain associated with multiple sclerosis: Systematic review and proposed classification. *Pain, 137*(1), 96–111. doi:10.1016/j.pain.2007.08.024

Oken, B. S., Flegal, K., Zajdel, D., Kishiyama, S. S., Lovera, J., Bagert, B., & Bourdette, D. N. (2006). Cognition and fatigue in multiple sclerosis: Potential effects of medications with central nervous system activity. *Journal of Rehabilitation Research and Development, 43*(1), 83–90. doi:10.1682/jrrd.2004.11.0148

Ostwald, S. K., Wasserman, J., & Davis, S. (2006). Medications, comorbidities, and medical complications in stroke survivors: The CAReS study. *Rehabilitation Nursing, 31*(1), 10–14. doi:10.1002/j.2048-7940.2006.tb00004.x

Owen, A. M., Schiff, N. D., & Laureys, S. (2009). A new era of coma and consciousness science. *Progress in Brain Research, 177*, 399–411. doi:10.1016/S0079-6123(09)17728-2

Padilla, R. (2011). Effectiveness of environment-based interventions for people with Alzheimer's disease and related dementias. *American Journal of Occupational Therapy, 65*(5), 514–522. doi:10.5014/ajot.2011.002600

Paillard, T., Rolland, Y., & de Souto Barreto, P. (2015). Protective effects of physical exercise in Alzheimer's disease and Parkinson's disease: A narrative review. *Journal of Clinical Neurology, 11*(13), 212–219. doi:10.3988/jcn.2015.11.3.212

Parkinson's Disease Foundation. (2017). Understanding Parkinson's. Retrieved from http://parkinson.org/understanding-parkinsons

Peat, S. (2010). Using cannabinoids in pain and palliative care. *International Journal of Palliative Nursing, 16*(10), 481–485. doi:10.12968/ijpn.2010.16.10.79211

Pendergast, T. (2002). Palliative care in the intensive care unit setting. In A. Berger, R. Portenoy, & D. Weissman (Eds.), *Principles and practice of palliative care and supportive oncology* (2nd ed., pp. 1086–1104). Philadelphia, PA: Lippincott Williams & Wilkins.

Pfeiffer, R. F. (2000). Gastrointestinal dysfunction in Parkinson's disease. *Clinical Neuroscience, 5*, 136–146.

Poppe, L., Rue, L., Robberecht, W., & Van Den Bosch, L. (2014). Translating biological findings into new treatment strategies for amyotrophic lateral sclerosis (ALS). *Experimental Neurology, 262*, 138–151. doi:10.1016/j.expneurol.2014.07.001

Posner, J. B., Saper, C. B., & Schiff, N. (2007). *Plum and Posner's diagnosis of stupor and coma* (4th ed.). Cary, NC: Oxford University Press.

Qian, F., Fonarow, G. C., Smith, E. E., Xian, Y., Pan, W., Hannan, E. L.,... Bhatt, D. L. (2013). Racial and Ethnic Differences in Outcomes in Older Patients With Acute Ischemic Stroke. *Circulation: Cardiovascular Quality and Outcomes, 6*, 284–292.

Querfurth, H. W., & LaFerla, F. M. (2010). Alzheimer's disease. *New England Journal of Medicine, 362*(4), 329–344. doi:10.1056/NEJMra0909142

Ramachandrannair, R., Sharma, R., Weiss, S. K., & Cortez, M. A. (2005). Reactive EEG patterns in pediatric coma. *Pediatric Neurology, 33*(5), 345–349. doi:10.1016/j.pediatrneurol.2005.05.007

Reilly, P. L., Simpson, D. A., Sprod, R., & Thomas, L. (1988). Assessing the conscious level in infants and young children: A paediatric version of the Glasgow Coma Scale. *Child's Nervous System, 4*(1), 30–33. doi:10.1007/BF00274080

Rocca, M. A., Amato, M. P., De Stefano, N., Enzinger, C., Geurts, J. J., Penner, I. K.,... Filippi, M. (2015). Clinical and imaging assessment of cognitive dysfunction in multiple sclerosis. *Lancet Neurology, 14*(3), 302–317. doi:10.1016/S1474-4422(14)70250-9

Rothenberg, L. R., Doberman, D., Simon, L. E., Gryczynski, J., & Cordts, G. (2014). Patients surviving in hospice care: Who are they? *Journal of Palliative Medicine, 17*(8), 899–905. doi:10.1089/jpm.2013.0512

Rubenfeld, G., & Crawford, S. (2001). Principles and practices of withdrawing life-sustaining treatment in the ICU. In J. Curtis & G. Rubenfeld (Eds.), *Managing death in the intensive care unit* (pp. 127–147). New York, NY: Oxford University Press.

Sasegbon, A., & Hamdy, S. (2017). The anatomy and physiology of normal and abnormal swallowing in oropharyngeal dysphagia. *Neurogastroenterology and Motility, 29*(11). doi:10.1111/nmo.13100.

Shagam, J. Y. (2008). Unlocking the secrets of Parkinson disease. *Radiologic Technology, 79*(3), 227–239; quiz 40.

Shapiro, J., & Downe, L. (2003). The evaluation and management of swallowing disorders in the elderly. *Geriatric Times, 4*(6). Retrieved from www.cmellc.com/geriatrictimes/g031217.html

Simon, R. (2000). Coma and disorders of arousal. In L. Goldman (Ed.), *Cecil textbook of medicine* (21st ed., pp. 2023–2026). Philadelphia, PA: Saunders.

Simons, J. A. (2017). Swallowing dysfunction in Parkinson's disease. *International Review of Neurobiology, 134*, 1207–1238. doi:10.1016/bs.irn.2017.05.026

Sperling, R. A., Aisen, P. S., Beckett, L. A., Bennett, D. A., Craft, S., Fagan, A. M.,... Phelps, C. H. (2011). Toward defining the preclinical stages of Alzheimer's disease: Recommendations from the National Institute on Aging -Alzheimer's Association workgroups on diagnostic guidelines for Alzheimer's disease. *Alzheimer's Dementia, 7*(3), 280–292. doi:10.1016/j.jalz.2011.03.003

Studenski, S. A., Lai, S. M., Duncan, P. W., & Rigler, S. K. (2004). The impact of self-reported cumulative comorbidity on stroke recovery. *Age and Ageing, 33*(2), 195–198. doi:10.1093/ageing/afh056

Subramanian, S., & Surani, S. (2007). Patient handout: Sleep disorders in the elderly. *Geriatrics, 62*(12), following 32.

Sura, L., Madhavan, A., Carnaby-Mann, G., & Crary, M. A. (2012). Dysphagia in the elderly: Management and nutritional considerations. *Clinical Interventions in Aging, 7*, 287–298. doi:10.2147/CIA.S23404

Takahashi, R. H., Nagao, T., & Gouras, G. K. (2017). Plaque formation and the intraneuronal accumulation of β-amyloid in Alzheimer's disease. *Pathology International, 67*, 185–193. doi:10.1111/pin.12520

Teri, L., Gibbons, L. E., McCurry, S. M., Logsdon, R. G., Buchner, D. M., Barlow, W. E.,... Larson, E. B. (2003). Exercise plus behavioral management in patients with Alzheimer disease: A randomized controlled trial. *Journal of the American Medical Association, 290*(15), 2015–2022. doi:10.1001/jama.290.15.2015

Truog, R. D., Cist, A. F., Brackett, S. E., Burns, J. P., Curley, M. A., Danis, M.,... Hurford, W. E. (2001). Recommendations for end-of-life care in the intensive care unit: The Ethics Committee of the Society of Critical Care Medicine. *Critical Care Medicine, 29*(12), 2332–2348. doi:10.1097/00003246-200112000-00017

Turner, A. P., Alschuler, K. N., Hughes, A. J., Beier, M., Haselkorn, J. K., Sloan, A. P., & Ehde, D. M. (2016). Mental health comorbidity in MS: Depression, anxiety, and bipolar disorder. *Current Neurology and Neuroscience Reports, 16*(12), 106. doi:10.1007/s11910-016-0706-x

United States President's Commission for the Study of Ethical Problems in Medicine and Biomedical and Behavioral Research. (1981). Defining death: A report on the medical, legal and ethical issues in the determination of death. Washington, DC. Retrieved from https://bioethicsarchive.georgetown.edu/pcbe/reports/past_commissions/defining_death.pdf

Van Cauwenberghe, C., Van Broeckhoven, C., & Sleegers, K. (2016). The genetic landscape of Alzheimer disease: Clinical implications and perspectives. *Genetics in Medicine, 18*(5), 421–430. doi:10.1038/gim.2015.117

van Es, M. A., Hardiman, O., Chio, A., Al-Chalabi, A., Pasterkamp, R. J., Veldink, J. H., & van den Berg, L. H. (2017). Amyotrophic lateral sclerosis. *Lancet, 390*(10107), 2084–2098. doi:10.1016/S0140-6736(17)31284-4

Veerbeek, J. M., van Wegen, E., van Peppen, R., van der Wees, P. J., Hendriks, E., Rietberg, M., & Kwakkel, G. (2014). What is the evidence for physical therapy poststroke? A systematic review and meta-analysis. *PLOS ONE, 9*(2), e87987. doi:10.1371/journal.pone.0087987

Verkaik, R., Nuyen, J., Schellevis, F., & Francke, A. (2007). The relationship between severity of Alzheimer's disease and prevalence of comorbid depressive symptoms and depression: A systematic review. *International Journal of Geriatric Psychiatry, 22*(11), 1063–1086. doi:10.1002/gps.1809

Vestergaard, K., Andersen, G., Gottrup, H., Kristensen, B. T., & Jensen, T. S. (2001). Lamotrigine for central poststroke pain: A randomized controlled trial. *Neurology, 56*(2), 184–190. doi:10.1212/WNL.56.2.184

von Gunten, C., & Weissman, D. (2001). Fast facts and concepts #34: Symptom control for ventilator withdrawal in the dying patient. Retrieved from https://www.mypcnow.org/blank-dthim

Vucic, S., Rothstein, J. D., Kiernan, M. C. (2014). Advances in treating amyotrophic lateral sclerosis: insights from pathophysiological studies. *Trends in Neurosciences, 37*(8), 433–442.

Walsh, K. (2001). Management of shoulder pain in patients with stroke. *Postgraduate Medical Journal, 77*(912), 645–649. doi:10.1136/pmj.77.912.645

Weintraub, D., & Claassen, D. O. (2017). Impulse control and related disorders in Parkinson's disease. *International Review of Neurobiology, 133*, 679–717. doi:10.1016/bs.irn.2017.04.006

Welschehold, S., Boor, S., Reuland, K., Beyer, C., Kerz, T., Reuland, A., & Müller-Forell, W. (2012). CT angiography as a confirmatory test in brain death. *Acta Neurochirurgica, 114*(Suppl.), 311–316. doi:10.1007/978-3-7091-0956-4_60

Westergren, A., Ohlsson, O., & Hallberg, I. R. (2002). Eating difficulties in relation to gender, length of stay, and discharge to institutional care, among patients in stroke rehabilitation. *Disability and Rehabilitation, 24*(10), 523–533. doi:10.1080/09638280110113430

Wharton, T., & Ford, B. K. (2014). What is known about dementia care recipient violence and aggression against caregivers? *Journal of Gerontological Social Work, 57*(5), 460–477. doi:10.1080/01634372.2014.882466

White, G. N., O'Rourke, F., Ong, B. S., Cordato, D. J., & Chan, D. K. (2008). Dysphagia: Causes, assessment, treatment, and management. *Geriatrics, 63*(5), 15–20.

Wilson, R. S., Bennett, D. A., Gilley, D. W., Beckett, L. A., Schneider, J. A., & Evans, D. A. (2000). Progression of parkinsonian signs in Alzheimer's disease. *Neurology, 54*(6), 1284–1289. doi:10.1212/WNL.54.6.1284

Yetimalar, Y., Gürgör, N., & Basoglu, M. (2004). Clinical efficacy of gabapentin for paroxysmal symptoms in multiple sclerosis. *Acta Neurologica Scandinavica, 109*(6), 430–431. doi:10.1111/j.1600-0404.2004.00276.x

Yevchak, A. M., Steis, M. R., & Evans, L. K. (2012). Sundown syndrome: A systematic review of the literature. *Research in Gerontological Nursing, 5*(4), 294–303. doi:10.3928/19404921-20120906-04

Debra J. Hain

End-Stage Renal Disease

CHAPTER

17

KEY POINTS

- Although the incidence and prevalence of end-stage renal disease (ESRD) have increased over the past decade, especially in those 65 years and older, recently there has been a decline in the incidence rate. This may be in part due to the increasing number of individuals receiving pre-ESRD care. Although the incidence rate may have declined, the prevalence rate remains stable, with over 678,383 cases.
- Adults with ESRD often have a high symptom burden along with multiple comorbid chronic conditions.
- Adults with ESRD have a shortened life expectancy compared to the general population. Individuals undergoing dialysis are expected to live less than one-third as long as those without ESRD, and in those over 80 years old, the life expectancy is about one-half. The main cause of mortality in this population is cardiovascular disease. Age is a key predictor for mortality, with the survival rate for those older than 75 years of about 17%; however, the life expectancy for children with ESRD has greatly improved.
- Hospice is underutilized by patients with ESRD. About 19.2% of patients with Medicare Parts A and B as the primary care provider received hospice care at the time of death. This was highest among those 85 and older (29.4%) and lowest among the 20- to 44-year-old age group (7.0%). Despite a high symptom burden, the rate of palliative care (PC) and hospice use by patients with ESRD is well below that of the general population.
- Information is now available that suggests that patients who are typically expected to do poorly on dialysis may benefit as much from conservative management and PC, an option referred to as nondialysis, as they would from dialysis.

CASE STUDY

Jim, a 72-year-old black male, had a history of chronic kidney disease (CKD) Stage 5 secondary to diabetic kidney disease. After several years of living with CKD, his healthcare provider informed him that he had ESRD and would need kidney replacement therapy (KRT) to survive. Years of poorly controlled type 2 diabetes mellitus (DM) had caused damage to both the glomeruli and tubules of the kidneys. Like many patients who first learn they will need KRT (hemodialysis, peritoneal dialysis [PD], or transplantation) to survive, he initially declined dialysis because he simply could not see how, at age 72 years, he could tolerate receiving any type of technological life-sustaining treatment. After receiving kidney disease education from a nurse practitioner, he agreed to a time-limited trial of dialysis. After starting in-center hemodialysis, Jim was able to incorporate the dialysis regimen into his daily living and remained on dialysis for many years.

He and his family adjusted to the 4-hour treatments three times a week. His wife became an expert in managing the various aspects of therapy required to live a healthy life with ESRD. Both were kind and supportive to the other patients undergoing dialysis at the same time. They were deeply religious people who brought a sense of grace and peace to the dialysis setting.

At age 80, Jim told his family and the dialysis staff that he could no longer tolerate dialysis. He was experiencing severe, uncontrolled osteoarthritic pain that worsened when he was undergoing dialysis. He had fallen three times in the past year, and with the third fall he sustained a hip fracture. He was losing his independence and was using a walker for ambulation. After the fourth fall with minor injury, he became wheelchair bound and was having difficulty participating in church and family events, which made his quality of life (QOL) unacceptable to him. Each time he had to come in for dialysis, he experienced more pain than was tolerable, and he was experiencing increased pain due to leg and foot ulcerations from ischemia. It became clear from his lab values that he was not eating adequately (albumin: 3.1 g/dL; blood urea and nitrogen [BUN]: 30 mg/dL; PO_4: 3.0 mg/dL—these values should be higher in patients undergoing dialysis).

The healthcare team (physician, nurse, dietitian, and social worker), Jim, and his wife engaged in shared decision making, where Jim's preferences and wishes for care were central to the conversation. Jim had advance directives with a healthcare proxy designating his wife as the healthcare agent. One of the important issues to consider before a patient withdraws from dialysis is whether or not the patient is depressed or whether there are other strategies that could effectively control his pain. A thorough psychological assessment indicated that Jim was not depressed. So the next step was to consider nonpharmacological and pharmacological treatments for pain management. He was offered a trial of several different types of pain control medications, including oxycontin and fentanyl lozenges for breakthrough pain. Jim agreed to try these therapies for 1 month. If there was no relief at the end of that period, he wanted to withdraw from treatment. He also said that he wanted to dialyze only twice weekly.

By the end of the month, the pain, with the help of powerful analgesics, had lessened greatly. Circulation to his legs also improved sufficiently for the ulcers to begin to heal. Jim was able to resume some of his church and family activities. He even decided to dialyze three times weekly. A good prognostic indicator was that his appetite and lab values improved. Unfortunately, in a short period of time, Jim fell again and this time sustained a more serious head injury. After a lengthy hospitalization he was discharged to a rehabilitative center, where he was confused and experienced severe uncontrolled pain, so the decision was made to enroll him in hospice and withdraw from dialysis.

Diagnosis of ESRD can be difficult for patients and families to hear because this means they will need some form of KRT to survive (hemodialysis, PD, or transplantation). ESRD means a patient has severe end-organ kidney damage and failure. Individuals with CKD can progress to the point where they require KRT or they can choose supportive therapy with no dialysis (depending on the age and the level of residual kidney function, death will occur in a relatively short period of time). CKD can be defined as kidney damage or estimated glomerular filtration rate (eGFR) less than 60 mL/min/1.73 m² for 3 months or longer. Markers of kidney damage (irrespective of specific pathology) include abnormalities in the blood, urine tests, or imaging studies (Kidney Disease: Improving Global Outcomes [KDIGO], 2013). There is emerging evidence that indicates that even though an individual over age 65 has an eGFR of less than 60 mL/min/1.73 m², without albuminuria or other markers of kidney damage, he or she may not have CKD. Glassrock, Delanaye, and El Nahas (2015) suggest that in persons over age 65 years, an eGFR less than 45 mL/min/1.73 m² may be a more accurate reflection of CKD. CKD should be classified based on the level of kidney function. This classification system is based on eGFR and categories of albuminuria (Kidney Disease Improving Global Outcomes [KDIGO], 2012; see Exhibit 17.1). The classification of G1 includes those with normal kidney function but with markers of kidney damage. G2 is considered a mild decrease in kidney function (e.g., individuals with diabetes with albuminuria). G3 has been further divided into 3A (eGFR between 45 and 59 mL/min/1.73 m²) and 3B (eGFR between 30 and 44 mL/min/1.73 m²); this is in consideration of the increased complications associated with advanced CKD.

Exhibit 17.1
Functions of the Kidneys

1. *Chemical and water equilibrium:* Kidneys regulate the volume and osmolarity of fluid in the body, as well as electrolyte content and acidity, by varying the excretion of ions and water in the urine. Electrolytes excreted or preserved by the kidneys include sodium, potassium, chloride, calcium, magnesium, and phosphate. Numerous bodily functions depend on the maintenance of optimal body fluid composition and volume, such as:
   a. Cardiac output
   b. Blood pressure
   c. Most enzymes that function best within a narrow range of pH
   d. K^+ concentration, which directly affects cell membrane potentials
   e. Membrane excitability, which depends on calcium concentration in the body fluid
2. *Excretion of metabolic end products and foreign substances:* Kidneys excrete urea and creatinine as well as the end products of metabolized drugs and toxins
3. *Production and secretion of enzymes and hormones:*
   a. Renin is a catalyst in the formation of angiotensin and a potent vasoconstrictor involved in sodium balance and blood pressure regulation
   b. Erythropoietin stimulates the maturation of erythrocytes in bone marrow and, when absent, causes anemia of chronic renal disease
   c. 1,25-Dihydroxyvitamin D3 is a steroid integral in parathyroid hormone (PTH) function and in regulating calcium and phosphorus

Source: Adapted from Schena, F. P. (2001). *Nephrology.* Milan, Italy: McGraw-Hill International.

The nursing care of individuals with ESRD is complex, as they typically have multiple comorbidities that can result in serious complications. This population has a high risk for cardiovascular disease (CVD). In fact, CVD is the leading cause of death in people with ESRD and is recognized as an independent risk factor for cardiovascular disease (Briasoulis & Bakris, 2013). There are many CVD conditions, such as stable atherosclerotic heart disease (ASHD), acute myocardial infarction (AMI), congestive heart failure (CHF), stroke, peripheral vascular disease, atrial fibrillation, and sudden cardiac arrest, that increase the risk of premature death. Other comorbid conditions that can impact the health and well-being of individuals with ESRD include DM, hypertension, osteoarthritis, and cognitive impairment. Considering the disease burden associated with multiple comorbidities, the risk of functional decline (especially in the older adult ESRD population), and the demands of undergoing a life-sustaining treatment, patients and families often experience many challenges in care management. Therefore, the most important role of the nurse is collaborating with the nephrology team to discover strategies aimed at improving health outcomes. It is also essential that nurses are truly present to engage in discussions regarding end-of-life (EOL) issues if the person expresses the desire to withdraw from dialysis.

When confronted with the extensive list of medical and psychological problems often associated with patients with ESRD, healthcare professionals often focus on treating the medical issues by implementing strategies to address abnormal laboratory values and treating comorbid conditions. Although these are essential for promotion of health, it is critical to consider the person living with ESRD and his or her QOL. The goal for patients with ESRD cannot be simply to preserve life but also to promote QOL. In addition, it is critical that a person-centered approach to care is central to decision making regarding the management of ESRD. Taking this approach necessitates the presence of a holistic interprofessional team committed to a shared decision-making approach, the importance of which is discussed later in the chapter. It is this approach that should prevail throughout the course of ESRD up to and including EOL care.

In this chapter, palliative care (PC) will be discussed in relation to three groups of patients with ESRD: (1) undergoing dialysis, (2) choosing conservative management, and (3) withdrawing from dialysis. In reading this chapter, the following questions should be considered: (a) What is the role of PC in improving health outcomes for individuals with ESRD? and (b) What are the best care practices for those who withdraw from dialysis?

■ INCIDENCE AND PREVALENCE

CKD is now considered a global health problem that is increasing worldwide (Levey & Coresh, 2012). In the United States, too, the incidence and prevalence continues to increase. In 2014, there were almost 121,000 new cases (an increase of 1.1% compared to 2013) and the prevalence was at 678,383 (up by 3.5% from 2013; Saran et al., 2017). Despite the fact that since 2010 the number of new cases of ESRD has plateaued, there continues to be a rise in prevalent cases of approximately 21,000 each year (Saran et al., 2017). The highest incidence rate is of individuals 75 and older, but the prevalence is the highest among those 65 to 74 years of age. In part, this is related to the high mortality risk of adults 75 and older (Saran et al., 2017). As expected, ESRD rates are being driven up proportionate to the overall rate of increase in kidney disease but at a slower overall rate than in the past (U.S. Renal Data System [USRDS], 2012). The scope of the problem is significant given that there is an anticipated increase in the number of older adults with diabetes, which is the number one reason for CKD in the United States. A substantial number of these patients will progress to ESRD.

The increase in ESRD is also of concern for economic reasons, as it is the only disease entity in the United States that is reimbursed primarily with public funds. Medicare pays for 80% of all costs of care for patients diagnosed with ESRD, if they have contributed to the Medicare fund or if a child has a parent who has contributed. A year of hemodialysis can be about $72,000 and PD costs approximately $53,000 per year. Those who are not eligible for Medicare may meet the criteria for Medicaid; however, the reimbursement is substantially less than that in Medicare. Undocumented immigrants pose other challenges, such as suboptimal care and adding to the current financial burden within the U.S. healthcare system. Many of these people will visit the emergency department to receive care (Saran et al., 2017).

Ethnic minorities (i.e., Hispanics, African Americans, Asian Americans) have a high risk of ESRD. In 2014, the incidence of ESRD was about 35% higher compared to that in the non-Hispanic population. The prevalence continues to rise among all ethnic groups except Native Americans, in whom there has been a decline. The prevalence remains high among blacks compared to any other racial group at nearly 2.6-fold higher than that in Native Americans and Asians, and 3.7-fold higher than that in whites (Saran et al., 2017).

There is a trend where adults are choosing home dialysis over in-center treatments with an overall 73% increase in use since 2007. In 2014 as compared to 2007, home hemodialysis increased by 72% and PD by 12%. Even though there has been a substantial increase in home modalities, they only represent about 3.4% of the dialysis population, with the majority choosing in-center hemodialysis.

■ PATHOPHYSIOLOGY

ESRD can be caused by any disease process that can damage the kidney; however, some diseases are more likely than others to cause irreversible damage and kidney failure. We know that glomerular diseases that attack the glomeruli of the kidney are the main cause of CKD that progresses to ESRD. Primary glomerular diseases originate from the kidney and secondary from systemic diseases (i.e., lupus nephritis, DM). When the glomeruli are damaged, protein and red blood cells (RBCs) can be seen in the urine. In fact, the first sign of kidney damage, even before seeing changes in blood laboratory studies, is microalbuminuria, proteinuria, and/or RBCs in the urine (Mahaffey, 2017). The most common glomerulonephritis (collection of glomerular diseases) is caused by immunological pathogenic mechanisms. Chronic glomerulonephritis can be the result of diseases, such as DM, amyloidosis in older adults, and IgA nephropathy in adults also associated with lupus nephritis. Glomerulosclerosis (scarring and hardening of the blood vessels within the glomeruli) is not caused by a single disease but common causes are infection, drug toxicity, and systemic diseases such as diabetes, HIV, or lupus nephritis.

Tubulointerstitial disease of the kidney involves structures outside the glomeruli and can be acute or chronic. Chronic tubulointerstitial nephritis can be caused by prolonged exposure to environmental conditions or medications (i.e., lithium, NSAIDs, diuretics) or therapeutic agents as well as systemic disease. Other causes of CKD are hypotensive nephrosclerosis and renal artery stenosis. Polycystic kidney disease (PKD) is the most common inherited disorder that can cause CKD. PKD accounts for about 2.0% of the ESRD population. Recurrent urinary tract infections can also cause kidney damage.

Although there are many risk factors for CKD such as race/ethnicity, age, and renal cell carcinoma, the primary cause for ESRD is DM with the second most common cause being hypertension. The highest rate of diabetic kidney disease and/or hypertension as a diagnosis for ESRD is among adults 75 and older followed by those 65 to 74 years old (Saran et al., 2017). In the case of both diabetes and hypertension, if they had been treated aggressively in the early-onset phase of the disease, most patients would not eventually be diagnosed with ESRD. Given that diabetes accounts for almost 50% of the cases of ESRD, the really alarming statistic is that the incidence of diabetes is increasing exponentially worldwide. Recent statistics set the rate of diabetes in the United States at 25.8 million, or slightly over 8.3% of the population (Centers for Disease Control and Prevention [CDC], 2010).

The underlying renal pathology of ESRD varies according to the etiology. For example, in the case of diabetic kidney disease, the renal lesion includes changes in the afferent and efferent arteries, tubular fibrosis, and thickening of the basement membrane with impingement on the filtration surfaces of the glomerulus. These changes progress as hyperglycemia persists and the resultant proteinuria contributes to hyperfiltration and high GFR, and ultimately to GFR decline (Eberhard & Wolf, 2010). Each disorder that causes ESRD will have a different histopathology, but all will have one thing in common; that is, sufficient destruction of the nephron in one form or another that, if left unchecked, will cause cellular death with CKD that progresses to ESRD.

In the pediatric population, the most common diagnoses that lead to ESRD differ from those of adults. They include, in the order of frequency, glomerular-nephritis (GN), vasculitis, and familial, including cystic, disease, with GN having the best prognosis. The mortality rate for children regardless of cause is 55.3/1,000 patient-years, which is better than that for adults (226/1,000 patient-years). The most recent statistics demonstrate an encouraging trend of progress in the 5-year survival rate for children. As with adults, the most common cause of death for children with ESRD was cardiovascular disease, at 25% (USRDS, 2012).

■ DISEASE TRAJECTORY

Evidence supports that the disease trajectory in some adults with ESRD includes stable periods followed by intervals of steady decline and death usually within 5 years of starting dialysis (Holley, 2007). In older adults, functional decline may be a more important predictor of the disease trajectory than age itself. This population often experiences a functional decline that is most noticeable 1 to 2 months before death (Murtagh et al., 2010). Individuals with advanced CKD and ESRD (before starting dialysis) have variability in the disease trajectory (Sumida & Kovesky, 2017). It appears that the risk of early mortality is the highest in the first 4 weeks of dialysis and then begins to decline. Some factors that contribute to mortality include dialysis access (highest risk is having a dialysis catheter), cause of CKD, presence of acute kidney injury, cardiovascular risk factors, rapid fluid and electrolyte removal, nosocomial-related infections, and patient-related behavioral factors (Foley, 2017; Sumida & Kovesky, 2017).

Individuals with ESRD have shown different patterns of disease trajectory because of several factors that include diabetes, age, hypertension, and race/ethnicity (Sumida & Kovesky, 2017). Adults with ESRD have the traditional cardiovascular risk factors (e.g., hyperlipidemia, hypertension) along with nontraditional risk factors such as inflammation, oxidative stress, secondary hyperparathyroidism, and endothelial dysfunction (Sameiro-Faria et al., 2013). The most common cause of death in adults with ESRD is related to cardiovascular events such as myocardial infarction (MI) and premature arterial aging, which results in aortic stiffening. It is also well documented that patients on dialysis are immune suppressed and therefore more prone to serious infection (Hauser et al., 2008), develop genitourinary tumors at a disproportionate rate (Mandayam & Shahinian, 2008), and are considered to be in a constant prothrombotic/proinflammatory state (Henrich, 2009). Adults with ESRD also develop chronic kidney disease–mineral and bone disorder (CKD–MBD), which increases cardiovascular risk factors. CKD–MBD is a disorder that involves an imbalance of calcium, phosphorus, vitamin D, and PTH. In addition, the population of patients with CKD–MBD can develop a rare but devastating condition called calciphylaxis. Severe painful, poorly healing skin lesions are the most common manifestation. Individuals will also have vascular calcification in the vascular bed, skeletal muscle, brain, lungs, intestines, eyes, and mesentery (Nigwekar et al., 2015). It is important when discussing kidney replacement options (i.e., dialysis, transplantation, conservative care) to first and foremost take a person-centered approach by determining what matters most to the individual and family. This includes making sure the person understands the risks and benefits of available options. Anecdotal evidence supports that many people say that they don't want dialysis when first being told they have ESRD. However, if given the opportunity to truly understand what the options are, people will choose dialysis. Many patients report improved QOL after starting dialysis (D. J. Hain, personal communication, November 20, 2017). In some cases, the person who is uncertain about undergoing dialysis may choose a time-limited trial, which is defined as "a goal-directed trial of dialysis that is limited by predetermined outcomes that are evaluated at planned intervals" (Scherer & Holley, 2015, p. 1). Considering disease trajectory and the variability of ESRD, it is challenging to provide an accurate prognosis, so taking an evidence-based approach that considers the best available evidence, patient/family wishes and preferences, and clinician's expertise is critically important when discussing treatment options.

Dying Trajectory

As expected, the dying trajectory for individuals with ESRD is characterized by symptoms of uremia, which is a clinical syndrome characterized by fluid and electrolyte and hormone imbalances along with metabolic abnormalities. Toxins that the kidneys normally eliminate, such as urea, excess phosphorus, potassium, acids, hormonal and protein by-products, sodium, and water, begin to accumulate. Symptoms from this abnormal systemic state cause discomfort as fluid and toxins build up. For example, if a person with ESRD is dying and is volume overloaded, dyspnea is almost certain. Knowing this, PC providers encourage fluid restriction and recommend that fluids be given only to provide comfort from thirst and dry mouth; however, it is important to determine if the person has urine output and to avoid dehydration.

Uremic pruritus can become unbearable, and treatment should be performed liberally. (See the PC issues section in this chapter for specific treatment.) Anorexia, nausea, vomiting, and diarrhea are common and should be treated symptomatically, as described in other sections of the text. Hyperkalemia commonly occurs and can be the ultimate cause of death. Hyperkalemia first results in hyperreflexia and muscle fasciculation, eventually progressing to muscle weakness, paralysis, cardiotoxicity, and finally death, as cells are no longer able to sustain normal electrical activity. One rare but significant symptom that can cause discomfort is hypothermia, which should be treated symptomatically with warm blankets and a heating pad (Henrich, 2009).

The final phase of the ESRD dying trajectory is due to the effect of uremic toxins on the brain, causing mental and behavioral changes. Memory deficits including amnesia, accompanied by lethargy and drowsiness, are common early symptoms. Gait disturbances, paraesthesias, organic psychosis, and finally coma can be seen in the later stages of dying. The neurotoxicity can lead to seizures, something that may be difficult for families to witness. Families benefit greatly by being informed of the risk prior to the occurrence of these symptoms (Henrich, 2009).

■ COMMON SIGNS AND SYMPTOMS OF ESRD

In the earlier stages of CKD (Stages 1–3), there may be few, if any, noticeable symptoms of disease. Even in the later stages (Stages 4–5), people may not endorse symptoms that can occur as the kidney function declines. Patients adjust to the gradual onset of symptoms that occur as CKD progresses to ESRD. In fact, progression to ESRD is often so insidious that patients do not realize that they have kidney disease until it is quite advanced. It is commonly revealed for the first time when patients have laboratory work done for other purposes. Even after diagnosis of CKD, the movement to ESRD can be so gradual that patients may be unaware of how badly they feel until they are dialyzed for several weeks and symptoms of uremia subside. Symptoms increase in severity as renal function (GFR) decreases. Many patients do not develop life-limiting symptoms of CKD until their GFR is below 10 mL/min or at the point at which they have lost 90% of their kidney function. Patients who have CKD Stage 5 with uremic symptoms, or who are underdialyzed or who opted to stop dialysis, will develop the manifestations of uremia, found in the second list that follows. Signs and symptoms include the following:

Early Signs and Symptoms:
■ Hyperparathyroidism
■ Anemia
■ Hypertension
■ Leg cramps, joint pain, gout, arthritis, muscular pains, muscle weakness
■ Pitting edema
■ Gains in weight with fluid retention
■ Weakness and fatigue

Late Signs and Symptoms (Uremic Indicators):
■ Dry scaly skin and pruritus
■ Frequent headaches
■ Heat or cold intolerance
■ Ammonia or urine smell to breath
■ Metallic taste in mouth, causing food to taste different
■ Poor healing of cuts, abrasions
■ Chest pain or palpitations
■ Dyspnea, orthopnea, paroxysmal nocturnal dyspnea
■ Pericardial friction rub
■ Easy bruising, purpura, or bleeding
■ Anorexia
■ Weight loss or gain
■ Nausea and vomiting
■ Fainting or seizures
■ Peripheral neuropathy
■ Decreased concentration and memory
■ Mood swings and depression
■ Grayish-bronze skin color with underlying pallor
■ Uremic frost, coma, death (Henrich, 2009)

■ COMORBIDITIES AND COMPLICATIONS

This section combines comorbidities and complications of ESRD, as they are intimately connected. Proper management of both determines life expectancy and QOL for individuals with ESRD. Comorbidities and complications associated with ESRD develop because the kidneys decline in function. Treatments of ESRD (dialysis and transplantation) are imperfect replacements for kidney function. The need for such interventions is a point that may be difficult for patients to comprehend, and many patients believe a transplant is the cure. However, there is no cure for kidney disease. Even with a transplant, the person still has kidney disease although he or she may not need dialysis. When rejection occurs, the person will need to receive a second kidney transplant. In many cases, patients will obtain a second, even third transplant.

Adults with CKD often live with multiple chronic health conditions for years before being diagnosed with ESRD, which contributes to their high mortality rate. Most recent USRDS data suggests that about 40% of individuals have DM, 32% hypertension, and 40% self-reported cardiovascular disease. Unfortunately, any of these chronic health conditions increases the risk for CKD; not many people are aware they have kidney disease until it is at an advanced stage (Saran et al., 2017). The absence of symptoms in early stages of CKD limits self-awareness of kidney disease (Chen & Harris, 2015). Unfortunately, the overall percentage of people that are even aware they have CKD has not changed much since 1999 (USRDS, 2017). Therefore, healthcare professionals, especially nurses, play a key role in educating patients about risk factors for kidney disease and the importance of being screened when at risk. This is important because early identification and treatment of comorbid conditions by a nephrology team can help delay ESRD and, when dialysis is required, help the person arrive at that point in reasonably good health. Early referral to nephrology supports preservation of kidney function, reduced mortality, and delaying the onset of debilitating complications. Individuals with CKD Stage 4 are more likely to visit a primary care provider than see a nephrologist until they have a more advanced disease (USRDS, 2017). However, it is important to see a nephrologist earlier in the disease because aggressive treatment of hyperglycemia, hypertension, anemia, CKD–MBD, and lipid disorders prior to the onset of ESRD improves survival statistics. Nephrologists and other nephrology advanced practitioners (nurse practitioner, physician assistant) are aware of this and are motivated to act accordingly.

In the presence of multimorbidity (two or more chronic health conditions), many adults with CKD experience an increased disease management burden especially when attempting to engage in self-management activities (dietary restrictions and managing multiple medications) and interacting with healthcare professionals, all of which impact their QOL (Fraser et al., 2015). About 25% of adults with CKD have three or more comorbidities, including diabetes, hypertension, chronic heart failure, atrial fibrillation, peripheral vascular disease, stroke, constipation, chronic pain, or depression (Tonelli et al., 2015). This is important to note because the greater the number and severity of the comorbidities, the lower the survival rate, increased risk of hospitalizations, and higher healthcare costs.

Although age is not a sole predictor for potential poor health outcomes, it plays a substantial role in the type of complications and health-related outcomes for people with ESRD. Both children and older adults with ESRD present special challenges because of the unique comorbid conditions and ESRD-related complications that are superimposed upon the normal anatomic and physiologic changes associated with those age groups. For example, pediatric patients with ESRD almost universally have growth failure, often necessitating the use of growth hormone, which has complications associated with it. Disease management for pediatric patients with ESRD is also so specialized that adult nephrologists are often ill prepared to care for this age group; therefore, to improve outcomes, a distinct subspecialty of pediatric nephrology has emerged. Pediatric nephrology involves caring for children of all ages with a broad range of conditions ranging from congenital anomalies of the kidney and urinary tract to glomerulopathies. The impact of living with ESRD that requires KRT can have a significant negative impact on QOL (Selewski et al., 2014). Older adults often have age-related health conditions, which put them at risk for complications. For example, older adults have a high risk of osteoporosis that coexists with CKD–MBD, which increases fracture risks. As a person ages, he or she has risks for cognitive impairment, a condition that is common among adults undergoing dialysis. Having cognitive impairment can make it difficult to effectively engage in self-management of a complex medical regimen. Therefore, nurses should consider cognitive impairment as a contributing factor when patients are not taking medications as prescribed rather than labeling them as non-adherent.

Finally, an important component of reducing ESRD-related complications in those undergoing dialysis is to achieve dialysis adequacy. At this time, determining adequacy requires specific patient parameters (pre-/post-dialysis BUN, individual's body weight, type of dialyzer, and vascular access). If patients are adequately dialyzed, they should experience reduced complications and an overall improved well-being and QOL. It is also essential to inquire about how the individual is tolerating the treatment and its impact on everyday living. In addition, having multiple coexisting chronic health conditions can result in other nondialysis-related complications that should be considered when attempting to improve health-related outcomes. Dialysis adequacy is improved when patients have functional dialysis vascular access, receive their full treatment as scheduled, and are dialyzed with the most appropriate dialyzer for that person. A brief review of the major comorbidities and complications associated with ESRD and available palliative treatment options for this population will be discussed in the final portion of this chapter. Treatment of these health conditions would be appropriate for patients who either are receiving dialysis or choose conservative management instead of KRT. If a decision is made to withdraw dialysis, then it would not be reasonable to treat some of the conditions discussed in this section unless there is some residual renal function or it is for symptom management. In those who choose conservative care, slowing the progression of CKD to ESRD and symptom management is essential. Those withdrawing from dialysis usually survive for 7 days or less, and therefore hospice care should be considered. However, even though the percentage of individuals receiving hospice care has increased over the past decade, hospice services continue to be underutilized. Some people undergoing dialysis are not prepared to withdraw despite having increased complications and poor QOL. In these cases, hospice care—while still undergoing dialysis—may provide the much-needed support for patients and families to make this EOL transition. Only if the person has another terminal illness that meets hospice criteria (i.e., cancer, heart failure [HF]), as determined by the hospice physician, can he or she use the ESRD Medicare benefit along with the hospice benefit. A major barrier to this is variability among hospice services; some do not provide this service, while others may.

Disorders of Calcium, Phosphorus, and Bone

The calcium–phosphorus imbalance associated with ESRD can lead to pruritus, bone disease, proximal myopathy, and soft tissue calcifications (vascular, visceral, periarticular, and cutaneous calcifications). The most common calcium–phosphorus disorder is a type of bone disease referred to as CKD–MBD, which involves disturbances in mineral and bone metabolism that occur as kidney function declines (Cahill & Haras, 2017). Current evidence supports that this may be occurring long before a change in laboratory studies indicates an imbalance.

This is a complex process that for purposes of this chapter will be briefly discussed. Initially, serum calcium levels fall as pathologic changes associated with advancing CKD cause retention of phosphorus. The high levels of serum phosphorus cause calcium to couple with phosphorus and become less available to the cells. This upregulates the parathyroid glands to secrete PTH, which stimulates calcium retention and normal reabsorption by the kidney. However, the diseased kidney cannot retain calcium, so the feedback system fails to accomplish the goal of raising serum calcium levels.

Another major cause of secondary hyperparathyroidism is that calcitriol (1,25-dihydroxyvitamin D3) production is suppressed. Calcitriol is synthesized in the kidney and acts on cells in the parathyroid gland to reduce PTH synthesis when there is adequate calcium absorption. So the normal response to low serum calcium is to upregulate calcitriol. Unfortunately, in the presence of reduced kidney function, calcitriol is less available (cannot be synthesized) and the calcitriol receptors in the parathyroid glands become reduced in number and less sensitive to calcitriol. The combination of low calcium levels and insufficient calcitriol then causes the parathyroids to produce more PTH. Continued PTH stimulation leads to hyperplasia and proliferation of parathyroid cells, resulting in secondary hyperparathyroidism.

Further, hyperphosphatemia, which occurs in later stages of CKD and ESRD, directly stimulates PTH secretion. Without medical and dietary intervention, these events cause the glands to enlarge and continue to increase the production of PTH. The constant, high levels of phosphorus and PTH and low levels of serum calcium cause calcium to be leeched from the bone, thereby causing the unique form of bone thinning and weakening seen in ESRD (Henrich, 2009). It is a complex cycle that requires aggressive intervention, or QOL becomes drastically reduced as bone pain, fractures, and decreased mobility occur.

One of the rare, but most devastating complications of the calcium–phosphorus imbalance associated with ESRD is metastatic calcification or calciphylaxis. Prolonged elevation of PTH, as well as calcium–phosphorus, leads to calcium–phosphorus being deposited in blood vessels, tissues, organs, and joints. In severe cases, the calcium deposits inflame the conjunctiva and produce palpable deposits under the skin that can become infected and cause tissue breakdown. This can be extraordinarily painful and is difficult to treat. The best treatment for calciphylaxis is prevention, which involves maintaining calcium and phosphorus balance through diet and the use of phosphate binders that prevent absorption of phosphorus. There are several different types of binders that should be taken with food. Calcium-based binders (calcium carbonate [Tums], calcium acetate) are mostly recommended for individuals with hypocalcemia and have no evidence of vascular calcifications. Non-calcium-based binders such as sevelamer hydrochloride (Renagel), sevelamer carbonate (Renvela), and lanthanum are most commonly used. Newer iron-based binders provide an additional option for patients who are either unable to tolerate the other binders or are not achieving the desired effect. Ferric citrate (Auryxia) has the additional benefit of providing the much-needed iron in the management of anemia. The other binder is sucroferric oxyhydroxide, which, although iron based, does not affect iron stores. Foods high in phosphorus include dairy products, meats, legumes, nuts, whole-grain breads and cereals, and many soft drinks. Collaboration with a dietitian can help establish a person-centered plan of care that considers the stage of CKD and nutritional needs, and honors patient preferences and wishes. Prior to dialysis, there is a Medicare benefit called Medical Nutritional Therapy, where a dietitian can educate and consult with patients with CKD Stages 3 to 5 who are not on dialysis. Once on dialysis, Medicare mandates that a dietitian be a member of the healthcare team. When someone has secondary hyperparathyroidism, the PTH levels can be maintained within the target range with the use of man-made active form of vitamin D (calcitriol), vitamin D analogs, calcimimetics, or a combination. Cinacalcet (Sensipar) is an oral CaSR agonist, and etelcalcetide (Parsabiv) is a new and exciting D-amino peptide calcimimetic for treating secondary hyperparathyroidism that is given IV at the end of the dialysis treatment. In severe cases, when the glands are hypertrophied from continued stimulation due to serum phosphorus levels and have become desensitized, available medications that treat secondary parathyroidism, or a parathyroidectomy, become the treatments of choice. However, this is a last resort because postoperative complications of parathyroidectomy, such as hypocalcemia, can be life threatening and create a treatment challenge for months after surgery (Henrich, 2009).

Anemia of Chronic Kidney Disease

Normocytic, normochromic anemia is one of the most common complications of CKD with increasing prevalence in advanced CKD. It is related to a decrease in erythropoietin (EPO) production. In ESRD, other factors contributing to anemia include iron deficiency, infection, inflammation, occult blood loss, oxidative stress, inadequate dialysis, and hyperparathyroidism. Before the advent of commercially manufactured erythropoiesis-stimulating agents (ESAs), individuals undergoing dialysis were frequently transfused with blood products, exposing them to bloodborne diseases, transfusion reactions, viral infections, iron overload, and immune sensitization. The development of injectable ESAs was a tremendous breakthrough in the treatment of anemia of kidney disease.

Treatment of anemia with an ESA should begin once the person is diagnosed and other causes of anemia are ruled out. Almost all individuals undergoing dialysis will require an ESA to maintain their hematocrit and to avoid complications associated with anemia. For example, adequate anemia management can help prevent left ventricular hypertrophy (LVH), the development of which increases morbidity and mortality for all patients.

When the hemoglobin (Hb) concentration drops below 10 g/dL, patients are particularly prone to develop LVH as well as CHF. So vigilance in diagnosing and aggressively treating anemia may be life preserving. Anemia may be present years before the initiation of dialysis. Therefore, to improve health outcomes, evaluation and treatment for anemia should be done in those with CKD. Anemia management with an ESA and iron supplementation, which is started when a person has CKD and is not on dialysis, often is continued once dialysis is initiated. This is something that requires further evaluation at the start of dialysis and continuous monitoring as per protocol (usually about every 2 weeks, a Hb is obtained). Interestingly, the recommended optimal Hb for individuals receiving an ESA has recently changed as studies have shown that normal or higher Hb levels may predispose people with ESRD to worse outcomes compared to those with lower Hb levels. Recent guidelines from the KDIGO initiative recommend a target Hb range of 10 to 11.5 g/dL, which is well below the normal adult range. The reason for this is evidence of increased thromboembolic events when the effort is made to normalize the Hb with an ESA. There is no lower parameter for Hb, but rather the goal of anemia management, especially for those who are attempting to receive a kidney transplant, is avoidance of blood transfusions. ESAs can be given subcutaneously or intravenously, and side effects include worsening of hypertension, seizures, thromboemboli, and dialysis access clotting. It is recommended to avoid treating patients with a known cancer diagnosis with an ESA.

When assessing patients for causes of anemia, it is essential to evaluate for blood loss, which could be due to menstrual or gastrointestinal bleeding. Laboratory studies include complete blood count with RBC indices and B_{12}, folate, and iron studies (transferrin saturation [TSAT]). Iron is needed for RBC production, and when there are inadequate stores, there will be minimal response to ESA administration. Iron deficiency can occur because of blood loss but most commonly due to impaired iron absorption in people with CKD. If patients with CKD have iron deficiency, a trial of oral iron is given; if this provides an inadequate response, then intravenous (IV) iron can be administered during dialysis or in those with CKD in an infusion center. Another important fact is that people undergoing dialysis lose a small amount of blood each treatment. Finally, any inflammatory process, such as infection or cancer, can result in ESA hyporesponsiveness and can impair the release of iron from storage sites. Hepcidin production, which regulates iron homeostasis in anemia, is increased when the person has iron that is available. Hepcidin is increased when iron is stored and ready for use, in the presence of inflammation or increased erythropoietic activity or hypoxia. Increased levels contribute to ESA hyporesponsiveness. Hyperparathyroidism can also cause erythropoietin resistance, which is another reason to actively control this disorder.

Cardiovascular Disease

CVD is the leading cause of death among individuals with CKD and ESRD undergoing dialysis. CKD is an independent risk factor for CVD similar to that of DM. In adults 65 and older, the prevalence of CVD is significantly higher (65.8%) compared to those without CKD (31.9%). The more advanced the stage of CKD is, the higher the risk of mortality due to CVD. In fact, many adults in the later stages of CKD never progress to ESRD because of CVD-related death (USRDS, 2017). A declining GFR is linked to the development of atherosclerotic CVD (Muntner et al., 2005). This population has the traditional CVD risk factors such as physical inactivity, hypertension, DM, smoking, LVH, family history, and dyslipidemia along with nontraditional risk factors, which include endothelial dysfunction, vascular medial hyperplasia, sclerosis, calcification, volume overload, CKD–MBD, anemia, malnutrition, inflammation, oxidative stress, and autonomic imbalance. Adults with CKD are at risk for AMI, which over time results in premature death. Two-year survival after experiencing AMI in those without CKD is about 81%, with CKD Stage 1 to 2 about 71%, and CKD Stage 4 to 5 about 56% (USRDS, 2017). HF is the most common CVD in the CKD population. In adults 65 and older, the prevalence of HF is about 30% compared to those without CKD (6%; USRDS, 2017). Atrial fibrillation that is associated with a very high mortality and morbidity rate frequently occurs in adults with CKD. Individuals undergoing dialysis do not seem to have classic atherosclerotic coronary artery disease (CAD) but rather develop a cardiomyopathy that has medial vascular calcifications, microvascular disease, or interstitial fibrosis of the myocardium, as well as LVH (Briedthardt & McIntrye, 2011). This puts the person with ESRD at risk for experiencing hemodialysis-related myocardial stunning, which is basically transient ischemia not caused by CAD. Myocardial stunning is emerging as a major contributing factor for the high CVD mortality rate in the ESRD population. Most often, it is related to ultrafiltration rate (fluid removal) and hemodynamic instability during dialysis (Brown et al., 2015). Discussion about fluid removal and intradialytic hypotension will be discussed later in the chapter.

Living with CVD can substantially impact mortality, morbidity, and QOL; thus, it is crucial that person-centered interventions are focused on prevention and the most appropriate treatment for the individual. KDIGO Clinical Practice Guidelines (CPGs; Sarnak & Levey, 2000) recommend the evaluation of risk factors for treatment includes screening for LVH and CAD; treating hypertension and hyperlipidemia using goals for patients who have preexisting CAD; low-sodium and low-fat diets; fluid restrictions; maintaining a calcium/phosphorus product below 55, which is obtained by multiplying the serum calcium number by the serum phosphorus number; as well as counseling for smoking cessation, exercise, and aggressive treatment of DM. For patients with CAD, attention to maintaining the hematocrit above 30 can help alleviate anginal symptoms in some cases. Dialysis patients also have increased risks for endocarditis, pericarditis, and arrhythmias, especially if they are inadequately dialyzed. Sudden death risk is increased and has been linked to hyperkalemia, usually related to dietary intake (Henrich, 2009).

Dialysis Access

Individuals undergoing hemodialysis require a vascular access such as an arteriovenous fistula (AVF), in which a native artery and vein are surgically joined together to produce one large vessel; an arteriovenous graft (AVG), in which a synthetic material is used to create a large conduit between an artery and a vein; or a venous catheter (VC), in which a double lumen catheter is placed in a vein, usually in the internal jugular, but in some cases is temporarily placed in the femoral vein. It is important to avoid using the subclavian vein due to an increased risk for central stenosis, which may impact AVF maturation. The AVF is the preferred vascular access; however, a subset of patients (i.e., older adults, people with DM) will have better health outcomes with another type of vascular access. Age, comorbidities, and gender are factors to consider when determining the best vascular access to be created or placed (Inglese, 2017). In the case of both the old and the young, successful access placement and maintenance for dialysis can be complicated by anatomy and physiology. Older adults frequently have peripheral vascular calcification or narrowing caused by diabetes, hyperlipidemia, high phosphorus levels, or hypertension. The placement of vascular access in calcified vessels increases the rate of ischemia and thrombosis. In children, blood vessels are often too small, necessitating the use of the PD modality.

VCs are considered short-term, nontunneled noncuffed or long-term, tunneled cuffed catheters. The short-term catheter is shorter in length and more rigid than the long-term catheter and is used only temporarily. The long-term catheter is tunneled under the skin from the point of insertion before entering a large vein and then is threaded toward the heart to the right atrium (Pryor & Brouwer-Maier, 2017). Long-term catheters are used in those patients for whom an AVF is maturing or in those who are not good candidates for AVF or AVG. The goal is to avoid catheter use, or, if necessary, use it only for a short period of time. In some cases, patients will have a catheter because of coexisting health conditions or poorly maturing AVF or because they are not a surgical candidate for AVF or AVG. In rare circumstances, when no other access is available, a patient may have a long-term femoral catheter placed. Individuals undergoing PD will have a catheter placed through the abdominal wall into the peritoneal space and dialysis fluid infused into the peritoneal space and drained out through the catheter after an exchange of electrolytes and systemic toxins.

AVFs are the safest type of access and have the lowest infection rate as compared to dialysis catheters or AVGs. A problem is that AVFs can't be used immediately after being created; it takes about 3 months to mature and be ready for needle cannulation. For this reason, The Fistula First Catheter Last Initiative recommends patients be assessed for AVF evaluation no later than CKD Stage 4, which should give the AVF time to mature and be ready for use once the person reaches ESRD. Before an AVF is surgically created, vessel mapping is done, usually with an ultrasound to study and evaluate the arterial and venous vasculature to determine the best site for AVF or AVG. Even though AVFs are least likely to have complications compared to other venous accesses, some potential complications exist that increase morbidity and mortality. These complications include: (a) stenosis (narrowing or stricture); (b) thrombosis (formation of blood clot); (c) bleeding that can occur postoperatively or post dialysis treatment; (d) infections (not common); (e) steal syndrome; and (f) aneurysms (weakened areas of the blood vessel that enlarge and may lead to clotting). Steal syndrome is when blood supply is routed away from the hand of the access arm, causing ischemic pain. Infection rates are highest in patients who have dialysis catheters, but can also occur with grafts. Graft infections can be superficial, or, worse, they may be deep seated. Catheter-related infections are common and significantly contribute to morbidity and mortality (Deaver & Counts, 2015). Both catheter and graft infections can lead to sepsis and require surgical removal or, worse, death from profound infection (Ahmad, 2009). Therefore, it is critical that only nurses who receive education and training and are competent should cannulate an AVF or AVG or access a dialysis VC.

The most common and serious complication of PD is peritonitis. Other complications include: (a) catheter obstruction, which is usually caused by mechanical blockage (clamps or kinks in tubing) and catheter tip migration or entrapment by omentum or adhesions; (b) internal or external leaks; and (c) exit-site or tunnel infections (Payton & Kennedy, 2017). Internal and external PD fluid leaks can occur at any time. Common signs of internal leaks are edema of the labia, scrotum, penis, or the soft tissue planes of the catheter insertion site, or a preexisting hernia. Hydrothorax is a rare and life-threatening complication that can occur. External leaks are detected when fluid drains out around the catheter. Treatment of leaks is beyond the scope of a non-nephrology nurse, so if a problem is identified, discussion and referral to the PD nurse is essential. The nephrology team will assess the patient and determine the best evidence-based treatment, which may include switching to hemodialysis (HD).

PD-Related Peritonitis

Peritonitis (inflammation of the peritoneal cavity primarily caused by infection) is a leading complication associated with PD. Exit-site and catheter-tunneled infections are the major factors that contribute to PD-related peritonitis. For this reason, prevention includes: (a) using systemic prophylactic antibiotics before insertion of the catheter; (b) routine exit-site care that may include daily application of antibiotic cream or ointment to the catheter exit site; (c) educating and training patients and family members about PD exit-site care and meticulous hand hygiene during dialysis exchange (draining the dialysate from abdomen and filling with fresh solution to dwell for a specified period of time); and (d) the best practices to assess for peritonitis (Kelman & Watson, 2017).

Peritonitis is diagnosed if two of the three are present: (a) clinical feature of peritonitis (i.e., abdominal pain and/or cloudy dialysis effluent [drained dialysate]); (b) dialysis effluent count greater than 100 µL or greater than $0.1 \times 109/L$ (after a dwell time of at least 2 hours) with greater than 50% polymorphonuclear; and (c) positive dialysis effluent culture (Kelman & Watson, 2017). Patients may also have a fever, nausea, or vomiting. It is important to note that patients with peritonitis may present with no abdominal pain to mild pain and cloudy effluent to extreme abdominal pain with rebound tenderness.

Early diagnosis and treatment with antibiotics provide the best chance for cure and preserving the access. Repeated infections can cause scarring of the peritoneum, which may cause failure of this dialysis modality and lead to a rare complication, known as sclerosing encapsulating peritonitis. In this disorder, the abdominal organs become wrapped in a fibrous cocoon, causing excruciating pain. Surgery is often required to release the bands and the disorder is often fatal. Treatment includes intraperitoneal (IP) antibiotics, pain management, one or two optional flushes for pain symptoms prior to IP antibiotics, and, of course, psychological support for the patient and family or friend who may experience feelings of guilt and distress (Kelman & Watson, 2017). Catheter removal may be necessary if the infection cannot be cleared with it in place, or when there is relapsing peritonitis or fungal peritonitis. Patients can consider having a catheter replacement at a later time, but until then they will have to undergo HD.

Intradialytic Hypotension

Intradialytic hypotension (IDH; low blood pressure [BP] during dialysis treatment) is a serious complication of undergoing hemodialysis that can lead to vascular access thrombosis, inadequate dialysis clearance, and mortality (Flythe, Hui, Lynch, Curhan, & Brunelli, 2015). The occurrence ranges from 15% to 50% of hemodialysis

done in an ambulatory dialysis center. This wide range is because there is variability in the definition, but what is known is that IDH can impact health outcomes. One research study's findings support researchers' conclusions that SBP lower than 90 mmHg pose the biggest risk for mortality (Flythe et al., 2015). However, based on anecdotal evidence, it is extremely important to pay attention to the individual patient's responses to dialysis treatment. Some patients have SBP readings well below 90 mmHg before they even start the dialysis treatment or may be asymptomatic with SBP less than 90 mmHg. Complications of intradialytic hypotension include seizures; thrombotic events, such as cerebrovascular accidents, myocardial ischemia, and infarction; and thrombosis of the dialysis access (Henrich, 2009).

Any person undergoing hemodialysis can experience intradialytic hypotension but for older adults, this is especially true when attempting to ultrafiltrate even if it is to the target weight. In part, this is due to their underlying cardiovascular disease. If fluid is removed from the intravascular space too rapidly, it can exceed the plasma filling capacity. When combined with an inability to increase peripheral vascular resistance and the host of drugs that people with ESRD are prescribed, abrupt hypotension can occur. In some cases, people have IDH because they have gained lean muscle mass, and the target weight (established weight without extra fluid) may need to be increased. In other cases, the person may have the extra fluid but the ultrafiltration (UF) goal is more than the person can tolerate for that one dialysis treatment. Postprandial hypotension is also common and occurs because of increased blood flow to the stomach and gut to digest food when patients eat during treatment. Dialysis can interfere with mealtimes for many patients, so they want to eat during the treatment. However, this is strongly discouraged; they must skip meals to avoid hypotension. Many dialysis centers prohibit eating and drinking during dialysis to avoid IDH; instead, asking the person to bring a snack to eat post treatment may be a better option for those who cannot wait until they go home to eat.

The optimal treatment is preventing too much or too rapid fluid removal. However, maintaining the recommended fluid restrictions can be difficult for many. The goal is to achieve euvolemia and have BP within the acceptable range. This requires a balance between sodium intake, water intake, urine output, and UF during dialysis. The majority of patients will be instructed to decrease sodium intake and not gain more than 1 kg per day. If a person has residual kidney function (still have urine output), it is essential to try to preserve this by reducing IDH and nephrotoxic agents. During the dialysis treatment, the dialysis team will monitor the tolerance to fluid removal, but sometimes patients have symptoms after the treatment once they go home. Patient education can help people gain knowledge to avoid high interdialytic weight gain (the weight gained in between the dialysis treatments due to fluid intake), but in many education alone may not be enough, thus calling for further behavioral research. Immediate treatment for symptomatic intradialytic hypotension consists of volume replacement with normal saline, lowering or stopping the UF goal, and placing the patient in a recumbent position. Vigilance by the dialysis staff during treatment is required to identify hypotension as soon as there are detectable signs and to then treat it quickly. Older patients typically cannot tolerate as much fluid removal as younger patients. Hypotensive episodes are avoided, if at all possible, due to reasons cited previously and because they can leave patients weak, contribute to falls, cause cramping during and after treatment, and decrease QOL (Henrich, 2009).

Some patients cannot take any antihypertensive medication before dialysis, even if their BPs are elevated, or they will have severe hypotension during treatment. Using shorter-acting medications in the evening prior to dialysis can help the patient arrive at a treatment with a more acceptable BP without the risk of intradialytic hypotension (Schena, 2001).

Hyperkalemia

The development of hyperkalemia (≥5.5 mmol/L) among individuals undergoing dialysis results from reduced or absent renal excretion of potassium in combination with normal or increased intake of potassium in the diet. People undergoing dialysis are in a positive potassium balance between the dialysis sessions and then a negative balance during dialysis. Reasons for hyperkalemia include increased potassium dietary intake, insufficient removal of potassium during dialysis, increased release of potassium from cells (i.e., metabolic acidosis, trauma, hemolysis), pseudohyperkalemia (hemolysis during blood collection), and poorly controlled constipation. Individuals undergoing dialysis may be asymptomatic with potassium levels above the normal range. People with ESRD tend to tolerate much higher serum potassium levels than the population at large, but even they have an upper limit beyond which symptoms and death occur. Cardiac and neuromuscular symptoms can occur, especially with more severe hyperkalemia. Symptoms include weakness, fatigue, paraesthesia, depression of deep tendon reflexes, palpitations, and cardiac arrhythmias. ECG changes parallel to the degree of hyperkalemia. There can be initial tenting of the T wave, then P-wave flattening, widening of the QRS complex, and development of a deep S wave. Ventricular fibrillation is usually the cause of death when hyperkalemia is severe (Schena, 2001).

Hemodialysis is the best way to treat hyperkalemia in the ESRD population. The amount removed depends on how many hours the person is undergoing dialysis, blood flow rate, dialysate flow, and potassium and buffer concentrations of the dialysate and dialyzer. Even though dialysis is the preferred way to reduce potassium, other treatment options must be considered when it is not available. In emergency situations, IV calcium insulin and sodium bicarbonate are commonly used as mechanisms to drive potassium from the serum into the cell where the effects are neutralized. Cation-exchange resins such as sodium polystyrene sulfate (Kayexalate), in which there is uptake of potassium and releases of sodium in the gut (someone without a functioning gut should not be given kayexalate), is given in non-emergency situations. A newer nonabsorbed cation-exchange polymer is Veltassa (patiromer), which binds with magnesium in the gut. It is important that patients take it with food and should take other medications 3 hours before or after Veltassa. In addition, magnesium levels should be monitored because hypomagnesemia may occur. These two medications should not be considered in an emergency; rather, following the protocol for emergency hyperkalemia (insulin, calcium, sodium bicarbonate) should be considered.

It can be challenging for many people undergoing dialysis to follow a low-potassium diet, so it is extremely important to collaborate with the dietitian at the dialysis center to develop a diet plan that fits a person's lifestyle and food preferences. In those who have residual kidney function, potassium may not be as much of a problem, but as kidney function continues to decline, this may require adjustment in dietary intake. Potassium is obtained at least on a monthly basis in the dialysis centers, so potassium levels should be reviewed before recommending a low-potassium diet because in some circumstances diets are liberalized due to potassium values at the lower end or below normal.

■ GENERAL MANAGEMENT—TREATMENT OPTIONS

The following section will address general PC management and broad treatment options for individuals with ESRD. Implementing evidence-based strategies will most likely yield the best health outcomes for this population. However, at this time, as a growing body of evidence emerges, there is a paucity of scientific evidence to inform practice initiatives. There is a deliberate focus on the part of nephrology professionals to conduct rigorous studies regarding PC for people with CKD. At the end of the section, there is a discussion of the nontreatment option, also known as the nondialysis option, which includes conservative management, or withholding or withdrawing of dialysis.

Care management should be designed to give patients with ESRD the best possible physical, psychological, spiritual, and social outcomes by using a person-centered approach that involves shared decision making. This approach is compatible with a PC philosophy that supports collaboration among all members of the healthcare team with patients or families to achieve optimal treatment goals. The main emphasis is on the alleviation of symptoms and prevention of complications that affect longevity and QOL. Ideally, with shared decision making, patients and providers mutually understand diagnosis and prognosis, and develop potentially attainable treatment goals. Healthcare professionals should be aware of the relevance of individualizing an approach to care that considers personal information, such as medical and social history, as well as the patient's wishes and preferences for care, which include advanced care planning. The intent of shared decision making is to engage in a dialogue about what matters most to the person and family, incorporate the patient's wishes and preferences, and integrate the best available evidence as well as the healthcare professional's expertise in care of individuals with ESRD to mutually establish goals to achieve desired outcomes. This is true whether the treatment goals are designed to preserve life or to support the patient's wishes to not undergo dialysis or withdraw while experiencing the end of life without suffering and with dignity.

The Renal Physicians Association/American Society of Nephrology (RPA/ASN) work group established a 10-step process for shared decision making to be used with adults with ESRD during the initial discussion of treatment options for ESRD. It focuses primarily on candid communication regarding diagnosis and prognosis and culminates in encouraging patients to explore EOL planning with family and friends (RPA/ASN, 2000).

Included in general palliative treatment strategies are the different dialysis modalities. Dialysis can be considered a palliative treatment option. As previously mentioned, KRT options for ESRD include PD, hemodialysis, or kidney transplant. Conservative/supportive care with no KRT should be included in the discussion regarding best KRT for an individual. The KRT modality should be a major focus and lends itself particularly well to the shared decision-making approach. The type of KRT should be decided well in advance of the need for dialysis. In this chapter, transplantation will not be discussed in any depth, as it is a highly specialized field and people who have received a transplant have very specific PC issues that overlap with the discussion of ESRD only if the transplant fails. Once this occurs, the PC needs are the same as those with ESRD. A common question asked by patients and families is when to start dialysis. The response may vary among nephrology providers but generally it is when people have uremic symptoms that can't be controlled with medical management. Laboratory values like eGFR, although they play a substantial role, are not necessarily the only indictor of when to start dialysis. Even though individuals may not report symptoms of uremia, most likely because of the chronicity of CKD, it is important to investigate the presence of symptoms. Patients have reported not being aware that they were that sick until they started to feel better upon undergoing dialysis. The first response from many people when told they have ESRD and should consider dialysis as an option is to decline; however, it is very important that they understand what dialysis is to truly make an informed decision. Once starting dialysis, many patients choose to continue until circumstances like high symptom burden occur. According to government data, withdrawal of dialysis is utilized in approximately 20% of cases. In the older dialysis population, withdrawal is the second most common reason for death. In the younger dialysis population, death is usually caused by a secondary disease process (USRDS, 2012).

Interestingly, African American patients are 50% to 66% less likely to stop dialysis than white patients (Oreopoulos, Hazzard, & Luke, 2000). It is not known why there is such a discrepancy associated with race. The most likely patients to withdraw from dialysis are white female nursing home residents older than 65 years of age. Further, they are more likely to have other chronic diseases, such as dementia or malignancy. Patients who perform their own HD at home are more likely to withdraw from dialysis when compared to patients that have in-center HD. Patients elect withdrawal from dialysis most commonly in their third month of treatment (Leggat, Bloembergen, Levine, Hulbert-Shearon, & Port, 1997). Implications for caregivers and management of patients who opt to not start or to withdraw from dialysis are discussed in the next section.

Symptoms that indicate the need to begin dialysis in all age groups include confusion and lethargy (which may indicate uremic encephalopathy), pericarditis, gastritis as manifested by nausea and vomiting, fatigue, accumulation of fluid and dyspnea, anorexia, severe anemia, or hyperkalemia. Patients without symptoms are usually started at an eGFR of 10 mL/min or 12 mL/min if they are diabetic, but once again this depends on many factors such as patient/family preferences.

Indications for choosing one dialysis modality (HD vs. PD) over another include lifestyle choice by the patient, healthcare providers' preferences, distance to the nearest dialysis center (urban vs. rural), and concurrent illnesses and associated symptoms. In rural areas, PD or home hemodialysis with the NxStage⁻ machine may be the best option because the closest dialysis center may be miles away, thus making it challenging for a person to get to the center three times a week. Either type of dialysis can generally be used. However, in the United States, HD is the most frequent form of KRT for adults. In pediatric populations, due to limited vascular access, PD is the most common modality used. Internationally, HD and PD are used in equal proportions (Henrich, 2009). Although older adults may have more complications with HD than with PD, age is not the only criterion for choosing this modality. Older adults with ESRD, regardless of the modality selected, have a high risk for malnutrition for a variety of reasons, including low income, missing teeth, malabsorption, and impaired gastric motility. Older patients predictably are hospitalized more frequently than younger patients (Berns, 2012). Recent evidence comparing complications and survival rate among older adults (≥70 years) choosing KRT versus conservative care indicated that there really wasn't a difference in outcomes, thus making conservative care a viable option for this population (Brunori et al., 2007; Verberne et al., 2016). As previously mentioned, in some circumstances, a time-limited trial of dialysis may be the best option for those who have uncertainty about undergoing or foregoing dialysis. In the renal PC guidelines issued by the Australian nephrology community, Crail, Walker, and Brown (2013) write:

> Not surprisingly, nephrologists, dialysis nurses and allied staff, along with patients and families are becoming less certain that dialysis will be the right choice for patients with multiple comorbidities, poor quality of life, nutrition or functional status .... Many nephrologists have already made it part of their usual practice to offer a non-dialysis pathway to selected patients. (p. 1)

In all age groups, as a person's physical and emotional health declines, or when the person decides or circumstances dictate that dialysis is no longer desirable, and when appropriate hospice care becomes crucial to preserve QOL, reduce symptom burden, and promote EOL comfort care, PC is important. The problem at this time is that hospice is underutilized in this population. In part, this is due to the lack of knowledge of nephrology providers as well as of patients and family members. There has been a concerted effort of many nephrology professionals to increase awareness of hospice as a feasible option. In some situations, when the patient has another terminal diagnosis that meets hospice criteria, he or she may be eligible to use both the Medicare hospice benefit and the ESRD benefit. Much depends on the hospice service that is available for the patient. When both benefits are used, it allows the patient to have the support from both hospice and nephrology teams, which also includes spiritual support. Palliative and hospice care are morally valid options, especially for patients with a high symptom burden. Healthcare practitioners should be prepared to discuss conservative care that includes no dialysis as part of the decision-making process. In addition, it is very important to make sure that the person does not have depression and/or suicidal ideations (Hain, Diaz, & Paixao, 2016). Fortunately, the nephrology team includes a social worker and often a nurse practitioner; both are capable of performing an evaluation of mood and addressing potential factors contributing to a depressed mood (i.e., uncontrolled pain). It is also important to consider the individual's cognitive ability to make informed decisions. Nephrology providers should start by asking the patient to explain the benefit and risks of continuing or discontinuing dialysis, and in some circumstances a formal evaluation of the person's cognitive status may be warranted. If it is determined that the person may lack the cognitive ability to engage in informed decision making, a designated representative

(i.e., healthcare surrogate) should make a decision that is in the patient's best interest (honors the person's wishes). If there is uncertainty about the best option, a time-limited trial of dialysis can be suggested with clear stopping points established with the patient, such as the time to feel well or finish family or personal business (Robert Wood Johnson [RWJ] Foundation, 2002; RPA/ASN, 2000). The patient who is not cognitively competent to make informed decisions places the provider in a more difficult situation. Unless the person has advance directives with a designated healthcare proxy, finding the appropriate decision maker and involving the patient in a reasonable way is most important. In cases where there is no designated decision maker, involving the social worker and an ethics consult team, as needed, can be of value in discussing the legal and ethical implications of deciding for or against dialysis. The primary question to ask is how would the patient decide if he or she were competent and how would a reasonable person decide given the same circumstances.

Ethical principles that guide shared decision making about initiating or withdrawing from dialysis include: (a) autonomy (self-determination); (b) nonmaleficence; (c) beneficence; and (d) justice. Autonomy is the right for human dignity, where a person is involved in the decision-making process to determine what is best for him or her, in other words, providing informed consent (knowing risks vs. benefits of undergoing dialysis). Nonmaleficence means "do no harm." Providing dialysis when not medically indicated, when the risks outweigh the benefits, or putting undue pressure on the person to make a decision that the healthcare professionals think is correct, are considered a violation of this principle. Beneficence is the duty to do good. In circumstances where the person is not able to make an informed decision, having a surrogate who honors the person's wishes is an important aspect of this ethical principle. Lastly, justice can be considered in the decision-making process by making sure all people, regardless of age, gender, or race or ethnicity, receive equal treatment and that appropriate use of scarce resources is addressed (Hain et al., 2016).

◼ PALLIATIVE CARE PRINCIPLES

Modern PC has benefited from the efforts of professional groups that have promoted the establishment of CPGs that are both general and specific to particular patient populations like ESRD. General PC guidelines include American Association of Colleges of Nursing Guidelines for End-of-Life Care, Hospice and Palliative Care Nursing Competencies, National Quality Forum Guidelines and Preferred Practice for Quality Palliative Care, and Liverpool Care Pathway for the Dying Patient. Guidelines specific to care of ESRD patients include those from the American Society of Nephrology entitled *Shared Decision Making in the Appropriate Initiation and Withdrawal*

From Dialysis (RPA/ASN, 2000). This guideline was designed to help nephrology professionals decide who will truly benefit from dialysis. A second guideline is the "End-Stage Renal Disease Workgroup—Recommendations to the Field," which was developed in affiliation with the RWJ Foundation's national program of Promoting Excellence in End-of-Life Care (RWJ Foundation, 2002). In addition, the Coalition for Supportive Care of Kidney Patients (www.kidneysupportivecare.org) offers nurses evidence-based information and recommendations to improve QOL and alleviate suffering in people with advanced CKD/ESRD.

The RWJ workgroup in particular has been instrumental in moving forward the effort to improve PC services for those with ESRD. This group identified the gaps, the lack of consensus, and the absence of available research specific to ESRD PC and made recommendations to address these needs to all involved parties. Based on these recommendations, a demonstration project, the Renal Palliative Care Initiative (RPCI), was developed by eight dialysis clinics and the Baystate Medical Center in Springfield, Massachusetts, with the cooperation of a large nephrology practice. Physicians, nurses, and social workers established a group that became educated in techniques of PC, developed programs to implement PC, and introduced them to the routines of dialysis patient care in the hospital and dialysis units. They also established survey instruments to ask family and patients about the quality of dying (Dialysis Quality of Dying Apgar [DQODA]; Cohen, Poppel, Cohn, & Reiter, 2001) and programs to support bereaved families.

The RPCI developed initiatives to holistically address the needs of patients, families, and the care team as they grappled with the challenges of renal disease, dialysis, and transplantation. They incorporated strategies to help with confronting the inevitability of eventual early death in the ESRD population even while continuing with KRT. The group found that the initiatives' measures enabled providers to become more likely to address palliative needs of people with ESRD and they became more proficient in doing so (Poppel, Cohen, & Germain, 2003). Gaps still exist, but the RWJ ESRD workgroup provided a well-thought-out plan to improve the QOL and dying for people with ESRD. Over the last decade, nephrology professionals have worked very hard to move research and clinical practice initiatives focused on PC in people with CKD forward. In fact, a recent KDIGO executive summary for supportive care in CKD was published to provide recommendations for assessment and management of symptoms and strategies to improve QOL (Davison et al., 2015). The summary recommends assessment and stepwise management of symptoms with nonpharmacological strategies as the first line, followed by pharmacological interventions (Davison et al., 2015). As nephrology experts witness the substantial growth of an aging CKD population, there is an expected increased focus on the valuable role PC has in improving health outcomes among individuals with advanced CKD.

Withholding or Withdrawing Dialysis

Although previously discussed under general PC options, the nontreatment option is reexamined here in more detail to reiterate the need to consider it carefully when treatment possibilities are being developed. As previously stated, the RPA/ASN (2000) responded to a request by the Institute of Medicine to issue guidelines for evaluating patients for whom the burdens of KRT may substantially outweigh benefits. The report is intended to provide direction to providers who frequently find themselves confronting EOL issues in the ESRD population (Levine, 2001). At the core of the report is the belief that initiation of and withdrawal from dialysis involve shared decision making where the individual makes an informed decision (RPA/ASN, 2000). A person-centered approach where the individual's EOL wishes and preferences are honored is essential. Engaging in advanced care planning should be started well before the person initiates KRT with strategic reevaluations (i.e., annually or when there is a change in the condition that warrants consideration of withdrawing) incorporated in the plan.

When discussing the option of withholding or withdrawing from dialysis with patients and families, candor is a most prized professional trait. Candor associated with death is regrettably somewhat rare institutionally and culturally in the United States. This is partially because American patients and families have an idealized view of the capabilities of medicine. As ethicist Daniel Callahan writes,

> We expect medicine to devise ever more ingenious ways to save our lives. That is why the NIH budget has always risen, budget crisis or not …. Why should anyone be astonished … that the other message many are trying to deliver—the need to stop treatment—has such a hard time getting through? (Callahan, 1987, p. 25)

If the illusion is allowed to remain that medicine has an unlimited ability to preserve life, patients suffer as inappropriate care is opted for. Candor regarding QOL, prognosis, and life expectancy is crucial to patients who are considering either withdrawal of dialysis or not starting treatment in the first place. However, it is also very important to consider the challenges of current predictive models and survival or mortality scores that are available for decision making in this population. Nephrology professionals should use the following when considering withholding dialysis in patients 75 and older: (a) ask the surprise question "Would I be surprised if my patient died within the next 12 months?"; (b) have a high comorbidity score (i.e., Modified Charlson Score ≥8); (c) have a marked functional impairment; or

(d) suffer from severe chronic malnutrition. Having two or more of the aforementioned may warrant withholding KRT; however, it is imperative to involve the patient in the decision-making process.

Openness with patients and families who are considering the nontreatment option is a deeply important part of the holistic care and shared decision making that enables the best, most well-informed decisions to be made by a person with ESRD. When the limits of medicine and technology are reached, patients are best served when they are accurately informed and all those who are significant to them work toward agreement on a plan of care. This means that the team begins the important work of care and comfort both for the dying and for those who remain after the patient's death. The ability to adjust thinking from the preservation of life to care of the dying is crucial for the provision of full-spectrum therapy, especially when working with a high-risk population, such as those with ESRD. Any lag time in this transition of thought and deed can create both psychological and physical suffering for all involved. When patients indicate a readiness to think of and speak about their death, the proper approach at that point is discussion of hospice care when indicated, available general support, and recognition of the importance of therapeutic presence. Unlike those who withdraw from dialysis, where life expectancy is about 7 days, uncertainty exists as to how long a person will survive if choosing to withhold KRT.

A systematic review (O'Connor & Kumar, 2012) reported that adults with ESRD, depending on comorbidities, who are treated conservatively with no dialysis, survived about 6.3 to 23.4 months once eGFR was below 15 mL/min/m². Regardless of the survival rate, symptom management, spiritual and psychological support, and helping prepare the person for hospice care when he or she meets a prognosis of 6 months or less are crucial for improving QOL (see Table 17.1 for hospice criteria).

Some evidence suggests that in some cases QOL and life expectancy for individuals with ESRD is equivalent whether dialysis is utilized or not (Brunori et al., 2007). There are patients for whom dialysis provides no survival benefit, and even if a survival benefit exists, it may be tempered by comorbidities such as heart disease and poor QOL (Davison, 2012; Murtagh, Cohen, & Germain, 2007; Schell, Da Silva-Gane, & Germain, 2013). Included in this group are patients with poor functional status and high numbers of comorbidity. One possible reason for this finding is that there have been improvements in the area of renal supportive care, and there are now sound resources available to guide clinicians in their care of this patient population if the nondialysis option is chosen (Chambers & Brown, 2010). It is important to note that this term is associated with, but not limited to, EOL care as patients may survive for months with adequate supportive care, which includes excellent symptom management. The focus of this care is on preserving what limited renal function exists, actively managing symptoms, and effectively using advanced care planning (Davison, 2012).

Renal Supportive Care: Symptom Management

Patients with ESRD have unique PC needs often years before death (Davison, 2012). Over 90,000 patients, or 24% of the total dialysis population, died in 2009 (USRDS, 2012), and statistics suggest that less than 22% of ESRD patients are enrolled in hospice or PC programs when dialysis is discontinued (Holley, 2013). USRDS data (2017) indicates that there has been an increase from 11% to 27% in the use of hospice services in this population, especially among those 85 and older. The highest use of hospice services has been in whites (22.7%) and other ethnic/racial groups have the lowest

---

TABLE 17.1. CMS Hospice Criteria, Benefits, and Eligibility Specific for Kidney Failure
CMS Hospice Criteria for Kidney Failure as a Terminal Diagnosis
■ Serum creatinine 8 mg/dL or greater (6 mg/dL or greater in patients with diabetes)   or   ■ Creatinine clearance is less than 10 mL/min/1/73 m² (less than 15 mL/min for individuals with diabetes)   or   ■ Symptoms of progressive uremia present (confusion, pruritus, oliguria, hyperkalemia, etc.)
CMS Hospice Benefits and Eligibility Specific for Kidney Failure
Home Health and Hospice Benefits Available for ESRD Beneficiaries, tagline 50.6.1   ■ "Medicare beneficiaries can receive care under both ESRD benefit and the home health or hospice benefits. The key is whether or not the services are related to ESRD"   ■ "If the patient's terminal condition is not related to ESRD, the patient may receive covered services under both ESRD benefit and the hospice benefit. A patient does not need to stop dialysis treatments to receive care under the hospice benefit"

CMS, Centers for Medicare and Medicaid; ESRD, end-stage renal disease.

use of hospice services (7.7%), with non-Hispanic versus Hispanic being higher (20.2% vs. 15.5%). Those undergoing dialysis had the highest hospice service (19.3%) compared to PD (18.6%) and transplant (18.3%). Once dialysis is stopped, death usually occurs in 6 to 8 days but can range over weeks to months if there is residual kidney function (Holley, 2007). The work groups and organizations trying to address gaps in the use of PC and hospice services when appropriate all agree that a good QOL until death is a priority. The only way this can be accomplished is through the provision of excellent PC. Cohen et al. (2001) surveyed patients with ESRD and families who withdrew from dialysis and asked what a good death would consist of for them. Their findings were that patients and families defined a good death as one that was pain free, peaceful, and brief. The researchers developed a tool to evaluate the quality of dying in the ESRD group, known as the Dialysis Discontinuation Quality of Dying (DDQOD) tool, as well as a second tool, the DQODA, which measures the quality of dying of patients with ESRD who did not discontinue dialysis (Cohen et al., 2001). As is the case with other dying patients, families believed that the most distressing symptoms at the end of life were pain, weakness, and dyspnea (Cohen, Germain, Woods, Mirot, & Burleson, 2005). To underscore the importance of adequate symptom management, evidence exists that patients dying from uremia have a symptom burden equivalent to that of patients dying from cancer or HF (Murtagh et al., 2007). Several EOL symptoms and their treatment will be reviewed next.

Anorexia, Nausea, and Vomiting

If dialysis is withdrawn, or never started, or it becomes difficult to dialyze patients adequately for any reason, patients eventually revert to a uremic state where uremic toxins accumulate and can cause chemically induced anorexia, nausea, and vomiting. These symptoms are reported as highly distressing by people who experience them (Neely & Roxe, 2000). The mechanism of nausea associated with uremia is stimulation of the central nervous system (CNS) referred to as the chemoreceptor trigger zone (CTZ). Blocking receptors in this zone, located in the fourth ventricle of the brain, seems to be the most effective pharmacologic therapy for the treatment of metabolically induced nausea and vomiting (Mannix, 2010). The tool recommended by the ESRD workgroup for the assessment of the symptom of nausea is the Edmonton Symptom Assessment Scale (Bruera, Kuehn, Miller, Selmser, & Macmillan, 1991). A modified version is available for use in those undergoing dialysis (Davison, Jhangri, & Johnson, 2006).

Antiemetics and management of associated acidosis is important in symptom management. Haloperidol and prochlorperazine are two agents that effectively block the CTZ. Haloperidol, which can also treat the delirium (acute confusion) that may be present if the patient is close to end of life, is given at 1.5 to 5 mg daily by mouth or subcutaneously but may cause extrapyramidal side effects such as dystonia, dyskinesia, and akathisia at higher doses. Promotility agents, such as metoclopramide, may be used with caution, or serotonergic antagonists like ondansetron may be useful to treat the nausea of uremia as well (Mannix, 2010). Metoclopramide, which requires renal dosing, is a dopamine antagonist that has both antiemetic and prokinetic properties and is effective in treating gastroparesis- and uremia-associated anorexia, nausea, and vomiting. Even though treatment is available, further research is still needed to assess and treat uremic anorexia, nausea, and vomiting effectively, as the current treatments have side effects that make them less than desirable.

Consider nonpharmacological treatments such as good oral hygiene; smaller, more frequent meals; minimizing aromas; avoiding greasy, spicy, or excessive sweet foods; sitting in an upright position; and wearing relaxing clothes (Davison & Jassal, 2016). Consultation with a dietitian may help determine food and fluid choices that are best for the person. Complementary therapies such as relaxation, guided imagery, acupressure, or acupuncture are other options that may help alleviate symptoms.

Pain

Pain is very common and distressing and requires a comprehensive assessment and individualized plan of care for people with ESRD. Pain can be related to the progression of CKD or due to concurrent comorbid conditions such as diabetic neuropathy, peripheral vascular disease, and osteoarthritis. Secondary causes of pain due to complications of ESRD include calciphylaxis and bone pain. Pain is the symptom that is most frequently reported by patients with ESRD who are dying, which can negatively affect QOL and contribute to depressive indications (Cohen, Germain, Poppel, Woods, & Kjellstrand, 2000; Koncicki, Unruh, & Schell, 2017).

There are many barriers to pain management in this population. First, although over 70% of nephrologists report confidence in treating pain, only about 37% actually do so on a regular basis. In part, this may be due to lack of pain management training, so referring to a pain specialist may be beneficial to assure maximum pain relief (Koncicki et al., 2017). Second, considering the current opioid epidemic, many providers are reluctant to prescribe opiates even though it might be the best form of treatment for the patient.

The first step in pain management is conducting a comprehensive pain assessment. This includes determining the type of pain: either nociceptive (stimulation of receptors when tissue damage occurs) or neuropathic (lesion of disease of the somatosensory system). Nociceptive pain can further be categorized as somatic (caused by inflammation of tissue and localized to one area) or visceral (precipitated by pathology of internal organs). Obtaining a pain history using the PQRST mnemonic can help identify the type of pain and its possible causes. *P* is precipitating or palliating factors; *Q* is quality of pain; *R* is region or radiation; *S* is severity; and *T* is timing (when did it start and whether it is constant or intermittent; Koncicki et al., 2017). Asking if the person has ever experienced pain, what has worked, and what has not worked is also very important. There are a few important points to be made in the case of pain palliation in ESRD. For hospice patients, analgesics should be used on a regular schedule using the World Health Organization (WHO) analgesic ladder as guidance for the management of pain in ESRD. Even so, there are some drugs that should not be used, and there are some drugs for which dosing should be monitored because their metabolites can accumulate in renal failure and cause unwanted side effects. Opioids are generally metabolized in the liver but some accumulate. For example, demerol should not be used for pain control in ESRD because the metabolite normeperidine accumulates and leads to seizures and neuro-excitation. Propoxyphene is another opioid narcotic that should not be used because of the accumulation of metabolites. Morphine has a distinct place in ESRD pain management and EOL care for short-term use because of the analgesic effect and the positive effect on dyspnea, but it can accumulate; therefore, side effects such as myoclonus should be carefully monitored (Cohen, Moss, Weisbord, & Germain, 2006). If myoclonus occurs, it can be treated with benzodiazepines such as clonazepam, which may help anxiety as well (Holley, 2007). There is anecdotal evidence that alternative strong opioids (hydromorphone, methadone, and fentanyl) are better tolerated, but there is inadequate research to support this presently (Davison, 2007). Many patients with ESRD are given tramadol even though the extended release form has not been studied in this population. Many pain medications have not been studied in the ESRD population, so regardless of whatever medication is used, it is important to monitor for desired or adverse effects. Factors that contribute to adverse effects (sedation, respiratory depression, or falls) are: (a) age 55 or older; (b) obesity with BMI greater than 30 kg/m^2; (c) untreated obstructive sleep apnea; (d) neck circumference over 17.5 inches; (e) preexisting pulmonary or cardiac disease; (f) concurrent use of CNS depressants; (g) opioid-naïve patients; (h) use of greater than 50 morphine-equivalent dosage; (i) cognitive impairment/dementia; and (j) gait unsteadiness (Koncicki et al., 2017).

Neuropathic pain is often related to diabetes or dialysis (i.e., secondary amyloid). First-line treatments are medications like gabapentin and pregabalin, tricyclic antidepressants (TCA), and serotonin and norepinephrine reuptake inhibitors. Topical lidocaine can be used as a concurrent treatment. Gabapentin and pregabalin have been shown to be effective in this population, and

therefore, with renal dose adjustments, they are preferred agents. TCA are more effective compared to serotonin and norepinephrine reuptake inhibitors but have anticholinergic effects that limit their use, especially in older adults (Koncicki et al., 2017).

Always think of nonpharmacological interventions like cognitive behavioral therapy, relaxation therapies, and mindfulness as adjunctive therapies.

Dyspnea

People with ESRD often have multiple comorbid conditions (i.e., HF, pulmonary hypertension) that add to the complexity of EOL care. Dyspnea, tachypnea, cough, and breathlessness may be common EOL symptoms experienced by patients with ESRD. These are typically the result of hypervolemia, CHF, and pleural effusion or pulmonary edema. Relief of these symptoms is crucial to providing comfort and palliation, especially at the end of life. Prevention is highly desirable and is best accomplished by limiting fluid intake as appropriate, yet providing mouth care and even over-the-counter saliva substitutes such as Biotene Oral Balance to prevent thirst and dry mouth are recommended.

One of the most potent causes of dyspnea is pleural effusion. It may be necessary to remove fluid from the chest by pleural aspiration to relieve air hunger and promote comfort regardless of the phase of the dying trajectory. This procedure can effectively improve symptoms and lessen air hunger, even if death is imminent.

Pruritus

Pruritus is one of the most bothersome symptoms of ESRD. An estimated 40.6% to 60% of patients with ESRD experience it. The characteristics, causes, and treatments widely vary; multiple reasons that are proposed are hyperphosphatemia, hypercalcemia, hyperparathyroidism, inadequate dialysis, anemia, iron deficiency, allergy to the dialyzer materials, allergies to medications, other allergies, contact dermatitis, and chronic xerosis (Cohen et al., 2006; Davison & Jassal, 2016). Palliative treatment should be preventive and should treat symptoms. Prevention includes adequate dialysis and treating CKD–MBD by achieving target phosphorus, calcium, and PTH levels through a well-controlled diet and medications (treatment of CKD–MBD was discussed earlier in the chapter). Prevention is not always achievable, so symptom management includes nonpharmacological strategies as well as pharmacological interventions. Nonpharmacological strategies include promoting good skin care, avoiding soaps that may irritate the skin, avoiding excessive bathing or bathing with hot water that can dry the skin, using emulsifying lotions in the bath, avoiding scratching (massage instead) and keeping nails short, wearing gloves at night, and maintaining a humid environment especially in cold winter climates. Topical emollients are a first-line treatment (should have high water content and be free of fragrances and additives). If these are not helpful, adding pharmacological agents such as low-dose gabapentin (starting at 50–100 mg post dialysis) or TCA doxepin 10 mg at bedtime can be effective (Davison & Jassal, 2016).

Because itching from renal failure is thought to be the result of uremic toxin accumulation, it makes sense that in the face of dialysis withdrawal, uremia increases and itching may worsen. Logically, in the hospice setting, continuing to give phosphate-binding drugs may be useful to control this uncomfortable symptom. However, these drugs are notorious for their gastrointestinal side effects such as bloating and nausea, and monitoring for these symptoms is important. Other interventions include a 0.5% to 2% phenol solution, Sarna, or other menthol phenol creams and pramoxine topically, as well as systemic therapies such as antihistamines. It is imperative to find at least one intervention that will be effective because pruritus is described as one of the more miserable symptoms to endure (Oreopoulos et al., 2000; Seccareccia & Gebara, 2011).

Fatigue

Fatigue is a common symptom experienced by people with ESRD with a prevalence of about 45% to 97% in those undergoing HD and 30% to 70% in people receiving PD. It is very challenging to treat but warrants assessment and attempts at symptom management. Depression can be a significant contributing factor and should be considered in the assessment and treatment of fatigue. Anemia, inadequate dialysis, vitamin D deficiency, metabolic acidosis, tertiary hyperparathyroidism, hypothyroidism, dialysis treatment (i.e., fluid removal), sleep disorders, polypharmacy, and malnutrition are other potential causes of fatigue in this population. The first step is assessing for and treating modifiable contributing factors. In postdialysis fatigue, determining if treatment modifications should be done is important. Encouraging the patient to engage in physical activity, such as low-intensity resistance and aerobic exercise, if appropriate, and assuring proper supportive systems are in place (i.e., assistance with activities of daily livings [ADLs] and instrumental activities of daily living [IADLs]) can be beneficial (Davison & Jassal, 2016).

Pediatric End-Stage Renal Disease

In the United States, over 40,000 children die from trauma, lethal congenital conditions, or acquired illnesses every year. ESRD falls mostly into the latter category. Pediatric ESRD is devastating but rare. The number of children and adolescents with ESRD has decreased over the past decade. In 2015, the number and rate of incident cases varied by age group; there were 211 cases in those aged 0 to 4 years, 117 aged 5 to 9, 163 aged 10 to 13, 336 aged 14 to 17, and 548 aged 18 to 21, for a total of 1,375 children with incident ESRD. Within these age-based cohorts, incidence rates in 2015 were 9.3 PMP per year for 0- to 4-year-olds, 4.8 for 5- to 9-year-olds, 8.6 for 10- to 13-year-olds, 18.4 for 14- to 17-year-olds, and 29.8 for 18- to 21-year-olds (USRDS, 2017).

The cause of ESRD and the primary cause of mortality in pediatrics differ from those of adults. The leading cause of CKD is congenital abnormalities of the kidney and urinary tract (22%), then primary glomerular disease (21.8%), followed by cystic/heredity/congenital disorders (12.5%) and finally secondary glomerular disease/vasculitis (10.7%; USRDS, 2017).

PKD and two congenital abnormalities, posterior urethral valves (PUVs) and hypoplastic/dysplastic kidneys, as well as GN of different types, are the primary causes of long-term kidney failure in children. Mortality rates for children are significantly lower than for adults and have declined over the past several years. During 2010 to 2014, the 1-year-adjusted all-cause mortality rate was 27 per 1,000 patient-years, a decrease of 30.8% from the 39 per 1,000 patient-years seen from 2005 to 2009. Reduced mortality was reported in almost all age categories, with the greatest point estimate of reduced mortality by 41.6% in children age 0 to 4 years. The improvement in the 1-year mortality in the 0 to 4 age group was mostly in infants less than 2 years of age at the onset of ESRD (age <2 years: 45% vs. age 2 to <5: 32% reduction in mortality; USRDS, 2017).

Children account for only a fraction of the total number of patients undergoing dialysis in the United States. Children who develop ESRD have a much greater likelihood (at least 30 times higher) of dying than the general pediatric population. Until recently, there were no gains in pediatric ESRD mortality rates. Five-year survival rate is around 80%—much better than in the adult ESRD population (Mitsnefes, Laskin, Dahhou, Zhang, & Foster, 2013). Even so, PC is still an important intervention for children with ESRD, but as in the case of adult ESRD, it is underutilized.

The issue of PC as it relates to children with ESRD is similar to the issue of PC in adult ESRD in that both children and adults with ESRD may need PC not only as a treatment to promote a good death but also to alleviate symptoms during life—or while a cure (transplantation) is being pursued. The American Academy of Pediatrics (AAP, 2000) supports PC throughout the course of a wide range of illnesses and, due to the high symptom burden in ESRD, believes it to be appropriate whether cure is possible or not (AAP, 2000; Himelstein, Hilden, Boldt, & Weissman, 2004). Both curative treatments, which seek to reverse the illness, and palliative treatments that are focused on relieving symptoms have a place in the care of pediatric ESRD patients. According to the AAP, pediatric ESRD falls into a category of conditions for which PC is appropriate and requires intensive long-term treatment aimed at maintaining QOL (Himelstein et al., 2004). Unfortunately, there is little research available on the QOL outcomes of PC in this age group.

Pediatric Palliative Care Issues

The use of PC and hospice services is relatively low in ESRD in general, but especially so in children. The younger the patient, the less likely is referral for palliation and hospice care. The presumed reason is that attempted curative care is ongoing in the case of pediatric patients, and providers and parents are less willing to move in the direction of stopping treatment or withdrawing dialysis. These two goals do not have to be at odds. The AAP has a helpful position on this dilemma. They recommend the availability of PC to children with a broad range of illnesses even when cure remains a possibility. The components of PC should be offered at diagnosis and continued throughout the course of illness, whether the outcome ends in cure or death. Himelstein et al. (2004) writes that "Pediatric PC should ... intersect with the aims of curing and healing ... improving the quality of life ... maintaining dignity and ameliorating the suffering of seriously ill or dying children" (p. 1752). The main issue associated with pediatric PC is helping the patient and family confront the reality of the illness with compassion and hope so that the treatment approach is appropriately (not overly) aggressive. With this approach, the topic of palliation and hospice can be introduced.

■ CONCLUSION

ESRD is a chronic disease that is characterized by steady functional decline, a 20% yearly mortality rate, and premature death for many patients. It is increasing in incidence and prevalence in all age groups in the United States and globally but to the greatest extent in the 75 and older age group. It is a disease with a high symptom burden that can take a toll on patients and families alike and for which PC is crucial to foster QOL, reduce symptom burden, and, when appropriate, encourage use of hospice services.

A person-centered approach that incorporates shared decision making, where the person's wishes, values, and preferences for care are honored, is critical. In addition, effective symptom management and psychological and spiritual support across the life span for the patient and his or her family are essential. It is important to note that recent evidence suggests that for patients with multiple comorbidities, advanced age, and limited functional ability, conservative or supportive management may be as efficacious as KRT. Discussion of withholding dialysis as an option is important in all patients, but more important is assuring that the person comprehends the risks and benefits of all treatment options. Making sure patients understand what dialysis is by having them meet someone undergoing dialysis or visiting a dialysis center can be helpful. People may fear what they don't know and understand, so in order to make an informed decision they must clearly understand what each option entails. Full integration of PC principles and standards can provide support for patients with ESRD as they attempt to make difficult decisions as to whether to withhold dialysis or to withdraw from dialysis once it has been started. PC can offer guidance during the process of living with ESRD and EOL care and experiencing a "good death."

As nurses, we have the responsibility to consider ethical principles as we engage in the dialogue regarding best treatment options. Infusing your personal beliefs into the conversation should be avoided; instead, providing the best available evidence along with your clinical expertise while taking a person-centered approach can help the patient and his or her family make decisions that are best for the patient.

DISCUSSION QUESTIONS

How can PC improve QOL for the patient with ESRD?
ESRD is a chronic illness with a high symptom burden and the potential to greatly diminish QOL. This is true whether patients are undergoing dialysis, have chosen a conservative/supportive nondialysis option, or have decided to withdraw from treatment. QOL in all of these circumstances can be poor. It is becoming increasingly clear that palliative treatment strategies are beneficial to people with ESRD as they emphasize person-centered care; informed, holistic, and collaborative decision making; advanced care planning; assessment of adequate treatment of symptoms; and appropriate comfort care of the dying. Given the premature life expectancy of many living with ESRD, early referral to PC is a reasonable treatment option.

What makes ESRD unique regarding withdrawal of treatment and PC?

When a patient reaches the ESRD level of CKD, the decision not to select a form of KRT most often means that death is inevitable sooner rather than later. The exception to this would be some patients who can be managed for a while using conservative treatment strategies because they have residual kidney function, which is important to maintain. If the person makes a decision that withholding dialysis or withdrawing from dialysis is the best option, they should understand that this means death will be eminent. In the case of withdrawal, this will be in about 7 to 8 days, and withholding is about 6 months to a year (some people will live beyond this time frame). Comorbid conditions such as cardiovascular disease significantly contribute to when death will occur. For example, someone may die from a fatal arrhythmia due to hyperkalemia. Patients are often alert and awake when they make this decision and are actively choosing death rather than extending life. It is important for healthcare providers to support this choice as a legitimate option for patients who have the cognitive capacity to make this high-level decision. This can be exceedingly difficult for the family and the healthcare staff; the support of the PC and hospice team is instrumental in adhering to and honoring the patient's wishes.

CASE STUDY *Conclusion*

Before dialysis was discontinued, Jim achieved adequate pain control and his cognitive status improved. Considering this change in his condition, the decision to withdraw from dialysis was stopped. Jim's improvement continued for approximately 3 months, until after Christmas, when he began to experience nosebleeds from the Coumadin, deterioration in the perfusion to his legs, and the return of pain.

Jim told his family that he was ready to stop dialysis; he was unwilling to tolerate the current symptoms, and the pain and disability were just too great. He wanted to die at home and his family was committed to granting this last request.

The PC team engaged home hospice services to provide comfort and supportive care. The dialysis team agreed to provide dialysis for fluid removal and comfort on an as-needed basis. This provision was unnecessary because he never returned to the dialysis center. Those who had cared for him over the years stayed in touch with his wife during the 10-day process of his death. Some nurses visited the home to say good-bye.

He remained committed to not having any more invasive therapy and never wavered from this final decision. Jim spent his last days with his family, his friends, pastors from his church, and the healthcare professionals who knew him best. As symptoms of uremia emerged, the hospice team treated them. His family faithfully followed directions to not overload him with fluids, as this would almost certainly add to his discomfort.

In the end, he died quietly at night with his wife of almost 35 years at his side. He had assured her that day that he was ready to die, reliant to the last on his faith. He whispered to her that he would see her again. His loss was difficult for the family, but Jim's faith and conviction eased the pain. The dialysis staff loved him. He was a quiet, respectful man with a smile that illuminated the room. His family was devoted to him as he was to them. He was 73 when he died. The funeral was a tribute to a life well lived. As providers, we gathered with family and friends in the church one last time on his behalf.

Jim's case is paradigmatically significant because of not only what happened and how events occurred but also what did not happen as well. Jim did not die in a hospital cared for by strangers; there were no IV drips, tube feedings, and futile attempts to preserve life when the body was clearly unable to sustain it. All talked, agreed, and were sad but comfortable with the decision. Essentially, this is an example of the beneficial effect of open dialogue and shared decision making around emotionally difficult topics such as death. Desirable outcomes occur when all involved are willing to speak candidly about prognosis and death with patients and their families and think about death as a part of the care continuum and not as a failed therapy.

CASE STUDY

AN INTERPROFESSIONAL PERSPECTIVE

Dianne Sandy, MD, Nephrologist

The ESRD population in the United States has become progressively older and patients typically carry a high chronic disease burden at the time of initiation of dialysis. Our elderly patients may start dialysis with complications of diabetes and hypertension, emphysema, cardiovascular disease, malignancy, severe arthritis, or dementia. These frail patients often do not tolerate the hemodynamic fluctuations associated with hemodialysis and may be plagued by crippling fatigue and frequent hospitalizations. Even if dialysis is well tolerated, the progression of comorbid disease may cause an intolerable decrease in the QOL. In particular, the presence of malignancy or a disease that severely restricts mobility, causes chronic pain, or leads to worsening cognitive deficits often leads the patient, family, and healthcare team to confront the hard choices about EOL care. This dilemma is not uncommon as approximately 25% of adults with ESRD patients in the United States withdraw from dialysis prior to their death.

Every request to withdraw dialysis should be considered carefully and with utmost respect for the patient's autonomy, and recognition of his or her central role in shared decision making. Some patients may have lost their ability to make decisions, and in that case, it is important that family members and healthcare surrogates, as well as all members of the healthcare team, come together to determine what is in the patient's best interest. The presence of advance directives makes this process much easier. A psychiatrist may be needed to determine competency and to rule out depression. In a patient who is competent and not depressed, we should look then for any possible reversible factors that may improve QOL. Once it is clear that withdrawal of dialysis is appropriate, palliative and hospice services help ensure a smooth and painless transition to comfort care. This is often a stressful and emotional time for the patient, family, and interprofessional team and requires frequent and open communication. As a nephrologist, I am frequently involved in these EOL situations, and for the most part, while emotionally draining, they can be very rewarding. They represent the natural culmination of a long-term doctor–patient relationship, in which my role has been to provide the care that is needed to maximize QOL at all stages of CKD, to recognize when this care has become futile, and to assist the patient and family in making decisions that ensure a comfortable and dignified EOL process.

Evidence-Based Practice

Brown, M. A., Collet, G. K., Josland, E. A., Foote, C., Li, Q., & Brennan, F. P. (2015). CKD in elderly patients managed without dialysis: Survival, symptoms, and quality of life. *Clinical Journal of Nephrology, 10,* 260–268. doi:10.2215/CJN.03330414

Study Aims
Uncertainty that surrounds survival, symptom burden, and QOL of older adults who choose conservative care versus dialysis prompted this study. The study's aim was to examine the differences between survival, QOL, and symptoms of older adults with advanced CKD who weren't planning on starting dialysis and those who had initiated dialysis.

Methodology

A prospective, observational study recruited participants from renal clinics and dialysis centers in Sydney. The renal clinics were staffed with PC experts, which included a nurse. Symptoms were measured using the Memorial Symptom Assessment Scale (MSAS-SF) and the Palliative Care Outcome Scale (POS-S) for those recruited from the renal clinics. QOL was measured using the Short Form 36 (SF-36) and survival was defined as the time to death and the percentage to 12-month survival.

Findings

The nondialysis (not choosing dialysis) group was significantly older compared to the predialysis group (mean of 82 years compared to 67 years; $p < .001$), but had similar eGFR at the first visit. Of those who chose dialysis, about 92 (34%) started dialysis. The death rate was lower for those in the predialysis group who didn't require dialysis (hazard ratio: 0.23; 95% CI: 0.12–0.41) and those requiring dialysis (0.30; 0.13–0.67), but not those who were undergoing dialysis who had not received care at the renal clinics (0.60; 0.35–1.03). Factors associated with survival were age, weight, body mass index, hemoglobin, serum albumin, corrected calcium, serum creatinine, and the presence of any comorbidity. Stability and/or improvement in symptoms occurred across all three groups with no statistical difference ($p > .01$). There was no statistical differences in physical or mental health QOL in the predialysis group compared to the conservative care group ($p > .01$), and there was no correlation between stable or improved QOL and stable or worsening eGFR.

Conclusion and Implications

The study findings support that conservative care within a renal clinic that has PC experts is a viable option for many older adults with advanced CKD. Survival rates, QOL, and symptom management may best be addressed within a nephrology or PC team model of care. Involving the patient and family in decision making is essential as is recognition and control of symptoms. Regardless that the nondialysis group was several years older than the predialysis group, all individuals with advanced CKD should have the opportunity to gain knowledge regarding best treatment options (pros/cons). This is essential as nurses and patients and their families engage in shared decision making. The findings from this study offer much-needed evidence for future research exploring the best way to provide care to older adults with advanced CKD and the outcomes related to collaboration between PC and nephrology interprofessional teams. There are many practice implications, but an important one is making sure patients understand the potential outcome of their choices and that they can change their mind anywhere along the disease trajectory (i.e., choosing no dialysis to choosing dialysis).

■ **Acknowledgment.** The editors would like to thank Lynn R. Noland, PhD, FNP for her contribution to the previous edition.

■ REFERENCES

Ahmad, S. (2009). *Manual of clinical dialysis* (2nd ed.). New York, NY: Springer.

American Academy of Pediatrics. (2000). Committee on bioethics and committee on hospital care. Palliative care for children. *Pediatrics, 106*(2 Pt. 1), 351–357. doi:10.1542/peds.106.2.351

Berns, J. S. (2012). Complications of hemodialysis in the elderly patient. Retrieved from uptodate.com

Breidthardt, T. & McIntyre, W. (2011). Dialysis induced myocardial stunning: The other side of the cardiorenal syndrome. *Reviews in Cardiovascular Medicine, 12*, 13–20. doi:10.3909/ricm0585

Briasoulis, A., & Bakris, G. L. (2013). Chronic kidney disease as a coronary artery disease equivalent. *Current Cardiology Reports, 15*(3), 340. doi:10.1007/s11886-012-0340-4

Brown, M. A., Collet, G. K., Josland, E. A., Foote, C., Li, Q., & Brennan, F. P. (2015). CKD in elderly patients managed without dialysis: Survival, symptoms, and quality of life. *Clinical Journal of Nephrology, 10*, 260–268.

Bruera, E., Kuehn, N., Miller, M. J., Selmser, P., & Macmillan, K. (1991). The Edmonton Symptom Assessment System: A simple method for the assessment of palliative care patients. *Journal of Palliative Care, 7*(2), 6–9.

Brunori, G., Viola, B. F., Parrinello, G., De Biase, V., Como, G., Franco, V., … Cancarini, G. C. (2007). Efficacy and safety of a very-low-protein diet when postponing dialysis in the elderly: A prospective randomized multicenter controlled study. *American Journal of Kidney Diseases, 49*(5), 569–580. doi:10.1053/j.ajkd.2007.02.278

Cahill, M., & Haras, M. S. (2017). Disorders of calcium and phosphorus metabolism. In S. M. Bodin (Ed.), *Contemporary nephrology nursing* (pp. 403–424). Pitman, NJ: American Nephrology Nurses Association.

Callahan, D. (1987). *Setting limits: Medical goals in an aging society*. New York, NY: Simon and Schuster.

Centers for Disease Control and Prevention. (2010). National diabetes surveillance system. Retrieved from http://www.cdc.gov/diabetes/surveillance

Chambers, E. J., & Brown, E. (2010). *Renal supportive care*. Oxford, UK: Oxford University Press.

Chen, T. & Harris, D. C. (2015). Challenges of chronic kidney disease prevention. *Medical Journal of Australia, 203*(5), 209–210. doi:10.5694/mja15.00241

Cohen, L. M., Germain, M. J., Poppel, D. M., Woods, A., & Kjellstrand, C. M. (2000). Dying well after discontinuing the life support treatment of dialysis. *Archives of Internal Medicine, 160*, 2513–2518. doi:10.1001/archinte.160.16.2513

Cohen, L. M., Germain, M. J., Woods, A. L., Mirot, A., & Burleson, J. A. (2005). The family perspective of ESRD deaths. *American Journal of Kidney Diseases, 45*(1), 154–161. doi:10.1053/j.ajkd.2004.09.014

Cohen, L. M., Moss, A. H., Weisbord, S. D., & Germain, M. J. (2006). Renal palliative care. *Journal of Palliative Medicine, 9*(4), 977–992. doi:10.1089/jpm.2006.9.977

Cohen, L. M., Poppel, D. M., Cohn, G. M., & Reiter, G. S. (2001). A very good death: Measuring quality of dying in end-stage renal disease. *Journal of Palliative Medicine, 4*(2), 167–172. doi:10.1089/109662101750290209

Crail, S., Walker, R., & Brown, M.; Renal Supportive Care Working Group. (2013). Renal supportive and palliative care: Position statement. *Nephrology, 18*(6), 393–400. doi:10.1111/nep.12064

Davison, S. N. (2007). The prevalence and management of chronic pain in end-stage renal disease. *Journal of Palliative Medicine, 10*(6), 1277–1287. doi:10.1089/jpm.2007.0142

Davison, S. N. (2012). The ethics of end-of-life care for patients with ESRD. *Clinical Journal of the American Society of Nephrology, 7*(12), 2049–2057. doi:10.2215/CJN.03900412

Davison, S. N., Levin, A., Moss, A. H., Jha, V., Brown, E. A., Brennan, F., … Obrador, G. T. (2015). Executive summary of the KDIGO Controversies Conference on Supportive Care in Chronic Kidney Disease: developing a roadmap to improving quality care. *Kidney International, 88*(3), 447–459. doi:10.1038/ki.2015.110

Davison, S. N., & Jassal, S. V. (2016). Supportive care: Integration of patient-centered kidney care to manage symptoms and geriatric syndromes. *Clinical Journal of American Society of Nephrology, 11*(10), 1882–1891. doi:10.2215/CJN.01050116

Davison S. N., Jhangri G. S., Johnson J. A. (2006). Cross-sectional validity of a modified Edmonton symptom assessment system in dialysis patients: a simple assessment of symptom burden. *Kidney International, 69*(9), 1621–1625. doi:10.1038/sj.ki.5000184

Deaver, K., & Counts, C. (2015). Central venous catheters. In C. S. Counts (Ed.), *Core curriculum for nephrology nursing: Module 3. Treatment options for patients with chronic kidney failure* (6th ed., pp. 206–214). Pitman, NJ: American Nephrology Nurses Association.

Eberhard, R., & Wolf, G. (2010). Pathogenesis, clinical manifestations, and natural history of diabetic nephropathy. In J. Floege, R. Johnson, & J. Feehaly (Eds.), *Comprehensive clinical nephrology* (4th ed., pp. 350–360). St. Louis, MO: Elsevier.

Flythe, J. E., Hui, X., Lynch, K. E., Curhan, G. C., & Brunelli, S. M. (2015). Association of mortality risk with variable definitions of intradialytic hypotension. *Journal of American Society of Nephrology, 26*, 724–734. doi:10.1681/asn.2014020222

Foley, R. N. (2017). Epidemiology and risk factors for early mortality after dialysis initiation. *Seminars in Nephrology, 37*, 114–119.

Fraser, S. D. S., Roderick, P. J., May, C. R., McIntyre, N., McIntyre, C., Fluck, R. J., … Taal, M. W. (2015). The burden of comorbidity in people with chronic kidney disease stage 3: a cohort study. *British Medical Nephrology, 16*(1), 193–202. doi:10.1186/s12882-015-0189-z

Glassrock, R. Delanaye, P., & El Nahas, M. (2015) An age-calibrated classification of chronic kidney disease. *Journal of American Medical Association, 314*(6), 559–560. doi:10.1001/jama.2015.6731

Hain, D.J., Diaz, D., & Paixao, R. (2016). What are the ethical issues when honoring an older adult's decision to withdraw from dialysis? *Nephrology Nursing Journal, 43*, 429–434.

Hauser, A. B., Stinghen, A. E., Kato, S., Bucharles, S., Aita, C., Yuzawa, Y., & Pecoits-Filho, R. (2008). Characteristics and causes of immune dysfunction related to uremia and dialysis. *Peritoneal Dialysis International, 28* (Suppl. 3), S183–S187.

Henrich, W. L. (2009). *Principles and practice of dialysis* (3rd ed.). Philadelphia, PA: Lippincott Williams & Wilkins.

Himelstein, B. P., Hilden, J. M., Boldt, A. M., & Weissman, D. (2004). Pediatric palliative care. *New England Journal of Medicine, 350*(17), 1752–1762. doi:10.1056/NEJMra030334

Holley, J. L. (2007). Palliative care in end-stage renal disease: Illness trajectories, communication, and hospice use. *Advances in Chronic Kidney Disease, 14*(4), 402–408. doi:10.1053/j.ackd.2007.07.002

Holley, J. L. (2013). Palliative care in end stage renal disease. Retrieved from https://www.uptodate.com/contents/palliative-care-end-stage-renal-disease

Inglese, M. (2017). Arteriovenous fistula. In S. M. Bodin (Ed.), *Contemporary nephrology nursing* (pp. 317–333). Pitman, NJ: American Nephrology Nurses Association.

Kelman, E. & Watson, D. (2017). Peritoneal dialysis. In S.M. Bodin (Ed.). *Contemporary nephrology nursing* (pp. 209–285). Pitman, NJ: American Nephrology Nurses Association.

Kidney Disease Improving Global Outcomes. (2012). Clinical practice guideline for anemia in chronic kidney disease. *Kidney International Supplement, 2*(4), 279–341. Retrieved from http://www.kdigo.org/clinical _practice_guidelines/pdf/KDIGO-Anemia%20GL.pdf

Kidney Disease Improving Global Outcomes (KDIGO) CKD Work Group. (2013). KDIGO 2012 Clinical Practice Guideline for the Evaluation and Management of Chronic Kidney Disease. *Kidney International, 3*(1, Suppl.), 1–150. doi:10.1038/kisup.2012.73

Koncicki, H. M., Unruh, M., & Schell, J. O. (2017). Pain management in CKD: A guide for nephrology providers. *American Journal of Kidney Disease, 69*, 451–460. doi:10.1053/j.ajkd.2016.08.039

Leggat, J. E., Bloembergen, W. E., Levine, G., Hulbert-Shearon, T. E., & Port, F. K. (1997). An analysis of risk factors for withdrawal from dialysis before death. *Journal of the American Society of Nephrology, 8*(11), 1755–1763.

Levey, A. S., & Coresh, J. (2012). Chronic kidney disease. *Lancet, 379*, 165–180. doi:10.1016/S0140-6736(11)60178-5

Levine, D. Z. (2001). Nephrology ethics forum. Shared decision making in dialysis: The new RPA/ASN guideline on the appropriate initiation and withdrawal of treatment. *American Journal of Kidney Diseases, 37*, 1081–1091. doi:10.1016/S0272-6386(05)80027-7

Mahaffey, L. E. (2017). Diseases of the kidney. In S. Bodin (Ed.), *Contemporary Nephrology Nursing* (3rd ed., pp. 79–100). Pitman NJ: American Nephrology Nurses Association.

Mandayam, S., & Shahinian, V. B. (2008). Are chronic dialysis patients at increased risk for cancer? *Journal of Nephrology, 21*(2), 166–174.

Mannix, K. A. (2010). Palliation of nausea and vomiting. In G. Hanks, N. I. Cherney, N. A. Christakis, & N. MacDonald (Eds.), *Oxford textbook of palliative medicine* (4th ed., pp. 801–812). Oxford, UK: Oxford University Press.

Mitsnefes, M. M., Laskin, B. L., Dahhou, M., Zhang, X., & Foster, B. J. (2013). Mortality risk among children initially treated with dialysis for end-stage kidney disease, 1990–2010. *Journal of the American Medical Association, 309*(18), 1921–1929. doi:10.1001/jama.2013.4208

Murtagh, F. E., Addington-Hall, J., Edmonds, P., Donohoe, P., Carey, I., Jenkins, K., & Higginson, I. J. (2010). Symptoms in the month before death for Stage 5 chronic kidney disease patients managed without dialysis. *Journal of Pain and Symptom Management, 40*(3), 342–352. doi:10.1016/j.jpainsymman.2010.01.021

Murtagh, F. E., Cohen, L. M., & Germain, M. J. (2007). Dialysis discontinuation: Quo vadis? *Advances in Chronic Kidney Disease, 14*(4), 379–401. doi:10.1053/j.ackd.2007.07.008

Muntner, P., He, J., Astor, B.C, Folsom, A.R., & Coresh, J. (2005). Traditional and Nontraditional risk factors predict coronary artery disease in chronic kidney disease: Results from the atherosclerosis risk in community study. *Journal of the American Society of Nephrology, 16*, 529–538. doi:10.1681/asn.2004080656

Neely, K. J., & Roxe, D. M. (2000). Palliative care/hospice and the withdrawal of dialysis. *Journal of Palliative Medicine, 3*(1), 57–67. doi:10.1089/jpm.2000.3.57

Nigwekar, S. U., Kroshinsky, D., Nazarian, R. M., Goverman, J., Malhotra, R., Jackson V.A., … Thadhani, R. I. (2015). Calciphylaxis: Risk factors, diagnosis, and treatment. *American Journal of Kidney Disease, 66*(1), 133–146. doi:10.1053/j.ajkd.2015.01.034

O'Connor, N. R. & Kumar, P. (2012). Conservative management of end-stage-renal disease without dialysis: A systematic review. *Journal of Palliative Medicine, 15*, 228–235. doi:10.1089/jpm.2011.0207

Oreopoulos, D. G., Hazzard, W. R., & Luke, R. (Eds.). (2000). *Nephrology and geriatrics integrated.* Dordrecht, The Netherlands: Kluwer Academic.

Payton, J., & Kennedy, S. K. (2017). Peritoneal Dialysis Access. In S. M. Bodin (Ed.), *Contemporary nephrology nursing* (pp. 363–375). Pitman, NJ: American Nephrology Nurses Association.

Poppel, D. M., Cohen, L. M., & Germain, M. J. (2003). The renal palliative care initiative. *Journal of Palliative Medicine, 6*(2), 321–326. doi:10.1089/109662103764978650

Pryor, L. A., & Brouwer-Maier, D. (2017). Central Venous Catheter. In S. M. Bodin (Ed.), *Contemporary nephrology nursing* (pp. 349–362). Pitman, NJ: American Nephrology Nurses Association.

Renal Physicians Association/American Society of Nephrology. (2000). *Shared decision making in the appropriate initiation and withdrawal from dialysis. Clinical practice guide.* #2. Washington, DC: Author.

Robert Wood Johnson Foundation. (2002). Promoting excellence in end of life care: End stage renal disease workgroup-recommendations to the field. Retrieved from http://www.promotingexcellence.org

Sameiro-Faria, M., Ribeiro, S., Costa, E., Mendonca, D., Teixeira, L., Rocha-Pereira, P., … Santos-Silva, A. (2013). Risk factors for mortality yin hemodialysis patients: two-year follow-up study. *Disease Markers, 35*, 791–798. doi:10.1155/2013/518945

Saran, R., Robinson, B., Abbott, K. C., Agodoa, L. Y., Albertus, P., Ayanian, J., … Shahinian, V. (2017). US Renal Data System 2016 Annual Data Report: Epidemiology of kidney disease in the United States. *American Journal of Kidney Diseases, 69*(3 Suppl. 1), A7–A8. doi:10.1053/j.ajkd.2016.12.004

Sarnak, M. J., & Levey, A. S. (2000). Cardiovascular disease and chronic renal disease: A new paradigm. *American Journal of Kidney Diseases, 35*(4 Suppl. 1), S117–S131. doi:10.1016/S0272-6386(00)70239-3

Schell, J. O., Da Silva-Gane, M., & Germain, M. J. (2013). Recent insights into life expectancy with and without dialysis. *Current Opinion in Nephrology and Hypertension, 22*(2), 185–192. doi:10.1097/MNH.0b013e32835ddb69

Schena, F. P. (2001). *Nephrology.* Milan, Italy: McGraw-Hill International.

Scherer, J. S., & Holley, J. L. (2015). The role of time-limited trials in dialysis decision making in critically ill patients. *Clinical Journal of American Society of Nephrology, 11*(2), 344–353. doi:10.2215/CJN.03550315

Seccareccia, D., & Gebara, N. (2011). Pruritus in palliative care: Getting up to scratch. *Canadian Family Physician Médecin de famille canadien, 57*(9), 1010–1013, e316.

Selewski, D. T., Massengill, S. F., Troost, J. P., Wickman, L., Messer, K. L., Herreshoff E., … Barletta, G. M. (2014). Gaining the patient reported outcome measurement information system (PROMIS) perspective in chronic kidney disease: A Midwest pediatric nephrology consortium study. *Pediatric Nephrology, 29*, 2347–2356. doi:10.1007/s00467-014-2858-8

Sumida, K., & Kovesdy, C. P. (2017). Disease trajectory before ESRD: Implications for clinical management. *Seminars in Nephrology, 37*, 132–143. doi:10.1016/j.semnephrol.2016.12.003

Tonelli, M., Wiebe, N., Guthrie, B., James, M. T., Quan, H., Fortin M., … Hemmelgarn, B. R. (2015). Comorbidity as a driver of adverse outcomes in people with chronic kidney disease. *Kidney International, 88*, 859–866. doi:10.1038/ki.2015.228

U.S. Renal Data System. (2012). *Annual data report: Atlas of end stage renal disease in the United States*. Bethesda, MD: National Institutes of Health, National Institute of Diabetes and Digestive and Kidney Diseases.

U.S. Renal Data System. (2017). 2017 *USRDS annual data report: Epidemiology of kidney disease in the United States*. Bethesda, MD: National Institutes of Health, National Institute of Diabetes and Digestive and Kidney Diseases.

Verberne, W. R., Geers, A. B. M. T., Jellema, W. T., Vincent, H. H., van Delden, J. J. M., & Bos, W. J. M. (2016). Comparative survival among older adults with advanced kidney disease managed conservatively vs. dialysis. *Clinical Journal of Society of Nephrology, 11*(4), 633–640. doi:10.2215/CJN.07510715

Lissi Hansen & Anna Sasaki

End-Stage Liver Disease

KEY POINTS

- Chronic liver disease and cirrhosis is the 12th leading cause of death in the United States.
- Liver cancer is one of the fastest growing cancers in the world.
- Patients with end-stage liver disease (ESLD) present with malnutrition, muscle wasting, hyperlipidemia, fatigue, jaundice, and renal disease.
- Given trends in obesity, fatty liver disease may soon become the leading cause of liver cirrhosis.
- Nurses need to be aware of the pathophysiology and etiologies of liver disease.
- Nurses need to explore and acknowledge their assumptions and biases about patients with liver disease and their families.
- Nurses play a pivotal role in advocating for advance care planning and early palliative care for patients with ESLD and their families.
- Patients with liver disease benefit from physical, psychosocial, and spiritual interventions offered through palliative care.

CASE STUDY

J.R. was a 65-year-old man with a history of obesity, hypertension, and insulin-dependent diabetes. He had been seen in the ED with complaints of right upper quadrant pain and nausea. Bloodwork revealed normal liver function tests, normal renal function, and a platelet count of 100,000 µL. A CT revealed cirrhosis and a 4 cm lesion consistent with hepatocellular carcinoma (HCC). The HCC was treated with Y-90 and he was referred for liver transplantation. However, the HCC recurred. He was determined to no longer be a transplant candidate. Over the next 6 months, he developed decreasing liver function, had the onset of ascites, and had an episode of spontaneous bacterial peritonitis. He was referred to palliative care for treatment of symptoms of pain and itching as well as discussions of goals of care.

The liver is the largest solid organ and weighs 1,200 to 1,500 g (Curry & Bonder, 2017). It lies in the right upper quadrant protected by the ribs and is supplied by the common hepatic artery. The liver is unique in that 60% to 85% of oxygen and nutrients come to it through the portal vein, which drains the small and large intestine, the spleen, the stomach, and the pancreas. The portal vein, hepatic artery, and bile duct course together in a thin fibrous bundle, and the artery and vein branch into smaller and smaller diameter vessels while the small bile ductules coalesce into larger ducts and carry bile in the opposite direction. The blood in the smallest arterioles and venules percolate along cords of liver cells in the sinusoids (leaky capillary-like structures) and drain into the central veins. These join other central veins and finally form the hepatic vein, which carries blood to the inferior vena cava and then to the heart.

The liver performs a myriad of functions:

- Protein synthesis and secretion: almost all plasma proteins (except for gamma globulin), including alpha and beta globulins, albumin, and binding proteins for metals, toxins, hormones, and lipoproteins
- Excretion: bilirubin, bile salts, heavy metals, lipids, toxins
- Storage: iron, vitamin A, glycogen, lipid
- Immune: Kupffer cells, which traverse the sinusoids, engulfing bacteria, bacterial products, dead hepatocytes, and senescent red cells
- Nutrition: governs the fate of amino acids to be used as an energy source, to synthesize new proteins, or to be degraded to urea; stores and metabolizes glucose; synthesizes lipids and conjugates them to proteins for secretion and delivery to all cells in the body
- Metabolism: due to its blood supply, which carries blood from the gut, lipid-soluble toxins, both exogenous and endogenous, contact hepatocytes first and are extracted efficiently from the bloodstream. Lipid-soluble medications are transformed by the cytochrome P-450 system and are either excreted in the bile or metabolized to inactive molecules.

There are many chronic liver diseases that lead to cirrhosis, such as viral hepatitis, autoimmune hepatitis, primary biliary cholangitis (PBC), primary sclerosing cholangitis (PSC), nonalcoholic steatohepatitis, alcohol, some toxins, and inborn errors of metabolism (National Institute of Diabetes and Digestive and Kidney Diseases, 2014). Whatever the etiology, cirrhosis is the final common pathway, and a new set of concerns and problems develops.

■ DEFINITIONS RELATED TO LIVER DISEASE

1. Cirrhosis is a diffuse pattern of liver injury and repair that leads to fibrosis, changes in liver blood flow, and loss of liver cells.
2. Compensated cirrhosis is cirrhosis with normal liver function (Child's Class A, see Table 18.1).
3. Decompensated cirrhosis is cirrhosis with decreases in serum albumin and other proteins, an increase in the international normalized ratio (INR), and the presence of one or more complications of portal hypertension.
4. End-stage liver disease (ESLD) is decompensated cirrhosis with the involvement of other organ systems such as kidney, heart, or recurrent encephalopathy.
5. Hepatic encephalopathy is a decrease in the cognitive function often accompanied by a decline in the level of consciousness.
6. Hepatocellular carcinoma (HCC), a cancer that arises from hepatocytes, increases in patients with compensated and decompensated cirrhosis.

■ INCIDENCE AND PREVALENCE OF CHRONIC LIVER DISEASE

Approximately 5.5 million Americans are affected by chronic liver disease. The treatment for chronic liver disease costs more than the treatment for any other gastrointestinal-related condition (Peery et al., 2015). Each year it accounts for more than 290,000 emergency room visits and 240,000 hospitalizations (Peery et al., 2015). Cirrhosis is the result of chronic liver disease and affects an estimated 633,300 Americans (Scaglione et al., 2015). Cirrhosis is a progressive destruction of the liver parenchyma that leads to ESLD, the final stage of this destruction when damage to cells, tissues, and functions of the liver is irreversible, causing complete failure.

Chronic liver disease and cirrhosis is the 12th leading cause of death in the United States. In 2014, 38,170 Americans died from these conditions (Kochanek, Murphy,

TABLE 18.1 Child–Pugh–Turcotte Classification of Cirrhosis			
	1	2	3
Ascites	None	Slight	Intractable
Encephalopathy	None	Mild	Severe
Albumen	>3.3	2.8–3.3	<2.8
Bilirubin	<2	2–3	>3
INR	<1.7	1.7–2.4	>2.4

Child's Class (% 1-year survival): A = 5–6 (100%), B = 7–10 (81%), C = 11–15 (45%)

INR, international normalized ratio.

Source: Dunn, W., Jamil, L. H., Brown, L. S., Wiesner, R. H., Kim, W. R., Narayanan Menon, K. V., . . . Shah, V. (2005). MELD accurately predicts mortality in patients with alcoholic hepatitis. *Heptology, 41,* 353–358. doi:10.1002/hep.20503

Jiaquan, & Tejada-Vera, 2016), a 2.0% increase from the year before. The death rate among white and Hispanic men is double that of white and Hispanic women (Kochanek et al., 2016), but the rate is close to equal between Native American or Alaska Native men and women.

Worldwide, hepatitis C virus (HCV) is one of the major causes of liver cirrhosis, hepatocellular carcinoma (HCC), and death (Petruzziello, Marigliano, Loquercio, Cozzolino, & Cacciapuoti, 2016). Annually, approximately 399,000 individuals die from HCV infection. About 15% to 45% of people infected with HCV will spontaneously clear the virus without any treatment. However, of the remaining 55% to 85% who will develop chronic HCV infection, 15% to 30% are at risk for cirrhosis within 20 years of being infected (World Health Organization [WHO], 2017). In 2015, 71 million individuals were infected with HCV, but only 14 million were aware of their diagnosis (Cohen, 2017). Although newly developed but expensive antiviral medicines can cure more than 95% of individuals infected with HCV, access to diagnosis and treatment is low. These newly developed medications are more effective and better tolerated than older therapies were.

Over the next two decades the incidence of HCV infections is estimated to decrease in developed countries because of the new medications. In the United States, such a decrease in the incidence and related deaths is predicted to change to an increase in deaths from nonalcoholic fatty liver disease (NAFLD; Younossi, Koenig, Abdelatif, Henry, & Wymer, 2016). NAFLD is an increase in the stored fat in liver cells and is associated with a chronic inflammatory reaction. Nonalcoholic steatohepatitis (NASH) is a more severe form of NAFLD, with increased inflammation and fibrosis, and is now a major cause of liver cirrhosis (Satapathy & Sanyal, 2015). Both NAFLD and NASH are called "fatty liver disease." The term "fatty liver disease" is used when more than 5% to 10% of the liver's weight is made up of fat (American Liver Foundation, 2016). Fatty liver disease is prevalent in individuals who are overweight, or have diabetes or metabolic syndrome (Spengler & Loomba, 2015). In the United States, 30% to 40% of all adults have NAFLD and 3% to 12% have NASH (Spengler & Loomba, 2015).

■ SYMPTOMS ASSOCIATED WITH LIVER DISEASE

Liver disease is often silent, and symptoms may not develop until a complication of cirrhosis occurs. The most common symptom is fatigue, which brings the patient to medical attention, and laboratory and imaging investigation lead to the diagnosis of liver disease. Fatigue should be evaluated first as a separate condition, since it is a nonspecific complaint and other causes may have more specific therapies (e.g., sleep apnea). As liver disease

progresses, weakness, mental fog or outright confusion, abdominal swelling, and pruritus are common. The latter may be due to the liver disease itself (as in PBC or PSC, due to bile salts in the skin) or to thinning and drying of the skin due to age or poor nutrition. The patient's caregiver is often more astute in describing signs and symptoms than the patient.

■ PHYSICAL ASSESSMENT RELATED TO LIVER DISEASE

Abnormalities in the physical examination occur late in the course of the cirrhosis and include muscle wasting of the face, neck, and large muscle groups. Protuberance of the abdomen may indicate ascites. The veins over the abdomen can be prominent. There may be cutaneous red spots that blanch under pressure, known as spider angiomata. Jaundice—yellowing of the skin, sclerae, and tympanic membranes due to elevated bilirubin—occurs late in the disease. Experienced observers can detect bilirubin levels of 2.5 to 3 mg/dL in the sclerae, but patients and caregivers most often detect bilirubin in the 4 to 5 mg/dL or greater range.

A Mini-Mental Examination is a very important part of the physical assessment (Folstein, Folstein, & McHugh, 1975). Two other tests allow the detection of significant levels of encephalopathy: asterixis, a low-frequency forward "flap" ("hold up your hands like you are stopping traffic") and "serial sevens" ("count backward from 100 by 7s"). In the serial sevens test, the correct answer is not important, but the ability of the patient to concentrate on the subtraction will show whether he or she is encephalopathic.

It is important to remember that these physical findings occur late, and the patient may be quite ill, and not yet manifest them.

■ PROGNOSIS AND SCORING IN ESLD

Because it is usually the complications of cirrhosis that determine morbidity and mortality, it is often hard to predict prognosis in an individual patient. There are two scoring systems in current use that describe mortality: the Child–Pugh–Turcotte Score (Child & Turcotte, 1964; refer to Table 18.1) and the Model of End-Stage Liver Disease (MELD; Kamath et al., 2001).

The second scoring system is the MELD, which is a statistical formula used initially to predict 90-day mortality after a transjugular intrahepatic portosystemic shunt (TIPS). The MELD score considers the serum bilirubin, the INR, creatinine, and sodium. The 90-day mortality is predicted with a MELD of 10 (6%), a MELD of 20 (25%), a MELD of 30 (62%), and a MELD of 40 (89%; see Exhibit 18.1). It is important to remember that other factors play a role in assessing mortality, and a person

Exhibit 18.1

Encephalopathy and Ascites as Predictors of 90-Day Mortality

Encephalopathy	Ascites	90-Day Mortality Total # (%)	Mean ± SD
Yes	Yes	7/9 (78)	29 ± 9 (17–38)
No	Yes	7/33 (21)	17 ± 8 (6–36)
Yes	No	2/8 (25)	21 ± 8 (7–33)
No	No	0/23 (0)	10 ± (0–18)

Source: Dunn, W., Jamil, L. H., Brown, L. S., Wiesner, R. H., Kim, W. R., Narayanan Menon, K. V., ... Shah, V. (2005). MELD accurately predicts mortality in patients with alcoholic hepatitis. *Heptology, 41*, 353–358. doi:10.1002/hep.20503

with a MELD of 25 may have a lower mortality than someone with a MELD of 18 who has an infection or hemorrhage.

■ HEPATOCELLULAR CARCINOMA

Hepatocellular carcinoma (HCC) is one of the fastest growing cancers in the world, with the highest incidence in sub-Saharan Africa and Southeast Asia. In the United States, it is the 10th most common cancer; it is the estimated fifth leading cause of cancer death in men and eighth in women (American Cancer Society, 2017). Overall, the 5-year survival is 17% (American Cancer Society, 2016). Eighty percent of liver cancer comes from liver cells, 10% to 20% from the bile ducts (cholangiocarcinoma), and about 1% from blood vessels (angiosarcoma). Most patients who develop HCC have underlying cirrhosis, and people who have cirrhosis of any etiology are at a much higher risk of liver cancer; for example, in cirrhosis due to hepatitis C, the risk is 2% to 6% per year (Sangiovanni et al., 2004).

Patients who have known cirrhosis should be screened for liver cancer every 6 months with ultrasound, CT, or MRI. Early cancers can be detected and treatment started earlier. Liver cancer most often grows silently, and patients become symptomatic late in the course of the disease. Modalities of treatment include liver-directed therapies such as surgical resection, transarterial chemo-embolization (TACE), radio-frequency, microwave, or cryo-ablation, ethanol injection into the tumor, focused-beam radiation therapy, and/or systemic therapies such as sorafenib, an oral medication. A person with a small tumor or few tumors may be a candidate for liver transplantation. Only patients with HCC are currently candidates for transplantation because of the high risk of recurrence of cholangiocarcinoma or angiosarcoma post transplant.

Some patients with cirrhosis seen in palliative care may have well-preserved liver function, but have a liver cancer burden too high for liver transplantation. There are strict criteria for the size and number of HCCs, established to minimize the probability of recurrence of cancer post transplant. If a person's disease falls outside these criteria, transplant is no longer an option, but local intervention for the liver cancer can and often does continue, particularly if the patient is symptomatic. All therapies at this point are noncurative, an attempt to slow the growth of the tumor(s). The tumors ultimately spread such that liver-directed therapy is ineffective or metastasis to lung, brain, or bone occurs, usually late in the course of the disease.

One of the greatest challenges in treating people with liver cancer is that they may feel good and find it hard to believe that there is anything wrong. This is true even in patients referred for palliative care. They may opt for naturopathic remedies that seem less toxic (e.g., cannabis/CBD oil), but none has been shown to be effective in halting the progression of cancer. Patients may decide to undergo liver-directed therapies when subsequent imaging shows that naturopathic remedies have not halted the disease. But the cancer is often more difficult to treat.

■ MILAN CRITERIA OF HEPATOCELLULAR CARCINOMA

Early in the transplant era, HCC was thought to be completely confined to the liver in most cases, and there was enthusiasm for transplanting all patients who presented with liver cancer. Unfortunately, many cancers recurred post transplant and metastasized to bone, lung, and brain. Survival was measured in months to a few years. The experience of the larger transplant centers was examined, and Milan criteria were developed to minimize the recurrence of post-transplant cancer to under 10% to 20% (De Carlis et al., 1989). The presence of one cancer less than 5 cm in diameter, or no more than three cancers, none of which is greater than 3 cm, was thought to be within the Milan criteria to be considered for transplant. Subsequent studies suggested that the Milan criteria were too strict and modifications have developed that allow for tumors up to 6.5 cm and a total tumor burden of 8 cm (Yao et al., 2002).

■ COMPLICATIONS OF CIRRHOSIS

Complications of cirrhosis may be classified into those due to portal hypertension and those due to loss of liver cells.

Complications Due to Portal Hypertension

■ **Upper Gastrointestinal Bleeding.** Upper gastrointestinal (GI) bleeding may be due to the rupture of esophageal or gastric varices or due to portal hypertensive gastropathy. Signs of bleeding, often dramatic, include hematemesis or melena, and patients may develop hypotension or shock. Upper endoscopy is performed to diagnose the site of bleeding, and variceal banding or sclerotherapy may control the bleeding. If these are ineffective, a TIPS may be done. A TIPS is an internal stent connection between the portal vein and the hepatic vein that significantly reduces portal hypertension.

■ **Ascites.** Ascites occurs when fluid leaking into the peritoneal cavity from engorged intestinal veins overwhelms the ability of the lymph vessels to carry the fluid back into the vascular system. Initial treatment by sodium restriction and prescription of diuretics is usually effective, but as the cirrhosis progresses, these may become ineffective. Paracentesis can be performed on a regular basis in a day surgery or the ED. Albumin is given when the ascites volume exceeds 4 L to prevent rapid re-accumulation of ascites at the expense of the vascular space, leading to renal dysfunction (Runyon, 2009). TIPS is often done when the paracentesis frequency is 1 to 2 weeks and/or if the volume of the fluid is high. Usually a patient whose bilirubin is greater than 2.5 to 3 mg/dL is not a candidate for a TIPS because the risk of acute liver failure (from decreased blood flow to the liver parenchyma) is high. In a patient who has been referred to palliative care or hospice, an indwelling peritoneal catheter can be placed by a radiologist, and 500 to 1,000 mL can be drawn off every day. There is an increased risk of infection with the use of the catheter. It is most useful in bed-ridden patients or when paracentesis services are not readily available. Intake of fluid should not be restricted in order to decrease ascites, since the vascular compartment is compromised first in fluid restriction.

This can lead to lightheadedness and make the patient prone to falls and to a decrease in kidney function.

■ **Spontaneous Bacterial Peritonitis.** Spontaneous bacterial peritonitis occurs because there is increased bacterial translocation in a patient with decompensated cirrhosis, and ascites is an excellent culture medium for bacterial growth. There is a high mortality if the peritonitis is not recognized, but antibiotics are effective, usually within 2 to 3 days of initiation of the treatment. Signs and symptoms of peritonitis are often absent, but a more rapid accumulation of ascites than usual or symptoms of encephalopathy should lead to a diagnostic paracentesis and treatment if the absolute neutrophil count in the fluid is greater than 250. Gut organisms such as *E. coli*, *Klebsiella*, and *Enterococcus* are the most common pathogens (Sheer & Runyon, 2005).

■ **Hepatic Encephalopathy.** Hepatic encephalopathy is a nonspecific decrease in cognitive function and level of consciousness, which can progress to coma, and is a distressing condition for both the patient and the caregiver. The etiologic agent(s) have not been completely identified; however, gut bacteria or bacterial products are the most likely causes. Serum ammonia is often elevated, and patients and medical providers use the ammonia level to diagnose and treat hepatic encephalopathy. The ammonia per se should not be treated, but the trigger(s) should be sought and identified. Triggers can include constipation, upper GI bleeding, infection, dehydration, kidney dysfunction, hypokalemia, or an acute hepatitis due to virus, toxins, or medications. In the outpatient setting, constipation or dehydration are the two most common triggers of hepatic encephalopathy. Symptoms include confusion, mood swings, changes in sleep pattern, inability to do mathematics, and slower reaction times.

Studies have shown that many patients have minimal hepatic encephalopathy even when they lack signs and symptoms of overt cognitive dysfunction (Nardone et al., 2016). Unfortunately, the patients often do not recognize when they are developing mild encephalopathy, and this can lead to anger and arguments between the patient and the caregiver. Treatment of constipation consists of lactulose or other laxatives to rid the colon of bacterial toxins before they can be absorbed, or by killing the bacteria with a nonabsorbable antibiotic such as rifaximin. If the patient is treated with a laxative, there should be no more than four to five stools a day, and the patient should drink sufficient water to quench thirst since dehydration also can trigger encephalopathy. It is important to educate the patient and family that this is a delirium not a dementia, and is entirely reversible when treated.

Not all patients with cirrhosis who have decreased cognitive function have hepatic encephalopathy. Other agents that can mimic hepatic encephalopathy include uremia, drug overdose with opiates or benzodiazepines, post-seizure, alcohol intoxication, hypoxia, and increased intracranial pressure. It is important to rule these out if there is clinical suspicion because management is quite different. For instance, a patient with cirrhosis may fall and suffer an intracranial hemorrhage. Many patients with encephalopathy who are seen in the ED appropriately receive head CTs.

■ **Alteration in Drug Metabolism.** Alteration in drug metabolism is due to a combination of altered blood flow and decreased hepatocyte function. Drugs with a high first-pass clearance and those that are highly protein bound will have prolonged half-lives and thus greater or longer effect. For instance, intravenous (IV) morphine given to patients with decompensated cirrhosis had a half-life three times that of controls, and for oral morphine the half-life was 1.5 to 2 times greater (Hasselström et al., 1990).

■ **Miscellaneous Complications.** Miscellaneous complications include poor nutrition, pain (see the text that follows), an increased risk of infection of all types, sexual dysfunction, weakness, and fatigue. The patient should be encouraged to engage in some degree of activity every day, as much as possible, to prevent loss of strength, which can lead to falls.

Complications Due to Loss of Liver Cells

As cirrhosis progresses, protein synthesis decreases and the ability of the liver to metabolize and excrete toxins wanes. Bilirubin rises, causing jaundice, and the serum albumin and coagulation parameters decrease, causing the INR to rise. Other causes of bilirubin rise include infection, particularly with gram-negative organisms, and biliary obstruction due to liver cancer or gallstones. It is important to distinguish among these different causes, because infection and gallstone disease are treatable.

As cirrhosis becomes further decompensated, other organs also develop dysfunction. About 10% to 15% of patients with cirrhosis will develop hepatopulmonary syndrome, with shunting in the lungs and hypoxia, or portopulmonary syndrome, with right ventricular and pulmonary artery hypertension. The former is cured by liver transplant; the latter is not cured and is associated with increased perioperative mortality. The heart may develop a cirrhotic cardiomyopathy. As decompensation progresses, the work of the heart increases until it is no longer able to meet demands, leading to high-output cardiac failure. Decreased hepatic metabolism of vasoactive hormones leads to vasoconstriction of the renal arteries and renal dysfunction known as hepatorenal syndrome (HRS). Finally, episodes of hepatic encephalopathy become more frequent and difficult to treat.

HRS is common in ESLD and can be the primary driver of the MELD score. HRS-II is a chronic form of renal dysfunction and occurs over months, characterized primarily by rises in creatinine, particularly when the patient becomes somewhat dehydrated or is over-diuresed. HRS-I is an acute decompensation of renal function and is defined as doubling of the serum creatinine within 2 weeks and a creatinine greater than 2 mg/dL. It is important to rule out other causes of kidney disease such as hypovolemia or acute tubular necrosis, drug toxicity, and urinary obstruction. Prognosis of HRS-I is poor—up to 80% mortality within 2 weeks. Dialysis will stabilize the patient, but nephrologists are appropriately reluctant to dialyze a patient who is not a liver transplant candidate, since liver-related mortality is high.

■ LIVER TRANSPLANTATION

A patient with decompensated cirrhosis and a MELD of 14 to 15, a significant complication of the liver disease, or the development of HCC within the Milan criteria can be referred for liver transplantation. A preliminary investigation into the health of other organ systems, acceptable psychosocial health, and adequate caregiver support is performed first, and then the information is sent to a transplant center. Further workup is done at the center, the patient is discussed at a multidisciplinary conference, and the patient's suitability for the transplant is determined. If all concerns of the transplant program personnel are satisfied, the patient is placed on a liver transplant waiting list corresponding to his or her blood type. The position on the list is determined by the MELD score.

Liver transplantation is an acceptable form of treatment with first-year survival greater than 90%. It should not be considered a magical cure—patients take many medications at least initially, immunosuppression can lead to infection or cancer, complications can develop, and sometimes the original liver disease recurs. However, many patients do well in the long term and lead fulfilling lives post transplant. Unfortunately, the need for donor livers has far exceeded the number of potential recipients. This leads to long wait times and the potential for deterioration of the patient's medical condition or growth of liver cancer to the point that transplant is no longer possible. Waiting is very stressful for both the patient and the caregiver. Palliative care providers could play an important role in ameliorating both physical and psychological symptoms and improve quality of life during this time. In the United States, approximately 1,550 adults die each year while waiting (Organ Procurement and Transplantation Network, 2017b). In 2016, 7,841 patients received a liver transplant (Organ Procurement and Transplantation Network, 2017a). Approximately, twice as many are waiting, and in June 2017, 14,389 in April 2018, 13,944 persons were listed on the liver transplant waiting list.

Liver transplantation is not for everyone, and no one should be pressured into being considered for transplant. Some cannot give up smoking, street drugs, or alcohol;

others have tenuous relationships and find it difficult to obtain caregiver support. For others, personal or religious convictions keep them from accepting transplant as an option. Palliative care can provide the much-needed support and guidance to these patients and their families.

■ MALNUTRITION

Adequate nutrition is a key to maintaining high quality of life in a patient with cirrhosis even if he or she is in palliative care. A malnourished patient is more likely to become infected, and muscle loss leads to disabling weakness, increased fatigue, and loss of ability to perform activities of daily living or of activities that provide enjoyment.

Although not all studies support the idea that ingested protein may trigger encephalopathy in cirrhotic patients, there is still the perception by some healthcare professionals and even dietitians that meat should be eaten sparingly, particularly red meat. This can lead to significant muscle loss if protein intake is inadequate. However, studies have shown that patients with cirrhosis require more ingested protein than a normal patient (i.e., 1.2 gm/kg/d in patients with stable cirrhosis, up to 1.5 gm/kg/d in the presence of infection; Amodio et al., 2013; Huynh, Selvanderan, Harley, Holloway, & Nguyen, 2015). In the liver, the normal cycle of protein breakdown and protein synthesis is about 90% efficient. This efficiency drops significantly in cirrhosis, and more protein is needed for endogenous protein utilization. The type of protein is not important, but the patient should bear in mind that animal protein is more easily digested and absorbed than vegetable protein; 40% to 50% of vegetable protein can be inaccessible to pancreatic enzymes due to binding to cellulose. Nonetheless, vegetarians can consume adequate protein through milk products, eggs, tofu, and other easily digestible foods as well as complementary vegetable proteins.

In addition, because of the alterations in liver blood flow, there is less first-pass clearance of nutrients from the small intestine, leading to a discrepancy between nutrient absorption and secretion of insulin, glucagon, and other digestive hormones. This can lead to the potential for hypoglycemia and to a shift in metabolism from glycogen to muscle protein, which occurs as early as after 12 hours of fasting (this shift occurs in non-cirrhotic patients after about 3 days). Muscle protein, once lost, is very difficult to replace and muscle weakness results.

There are many reasons why patients with ESLD lose their desire to eat. Diets restricted in sodium or potassium may lead to food being tasteless. In a person who already has muscle wasting, weak muscles of mastication may cause fatigue after only a few bites of food. Ascites may limit the amount of food intake, and medications, such as spironolactone, may cause nausea and alteration of

taste. The endogenous breakdown of sulfur-containing proteins can lead to the peculiar "garlic breath" that can be distressing to patients and caregivers. The substance(s) associated with hepatic encephalopathy may also affect nerves associated with taste. Finally, hospitalization often leads to prolonged nil per os (NPO) status for various reasons, and the patients may leave the hospital more malnourished than on admission.

Malnutrition results in not only the loss of muscle strength but also in a decrease in the patients' ability to perform the activities of daily living and a loss of independence. Weakness of muscles of mastication and swallowing may lead to aspiration with subsequent pneumonia. And weakness of breathing muscles can limit coughing and make the person prone to pneumonia. It is important to encourage the patient and caregiver to be creative when preparing food and to experiment with seasonings to improve the taste of food. If a patient has been ingesting a lot of salt, and needs to decrease to a sodium level of less than 2,000 mg a day, it is better to do that in stages over several weeks. Frequent smaller feedings, including a bedtime snack and some nutritious food for breakfast, will block the shift in metabolism. Fluid should not be restricted unless specifically prescribed (see also the section on ascites).

■ PAIN

Although cirrhosis per se is usually painless, issues regarding pain are common. Research shows that patients with ESLD experience moderate-to-severe pain (Desbiens & Wu, 2000; Hansen, Leo, Chang, Zucker, & Sasaki, 2014; Roth, Lynn, Zhong, Borum, & Dawson, 2000). Large liver cancers can stretch the liver capsule and cause pain in the right upper quadrant, which can also be referred to other areas. Loss of muscle mass and strength leads to muscle pain as the patient tries to do usual activities of daily living. Other diseases such as pancreatitis, diverticulosis, or colonic distension can cause abdominal pain. Healthcare professionals are often reluctant to prescribe pain medication because of former addiction issues or concern for altered drug metabolism or triggering encephalopathy. The chronic use of NSAIDs, such as ibuprofen or naproxen, is contraindicated because they decrease platelet function, may cause gastric ulcers, and lead to a higher risk of interstitial nephritis in patients with cirrhosis (Dwyer, Jayasekera, & Nicoll, 2014). Acetaminophen, if the patient is not drinking excessive alcohol and has adequate nutrition, is the safest analgesic. Opioids can be prescribed starting with a lower dose (Boyd, Kimbell, Murray, & Iredale, 2012). Hope and Morrison (2011) recommend decreasing the typical starting dose of an opioid by 25% to 50%. Opioids should not be given to ameliorate abdominal pain due to lactulose, but rather there should be a change to a different laxative, which may be more effective.

■ PSYCHOSOCIAL AND SPIRITUAL ASSESSMENT OF PATIENTS WITH ESLD

The psychosocial and spiritual assessment of patients with ESLD may reveal the ongoing experience of loss. Patients may mourn the loss of former relationships with work, family members, and friends. Patients' independence changes to one of dependence as the illness progresses, and there is an increasing need to rely on care by family members (Brown, Sorrell, McClaren, & Creswell, 2006).

Patients may also experience losses due to body image and distress caused by a functional decline. The massive development of ascites causes the abdomen to balloon, shortness of breath, and swelling in legs and ankles leading to difficulty with balance and walking. This may result in a limitation in social interactions and activities. Male patients may also develop gynecomastia and impotence. In a study examining symptom distress in patients with ESLD, "having problems with sexual interest and activity" was rated by patients among of the 10 most frequently experienced symptoms (Hansen et al., 2015). Furthermore, patients may become more insecure and afraid of losing control due to anticipated development of hepatic encephalopathy.

Spirituality may play a significant role in patients' lives and be a source of strength in helping them cope with their liver disease. Learning the role spirituality has played through their lives and during the progression of disease in patients with ESLD may provide healthcare professionals with information about patients' strengths and areas of concern. Professionals should encourage patients to define what spirituality has meant and currently means to them and to express their fears and hopes at this late stage of disease progression. Building on patients' strengths, positive experiences, and prior successfully used coping strategies, professionals may facilitate patients' spiritual well-being and quality of life. Spiritual needs should be identified and addressed to enhance healthcare professionals' ability to appropriately help and support patients. Patients with ESLD may seek forgiveness from family members from whom they have been estranged due to addiction or mental illness. As a result of estrangement, these patients may have little support at the same time they may be struggling with self-forgiveness. Self-forgiveness may be the hardest (Hansen, Sasaki, & Zucker, 2010).

Family Caregivers of Patients With ESLD

The assessment of patients with ESLD should include an assessment of their family members/caregivers. First, it is critical for healthcare professionals to identify the patient's family. Some patients may have challenging or strained family relationships because of their prior and/ or current substance abuse. Family members may be angry and upset with the patient, believing that he/she caused the disease. Others may have alienated family members and friends over time. Their "family" may be a single person such as a neighbor or several unrelated individuals. Therefore, patients should determine who is significant in their lives and who they trust to participate in their care and well-being.

As the liver disease progresses, the involvement of family in the patients' care increases and the impact on family members becomes more and more burdensome. Research shows that informal caregivers of patients with ESLD experience significant caregiver strain (Bajaj et al., 2011; Miyazaki et al., 2010), are depressed (Malik et al., 2014), and feel overwhelmed (Kunzler-Heule, Beckmann, Mahrer-Imhof, Semela, & Handler-Schuster, 2016).

Families may also experience significant financial impact because of the patients' liver disease, including loss of income and draining of savings (Roth et al., 2000). In addition, patients' insurance status, perceived stigma, and their beliefs about their disease may serve as barriers to timely and effective healthcare (Mellinger et al., 2016; Vaughn-Sandler, Sherman, Aronsohn, & Volk, 2014). Because of the symptom burden experienced by both family members and patients, healthcare professionals should focus their assessment and interventions on both the patient and the family as the unit of care.

■ PALLIATIVE CARE

Given that the disease progression from ESLD is slow and involves intermittent acute exacerbations, predicting survival is difficult. Death from ESLD is relatively sudden and unpredictable until the last week of life (Roth et al., 2000). These uncertainties and challenges in prognostication are among several barriers for early referral of individuals with ESLD to palliative care or hospice. Individuals with ESLD often receive palliative care late in the disease trajectory (Antaki & Lukowski, 2007; Hansen et al., 2014; Poonja et al., 2014). Palliative care in other conditions has been associated with better end-of-life care by improving symptom control and quality of life (Bakitas et al., 2009; Barton, 2014; Follwell et al., 2009; Hui et al., 2014), as well as extending life and lowering healthcare resource utilization (Greer et al., 2012; Temel et al., 2010).

Individuals with ESLD tend to live in a state of poor and declining health, but often have a limited understanding of their disease severity and prognosis and, therefore, may not realize how close they are to death. As such, the introduction of end-of-life care conversations and referral to palliative care is often challenging for healthcare professionals. At the same time, healthcare professionals may lack training and experience in initiating end-of-life conversations, and may overestimate life expectancy (Christakis & Lamont, 2000), focusing on medical interventions (Rakoski & Volk, 2015).

Professionals may be concerned that palliative care referrals are alarming to patients and families (Smith et al., 2012). They may also be concerned about taking away patients' hope for a potential liver transplant and therefore postpone difficult end-of-life conversations. Patients and families may perceive that palliative care is similar to hospice and that professionals are "giving up" on them, rather than understanding that palliative care and hospice improve the quality of life until its end. In a study following patients with ESLD admitted to the intensive care unit for the treatment of liver complications, Hansen et al. (2012) found that the possibility of receiving a liver transplantation was the driving force for patients, family members, and healthcare professionals to continue life-sustaining treatments (Hansen et al., 2012). Although due to disease severity patients may become ineligible for a liver transplant, professionals often find the introduction of palliative care and hospice to be a difficult conversation. The result is that palliative care or hospice may begin within days of death, leaving little time to address end-of-life needs and concerns (Potosek, Curry, Buss, & Chittenden, 2014; Rossaro et al., 2004).

It is important to realize that palliative care can be introduced at any time in the illness trajectory to improve the quality of life of patients and families, with discussions of the goals of care, and the management of physical, emotional, and spiritual needs. Baumann et al. (2015) examined an early palliative care intervention for patients with ESLD during the patients' standard 1-week pre-transplant evaluation process. The intervention included symptom assessment and control as well as discussions of psychosocial well-being and spiritual health. Twenty-nine of the 50 patients who had the intervention completed a follow-up assessment within 6 months. The results indicated that the intervention improved symptoms of pruritus, appetite, anxiety, fatigue, and depression. This work supports the notion that palliative care interventions are beneficial to patients with ESLD, even those who are referred for a liver transplant evaluation and awaiting a transplant.

■ IMPLICATIONS FOR NURSING PRACTICE

Personal Assumptions and Biases Related to Patients With ESLD

When caring for individuals with ESLD, nurses must be honest with themselves and be aware of their own assumptions and biases about this population and their families. Hearing that an individual has ESLD may lead a nurse to make assumptions about the cause of the disease ("he or she is an alcoholic and/or drug user") and/or the individual's previous or current lifestyle. Nurses need to reflect on and explore such assumptions. It is important for nurses to acknowledge them so they do not interfere with the respect each individual and his or her family deserve. Nurses need to keep in mind that there are many causes for ESLD. Individuals should not be judged by their past but instead be supported as they move forward with a terminal illness potentially causing physical and psychological pain and suffering.

Research has shown that patients feel stigmatized from liver disease (Sogolow, Lasker, Sharim, Weinrieb, & Sass, 2010; Vaughn-Sandler et al., 2014). Vaughn-Sandler et al. (2014) examined the prevalence and consequences of stigma in patients with cirrhosis. Patients with higher levels of perceived stigma reported less social support, had worse quality of life, and were less likely to seek medical care. In a study by Sogolow et al. (2010), the stigma experienced by women with the autoimmune liver disease primary biliary cirrhosis was explored. The participating women completed a survey including measures of stigma and quality of life and open-ended questions related to stigmatizing experiences. Higher stigma scores were associated with more disease symptoms, greater disease uncertainty, and diminished mental and social dimensions of quality of life. Nearly one in five reported experiencing stigma that caused feelings of hurt and anger. In particular, stigmatizing behaviors came from healthcare professionals. Nurses and other healthcare professionals need to be knowledgeable about and sensitive to the consequences stigmatizing behaviors may have on patients with liver disease, irrespective of the etiology of the disease. Emotions experienced by patients often extend to family members as they provide support and care. Therefore, it is critical that nurses strive to understand family members' perceptions of stigmatization. Nurses should be cognizant of stigmatization and the sense of alienation and hopelessness experienced by patients with ESLD and their families, and provide effective and compassionate family-centered care.

Advance Care Planning and Early Palliative Care Referral

Nurses play a pivotal role in advocating for early palliative care and significantly influence the quality of care provided to patients with ESLD and their families. Nurses work with patients and their families in outpatient and inpatient care settings. In inpatient care settings, nurses care for patients during 8- or 12-hour shifts (Owens & Flom, 2005). They spend a lot of their time at their patients' bedside, which provides valuable opportunities to connect with both patients and families and to learn about their understanding of ESLD and what is important to them. Patients with ESLD are frequently admitted to inpatient care settings due to disease-related complications. This is often a time of crisis, making the introduction of end-of-life care and treatment decisions stressful if patients and families have had no prior or limited discussions about their hopes and fears and preferences regarding illness, dying, and surrogate decision making.

Nurses in outpatient care settings often care for patients earlier in the disease trajectory, which offers them the opportunity to introduce advance care planning to patients with ESLD and their families. Most of the care these patients receive is in the outpatient setting, stressing the importance of the role nurses play in this setting, with initiating advance care planning and helping and guiding patients and families to have honest and meaningful conversations about end-of-life treatment choices and death before a crisis occurs (Meier & Beresford, 2008; Rabow et al., 2013).

Advance care planning is the process of making such treatment choice decisions and about the care individuals with ESLD would want to receive should they become unable to speak for themselves. Advance care planning is particularly critical for individuals with ESLD because they often develop hepatic encephalopathy and are unable to make their own decisions. Approximately 30% of patients dying of ESLD experience significant hepatic encephalopathy (Roth et al., 2000). At an earlier stage of the liver disease, encephalopathy is reversible with treatment, but severe complications may occur unexpectedly and the patient may die within a short time frame. Therefore, early on in the disease trajectory, patients should identify who they would want to make not only healthcare decisions for them but also legal and financial decisions.

CASE STUDY

AN INTERDISCIPLINARY PERSPECTIVE

Anna Sasaki, MD, PhD

Caring for a patient with ESLD is challenging and best done by an interprofessional healthcare team familiar with the patient and able to follow closely. With the rising prevalence of obesity, the incidence of NASH will be the most common cause of liver cirrhosis in the future. Primary care providers should have a high index of suspicion for the often silent liver disease. Follow-up with laboratory values and imaging will allow early detection of complications of cirrhosis, especially HCC. Early detection of decompensated cirrhosis or HCC would be a perfect time to refer to palliative care. It could mean better symptom identification and management. As the disease progresses, symptoms become more complex, requiring frequent titration and changes in medications. In addition, patients with ESLD and families may need multifaceted spiritual and psychological support to maximize their quality of life. An interprofessional palliative care team is in a unique position to initiate discussions about goals of care and address physical, spiritual, and psychological needs of these patients and their families, each patient and family as a unit of care who may have had longstanding complicated relationships.

J.R. would have been better served by a palliative care consult at the time he was diagnosed with advanced liver disease, not just at the time it was determined that he no longer was a liver transplant candidate. With the support of the palliative care team, J.R.'s pain, itching, and ascites would have been better managed and his quality of life improved. His family's needs would have been assessed and addressed as well.

Evidence-Based Practice

Perri, G-A., Bunn, S., Oh, Y. J., Kassam, A., Berall, A., Karuza, J., & Khosravani, H. (2016). Attributes and outcomes of end-stage liver disease as compared to other noncancer patients admitted to a geriatric palliative care unit. *Annals of Palliative Medicine,* 5(2), 76–82. doi:10.21037/apm.2016.03.07

Background
End-stage liver disease (ESLD) is the 12th leading cause of death in North America. Because patients with ESLD often lack a "terminal phase" due to a gradual declining

disease trajectory challenged by unpredictable complications, these patients rarely are referred to palliative care or are referred late. These patients' late referral may be due to a longer perceived length of stay (LOS) in palliative care units (PCUs) compared to patients with other noncancer diagnoses, and therefore, patients with ESLD may not be given equitable access to such units. PCUs, a limited recourse, provide an option for continued care for patients with ESLD but are not able to accommodate patients with longer LOS. The aim of the study was to better characterize the illness experience of patients with ESLD on a geriatric PCU comparing ESLD patients and other noncancer patients in terms of admission Palliative Performance Score (PPS), estimated prognosis, and LOS.

Methods

From September 1, 2011, to April 10, 2015, retrospective medical record reviews were completed of all noncancer patients ($n = 235$) admitted to Baycrest Health Sciences PCU in Toronto, Canada. The Baycrest PCU is a 31-bed inpatient facility for patients with a prognosis of fewer than 3 months. Patients with ESLD were those excluded from liver transplantation. Data collection included demographics, admitting diagnosis, estimated prognosis, PPS score within 7 days of admission, LOS, and disposition (death or discharge location). The PPS is a scale measuring functional status among patients receiving palliative care. It includes 11 performance categories that are measured in decremental stages from 100% (no limitations on any aspects of daily life) to 0% (deceased). A higher score represents a higher functional status.

Results

Of the 235 noncancer patients admitted, 44 (19%) had ESLD. Patients with ESLD were significantly younger (mean age of 72 vs. 84, $p < .001$) compared to other noncancer patients and were admitted to the PCU with a significantly higher PPS. There were no significant differences in estimated prognosis, LOS, or disposition between the two groups. However, there was a nonsignificant trend toward a shorter LOS for patients with ESLD (mean LOS of 19 days vs. 32 days).

Conclusion/Implications

Study findings suggest that patients with ESLD in PCUs do not live longer than other noncancer patients despite a better admitting PPS. Patients should be admitted to PCUs based on their needs and not their diagnosis or prognosis.

■ REFERENCES

American Cancer Society. (2016). Cancer facts & figures. Retrieved from http://www.cancer.org/acs/groups/content/@research/documents/document/acspc-047079.pdf

American Cancer Society. (2017). Cancer facts & figures. Retrieved from https://www.cancer.org/content/dam/cancer-org/research/cancer-facts-and-statistics/annual-cancer-facts-and-figures/2017/leading-sites-of-new-cancer-cases-and-deaths-2017-estimates.pdf

American Liver Foundation. (2016). Non-alcoholic fatty liver disease. Retrieved from https://www.liverfoundation.org/for-patients/about-the-liver/diseases-of-the-liver/non-alcoholic-fatty-liver-disease/

Amodio, P., Bemeur, C., Butterworth, R., Cordoba, J., Kato, A., Montagnese, S., ... Morgan, M. Y. (2013). The nutritional management of hepatic encephalopathy in patients with cirrhosis: International Society for Hepatic Encephalopathy and Nitrogen Metabolism Consensus. *Hepatology, 58*, 325–336. doi:10.1002/hep.26370

Antaki, F., & Lukowski, A. (2007). The model for end-stage liver disease (MELD) predicts survival of liver cirrhosis patients after discharge to hospice. *Journal of Clinical Gastroenterology, 41*, 412–415. doi:10.1097/01.mcg.0000225594.01201.9b

Bajaj, J. S., Wade, J. B., Gibson, D. P., Heuman, D. M., Thacker, L. R., Sterling, R. K., ... Sanyal, A. J. (2011). The multi-dimensional burden of cirrhosis and hepatic encephalopathy on patients and caregivers. *American Journal of Gastroenterology, 106*, 1646–1653. doi:10.1038/ajg.2011.157

Bakitas, M., Lyons, K. D., Hegel, M. T., Balan, S., Brokaw, F. C., Seville, J., ... Ahles, T. A. (2009). Effects of a palliative care intervention on clinical outcomes in patients with advanced cancer: The Project ENABLE II randomized controlled trial. *Journal of the American Medical Association, 302*, 741–749. doi:10.1001/jama.2009.1198

Barton, M. K. (2014). Early outpatient referral to palliative care services improves end-of-life care. *CA: A Cancer Journal for Clinicians, 64*, 223–224. doi:10.3322/caac.21230

Baumann, A. J., Wheeler, D., James, M., Turner, R., Siegel, A., & Navarro, V. J. (2015). Benefit of early palliative care intervention in end-stage liver disease patients awaiting liver transplantation. *Journal of Pain and Symptom Management, 50*, 882–886. doi:10.1016/j.jpainsymman.2015.07.014

Boyd, K., Kimbell, B., Murray, S., & Iredale, J. (2012). Living and dying well with end-stage liver disease: Time for palliative care? *Hepatology, 55*, 1650–1651. doi:10.1002/hep.25621

Brown, J., Sorrell, J. H., McClaren, J., & Creswell, J. W. (2006). Waiting for a liver transplant. *Qualitative Health Research, 16*, 119–136. doi:10.1177/1049732305284011

Child, C. G., & Turcotte, J. G. (1964). The liver and portal hypertension. In C. G. Child (Ed.), *Surgery and portal hypertension* (pp. 50–64): Philadelphia, PA: Saunders.

Christakis, N. A., & Lamont, E. B. (2000). Extent and determinants of error in doctors' prognoses in terminally ill patients: Prospective cohort study. *BMJ, 320*, 469–472. doi:10.1136/bmj.320.7233.469

Cohen, J. (2017). New report halves the number of people infected with hepatitis C worldwide. Retrieved from http://www.sciencemag.org/news/2017/04/new-report-halves-number-people-infected-hepatitis-c-worldwide

Curry, M. P., & Bonder, A. (2017). Hepatomegaly: Differential diagnosis and evaluation. Retrieved from https://www.uptodate.com/contents/hepatomegaly-differential-diagnosis-and-evaluation

De Carlis, L., Belli, L. S., Romani, F., Aseni, P., Baticci, F., Sansalone, C. V., ... Belli, L. (1989). Selection criteria for liver transplantation: Preliminary experience of Niguarda Hospital, Milan. *Transplantation Proceedings, 21*, 2415–2416.

Desbiens, N. A., & Wu, A. (2000). Pain and suffering in seriously ill hospitalized patients. *Journal of American Geriatrics Society, 48*, S183–S186. doi:10.1111/j.1532-5415.2000.tb03130.x

Dunn, W., Jamil, L. H., Brown, L. S., Wiesner, R. H., Kim, W. R., Narayanan Menon, K. V., ... Shah, V. (2005). MELD accurately predicts mortality in patients with alcoholic hepatitis. *Heptology, 41*, 353–358. doi:10.1002/hep.20503

Dwyer, J. P., Jayasekera, C., & Nicoll, A. (2014). Analgesia for the cirrhotic patient: A literature review and recommendations. *Journal of Gastroenterology Hepatology, 29*(7), 1356–1360. doi:10.1111/jgh.12560

Follwell, M., Burman, D., Le, L. W., Wakimoto, K., Seccareccia, D., Bryson, J., ... Zimmermann, C. (2009). Phase II study of an outpatient palliative care intervention in patients with metastatic cancer. *Journal of Clinical Oncology, 27*, 206–213. doi:10.1200/JCO.2008.17.7568

Folstein, M. F., Folstein, S. E., & McHugh, P. R. (1975). "Mini-mental status." A practical method for grading the cognitive state of patients for the clinician. *Journal of Psychiatric Research, 12*, 189–198. doi:10.1016/0022-3956(75)90026-6

Greer, J. A., Pirl, W. F., Jackson, V. A., Muzikansky, A., Lennes, I. T., Heist, R. S., ... Temel, J. S. (2012). Effect of early palliative care on chemotherapy use and end-of-life care in patients with metastatic non-small-cell lung cancer. *Journal of Clinical Oncology, 30*, 394–400. doi:10.1200/JCO.2011.35.7996

Hansen, L., Leo, M., Chang, M., Atif, Z., Naugler, S., & Schwartz, J. (2015). Symptom distress in patients with end-stage liver disease toward the end of life. *Gastroenterology Nursing, 38*, 201–210. doi:10.1097/SGA.0000000000000108

Hansen, L., Leo, M. C., Chang, M. F., Zucker, B. L., & Sasaki, A. (2014). Pain and self-care behaviours in adult patients with end-stage liver disease: A longitudinal description. *Journal of Palliative Care, 30*, 32–40.

Hansen, L., Press, N., Rosenkranz, S. J., Baggs, J. G., Kendall, J., Kerber, A., ... Chesnutt, M. S. (2012). Life-sustaining treatment decision making in the ICU for patients with ESLD: A longitudinal investigation. *Research in Nursing and Health, 35*, 518–532. doi:10.1002/nur.21488

Hansen, L., Sasaki, A., & Zucker, B. (2010). End-stage liver disease: Challenges and practice implications. *Nursing Clinics of North America, 45*, 411–426. doi:10.1016/j.cnur.2010.03.005

Hasselström, J., Eriksson, S., Persson, A., Rane, A., Svensson, J. O., & Säwe, J. (1990). The metabolism and bioavailability of morphine in patients with severe liver cirrhosis. *British Journal of Clinical Pharmacology, 29*, 289–297. doi:10.1111/j.1365-2125.1990.tb03638.x

Hope, A. A., & Morrison, R. S. (2011). Integrating palliative care with chronic liver disease. *Journal of Palliative Care, 27*, 20–27.

Hui, D., Kim, S. H., Roquemore, J., Dev, R., Chisholm, G., & Bruera, E. (2014). Impact of timing and setting of palliative care referral on quality of end-of-life care in cancer patients. *Cancer Epidemiology, Biomarkers and Prevention, 120*, 1743–1749. doi:10.1002/cncr.28628

Huynh, D. K., Selvanderan, S. P., Harley, H. A., Holloway, R. H., & Nguyen, N. Q. (2015). Nutritional care in hospitalized patients with chronic liver disease. *World Journal of Gastroenterology, 21*, 12835–12842. doi:10.3748/wjg.v21.i45.12835

Kamath, P. S., Wiesner, R. H., Malinchoc, M., Kremers, W., Therneau, T. M., Kosberg, C. L., ... Kim, W. R. (2001). A model to predict survival in patients with end-stage liver disease. *Hepatology, 33*, 464–470. doi:10.1053/jhep.2001.22172

Kochanek, K. D., Murphy, S. L., Jiaquan, X., & Tejada-Vera, B. (2016). National vital statistics reports. Retrieved from https://stacks.cdc.gov/view/cdc/40133

Kunzler-Heule, P., Beckmann, S., Mahrer-Imhof, R., Semela, D., & Handler-Schuster, D. (2016). Being an informal caregiver for a relative with liver cirrhosis and overt hepatic encephalopathy: A phenomenological study. *Journal of Clinical Nursing, 25*, 2559–2568. doi:10.1111/jocn.13298

Malik, P., Kohl, C., Holzner, B., Kemmler, G., Graziadei, I., Vogel, W., & Sperner-Unterweger, B. (2014). Distress in primary caregivers and patients listed for liver transplantation. *Psychiatry Research, 215*(1), 159–162. doi:10.1016/j.psychres.2013.08.046

Meier, D. E., & Beresford, L. (2008). Outpatient clinics are a new frontier for palliative care. *Journal of Palliative Medicine, 11*, 823–828. doi:10.1089/jpm.2008.9886

Mellinger, J. L., Moser, S., Welsh, D. E., Yosef, M. T., Van, T., McCurdy, H., … Su, G. L. (2016). Access to subspecialty care and survival among patients with liver disease. *American Journal of Gastroenterology, 111*, 838–844. doi:10.1038/ajg.2016.96

Miyazaki, E. T., dos Santos, R. J., Miyazaki, M. C., Domingos, N. M., Felicio, H. C., Rocha, M. F., … Silva, R. C. M. A. (2010). Patients on the waiting list for liver transplantation: Caregiver burden and stress. *Liver Transplantation, 16*, 1164–1168. doi:10.1002/lt.22130

Nardone, R., Taylor, A. C., Höller, Y., Brigo, F., Lochner, P., & Trinka, E. (2016). Minimal hepatic encephalopathy: A review. *Neuroscience Research, 111*, 1–12. doi:10.1016/j.neures.2016.04.009

National Institute of Diabetes and Digestive and Kidney Diseases, U.S. Department of Health and Human Services. (2014). Cirrhosis. Retrieved from https://www.niddk.nih.gov/health-information/liver-disease/cirrhosis

Organ Procurement and Transplantation Network, U.S. Department of Health and Human Services. (2017a). Transplants by donor type; U.S. transplants performed: January 1, 1988–May 31, 2017. Retrieved from https://optn.transplant.hrsa.gov/data/view-data-reports/national-data/#

Organ Procurement and Transplantation Network, U.S. Department of Health and Human Services. (2017b). Removal reason by year. Retrieved from https://optn.transplant.hrsa.gov/data/view-data-reports/national-data

Owens, D., & Flom, J. (2005). Integrating palliative and neurological critical care. *AACN Clinical Issues in Critical Care Nursing, 16*, 542–550.

Peery, A. F., Crockett, S. D., Brritt, A. S., Dellon, E. S., Gangarosa, L. M., Jensen, E. T., … Sandler, R. S. (2015). Burden of gastrointestinal disease in the United States. *Gastroenterology, 149*, 1731–1741. doi:10.1053/j.gastro.2015.08.045

Perri, G-A., Bunn, S., Oh, Y. J., Kassam, A., Berall, A., Karuza, J., & Khosravani, H. 2016). Attributes and outcomes of end-stage liver disease as compared to other noncancer patients admitted to a geriatric palliative care unit. Annals of Palliative Medicine, 5(2), 76–82. doi:10.21037/apm.2016.03.07

Petruzziello, A., Marigliano, S., Loquercio, G., Cozzolino, A., & Cacciapuoti, C. (2016). Global epidemiology of hepatitis C virus infection: An update of the distribution and circulation of hepatitis C virus genotypes. *World Journal of Gastroenterology, 22*, 7824–7784. doi:10.3748/wjg.v22.i34.7824

Poonja, Z., Brisebois, A., Veldhuyzen van Zanten, S., Tandon, P., Meeberg, G., & Karvellas, C. J. (2014). Patient with cirrhosis and denied liver transplantation rarely receive adequate palliative care or appropriate management. *Clinical Gastroenterology and Hepatology, 12*, 692–698. doi:10.1016/j.cgh.2013.08.027

Potosek, J., Curry, M., Buss, M., & Chittenden, E. (2014). Integration of palliative care in end-stage liver disease and liver transplantation. *Journal of Palliative Medicine, 17*, 1271–1277. doi:10.1089/jpm.2013.0167

Rabow, M., Kvale, E., Barbour, L., Cassel, J. B., Cohen, S., Jackson, V., … Weissman, D. (2013). Moving upstream: A review of the evidence of the impact of outpatient palliative care [Review]. *Journal of Palliative Medicine, 16*, 1540–1549. doi:10.1089/jpm.2013.0153

Rakoski, M. O., & Volk, M. L. (2015). Palliative care for patients with end-stage liver disease: An overview. *Clinical Liver Disease, 6*, 19–21. doi:10.1002/cld.478

Rossaro, L., Troppmann, C., McVicar, J. P., Sturges, M., Fisher, K., & Meyers, F. J. (2004). A strategy for the simultaneous provision of pre-operative palliative care for patients awaiting liver transplantation. *Transplant International, 17*, 473–475. doi:10.1111/j.1432-2277.2004.tb00473.x

Roth, K., Lynn, J., Zhong, Z., Borum, M., & Dawson, N. V. (2000). Dying with end stage liver disease with cirrhosis: Insight from SUPPORT. *Journal of the American Geriatrics Society, 48*, S122–S130. doi:10.1111/j.1532-5415.2000.tb03121.x

Runyon, B. A. (2009). AASLD Practice Guidelines Committee. Management of adult patients with ascites due to cirrhosis: An update. *Hepatology, 49*, 2087–2107. doi:10.1002/hep.22853

Sangiovanni, A., Del Ninno, E., Fasani, P., De Fazio, C., Ronchi, G., Romeo, R., … Colombo, M. (2004). Increased survival of cirrhotic patients with a hepatocellular carcinoma detected during surveillance. *Gastroenterology, 126*, 1005–1014. doi:10.1053/j.gastro.2003.12.049

Satapathy, S. K., & Sanyal, A. J. (2015). Epidemiology and natural history of nonalcoholic fatty liver disease. *Seminars in Liver Disease, 35*, 221–235. doi:10.1055/s-0035-1562943

Scaglione, S., Kliethermes, S., Cao, G., Shoham, D., Durazo, R., Luke, A., & Volk, M. L. (2015). The epidemiology of cirrhosis in the United States. *Journal of Clinical Gastroenterology, 49*, 690–696. doi:10.1097/MCG.0000000000000208

Sheer, T. A., & Runyon, B. A. (2005). Spontaneous bacterial peritonitis. *Digestive Diseases, 23*, 39–46. doi:10.1159/000084724

Smith, C. B., Nelson, J. E., Berman, A. R., Powell, C. A., Fleischman, J., Salazar-Schicchi, J., & Wisnivesky, J. P. (2012). Lung cancer physicians' referral practices for palliative care consultation. *Annals of Oncology, 23*, 382–387. doi:10.1093/annonc/mdr345

Sogolow, E. D., Lasker, J. N., Sharim, R. R., Weinrieb, R. M., & Sass, D. A. (2010). Stigma and liver disease. *Illness, Crisis and Loss, 18*, 229–255. doi:10.2190/IL.18.3.e

Spengler, E. K., & Loomba, R. (2015). Recommendations for diagnosis, referral for liver biopsy, and treatment of nonalcoholic fatty liver disease and nonalcoholic steatohepatitis. *Mayo Clinic Proceeding, 90*(9), 1233–1246. doi:10.1016/j.mayocp.2015.06.013

Temel, J. S., Greer, J. A., Muzikansky, A., Gallagher, E. R., Admane, S., Jackson, V. A., … Lynch, T. J. (2010). Early palliative care for patients with metastatic non-small cell lung cancer. *New England Journal of Medicine, 363*, 733–742. doi:10.1056/NEJMoa1000678

Vaughn-Sandler, V., Sherman, C., Aronsohn, A., & Volk, M. L. (2014). Consequences of perceived stigma among patients with cirrhosis. *Digestive Diseases and Sciences, 59*, 681–686. doi:10.1007/s10620-013-2942-0

World Health Organization. (2017). Hepatitis C. Retrieved from http://www.who.int/mediacentre/factsheets/fs164/en

Yao, F. Y., Ferrell, L., Bass, N. M., Bacchetti, P., Ascher, N. L., & Roberts, J. P. (2002). Liver transplantation for hepatocellular carcinoma: Comparison of the proposed UCSF criteria with the Milan criteria and the Pittsburgh modified TNM criteria. *Liver Transplantation, 8*, 765–774. doi:10.1053/jlts.2002.34892

Younossi, Z. M., Koenig, A. B., Abdelatif, D. Y. F., Henry, L., & Wymer, M. (2016). Global epidemiology of nonalcoholic fatty liver disease-meta-analytic assessment of prevalence, incidence, and outcomes. *Hepatology, 64*, 73–84. doi:10.1002/hep.28431

Patrick Kenny, Carl A. Kirton, Anna Krakowski, &
Deborah Witt Sherman

Palliative Care and HIV/AIDS

CHAPTER 19

KEY POINTS

- In countries with advanced healthcare, HIV/AIDS is managed as a chronic illness, while in resource poor countries, individuals without access to care are continuing to die from AIDS.
- HIV and AIDS are not synonymous terms but, rather, refer to the natural history or progression of the infection, ranging from asymptomatic infection to life-threatening illness.
- The components of high-quality HIV/AIDS palliative care include competent, skilled practitioners; confidential, nondiscriminatory, and culturally sensitive care; flexible and responsive care; collaborative and coordinated care; and fair access to care.
- The control of pain and symptoms associated with HIV/AIDS enables the patient family to expend their energies on spiritual and emotional healing, and the possibility for personal growth and transcendence even as death approaches.
- Knowledge regarding HIV disease enables nurses to offer effective and compassionate care to patients and families at all stages of HIV disease.

CASE STUDY

Terry, a 42-year-old woman, began to have daily episodes of diarrhea. She was admitted to the hospital with fever, fatigue, anorexia, nausea and vomiting, and weight loss of 15 lbs over the past 3 weeks. Her significant other was diagnosed with HIV 8 years ago. She was offered antiretroviral therapy (ART) but was nonadherent due to active substance use and is currently not on therapy. She also reported having unprotected sex on several occasions to support her drug habit. Terry's CD4 count was 70 cells/mm^3 with a viral load (VL) of 140,000 copies/mL. Her laboratory work indicated anemia and an elevated alkaline phosphatase. *Mycobacterium avium complex* (MAC) was confirmed by biopsy with acid fast bacterial (AFB) stain. On physical examination, she had an enlarged spleen, and lymph nodes were palpable in her inguinal area. The diagnosis was advanced-stage AIDS. Terry was begun on an antiretroviral regimen consisting of a protease inhibitor (PI) plus two nonnucleoside reverse transcriptase inhibitors (nNRTIs). She was also treated for MAC with azithromycin and rifabutin. Terry's mother and sister, although close by, have a poor relationship with her. Terry has a 10-year-old son from a previous relationship; her mother is the legal guardian of her son.

Terry responded well following MAC treatment and her diarrhea improved. However, she still remained weak and found it difficult to climb the stairs of her three-story walk-up apartment. Although Terry is Catholic, she finds little comfort in her faith, believing that her illness is a punishment from God for an abortion she had 2 years ago. Terry is becoming increasingly depressed. The home health aide, which assisted her in the first few weeks after discharge, was no longer available. It became clear to Terry that her life was threatened by the disease and she may never see her child grow up.

Despite being on ART, there was little improvement in her CD4 counts or in the lowering of her VL. Terry began to stay in bed for long periods of time during the day. She feared that she was never going to recover and worried about who would care for her son. After some additional testing, the infectious disease physician, who she saw at the AIDS clinic, changed her initial regimen. Terry was also treated with an antidepressant, and within weeks her mood, as well as her appetite, improved.

Within 3 months, Terry's quality of life (QOL) improved because she was free of opportunistic infections. Although unemployed, she kept busy with household activities and the care of her son. Even though Terry has two friends, who live in her building, they have their own personal and health-related issues. Terry understands the fragility of her condition, and this time is adherent to her medication regimen. She needs ongoing management of symptoms related to the disease and its treatment, as well as emotional and spiritual support, as she faces her own mortality.

It has been more than 35 years since the beginning of the HIV/AIDS epidemic, yet there remains no cure for this disease that has affected global health. In countries with advanced healthcare, the development and accessibility of ART has significantly reduced the mortality from HIV and has transformed AIDS into a manageable chronic illness, where patients can live long and productive lives. The global expansion of access to HIV treatment ranks among the great recent achievements in public health. Out of approximately 36.7 million people living with HIV globally today, by mid-2016 an estimated 18.2 million people were receiving ART therapy (World Health Organization [WHO], 2016). Several countries, those with limited resources, have reached or are close to achieving "universal access" to ART. Because of easier access of ART and multiple prevention choices, new HIV infections fell by 35%, and AIDS-related death fell by 28% (WHO, 2016). HIV incidence and mortality rates have been trending down as well. In 2015, there were 1.1 million AIDS-related deaths, as compared to 1.7 million in 2011 (WHO, 2016).

In the past decade the trajectory of HIV/AIDS has changed significantly, shifting to a disease less like cancer and more like a chronic disease such as diabetes or heart disease. In response to that, the care for people with HIV/AIDS needed to change as well, bringing palliative care (PC) to the front along with other treatments. PC for patients with HIV/AIDS is an approach to care for patients not only in the advanced stage of the illness but also as an aspect of care that begins in the early stage of illness and continues as the disease progresses (Dahlin, 2013). The goal of PC is to minimize and prevent suffering for patients who are dealing with serious illness, including HIV/AIDS, at any stage of the disease. PC offers physical, emotional, social, and spiritual support to promote, maximize, and maintain good QOL of patients and their families. Despite the advent of effective pharmacological therapy and its availability, patients with HIV/AIDS still continue to experience a high burden of pain and other chronic symptoms through the disease trajectory, which presents many PC challenges (Merlins, Tucker, Saag, & Selvyn, 2013).

■ INCIDENCE AND PREVALENCE

AIDS has been characterized as a volatile and dynamic epidemic, which has spread globally. This epidemic is complex due to the virus's ability to mutate and cross all socioeconomic, cultural, political, and geographic boundaries. As a worldwide epidemic, HIV/AIDS has affected more than 36 million people. In 2015, an estimated 2.1 million people acquired HIV, with an estimated 1.1 million people dying from AIDS (WHO, 2016). In the United States, an estimated 1.2 million people are living with HIV infection, but 1 out of 8 of them do not know that they are infected (Centers for Disease Control and Prevention [CDC], 2016). Certain groups, including African Americans, Latinos, and gay and bisexual men of all races/ethnicities, continue to be disproportionately affected (CDC, 2016).

Perinatal transmission of HIV has seen a dramatic decline in the United States. This is largely due to a highly effective public health initiative focusing on prevention and early intervention for mothers with HIV. Prior to effective and timely treatment, more than 2,000 HIV-infected infants were born each year. Based on the most recent data, approximately 8,500 women living with HIV give birth annually. With such great advances in HIV research, prevention, and treatment, many women living with HIV virus can now give birth to their babies without transmitting the virus. An estimated 21,956 cases of perinatally acquired HIV infections were prevented between 1994 and 2010, with the average of about 1,372 new cases per year (CDC, 2017).

■ PATHOGENESIS OF HIV

The HIV virus survives by reproducing itself in a host cell, replacing the genetic machinery of that cell, and eventually destroying the cell. The HIV is a retrovirus whose life cycle consists of (a) attachment of the virus to the cell, which is affected by cofactors that influence the virus's ability to enter the host cell; (b) uncoating of the virus; (c) reverse transcription by an enzyme called reverse transcriptase, which converts two strands of viral RNA to DNA; (d) integration of newly synthesized proviral DNA into the cell nucleus, assisted by the viral enzyme integrase, which becomes the template for new viral components; (e) transcription of proviral DNA into messenger RNA; (f) movement of messenger RNA outside the cell nucleus, where it is translated into viral proteins and enzymes; and (g) assembly and release of mature virus particles out of the host cell (Fan, Conner, & Villarreal, 2011).

These newly formed viruses have an affinity for any cell that has the CD4 molecule on its surface, such as T lymphocytes and macrophages, and become major viral targets. Because CD4 cells are the master coordinators of the immune-system response, the chronic destruction of these cells severely compromises individuals' immune status, leaving the host susceptible to opportunistic infections and eventual progression to AIDS.

Since the identification of the first case of HIV in 1981, there has been significant scientific advancements made in the diagnosis and treatment of the disease; specifically, the virus has been identified; screening for HIV infection has been implemented; biological and behavioral cofactors have been identified related to infection and disease progression; prophylactic treatments are available to prevent opportunistic infections; HIV-RNA quantitative assays have been developed to measure VL; combination ARTs are available to treat the infection; and vaccines are being tested (Fan et al., 2011). Pre-exposure prophylaxis (PreEP) has become an important part of HIV prevention ever since it was approved by the U.S. Food and Drug Administration (FDA) in 2012. Daily regimen with tenofovir disoproxil fumarate (TDF) regimen recommended for sexually active adults at a substantial risk of HIV acquisition, men who have sex with men (MSM), heterosexually active men and women, adult injection-drug users, and heterosexually active women and men whose partners

are known to have HIV has shown to be effective up to 80% (CDC, 2014; Marrazzo, 2017). Current data on the efficacy and safety of PreEP is not sufficient for the population of adolescents (CDC, 2014).

■ DISEASE TRAJECTORY

HIV and AIDS are not synonymous terms but, rather, refer to the natural history or progression of the infection, ranging from asymptomatic infection to life-threatening illness characterized by opportunistic infections and cancers. Without treatment, this continuum of illness is associated with progressive immune-system dysfunction (as evidenced by a decrease in CD4 cell count) and persistent viral replication (as evidenced by a rise in plasma HIV-RNA levels).

The natural history of HIV infection begins with acute HIV infection in which the virus enters the body and replicates in large numbers in the host cell. As a result, there is a rapid depletion in the number of CD4 cells and a significant rise in viral replication (as measured by the VL) during the first 2 weeks of the infection. Within 5 to 30 days of infection, 70% of individuals experience flu-like symptoms, such as fever, sore throat, skin rash, lymphadenopathy, and myalgia. Other symptoms of primary HIV infection include fatigue, splenomegaly, anorexia, nausea and vomiting, meningitis, retro-orbital pain, neuropathy, and mucocutaneous ulceration (Pilcher, Eron, Galvin, Gay, & Cohen, 2004). Within 6 to 12 weeks of the initial infection, the production of HIV antibodies results in seroconversion. If tested at this time, the patient will be diagnosed as HIV positive.

Clinical latency refers to the chronic, clinically asymptomatic state in which there is a decreased VL and resolution of symptoms of acute infection. At this point, there is continuous viral replication in the lymph nodes with more than 10 billion copies of the virus being made every day.

After years of HIV infection, the individual enters a stage that is apparent by conditions indicative primarily of defects in cell-mediated immunity. Symptomatic infection generally occurs when CD4 counts fall below 500 cells/mm^3, which indicates the progression of HIV disease. Symptoms of advancing HIV infection include oral candidiasis and hairy leukoplakia as well as ulcerative lesions of the mucosa. Gynecological infections are common in women with HIV disease as well as dermatological manifestations, which include bacterial, fungal, viral, neoplastic, and other conditions such as exacerbation of psoriasis, severe pruritus, or the development of recurrent pruritic papules (CDC, 2013; Lazenby, 2012; Oramasionwu et al., 2012).

When the CD4 count drops below 200 cells/mm^3, HIV infection now meets one of the Centers for Disease Control and Prevention's definitions of AIDS (CDC, 2013). With AIDS, patients often experience several opportunistic infections or cancers (see the following discussion). When the CD4 cell count drops below 50 cells/mm^3, the immune system is so impaired that both HIV- and non-HIV-related infections become commonplace. With advanced disease, individuals may experience symptomatic health problems such as shortness of breath from pneumonia, difficulty swallowing from oral candidiasis, depression, dementia, skin infections, anxiety, incontinence, fatigue, isolation, bed dependency, wasting syndrome, and significant pain.

AIDS-Related Opportunistic Infections and Comorbidities

Opportunistic infections are the greatest cause of morbidity and mortality in individuals with HIV disease. Given the compromised immune system of HIV-infected individuals, there is a wide spectrum of pathogens that can produce primary, life-threatening infections, particularly when the CD4 cell counts fall below 200 cells/mm^3.

Given the weakened immune systems of HIV-infected persons, even previously acquired infections can be reactivated. Most of these opportunistic infections are incurable and can at best be palliated to control the acute stage of infection and prevent recurrence through long-term suppressive therapy. In addition, patients with HIV/AIDS often experience concurrent or consecutive opportunistic infections and various malignancies that are severe and cause a great number of symptoms. A large Veterans Aging Cohort Study that compared HIV-infected patients ($n = 30,564$) with uninfected patients ($n = 68,123$) showed that HIV-infected patients had a higher risk for non-AIDS-related diseases and cardiovascular, renal, and non-AIDS-defining cancers than the uninfected patients, but the onset of those diseases occurred at similar ages in both groups (Althoff et al., 2015). Also, the overall proportion of deaths that are attributed to non-AIDS diseases has not only remained significantly higher, but has increased, as opposed to deaths due to AIDS-related diseases. In a recent retrospective multicohort collaboration review of underlying causes of death in people with HIV between 1999 and 2011, Smith et al. (2014) found that only 29% of deaths were AIDS related, with the remaining causes contributing to non-AIDS-defining cancers (15%), liver disease (13%), and cardiovascular disease (11%). In 2014 only half of the deaths were related directly to HIV (CDC, 2016).

In 2015 almost 80% of patients diagnosed with HIV were aged 20 to 49, followed by patients aged 50 years and older (17%; CDC, 2016). Increasing age, comorbid conditions, and markers of functional status are more predictive of mortality than traditional HIV-prognostic variables (Justice, 2010; Piggott et al., 2013). AIDS involves multiple symptoms not only from the disease processes but also from the side effects of medications and other therapies. Patients with AIDS present with complex care issues because they experience bouts of severe illness and debilitation alternating with periods of symptom stabilization.

■ HIV/AIDS AND PALLIATIVE CARE

PC is the comprehensive management of the physical, psychological, social, spiritual, and existential needs of patients with incurable progressive illness (Dahlin, 2013). PC has become an important component of AIDS care from diagnosis to death, involving ongoing prevention, health promotion, and health maintenance to promote the patient's QOL throughout the illness trajectory. The components of high-quality HIV/AIDS PC, as identified by healthcare providers, include competent, skilled practitioners; confidential, nondiscriminatory, and culturally sensitive care; flexible and responsive care; collaborative and coordinated care; and fair access to care. Resources aimed at prevention, health promotion and maintenance, symptom surveillance, and end-of-life (EOL) care are essential (Gysels et al., 2013). The treatment of not only chronic debilitating conditions but also superimposed acute opportunistic infections and related symptoms is necessary to maintain a good QOL. As one example, health prevention measures, such as ongoing intravenous (IV) therapies to prevent blindness from cytomegalovirus (CMV) retinitis, must be available to patients with AIDS to maintain their QOL.

The precepts of PC include comprehensive care with respect for patient goals, preferences, and choices, and acknowledgment of caregivers' concerns (Dahlin, 2013). These precepts are fundamental in addressing the complex needs of patients and families with HIV/AIDS and require the coordinated care of an interprofessional PC team, involving physicians, advanced practice nurses, staff nurses, social workers, dietitians, physiotherapists, and clergy. Therapeutic interventions and decisions for patients with advanced AIDS should not only include the patient's expectations, preferences, and goals, but also the benefits and burdens of antiretroviral therapy, and advance care planning as part of the clinical discussions and planning for the future (Houben, Spruit, Groenen, Wouters, & Janssen, 2014). Healthcare personnel taking care of patients with advanced AIDS should, in addition to the medical management and providing adequate relief from pain, maintain hope while helping the patient and his or her family to confront the chronic and terminal nature of the illness. Healthcare providers and patients must determine the balance between aggressive and supportive efforts, particularly when increasing debility, wasting, and deteriorating cognitive function are evident in the face of advanced disease. As the unit of care is the patient and his or her family, the PC team offers support not only for patients to live as fully as possible until death but also for the family to help them to cope during the patient's illness and in their own bereavement (Dahlin, 2013).

Although the hospice and PC movement developed as a community response to those who were dying, primarily of cancer, the advent of the AIDS epidemic made it necessary for hospices to begin admitting patients with AIDS. This meant applying the old model of cancer care to patients with a new infectious, progressive, and terminal disease. Unlike the course of cancer, which is relatively predictable once the disease progresses beyond cure, AIDS patients experience a series of serious and sometimes life-threatening opportunistic infections. With appropriate treatment offered, there may be resolution of an AIDS-related illness or chronic therapy may be necessary. Therefore, the underlying goal of AIDS care remains one of palliation.

The predominant thinking is of HIV disease as a chronic illness. Both public and private third-party payers have reimbursed for EOL care when physicians have verified a life expectancy of less than 6 months. However, private third-party payers are not required to provide hospice or PC services. Yet, generally speaking, comprehensive AIDS care is publicly funded. While no studies exist that examine the cost of AIDS-related palliative or hospital care, the cost of care in cities with large HIV populations indicate that as CD4 cells decline, particularly less than 50 cells/mm^3, annual healthcare expenditures are 2.6 times greater than expenditures for patients with CD4 greater than 350 cells/mm^3. Early diagnosis of HIV and initiation of treatment leads to the prevention of complications. Although it does increase the lifetime costs of treating the illness, at the same time it reduces the number of new infections by 50% and improves length and QOL (Farnham et al., 2013).

An additional barrier to PC are the patients themselves. There is a need to shift the perception of PC as only EOL care and to promote PC as an aggressive approach to enhance QOL throughout the course of the illness. Over the years, there have been public initiatives and media campaigns to improve the care of the seriously ill in the United States and to inform patients and families about the availability of PC across healthcare settings.

A review of the evidence of barriers and inequality in HIV care by Harding et al. (2005) found that there is increased complexity in the balance of providing concurrent curative and palliative therapies given the prolongation of life span as a result of ART therapy. Harding and colleagues propose the need for multidimensional PC assessment for different populations; basic PC skills training for all clinical staff in standard assessments; the development of referral criteria and systems for patients with complex PC needs; and the availability of specialist consultation across all settings.

When patients are in the advanced stage of AIDS, the following criteria are considered regarding the admission to hospice: CD4 count of less than 25 cells/mm^3, persistent VL of more than 100,000 copies/mL, history of opportunistic infections, functional status, and statistical prognosis (HIV Disease, 2017). These criteria give a better understanding of the patient's prognosis and needs. Hospices are offering the necessary support to patients with AIDS at the end of life. Different models of PC are being developed, including partnerships with community hospitals or agencies.

Assessment of Patients With HIV/AIDS

Throughout the course of their illness, individuals with HIV disease require primary care services to identify early signs of opportunistic infections and to minimize related symptoms and complications. This includes a complete health history, physical examination, and laboratory data including determination of immunological and viral status.

■ **Health History.** In the care of patients with HIV/AIDS, the health history should include the following (Sherman, 2006):

- History of present illness, including a review of those factors that led to HIV testing
- Past medical history, particularly those conditions that may be exacerbated by HIV disease or its treatments, such as diabetes mellitus, hypertriglyceridemia, or chronic or active hepatitis B infection
- Childhood illnesses and vaccinations for preventing common infections such as polio, DPT, or measles
- Medication history, including the patient's knowledge of the types of medications, side effects, adverse reactions, drug interactions, and administration recommendations
- Sexual history, regarding sexual behaviors and preferences and the history of sexually transmitted diseases, which can exacerbate HIV disease progression
- Lifestyle habits, such as the past and present use of recreational drugs, including alcohol, which may accelerate progression of disease, and cigarette smoking, which may suppress appetite or be associated with opportunistic infections such as oral candidiasis, hairy leukoplakia, and bacterial pneumonia
- Dietary habits, including risks related to foodborne illnesses such as hepatitis A
- Travel history, to countries in Asia, Africa, and South America, where the risk of opportunistic infections increases
- Complete systems review, to provide indications of clinical manifestations of new opportunistic infections or cancers as well as AIDS-related complications from both the disease and its treatments

■ **Physical Examination.** A physical examination should begin with a general assessment of vital signs and height and weight as well as the overall appearance and mood. A complete head-to-toe assessment is important and may reveal various findings common to individuals with HIV/AIDS such as the following (Sherman, 2006):

- Oral cavity assessment may indicate candida, oral hairy leukoplakia, or Kaposi sarcoma (KS).
- Funduscopic assessment may reveal visual changes associated with CMV retinitis; glaucoma screening annually is also recommended.
- Lymph node assessment may indicate adenopathy detected at any stage of the disease.
- Dermatological assessment may indicate various cutaneous manifestations that occur throughout the course of the illness such as HIV exanthema, KS, or infectious complications such as dermatomycosis.
- Neuromuscular assessment may determine various central, peripheral, or autonomic nervous system disorders and signs and symptoms of conditions such as meningitis, encephalitis, dementia, or peripheral neuropathies.
- Cardiovascular assessment may reveal cardiomyopathy.
- Gastrointestinal assessment may indicate organomegaly, specifically splenomegaly or hepatomegaly, particularly in patients with a history of substance abuse as well as signs related to parasitic intestinal infections. Annual stool guaiac analysis and rectal examination, as well as sigmoidoscopy every 5 years, are also parts of health maintenance.
- Reproductive system assessment may reveal occult sexually transmitted diseases or malignancies, as well as vaginal candidiasis, cervical dysplasia, pelvic inflammatory disease, or rectal lesions in women with HIV/AIDS as well as urethral discharge and rectal lesions or malignancies in HIV-infected men. Health maintenance in individuals with HIV/AIDS also includes annual mammograms in women older than 40 years, as well as testicular examinations in men, and prostate screening examinations as per current recommendations.

■ **Laboratory Data.** Evaluation of these laboratory data is important in assisting the healthcare practitioner in making therapeutic decisions. The following laboratory tests performed during initial patient visits can be used to stage HIV disease and to select ART (Department of Health and Human Services [HHS], 2013):

- HIV antibody testing (if prior documentation is not available or if HIV-RNA is below the assay's limit of detection)
- CD4 T-cell count (CD4 count)
- Plasma HIV-RNA (VL)
- Complete blood count, chemistry profile, transaminase levels, blood urea nitrogen (BUN), and creatinine, urinalysis, and serologies for hepatitis A, B, and C viruses
- Fasting blood glucose and serum lipids
- Genotypic resistance testing at entry into care, regardless of whether ART will be initiated immediately; for

patients who have HIV-RNA levels less than 500 to 1,000 copies/mL, viral amplification for resistance testing may not always be successful

The HHS's (2013) panel on clinical practices for the treatment of HIV recommends that the CD4 count and the VL be measured upon entry into care and every 3 to 6 months subsequently. Immediately before a patient is started on ART, the patient's HIV-RNA (VL) should be measured, and again 2 to 8 weeks after treatment is initiated, to determine the effectiveness of the therapy. With adherence to the medication schedule, it is expected that the HIV-RNA will decrease to undetectable levels (less than 50 copies/mL) in 16 to 24 weeks after the initiation of therapy (HHS, 2013). If a patient does not significantly respond to therapy, the clinician should evaluate adherence, repeat the test, and rule out malabsorption or drug–drug interactions.

The decision regarding laboratory testing is based on the stage of HIV disease, the medical processes warranting initial assessment or follow-up, and consideration of the patient benefit-to-burden ratio (Sherman, 2006). Complete blood counts are often measured with each VL determination or with a change in ART, particularly with patients on drugs known to cause anemia. Chemistry profiles are done to assess liver function, lipid status, and glycemia every 3 to 6 months or with a change in therapy, and are determined by the patient's ART, baseline determinations, and coinfections. Abnormalities in these profiles may occur as a result of ART. Increasing hepatic dysfunction is evident by elevations in the serum transaminases (aspartate aminotransferase [AST], alanine transaminase [ALT], and bilirubin). Blood work should also include hepatitis C serology (antibody), hepatitis B serology, and *Toxoplasma* immunoglobulin G (IgG) serology (HHS, 2013).

Urine analysis should be done annually unless the person is on ART, which may require more frequent follow-up to check for toxicity. Syphilis studies should be done annually; however, patients with low positive titers should have follow-up testing at 3, 6, 9, 12, and 24 months. Gonorrhea and chlamydia tests are encouraged every 6 to 12 months if the patient is sexually active. Annual Papanicolaou (Pap) smears are also indicated, with recommendations for Pap smears every 3 to 6 months in HIV-infected women who are symptomatic. In addition, HIV-infected persons should be tested for IgG antibody to *Toxoplasma* soon after the diagnosis of HIV infection to detect latent infection with *Toxoplasma gondii*. *Toxoplasma* seronegative persons who are not taking a primary care provider (PCP) prophylactic regimen known to be active against toxoplasma encephalitis (TE) should be retested for IgG antibody to *Toxoplasma* when their CD4$^+$ counts decline to less than 100 cells/mm^3 to determine whether they have seroconverted and are therefore at risk of TE (CDC, 2013).

Individuals should be tested for latent tuberculosis infection (LTBI) at the time of their HIV diagnosis, regardless of their TB risk category, and then annually if negative. LTBI diagnosis can be achieved with the use of tuberculin skin test (TST) or by interferon gamma release assay (IGRA) using the patient's serum. A TST is considered positive in patients with induration of greater than or equal to 5 mm. An IGRA is reported as positive or negative. Any positive test warrants chest radiograph for active disease and consideration of antituberculosis therapy based on history, laboratory, physical, and radiographic findings.

Management of HIV/AIDS

◼ **The Use of Antiretroviral Therapy.** The goal of ART is to slow the disease progression and limit the occurrence of opportunistic infections. ART is administered to maximize long-term suppression of HIV-RNA and restore or preserve immune-system function, thereby reducing morbidity and mortality and promoting QOL (HHS, 2016). Historically, the assessment of CD4 cell count was used to determine the initiation of ART, with ART primarily reserved for CD4 counts below 350 cells/mm^3. Currently, HIV therapy is recommended for all HIV patients regardless of CD4 cell count (HHS, 2013). When initiating therapy, consideration must be given to toxicities associated with certain antiretroviral medications, such as elevations in serum levels of triglycerides and cholesterol, alterations in fat distribution, or insulin resistance and diabetes mellitus. However, the benefits of early therapy include earlier suppression of viral replication, preservation of the immune-system functioning, prolongation of disease-free survival, and a decrease in the risk of HIV transmission (HHS, 2013).

Classifications of Antiretroviral Therapies and Recommendations

Antiretroviral drugs are broadly classified by the phase of the retrovirus life cycle that the drug inhibits. Specifically, they act in the following ways:

- Nucleoside reverse transcriptase inhibitors (NRTIs) interfere with the action of an HIV protein called reverse transcriptase, which the virus needs to make new copies of itself.
- Non-nucleoside reverse transcriptase inhibitors (NNRTIs) inhibit reverse transcriptase directly by binding to the enzyme and interfering with its function.
- PIs target viral assembly by inhibiting the activity of protease, which is an enzyme used by HIV to cleave nascent proteins for final assembly of new virions.
- Integrase inhibitors inhibit the enzyme integrase, which is responsible for the integration of viral DNA into the DNA of the infected cell.
- Entry inhibitors (fusion inhibitors and CCR5 antagonists) interfere with binding, fusion, and entry

of HIV-1 to the host cell by blocking one of several targets. Maraviroc and enfuvirtide are the two currently available agents in this class.

When patients are naïve to ART, it is recommended that they begin a combination antiretroviral regimen. Preferred regimens are either nNRTI based, PI based, or integrase inhibitor based. The exact combinations recommended change based on the emergence of high-quality evidence that supports its use. The reader should refer to the HHS website to obtain the latest recommendations (aidsinfo.nih.gov/guidelines). The goal of the therapy is maximal VL suppression.

If there is insufficient viral suppression, which is evidenced by an increase in VL, inadequate increase in CD4 cell counts, evidence of disease progression, adverse clinical effects of therapy, or compromised adherence caused by the inconvenience of difficult regimens, it is appropriate to consider a change in the medication regimen. The decision to change therapy involves the consideration of whether other drug choices are available, the results of baseline resistance assays, and the patient's commitment to adhere to the therapy.

The criteria for considering changing a patient's antiretroviral regimen include the following (HHS, 2013):

- When there is virologic or incomplete failure; when the HIV VL fails to fall to a level less than 200 copies/mL or less than 50 copies/mL by 48 weeks after starting therapy; when there is virologic rebound, that is, when there is HIV-RNA greater than 200 copies after complete suppression
- When there is immunologic failure, persistent decline in CD4 cell, or failure to achieve an adequate CD4 response despite virologic suppression
- The occurrence or recurrence of HIV-related events after at least 3 months on an antiretroviral regimen (excluding immune reconstitution syndrome)

A change in an antiretroviral regimen can also be guided by drug-resistance tests, such as genotyping and phenotyping assays. Consultation with an HIV specialist is often of value.

Considerations Relevant to Antiretroviral Therapy in Palliative Care

Clinicians must consider possible drug interactions with the administration of drugs in the treatment of HIV/AIDS and relief of symptoms. Pharmacokinetic interactions occur when the administration of one agent changes the plasma concentration of another agent. Pharmacodynamic interactions also occur when a drug interacts with the biologically active sites and changes the pharmacological effect of the drug without altering the plasma concentration. In PC, drug interactions have been reported for patients who are receiving methadone for pain management and who begin therapy with an nNRTI, nevirapine. These individuals have reported symptoms of opioid withdrawal within 4 to 8 days of beginning nevirapine due to its effect on the cytochrome P-450 (CYP) metabolic enzyme CYP3A4 and its induction of methadone metabolism (HHS, 2013, 2016).

Furthermore, patients and healthcare providers should discuss the continuation of ART in hospice or palliative settings. Such decisions are often contingent on the feelings of patients regarding the therapy. Patients may be asked such questions as "How do you feel when you take your antiretroviral medications?" Patients who enter hospice may have a greater acceptance of their mortality and may wish to stop antiretrovirals because of the side effects. However, patients may wish to continue ART because of its symptom relief and the prevention of future symptoms related to opportunistic infections. Alexander (2011) has recommended that antiretrovirals be discontinued if the drugs cause burdensome symptoms or the patient no longer wants to use the drug. However, if the patient is asymptomatic and wishes to continue with ART, medications should be continued with close clinical assessment. Facilitating discussion of benefits and burdens of ART is an important aspect of PC, and the decision to discontinue ART for hospice patients with AIDS should be a part of comprehensive PC.

In the hospice and PC settings, it is important for clinicians to discuss with patients and families their goals of care to make important decisions regarding the appropriateness of curative, palliative, or both types of interventions. More specifically, examples of clinical decisions regarding PC or disease-specific treatment include: (a) consideration of risks versus benefits of treatments, like the use of blood transfusions; (b) the use of psychostimulants, or corticosteroids, to treat fatigue in patients with late-stage AIDS; (c) the use of aggressive antiemetic therapy for PI-induced nausea and vomiting; (d) continuation versus discontinuation of ARTs that may result in severe side effects; (e) continuation of suppressive therapy; and (f) the use of prophylactic medications in dying patients.

Symptom Management in HIV Disease

Patients with HIV/AIDS require symptom management not only for chronic debilitating opportunistic infections and malignancies but also for the side effects of treatments and other therapies. Personal characteristics that interact with both HIV diagnosis and its medical management can influence symptom experience. The most prevalent symptoms in the AIDS population are fatigue (54%–85%), pain (63%–80%), nausea (43%–49%), and constipation (34%–35%); other symptoms include depression, breathlessness, insomnia, diarrhea, anorexia, and anxiety (Solano, Gomes & Higginson, 2006). In a prospective longitudinal study, 317 men and women living with HIV/AIDS in the San Francisco Bay Area completed the Memorial Symptom Assessment Scale, which is designed to estimate the prevalence, severity, and distress of each symptom and global symptom burden. The median number of symptoms was nine, and symptoms experienced by more than half the sample population included lack of energy (65%), drowsiness (57%), difficulty sleeping (56%), and pain (55%). Global symptom burden was unrelated to age or CD4 cell count. Those with an AIDS diagnosis had significantly higher symptom burden scores as did those currently receiving ART. According to Lee et al. (2009), African Americans reported fewer symptoms than whites or mixed/other race, and women reported more symptom burden after controlling for AIDS diagnosis and race.

Symptom and comfort measures at the end of life for HIV-infected patients share many of the features seen in non-HIV-infected patients at the end of life because a large percentage of late-stage AIDS patients are now dying of non-AIDS-defining illnesses. Therefore, the translation of basic principles in pain and symptom management should be used for HIV-infected patients at the end of life (Fausto & Selwyn, 2011).

The five broad principles fundamental to successful symptom management have not changed since first described and published by Newshan and Sherman in 1999. These principles are: (a) taking the symptoms seriously, (b) assessment, (c) diagnosis, (d) treatment, and (e) ongoing evaluation (Newshan & Sherman, 1999). Patient's self-report of symptoms should be taken seriously by the practitioner and acknowledged as a real experience of the patient. An important rule in symptom management is to anticipate the symptom and attempt to prevent it. The assessment and diagnosis of signs and symptoms of disease and treatment of side effects require a thorough history and physical examination. Questions as to when the symptom began and its location, duration, severity, and quality, as well as factors that exacerbate or alleviate the symptom, are important to ask. Patients can also be asked to rate the severity of a symptom by using a numerical scale from 0 to 10, with 0 being *no symptom* to 10 being *extremely severe*. Such scales can also be used to rate how much a symptom interferes with activities of daily life, with 0 meaning *no interference* and 10 meaning *extreme interference*. One of the most frequently used tools to assess symptoms is the Edmonton Symptom Assessment Scale (ESAS), a validated and reliable instrument to assist in the assessment of nine common symptoms: pain, tiredness, drowsiness, nausea, appetite, shortness of breath, depression, anxiety, and well-being. When using this tool, patients who score greater than seven have a self-defined symptom burden, meaning that their symptoms significantly impact their physical, emotional, and social functioning. Use of this tool is a simple and effective method of assessing the impact of select symptoms on individual QOL (Selby et al., 2011). When a patient seeks medical care for a specific symptom, the clinician should conduct a focused history including any past medical illnesses that may exacerbate HIV disease, a comprehensive physical examination, and judicious diagnostic testing. A detailed assessment of current medications, chemotherapy and radiation therapy, or complementary therapies such as biofeedback, herbal therapies, or yoga should also be ascertained to determine the effects and side effects of treatment, and to prevent drug interactions. In the case of extremely advanced disease, practitioners must reevaluate the benefits versus burden of diagnostic testing and treatments, particularly the need for daily blood draws or more invasive and uncomfortable procedures. When the decision of the practitioners, patient, and family is that all testing and aggressive treatments are more burdensome than beneficial, their discontinuation is warranted. Ongoing evaluation of the effectiveness of traditional, experimental, and complementary therapies is the key to symptom management. Changes in therapies are often necessary because concurrent or sequential illness or conditions occur.

In an article regarding the symptom experience of patients with HIV/AIDS, Holzemer (2002) emphasized a number of key tenets, specifically (a) the patient is the gold standard for understanding the symptom experience; (b) patients should not be labeled *asymptomatic* early in the course of the infection because they often experience symptoms of anxiety, fear, and depression; (c) nurses are not necessarily good judges of patients' symptoms, as they frequently underestimate the frequency and intensity of HIV signs and symptoms; however, following assessment, they can answer specific questions about a symptom, such as location, intensity, duration, and so forth; (d) nonadherence to treatment regimens is associated with greater frequency and intensity of symptoms; (e) greater frequency and intensity of symptoms leads to lower QOL; (f) symptoms may or may not correspond with physiological markers; and (g) patients use few self-care symptom management strategies other than medication.

Pain in HIV/AIDS

Pain syndromes in patients with AIDS are diverse in nature and etiology. For patients with AIDS, pain is a common symptom, which often becomes chronic in nature and can occur in more than one site. Patients may experience neuropathic pain, such as peripheral neuropathy resulting from the use of ARTs, or from nerves directly damaged by HIV itself, as well as pain in the abdomen, oral cavity, esophagus, skin, perirectal area, chest, joints, muscles, and headache. A systematic review completed by Parker, Stein, and Jelsma (2014) reports that pain in the lower limbs is the most frequently reported pain, followed by headache and neck pain. In terms of the intensity of the pain, most patients reported moderate-to-severe pain, which had significant impact on their QOL (Parker et al., 2014). Pain can also be related to HIV/AIDS therapies

such as antibacterials (e.g., isoniazid, ethambutol), chemotherapy, radiation, surgery, and procedures (Lorenz, Cunningham, Spritzer, & Hays, 2006). Patients may be suffering from inflammatory or infiltrative processes and somatic and visceral pain. Studies have also shown that patients with moderate-to-severe chronic pain are more likely to be severely depressed and are more likely to be taking antidepressant medications and prescription opioids (Uebelacker et al., 2015). Frequent reassessment of pain to evaluate the effectiveness of pain therapy is very important in providing quality PC.

Following a complete assessment, including a history and physical examination, an individualized pain management plan should be developed to treat the underlying cause of the pain, often arising from underlying infections associated with HIV disease. The principles of pain management in the PC of patients with AIDS are the same as for patients with cancer and include regularity of dosing, individualization of dosing, and the use of combinations of medications. The three-step guidelines for pain management as outlined by WHO should be used for patients with HIV disease. This approach advocates for the selection of analgesics based on the severity of pain. For mild-to-moderate pain, anti-inflammatory drugs such as nonsteroidal anti-inflammatory drugs (NSAIDs) or acetaminophen are recommended. However, the use of NSAIDs in patients with AIDS requires the awareness of toxicity and adverse reactions because they are highly protein bound, and the free fraction available is increased in AIDS patients who are cachectic or wasted. For moderate-to-severe pain that is persistent, opioids of increasing potency are recommended, beginning with opioids such as codeine, hydrocodone, or oxycodone, each available with or without aspirin or acetaminophen, and advancing to more potent opioids such as morphine, hydromorphone (Dilaudid), methadone (Dolophine), or fentanyl either orally, intravenously, or transdermally. In conjunction with NSAIDs and opioids, adjuvant therapies are also recommended (Trescot et al., 2008), such as the following:

- Tricyclic antidepressants, heterocyclic and noncyclic antidepressants, and serotonin reuptake inhibitors for neuropathic pain
- Psychostimulants to improve opioid analgesia and decrease sedation
- Phenothiazine to relieve associated anxiety or agitation
- Butyrophenones to relieve anxiety and delirium
- Antihistamines to improve opioid analgesia and relieve anxiety, insomnia, and nausea
- Corticosteroids to decrease pain associated with an inflammatory component or with bone pain
- Benzodiazepines for neuropathic pain, anxiety, and insomnia

Caution is noted, however, with use of PIs because they may interact with some analgesics. For example, ritonavir has been associated with potentially lethal interactions with meperidine, propoxyphene, piroxicam, codeine, hydrocodone, oxycodone, and methadone, increasing their levels, resulting in drug toxicity. Furthermore, for patients with HIV disease who have high fever, the increase in body temperature may lead to an increased absorption of transdermally administered fentanyl, leading to toxic levels of drug.

To ensure appropriate dosing when changing the route of administration of opioids, or changing from one opioid to another, the use of an equianalgesic conversion chart is suggested (see Table 20.8). As with all patients, oral medications should be used, if possible, with around-the-clock (ATC) dosing at regular intervals, and the use of rescue doses for breakthrough pain. Often, controlled-release morphine or oxycodone are effective drugs for patients with chronic pain from HIV/AIDS. Taking under consideration that patients with HIV infection take several medications per day, minimizing the number of medications is the best option. Sustained-release opioids can provide 8 to 12 hours of analgesia, whereas transdermal opioids do not require taking the pills at all. In the case of neuropathic pain, often experienced with HIV/AIDS, tricyclic antidepressants such as amitriptyline, or anticonvulsants such as Neurontin, can be very effective (Trescot et al., 2008). However, the use of neuroleptics must be weighed against an increased sensitivity of AIDS patients to the extrapyramidal side effects of these drugs. In addition to opioids and adjuvant medications, such as tricyclic antidepressants or anticonvulsants, the use of cannabis has shown symptom-relieving benefits from neuropathic pain, stress, and anorexia (Harris et al., 2014). Unfortunately, the use of cannabis for medical purposes, especially for patients with HIV/AIDS, poses many challenges, because of the significant overlap between the use of medicinal cannabis versus recreational use that may precede the HIV diagnosis (Harris et al., 2014).

If the cause of pain is the increasing tumor size, radiation therapy can also be very effective in pain management by reducing the tumor size as well as the perception of pain. In cases of refractory pain, nerve blocks are available through neurosurgical procedures for pain management. Increasingly, epidural analgesia is an additional option that provides continuous pain relief.

In addition to pharmacological management of pain and other symptoms, clinicians may consider the value of nonpharmacological interventions such as bed rest, simple exercise, heat or cold packs to affected sites, massage, transcutaneous electrical stimulation (TENS), and acupuncture. Psychological interventions to reduce pain perception and interpretation include hypnosis, relaxation, imagery, biofeedback, distraction, art therapy, and patient education.

Patients with HIV disease seek complementary therapies to treat symptoms, slow the progression of the disease, and enhance their general well-being. Milan et al. (2008) found that more than 90% of inner-city, middle-aged, heterosexual women and men ($n = 93$) who were at risk for or who had HIV infection reported the use of complementary and alternative therapies in the prior 6 months. The 10 most commonly used complementary therapies and activities reported by 1,106 participants in the alternative medical care outcomes in AIDS study were aerobic exercise (64%), prayer (56%), massage (54%), needle acupuncture (48%), meditation (46%), support groups (42%), visualization and imagery (34%), breathing exercises (33%), spiritual activities (33%), and other exercises (33%; Milan et al., 2008). Nurses' knowledge, evaluation, and recommendations regarding complementary therapies are important aspects of holistic care.

■ HEALTH PROMOTION RELATED TO HIV/AIDS

With no current cure, the health management of patients with HIV/AIDS is directed toward controlling HIV disease and prolonging survival, while maintaining QOL (Burgoyne & Tan, 2008). QOL is associated with health maintenance for individuals with HIV/AIDS, particularly as it relates to physical and emotional symptoms and functioning in activities of daily living as well as social functioning (Vigneshwaran, Padmanabhareddy, Devanna, & Alvarez-Uria, 2013). QOL is based on the patient's perceptions of his or her ability to control the physical, emotional, social, cognitive, and spiritual aspects of the illness. In a study regarding the functional QOL of 142 men and women with AIDS, Vosvick et al. (2003) concluded that maladaptive coping strategies were associated with lower levels of energy and social functioning and that severe pain interfered with daily living tasks and was associated with lower levels of functional QOL (physical functioning, energy/fatigue, social functioning, and role functioning). Therefore, health-promotion interventions should be aimed at developing adaptive coping strategies and improving pain management.

Health Promotion

In the management of HIV/AIDS, it is important to prevent or decrease the occurrence of opportunistic infections and AIDS-indicator diseases. HIV management therefore involves health promotion and disease prevention. In addition to the treatment of AIDS-related diseases and associated symptoms, PC involves prophylactic interventions and the prevention of behaviors that promote disease expression (Bolin, 2006).

Through all stages of HIV disease, health can be promoted and maintained through diet, micronutrients, exercise, reduction of stress and negative emotions, symptom surveillance, and the use of prophylactic therapies to prevent opportunistic infections or AIDS-related complications. A health-promoting diet is essential for optimal functioning of the immune system. Cell-mediated immunity, phagocytic function, and antibody response are impaired by deficiencies in diet, including low protein intake. Alteration in nutrition leads to secondary infections, disease progression, psychological distress, and fatigue. In patients with AIDS, common nutritional problems are weight loss, vitamin and mineral deficiencies, loss of muscle mass, and loss or redistribution of fat mass. With the administration of ART, there is the possibility of redistribution of fat, characterized by increased abdominal girth, loss of fat from the face, and a "buffalo hump" on the back of the neck (Keithley, Swanson, Murphy, & Levin, 2000). Diseases of the mouth and oropharynx, such as oral candidiasis, annular cheilitis, gingivitis, herpes simplex, and hairy leukoplakia, may limit oral intake. Diseases of the GI tract that can cause malabsorption include CMV, MAC, cryptosporidiosis, and KS. These diseases are experienced in individuals with CD4 counts of 50 cells or less and may adversely affect their nutritional status (Crum-Cianfione, 2010). Metabolic alterations may be due to HIV infection or secondary infections as well as abnormalities in carbohydrate, fat, and protein metabolism (Vosvick et al., 2003). A good diet is one of the simplest ways to delay HIV progression and will bolster immune-system function and energy levels and help patients live longer and more productive lives (Hussein, 2003). It is recommended to have 2 or 3 servings daily from the protein and dairy groups, 7 to 12 servings from the starch and grain group, 2 servings of fruits and vegetables rich in vitamin C, as well as 3 servings of other fruits and vegetables (Grobler, Siegfried, Visser, Mahlungulu, & Volmink, 2012).

Multivitamin supplementation is a good preventive measure (Mehta & Fawzi, 2007). Vitamin B, C, E, and folic acid have been shown to delay the progression of HIV. Supplementation with selenium, N-acetyl cysteine, probiotics, and prebiotics has considerable potential, but the evidence needs to be further substantiated. Vitamin A, iron, and zinc have been associated with adverse effects and caution is warranted for their use (Hummelen, Hemsworth, & Reid, 2010).

Exercise is also important for health promotion in patients with HIV/AIDS. Obrien, Nixon, Tyan, and Glazier (2010) examined the safety and effectiveness of aerobic exercise interventions on immunologic and virologic, cardiopulmonary, and psychologic outcomes and strength, weight, and body composition in adults living with HIV. Performing constant or interval aerobic exercise, or a combination of constant aerobic exercise and progressive resistive exercise for at least 20 minutes at least three times per week for at least 5 weeks, appears to be safe and may lead to significant improvements in selected outcomes of cardiopulmonary fitness (maximum oxygen consumption), body composition (leg muscle area, percent body fat), and psychological status (depression–dejection symptoms).

Summarizing the importance of exercise in HIV disease, Hand, Lyerly, Jaggers, and Dudgeon (2009) concluded that moderate- to high-intensity aerobic exercise combined with a resistance exercise regimen is safe and favorable and results in changes in body composition, muscular strength, improved depression and anxiety, and improving QOL.

Stress and negative emotions are also associated with immune suppression and increase an individual's vulnerability to infections. For patients living with HIV/AIDS, there is stress related to the uncertainty regarding illness progression and prognosis, stigmatization, discrimination, financial concerns, and increased disability as the disease progresses. Individuals with AIDS frequently cite the avoidance of stress as a way of maintaining a sense of well-being (Antoni, 2003). Based on a study of 96 HIV-infected homosexual men without symptoms or antiretroviral medication use, Leserman et al. (2002) reported that higher cumulative average stressful life events, higher anger scores, lower cumulative average social support, and depressive symptoms predicted a faster progression to both the CDC AIDS classification and a clinical AIDS condition. In a study of QOL of women with AIDS, cognitive-behavioral interventions have been shown to improve cognitive functioning, health distress, and overall health perceptions, yet there were no changes in energy/fatigue, pain, or social functioning (Lechner et al., 2003). There is some evidence to support the use of massage therapy to improve QOL for people living with HIV/AIDS, particularly in combination with other stress-management modalities, and that massage therapy may have a positive effect on immunological function (Hiller, Louw, Morris, Uwimana, & Statham, 2010). A further consideration is the use of recreational drugs such as alcohol, chemical stimulants, tobacco, and marijuana, which increases physical and emotional stress. In patients with HIV/AIDS, physical and emotional stress are associated with these agents, as they have an immunosuppressant effect and may interfere with health-promoting behaviors. Substance use may also have a negative effect on interpersonal relationships and is associated with a relapse to unsafe sexual practices (Lambert et al., 2011). Patients who have substance abuse problems are encouraged to participate in self-health groups and harm-reduction programs to promote their health and QOL.

Research further suggests that the promotion of health involves positive emotional coping, such as having a strong will to live, positive attitudes, feeling in charge, a strong sense of self, expressing their needs, and a sense of humor. Based on a sample of 103 HIV/AIDS patients (Cohen, 2001), the relationship between the use of humor to cope with stress (coping humor) and perceived social support, depression, anxiety, self-esteem, and stress was examined. Although patients who used more coping humor were less depressed, expressed higher self-esteem, and perceived greater support from friends, humor did not buffer stress, anxiety, or immune-system functioning. Other health-promotion strategies frequently used by these patients included remaining active, seeking medical information, talking to others, socializing and pursuing pleasurable activities, taking good medical care, and counseling. It is recognized that stress can also be associated with the financial issues experienced by patients with HIV/AIDS. Financial planning, identification of financial resources available through the community, and public assistance offered through Medicaid were important in reducing stress.

In addition, health promotion for patients with HIV/AIDS includes avoidance of exposure to organisms in the environment and thereby prevention of the development of opportunistic infections. The immune system can be supported and maintained through the administration of prophylactic and/or suppressive therapies, which decrease the frequency or severity of opportunistic infections (Panel on Opportunistic Infections in HIV-Infected Adults and Adolescents, n.d.). The administration of a pharmacological agent to prevent the initial infection is known as primary prophylaxis, while the administration of a pharmacological agent to prevent future occurrences of infection is referred to as secondary prophylaxis (Panel on Opportunistic Infections in HIV-Infected Adults and Adolescents, n.d.). There has been a significant decrease in the incidence of opportunistic infections due to the effectiveness of ART. Prophylaxis for life for HIV-related coinfections is no longer necessary in many cases. With the restoration of immune-system function, as evidenced by a rise in CD4 counts, clinicians may consider discontinuation of primary prophylaxis under defined conditions (CDC, 2013). Ending preventive prophylaxis for opportunistic infections in selected patients may result in a decrease in drug interactions and toxicities, lower cost of care, and greater adherence to highly active antiretroviral therapy (HAART) regimens. However, prophylaxis remains important to protect against opportunistic infections in the late symptomatic and advanced stages of HIV disease, when CD4 counts are low. Therefore, throughout the illness trajectory, and even in hospice settings, patients may be taking prophylactic medications, requiring sophisticated planning and monitoring. The recommendation is that prophylaxis and suppressive therapy continue in hospice care/PC if the patient is clinically stable and wants to continue prophylaxis drug therapy (Alexander, 2011). However, if side effects occur, and the patient continues to be otherwise stable, alternative regimens should be considered. Furthermore, if the patient is intolerant of prophylaxis and/or the regimens are burdensome, medications should be discontinued. In addition, HIV-infected individuals are at a risk of severe diseases such as hepatitis B, tetanus, influenza, pneumococcal disease and measles, rubella, and mumps. Therefore, it is important to offer such vaccinations as a component of health promotion and disease prevention.

■ PSYCHOSOCIAL ISSUES FOR PATIENTS WITH HIV/AIDS AND THEIR FAMILIES

Many practitioners focus on the patient's physical functioning and performance status as the main indicators of QOL, rather than on the symptoms of psychological distress such as anxiety and depression. Based on a sample of 203 patients with HIV/AIDS, Farber, Mirsalimi, Williams, and McDaniel (2003) reported that the positive meaning of the illness was associated with a higher level of psychological well-being and lower depressed mood, and contributed more than problem-focused coping and social support to predicting both psychological well-being and depressed mood. Sherman et al. (2006), in a 2-year longitudinal pilot study regarding QOL for patients with advanced cancer and AIDS, found that while patients with advanced AIDS ($n = 63$) reported a total lower QOL as compared to patients with advanced cancer ($n = 38$), AIDS caregivers ($n = 43$) reported greater overall QOL, psychological well-being, and spiritual well-being than did cancer caregivers ($n = 38$). Sherman et al. posited that even as death approaches, health professionals can identify changes in QOL and appropriate interventions to improve QOL outcomes for HIV/AIDS patients.

Uncertainty is also a source of psychological distress for persons living with HIV disease, particularly as it relates to ambiguous symptom patterns, exacerbation and remissions of symptoms, selection of optimal treatment regimens, the complexity of treatments, and the fear of stigma and ostracism. Slater et al. (2013) identified the determinants of QOL in a sample of 60 older gay individuals with HIV/AIDS. Age, social support, and problem-focused coping were significantly and positively correlated with QOL, while medical comorbidities, social stigma, and emotion-focused coping were all significantly and negatively associated with QOL ($p < .01$). In stepwise linear regression analysis, emotional/ informational support remained as a significant positive predictor, and medical comorbidities, HIV stigma, and emotion-focused coping remained as significant negative predictors, accounting for 64% of the variance in QOL. The prevalence of major depression disorder (MDD) in patients diagnosed with HIV/AIDS has been estimated at 36%, 27% with dysthymic disorder, and 21% with both MDD and dysthymic disorder and is characterized by depressed mood, low energy, sleep disturbance, anhedonia, inability to concentrate, loss of libido, weight changes, and possible menstrual irregularities (Bing et al., 2001). In patients experiencing depression, clinicians also should assess their use of alcohol, drugs, and opioids.

The psychosocial issues experienced by patients with HIV/AIDS include multiple losses, complicated grief, substance abuse, stigmatization, and homophobia, which contribute to patients' sense of alienation, isolation, hopelessness, loneliness, and depression (Sherman, 2006). Such emotional distress often extends to the patient's family caregivers as they attempt to provide support and lessen the patient's suffering, yet experience suffering themselves.

Psychosocial assessment of patients with HIV disease is important throughout the illness trajectory, particularly as the disease progresses, and there is increased vulnerability to psychological distress. Psychosocial assessment includes the following (Sherman, 2006):

- Past social, behavioral, and psychiatric history, which includes the history of interpersonal relationships, education, job stability, career plans, substance use, preexisting mental illness, and individual identity
- Crisis points related to the course of the disease as anxiety, fear, and depression intensify, creating a risk of suicide
- Life-cycle phase of individuals and families, which influences goals, financial resources, skills, social roles, and the ability to confront personal mortality
- Influence of culture and ethnicity, including knowledge and beliefs associated with health, illness, dying, and death, as well as attitudes and values toward sexual behaviors, substance use, health promotion and maintenance, and healthcare decision making
- Past and present patterns of coping, including problem-focused and/or emotion-focused coping
- Social support, including sources of support, types of supports perceived as needed by the patient/family, and perceived benefits and burdens of support
- Financial resources, including healthcare benefits, disability allowances, and the eligibility for Medicaid/ Medicare

Patients diagnosed with depression should be treated with antidepressants to control their symptoms (Repetto & Petitto, 2008). Selective serotonin reuptake inhibitors (SSRIs) are as effective as tricyclic antidepressants but are better tolerated because of their more benign side-effect profile. SSRIs may interact with such antiretroviral medications as PIs and nNRTIs; therefore, initial SSRI dosage should be lowered with careful upward titration and close monitoring for toxic reactions (Repetto & Petitto, 2008). Serotonin and norepinephrine reuptake inhibitors (SNRIs), such as venlafaxine and duloxetine, are newer antidepressants that also are useful in treating chronic pain. Tricyclic antidepressants are indicated for treating depression only in patients who do not respond to newer medications. It is noted that monoamine oxidase inhibitors (MAOIs) may interact with multiple medications used to treat HIV disease and, therefore, should be avoided. Medication interaction and liver function profiles should be considered before antidepressant therapy is initiated.

Another psychological symptom experienced by persons with HIV/AIDS is anxiety. Anxiety may also result from the medications used to treat HIV disease, such as anticonvulsants, sulfonamides, NSAIDs, and corticosteroids. Manifestations of generalized anxiety disorder include worry, trouble falling asleep, impaired concentration, psychomotor agitation, hypersensitivity, hyperarousal, and fatigue (Arriendel, 2003). The treatment for patients with anxiety is based on the nature and severity of the symptoms and the coexistence of other mood disorders or substance abuse. Short-acting anxiolytics, such as lorazepam (Ativan) and alprazolam (Xanax), are beneficial for intermittent symptoms, while buspirone (BuSpar) and clonazepam (Klonopin) are beneficial for chronic anxiety (Gallego, Barreiro, & López-Ibor, 2012).

Significant stress is also associated with sharing information related to the diagnosis, and particularly when such disclosures occur during the stage of advanced disease. The need for therapeutic communication and support from all health professionals caring for the patient and his or her family exists throughout the illness continuum. For many patients experiencing psychological distress associated with HIV disease, therapeutic interventions such as skill building, support groups, individual counseling, and group interventions using meditation techniques can provide a sense of psychological growth and a meaningful way of living with the disease (Hanrahan et al., 2011). Fear of disclosure of the AIDS diagnosis and stigmatization in the community often raise concern in the family about the diagnosis stated on death certificates. Practitioners may therefore write a nonspecific diagnosis on the main death certificate and sign section B on the reverse side to signify to the registrar general that further information will be provided at a later date.

Spiritual Issues in HIV/AIDS

The assessment of patients' spiritual needs is an important aspect of holistic care. Nurses must assess patients' spiritual values, needs, and religious perspectives, which are important to understand patients' perspectives regarding their illness and their perception and meaning of life. Patients living with and dying from HIV disease have the spiritual needs of meaning, value, hope, purpose, love, acceptance, reconciliation, ritual, and affirmation of a relationship with a higher being (Kylmä, Vehviläinen-Julkunen, & Lähdevirta, 2001). Assisting patients to find meaning and value in their lives, despite adversity, often involves a recognition of past successes and their internal strengths. Encouraging open communication between the patient and his or her family is important to work toward reconciliation and the completion of unfinished business.

As with many life-threatening illnesses, patients with AIDS may express anger with God. Some may view their illness as a punishment or be angry that God is not answering their prayers. Expression of feelings can be a source of spiritual healing. Clergy can also serve as valuable members of the PC team in offering spiritual support and alleviating spiritual distress. The use of meditation, music, imagery, poetry, and drawing may offer outlets for spiritual expression and promote a sense of harmony and peace.

For all patients with chronic life-threatening illness, hope often shifts from hope that a cure will soon be found to hope for a peaceful death with dignity, including the alleviation of pain and suffering, determining one's own choices, being in the company of family and significant others, and knowing that their EOL wishes will be honored. Often, the greatest spiritual comfort offered by caregivers or family for patients comes from active listening and meaningful presence. Simple gestures like sitting and holding the patient's hands may have a great impact on the patient's well-being and them not feeling abandoned.

Spiritual healing may also come from life review, as patients are offered an opportunity to reminisce about their lives, reflect on their accomplishments and misgivings, and forgive themselves and others for their imperfections. Indeed, such spiritual care conveys that even in the shadow of death, there can be discovery, insight, the completion of relationships, the experience of love of self and others, and the transcendence of emotional and spiritual pain. Often, patients with AIDS, by their example, teach nurses, family, and others how to transcend suffering and how to die with grace and dignity.

Advanced Care Planning

Advanced planning is another important issue related to EOL care for patients with HIV/AIDS. First, the healthcare provider must assess the patient's competency to participate in his or her own plan of care. In assessing the patient's competency, the healthcare provider must question whether the decision maker knows the nature and effect of the decision to be made and understands the consequences of his or her actions, and determine if the decision is consistent with an individual's life history, lifestyle, previous actions, and best interests. When an individual is competent, and in anticipation of the future loss of competency, he or she may initiate advance directives such as a living will and/or the designation of a healthcare proxy who will carry out the patient's healthcare wishes or make healthcare decisions in the event that the patient becomes incompetent. The patient may also give an individual the power of attorney regarding financial matters and care or treatment issues. Advance directives include the patient's decisions regarding such life-sustaining treatments as cardiopulmonary resuscitation, use of vasoactive drips to sustain blood pressure and heart rate, dialysis, artificial nutrition and hydration, and the initiation or withdrawal of ventilatory support. The signing of advance directives in the form of a healthcare proxy must be witnessed by two individuals who are not related to the patient or involved in the patient's treatment. Individuals who are mentally competent

can revoke at any time their advance directives. If a patient is deemed mentally incompetent, state statutes may allow the court to designate a surrogate decision maker as the legal guardian to make decisions for the patient.

Up until a few years ago, the majority of patients with AIDS usually had not discussed with their physicians the kind of care they want at the end of life for a variety of reasons, although more gay men have executed an advance directive than injection-drug users or women (Curtis, Patrick, Caldwell, & Collier, 2000). White patients were more likely to believe that their doctor was an HIV/AIDS expert and good at talking about EOL care, recognize they have been very sick in the past, and that such discussions are important. By contrast, nonwhite patients with AIDS report that they do not like to talk about the care they would want if they were very sick and are more likely to feel that if they talk about death it will bring death closer (Curtis et al., 2000).

In addition to the discussion of goals of care and the completion of advance directives, healthcare providers can also assist patients and families by discussing the benefits of social support programs, unemployment insurance, worker's compensation, pension plans, insurance, and union or association benefits. In addition, they may emphasize the importance of organizing information and documents so that they are easily located and accessible, and suggest that financial matters be in order, such as power of attorney or bank accounts, credit cards, property, legal claims, and income tax preparation. Health professionals may also discuss matters related to the chosen setting for dying and the patient's wishes regarding his or her death.

Care of the Dying

Dying is a natural part of life, and many people do not know what to expect when that moment comes. They have to learn to navigate through the unfamiliarity of the situation and simultaneously deal with their own grief. It is not uncommon to experience a wide range of emotions during the last months, weeks, or days as patient and/or family caregiver. The dying process is unique to each person, but for patients with advanced AIDS, it is commonly marked by increasingly severe physical deterioration, decrease in appetite followed by muscles wasting, decrease in energy, and a bedbound state. At the end of life, common symptoms include pain, dyspnea, and pressure ulcers. Febrile states and changes in mental status often occur as death becomes more imminent. Maintaining the comfort and dignity of the patients becomes a nursing priority. Frequent and thorough reassessment, addressing and treating physical, emotional, and psychosocial symptoms, should be continued throughout the dying process since even obtunded patients may feel pain and other symptoms.

Because PC also addresses the needs of family, it is important to consider the vulnerability of family members to patients' health problems at the end of life. As illness progresses, health professionals should encourage patients and family members to express their fears and EOL wishes. Encouraging patients and families to express such feelings as "I love you," "I forgive you," "Forgive me—I am sorry," "Thank you," and "Good-bye" is important to the completion of relationships (Byock, 1997). Peaceful death can also occur when families give patients the permission to die and assure them that they will be remembered.

Loss, Grief, and Bereavement for Persons With HIV/AIDS and Their Survivors

Patients with HIV disease experience many losses across the illness trajectory: a sense of loss of identity; loss of control over health and function; loss of roles as the illness progresses; loss of body image due to skin lesions, changes in weight, and wasting; loss of sexual freedom because of the need to change sexual behaviors to maintain health and prevent transmission to others; loss of financial security through possible discrimination and increasing physical disability; and loss of relationships through possible abandonment, self-induced isolation, and the multiple deaths of others from the disease (Sikkema, Kochman, DiFranceisco, Kelly, & Hoffmann, 2003). Each occurrence of illness may pose new losses and heighten the patient's awareness of mortality. Illness experiences are opportunities for health professionals to respond to patients' cues in addressing their concerns and approaching the subject of loss, dying, and death. Given that grief is the emotional response to loss, patients living with and dying from AIDS may also manifest the signs of grief, which include feelings of sadness, anger, self-reproach, anxiety, loneliness, fatigue, shock, yearning, relief, and numbness; physical sensations such as hollowness in the stomach, tightness in the chest, oversensitivity to noise, dry mouth, muscle weakness, and loss of coordination; cognitions of disbelief and confusion; and behavior disturbances in appetite, sleep, social withdrawal, loss of interest in activities, and restless overactivity (Mallinson, 2013).

The bereavement time begins upon the death of their loved one. Bereavement is a state of having suffered a loss, which is often a long-term process of adapting to life without the deceased (Mallinson, 2013). Family and significant others may experience signs of grief, including a sense of presence of the deceased, paranormal experiences or hallucinations, dreams of the deceased, a desire to have cherished objects of the deceased, and visit places frequented by the deceased. Grief work is a dynamic process that is not time limited and predictable (Mallinson, 2013). Those left behind might never "get over" the loss but, rather, find a place for it in their life and create a new relationship with their loved one through memories.

Families and partners of patients with AIDS may experience disenfranchised grief, defined as the grief that persons experience when they incur a loss that is not openly acknowledged, publicly mourned, or socially supported (Doka, 2002; Mallinson, 2013). Support is not only important in assisting families in the tasks of grieving, but is also important for nurses who have established valued relationships with their patients. Disenfranchised grief may also be experienced by nurses who do not allow themselves to acknowledge their patient's death as a personal loss, or who are not acknowledged by others, such as the patient's family or even professional colleagues, for having suffered a loss.

Worden (2008) has identified the tasks of grieving as accepting the reality of the death; experiencing the pain of grief; adjusting to a changed physical, emotional, and social environment in which the deceased is missing; and finding an appropriate emotional place for the person who died in the emotional life of the bereaved. Mallinson (2013) recommends the following nursing interventions to facilitate grief work:

- Accept the reality of death by speaking of the loss and facilitating emotional expression
- Work through the pain of grief by exploring the meaning of the grief experience
- Adjust to the environment without the deceased by acknowledging anniversaries and the experience of loss during holidays and birthdays; help the bereaved to solve problems and recognize their own abilities to conduct their daily lives
- Emotionally relocate the deceased and move on with life by encouraging socialization through formal and informal avenues

The complications of AIDS-related grief often come from the secrecy and social stigma associated with the disease. Reluctance to contact family and friends can restrict the normal support systems available for the bereaved. The death of patients with AIDS may therefore result in complicated grief for the bereaved. Complicated grief may also occur when death occurs after lengthy illness and the relationship has been ambivalent. Culturally sensitive and truthful communication is important as health professionals offer support to families in their grief.

■ CONCLUSION

PC offers a comprehensive approach to address the physical, emotional, social, and spiritual needs of individuals with incurable progressive illness throughout the illness trajectory until death and into the bereavement period for families. For patients with HIV/AIDS, PC offers a combination of disease-modifying and supportive interventions throughout the disease trajectory to relieve the suffering associated with opportunistic infections and malignancies. Knowledge regarding HIV disease is important so that nurses can offer effective and compassionate care to patients and help to alleviate physical, emotional, social, and spiritual suffering at all stages of HIV disease. By establishing a partnership with their healthcare professionals in planning and implementing their healthcare, patients can maintain a sense of control during the illness experience. Through advanced care planning, patients can ensure that their EOL preferences and wishes are honored. The control of pain and symptoms associated with HIV/AIDS enables the patient and his or her family to expend their energies on spiritual and emotional healing, and the possibility for personal growth and transcendence even as death approaches (Sherman, 2006). PC preserves patients' QOL by protecting their self-integrity, reducing a perceived helplessness, and lessening the threat of exhaustion of coping resources. Through effective and compassionate nursing care, patients with AIDS can achieve a sense of inner well-being even at death, with the potential to make the transition from life as profound, intimate, and precious an experience as their birth (Byock, 1997).

CASE STUDY *Conclusion*

Within 6 months, Terry experienced night sweats, fever, and diarrhea due to an exacerbation of MAC. This resulted in severe dehydration. The PC team was asked for a consultation by the AIDS specialist. The advanced practice nurse developed a very supportive relationship with Terry and her significant other. She listened attentively and offered a comforting presence. The PC nurse provided effective symptom management and lessened their anxiety by developing together a plan of care based on Terry's wishes and preferences. They discussed her relationship with her mother and sister. Terry decided to reach out and call her sister to tell her about her hospitalization. Her sister came to the hospital to visit. Over the next few weeks, a closeness was reestablished and her sister told her that she would be the guardian of her little boy. This conversation was facilitated by the advanced practice nurse. Terry was coming to terms with her diagnosis and confided that she wanted to speak to a priest for confession. An intimate conversation with the nurse was of comfort and a visit by the chaplain was arranged.

Terry never left the hospital as her fever began to rise, and she became delirious. Several tests were conducted to identify other potential sources of the infection and other possible reasons for the delirium. Her symptoms were treated with Haldol and antipyretics. However, within the next day, Terry slipped into a coma. Her breathing was labored and she was given low doses of morphine to increase her comfort. With support from the advanced practice nurse, Terry's little boy visited his mother. He kissed her hand and hung a picture he drew from the bedrail. With her mother, sister, and significant other at the bedside, tears flowed. Terry left a letter to her family in the nightstand. She reminded her son of her strong love for him and promised to watch over him from above. Terry thanked her mother and sister for their promise to protect and care for her child. To her partner, she expressed a love and wish that things were different. She asked the PC nurse to offer ongoing support to her family and thanked her for her loving and supportive care.

CASE STUDY

AN INTERPROFESSIONAL PERSPECTIVE

Luis Padilla, MD

PC is supportive, symptoms-oriented, and patient- and his or her family-centered care. Its goal is to optimize QOL for patients dealing with life-threatening illnesses through anticipation, prevention, and treatment of suffering (physical, emotional, spiritual, and psychosocial). An interdisciplinary approach is essential for excellent PC. The care for patients with HIV/AIDS requires a balance between treatment directed at AIDS-related illnesses, symptoms management throughout the illness trajectory, and when patients approach the end of their lives. With the growth and expansion of PC services throughout the country (both as inpatient/outpatient and as community), we will hopefully see a trend toward earlier rather than later referral to PC.

In the case study, Terry had multiple issues that could have been prioritized and dealt with much earlier in her disease trajectory if she had an early referral to PC. It is evident that over time, multiple issues contributed to her distress and suffering, such as social issues (history of drug abuse, unprotected sex), emotional issues (depression, loss of the role as a mother and caregiver, loss of a role as a provider, potential loss of parent rights of her child, poor family support), and spiritual issues (little comfort in faith). Terry had little emotional or practical support from her family or community. Early referral to PC could have helped Terry cope with her illness and offer support to her children. Health education and close monitoring could result in the early detection of opportunistic infections. PC involvement, even though it came at the end of Terry's life, significantly improved her QOL.

In conclusion, with advancement in the treatment of HIV/AIDS, patients can live longer and have much better lives. Every patient has a unique life situation and needs, but a healthy lifestyle and early treatment can slow the progression from HIV to AIDS. Early referral to PC addresses the physical, emotional, social, and cultural needs of patients with HIV/AIDS and their families. As opposed to considering it a death sentence, patients are learning to live with HIV/AIDS as a chronic illness. The interprofessional approach offered by PC practitioners offers a whole-person approach to care, improving the QOL across the illness trajectory.

Evidence-Based Practice

Slater, L. Z., Moneyham, L., Vance, D E., Raper, J. L., Mugavero, M. J., & Childs, G. (2015). The multiple stigma experience and quality of life in older gay men with HIV. *Journal of the Association of Nurses in AIDS Care*, 26(1), 24–35. doi:10.1016/j.jana.2014.06.007

Background
With the life expectancy for persons living with HIV increased due to antiretroviral therapy, multiple issues have emerged for older HIV-infected gay men that can negatively affect their QOL. Issues related to sexual orientation (homonegativity), HIV stigma, and age (ageism) have become an emerging concern for older gay men with HIV, who comprise more than 50% of older adults living with HIV in the United States.

Purpose
The purpose of this study was to examine the multiple stigma experience (homonegativity, internalized HIV stigma, and ageism) and its effect on QOL in older gay men with HIV.

Design
Secondary analysis of data collected for a quantitative, cross-sectional study that examined stigma, support, coping health, and QOL in 60 gay men ages 50 to 65 (Slater et al., 2013).

Results
Age- and emotion-focused coping were predictors of homonegativity, accounting for 28% of its variance. Age, HIV support group participation, total medications, availability

of support, and emotion-focused coping were predictors of internalized HIV stigma accounting for 35%. Problem-focused coping predicted ageism and accounted for 7% of its variance in QOL. Multiple stigmas have a much higher effect on QOL on populations with multiple health disparities.

Conclusion
Study findings demonstrate that social support, HIV support group participation, and the use of problem-focused coping strategies may help decrease homonegativity, internalize HIV stigma and ageism, and at the same time improve QOL in this population.

■ REFERENCES

Alexander, C. (2011). HIV/AIDS. In L. L. Emanuel & S. L. Librach (Eds.), *Palliative care: Core skills and clinical competencies* (2nd ed., pp. 372–390). Philadelphia, PA: W. B. Saunders.

Althoff, K. N., McGinnis, K. A., Wyatt, C. M., Freiberg, M. S., Gilbert, C., Oursler, K. K., . . . Justice, A. C. (2015). Comparison of risk and age at diagnosis of myocardial infarction, end-stage renal disease, and non-AIDS-defining cancer in HIV-infected versus uninfected adults. *Clinical Infectious Diseases, 60*(4), 627–638. doi:10.1093/cid/ciu869

Antoni, M. H. (2003). Stress management effects on psychological, endocrinological, and immune functioning in men with HIV infection: Empirical support for a psychoneuroimmunological model. *Stress, 6*(3), 173–188. doi:10.1080/1025389031000156727

Arriendel, J. (2003). Differential coping strategies, anxiety, depression, and symptomatology among African–American women with HIV/AIDS. *Dissertation Abstracts International. Section B: The Sciences and Engineering, 64*, 1481.

Bing, E. G., Burnam, M. A., Longshore, D., Fleishman, J. A., Sherbourne, C. D., London, A. S., ... Shapiro, M. (2001). Psychiatric disorders and drug use among human immunodeficiency virus-infected adults in the United States. *Archives of General Psychiatry, 58*(8), 721–728. doi:10.1001/archpsyc.58.8.721

Bolin, J. N. (2006). Pernicious encroachment into end-of-life decision making: Federal intervention in palliative pain treatment. *American Journal of Bioethics, 6*(5), 34–36; discussion W30. doi:10.1080/15265160600861967

Burgoyne, R. W., & Tan, D. H. (2008). Prolongation and quality of life for HIV-infected adults treated with highly active antiretroviral therapy (HAART): A balancing act. *Journal of Antimicrobial Chemotherapy, 61*(3), 469–473. doi:10.1093/jac/dkm499

Byock, I. (1997). *Dying well: The prospect for growth at the end of life.* New York, NY: Riverhead Books.

Centers for Disease Control and Prevention. (2013). *HIV surveillance report, 2011* (Vol. 23). Retrieved from http://www.cdc.gov/hiv/topics/surveillance/resources/reports

Centers for Disease Control and Prevention. (2014). Preexposure prophylaxis for the prevention of HIV infection in the United States-2014. Clinical providers' supplement. Retrieved from https://www.cdc.gov/hiv/pdf/prepprovidersupplement2014.pdf

Centers for Disease Control and Prevention. (2016). *HIV surveillance report, 2016* (Vol. 27). Retrieved from https://www.cdc.gov/hiv/statistics/overview/ataglance.html

Centers for Disease Control and Prevention. (2017). HIV among pregnant women, infants and children/fast facts, 2017. Retrieved from https://www.cdc.gov/hiv/group/gender/pregnantwomen

Cohen, M. (2001). The use of coping humor in an HIV/AIDS population. *Dissertation Abstracts International, 61*, 4976.

Crum-Cianfione, N. (2010). HIV and the gastrointestinal tract. *Infectious Disease in Clinical Practice, 18*(5), 283–285. doi:10.1097/IPC.0b013e3181f1038b

Curtis, J. R., Patrick, D., Caldwell, E., & Collier, A. (2000). The attitudes of patients with advanced AIDS toward use of the medical futility rationale in decisions to forgo mechanical ventilation. *Archives in Internal Medicine, 60*, 1597–1601. doi:10-1001/pubs.Arch Intern Med

Dahlin, C. (Ed.). (2013). *Clinical practice guidelines for quality palliative care* (3rd ed.). Pittsburgh, PA: National Consensus Project for Palliative Care. Retrieved from http://nationalconsensusproject.org

Department of Health and Human Services. (2013). Panel on antiretroviral guidelines for adults and adolescents. Guidelines for the use of antiretroviral agents in HIV-1-infected adults and adolescents. Retrieved from http://aidsinfo.nih.gov/contentfiles/lvguidelines/AdultandAdolescentGL.pdf

Department of Health and Human Services. (2016). Panel on antiretroviral guidelines for adults and adolescents. Guidelines for the use of antiretroviral agents in HIV-1-infected adults and adolescents. Retrieved from https://aidsinfo.nih.gov/contentfiles/lvguidelines/AA_Recommendations.pdf

Doka, K. (2002). *Disenfranchised grief: New directions, challenges and strategies for practice.* Champaign, IL: Research Press.

Fan, H., Conner, R. F., & Villarreal, L. P. (2011). *AIDS: Science and society* (pp. 41–66). Burlington, MA: Jones & Bartlett.

Farber, E. W., Mirsalimi, H., Williams, K. A., & McDaniel, J. S. (2003). Meaning of illness and psychological adjustment to HIV/AIDS. *Psychosomatics, 44*(6), 485–491. doi:10.1176/appi.psy.44.6.485

Farnham, P. G., Gopalappa, Ch., Sansom, S. L., Hutchinson, A. B., Brooks, J. T., Weidle, P. J., ... Rimland, D. (2013). Updates of lifetime costs of care and quality-of-life estimates for HIV-infected persons in the United States: Late vs. early diagnosis and entry into care. *Journal of Acquired Immune Deficiency Syndrome, 64*(2), 183–189. doi:10.1097/QAI.0b013e3182973966

Fausto, J. A., & Selwyn, P. A. (2011). Palliative care in the management of advanced HIV/AIDS. *Primary Care, 38*(2), 311–326, ix. doi:10.1016/j.pop.2011.03.010

Gallego, L., Barreiro, P., & López-Ibor, J. J. (2012). Psychopharmacological treatments in HIV patients under antiretroviral therapy. *AIDS Reviews, 14*(2), 101–111.

Grobler, L., Siegfried, N., Visser, M. E., Mahlungulu, S. S., & Volmink, J. (2013). Nutritional interventions for reducing morbidity and mortality in people with HIV. *Cochrane Database of Systematic Reviews,* (2), CD004536. doi:10.1002/14651858.CD004536.pub3

Gysels, M., Evans, N., Meñaca, A., Higginson, I. J., Harding, R., & Pool, R.; Project PRISMA. (2013). Diversity in defining end of life care: An obstacle or the way forward? *PLOS ONE, 8*(7), e68002. doi:10.1371/journal.pone.0068002

Hand, G. A., Lyerly, G. W., Jaggers, J. R., & Dudgeon, W. D. (2009). Impact of aerobic and resistance exercise on the health of HIV-infected persons. *American Journal of Lifestyle Medicine, 3*(6), 489–499. doi:10.1177/1559827609342198

Hanrahan, N. P., Rolin-Kenny, D., Roman, J., Kumar, A., Aiken, L., & Blank, M. (2011). Promoting self-care management among persons with serious mental illness and HIV. *Home Health Care Management and Practice, 23*(6), 421–427. doi:10.1177/1084822311405457

Harding, R., Easterbrook, P., Higginson, I. J., Karus, D., Raveis, V. H., & Marconi, K. (2005). Access and equity in HIV/AIDS palliative care: A review of the evidence and responses. *Palliative Medicine, 19*(3), 251–258. doi:10.1191/0269216305pm1005oa

Harris, G. E., Dupuis, L., Mugford, G. J., Johnston, L., Haase, D., Page, G., & Dow, G. (2014). Patterns and correlates of cannabis use among individuals with HIV/AIDS in Maritime Canada. *Canadian Journal of Infectious Diseases and Medical Microbiology, 25*(1), e1–e7. doi:10.1155/2014/301713

Hiller, S. L., Louw, Q., Morris, L., Uwimana, J., & Statham, S. (2010). Massage therapy for people with HIV/AIDS. *Cochrane Database of Systematic Reviews,* (1), CD007502. doi:10.1002/14651858.CD007502.pub2

HIV Disease. (2017). Indicators and limitations of coverage and/or necessity. Retrieved from https://www.arborhospice.org/healthcare-professionals/disease-indicators/hivaids

Holzemer, W. L. (2002). HIV and AIDS: The symptom experience. What cell counts and viral loads won't tell you. *American Journal of Nursing, 102*(4), 48–52.

Houben, C., Spruit, M. S., Groenen, M. T., Wouters, E. F., & Janssen, D. J. (2014). Efficacy of advance care planning: A systematic review and meta-analysis. *Journal of the American Medical Directors Association, 15*(7), 477–489. doi:10.1016/j.jamda.2014.01.008

Hummelen, R., Hemsworth, J., & Reid, G. (2010). Micronutrients, N-acetyl cysteine, probiotics and prebiotics, a review of effectiveness in reducing HIV progression. *Nutrients, 2*(6), 626–651. doi:10.3390/nu2060626

Hussein, R. (2003). Current issues and forthcoming events. *Journal of Advanced Nursing, 44*, 235–237.

Justice, A. C. (2010). HIV and aging: Time for a new paradigm. *Current HIV/AIDS Reports, 7*(2), 69–76. doi:10.1007/s11904-010-0041-9

Keithley, J., Swanson, B., Murphy, M., & Levin, D. (2000). HIV/AIDS and nutrition implications for disease management. *Nursing Case Management, 5*, 52–62.

Kylmä, J., Vehviläinen-Julkunen, K., & Lähdevirta, J. (2001). Hope, despair and hopelessness in living with HIV/AIDS: A grounded theory study. *Journal of Advanced Nursing, 33*(6), 764–775. doi:10.1046/j.1365-2648.2001.01712.x

Lambert, G., Cox, J., Hottes, T. S., Tremblay, C., Frigault, L. R., Alary, M., ... Remis, R. S.; M-Track Study Group. (2011). Correlates of unprotected anal sex at last sexual episode: Analysis from a surveillance study of men who have sex with men in Montreal. *AIDS and Behavior, 15*(3), 584–595. doi:10.1007/s10461-009-9605-3

Lazenby, G. B. (2012). Opportunistic infections in women with HIV AIDS. *Clinical Obstetrics and Gynecology, 55*(4), 927–937. doi:10.1097/GRF.0b013e3182718e0d

Lechner, S. C., Antoni, M. H., Lydston, D., LaPerriere, A., Ishii, M., Devieux, J., ... Weiss, S. (2003). Cognitive-behavioral interventions improve quality of life in women with AIDS. *Journal of Psychosomatic Research, 54*(3), 253–261. doi:10.1016/S0022-3999(02)00480-4

Lee, K. A., Gay, C., Portillo, C. J., Coggins, T., Davis, H., Pullinger, C. R., & Aouizerat, B. E. (2009). Symptom experience in HIV-infected adults: A function of demographic and clinical characteristics. *Journal of Pain and Symptom Management, 38*(6), 882–893. doi:10.1016/j.jpainsymman.2009.05.013

Leserman, J., Petitto, J. M., Gu, H., Gaynes, B. N., Barroso, J., Golden, R. N., ... Evans, D. L. (2002). Progression to AIDS, a clinical AIDS condition and mortality: Psychosocial and physiological predictors. *Psychological Medicine, 32*(6), 1059–1073. doi:10.1017/S0033291702005949

Lorenz, K. A., Cunningham, W. E., Spritzer, K. L., & Hays, R. D. (2006). Changes in symptoms and health-related quality of life in a nationally representative sample of adults in treatment for HIV. *Quality of Life Research, 15*(6), 951–958. doi:10.1007/s11136-005-6010-x

Mallinson, R. K. (2013). Grief in the context of HIV: Recommendations for practice. *Journal of the Association of Nurses in AIDS Care, 24*(1 Suppl.), S61–S71. doi:10.1016/j.jana.2012.08.012

Marrazzo, J. M. (2017). HIV prevention: Opportunities and challenges. *HIV Prevention, 24*(4). Retrieved from http://www.iasusa.org/sites/default/files/tam/24-4-123.pdf

Mehta, S., & Fawzi, W. (2007). Effects of vitamins, including vitamin A, on HIV/AIDS patients. *Vitamins and Hormones, 75*, 355–383. doi:10.1016/S0083-6729(06)75013-0

Merlins, J. S., Tucker, R. O., Saag, M. S., & Selvyn, P. A. (2013). The role of palliative care in the current HIV treatment era in developed countries. *Topics in Antiviral Medicine, 21*(1), 20–26.

Milan, F. B., Arnsten, J. H., Klein, R. S., Schoenbaum, E. E., Moskaleva, G., Buono, D., & Webber, M. P. (2008). Use of complementary and alternative medicine in inner-city persons with or at risk for HIV infection. *AIDS Patient Care and STDs, 22*(10), 811–816. doi:10.1089/apc.2007.0159

Newshan, G., & Sherman, D. W. (1999). Palliative care: Pain and symptom management in persons with HIV/AIDS. *Nursing Clinics of North America, 34*(1), 131–145.

O'brien, K., Nixon, S., Tyan, A. M., & Glazier, R. (2010). Aerobic exercise interventions for adults living with HIV/AIDS. *Cochrane Database of Systematic Reviews,* (8), CD001796. doi:10.1002/14651858.CD001796.pub3

Oramasionwu, C. U., Koeller, J. M., Lawson, K. A., Brown, C. M., Morse, G. D., & Frei, C. R. (2012). The state of disparities in opportunistic infection prophylaxis for blacks with HIV/AIDS. *Medical Care, 50*(11), 920–927. doi:10.1097/MLR.0b013e31826c85d1

Panel on Opportunistic Infections in HIV-Infected Adults and Adolescents. (n.d.). Guidelines for prevention and treatment of opportunistic infections in HIV-infected adults and adolescents: Recommendations from the Centers for Disease Control and Prevention, the National Institutes of Health, and the HIV Medicine Association of the Infectious Diseases Society of America. Retrieved from http://aidsinfo.nih.gov/contentfiles/lvguidelines/adult_oi.pdf

Parker, R., Stein, D. J., & Jelsma, J. (2014). Pain in people living with HIV/AIDS: A systemic review. *Journal of the International AIDS Society, 17,* 18719. doi:10.7448/IAS.17.1.18719

Piggott, D. A., Muzaale, A. D., Mehta, S. H., Brown, T. T., Patel, K. V., Leng, S. X., & Kirk, G. D. (2013). Frailty, HIV infection, and mortality in an aging cohort of injection drug users. *PLOS ONE, 8*(1), e54910. doi:10.1371/journal.pone.0054910

Pilcher, C. D., Eron, J. J., Galvin, S., Gay, C., & Cohen, M. S. (2004). Acute HIV revisited: New opportunities for treatment and prevention. *Journal of Clinical Investigation, 113*(7), 937–945. doi:10.1172/JCI21540

Repetto, M. J., & Petitto, J. M. (2008). Psychopharmacology in HIV-infected patients. *Psychosomatic Medicine, 70,* 585–592. doi:10.1097/PSY.0b013e3181777190

Selby, D., Chakraborty, A., Myers, J., Saskin, R., Mazzotta, P., & Gill, A. (2011). High scores on the Edmonton Symptom Assessment Scale identify patients with self-defined high symptom burden. *Journal of Palliative Medicine, 14*(12), 1309–1316. doi:10.1089/jpm.2011.0187

Sherman, D. W. (2006). Patients with acquired immunodeficiency syndrome. In B. Ferrell & N. Coyle (Eds.), *Textbook of palliative nursing* (2nd ed., pp. 671–712). New York, NY: Oxford University Press.

Sherman, D. W., Ye, X. Y., McSherry, C., Parkas, V., Calabrese, M., & Gatto, M. (2006). Quality of life of patients with advanced cancer and acquired immune deficiency syndrome and their family caregivers. *Journal of Palliative Medicine, 9*(4), 948–963. doi:10.1089/jpm.2006.9.948

Sikkema, K. J., Kochman, A., DiFranceisco, W., Kelly, J. A., & Hoffmann, R. G. (2003). AIDS-related grief and coping with loss among HIV-positive men and women. *Journal of Behavioral Medicine, 26*(2), 165–181. doi:10.1023/A:1023086723137

Slater, L. Z., Moneyham, L., Vance, D. E., Raper, J. L., Mugavero, M. J., & Childs, G. (2013). Support, stigma, health, coping, and quality of life in older gay men with HIV. *Journal of the Association of Nurses in AIDS Care, 24*(1), 38–49. doi:10.1016/j.jana.2012.02.006

Smith, C. J., Ryom, L., Weber, R., Morlat, P., Pradier, C., Reiss, P., ... Kirk, O. (2014). Trends in underlying causes of death in people with HIV from 1999 to 2011: A multicohort collaboration. *The Lancet, 384*(9939), 241–248. doi:10.1016/S0140-6736(14)60604-8

Solano, J. P., Gomes, B., & Higginson, I. J. (2006). A comparison of symptom prevalence in far advanced cancer, AIDS, heart disease, chronic obstructive pulmonary disease and renal disease. *Journal of Pain and Symptom Management, 31*(1), 58–69. doi:10.1016/j.jpainsymman.2005.06.007

Trescot, A. M., Helm, S., Hansen, H., Benyamin, R., Glaser, S. E., Adlaka, R., & Manchikanti, L. (2008). Opioids in the management of chronic non-cancer pain: An update of American Society of the Interventional Pain Physicians' (ASIPP) Guidelines. *Pain Physician, 11*(2 Suppl), S5–S62.

Uebelacker, L. A., Weisberg, R. B., Herman, D. S., Bailey, G. L., Pinkston-Camp, M. M., & Stein, M. D. (2015). Chronic pain in HIV-infected patients: Relationship to depression, substance use, and mental health and pain treatment. *Pain Medicine, 16*(10), 1870–1881. doi:10.1111/pme.12799

Vigneshwaran, E., Padmanabhareddy, Y., Devanna, N., & Alvarez-Uria, G. (2013). Gender differences in health related quality of life of people living with HIV/AIDS in the era of highly active antiretroviral therapy. *North American Journal of Medical Sciences, 5*(2), 102–107. doi:10.4103/1947-2714.107526

Vosvick, M., Koopman, C., Gore-Felton, C., Thoresen, C., Krumboltz, J., & Spiegel, D. (2003). Relationship of functional quality of life to strategies for coping with the stress of living with HIV/AIDS. *Psychosomatics, 44*(1), 51–58. doi:10.1176/appi.psy.44.1.51

Worden, J. (2008). *Grief counseling and grief therapy: A handbook for the mental health practitioner* (4th ed.). New York, NY: Springer.

World Health Organization. (2016). HIV/AIDS: Fact sheet. Retrieved from http://www.who.int/mediacentre/factsheets/fs360/en

Physical Health: Symptom Management

IV

Rose Anne Indelicato & Mary Layman-Goldstein

20

Pain: Assessment and Treatment Using a Multimodal Approach

KEY POINTS

- Pain remains a common symptom experienced in the palliative care patient population.
- Despite advances in pain management, patients remain at risk for inadequate relief, especially at end of life.
- Pain is multidimensional, multifactorial, and rarely occurs in isolation from other symptoms.
- In order to provide quality pain relief, nurses must possess appropriate knowledge regarding assessment and treatment including pharmacological and nonpharmacological interventions.
- Certain patient populations including children, the elderly, those with a history of substance abuse, and those with impaired communication are especially at risk of poorly managed pain.
- Nurses and other healthcare providers should consider whether a particular intervention will need high or low levels of patient or caregiver involvement at a time when both may be unable to participate at the level necessitated for success of the intervention.
- Nurses play a crucial role in the recognition of pain and its management through the illness continuum, especially for patients at the end of life.

CASE STUDY

Ms. T. is a 44-year-old woman who is being seen at the outpatient palliative care practice for pain management. Four years ago, she was diagnosed with rectal cancer and underwent a surgical resection. When her disease recurred 2 years later, she decided to seek holistic and herbal treatments which were unsuccessful. Unfortunately, she experienced an intestinal obstruction, and underwent surgery (transverse colostomy), chemotherapy, and radiation. In addition to her cancer pain, Ms. T. has chronic pain related to rheumatoid arthritis and degenerative disc disease in her spine. She reports continuous pain in her lower abdomen and lower buttock, which is described as throbbing and stabbing. She rates her pain as 7/10 at its worst and 2/10 at its best. The pain is now constant, exacerbated by standing and has been getting worse over the past few weeks. Her pain management includes a combination of extended-release morphine 90 mg po q12h, immediate-release morphine 15 mg po q4h prn (6 tabs/d) with docusate and senna as a bowel regimen. Ms. T. reports that this regimen had been working well, without any side effects, but now she experiences only 50% relief. Recently, she needed to go on disability from her cashier's job because the pain "just gets so bad." Based on her report, the medication regimen is changed to include extended-release morphine 150 q12h, immediate-release morphine 30 mg po q4h prn, and the addition of gabapentin 300 mg po at night, with titration up to 600 mg po TID. What types of pain is Ms. T. experiencing? What principles of opioid and co-analgesic management were demonstrated in this case? What would you add, if anything, to her analgesic regimen?

Few things are of more concern to palliative care (PC) patients at end of life (EOL) and to their families than that pain will be well controlled (D'Arcy, 2012; Ferrell & Coyle, 2010; Hospice and Palliative Nurses Position Statement, 2016; Institute of Medicine [IOM], 2014; National Cancer Institute at the National Institutes of Health, 2013b). In the words of one patient, "I can't emphasize enough that pain blinds you to all that is positive—I mean the real bad pain. It just closes you down." Unrelieved pain can consume the attention and energy of those who are dying, and create an atmosphere of impotency and despair in their families and caretakers (Hospice and Palliative Nurses Position Statement, 2016). The fear of unrelieved pain expressed by patients and their families is sadly often reflective of what they have or will experience (American Geriatrics Society, 2013; Connors et al., 1995; IOM, 2014). With the knowledge and art that is now available, we have the ability to relieve the majority of pain including pain at the EOL (American Nurses Association [ANA], 2016a, 2016b).

The intent of this chapter is to provide nurses with a basic overview of the principles of pain assessment and pharmacological management throughout the illness continuum and at EOL. The needs of special populations who have been identified as "at risk" of inadequate pain control are highlighted, including older adults, children, persons with communication impairment, patients with a history of substance abuse, and cancer survivors. These groups represent those in whom pain is often unrecognized, not respected, or not believed.

■ SECTION 1: PAIN ASSESSMENT AND BARRIERS TO PAIN RELIEF

Pain in patients with advanced illness varies by diagnosis and other factors. Between 11% and 88% of patients with cancer or other life-threatening illness will experience pain at some point (Bennett et al., 2012; IOM, 2011; Moens, Higginson, & Harding, 2014). Pain in the cancer population has been widely studied and is a valuable model for assessment and management (National Cancer Institute at the National Institutes of Health, 2013c). Therefore, it will be used as the framework for this chapter. It is recognized that pain associated with

a serious illness may be superimposed on many other chronic pain syndromes, including musculoskeletal pain such as osteoarthritis and low back pain. The principles outlined in this chapter can be applied to any pain situation.

Barriers to Pain Relief

Numerous clinician-, institutional-, and patient- and family-related barriers have been identified that consistently interfere with adequate pain management even at the EOL. In addition, there is growing research on the influence of and gender on the experience of pain and response to treatment (Fink, Gates, & Montgomery, 2015; Hurley & Adams, 2009).

Clinician-related barriers include inadequate knowledge of pain management, incomplete assessment of pain, concern about regulation of controlled substances, fear of causing patient addiction, concern about analgesic side effects, and concern that if strong opioids are used "too early" they will be ineffective later when the need is greatest. In addition, a failure of clinicians to evaluate or appreciate the severity of the pain problem and to appreciate the impact of pain on the patient's day-to-day existence is likely to be a major predictor of inadequate relief (Paice, 2015).

Healthcare setting–related barriers include lack of pain visibility; lack of a common, consistent language to describe pain; lack of commitment to prioritize pain management; and failure to use validated pain measurement tools in clinical practice. Use of the appropriate tool in the appropriate setting can improve pain and patient outcomes. The healthcare provider should be knowledgeable to choose the best tool given the patient population. The Critical-Care Observation Tool (CCOT); Faces Legs, Arms, Cry, Consolability (FLACC); Faces, Pain Scale-Revised (FPS-R); Visual Analog Scale (VAS); Numerical Rating Scale (NRS); Behavioral Pain Scale (BPS); Nonverbal Pain Indicators (CNPI); Nonverbal Pain Scale (NVPS); Critical Care Pain Observation Tool (CPOT); Multidimensional Observation Pain Assessment Tool (MOPAT); and Behavioral Pain Assessment Tool (BPAT) are examples of valid and reliable pain assessment tools (Gélinas, Puntillo, Levin, & Azoulay, 2017; McGuire, Kaiser, Haisfield-Wolfe, & Ivamu, 2016;

Pasero & McCaffery, 2011). Economic factors and drug availability are further impediments to adequate pain treatment, especially in underserved and minority communities and when pain is to be managed in the home (Hazin & Giles, 2011; National Comprehensive Cancer Network, 2017; Voelkner, 2010).

Patient-related barriers have many similarities to clinician-related barriers and include reluctance to report pain, reluctance to follow treatment recommendations, fears of tolerance and addiction, concern about treatment-related side effects, fears regarding disease progression, and belief that pain is an inevitable part of cancer and must be accepted (International Association for the Study of Pain [IASP], 2009; Paice, 2015).

Family-related barriers to pain management are extremely important to understand (National Cancer Institute at the National Institutes of Health, 2013c). Frequently, it is a family member who is the primary care provider in the home and it is a family member who will be assessing pain and administering the pain medications (Ferrell, Hanson, & Grant, 2013). An early small descriptive study investigated the experience of managing pain at home from the perspectives of the patient, the primary family caregiver, and the home care nurse, and it encapsulated many of the important areas that still affect pain management in the home (Vallerand, Collins-Bohler, Templin, & Hasenau, 2007). Areas of decision making and conflict mainly focus on the use of medications. Patients were preoccupied with decisions about the choice, dose, and frequency of analgesics. Negative side effects and the meaning ascribed to these medications contributed to conflicts in the patient's mind as to whether he or she was doing the "right thing" in taking the analgesic. Nearly all the patients assumed their pain would increase with impending death. Patients' decisions about how to live with and cope with their pain included considerations of how their words and actions affected their family members and healthcare professionals. Sometimes, these factors continued to lead the patients to deny the presence of pain (National Cancer Institute at the National Institutes of Health, 2013b). Similarly, the decisions and conflicts that arose most frequently for family caregivers also related to pain medication and having to make decisions about which pill to give and when. Compounding these decisions were the concerns related to overdosing, adverse side effects, and addiction. These fears were reaffirmed in a recent study evaluating outpatient oncology patients and their families (Valeberg, Miaskowski, Paul, & Rustøen, 2016).

A variety of approaches and specific programs have been developed to address these barriers; for example, making pain visible within an institution by incorporating a pain measurement tool into daily clinical practice and introducing broad educational efforts to change attitudes, behaviors, and knowledge deficits in patients, clinicians, and facilities (The Joint Commission [TJC], 2012). TJC standards on pain management have been helpful in

making institutions accountable for assessment and management of pain across care settings (TJC, 2012). With the recent concerns regarding opioid misuse and abuse, TJC is revising these standards to include a focus on patient functionality and the importance of nondrug pain-relieving factors (Baker, 2017). In addition, various professional organizations have developed and regularly update clinical practice guidelines for the assessment and management of pain. These organizations include the American Pain Society (APS), the American Society for Pain Management Nursing, the National Comprehensive Cancer Network (NCCN), the American Geriatric Society, and the National Consensus Guidelines for Quality Palliative Care. Clinical practice guidelines, as well as major national professional educational efforts on EOL care (End of Life Nursing Education Consortium [ELNEC] and Education for Physicians on End-of-Life Care [EPEC]), and Initiative for Pediatric Palliative Care (IPPC) are providing ongoing efforts to improve care of the dying and address the problem of inadequate pain control (American Association of Colleges of Nursing, 2016; Education for Physicians on End-of-Life Care, 2017; IPPC, 2014). Since the initiation of these organizations, the field of PC has expanded to include pediatrics, geriatrics, veterans, critical care, and advance practice nurse specialties. ELNEC has provided international educational programs for nurses, extending its impact to 90 countries throughout the world.

Pain in Non-Oncologic Populations Facing Life-Threatening Illness

The pain experience for patients with non-cancer diagnoses has not been well defined in the literature, but what is known highlights the frequency of suffering within this population (Alpert, Smith, Hummel, & Hummel, 2017; Koncicki, Unruh, & Schell, 2017; Lilly & Senderovich, 2016). As in cancer, these patients may experience pain related to their underlying diagnosis, as an outcome of treatment modalities, or as a consequence of living longer with a chronic illness. Currently, the literature suggests providers utilize the World Health Organization (WHO) analgesic ladder when considering pain alleviating therapies in these patient groups (Phongtankuel, Amorapanth, & Siegler, 2016).

Further research and expansion of evidence-based practices are critical in better defining pain assessment and management for these populations (Paice, 2016). The following information should provide the nurse with an important foundation in addressing pain in patients with cardiovascular, neurological, and other non-cancer–related diagnoses.

■ **Pain in Congestive Heart Failure (CHF).** On average, more than 50% of patients with heart failure experience pain. Pain intensity worsens with progression of heart failure, affecting up to 89% with NYHA Class IV disease (Alpert et al., 2017). Separate from angina, the most common types of pain in this population include musculoskeletal as well as neuropathic due to comorbidities such as diabetes. Treatment of these pain etiologies can be difficult, since medications such as nonsteroidal anti-inflammatory drugs (NSAIDs), anticonvulsants, and antidepressants can cause adverse side effects including fluid retention, Q-T wave prolongation, and renal complications (Phongtankuel et al., 2016). Acetaminophen and topical NSAID preparations are considered safe treatment strategies in CHF patients. Although there are limited data regarding the use of opioid analgesics, tramadol, oxycodone, hydromorphone, and fentanyl have been identified as being the most appropriate medications for this patient population. Morphine and codeine should be avoided, as there may be accumulation of active metabolites which may precipitate problematic side effects (Light-McGroary & Goodlin, 2013).

■ Chronic Obstructive Pulmonary Disease (COPD).

A recent systematic review by van den Heuvel et al. (2017) revealed pain prevalence in COPD patients ranging from 21% to 77%. The potential underlying pain mechanisms in this patient population include: activation of cytokines which can lead to neuropathic pain, musculoskeletal conditions caused by limited chest wall movement and osteoporosis, and other conditions such as arthritis (van den Heuvel et al., 2017). As in other non-cancer diagnoses, pain in COPD patients can be addressed by using the WHO analgesic ladder (Lilly & Senderovich, 2016).

■ HIV/AIDS.

As in the oncology patient, those with HIV/AIDS can experience pain directly related to the virus (e.g., opportunistic infections: progressive multifocal leukoencephalopathy; malignancies: Kaposi sarcoma), its treatment (neuropathies as a side effect of antiviral medications), or other chronic comorbidities (Wentlandt & Zimmermann, 2016). With improvement in treatment options, patients with HIV/AIDS are living longer, putting them at risk of developing pain-related problems. The prevalence of moderate-to-severe pain in this population has been noted to be between 54% and 83% (Parker, Stein, & Jelsma, 2014). Since pain in these patients tends to be neuropathic in nature, use of co-analgesics and opioids can provide adequate relief (Wentlandt & Zimmermann, 2016).

■ Liver Disease.

Patients with end-stage liver disease experience pain due to abdominal distention related to ascites, peritonitis, or hepatic cell carcinoma. If pain is mild, low-dose acetaminophen (max 2 gm/d) can be used. Opioid analgesics, especially short-acting preparations, can be prescribed for moderate-to-severe pain, but dosing should be adjusted for impaired hepatic function. The use of steroids such as dexamethasone can be a potent co-analgesic in the management of pain due to capsular distention (Medici & Meyers, 2016).

■ Neurological Disorders.

Amyotrophic Lateral Sclerosis (ALS): Patients with ALS may experience pain due to immobility, spasticity, or contractures. Pain management can include co-analgesics, anti-inflammatory agents, or low-dose opioid analgesics, as well as nondrug interventions such as physical therapy (Walbert, 2016).

Multiple Sclerosis (MS): Pain affects between 50% and 75% of patients who have pain related to MS and the etiology is usually neuropathic in nature, often affecting the lower extremities. Management includes the use of co-analgesics such as carbamazepine or other anticonvulsants as well as tricyclic antidepressants (Walbert, 2016).

Stroke: Patients who suffer from a cerebral vascular accident (CVA) are at risk of developing poststroke pain syndromes (Phongtankuel et al., 2016). With a prevalence between 4% and 66%, these syndromes include both musculoskeletal and neuropathic etiologies (e.g., central poststroke pain, muscle spasticity, and poststroke shoulder pain; Hansen et al., 2012; Jonsson, Lindgren, Hallstrom, Norrving, & Lindgren, 2006; O'Donnell et al., 2013). NSAIDs including topical formulations as well as co-analgesics such as antidepressants (amitriptyline) and anticonvulsants (lamotrigine) can be beneficial in managing these pain syndromes (Walbert, 2016).

Renal Disease: Pain affects roughly 58% to 65% of patients with renal disease, including those patients receiving hemodialysis (Koncicki et al., 2017; Phongtankuel et al., 2016). As with other chronic illnesses, the etiology of pain in renal disease is multifactorial. Chronic kidney disease mineral and bone disorder (CKD-MBD) can precipitate bony pain, calciphylaxis can result in painful skin lesions due to decreased vascular perfusion, and polycystic kidney disease (PCKD) can cause abdominal, back, and flank pain. Additionally, these patients experience pain due to dialysis therapy (e.g., cramping or headaches) or from other chronic illnesses such as diabetic neuropathy (Koncicki et al., 2017).

Given that many analgesics are renally excreted, managing pain in this patient population can be particularly challenging. As with other non-cancer diagnoses, providers should adapt the WHO analgesic ladder to address pain relief in these patients. Dose reduction of non-opioids, opioids, and co-analgesics should be considered in patients with impaired renal function. Acetaminophen and time-limited use of NSAIDs can be prescribed for mild pain. Tramadol in a reduced dose may be useful in the management of moderate pain. Morphine should be avoided due to the potential accumulation of active metabolites, which can lead to serious adverse side effects such as myoclonus and seizures. Other opioids such as fentanyl and methadone do not have active metabolites; therefore, they may offer a better choice for the management of severe pain in end-stage renal disease patients (Davison & Hui, 2016; Koncicki et al., 2017).

Basic Principles of Pain Assessment

Pain assessment is the underpinning of pain management. The goals of pain assessment are to prevent pain if possible and to identify pain immediately should it occur. These objectives can be facilitated by standardized screening of all patients for pain on a routine basis and across care settings (TJC, 2012). Standardized screening for pain can be as simple as asking the patient, "Do you have pain?" A comprehensive assessment of pain follows if a patient reports pain that is not being addressed or adequately managed. TJC's *Speak Up* series is a consumer publication urging the patient to take a more active role in pain management (TJC, 2015). The Centers for Medicare and Medicaid Services (CMS, 2015) integrated questions regarding pain management into the HCAHPS survey which evaluates patient satisfaction during recent hospitalization.

Pain is always subjective and is defined by the IASP (2012) as "an unpleasant sensory and emotional experience associated with actual or potential tissue damage or described in terms of such damage." This definition clarifies the multidimensionality of pain. McCaffery's definition of pain, 'Whatever the person says it is, existing whenever he or she say it does' (Pasero & McCaffery, 2011), further supports the subjectivity of pain. The patient is acknowledged as the expert on the severity of his or her pain and of the adequacy of relief obtained. The interprofessional team's expertise is in identifying the different etiologies of the pain and arriving at effective management strategies with the patient and/or family. Although verbal report of pain and adequacy of pain relief is considered the gold standard, some individuals at EOL are unable to communicate verbally (McGuire et al., 2016). In these situations, other behavioral measures for assessing pain are required. The American Society for Pain Management Nursing's position statement (2015) promotes that in the presence of a pathology that is known to cause pain, a practitioner can "assume pain is present" and an analgesic trial should be implemented. For example, patients who are semiconscious or in a coma may moan or cry out or exhibit other signs of distress when moved. Although these behaviors are not necessarily associated with pain, the likelihood of pain should be strongly considered. If the decision is made to medicate the patient for pain, subsequent signs of diminished distress on movement may indicate that pain was present. If such a patient was on an analgesic regimen prior to diminution of consciousness, analgesics should be continued or increased until the patient shows signs of comfort.

Assessment of pain at EOL is often complicated by the presence of multiple other symptoms that are common during the dying process, including cognitive impairment (Gao et al., 2013; refer to Table 20.1). In addition,

TABLE 20.1 Challenges When Assessing Pain in the Advanced Palliative Care Patient

- Multiple concurrent medical problems.
- Multiple symptoms and symptom clusters.
- Hepatic and renal failure and susceptibility to drug accumulation and adverse side effects.
- Prevalence of delirium when close to death.
- Requires more time than patients who are less ill.
- Patients become easily fatigued and may be short of breath.
- May be in "too much pain" or bothered by other symptoms to answer questions.
- Possible tendency of family members to answer questions on patient's behalf.

the suffering that patients experience at the EOL is not necessarily related to the severity of the symptom. Mild symptoms may cause considerable distress to some patients due to the personal meaning of the pain or because the individual has not yet come to terms with dying (National Cancer Institute at the National Institutes of Health, 2012). Unrelieved pain and suffering can become the primary focus for patients and their families, thereby depriving them of quality time for communication and reconciliation. Nurses have an extraordinary responsibility to be patient advocates in the assessment and management of pain throughout the course of a disease process, but especially at the EOL (ANA, 2016a, 2016b). Due to its complexity, the assessment of pain is enhanced by a multidimensional and interprofessional approach (IOM, 2011; Wong & Reddy, 2016). The tissue damage response leading to the complaint of pain, the suffering component of the pain, and the meaning of the pain to the individuals and their families all need to be addressed. Although this comprehensive pain assessment is usually interprofessional, it is the nurse who brings that assessment and plan to the bedside. The assessment of pain is carried out within the framework of goals of care, patient and family values, knowledge of the disease process, and nearness of the individual to death.

Types of Pain—Neurophysiological Mechanisms of Pain

Two major types of pain, *nociceptive pain* (which includes somatic and visceral pain) and *neuropathic pain*, have been described in the cancer and non-cancer palliative care populations (Alpert et al., 2017; Koncicki et al., 2017; National Comprehensive Cancer Network, 2017; Phongtankuel et al., 2016). *Somatic pain* occurs as a result of activating pain-sensitive structures, or nociceptors, in the cutaneous and deep musculoskeletal tissues. This pain is typically well localized and may be felt in the superficial cutaneous or deeper musculoskeletal structures. Examples of somatic pain include bone metastases, postsurgical incisional pain, and pain accompanying myofascial or musculoskeletal inflammation or spasm. Somatic pain is responsive to NSAIDs, opioid drugs, and steroids (Portenoy, Ahmed, & Keilson, 2017).

Visceral pain results from infiltration, compression, distention, or stretching of thoracic or abdominal viscera. This type of pain is poorly localized; often described as deep, squeezing pressure; and may be associated with nausea, vomiting, and diaphoresis (especially when acute). Visceral pain is often referred to cutaneous sites that may be remote from the site of the lesion; for example, shoulder pain associated with diaphragmatic irritation. Tenderness and pain on touching the referral cutaneous site may occur (Portenoy & Dhingra, 2015). Visceral pain is responsive to NSAIDs, opioid drugs, and steroids (Portenoy et al., 2017; Portenoy, Mehta, & Ahmed, 2017a; 2017b).

Neuropathic pain results from injury to the peripheral or central nervous system (CNS). In the cancer patient, neuropathic pain most commonly occurs as a consequence of the tumor compressing or infiltrating peripheral nerves, nerve roots, or the spinal cord. In addition, this type of pain may result from surgical trauma and chemical or radiation-induced injury to peripheral nerves or the spinal cord from cancer therapies. Examples of common neuropathic pain syndromes include metastatic or radiation-induced brachial or lumbosacral plexopathies, epidural spinal cord or cauda-equina compression, postherpetic neuralgia (PHN), diabetic retinopathy, and painful chemotherapy-induced neuropathies. Neuropathic pain is often described as having sharp, shooting, electric shock–like qualities that are unfamiliar to the patient. It can also be described as a constant dull ache, sometimes with a pressure or vise-like quality with episodic paroxysms of burning or electric shock–like sensations. Neuropathic pain is often severe, very distressing to the patient, and sometimes difficult to control (Portenoy & Dhingra, 2015). Although partially responsive to the opioid drugs, neuropathic pain is also responsive to adjuvant drugs or co-analgesics such as antidepressants, anticonvulsants, steroids, local anesthetics, and N-methyl-D-aspartate (NMDA) antagonists such as ketamine (Portenoy et al., 2017a, 2017b).

Temporal Pattern of Pain

Pain can also be defined on a temporal basis; for example, acute pain and chronic pain. Patients with serious illness, especially at the EOL, frequently have a combination of both acute and chronic pain (Broglio & Portenoy, 2016).

Acute pain is characterized by a well-defined pattern of onset. Generally, the cause of the pain can be identified and the pain may be accompanied by physiological signs of hyperactivity of the autonomic nervous system

such as a rapid pulse and elevated blood pressure. Acute pain usually has a precipitating cause; for example, small bowel obstruction, a painful dressing change, or a pathological fracture. The pain tends to be time-limited and responds to analgesic drug therapy and, where possible, treatment of the precipitating cause. Acute pain can be further subdivided into subacute pain and intermittent or episodic types (Pasero & McCaffery, 2011).

Subacute pain describes pain that comes on over several days, often with increasing intensity, and may be associated with a variety of causes such as a progressive pathological process or an analgesic regimen that has not been titrated upward to accommodate for disease progression. Episodic pain refers to pain that occurs during defined periods of time on a regular or irregular basis (Pasero & McCaffery, 2011). Intermittent pain is an alternative way to describe episodic pain. Such pain may be associated with movement, dressing changes, or other activities. Because the trigger for intermittent pain often can be identified, the nurse, through appropriate use of analgesics prior to the pain-provoking event, can have a significant impact on decreasing these painful episodes for the patient. The fear of pain associated with these activities is therefore lessened for the patient (National Comprehensive Cancer Network, 2017).

Chronic pain differs from acute pain in its presentation. These differences are essential for the nurse to understand because patients with chronic pain are at risk of having their pain unrecognized, untreated, or undertreated. Chronic pain is defined as pain that persists for more than 3 months (Pasero & McCaffery, 2011). Adaptation of the autonomic nervous system occurs and the patient does not exhibit the objective signs of pain found so frequently in those with acute pain (e.g., there is no rapid pulse or elevated blood pressure). Poorly relieved chronic pain at the EOL can contribute to fatigue, depression, insomnia, general despair, withdrawal from interaction with others, and desire for death (National Cancer Institute at the National Institutes of Health, 2013b; Pasero & McCaffery, 2011).

Breakthrough pain is defined as a transient increase in pain to greater than moderate intensity, occurring on a baseline pain of moderate intensity or less (National Comprehensive Cancer Network, 2017). Breakthrough pain has a diversity of characteristics. In some patients, for example, it is characterized by marked worsening of pain at the end of the dosing interval of regularly scheduled analgesics, known as end-of-dose failure (Hall & O'Lenic, 2012). In other patients, it occurs by the action of the patient or the nurse (e.g., when turning or having a dressing change), and is referred to as incident pain. Patients frequently have a combination of these different types of pain; noting the patterns of pain in a particular individual is an essential component of pain assessment. Attention to such details is the essence of symptom control at the EOL. A pain diary or log, kept by the patient or family, can help identify the pattern of pain. The log can indicate, over the course of the day, the patient's pain rating, medication taken, activity level, and/or the use of any other pain relief measures.

Clinical Assessment of Pain

The previously described mechanisms of pain and types of pain that can be experienced by patients with advanced progressive disease are a useful background from which to start a clinical pain assessment. The clinical assessment is based on a process of both observation and interview. The basic principles of a pain assessment are outlined in Table 20.2. It is based on the premise that the person experiencing the pain is the expert on his or her pain (Herr, Coyne, McCaffery, Manwarren, & Merkel, 2011; National Comprehensive Cancer Network, 2017). The clinician's role is to sort out the etiology of the pain complaint and arrive at a targeted management approach with the patient and family. If the patient is too ill or cognitively impaired to respond to the questions, a family member or care provider is asked to give the pain history as best as he or she can.

A variety of validated pain assessment tools are available for use in the hospital or home setting. Ideally, any pain assessment tool includes intensity of pain, relief of pain, psychological distress, and functional impairment. For the patient with severe cognitive impairment, various assessment tools are also available (McGuire et al., 2016). In the terminally ill patient when multiple symptoms are common, it can be useful to follow the intensity of pain and other symptoms in graph form longitudinally.

Taking a focused pain history involves assessing the following parameters:

■ **Onset.** Have the patient describe when the pain first began. Was it associated with a particular activity or known medical event? Did other symptoms accompany the onset of pain such as nausea or vomiting?

■ **Site(s).** Ask the patient to point to the site or sites of pain. Frequently, individuals with pain have multiple sites of pain. Each site needs to be examined and assessed as the management approach may differ depending on the etiology of the pain.

TABLE 20.2 Clinical Assessment of Pain: Basic Principles

■ Accept the patient's complaint of pain. The patient is the expert on the pain being experienced. The multidisciplinary staff are the experts in determining the etiology of the pain.

■ Take a careful history of the pain complaint and place it within the context of the patient's medical history and goals of care. If the patient is unable to communicate verbally, obtain a history from those most involved in the patient's care, both family and other informal and formal healthcare providers.

■ Observe the patient for nonverbal communication regarding pain; for example, guarding, wincing, and moaning, as well as bracing or crying out when turned or moved.

■ Recognize that the patient near the end of life may have multiple symptoms complicating pain assessment.

■ Assess the characteristics of each pain, including the site, pattern of referral, what makes it better and what makes it worse, and the impact of the pain on the individual's activities of daily living and quality of life; for example, mood, sleep, movement, and interaction with others.

■ Clarify the temporal aspects and pattern of the patient's pain; for example, acute, chronic, baseline, intermittent, breakthrough, or incident.

■ Assess the psychological state of the patient and the meaning of the pain to the patient and his or her family.

■ Examine the site of the pain for presence of pathology.

■ Based on the goals of care, facilitate appropriate diagnostic testing, assuring that the patient's pain is adequately managed during the workup.

■ Provide continuity of care for the patient and family during ongoing pain assessment and management.

■ Assess and reassess the effectiveness of the pain management regimen both for baseline pain and breakthrough pain and make adjustments accordingly.

■ Give a time frame where you would expect to see evidence of patient comfort after the start or adjustment of a pain management approach. If pain relief is not evident, reassess the patient. Ongoing reassessment is essential in the setting of a complex patient with multiple symptoms.

■ Assess and reassess patients for the presence of adverse side effects from the pain management regimen.

■ **Quality of the Pain.** Have the patient describe the quality of each pain. Word descriptors used by patients to describe their pain help the clinician to arrive at an inferred pain mechanism. This, in turn, influences the choice of pharmacotherapy. For example, sharp, shooting, electric shock–like descriptions of pain, often described by the patient as "unfamiliar," suggests a neuropathic component to the pain (Pasero & McCaffery, 2011). Such pain may be responsive to co-analgesic/adjuvant drugs as well as to opioid analgesics.

■ **Severity of the Pain.** Have the patient describe the severity of each pain. It is particularly important that the nurse recognize the significance of escalating pain within the context of that particular patient's disease process, value system, goals of care, and nearness to death. Treatment decisions take all of these factors into account. As previously described, a variety of tools for measuring pain are available for use in the hospital or home setting. Ask the patient the amount of distress caused by each site of pain. In this way, each pain can be prioritized.

Although numerical estimates are the most frequently used methods for assessing pain severity and adequacy of pain relief, some patients cannot use a numerical estimate. In these cases, one of the other tools may be more appropriate. Consistency in using a particular assessment tool with an individual patient is likely to enhance communication among team members regarding the efficacy of a pain management approach. Some patients will underreport their pain. The reasons are varied but include a patient's appraisal of the consequences of reporting pain (National Cancer Institute at the National Institutes of Health, 2012). For example, having an opioid dosage increased may lead to fear of increased constipation. This potential outcome may not be acceptable to the patient and therefore he or she chose not to report the pain. Other patients do not report escalating pain because previous reports of pain have led to ineffective management. In other words, they "give up" trying.

■ **Assess Pain Severity at Times of Different Activity.** Pain intensity should be assessed at rest, on movement, and in relation to daily activity and the patient's analgesic schedule. Asking certain questions helps establish if the appropriate drug has been selected, dose efficacy, and if the time interval between doses for this patient is correct: "How much pain is relieved when you take the pain medication?", "How long does the relief last?" and "Are side effects present?" A more global 24-hour assessment of the adequacy of pain management in general includes asking the patient his or her pain scores—"right now," "at its best," "at its worst," and "on average" (National Cancer Institute at the National Institutes of Health, 2012).

■ **Exacerbating and Relieving Factors.** Identifying factors that increase or relieve the patient's pain can be helpful in arriving at a pain diagnosis and in giving the nurse the opportunity to reinforce techniques that the patient has found useful in the past to relieve pain. Cancer patients who report rapidly escalating back pain with a band-like quality that is worse when lying in bed and better when standing is considered to have cord compression until proved otherwise (Huff & Brenner, 2012). Early recognition of cord compression and treatment, frequently with steroids, radiation therapy, or both, may prevent paraplegia in the last few weeks or months of a patient's life. Escalating back pain may be the only sign of the impending cord compression. It is critical that the nurse who is caring for a patient at the EOL recognizes the significance of escalating pain within the construct of that particular patient's disease process and goals of care.

■ **Impact of the Pain on the Patient's Psychological State.** The interface between pain and suffering has been well described (Cherney, 2010; Cherney & Coyle, 1994; Saunders, 1967). In clinical situations, when patients are asked, "What does this pain mean to you?" and "What do you think is causing the pain?" a flood of suffering and fear is often expressed. Patients are fearful of what their dying will be like, of uncontrolled and excruciating pain, of being a burden on their family, and of being "drugged out." The same questions may be asked by the patient and family time and time again, and need to be responded to in a sensitive, accurate, and reassuring manner. Some clinicians, when meeting a patient in severe pain for the first time, ask if the pain has ever been so bad that the individual has thought of harming himself or herself. Again, the response may indicate that suicide has been considered as an option if the pain is not controlled or if things get "too bad." These are important questions for an experienced clinician to ask so that the patient's vulnerabilities and anxieties are verbalized, suicide vulnerability factors are identified, and education and support from other members of the interprofessional pain team, including psychiatrists, psychologists, social workers, and chaplains, are mobilized (Rosenblatt & Meyer, 2017). All of the patient's worries and fears need to be addressed if the pain is to be adequately controlled. This is an ongoing process.

■ **Pain Treatment History and Responses to Previous and Current Analgesic Regimens.** The patient needs to be asked very specifically about what approaches have been used to manage pain in the past—both pharmacological (including over-the-counter medication) and nonpharmacological—and the subsequent amount of relief. Included should be analgesics that have been previously prescribed, dosages, time intervals, routes of administration, effects, side effects, and the reasons why a particular approach was discontinued. Additionally, discussion of previous use of opioid analgesics can assist the practitioner to determine tolerance and risk for misuse and abuse (National Comprehensive Cancer Network, 2017). Fear of recurrence of previously experienced side effects (e.g., sedation, nausea, mental haziness, and constipation) may make a patient reluctant to start a new analgesic regimen. Focusing attention on his or her concerns and a clear explanation of how side effects will be managed if they do occur can do much to allay these fears. This is a commitment that will require close monitoring of the patient's response to therapy and a rapid response to the management of any adverse side effects should they occur.

■ **Examine the Patient and the Site of the Pain.** Examining the site of the pain and possible referral sites may help identify the source of the pain (Herr et al., 2011). This is always done within knowledge of the patient's disease process, extent of disease, possible referral sites of pain, and goals of care. The source of the pain may be obvious. For example, pain may be due to a distended abdomen associated with a full bladder, bowel obstruction or liver distention, a prior skin eruption with PHN, a bony deformity or inability to use a limb due to a pathological fracture, or an open fungating infected wound. In the patient with advanced illness, the cause of pain is frequently multifactorial requiring a multimodal approach (National Cancer Institute at the National Institutes of Health, 2012). Whenever possible, within the constraints of nearness to death and goals of care, an attempt is made to treat the cause of the pain as well as the pain itself. The extent of the diagnostic workup depends on the goals of care and the likely impact these test results will have on the patient's treatment plan and overall quality of life (QOL). The benefit-to-burden ratio to the patient is of upmost concern and needs to be discussed fully with the patient and family or the patient's healthcare agent (IOM, 2014). Although most pain can be adequately controlled to the patient's satisfaction, the complete absence of pain may not be possible. Realistic goal setting with the patient to establish an acceptable pain level that would not interfere with function or QOL is part of the assessment. The balance is to achieve maximum pain relief and minimal adverse effects of treatment. Realistic goal setting is likely to diminish later frustration and loss of trust in the clinician's competence.

Components of Pain Management

Pain is a multidimensional experience that involves sensory, affective, cognitive, behavioral, and sociocultural components (Huijer, Miaskowski, Quinn, & Twycross, 2013). Table 20.3 illustrates factors that contribute to the concept of "total pain" at EOL and its multidimensional nature. Effective management involves treating the underlying cause if possible and systematically utilizing appropriate treatment modalities.

TABLE 20.3 Factors Contributing to a Patient's "Total Pain" or "Existential Distress"

Tissue damage response associated with the disease or its treatment causing pain
  Nociceptive pain
  Neuropathic pain
  Mixed pain syndrome

Multiple other disease-related or treatment-related distressing symptoms
  Psychological, spiritual, and social distress

Anxiety, fear, and spiritual distress associated with
  Worsening pain representing progression of disease
  Uncontrolled pain or other symptoms
  Perceived loss of dignity
  Loss of bodily control
  Uncertainty about the future
  Uncertainty about God
  Fear of death
  Fear of abandonment (by God, family, friends, the medical team)
  Worry about exhausting and burdening the family, friends, and medical team
  Worry about how he or she will be remembered
  Worry about finances and financially depleting the family

Depression associated with
  Loss of sense of "self"
  Loss of social position and role in the family
  Loss of control
  Sense of helplessness and demoralization
  Perceived loss of dignity
  Loss of meaning and purpose in continued life
  Loss of hope

Anger associated with
  Delays in diagnosis resulting in late diagnosis and diminished hope for a cure
  Bureaucratic bungling
  Therapeutic failures
  Insensitive communication
  Friends who do not visit

Of note, the previous factors are interrelated. Their interrelatedness is dynamic and nonlinear. When one factor changes it influences other factors. The impact of each factor varies from patient to patient and within one patient at any given time. This list is not all-inclusive.

Although pharmacotherapy is the foundation of pain management, pharmacotherapy alone will not be an effective approach to pain control in the PC patient. A multimodal approach, such as described in Table 20.4, is usually required, including attention to the suffering and spiritual or existential component to the patient's pain (Okon, 2016; Saunders, 1967). In addition, the needs of the family must be addressed (National Cancer Institute at the National Institutes of Health, 2013a; National Comprehensive Cancer Network, 2017).

TABLE 20.4 Multimodal Components of Pain Management
Pharmacological: Acetaminophen and nonsteroidal anti-inflammatory drugs Opioid drugs Co-analgesic or adjuvant analgesics
Interventional: Surgical management Injection therapies Neural blockage Implanted therapies Neurodestructive techniques
Neurostimulation: Transcutaneous Transcranial Percutaneous peripheral nerve and spinal cord/route stimulation Neurodestructive techniques
Rehabilitative: Positioning and movement Therapeutic exercise Hydrotherapy Supportive orthotic devices Physical modalities: heat and cold Therapies of specific disorders (such as lymphedema)
Psychological: Psychoeducational interventions Cognitive behavioral interventions ■ Pain diary ■ Relaxation therapy, guided imagery, other types of stress management ■ Mindfulness ■ CBT ■ PCST
Integrative Treatments: Acupuncture Hypnosis Massage Music

CBT, cognitive behavioral therapy; PCST, pain coping skills training.

Sources: Adapted from Portenoy, R. E., & Ahmed, E. (2014). Principles of opioid use in cancer pain. *Journal of Clinical Oncology, 32*(16), 1662–1670. doi:10.1200/JCO.2013.52.5188; Paice, J. A., Portenoy, R. K., Lacchetti, C., Campbell, T., Cheville, A. Citron, M., … Bruera, E. (2016). Management of chronic pain in survivors of adult cancers: American Society of Clinical Oncology clinical practice guideline. *Journal of Clinical Oncology, 34*(27), 3325–3345. doi:10.1200/JCO.2016.68.5206

CASE STUDY *Continued*

During a follow-up call a few days later, Ms. T. reports 75% pain relief with the medication changes. She has noticed some constipation, so Miralax is added to her bowel regimen. You ask Ms. T. to contact you after she sees her oncologist later that month. When she calls you, Ms. T. is tearful on the phone. Her rectal cancer has recurred and she is scheduled to undergo a (total abdominal hysterectomy and bilateral salpingo-oophorectomy) TAHBSO, with a plan for chemotherapy after surgery. She shares with you that undergoing a hysterectomy only brings back memories of a stillbirth she experienced 7 years ago. Due to the financial strains of being on disability, she's now living in her childhood home with her husband, Brian. She says that her pain is worse and she is not able to sleep at night, because "my mind just keeps racing." Ms. T. comes into the outpatient practice the next day for a follow-up visit. She rates her pain as 6/10 and has been taking a total of 420 mg of morphine per day (300 mg extended release and 120 mg immediate release). She asks if there is another way to manage her pain so that she wouldn't need to take "all these pills." A decision is made to switch her regimen to transdermal fentanyl 100 mcg/h patch q72h and hydromorphone 8 mg po q4h prn.

In addition to reviewing her pain medication regimen, what other assessment questions would you ask? Are other symptoms exacerbating her pain experience? What other medications and nonpharmacological interventions might be useful?

■ SECTION 2: PHARMACOLOGICAL TREATMENTS

Inadequate knowledge of analgesic pharmacotherapy is one of the most commonly cited reasons for undertreatment of pain (Paice, 2015). Developing expertise in the use of analgesic drugs is an integral part of nursing care for PC patients throughout the continuum of illness.

Over two decades ago, an expert committee convened by the cancer unit of the WHO developed a three-step "analgesic ladder" approach to the selection of drugs for the treatment of cancer pain (WHO, 2010). Drug categories in the three-step ladder included NSAIDs, opioids, and co-analgesics or adjuvant drugs. While this strategy remains the foundation for the treatment of pain in cancer and PC patients, changes to the ladder diagram have been proposed to either eliminate the middle step ("weak opioid") treatments or to include a fourth step for interventional procedures (Vargas-Schaffer, 2010; see Figure 20.1). The following text will include the rationale for selection, dose titration, routes of administration, and side effect management for these groups of drugs.

Acetaminophen and Nonsteroidal Anti-Inflammatory Drugs

■ **Acetaminophen.** Although lacking in significant anti-inflammatory effects, acetaminophen is a useful analgesic in the management of mild pain or in combination with an opioid for the management of moderate-to-severe pain. Acetaminophen has fewer adverse effects than the NSAIDs. Gastrointestinal (GI) toxicity is rare, and there are no adverse effects on platelet function or cross-reactivity in patients with aspirin hypersensitivity (Risser, Donovan, Heintzman, & Page, 2009). Hepatic toxicity can occur, however, and patients with chronic alcoholism and liver disease can develop severe hepatotoxicity even when the drug is taken in usual therapeutic doses (Chandok & Watt, 2010). The U.S. Food and Drug Administration (U.S. FDA, 2011) limited the amount of acetaminophen in each tablet or capsule to no more than 325 mg and a 24-hour maximum dose not to exceed 4,000 mg. McNeil Consumer Healthcare, a division of Johnson & Johnson, the maker of the brand Tylenol, changed its packaging to recommend the daily dose not to exceed 3,000 mg in a 24-hour period (Nordqvist, 2011). Reduced doses or avoidance of acetaminophen is recommended in the face of renal insufficiency or severe liver compromise (Chandok & Watt, 2010). Offirmex, a parenteral form of acetaminophen, has been introduced in the United States, but its cost may prohibit its use in some PC settings (Paice, 2016).

■ **Nonsteroidal Anti-Inflammatory Drugs.** The NSAIDs include many subclasses, are frequently used in all steps of the "analgesic ladder" (National Cancer Institute at the National Institutes of Health, 2013a), and are analgesic, antipyretic, and anti-inflammatory. Aspirin is the prototype of the NSAIDs. These drugs are most effective in treating mild-to-moderate pain when there is an inflammatory component in Step 1 of the analgesic ladder while acting as a co-analgesic in Steps 2 and 3 (Wong & Reddy, 2016). The NSAIDs can be extremely effective when combined with an opioid drug in treating bone pain in cancer patients since prostaglandins, which are rich in the periosteum of the bone, are implicated in pain modulation. Unlike the opioid drugs, NSAIDs have a ceiling effect, that is, a dose beyond which added analgesia is not obtained (Portenoy, Ahmed, & Keilson, 2015). These drugs do not produce tolerance or physical dependence and are not associated with psychological dependence (addiction; Becker, 2010). This class of drugs may also have an opioid-sparing effect in some patients.

Mechanism of Action

The NSAIDs mainly affect analgesia by reducing the biosynthesis of prostaglandins, inhibiting the cascade of inflammatory events that lead to nociception (Wong & Reddy, 2016).

Adverse Effects and Their Management

Patients with cancer and other serious illnesses are very susceptible to adverse side effects of pharmacotherapy. A careful balance is needed between achieving the desired effect of the selected drug for the patient and the potential for adverse effects. This balance is particularly important with NSAIDs. Unlike the opioids where the adverse effects are usually dose-dependent and controllable, NSAIDs have a largely "hidden" side effect profile (Becker, 2010). Although they occur in a minority of patients, these adverse effects are often "silent," that is, not producing symptoms until a major event, such as GI

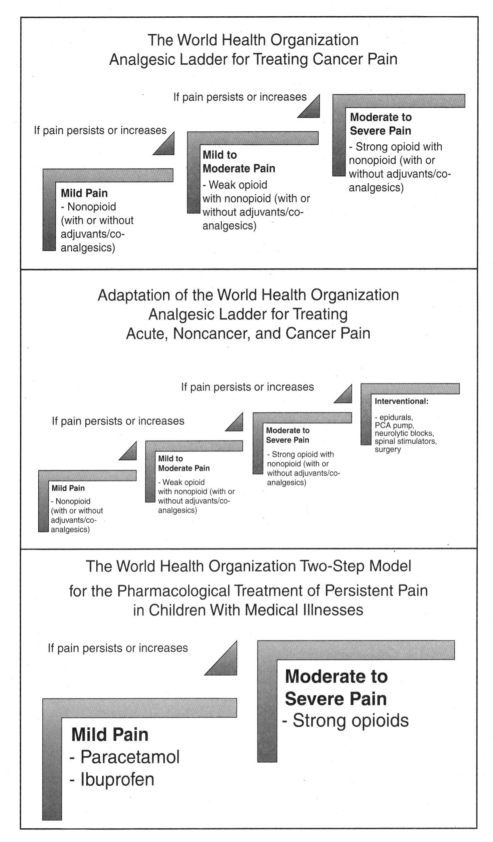

FIGURE 20.1 The World Health Organization analgesic ladder with variations.

PCA, patient-controlled analgesia.

bleeding, occurs without prior warning. The nurse is an active participant in assessing this risk/benefit ratio for the patient and needs to become familiar with the relative side effect profile for each of the drugs within this category. The potential adverse effects of the NSAIDs include those affecting the cardiovascular, GI, hematological, hepatic, and renal systems (Portenoy et al., 2015). The selective Cox-2 inhibitors differ in their side effect profile from other NSAIDs in relation to potential for less gastric irritation (at least with short-term use) and interference with platelet aggregation. However, renal adverse effects are similar and concern about cardiovascular risks suggests that they should be used with caution in "at-risk" patients (Becker, 2010).

Principles of Administration of Nonsteroidal Anti-Inflammatory Drugs

■ **Drug Selection.** A careful medical and pain history provides the nurse with information about potential benefits and risks for a patient about to receive a NSAID. An analgesic history should illuminate the patient's prior exposure to the NSAIDs, including frequency of administration, analgesic effects, and side effects. Information regarding the timing interval of other analgesics is important so that a prescribed NSAID regimen fits in with the patient's total analgesic plan. For example, if a patient was on an 8- or 12-hour dosing regimen of a controlled-release morphine preparation, an NSAID with a similar dosing profile would be appropriate. This may aid in compliance by reducing the patient's perception of needing to take frequent doses of medication. For chronic NSAID use, the addition of a proton pump inhibitor may be helpful in reducing the potential for GI bleeding (Paice, 2016).

■ **Choice of Starting Dose and Dose Titration.** An NSAID is combined with an opioid drug in Steps 2 and 3 of the analgesic ladder. Doses are often started at the lower end of the recommended scale in these medically fragile individuals who are coming to the end of their lives and are increased as needed. Although several weeks are needed to evaluate the efficacy of a dose, when NSAIDs are used in the treatment of grossly inflammatory conditions such as arthritis, clinical observation suggests that a shorter time period, usually a week, is adequate for pain relief in a patient with cancer or other life-limiting illnesses. Pain and other symptoms should be monitored before and after starting the NSAIDs to document any improvement or adverse effects. If no benefit is seen or if adverse effects are noted, consideration should be given to discontinuing the drug or switching to an alternate NSAID, as marked variability has been noted in patients' response to different NSAIDs. Indicators of an effective response would be either a significant improvement in pain or a significant decrease in opioid use with a subsequent reduction in opioid-related side effects. The degree of monitoring for adverse effects from the NSAIDs should be individualized to the patient. Tables 20.5 and 20.6 provide guidelines for common NSAID selection and dosing.

Opioid Drugs and Related Definitions

In order to break down the pervasive barriers that stigmatize opioid analgesic use, nurses must possess a clear understanding and working knowledge of the role that tolerance, physical dependence, and psychological dependence (addiction) play in pain management for the PC patient (refer to Table 20.7).

Tolerance is the phenomenon characterized by the need for increasing dose to maintain the same drug effect (Pasero & McCaffery, 2011). Usually, the reason for dose escalation, particularly at the EOL, occurs in the setting of increasing pain associated with progressive disease (National Cancer Institute at the National Institutes of Health, 2013a). Patients with stable disease do not usually require increasing opioid doses (Pasero & McCaffery, 2011). This observation, integrated with the knowledge that there is no "ceiling" effect to the opioid drugs, implies the following: (a) Concern about tolerance to analgesic effects should not impede the use of opioids early in the course of the disease and (b) worsening pain in a patient on a stable dose of opioids is assumed to be evidence of disease progression until proven otherwise (National Comprehensive Cancer Network, 2017).

TABLE 20.5 Key Points in the Selection and Use of NSAIDs and Acetaminophen
■ The older adult with chronic heart failure, renal insufficiency, cirrhosis with ascites, significant atherosclerotic disease, or multiple myeloma is at risk of NSAID-induced renal failure or gastrointestinal bleeding.
■ Unlike opioids, the adverse side effects of NSAIDs often do not produce obvious symptoms until a major event such as a GI bleed occurs.
■ Selective Cox-2 inhibitors differ in their side effect profile from nonselective NSAIDs in relation to potential for gastric irritation and interference with platelet aggregation. However, selective Cox-2 inhibitors have similar adverse effects (e.g., sodium retention, edema, hypertension) to the nonselective NSAIDs.
■ Avoid NSAIDs if possible in patients with gastroduodenopathy, bleeding diathesis, renal insufficiency, hypertension, severe encephalopathy, and cardiac failure.
■ NSAIDs should not be used concomitantly with other drugs that have the potential to cause gastric erosion (e.g., corticosteroids).
■ In patients without renal or hepatic failure, the daily dose of acetaminophen should not exceed 3,000 mg/24 h. In patients with renal or hepatic failure, the daily dose of acetaminophen should not exceed 2,000 mg/24 h.

GI, gastrointestinal; NSAIDs, nonsteroidal anti-inflammatory drugs.

TABLE 20.6 Commonly Prescribed NSAIDs

Drug	Dosing
Acetaminophen	325–650 mg every 4–6 hours Maximum daily dose: 2,000–3,000 mg/d
Salicylates Aspirin Diflusinal Choline magnesium trisalicylate Salsalate	325–650 mg every 4–6 hours Maximum daily dose: 4,000 mg/d (Causes irreversible platelet function for 7–10 days) 250–500 mg every 8–12 hours Maximum daily dose: 1,500 mg/d 500–750 mg every 8–12 hours Maximum daily dose: 3,000 mg/d 500–1,000 mg every 8–12 hours Maximum daily dose: 3,000 mg/d
Propionic Acids Naproxen Ibuprofen Ketoprofen Oxaprozin	250–550 mg every 12 hours Maximum daily dose: 1,250–1,375 mg/d (acute usage) 1,000–1,100 mg/d (chronic usage) 400–800 mg every 4–6 hours Maximum daily dose: 3,200 mg/d (acute usage) 2,400 mg/d (chronic usage) 50–75 mg every 6–8 hours Maximum daily dose: 300 mg/d 1,200 mg once daily
Acetic Acids Diclofenac Indomethacin Tolmetin Sulindac	25–75 mg every 8 hours Maximum daily dose: 150 mg/d 25–50 mg every 8–12 hours (immediate release) 75 mg once or twice a day (extended release) Maximum daily dose: 150 mg/d 400–600 mg every 8 hours Maximum daily dose: 1,800 mg/d 150–200 mg every 12 hours Maximum daily dose: 400 mg/d
Oxicams Meloxicam Prioxicam	7.5–15 mg once a day Maximum daily dose: 15 mg/d 10–20 mg once a day Maximum daily dose: 20 mg/d
Fenamates Meclofenamate Mefenamic acid	50 mg every 4–6 hours Maximum daily dose: 400 mg/d 250 mg every 6 hours Maximum daily dose: 1,000 mg/d
Nonacidic Nabumetone	500–750 mg every 8–12 hours or 1,000–1,500 mg once daily Maximum daily dose: 2,000 mg/d
Selective Cox-2 Inhibitors Celecoxib	100 mg every 12 hours or 200 mg once daily Maximum daily dose: 200 mg/d

NSAIDs, nonsteroidal anti-inflammatory drugs.

Sources: Adapted from Pasero, C., & McCaffery, M. (2011). *Pain assessment and pharmacologic management*. St Louis, MO: Mosby Elsevier; Portenoy, R. K., Ahmed, E., & Keilson, Y. Y. (2015). Cancer pain management: Use of acetaminophen and nonsteroidal anti-inflammatory drugs. *Up To Date*. Retrieved from https://www.uptodate.com/contents/cancer-pain-management-use-of-acetaminophen -and-nonsteroidal-antiinflammatory-drugs

TABLE 20.7 Clarification of Terms
■ **Tolerance** is a state of adaptation in which exposure to a drug induces changes that result in diminution of one or more of the drug's effects over time. Note: Need for opioid escalation in a patient with cancer is usually associated with progressive disease rather than tolerance per se.
■ **Physical dependence** is a state of adaptation that is manifested by a drug class-specific withdrawal syndrome that can be produced by abrupt cessation, rapid dose reduction, decreasing blood level of the drug, and/or administration of an antagonist.
■ **Psychological Dependence/Addiction** is a primary, chronic, neurobiological disease, with genetic, psychosocial, and environmental factors influencing its development and manifestations. It is characterized by behaviors that include one or more of the following: impaired control over drug use, compulsive use, continued use despite harm, and craving.
■ **Pseudo-addiction** is the mistaken assumption of addiction in a patient seeking pain relief.
■ **Diversion** is the shifting of legally obtainable drugs into illegal channels or the acquisition of a controlled substance by an illegal method

Physical dependence is an altered physiological state that occurs in patients who use opioids on a long-term basis (APS, 2008). If the drug is stopped abruptly or an antagonist, such as naloxone, is given, the patient exhibits signs of withdrawal. These signs include anxiety, alternating hot flashes and cold chills, salivation, rhinorrhea, diaphoresis, piloerection, nausea, vomiting, abdominal cramping, and insomnia (Gordon & Dahl, 2011). The time frame of the withdrawal syndrome depends on the half-life of the drug. For example, abstinence from drugs with a short half-life such as morphine and hydromorphone may occur within 6 to 12 hours of stopping the drug and be most severe after 24 to 72 hours. After withdrawal of drugs with a long half-life such as methadone, the symptoms may not occur for a day or longer (Gordon & Dahl, 2011). Gradual reduction of the opioid dose in the physically dependent patient who no longer has pain will prevent the withdrawal syndrome (Gowing, Farrel, Ali, & White, 2009). Clinical experience suggests that administering 25% of the previous analgesic dose will prevent the withdrawal syndrome in most patients (Gordon & Dahl, 2011). However, patients must be closely monitored during the tapering process to be sure they are not experiencing symptoms of withdrawal. A small proportion of patients require an extremely slow opioid taper because of persistent withdrawal symptoms. If withdrawal symptoms persist, they can be managed with the addition of an alpha-2-agonist, such as clonidine (Pasero & McCaffery, 2011).

The use of an antagonist such as naloxone in the physically dependent patient will precipitate acute withdrawal symptoms unless carefully titrated (Pasero & McCaffery, 2011). If a drug overdose is suspected in a patient who has received opioids for more than a few days, a dilute solution of naloxone can be used (0.4 mg in 10 mL of normal saline solution; National Comprehensive Cancer Network, 2017). This may be administered in 1 mL bolus injections every 1 to 3 minutes until the patient becomes responsive. The goal is to reverse respiratory depression and not reverse the analgesic effect of opioids.

It is reiterated that the need to use naloxone to reverse opioid-induced respiratory depression at EOL is exceedingly rare (National Cancer Institute at the National Institutes of Health, 2013a). Further discussion regarding respiratory depression will be highlighted later in this chapter.

Psychological dependence (addiction) is defined as a pattern of compulsive drug use characterized by a continued craving for an opioid, loss of control, and continued use despite harm (Rinaldi, Steindler, Wilford, & Goodwin, 1988). The current prevalence of substance abuse disorder in oncology patients remains unknown (Compton & Chang, 2017). Older studies have reported opioid abuse in cancer patients at rates near 8% (Ballantyne & LaForge, 2007). A recent study revealed that cancer pain patients have a risk profile for substance misuse similar to the chronic pain patient population (Price, Hawkins, & Passik, 2015). Concerns about this outcome, however, continue to be a reason for undertreatment of pain (Oliver et al., 2012). In a patient who does have a history of previous drug abuse, pain can still be well managed using opioid analgesics. The management of pain in patients with a history of drug abuse will be further discussed in the chapter section on special populations.

Pseudo-addiction describes drug-seeking behavior reminiscent of addiction that occurs in the setting of inadequate pain relief and is eliminated by improved analgesia (Weissman, 2009). For the most part, this behavior signifies inadequate pain relief. Patients and their families need to be reassured that use of opioid drugs in the amount that is needed to control pain, regardless of what that amount is, is unlikely to cause addiction if an individual does not have a history of drug abuse. In the setting of poorly relieved pain, "aberrant" drug-seeking behavior such as clock-watching requires careful nursing assessment.

Diversion is the "illegal distribution or abuse of prescription drugs or their use for purposes not intended by the prescriber (e.g., recreation, addiction, or financial gain)" (Centers for Medicare and Medicaid Services [CMS], 2016).

■ Opioids and the Three-Step Analgesic Ladder.

Opioid analgesics are the mainstay of pain treatment for PC patients. These drugs are used for moderate-to-severe pain in Steps 2 and 3 of the WHO analgesic ladder. They are frequently combined with acetaminophen or an NSAID (Wong & Reddy, 2016). When formulated with an NSAID drug, dose escalation is limited by reaching the maximum recommended daily dose of the NSAID. When formulated as a single agent, however, there appears to be no ceiling effect (Motov, 2008). Dose escalation may be limited by adverse effects such as sedation, confusion, nausea, vomiting, myoclonus, and (rarely) respiratory depression (Portenoy et al., 2017a; 2017b). Dose escalation is governed by the balance between pain relief and intolerable, unmanageable side effects (Fine & Portenoy, 2011). This balance can be determined only by ongoing assessment and documentation of the effects and side effects produced by the opioid.

Mechanism of Action

Opioids produce their effects through binding to receptors in the brain and spinal cord to prevent the release of neurotransmitters involved in pain transmission (Pasero & McCaffery, 2011). Opioids can also have a peripheral site of action in the presence of inflammation (Sehgal, Smith, & Manchikanti, 2011). In addition, opioid receptors are present in immunocompetent cells that migrate to inflamed tissue (APS, 2008). The opioids can be divided into agonists, agonist–antagonists, and antagonist classes based on their interactions with the receptor types. Pure opioid agonists (e.g., morphine, hydromorphone, oxycodone, fentanyl, and methadone) bind primarily to the mu receptors.

Partial agonists and mixed agonist–antagonists either block or remain neutral at the mu-opioid receptors while activating kappa-opioid receptors (Pasero & McCaffery, 2011). Historically, partial agonists, for example, have limited use in PC due to their ceiling effect and precipitation of withdrawal in patients receiving pure agonists such as morphine (National Cancer Institute at the National Institutes of Health, 2013a; National Comprehensive Cancer Network, 2017). The incidence of psycho-mimetic effects (agitation, dysphoria, confusion) from the mixed agonist–antagonist is greater than that of pure agonists like morphine (Pasero & McCaffery, 2011). Recently, there has been regained interest in these medications and their potential to provide pain relief, as demonstrated by studies evaluating the role of buprenorphine in the management of cancer-related pain (Pergolizzi et al., 2009).

The opioid antagonist drugs include naloxone and naltrexone. These drugs bind to opioid receptors and block the effect of morphine-like agonists. As previously mentioned, these drugs are rarely used in PC patients except for the management of opioid-induced constipation (Ford, Brenner, & Schoenfeld, 2013).

Commonly Used Opioids in Palliative Care

Morphine is the prototype of the pure opioid agonist. The WHO placed morphine on the essential drug list and requested that it be made available throughout the world for cancer pain relief (WHO, 2011). Morphine is available in tablet, elixir, suppository, and parenteral form. Various oral controlled-relief preparations provide analgesia with duration of 8 to 12 to 24 hours. Alternate routes of drug administration are available for patients who are unable to use the oral or rectal route.

Patients with severe pain are initially titrated with immediate-release morphine, or if in a hospital setting with parenteral opioids, and once stabilized are converted to a controlled-release preparation. To manage breakthrough pain or incident pain, prn immediate-release morphine should be made available to all patients receiving controlled-release preparations. In most patients, this prn dose should equal 5% to 15% of the total daily dose of the controlled-release preparation (APS, 2008). Absorption of morphine after oral administration occurs mostly in the upper small bowel. The average bioavailability for oral morphine is 20% to 30% (National Cancer Institute at the National Institutes of Health, 2013a). This explains why there is a need to increase the patient's opioid dose when changing from the parenteral to the oral route of drug administration. In patients with normal renal function, the average plasma half-life is 2 to 3 hours, whereas the average duration of analgesia is about 4 hours (Smith, 2009). Morphine-3-glucuronide (M-3-G), an active metabolite of morphine, may accumulate in patients with impaired renal function. This accumulation may contribute to myoclonus, seizures, and hyperalgesia (increasing pain) in patients with marked renal impairment (Kullgren, Le, & Wheeler, 2013). Because of these and other factors, the nurse must take note of the patient's renal status, especially in the older adult, when administering morphine and monitor accordingly for signs of opioid toxicity. If adverse effects exceed the analgesic benefit of the drug, the patient should be rotated to a different opioid. The comparative potency of the opioid drugs and bioavailability dependent on route of administration underscores the need for nurses to be competent in the use of the equianalgesic table (Table 20.8). Additional information regarding opioid rotation will be discussed later in this chapter.

Hydromorphone is a semisynthetic, short half-life opioid and is a useful alternative to patients who develop intolerable side effects with morphine. Hydromorphone is more potent, when compared milligram to milligram, than morphine and can be administered by the oral, rectal, parenteral, subcutaneous, and intraspinal routes.

TABLE 20.8 Equianalgesic Dose Table: Relative Potencies of Commonly Used Opioid Analgesics

Drug	Equianalgesic Parenteral Dose (mg)	Equianalgesic Enteral Dose (mg)	Comment
Morphine	10	30	Standard of comparison for opioid analgesics. Multiple routes of administration. Controlled-release available. M-3-G accumulation in patients with renal failure. Lower doses for the elderly.
Oxymorphone	1	10	Available in suppository form as Numorphan.
Hydromorphone	1.5	7.5	Useful alternative for morphine. H-3-G accumulation in patients with renal failure. Multiple routes available.
Methadone	*	*	Long half-life. For dosing, consult with a palliative care specialist.
Levorphanol	2	4	Long half-life.
Fentanyl	—	—	Short half-life when used acutely. Parenteral use via infusion. Clinical experience suggests 4 mg IV morphine sulfate/hour = 100 mcg transdermal patch. Patches available to deliver 12.5, 25, 50, 75, and 100 mcg/hr. Transmucosal delivery systems available.
Oxycodone	Not available	20	Available in liquid or tablet preparation, and in combination with a non-opioid. Controlled-release also available.
Codeine	130	200	Used orally for less severe pain. Usually combined with a non-opioid.
Hydrocodone	Not available	20–30	Usually combined with a non-opioid.

*See text and Table 20.9.

Note: This table should be used as a guide only and not replace a more in-depth review. Individual dosing and drug selection depends on each patient's particular situation and comprehensive assessment. These ratios are useful guides when switching drugs or routes of administration (see text). In clinical practice, the potency of the intramuscular (IM) route is considered to be identical to the IV and subcutaneous routes. References cited in the section of the text discussing use of opioid drugs.

H-3-G, hydromorphone-3-glucuronide; IV, intravenous; M-3-G, morphine-3-glucuronide.

The half-life of hydromorphone of 30 minutes to 3 hours is slightly shorter than that of morphine, and it has an oral bioavailability of 30% to 40% (National Cancer Institute at the National Institutes of Health, 2013a). The main metabolite of hydromorphone, hydromorphone-3-glucuronide, may lead to CNS toxicity, including myoclonus, hyperalgesia, and seizure, especially in the setting of renal failure (Kullgren et al., 2013). Personal clinical experience suggests that these adverse effects usually occur in the setting of high parenteral doses being administered by continuous infusion. Hydromorphone is available in a controlled-release formulation known as Exalgo.

Oxycodone is a semisynthetic opioid. The equianalgesic ratio to that of morphine is approximately 20–30:30. It has a half-life of 2 to 4 hours and is mainly excreted by the kidneys. Oxycodone is available in combination with aspirin (Percodan) or acetaminophen (Percocet), oral solution (Oxydose, Oxyfast, or Roxicodone Intensol), or as a single immediate-release or controlled-release tablet. The controlled-release tablet (OxyContin) provides the patient with analgesia for 8 to 12 hours. Both hydromorphone and oxycodone are used in Steps 2 and 3 of the analgesic ladder. Oxycodone is not available in parenteral form in the United States.

Fentanyl is a lipid-soluble potent opioid that is being used with increasing frequency in PC, especially in the transdermal form. Because of its potency, fentanyl dosing is usually in micrograms. Clinical experience with cancer patients suggests that a 100 mcg/hr fentanyl patch is equianalgesic to 2 to 4 mg of parenteral morphine per hour (Twycross, 2012). Based on this calculation, the switch to transdermal fentanyl often does not require the dose reduction that is undertaken when rotating to other opioid analgesics. Although most patients maintain satisfactory pain control with a patch change every 72 hours, some patients require the patch to be changed after 48 hours. Careful monitoring of adequacy of pain relief and evidence of end of dose failure will guide the nurse in the needs of the particular patient. It is important that the nurse also realizes that there is a lag in absorbing fentanyl through the skin. It takes 12 to 16 hours for the patient to see a substantial therapeutic effect (Twycross, Prommer, Mihaly, & Wilcock, 2012). Availability of a different route of drug administration is therefore necessary during the 12 to 16 hours following the initial patch placement. An alternate route of drug administration is also required for breakthrough pain medication. Significant concentrations of fentanyl remain in the plasma for about 24 hours after removal of the patch because of delayed release from the tissues and subcutaneous depots. Drug side effects (if present) may persist for that length of time. Fever, cachexia, obesity, edema, and ascites may all have a significant effect on absorption and clinical results (Hesselgard, Reinstrup, Stromblad, Undén, & Romner, 2007). Patches range in strength from 12.5 to 100 mcg. A 12.5 mcg patch releases 12.5 mcg of fentanyl per hour while a 100 mcg patch releases 100 mcg of fentanyl per hour.

Oral transmucosal fentanyl citrate (OTFC) provides a useful mode of delivering a potent, short-half-life opioid to a patient who requires a potent drug with a rapid onset of action and short duration of effect for severe breakthrough pain (APS, 2008; Zeppetella, 2008). OTFC (Actiq®) is approved for breakthrough pain treatment in opioid-tolerant cancer patients only but has proven safe in severe nonmalignant pain with the recommendation that the product is only to be used in patients who are opioid tolerant and who are receiving the equivalent of no less than 60 mg of oral morphine a day or transdermal fentanyl 50 mcg every 3 days. OTFC differs from other breakthrough pain medication in that there is no relationship between the baseline dose of the patient's pain medication and the microgram dose of OTFC required to relieve breakthrough pain (APS, 2008; Coluzzi et al., 2001). In all other opioid drugs, there is a relation between the two. With OTFC, the smallest available dose is initially chosen (200 mcg) and titrated up depending on the patient's response (available strengths range from 200 to 1,600 mcg/unit). Pain relief can usually be expected in about 5 minutes after beginning use (Gordon & Schroeder, 2008). Patients should use OTFC over a period of 15 minutes because too rapid use will result in more of the agent being swallowed than absorbed transmucosally. The use of OTFC has been associated with the development of dental caries (Pasero & McCaffery, 2011).

Buccal fentanyl tablets, when compared with OTFC, may provide more rapid onset of pain relief and greater extent of absorption (Darwish, Kirby, Robertson, Tracewell, & Jiang, 2007). The adverse effects are similar to those of other opioids. A small group of patients cannot tolerate the sensation of the tablet effervescing in the buccal space. For patients who are unable to place the tablet buccally

(between the gum and cheek pouch), sublingual (under the tongue) absorption appears to be comparable (Darwish, Kirby, Jiang, Tracewell, & Robertson, 2008). Buccal fentanyl (Fentora©) has a bioavailability approximately half of the transdermal route (Gordon & Schroeder, 2008). OTFC and buccal fentanyl should not be referred to as a lollipop or sucker to minimize the attraction to children (Pasero & McCaffery, 2011).

Methadone is another useful synthetic opioid for the management of pain in the PC patient. It is particularly useful for patients who have not done well on other opioids (Mannino, Coyne, Swainey, Hansen, & Lyckholm, 2006). Patients, however, may be reluctant to use methadone for pain because of its association with addiction. Methadone is primarily metabolized by cytochrome P450 (CYP) enzymes. Drugs that induce CYP enzymes, for example, dexamethasone, carbamazepine, phenytoin, and barbiturates, may accelerate the metabolism of methadone, resulting in decreased plasma levels of the drug and decreased pain relief. Conversely, drugs that inhibit CYP enzymes, for example ketoconazole, omeprazole, and selective serotonin reuptake inhibitor (SSRI) antidepressants, may potentially slow down the metabolism of methadone, leading to sedation and the possibility of respirator depression (Paice & Ferrell, 2011). Awareness by the nurse of any changes in the patient's medication regimen and the potential effect on the patient's pain relief or development of adverse effects is an integral aspect of pain management. Methadone in inexperienced hands is a potentially dangerous drug because of its variable long half-life (range, 13 hours to over 100 hours; Coyle & Layman-Goldstein, 2007) and a discrepancy between drug half-life and the duration of analgesic effect (4–8 hours). Patients are at increased risk of drug accumulation and subsequent toxicity when treatment is initiated, the dose is increased, or multiple organ failure develops. Warning signs of drug accumulation are, for example, a patient who becomes confused and increasingly sedated during the titration phase. Because of this risk, methadone should only be prescribed by experienced clinicians (Coyle & Layman-Goldstein, 2007).

The equianalgesic dose ratio of morphine to methadone has been a matter of controversy, with a confusing lack of clarity for clinicians (Knotkova, Fine, & Portney, 2009). Available data indicate that the ratio correlates with the total opioid dose administered before switching to methadone (Chou et al., 2014; Plonk, 2005; Walker et al., 2008; Weschules & Bain, 2008).

For example, when rotating a patient from morphine to methadone, the higher the current 24-hour dose of morphine the patient has been receiving, the larger the conversion ratio needs to be to provide pain relief. For example, if a patient is receiving from 30 to 90 mg morphine in 24 hours, the morphine to methadone ratio is 4:1. If the patient has been receiving 91 to 300 mg of morphine in 24 hours, the morphine to methadone ratio is 9:1, and if the patient has been receiving greater than 300 mg of morphine in

24 hours, the morphine to methadone ratio is 12:1 or higher (Benítez-Rosaria, Salinas-Martín, Aguirre-Jaime, Pérez-Méndez, & Feria, 2009; refer to Table 20.9). Questions have been raised regarding the effect of methadone on cardiac conduction. Prolonged QTc intervals have been reported in patients receiving both oral and parenteral methadone and may require ECG monitoring (Chou et al., 2014). Additionally, patients who receive greater than 40 mg of oral methadone per day have been found to be at higher risk of experiencing hypoglycemia, prompting the need for ongoing serum glucose testing (Flory, Wiesenthal, Thaler, Koranteng, & Moryl, 2016).

TABLE 20.9 Guide for Rotation to Methadone From Morphine

■ If oral morphine is less than 40–60 mg/d, change to methadone 2.5 mg q8h and discontinue previous opioid. Titrate dose by a maximum of 5 mg q 5–7 days.

■ If oral morphine is less than 100 mg/24 hours, use 3-day rotation period:
  – Day 1—reduce oral morphine dose by 30%–50% and replace with methadone using a 10:1 ratio. Administer methadone every 8 hours
  – Day 2—Reduce oral morphine by another 30%–50% of original dose and increase methadone if pain is moderate to severe. Supplement with short-acting opioids
  – Day 3—Discontinue oral methadone and titrate methadone dose daily

Alternate approach when rotating morphine to methadone. Conversion can be accomplished in one step using the following morphine to methadone ratios:

■ Morphine 30–90 mg/24 hours, use 4:1 ratio
■ Morphine 91–300 mg/24 hours, use 8:1 ratio
■ Morphine greater than 300 mg/24 hours, use 12:1 ratio

(Higher doses require higher ratios)

Sources: Chou, R., Cruciani, R. A., Fiellin, D. A., Compton, P., Farrar, J. T., Haigney, M. C., ... Zeltzer, L. (2014). Methadone safety: A clinical practice guideline from the American Pain Society and College on Problems of Drug Dependence, in collaboration with the Heart Rhythm Society. *Journal of Pain, 15*(4), 321–337. doi:10.1016/j.jpain.2014.01.494; Coyle, N., & Layman-Goldstein, M. (2007). Pharmacologic management of adult cancer pain. *Oncology, 21*(2), 1–17; Cruciani, R. A. (2008). Methadone: To EKG or not to EKG—That is still the question. *Journal Pain and Symptom Management, 36*(5), 545–552; Knotkova, H., Fine, P. G., & Portney, R. K. (2009). Opioid rotation: The science and limitations of equianalgesic dose table. *Journal of Pain and Symptom Management, 38*(3), 426–439. doi:10.1016/j.jpainsymman.2009.06.001; Paice, J. A., & Ferrell, B. (2011). The management of cancer pain. *CA: A Cancer Journal for Clinicians, 61*(3), 157–182. doi:10.3322/caac.20112; Plonk, W. (2005). Simplified methadone conversion. *Journal of Palliative Medicine, 8*(3), 478–479. doi:10.1177/1049909110373508; Walker, P. W., Palla, S., Pei, B., Kaur, G., Zhang, K., Hanohano, J., ... Bruera, E. (2008). Switching from methadone to a different opioid: What is the equianalgesic dose ratio? *Journal of Palliative Medicine, 11*(8), 1103–1108. doi:10.1089/jpm.2007.0285; Weschules, D. J., & Bain, K. T. (2008). A systematic review of opioid conversion rations used with methadone for the treatment of pain. *Pain Medicine, 9*(5), 595–612. doi:10.1111/j.1526-4637.2008.00461.x.

Other Opioids

Codeine, hydrocodone, and levorphanol are other opioids available for pain management in the United States. Additional information regarding dosing can be found in Table 20.8.

Oxymorphone (Opana, Opana ER) is a semisynthetic highly lipophilic opioid available in parenteral and more recently oral immediate-release and controlled-release formulations in the United States. Its safety and efficacy profile is similar to other opioids. Its milligram potency is double that of oxycodone (Palangio et al., 2002). Due to recent concerns regarding the drug's abuse potential, the FDA has removed Opana ER from the U.S. market (www.fda.gov).

Tramadol (Ultram) acts as both a weak opioid and a serotonin–norepinephrine reuptake inhibitor (SNRI). It is available in oral formulations including an orally disintegrating tablet (ODT; Paice, 2016). Tapentadol (Nucynta), which acts as both an opioid and a norepinephrine reuptake inhibitor, was approved by the FDA for moderate-to-severe acute pain (Fidman & Nogid, 2010). Since tramadol and tapentadol are not pure mu agonists, the drugs' effects are not completely reversed with the administration of naloxone (Paice, 2016).

Meperidine is *not* indicated for the management of chronic pain neither earlier in the disease process nor at the EOL. Meperidine has an active metabolite, normeperidine, that is twice as potent as a convulsant and half as potent as an analgesic as its parent compound (Simopoulos, Smith, Peeters-Asdourian, & Stevens, 2002). Meperidine's effect on rigors and shivering has shown benefits in both hypothermic and normothermic patients, especially in the postanesthesia care area. Administration of naloxone, a mu antagonist, does not reverse meperidine-induced seizures, but could potentially precipitate seizures by blocking the depressant effects of meperidine and allowing manifestation of the convulsant effects of normeperidine (O'Connor, Schug, & Cardwell, 2000).

Opioid Side Effects and Their Management

Close monitoring of the patient's response to therapy and rapid attention to the management of any adverse side effects is an important aspect of a patient's pain medication regimen. The nurse plays an integral role in the ongoing assessment and management of these untoward effects.

■ **Constipation.** Constipation in the PC patient is common and usually multifactorial (National Cancer Institute at the National Institutes of Health, 2013a). It is the most frequently encountered side effect experienced during opioid therapy and the one to which patients rarely develop tolerance. Opioid binding to peripheral receptors in the gut prolongs colon transit time by increasing or decreasing segmental contractions and decreasing propulsive peristalsis (Coyle & Layman-Goldstein, 2007). Because the likelihood of constipation is so great in patients who are receiving opioid therapy, laxative medications should be prescribed in a preemptive manner (National Cancer Institute at the National Institutes of Health, 2012). Most clinicians recommend a laxative with or without a stool softener (such as docusate) prophylactically (Tarumi, Wilson, Szafran, & Spooner, 2013). Bulking agents (e.g., psyllium) should be avoided as they tend to cause a large bulkier stool. In addition, debilitated patients are rarely able to take in sufficient fluids to facilitate the action of bulking agents (National Comprehensive Cancer Network, 2017). Metoclopramide can minimize nausea and increase motility to minimize constipation but is contraindicated in the presence of a bowel obstruction, bowel perforation, or GI bleeding. Oral naloxone has been found to be an effective therapy, but has the potential for precipitating withdrawal in patients on chronic opioid therapy (Ford et al., 2013). Polyethylene glycol (Miralax) is also well tolerated for opioid-induced constipation. A parenteral compound, methylnaltrexone (Relistor), has been shown to be effective in relieving opioid-induced constipation when given subcutaneously at doses of 0.15 mg/kg (Candy, Jones, Goodman, Drake, & Tookman, 2011). Additionally, lubiprostone, naloxegol, and naldemedine have been FDA approved for the treatment of opioid-induced constipation, but may be prohibitive for patient use due to cost (Portenoy et al., 2017; 2017a; 2017b).

■ **Sedation.** Some level of sedation is experienced by many patients at the initiation of opioid therapy and during significant dose escalation. Patients usually develop tolerance to this effect in days to weeks (Pasero & McCaffery, 2011). Should sedation persist at a level that is unacceptable to the patient, a careful assessment by the nurse is needed. Confounding factors such as other sedating drugs, metabolic disturbances, sleep deprivation, and the somnolence that may occur at EOL must be identified. Management steps include elimination of nonessential drugs with CNS depressant effects, reduction of the opioid dose if feasible, changing to an alternate opioid drug, and, if necessary, adding a psychostimulant such as modafinil or methylphenidate (Paice, 2015).

■ **Confusion and/or Delirium.** Like sedation, mild cognitive impairment is common after initiation of opioid therapy. Patients may express this as feeling "mentally hazy" or "not as sharp as before." Patients should be reassured that these effects are transient in most individuals and last from a few days to a week or two (Swegle & Logemann, 2006). Persistent confusion attributable to opioids alone is uncommon. More often confusion or delirium in patients, especially at EOL, is multifactorial and includes electrolyte disorders, neoplastic involvement of the CNS, sepsis, vital organ failure, and hypoxia (Bush, 2016). If confusion or delirium persists, opioid rotation may be warranted, especially if the current opioid has active metabolites that may be contributing to the delirium (Wong & Reddy, 2016). A common example of this clinical situation would be an elderly patient with renal impairment who is receiving escalating doses of morphine to manage the pain.

■ **Nausea and Vomiting.** Nausea and vomiting are common at the start of opioid therapy. Tolerance to this effect typically develops within days to weeks and the need for scheduled antiemetics decrease but should be made available on an as-needed basis (Portenoy et al., 2017; 2017a; 2017b). Both peripheral and central mechanisms are thought to be involved. Opioids stimulate the medullary chemoreceptor trigger zone and increase vestibular sensitivity. Direct effects on the GI tract include increased gastric antral tone, diminished motility, and delayed gastric emptying. Constipation may also be a contributing factor (Portenoy et al., 2017; 2017a; 2017b).

Establishing the pattern of nausea may clarify the etiology of the symptom and guide management approaches. Depending on the pattern of the nausea and presumed underlying mechanism, a combination of cognitive and pharmacological approaches is frequently used (National Cancer Institute at the National Institutes of Health, 2013a). Cognitive techniques might include relaxation training with focused breathing, guided imagery, and distraction. For nausea associated with early satiation and bloating, metoclopramide is often the initial pharmacological approach. If vertigo or movement-induced nausea is the predominant feature, the patient may benefit from an antivertiginous drug such as scopolamine (transdermal) or meclizine. Scopolamine should be used cautiously in the elderly or frail patient as it may cause confusion. Other options include trials of alternative opioids, treatment with an antihistamine (e.g., hydroxyzine or diphenhydramine), a neuroleptic (e.g., haloperidol or chlorpromazine), a benzodiazepine (e.g., lorazepam), or a steroid (e.g., dexamethasone; National Comprehensive Cancer Network, 2017). The role of serotonin antagonists (e.g., ondansetron) is primarily in chemotherapy-induced nausea, but it has been used in the PC patient to manage opioid-related nausea and vomiting (Wong & Reddy, 2016). Although an effective antiemetic, ondansetron has the potential to cause constipation; therefore, it should be used cautiously in this patient population (Wald, 2016).

■ **Multifocal Myoclonus.** Mild and infrequent multifocal myoclonus can occur with all opioids (Pasero & McCaffery, 2011). The effect is usually dose related, can occur in the presence of renal impairment, and/or is related to glucuronide toxicity from morphine and hydromorphone metabolism (Kullgren et al., 2013). Myoclonus is extremely distressing to the patient, where the uncontrolled, abrupt, jerking movements of the patient's limbs or torso can increase already existing pain. The clinician may interpret the movements as increased signs of pain, escalating the dose or frequency of the opioid, further adding to the involuntary movements. Myoclonus can be a sign of opioid toxicity and is a reason to switch to an alternate opioid (Kullgren et al., 2013). Carefully reviewing the patient's renal function can assist in choosing the best opioid. If myoclonus persists despite opioid rotation, the addition of clonazepam can often provide symptom relief (Paice, 2015).

■ **Opioid-Induced Hyperalgesia (OIH).** OIH is believed to be a rare phenomenon that can occur when patients receive chronic opioid therapy. It is best described as increased pain during aggressive opioid dose titration (Portenoy et al., 2017; 2017a; 2017b). In addition to worsening intensity, patients may also develop a pain response to non-painful stimuli, also known as allodynia. OIH is thought to be caused by changes in both the peripheral and central nervous systems, which in turn produce pain or increase a patient's sensitivity to pain over time (Pasero & McCaffery, 2011). It differs from physical tolerance. In tolerance, patients may require higher doses of opioids to achieve pain relief. In OIH, despite increasing opioid dosing, patients experience worsening pain (Cooney & Broglio, 2017). The incidence and clinical impact of OIH in pain management continues to be debated in the literature (Eisenberg, Suzan, & Pud, 2015). The suggested management of OIH includes opioid rotation or the initiation of adjuvant analgesic therapy.

■ **Urinary Retention.** Urinary retention can occur in patients receiving opioid drugs, especially in those who require rapid escalation of the drug, while receiving other drugs with anticholinergic effects (e.g., tricyclic antidepressants), or have compromised bladder function. Older men with an enlarged prostate are particularly at risk. Opioids increase smooth muscle tone and infrequently cause bladder spasm or an increase in sphincter tone, which may lead to urinary retention. Although prophylactic interventions have not been identified, management of urinary retention may require catheterization, reduction/rotation of the opioid analgesic, or dose reduction of the anticholinergic drug (Portenoy et al., 2017; 2017a; 2017b).

■ **Pruritus.** Pruritus can occur with any opioid, is associated with histamine release, and is most commonly seen with morphine use (Paice, 2015). Fentanyl and oxymorphone may be associated with less histamine release (APS, 2008). Prescribing an antihistamine such as diphenhydramine or mirtazapine can minimize the side effect (Wong & Reddy, 2016). Ondansetron has also been reported to be effective in the management of opioid-related pruritus (Paice, 2015).

■ **Respiratory Depression.** Respiratory depression is rarely a clinically significant problem in an opioid-tolerant patient. Increased sedation precedes respiratory depression and can be identified early if a comprehensive assessment is completed (National Comprehensive Cancer Network, 2017). However, fear of respiratory depression is a frequently cited concern among medical and nursing staff when initiating opioid therapy or when rapidly increasing opioids to control pain or dyspnea in a debilitated patient at the EOL. Clinically significant respiratory depression is always accompanied by other signs of CNS depression, such as sedation and mental clouding, and is unusual in the patient receiving chronic opioid therapy unless other contributing factors are present. Pain antagonizes CNS depression, and respiratory effects are unlikely to occur in the presence of severe pain. With repeated administration of an opioid, tolerance develops rapidly to the respiratory depressant effects of the drug (Portenoy et al., 2017; 2017a; 2017b). Unwarranted fears of respiratory depression should not interfere with appropriate upward titration of opioids to relieve pain (APS, 2008; Spathis & Booth, 2008). Capnography and end-tidal carbon dioxide monitoring ($ETCO_2$) can be used for patients who are at risk of respiratory depression or apnea (Burton, Harrah, Germann, & Dillon, 2008). The onset or exacerbation of existing sleep apnea in patients taking opioids for pain has been reported (APS, 2008). Risk factors appear to be the use of methadone, concomitant use of benzodiazepines or other sedative agents, respiratory infections, and obesity.

Occasionally, staff unfamiliar with the dying process and the altered breathing pattern that so frequently occurs at this time become concerned that continued use of opioids will hasten death, especially in the higher doses sometimes required to control pain at EOL. The input and mentoring by a nurse who is knowledgeable in pain and PC will help refocus the more inexperienced staff on appropriate dosing strategies in the symptomatic dying patient. The principle of double effect can minimize the fears of the nurse while ensuring adequate pain at the EOL (D'Arcy, 2012). This ethical tenet supports the nurse's administration of opioid analgesics to manage pain or other symptoms at the EOL, even if the unintended outcome is the patient's death. In this scenario, the nurse's intent is not to hasten death but instead to alleviate uncontrolled pain and suffering. This doctrine is supported by professional organizations, including the ANA (2016a, 2016b).

Principles of Opioid Selection and Administration

Numerous factors, both patient-related and drug-related, must be considered in the selection of an appropriate opioid for a patient (Pasero & McCaffery, 2011). The opioid should be compatible with the patient's pain severity, age, dosing and route requirements, underlying illness, and metabolic state. Selection of an opioid that is available as a controlled-release formulation, such as morphine or oxycodone, may be an important consideration for some patients. In addition, cost may be a factor for patients being cared for at home. For the older adult or those who have major organ dysfunction, an opioid without known active metabolites and with a short half-life, such as fentanyl, hydromorphone, or oxycodone, may be preferable (Portenoy et al., 2017; 2017a; 2017b).

The potential for additive side effects and serious toxicities from drug combinations must be recognized by the nurse each time a new drug is added to a patient's regimen (Chau, Walker, Pai, & Cho, 2008). Patients frequently have many distressing symptoms and are receiving multiple drugs. The impact of each new drug added to the patient's regimen must be carefully weighed for benefit versus burden.

■ **Opioid Rotation.** Sequential trials of opioid drugs may be needed to find the most favorable balance for the patient between pain relief and adverse effects (Wong & Reddy, 2016). The patient and family should be warned that these trials are a common occurrence so that they do not become discouraged during the process. Usually if one or two side effects are present and pain control is good, an attempt is made to treat the side effects and maintain the current opioid. If more than two side effects are present (excluding constipation), opioid rotation is probably warranted (refer to Table 20.10). The steps followed when rotating opioids are based on the following assessment:

1. Is the pain control good but significant side effects present? If so, reduce the equianalgesic dose of the new opioid by 50% (to accommodate for incomplete cross-tolerance) and continue to monitor the patient for resolution of adverse side effects and adequacy of pain control. Frequent rescue doses should be available to the patient.
2. Is the pain control poor and are significant side effects present? If so, reduce the equianalgesic dose by 25% to 50% and continue to monitor the patient closely for resolution of adverse side effects and improvement in pain control. Frequent rescue doses should be available to the patient.
3. Is the plan to convert the patient to methadone? If so, the around-the-clock (ATC) equianalgesic dose of methadone should be decreased by 90%, with provision for frequent rescue doses and careful monitoring of the patient for signs of drug accumulation and toxicity, especially sedation (Table 20.9).

Because of the large interpatient variability, in all instances when an opioid dose is decreased or the drug is changed, the patient must be closely monitored for adequacy of pain relief or presence of adverse side effects. Additionally, geriatric patients may require greater dose reductions to account for reduced fat stores, hepatic and/or renal insufficiency that comes with increasing age (Fine, 2012).

TABLE 20.10 Guidelines When Switching From One Opioid to Another—Opioid Rotation

- If one or two side effects are present and pain control is good, treat the side effects and maintain the present opioid.
- If more than two side effects are present, refer to the equianalgesic dose table (Table 20.8) prior to switching the opioid.
- In a minority of patients, two to three different opioids will need to be tried before a balance is reached between adequate pain relief and manageable side effects.
- A large interpatient variability is present in the way opioids are metabolized.
- If the pain control is good but significant side effects are present, reduce the equianalgesic dose of the new opioid by 50% (accommodates for incomplete cross-tolerance). Continue to monitor the patient for reduction in adverse side effects and adequacy of pain relief. Provide for rescue doses.
- If pain control is poor and significant side effects are present, rotate opioids and reduce the equianalgesic dose of the new opioid by 25% to 50%. Continue to monitor the patient for reduction in adverse side effects and adequacy of pain relief. Provide for rescue doses.
- Geriatric patients may require greater dose reductions to account for physiological changes due to aging.
- If converting to methadone, refer to Table 20.9.
- Unlike other opioids, dose reduction is not required when switching to transdermal fentanyl.
- In all situations of opioid rotation, monitor the patient closely for adequacy of pain relief and gradual clearing of adverse effects.

■ **Choice of Starting Dose and Dose Titration.** A patient who is relatively opioid-naive should generally begin treatment at an opioid dose equivalent to 5 to 10 mg of parenteral morphine every 4 hours (APS, 2008; NCCN, 2017). Lower doses may be required in geriatric patients or those patients with renal and/ or hepatic insufficiency. Titration of the opioid dose is usually necessary at the start of pain therapy and at different points during the disease course. It is important to understand that the metabolism of opioids can be affected by race, genetics, and medical condition of the patient (Smith, Kirsh, & Passik, 2009). At all times, inadequate relief should be addressed with dose escalation until relief is reported or until intolerable and unmanageable side effects occur. Integration of ATC dosing with supplemental rescue doses provides a rational stepwise approach to dose escalation and is appropriate to all routes of drug administration. Patients who require more than four to six rescue doses per day should generally undergo escalation of the baseline dose. In all cases, escalation of the baseline dose should be accompanied by a proportional increase in the rescue dose so that the size of the supplemental dose remains a constant percentage of the fixed dose (Table 20.11). As a guide, rescue doses are usually the equivalent of 5% to 15% of the total daily dose (APS, 2008). Nursing assessment of the patient's pattern of pain, rescue use, and level of pain relief is essential for appropriate dose titration. Table 20.12 summarizes the basic principles in the use of opioid drugs to manage pain.

■ **Selecting a Route.** The least invasive and safest route capable of producing adequate analgesia should be considered when selecting the route of administration. Clinical experience indicates that the majority of patients can use the oral route of drug administration throughout the course of their disease. However, some patients become unable to use this route and require an alternate approach (National Cancer Institute at the National Institutes of Health, 2013a). Nurses need to be skilled in selecting among the alternate routes to meet the needs of a particular patient. The most commonly used alternate routes include rectal, sublingual, transmucosal, transdermal, subcutaneous, IV, epidural, and intrathecal. IM administration should be avoided, as it causes pain at the injection site and leads to erratic drug absorption (APS, 2008).

A switch in route of opioid administration requires that the nurse have knowledge of relative potencies, to avoid overdosing or underdosing (refer to Table 20.8). During transition from one drug or route to another, the patient is at risk of pain escalation or the development of adverse side effects. Frequent assessment is therefore required during the transition period. The equianalgesic dose table provides a guide to dose selection when these changes are made. The calculated equianalgesic dose is usually reduced 25% to 50% when switching drugs to account for incomplete cross-tolerance (APS, 2008; NCCN, 2017). As noted previously, a much larger reduction (sometimes as much as 80% to 90%) is necessary when switching to methadone.

■ **Dosing Interval.** Patients with continuous or frequently occurring pain generally benefit from ATC dosing. This schedule provides a more stable plasma level of the drug and helps prevent pain from recurring. A rescue dose is offered on a prn basis and provides a means to treat pain that breaks through the fixed analgesic schedule. The drug used for breakthrough pain is usually the same as that administered on a regular basis. An alternative short-half-life drug is recommended when using methadone or transdermal fentanyl while waiting to reach steady state (Mercadante, Villari, Ferrera, Casuccio, & Gambaro, 2007). However, some clinicians prefer to use methadone as the rescue drug if a patient is already on methadone. The breakthrough or rescue dose should be 5% to 15% of the total 24-hour dose given every 1 to 2 hours as needed (APS, 2008). For example, for a patient receiving 60 mg of a controlled-release oral morphine preparation every 12 hours, the total 24-hour dose is 120 mg. The rescue dose or supplemental dose of 10 to 15 mg of immediate-release oral morphine should be available on a 1- to 2-hour basis as needed. The number of rescue doses used by the patient in a 24-hour period is a guide to titration of their ATC dosage.

■ **Patient-Controlled Analgesia (PCA).** PCA in the PC setting is a method that refers to parenteral drug administration in which the patient controls a pump that delivers analgesics according to parameters set by the nurse practitioner (NP) or physician. These parameters include concentration of the drug, basal infusion rate, and bolus dose with permitted intervals between doses for breakthrough pain (Portenoy et al., 2017; 2017a; 2017b). Use of a PCA device is fairly common in PC patients who require a parenteral route of drug administration or when severe pain needs to be brought rapidly under control. This technique can be managed safely at home by most patients, providing a system of education, monitoring, and support is in place. In the event the patient cannot use the function of the PCA, authorized agent controlled analgesia (AACA) is an alternative. Previously known as "PCA by Proxy," AACA involves the education of a competent person (i.e., nurse, family member, or caregiver) who is then authorized by the prescriber to administer a dose of medication

---

TABLE 20.11 Guidelines for Opioid Titration

Three choices are available when upward titration of an opioid dose is needed. The choice in approach is based on assessment of the patient's pain—both baseline pain and breakthrough pain.

- Increase the basal or ATC dose (oral, transdermal, subcutaneous, IV).
- Increase the rescue dose.
- Increase both the basal (ATC) dose and the rescue dose.

Most patients will require an increase in both the basal (ATC) dose and rescue dose.

- Calculate the number of rescue doses the patient has used in the past 24 hours.
- Increase the basal (ATC) dose by that amount or increase by 25% or 50% for moderate-to-severe pain.
- Also increase the rescue dose by 5%–15% of the new 24-hour dose.

Monitor closely for the effectiveness of the new dose and presence of adverse effects such as sedation and/or confusion.

ATC, around the clock; IV, intravenous.

Information based on APS Guidelines (2008); National Comprehensive Cancer Network, Clinical Guidelines—Pain (2017); and the clinical experience of the authors.

TABLE 20.12 Principles of Opioid Use in the Management of Pain

- Select analgesic(s) from Steps 1, 2, and/or 3 of the analgesic ladder appropriate to the patient's inferred pain mechanism(s), analgesic history, and severity of pain.

- Take into consideration the patient's age, metabolic state, presence of major organ failure (renal, hepatic, lung), and presence of coexisting disease.

- Consider pharmacological issues (e.g., potential accumulation of active metabolites, effects of concurrent drugs, and possible drug interactions).

- Know the drug class (e.g., agonist, agonist/antagonist), duration of analgesic effects, and pharmacokinetic properties.

- Be aware of the various drug formulations available for the opioid selected (e.g., immediate-release, controlled-release, liquid, transmucosal).

- Be aware of the available routes of administration for the opioid selected (e.g., oral, rectal, transdermal, transmucosal, subcutaneous, intravenous, epidural, intrathecal).

- Select the least invasive route to meet the patient's needs.

- Consider issues that may affect patient ability to follow the prescribed regimen (e.g., convenience, ease for home management, cost).

- Administer the analgesic on a regular basis for persistent pain. Make sure that "rescue" doses are available for breakthrough or incident pain.

- Titrate to achieve a favorable balance between good pain relief and minimal adverse effects.

- Use drug combinations where appropriate to provide added analgesia (e.g., NSAIDs and co-analgesics).

- Avoid drug combinations that increase sedation without enhancing analgesia.

- Anticipate and treat distressing side effects (e.g., constipation).

- If one or two distressing side effects are present, treat the side effects and continue on the current opioid. If more than two side effects are present (excluding constipation), consider opioid rotation.

- Prevent precipitation of an acute withdrawal syndrome through abruptly discontinuing an opioid in the patient who has been on an ATC regimen of an opioid for greater than 1 week. Taper the opioids if they are to be discontinued.

- Systematically evaluate the effectiveness of the analgesic regimen (e.g., amount of pain relief, duration of relief, frequency of breakthrough pain, frequency and pattern of "rescue" dose use, presence of adverse side effects, and satisfaction with mode of therapy).

- Teach the patient and family the principles of analgesic therapy. Address the frequently held misconceptions regarding addiction and tolerance.

ATC, around the clock; NSAIDs, nonsteroidal anti-inflammatory drugs.

by pushing the PCA button in response to the patient's demonstration of pain. This practice continues to be supported by the American Society of Pain Management Nurses (Cooney et al., 2013).

Safety Concerns Regarding the Use of Opioid Analgesics

The safe use of opioid analgesics has come under greater scrutiny due to the increase in prescription abuse and overdose-related deaths. In 2015, more than 33,000 deaths were related to opioid overdoses, four times those in 1999 (Laderman & Martin, 2017). Deemed an epidemic and a crisis in public health (Baker, 2017; U.S. Department of Health and Human Services, 2016), a number of

government initiatives have been pursued and expanded to address opioid abuse. In the United States, prescription drug monitoring (PDMP) programs are currently available in 49 states and the District of Columbia. These programs allow licensed prescribers access to databases regarding the dispensing of controlled substances (Wen, Schackman, Aden, & Bao, 2017). In 2011, the U.S. FDA introduced the Risk Evaluation and Mitigation Strategy (REMS) program for all transmucosal immediate-release fentanyl products (National Comprehensive Cancer Network, 2017).

A government effort to reduce the safety risks associated with Schedule II opioid medications, REMS requires the use of clinician–patient agreements, patient counseling, and continuing education for prescribers. Only licensed practitioners registered in the REMS program can prescribe REMS-regulated medications and REMS-regulated prescriptions can only be filled at REMS-registered pharmacies. This program was expanded in 2013 and now includes extended-release/long-acting opioids, sublingual buprenorphine, and tapentadol (National Comprehensive Cancer Network, 2017).

The use of universal precautions has been described in the literature as a strategy when prescribing opioid analgesics for pain management, including patients receiving palliative or hospice care (Covington-East, 2017; Walsh & Broglio, 2016). Initially recommended for primary care and pain specialists in 2005, this approach recognizes the challenge providers face in identifying patients who are at risk of opioid abuse and/or engaging in drug diversion. The implementation of universal precautions in patients receiving opioid therapy includes the following components: a thorough pain assessment and risk assessment for opioid abuse, identification of pain diagnoses, documentation of informed consent and of the treatment plan, identification of the patient's goals for opioid therapy, continual reassessment of opioid effects, and the implementation of drug screening. Using this strategy, all patients would be considered at risk of addiction. All patients are treated in the same manner, which has the potential to reduce individual patient stigma (Walsh & Broglio, 2016). The use of a risk mitigation tool (such as the Screener and Opioid Assessment for Patients with Pain [SOAPP]) can help clinicians identify patients at high risk of substance abuse. Work by Koyyalagunta et al. (2013) used the SOAPP-SF to evaluate cancer patients in the outpatient setting. Patients who were deemed to be at risk were younger, with higher pain ratings and higher frequencies of both depression and anxiety. These findings further supported those previously described in the literature.

Recently, the Centers for Disease Control and Prevention (CDC, 2016) published guidelines for the use of opioid analgesics in the management of chronic pain including 12 recommendations related to the selection, prescribing, and monitoring of drug use and abuse. While these recommendations excluded PC patients, the guidelines adapted from the CMS (2016) will only exclude patients with cancer or patients receiving hospice services. These activities have raised clinician concerns about providers' willingness to prescribe opioid analgesics, and thereby put many patients at risk of inadequate pain relief (Fisch & Chang, 2016). A thought-provoking essay written by Sally Glod (2017) explores these restrictive prescribing limitations, their negative impact, and their potential to cause undue suffering in patients with serious, life-limiting illness.

Co-Analgesic or Adjuvant Analgesics

Co-analgesic or adjuvant analgesics are those drugs that have a primary indication other than pain but are analgesic in certain pain states (Portenoy et al., 2017; 2017a; 2017b). They can be used at any step of the analgesic ladder. As with the institution of any pain-relieving regimen, the use of adjuvant analgesics is based on a careful assessment of the pain, inferred pain mechanism(s), and analgesic history. Co-analgesics or adjuvant drugs in the PC setting are typically used to enhance the effects of the opioid drugs or to allow for dose reduction because of adverse opioid side effects. It is useful to classify the adjuvant analgesics into three broad groups: multipurpose adjuvant analgesics, adjuvant analgesics used primarily for neuropathic pain, and adjuvant analgesics used for bone pain. Table 20.13 provides a guide to the commonly used co-analgesic/adjuvant drugs. As a general principle, low initial doses are suggested with dose titration until symptom relief is achieved.

■ **Multipurpose Analgesics.** *Corticosteroids* are used to treat various types of neuropathic pain resulting from tumor-infiltrating or compressing neural structures such as nerve, plexus, root, or spinal cord. Corticosteroids can be extremely useful in the acute management of a pain crisis when neural structures or bone are involved. Dexamethasone (16–24 mg/d), in combination with an opioid, may be used to treat bone pain, neuropathic pain, back pain associated with cord compression, headaches associated with brain tumors, and pain associated with liver capsule distension (APS, 2008). Pain relief is assumed to be associated with anti-inflammatory and antiedema effects (Vyvey, 2010). Adverse effects of corticosteroids include hyperglycemia, gastric irritation, dysphoria, delirium, and myopathy. Lower dose corticosteroids (2–4 mg dexamethasone) can improve mood and appetite. These drugs should not be used concurrently with an NSAID, and their chronic use should be combined with gastroprotective therapy. Be aware that a patient who is on steroids for reasons other than pain may experience increased pain or analgesic requirements if the steroid dose is tapered or reduced.

■ **Adjuvant Analgesics for Neuropathic Pain.** *Antidepressants* are nonspecific analgesics that are used predominantly for the continuous dysesthesic component of neuropathic pain. Analgesia can occur in the absence of mood changes, and the effective analgesic dose in the PC population is usually lower than that required to treat depression (Jefferies, 2010). Their analgesic effect appears to be related to inhibition of norepinephrine, serotonin, and dopamine (Portenoy et al., 2017; 2017a; 2017b). Common dose-related side effects include sedation, orthostatic hypotension, constipation, dry mouth, and dizziness. Tricyclic antidepressants (TCAs) are relatively contraindicated in patients with coronary disease in whom they can worsen ventricular arrhythmias (Kemp, Malhotra, Franco, Tesar, & Bronson, 2013). Current evidence-based guidelines recommend the use of TCAs and SNRIs as first-line options for the treatment of neuropathic pain (Moultry, 2009). In elderly patients, serotonin reuptake inhibitors seem to be safer and

TABLE 20.13 Co-Analgesic Medications

Drug Class	Indications	Drug Examples of Drugs Starting Dose (Range)	Adverse Effects
Antidepressants (PO)	Neuropathic pain (burning quality) ■ Added benefit for insomnia or depression	Amitriptyline 10–25 mg hs Nortriptyline 10–25 mg hs Desipramine 10–25 mg hs Venlafaxine 37.5 mg BID Duloxetine 30 mg BID	Anticholinergic effects (most prominent with Amitriptyline) Nausea, dizziness
Anticonvulsants (PO)	Neuropathic pain (sharp, shooting, electric shock–like quality)	Clonazepam 0.5–1 mg hs, BID or TID Carbamazepine 100 mg qd-TID Gabapentin 100 mg TID Pregabalin 50 mg BID-TID	Sedation, dizziness, LE edema—frail elders more at risk
Corticosteroids (PO, IV, SC)	Cord compression, bone pain, neuropathic pain, visceral pain, pain crisis	Dexamethasone 2–20 mg/d (give up to 100 mg IV for pain crisis) Prednisone 15–30 mg TID	"Steroid psychosis"—delirium, dyspepsia
Local anesthetics (PO, IV, SC, transdermal)	Neuropathic pain	Mexiletine 150 mg TID Lidocaine 1–5 mg/kg hourly Lidocaine patch 5% 12 h on 12 h off	Lightheadedness, tremor, paresthesia, arrhythmias, local irritation with transdermal patch
NMDA receptor antagonists (IV, SC, PO)	Neuropathic pain	Ketamine (IV: 0.1–0.2 mg/kg per h) (PO: 5 mg with titration to 10–15 mg q6h)	Delirium, nightmares, hallucinations
Alpha-2 adrenergic agonists (PO, intraspinal, transdermal)	Refractory pain. Can be used in combination with an intraspinal opioid	Clonidine transdermal patch 30 mcg/cm^2/d Tizanidine 2 mg po	
Bisphosphonates (IV)	Osteolytic bone pain	Pamidronate 90 mg	Pain flair over 2 h q 2–4 weeks
Antispasmodic (PO, IV)	Muscle spasms	Baclofen 10 mg (PO) qd-QID	Muscle weakness, cognitive changes
Calcitonin (SC, nasal)	Neuropathic pain, bone pain	Calcitonin 25 IU/d	Hypersensitivity reaction, nausea

BID, morning and night; IV, intravenous; LE, lower extremity; NMDA, N-methyl-d-aspartate; PO, by mouth; SC, subcutaneous; TID, three times a day.

better tolerated than the TCAs (Kahwam, Laurencic, & Malone, 2006).

Anticonvulsants are used to control the sharp, shooting, stabbing quality of neuropathic pain. Carbamazepine, phenytoin, valproate, gabapentin, and pregabalin have all been used in the management of neuropathic pain. Carbamazepine reduces pain by blocking sodium channels (Morisset, Davis, & Tate, 2013). Gabapentin (Neurontin) and pregabalin (Lyrica), a newer anticonvulsant, have been found to be useful in the management of both the dysesthetic and electric shock–like components of neuropathic pain and have a more favorable side effect profile than other anticonvulsants (Mishra, Bhatnagar, Goval, Rana, & Upadhya, 2012). Pregabalin was the first drug approved by the FDA for the treatment of fibromyalgia (U.S. FDA, 2007). Both gabapentin and pregabalin are hepatically metabolized. Pregabalin is distinguished

from gabapentin in that it is more efficiently absorbed through the GI tract, and the extent of absorption is proportional to the dose. Titration to the analgesic dose is likely to require just two or three steps rather than the multiple steps typically required with gabapentin (Bockbrader et al., 2010).

Gamma-aminobutyric acid (GABA) agonists include baclofen, an agonist at the GABA-B receptor. Baclofen is primarily used for spasticity but is potentially analgesic for lancinating or paroxysmal pains associated with neural injury of any kind (C. A. Lee, Kim, Kim, & Lee, 2016). Baclofen may interfere with mechanisms involved in neuropathic pain. Additionally, baclofen may have beneficial effects on singultus, commonly known as hiccups (J. H. Lee et al., 2010). The starting dose is 5 mg two to three times/ day, and the dose can be titrated upward to a range of 30 to 60 mg/d. The side effect profile includes dizziness, somnolence, feelings of confusion, and hallucinations. Slow upward dose titration is suggested in the PC setting. Abrupt discontinuation following prolonged use can result in a withdrawal syndrome (including delirium and seizures); therefore, doses should always be tapered before discontinuation.

Alpha-2 adrenergic antagonists include clonidine, the most commonly used alpha-2 adrenergic antagonist for neuropathic pain refractory to opioids and other co-analgesics or adjuvants. Systemic administration of clonidine via the oral or transdermal routes or intraspinal infusions have been used (Campbell et al., 2012; Engelman & Marsala, 2013). Tizanidine, which is also an alpha-2-adrenergic antagonist, has been shown to be beneficial in the treatment of pain due to spasticity (Chou, Peterson, & Helfand, 2004).

Muscle relaxants are used to control involuntary muscle spasms that can occur in some conditions such as cerebral palsy or MS. Benzodiazepines are effective in controlling the spasms but these centrally acting medications have questionable merit (van Tulder, Touray, Furlan, Solway, & Bouter, 2003). Carisoprodol (Soma), which is metabolized to the nonbarbiturate sedative hypnotic meprobamate, is not recommended; it has been abused and is a controlled substance in some states (van Tulder et al., 2003).

Local anesthetics are generally considered second-line drugs in the management of neuropathic pain. They can be given orally, topically, IV, subcutaneously, or spinally (Moulin et al., 2007). A brief IV infusion of lidocaine or procaine has been used to relieve severe neuropathic pain that has not responded promptly to an opioid and adjuvant drugs and requires immediate relief (Buchanan & MacIvor, 2010; Sharma et al., 2009; van den Heuvel et al., 2017). Oral local anesthetics used in neuropathic pain include tocainide, mexiletine, and flecainide. The analgesic effects of local anesthetics are thought to derive from suppression of aberrant electrical activity or hypersensitivity in neural structures involved in the pathogenesis of neuropathic pain (Hara & Sata, 2007). Local anesthetics produce dose-dependent adverse effects that involve the CNS and cardiovascular system including dizziness, tremor, unsteadiness, paresthesia, nausea, bradycardia, and other arrhythmias (Press, 2015). Their use should be avoided in patients with a history of cardiac arrhythmias or cardiac insufficiency.

Topical local anesthetics, for example, the eutectic mixture of local anesthetics (EMLA) cream, when applied locally, demonstrated mixed results in relieving pain due to PHN (Peppin et al., 2015). Lidocaine patches (Lidoderm; 5%) applied to the site of the pain—12 hours on and 12 hours off—has been approved for the management of pain in PHN and may be useful in treating other neuropathic pain conditions (Rosielle, 2015). Topical lidocaine in the form of a 5% lidocaine gel can also be effective in patients with PHN. The risk of toxicity from systemic absorption of a topical local anesthetic appears to be small.

Topical capsaicin may be useful to control the constant, burning, local, dysesthetic pain of PHN for some patients. Capsaicin is thought to lessen pain by reducing the concentration of small peptides (including substance P) in primary afferent neurons, which activate nociceptive systems in the dorsal horn of the spinal cord (Derry, Sven-Rice, Cole, Tan, & Moore, 2013). An unpleasant burning sensation, however, may follow topical application, making its use intolerable for some patients. This burning sensation may lessen or disappear after days or weeks of continued use. Topical transdermal capsaicin patches (Qutenza) were released in 2009 specifically for the treatment of PHN. Recently, a small observational study found Qutenza useful in managing ischemic pain due to peripheral vascular disease in end-stage renal patients (Aitken, McColl, & Kingsmore, 2017).

NMDA receptor antagonists are believed to block the binding of excitatory amino acids in the spinal cord. These antagonists, in combination with the opioids, are being increasingly used in the management of difficult to control neuropathic pain or when opioid dose reduction is the goal. Neuropathic pain includes a large number of diverse pain syndromes, some of which are thought to be mediated by NMDA receptors in the spinal cord (Woolf, 2011).

Ketamine, a potent analgesic at low dose and a dissociative anesthetic at higher doses, is included in this class of drugs (Paice, 2015). Ketamine's use in treatment is often limited by its side effect profile, which includes delirium, nightmares, hallucinations, and dysphoria (Okamoto et al., 2013). Assessment for these symptoms prior to initiating the infusion and on an ongoing basis is necessary. Haloperidol can be used to treat the hallucinations and scopolamine or glycopyrrolate may be needed to reduce the excess salivation sometimes seen with this drug (Amr, Shams, & Al-Wadani, 2013; Bickel & Arnold, 2009). Currently, the literature suggests that IV or oral ketamine can have a beneficial pain-relieving effect in children, adolescents, and adults (Bredlau, Thakur, Korones, & Dworkin, 2013; Carter & Brunkhorst, 2017). As with an infusion of local anesthetics, anesthesia members of the care team are usually involved in decisions surrounding a ketamine infusion in PC. A ketamine trial can be initiated at low doses of 0.1 to 0.15 mg/kg for a brief infusion or 0.1 to 0.15 mg/kg/hr for a continuous infusion (Moryl, Coyle, & Foley, 2008).

Adjuvant Analgesics for Bone Pain

Bone pain can be an extremely troublesome problem for cancer patients, especially those with advanced disease and multiple bone metastasis. As previously described, NSAIDs can be helpful in combination with the opioid drugs (Steps 2 and 3 of the analgesic ladder). Parenteral NSAIDs or corticosteroids can produce dramatic relief in difficult cases as previously reviewed; for example, the patient with bone pain who presents in a pain crisis.

Depending on the goals of care, a concentrated course of radiation should also be considered for patients with focal bone pain (National Comprehensive Cancer Network, 2017). Palliative radiation can be beneficial in managing pain in advanced malignancy. Painful osseous metastasis is common in oncologic practice. Although treatment can be effective for patients with mild, moderate, or severe pain, early intervention may be useful in maintaining QOL and minimizing side effects of analgesic medications (Kachnic & Di Biase, 2013).

Bisphosphonates inhibit osteoclast-mediated bone reabsorption and can reduce pain related to metastatic bone disease and multiple myeloma. Pamidronate disodium has been shown to reduce pain, hypercalcemia, and skeletal morbidity associated with breast cancer and multiple myeloma (Weinstein & Arnold, 2015). Dosing is generally repeated every 4 weeks with the analgesic effects occurring after 2 to 4 weeks. Zoledronic acid can relieve pain due to metastatic bone disease. A newer bisphosphonate, denosumab, has been prophylactic in preventing fractures, thereby preventing pain (Paice, 2015).

Radiopharmaceuticals such as strontium-89 and samarium-153 have been shown to be effective in reducing metastatic bone pain (Ogawa & Washiyama, 2012). Thrombocytopenia and leukopenia are relative contraindications to the use of strontium-89 (Portenoy & Koh, 2009). Because of the lag in response time to treatment of 2 to 3 weeks to beneficial effects, this approach is not appropriate for patients who are very close to death. Patients should be advised that a transient pain flair may occur following treatment and additional analgesia should be available as needed. Radium-223 dichloride can be considered a treatment option for the prevention of pathological fractures and the subsequent pain in patients with castration-resistant prostate cancer (Sartor et al., 2014).

Calcitonin is also an inhibitor of osteoclast-induced bone reabsorption and may be considered for patients with refractory bone pain or neuropathic pain although results are inconclusive (National Cancer Institute at the National Institutes of Health, 2013a). It can be administered via the subcutaneous or nasal route.

Hormone therapy is often prescribed in metastatic breast and prostate cancers (Riccio, Wodajo, & Malawer, 2007). Prostate cancer treatment with diethylstilbestrol has shown to reduce pain and improve the ability to ambulate in 40% to 70% of patients (Riccio et al., 2007).

Medicinal Use of Marijuana

While gaining state legalization for medicinal and recreational use, marijuana's role in pain management remains controversial. Cannabis has had a long-standing history as a therapeutic agent, first noted in 2000 BCE China as an anti-inflammatory, sleep aide, and pain reliever (Tateo, 2017). Marijuana was brought to the United States during the 1800s and was an accepted treatment for spasticity, headaches, and depression (Whiting et al., 2015) until its classification as a Schedule 1 substance in 1970 by the U.S. Drug Enforcement Administration (ANA, 2016a, 2016b). This designation has contributed to marijuana's stigma, thereby limiting the funding and support for its research (Paice, 2016). Currently, marijuana and cannabis have been legalized in 29 states and the District of Columbia for a number of medical conditions, including pain (National Conference of State Legislators, 2017). Research has identified tetrahydrocannabinol (THC) and cannabidiol (CBD) as the substances possessing analgesic properties, either by reducing inflammation or by acting as an anticonvulsant (Tateo, 2017).

In addition to its psychoactive side effects, inhaled cannabis can cause respiratory complications such as fungal infections, bronchitis, and lung cancer (Hospice and Palliative Nurses Association, 2014). In the United States, Nabilone (Cesamet®) and Dronabinol (Marinol®) are approved by the FDA for the treatment of chemotherapy-induced nausea and vomiting, but not for the management of pain (HPNA, 2014). A recent systematic review highlighted eight randomized controlled trials using newer formulations of cannabinoids, including a mucosal spray nabiximols (Sativex®) which is approved for treatment of MS-related spasticity in 20 other countries (Portenoy et al., 2017; 2017a; 2017b; Tateo, 2017). While all of the studies identified positive analgesic effects versus placebo, none of the results were statistically significant.

Numerous professional nursing organizations including the HPNA (2014), the ANA (2016a, 2016b), and the American Society for Pain Management Nursing (2015) have published position statements outlining the legal issues surrounding cannabis and supported the need for further research to define marijuana's role in pain management. The creation of the Center for Medical Cannabis Education and Research (CMCER) at Thomas Jefferson University in Philadelphia, Pennsylvania, hopes to begin to meet this need by providing impartial information to patients and providers regarding marijuana's role as a medicinal therapy (Thomas Jefferson University, 2016). Given the rapid expansion of medical marijuana in the United States, nurses should remain current regarding its evolving legality and its potential role in pain management so that they can best advocate for their patients.

■ SECTION 3: PROCEDURAL AND NONPHARMACOLOGICAL TREATMENTS

Interventional Treatments

Interventional or invasive interventions can be considered for a small percentage of palliative patients whose pain cannot be adequately controlled by pharmacological means. This population includes individuals whose pain is localized to one or two areas, is expected to persist, and who cannot achieve an acceptable balance between analgesia and intolerable, dose-limiting side effects from these analgesics.

When evaluating patients for invasive approaches, it is important to clarify that all feasible primary therapies that are likely to improve patient outcomes have been initiated, that the opioid dose has been titrated up to the maximal tolerated dose, that side effects have been treated with appropriate medication therapy or through opioid rotation, that appropriate adjuvant analgesics have been considered or tried, and that appropriate routes of drug administration have been instituted. Invasive interventions to relieve pain include nerve blocks, surgically implanted devices, or neurolytic agents and are performed by skilled specialists who can evaluate a patient for appropriateness.

Surgical management may be used to decrease pain (by treating the underlying cause) and increase functional status as in the case of orthopedic fractures. Although a palliative intervention, surgery should not be offered as an option for severely ill patients who have an extremely limited life expectancy, or if the procedure is in conflict with the patients' goals of care (Wolanczyk, Fakhrian, & Adamietz, 2016).

Injection therapies, such as soft tissue or joint injections, are frequently used for individuals with non-cancer chronic pain. Depending on the area affected by chronic pain, injections to the epidural space, facet joint, or sacroiliac joint may be appropriate. Individuals with painful malignant vertebral compressions may be candidates for kyphoplasty or vertebroplasty, as well as other injection therapies (Portenoy & Copenhaver, 2017).

Neural blockade is an anesthetic intervention for either temporary or permanent effect and is commonly called a nerve block. A local anesthetic (usually lidocaine or bupivacaine) is injected into or around a nerve. Nerve blocks can be considered diagnostic, prognostic, therapeutic, or preemptive/prophylactic. A *diagnostic nerve block* is done to determine the specific pain pathway and to aid in the differential diagnosis. A *prognostic nerve block* is one that is done to predict the efficacy of a permanent ablating procedure. A *therapeutic nerve block* is done to provide temporary pain relief in a pain crisis or to treat painful conditions that respond to these blocks (e.g., a celiac block for the relief of pain due to pancreatic cancer). A *preemptive/prophylactic nerve block* is done proactively to prevent the development of a chronic pain syndrome. Neurolysis, or nerve destroying, is a permanent procedure that interferes with the transmission of a painful stimulus by injection of a chemical substance such as alcohol or phenol to destroy or ablate the nerve (Miguel, 2000). This procedure has decreased in popularity with the advancement of spinal analgesia and the increase in life expectancy but it is still a viable option. QOL and side effects must be evaluated before proceeding. One of the distressing side effects of this intervention is sphincter weakness, which many patients find unacceptable (Miguel, 2000).

A successful prognostic nerve block may not always mean a successful neurolysis. This may be due to such things as analgesic and sedating premedications, placebo response, spread of local anesthetic to adjacent neural structures, or systemic absorption of local anesthetics. Contraindications to an individual undergoing a nerve block include infection, coagulopathies, ineffective prognostic block, inadequate patient and family preparation, patient refusal, inability to understand and sign informed consent, and inability to cooperate during the procedure. The use of ultrasound guidance—a more recent development that allows the anesthesiologist to position the needle more accurately and monitor the distribution of the local anesthetic medication—has improved both safety and efficacy of neural blockade (Marhofer & Chan, 2007; Marhofer, Greher, & Kapral, 2005).

General types of neural blockade are peripheral blocks (including brachial plexus, and cranial, intercostal, and sacral nerves), neuroaxonal blocks (including epidural and intrathecal), and sympathetic nerve blocks (including celiac plexus block and superior hypogastric block; Latifzai, Sites, & Koval, 2008). Specific nerve blocks are identified by the anatomical location where they are performed. Depending on the location of the block, some of the risks or complications include fatigue, over-sedation (if analgesics administered via other routes are not decreased in relation to decreased pain), sensory loss, motor weakness, altered bowel and bladder function, altered sexual function, intravascular injection, hematoma, and new pain. It is estimated that 14% to 30% of individuals undergoing peripheral neurolytic blockade will develop neuropathic pain as a result (Soloman, Mekhail, & Mekhail, 2010). Side effects from nerve blocks can include Horner's syndrome, characterized by constricted pupil, ptosis, "and decreased sweating resulting from interruption of the sympathetic pathways to the eye," numbness, weakness, increased warmth, diarrhea, and lowered blood pressure (Soloman et al., 2010). These effects are temporary, if done with a local anesthetic, or long-lasting or permanent, if done with alcohol or phenol (as with a neurodestructive block). A recent systematic review of neurological complications after regional anesthesia found a neurological complication rate of 0.04%, with permanent neurological injury rarely occurring (Brull, McCartney, Chan, & El-Beheiry, 2007). It is the responsibility of nurses caring for individuals undergoing these procedures to be knowledgeable about the side effects and alert to developing complications.

Implanted devices, such as an epidural or intrathecal drug delivery system, can facilitate safe, analgesic-effective, and cost-effective neuraxial infusion of opioids and local anesthetics via the spinal route if individuals have a life expectancy of months or greater. This targeted delivery system, involving an implanted, programmable infusion pump and a percutaneously tunneled spinal catheter, delivers the analgesics to the closest spinal segment that processes the pain. Prior to choosing this delivery device, a risk benefit analysis should take place to make certain that it is appropriate. Patients with sepsis, raised intracranial pressure, coagulopathy, or suspected mass at the surgical site are not candidates for implanted intraspinal pumps (Birthi & Sloan, 2013).

Neurodestructive techniques can include rhizotomy, the disruption of the cranial or spinal nerve root through chemicals or radio waves. Selective dorsal rhizotomy has been successful in the pediatric population to decrease spasticity from many neurological disorders (Hesselgard et al., 2007). *Cordotomy* is a neuroablative, rarely done, neurosurgical procedure that involves making a lesion in the anterior spinothalamic tract, contralaterally to the pain site, either percutaneously or with an open surgical approach, to destroy the function of a portion of the particular spinothalamic tract that innervates the site of pain. Individuals with severe, intractable visceral pain, on rare occasions, may be evaluated for dorsal punctate midline myelotomy (DPMM), which destroys the area that transmits visceral pain.

Neurostimulation Treatments

Examples of neurostimulatory interventions include transcutaneous electrical nerve stimulation (TENS), spinal cord stimulation (SCS), peripheral nerve stimulation, and transcranial stimulation. Conventional TENS involves noninvasive delivery of low voltage electrical currents to the skin surface, near a painful area, for the purpose of pain relief. SCS, a minimally invasive, reversible spinal neuromodulation system, can be used for individuals with chronic neuropathic pain following injury to a portion of the nervous system. Frequently, candidates for SCS will have a screening trial with an external pulse generator before undergoing permanent implantation (Cruccu et al., 2007). Recommendations for use of these recommendations are weak but the benefits are thought to outweigh the harm (Paice et al., 2016).

Rehabilitative Treatments

People with cancer and other serious, life-threatening illnesses can experience significant loss of function that impacts on their QOL and contributes to pain and other symptoms. The fact that pain is disabling is well established. Rehabilitative interventions can be helpful in the pain management plan and contribute to overall improved QOL. These interventions include positioning and movement, application of modalities such as heat and cold, therapeutic exercises, and the use of supportive orthotic devices. Physical rehabilitation professionals are the experts who strive to achieve mutually agreed upon goals that will allow patients to maintain or achieve their highest level of physical

function. In addition to their role in the maintenance and restoration of physical function and health, physical therapists are also involved in the promotion of health and wellness, prevention of physical dysfunction and disability, and public health initiatives (Ohtake, 2013). The rehabilitation expert, a useful member of some PC teams, looks at an individual with cancer or other life-limiting illness from four rehabilitation perspectives: (a) preventive—to minimize the effects of predictive disabilities; (b) adaptive—to assist the individual to adapt to definite changes; (c) maintenance—that is, maintaining the individual at the current level of functioning; and (d) palliative rehabilitation—keeping the individual functioning and involved in the environment (Barawid, Covarrubias, Tribuzio, & Liao, 2015). For nurses to set realistic, achievable goals with PC patients with pain, it is useful to consider these four possibilities as goals of care change and evolve.

Positioning and Movement

Healthy individuals are unconsciously and continuously initiating pain-relieving movements. A debilitated individual with pain may be in static positions for extraordinary lengths of time. This in itself can exacerbate existing pain or produce new pain, including pressure sores and painful joint conditions. Basic nursing texts give thorough overviews of the principles of positioning and movement that are so essential to good nursing care at the EOL. Family members and caregivers can be taught to move and position patients to maximize comfort. A nurse can assist patients and their caregivers to promote positions or postures that maintain or facilitate normal physiological function of the musculoskeletal system. When properly done, positioning places minimal stress on the joint capsule, tendons, and muscle structure (American Physical Therapy Association, 2014). For some patients, however, turning and repositioning is extremely painful. If patients experience pain with movement, every effort should be taken to medicate them prior to positioning. This will prevent unnecessary suffering and fear of movement (Czarnecki et al., 2011; Layman-Goldstein & Coyle, 2013). The American Society for Pain Management Nursing position statement on procedural pain is beneficial for the healthcare provider to understand management of painful procedures including turning and repositioning (Czarnecki et al., 2011).

For the bedbound PC patient who is not so close to death, range of motion (ROM), either active (AROM), active assisted (AAROM), or passive (PROM), can promote comfort and maintain or restore the integrity of muscles, ligaments, joints, bones, and nerves used in movement. It is hoped this will prevent the development of additional complications. AAROM or PROM can be used for patients who lack the energy for AROM and are neurologically impaired or unconscious.

Therapeutic Exercise

Because of methodological limitations of studies to date, the use of exercise to reduce chronic pain has not been firmly established (Brant, Keller, McLeod, Yeh, & Eaton, 2017). However, systematic implementation of a physical therapy program, based on an individual patient's performance status and specific rehabilitation goals, is unlikely to harm, and can enable that individual to achieve better function and decreased pain. A therapeutic exercise plan may include stretching, passive mobilization, and active exercise. Recently, De Groef and colleagues evaluated 18 studies which utilized physical therapy with patients who had undergone treatment for breast cancer. Their review showed that physical therapy improved upper limb ROM and decreased pain in this population (De Groef et al., 2015).

Hydrotherapy, useful in chronic conditions such as rheumatoid arthritis or ankylosing spondylitis, involves immersing the painful body part in a tank of warm water (less than 40°C). In this environment, patients with movement-related pain may be better able to undergo individually planned therapeutic exercise because the warm water provides both buoyancy and decreased joint stress. This, in turn, can increase their participation in therapy (American Physical Therapy Association, 2014).

Supportive Orthotic Devices

In attempting to decrease pain and increase functioning at the EOL, it may be helpful to consult with a physical therapist or rehabilitation medicine physician to evaluate the possible use of a supportive orthotic device such as a splint, sling, brace, or corset. Their use can immobilize or provide support to painful tissues and maximize the use of weakened tissues to promote functioning. Appropriate use of such a device may decrease incident or mechanical-type pain for certain patients (American Physical Therapy Association, 2014). Also, the use of certain devices for patients with bone metastasis may immobilize areas of potential fractures to prevent this painful complication (Jacox et al., 1994).

Assistive devices such as canes, walkers, and wheelchairs, when appropriately used, can promote mobility, decrease pain, and prevent injury (American Physical Therapy Association, 2014). Consulting with a rehabilitative specialist to obtain the correct assistive device for an individual patient and teaching the patient and the caregivers the proper use of such devices can be invaluable. Often, an evaluation of the home situation will be necessary to recommend the most appropriate device to maximize an individual's rehabilitation efforts.

Physical Modalities: Heat and Cold

Superficial heating or cooling can cause a decrease in pain sensitivity. There is a lack of well-controlled studies concerning the use of heat and cold. Most of the information discussed is based on clinical experiences presented in the literature. Patients with aching muscles, muscle spasm, joint stiffness, low back pain, or itching may benefit from the use of superficial heating or cooling. Their use seems to be most effective for well-localized pain (Jelinek & Barnden, 2012). It is important to consider patient safety and comfort when using these interventions. Cold should not be used in the following patient situations: if an individual has a history of peripheral vascular disease (such as Raynaud's disease); arterial insufficiency; cognitive or communication impairments; connective tissue disease; or impaired sensation of the skin (Jelinek & Barnden, 2012). Heat should not be used in the following patient situations: an inability to communicate, significant cognitive impairment, ischemia, bleeding disorders, neuropathic pain characterized by a hypersensitivity to touch, areas where the skin is broken, and recently irradiated skin (Strax, Gonzales, & Cuccurullo, 2004). In 2007, the FDA issued a warning that patients with transdermal fentanyl patches should not be exposed to external heat sources as this will increase the drug to be released and can be life-threatening (U.S. FDA, 2007).

Most hospitalized individuals will need an order or institutional protocol before the initiation of superficial heating or cooling. Care must be taken with both modalities to protect the skin with at least a layer of terry cloth or a pillowcase. Moisture increases the intensity of the heat or cold. Patients should be discouraged from lying on heat sources. The skin must be inspected at regular intervals for irritation, swelling, blistering, excessive redness that does not subside between treatments, or bleeding. Some patients develop a "hunting reaction," in which the skin alternatively blanches and turns red after the application of cold. If this occurs, the use of cold should be immediately discontinued. Extreme vigilance is necessary for patients with impaired or decreased sensation, cognitive impairment, or who are unconscious, as these may be considered relative contraindications. Treatment should be discontinued if the patient asks or if pain or any form of skin irritation occurs (Jacox et al., 1994; Jelinek & Barnden, 2012). Patient and family or caregiver education is needed before introducing these measures (van Middelkoop et al., 2011).

Therapies of Specific Disorders (Such as Lymphedema)

Lymphedema, a common and frequently painful secondary condition resulting from either cancer or its treatment (i.e., surgical lymph node dissection, or radiation therapy), is characterized by swelling and fluid retention in specific body areas which have a compromised lymph drainage system. This frequently occurs in either the upper or lower extremities but can also be found in other body sites such as the head and neck. Physical therapy for this specific disorder involves lymphatic drainage, massage, compression therapy, and exercises. These interventions seek to decrease swelling. Often the decreased swelling results in decreased pain and improved mobility and function. Patient and family education also includes trauma avoidance and meticulous skin care to prevent complications such as infections (Tacani et al., 2016).

Psychological Treatments

Successful, effective pain management includes interventions that address the body, mind, and emotions. Psychological interventions address these factors and enable an individual to gain a sense of control and build upon the interplay of physical and psychological variables in pain perception and response. These interventions can primarily be classified as psychoeducational, cognitive behavioral, mindfulness based, or psychotherapeutic. They can include such things as patient and family education, distraction, self-statements, relaxation techniques, guided imagery and hypnosis, patient pain diaries, and cognitive behavioral therapy (CBT). The NCCN Cancer Pain Guidelines for Adults (Version 2, 2017) encourage the use of psychosocial interventions for pain management early in the course of disease as part of a multimodal approach. Meta-analysis of psychosocial interventions for pain in individuals with cancer (including cancer survivors) demonstrated a statistically significant overall positive effect (Johannsen, Farver, Beck, & Zachariae, 2013; Sheinfeld et al., 2012). The nurse who is caring for an individual with a life-threatening illness may find that this person is well versed in using specific psychological approaches and is open to using these techniques to aid in coping with pain and other symptoms. On the other hand, the person for whom the nurse may be caring may be too weak, debilitated, and cognitively impaired to be taught or even to use a simple, previously utilized relaxation technique. A thorough assessment is key to developing a realistic plan. The intervention must match the specific problem with an appreciation for the patient's abilities and motivations.

Psychoeducational Interventions

Education about pain and its management is an important component of any pain management plan. Knowledge regarding pain management reviewed earlier should include pain and its etiology; the principles and methods of pain management; types of analgesics; potential side effects of analgesics and their management; equipment and devices used to deliver analgesics; the concepts of physical dependence, tolerance, and addiction; nonpharmacological interventions; and expected participation in pain management (NCCN, 2017). Recent work suggests that to implement a pain management regimen successfully at home, patients and families will also need other knowledge to assist them in problem solving to improve pain control.

Challenges include obtaining and processing further information, obtaining prescribed analgesics, applying prescribed regimens to their very individual situation, managing new or changed pain, and managing side effects and other concurrently occurring symptoms (Strouse, Flanagan, Kerrihand, Williams, & Wolcott, 2006). Knowledge of how to approach these challenges will enable individuals and their families to be active, informed participants in the plan of care. Knowledge deficits related to pain management encompass all dimensions of learning: cognitive, psychomotor, and affective. It is especially important to allay fears and concerns about opioid use, specifically, addiction, tolerance, and physical dependence. Individuals who need equipment to relieve their pain will need special opportunities for their families and themselves to practice with that equipment to gain confidence in its use (Reinhard, Given, Petlick, & Bernis, 2008).

Pain management education can be delivered in a variety of ways: standardized or individualized, in classes, on the web, or even over the phone. Nurses in various practice settings can coach patients and families to reinforce educational points. A recent systematic review of psychoeducational interventions reported that all these educational efforts are likely to be effective in contributing to chronic cancer pain relief (Eaton, Brant, McLeod, & Yeh, 2017).

Ideally, at the EOL, patients, their families, and their caregivers will be well informed about pain management. However, the nurse working with any patient, especially those who present with advanced disease, will often find that this is not the case. Regardless of the circumstances, it is necessary to maintain ongoing assessment and reinforcement of educational information as the clinical situation and patient's needs change.

Cognitive Behavioral Interventions

A *pain diary* is a tool that is especially useful when working with patients cared for in ambulatory settings but could also be used with other patients cared for in other settings. Clinicians can review this diary with patients over the phone, at home, or on clinic visits.

The diary can be as simple or sophisticated as the patient using it. The amount of information included often is a reflection of the patient's energy level. Essential information includes date and time of events, medication, dose of medication, and pain intensity before and after interventions. It is helpful if patients include their activities, periods of rest and sleep, pain quality, mood, and other symptoms, but this is up to the individual patient. Some prefer to use preprinted forms provided by pharmaceutical companies or other sources, whereas others prefer to use their computer or smartphone. Many free and low-cost applications are available on mobile devices that make real-time documentation possible. A pain diary can give a patient a sense of control and promotes communication about pain, putting words to feelings that he or she can share with family members and others. For high-risk patients, the use of a pain diary is recommended to help document opioid use (NCCN, 2017).

Relaxation therapy and other types of stress management techniques help individuals to decrease pain and anxiety, and improve their ability to cope with pain and other stressful situations. Use of distraction, self-statements/coping thoughts, and various relaxation techniques such as progressive muscle relaxation, focused breathing, meditation, guided imagery, and hypnosis can be appropriate additions to an individual's pain management program (Rini et al., 2017). Referrals to mental health professionals, trained in the use of these types of interventions, can help patients with pain learn how to utilize these interventions in a way that is appropriate to their individual situations (Melton, 2017).

There is a growing literature regarding the use of *mindfulness* in the comprehensive approach to pain management. Mindfulness has been defined in various ways but most definitions share the idea that it involves an individual "openly attending, with awareness, to one's present moment of experience" (Creswell, 2017, p. 493). This attention means that one deliberately focuses on his or her body sensations, emotional reactions, and thoughts. It is important that the person who is practicing mindfulness is nonjudgmental, actively accepting of whatever he or she is experiencing, moment by moment (Creswell, 2017; Kabat-Zinn, 2013). Mindfulness-based interventions have been classified into two general types, mindfulness-based stress reduction (MBSR) and mindfulness-based cognitive therapy (MBCT). Both work to help people deal with pain and distress from chronic health problems. MBCT builds on MBSR and adds cognitive techniques. It is not yet clear as to the mechanism of action for MBSR/MBCT but it is thought that its use can help people learn better ways of reacting to distressful situations (such as pain), thereby lessening an individual's distress (Alsubaie et al., 2017).

Doran's (2014) qualitative study evaluating the impact of mindfulness on chronic back pain illustrates the positive effects that this therapy can bring to a chronic pain situation. Study participants found that use of mindfulness enabled them to become more familiar with their patterns of pain and their usual reactions to their pain. It helped them to recognize the early signs of an upcoming pain flare and decreased maladaptive attitudes and approaches to their pain.

Cognitive behavioral therapy was originally developed by psychologists to treat anxiety, stress, and depression, by using some of the psychoeducational, cognitive, and behavioral techniques previously described. CBT has been used to treat individuals in a variety of situations with the goal of therapy based on the situation. For the individual with cancer-related pain, the goal of CBT is to enhance the sense of self-efficacy or personal control (Syrjala et al., 2014).

CBT has been successfully used with individuals with advanced cancer, helping to address both medical and psychological concerns. An example of this can be seen in the protocol developed by Greer, Park, and Safren (2010). This approach involves the use of four core modules: (a) psychoeducation and goal setting; (b) relaxation training; (c) coping with cancer fears; and (d) activity planning and pacing (Greer et al., 2010). It works best in a series of structured sessions that are flexible and modifiable, according to the developing needs of the individual, irrespective of the format.

Greer et al. (2010) suggest that there be clear and explicit goal setting and treatment goals. These goals are to be developed collaboratively by therapist and patient. Together, they look at the range of problems present and prioritize them. They review this list on a regular basis, and reprioritize goals as personal, social, and medical changes develop. Based on this list, appropriate, systematic interventions to address these problems are determined. The purpose of the interventions is to resolve specifically defined current problems and not long-term personality and social relations disturbances.

Ideally, work with CBT occurs early in the treatment phase of an illness. As disease progresses, an individual may experience cognitive impairment from a variety of causes that make it impossible to employ these techniques. When this occurs, it may be necessary to focus more on the family and caregivers with the goals to maximize their coping skills and increase their sense of control.

Pain coping skills training (PCST) may be the next addition to multimodal pain management, helping to combine pharmacological pain treatments with psychological pain interventions. PCST focuses on helping patients learn the skills they need to cope with and manage their pain, building on the principles of CBT. A PCST program will teach such things as progressive muscle relaxation, brief relaxation, activity/rest cycling, pleasant activity scheduling, negative thoughts identification, coping with negative thoughts, distraction techniques, problem solving, and strategies to maintain these skills (Rini et al., 2017).

Identified barriers to instituting PCST include healthcare providers being unfamiliar with PCST, and their concerns about overburdening patients. Patient barriers to PCST include ability and/or willingness to participate in such a program, and availability of accessible PCST programs. A recent pilot of a PCST computer-based program that attempted to address these concerns found that a web-based program was acceptable to both providers and patients. Future work needs to look at implementation of PCST programs in more diverse socioeconomic and ethnic populations including both in person and web-based study arms (Rini et al., 2017).

Integrative Treatments

Many adults with pain (some sources estimate up to 30%) will use approaches for pain relief that have been developed outside of mainstream, conventional medicine. These practices can be classified as "alternative" if they are used in place of conventional medicine or "complementary" if used together with conventional medicine. The National Center for Complementary and Integrative Health (NCCIH) uses the term "integrative" for complementary approaches that combine complementary and conventional treatments together in an integrative way (NCCIH, 2016). There is growing evidence that some of these complementary interventions help in the management of pain (Nahin, Boineau, Khalsa, Stussman, & Weber, 2016). A recent survey of oncology nurses demonstrated a strong interest in integrating complementary therapies into the care of their patients (Ben-Arye et al., 2017). When considering the addition of integrative modalities into a plan of care for pain management, the individual patient should be asked about his or her interest and comfort using these types of interventions. Additionally, counseling should be provided regarding the risks and benefits of these therapies (Deng et al., 2013).

NCCIH currently classifies integrative interventions into three main categories: (a) Natural Products, (b) Mind and Body Practices, and (c) Other Complementary Approaches. The following discussion will focus on acupuncture, hypnosis, massage therapy, and music therapy, the mind and body practices that have the strongest evidence for incorporation into pain management plans for cancer-related pain as identified by the Society for Integrative Oncology (SIO). SIO is an organization that evaluates which integrative treatments are safe and effective for patients with cancer. They systematically evaluate peer-reviewed randomized clinical trials and assign grades to therapies based on evidence strength. A grade "A" rating indicates the strongest recommendation. However, the only mind body interventions recommended by SIO for pain relief received "C" ratings. These interventions are recommended to be selectively offered to individual patients based on professional judgment and patient preferences because there is only "moderate certainty that the net benefit is small" (Greenlee et al., 2017, p. 198). This rating may be due to lack of study and could change in the future depending on the results of well designed, clinical trials. Despite the limited evidence for effectiveness in pain control, there is no clear indication of harm and clinicians should consider the use of these integrative strategies on a case by case basis (Eaton et al., 2017). The NCCIH has recognized the need for quality research regarding complementary and integrative interventions as outlined in their 2016 strategic plan. Nonpharmacological pain management approaches were given high priority, which may lead to future improvements in the identification of evidence-based treatment strategies (NCCIH, 2016).

Acupuncture, a treatment from traditional Chinese medicine (TCM), has been shown to treat pain, depression, nausea, and other health problems effectively (National Cancer Institute at the National Institutes of Health, 2013a). In TCM, it is thought that good health depends on the balance of energy in the body. Energy, called *chi* or *qi*, is thought to be constantly circulating in the body. Acupuncture acts to promote circulation of chi or qi vital energy. In this holistic, energy-based approach, thin, disposable needles, heat, pressure, and other treatments are applied to certain places on the skin to cause a change in the physical functions of the body (National Cancer Institute at the National Institutes of Health, 2013a). This is not on a disease-oriented, diagnostic treatment approach but an individualized, holistic, energy-focused approach. The fact that acupuncture causes a multitude of biological responses has been clearly demonstrated. Western medicine considers the proposed mechanisms of action for pain relief by acupuncture to include endorphin release, mediation of pain-producing neurotransmitters, and stress-induced analgesia (Kravitz, 2015).

Acupuncture is gaining more practitioners with Western medicine backgrounds and more general support from Western practitioners. Along with others, some nurses are going through extensive training to become licensed practitioners of acupuncture. Issues of training, licensure, and accreditation are in the process of being clarified. In the United States, educational standards have been developed for the training of practitioners. An agency recognized by the U.S. Department of Education has accredited many of the acupuncture educational programs. Physician acupuncturists can sit for a nationally recognized exam. Nonphysician acupuncturists can sit for an entry-level competency exam that is offered by the National Certification Commission for Acupuncture and Oriental Medicine (NCCAOM). Unfortunately, there is much variation from state to state. This includes differences in the requirements to obtain licensure and in the titles conferred. This variation leads to confusion and to less confidence in the qualifications of acupuncture practitioners. It is important that nurses be aware of the requirements and titles conferred in the states in which they practice in order to guide patients who desire a TCM evaluation for acupuncture to the most qualified, safe practitioners (NIH Consensus Conference Acupuncture, 1998).

A more detailed discussion of acupuncture and related acupuncture-based therapies, such as acupoint stimulation and electroacupuncture, are beyond the scope of this text. Nurse educators desiring to include more information about these techniques in the nursing curriculum are encouraged to seek out licensed practitioners of acupuncture for collaboration.

Hypnosis, often considered a psychological pain intervention, is a well-established approach that is being utilized more and more for control of pain, including procedural, acute, and chronic pain conditions. Through hypnosis, an individual is directed by a clinician to enter a state of deep relaxation and to use his or her imagination to alter both one's perception of and response to a symptom, such as pain. Healthy, intact individuals vary in their ability to utilize hypnosis. Debilitated individuals, especially at the EOL, may have less than their usual ability to utilize hypnosis. Hypnosis should only be done by specially trained professionals and will not be reviewed here in greater depth. It is important that entry into practice and advanced practice students be aware that hypnosis can enhance one's sense of self-efficacy in managing pain, enabling one to alter what he or she thinks, feels, and does in response to the pain. If a patient wishes to explore the use of hypnosis in his or her pain management plan, then a referral to a trained professional should be initiated (Cramer et al., 2015; Syrjala et al., 2014).

Massage has long been utilized to enhance health and healing since ancient times and involves the systematic manipulation of soft tissues by massage therapists and others involved with a patient's care. When considering massage, it is important for the nurse to consider the patient's comfort with touch, previous experiences with massage, and preferred techniques (Wells, Pasero, & McCaffery, 2008). Massage is contraindicated over sites of tissue damage (such as open wounds or tissue undergoing irradiation), in patients with bleeding disorders or thrombophlebitis, patients uncomfortable with touch, or those who might misinterpret touch as sexual (although this might be acceptable if the massager was a spouse or close partner). In working with cancer patients, light pressure is best, and deep or intense pressure is to be avoided (Deng, Cassileth, & Simon, 2004; Deng et al., 2007).

Providing massage therapy to the site of pain may or may not serve to decrease pain at that site. Debilitated patients may be unable to tolerate an extensive massage but may find massage of limited sites beneficial. For example, massage of the neck, back, or shoulders may be sufficient to promote comfort. Alternatively, some may find this massage too strenuous. For these patients, the nurse could consider massage to the hands or feet. Massage movements can include rhythmic stroking, kneading, or circular, distal-to-proximal movements. Effleurage, using slow, smooth, long strokes, is usually done to promote relaxation.

The patient should be involved in choosing the sites and massage movements that provide the most comfort along with how long the massage should last. It may be helpful to try different types of strokes with varying degrees of pressure in an effort to find what is most effective for an individual (Jacox et al., 1994; Wells et al., 2008). The patient may be sitting in a chair, or lying on his or her side, or prone on a bed or table. It is helpful to determine with the individual if the room will be quiet, if music will be played, or if conversation will take place during the massage (Wells et al., 2008).

During the actual massage, ideally both the nurse and the patient will be as relaxed as possible. The patient should be in a position that is supported and easy to maintain for the duration of the massage. The massager should be in a position that utilizes good body mechanics. Patient comfort and modesty are to be maintained with sheets, blankets, or towels. The use of a warmed, alcohol-free lotion will decrease friction. One hand should be on the patient at all times until the massage is over. For example, the right hand could begin its stroke as the left hand is completing its stroke. Removing both hands can communicate to the patient that the massage is over; patients may fall asleep during massage (Adams, White, & Beckett, 2010).

Feedback from the patient, if possible, is useful for future planning. If patients find massage helpful, it should be scheduled on a regular basis. Massage can be quite comforting to dying patients who are often deprived of human touch at the EOL. Family members and caregivers, if not overwhelmed or feeling overburdened, may wish to be instructed or included in this pain-relieving intervention. Massage therapy can provide pain relief and relaxation, can support a patient's emotional well-being and recovery, and can ultimately aid in the healing process for hospitalized patients (Adams et al., 2010).

Music has been shown to be an effective intervention for pain control through a variety of physiological and psychological effects. Affective, cognitive, and sensory processes can be engaged, activated, and altered by music. In PC, music therapy "strives to promote well-being and quality of life for patients and caregivers" (Magill, 2009, p. 37). This is done by processes such as use of prior skills, relaxation, distraction, alteration of mood, and improved sense of control. Physical effects include increasing or decreasing pulse and blood pressure (Cincinnati Children's Hospital Medical Center, 2012).

In using music with an individual, music therapists evaluate the patient's medical situation, the person's social and cultural history, and how emotions are affecting that person's pain. The music therapist can then utilize a variety of techniques to help ameliorate pain and suffering. Vocal techniques can include toning, chanting, singing precomposed songs, writing songs, and singing improvisations. Listening techniques and use of prerecorded or live instrumental music can provide opportunities for exploration and expression (Magill, 2009).

A patient's needs may change daily. Because of this, the music selection is best done with the individual on a day-to-day basis. "The aim is always to promote comfort, healing, and a decreased sense of pain" (Magill, 2009, p. 34). Working in collaboration with other pain modification approaches, music therapy can help soothe pain as well as heal suffering. Music therapy can promote wellness, manage stress, alleviate pain, express feelings, enhance memory, improve communication, and promote physical rehabilitation (Bradt, Dileo, Magill, & Teague, 2016; Gutgsell et al., 2013; Music Therapy Association, 2013).

CASE STUDY *Continued*

Despite surgery and chemotherapy, Ms. T. experiences progression of disease and has developed a perirectal fistula. She calls the outpatient clinic for an appointment and is seen urgently, as she reports her pain is constantly 10/10. She is found to have significant weight loss, anorexia, and generalized weakness. She admits to you that she has been taking more hydromorphone than has been prescribed just to be able to get some sleep and remains unwilling to take any medication for anxiety or depression. Because of her weakness, Ms. T. is having more difficulty caring for herself. She feels like her life is spinning out of control, as her husband has begun drinking again. She no longer finds support in being a practicing Jehovah's Witness. She is afraid of what the future holds and if she'll even live to see another holiday. Ms. T. is admitted to the inpatient palliative care unit for symptom management. Is Ms. T. demonstrating signs of addiction? Can opioid analgesics be prescribed in a safe manner? What other supports might help Ms. T. during her pain crisis?

■ SECTION 4: INTEGRATING MULTIMODAL THERAPY INTO COMPREHENSIVE PAIN MANAGEMENT PLANS

While a thorough and comprehensive assessment is critical in formulating a successful pain management plan, deciding on the appropriate pharmacological and nonpharmacological interventions should be based on the following palliative principles: when feasible, address the underlying cause of pain; discuss treatment options within the context of the patient's and family's goals of care; attempt to avoid new complications when implementing a pain management regimen; prepare the family and caregiver for possible treatment side effects; be cognizant of the potential burdens (either physical, psychological, social, or financial) of the proposed intervention; and consider if the treatment will be valuable for the patient (Indelicato, 2006).

The use of any intervention is based on the assessment of the patient. It is important to evaluate the individual carefully and apply what is appropriate for that individual in a particular situation. After the initiation of systemic analgesic therapy and treatment of underlying disease when possible, the next step would be to consider the addition of less invasive nonpharmacological treatments for pain management. While medical drugs are being used for treating the somatic (physiological) dimension of the pain, nonpharmacological therapies aim to treat the affective, cognitive, behavioral, and sociocultural dimensions of the pain to improve control and possibly improve the balance between analgesia and side effects (Demir, 2012). If these measures are not effective, the use of more invasive techniques can be considered. Palliative sedation, at EOL for intractable symptoms, is also an option.

Managing a Pain Crisis

A pain crisis can be defined as pain that is severe, uncontrolled, and distressing to the patient (Moryl et al.,

2008). It may be acute in onset or may have progressed gradually in severity. A pain crisis is considered a medical and nursing care emergency for those at the EOL. At the same time the pain is being managed, the probable etiology of the pain is assessed within the framework of the previous pattern of pain, probable cause of present pain crisis, goals of care, and the most effective long-term management approaches (Moryl et al., 2008).

In patients who do not respond to opioid titration, or who develop intolerable side effects, the following adjuvants should be considered: (a) a parenteral NSAID, for example, ketorolac, for no longer than 5 days, due to increased risk of GI bleeding (Portenoy et al., 2015). During this period, other longer-term approaches for pain relief should be considered; (b) parenteral steroids, for example, dexamethasone, with the dose being gradually tapered down to the lowest effective dose for the patient. Anecdotal experience has shown the use of parenteral NSAIDs or steroids to be effective in a pain crisis associated with bone pain and neuropathic pain; (c) if the pain is predominantly neuropathic, IV lidocaine or ketamine can be helpful for some patients (Broglio & Portenoy, 2016). The efficacy of a nerve block or spinal delivery system of drug administration for this particular clinical situation should be considered (Ferrell & Coyle, 2010).

Palliative Sedation at the End of Life

A proportion of patients at the EOL will experience refractory symptoms, including pain that is not possible to control in the absence of sedation, despite the use of state-of-the-art techniques. The number of patients involved is not clear. Palliative sedation at EOL is always an option for these individuals (Barathi & Chandra, 2013). Despite the lack of consensus regarding its definition, palliative sedation can be described as the use of benzodiazepines, barbiturates, or anesthetics to produce unresponsiveness with the intent to alleviate intolerable symptoms until death (Bobb, 2016; Cherney, 2017). Clear documentation and communication among the team members and with the family is essential when the plan is to provide palliative sedation at EOL to ease intractable symptoms. It should reflect the goals of care clearly stated in unambiguous terms with resuscitation status established; discussion with the patient or healthcare proxy with informed consent; symptom being treated and management approach selected; and endpoint to be achieved and monitoring parameters (Hospice and Palliative Nurses Association, 2016). Opioid or sedative drug dose escalation without clear indications should not occur.

■ PAIN MANAGEMENT IN SPECIAL, VULNERABLE POPULATIONS

Special Considerations for Older Adults

The world's population is aging. It is estimated that by 2050, one-fourth of the world's population will be more than 60 years old (Savvas & Gibson, 2016). The National Council on Aging (NCOA) estimates that approximately 92% of older adults have at least one chronic disease and 72% will have two or more in the future (NCOA, 2017). The probability is high that the older patient will experience pain at the EOL as pain prevalence increases significantly with age, due to both malignant and non-malignant causes. Despite its prevalence, pain is often overlooked and, in turn, undertreated in adults living with advanced illnesses (Phongtankuel et al., 2016).

Aggressive pain management is as necessary for older adults as it is for younger individuals. The approach to pain is the same, involving a thorough assessment and incorporating pharmacological and nonpharmacological interventions addressing the underlying cause, compatible with the individual goals of care. In elder patients, pain is frequently undertreated across all practice settings. The dying older patient may be cared for at home, in a nursing home, or in a hospital. In any setting, untreated pain can lead to loss of function and psychological complications in this vulnerable population.

Some older adults may be reluctant to report pain for fear of receiving an unfavorable diagnosis or fear of finding progression of disease (Malec & Shega, 2015; Savvas & Gibson, 2016). Other barriers to pain management in older adults include the following misconceptions: (a) Pain is a normal or expected part of aging; (b) if individuals do not complain of pain, they must not have much pain; and (c) the side effects from opioids make them too dangerous to use in elderly patients (American Geriatrics Society, 2009; Savvas & Gibson, 2016). Nurses need to reinforce that pain is not an inevitable part of aging and be committed to its evaluation and treatment (Malec & Shega, 2015; Savvas & Gibson, 2016).

In treating pain in the older adult, it is important to understand the effects of age on the pharmacokinetic and pharmacodynamic responses to analgesic medications including risk of drug accumulation. The general rule for using medications in the older adult is to "start low and go slow." Those caring for dying older patients with pain also need to be aware of the following (Abdulla et al., 2013; Brown, Kirkpatrick, Swanson, & McKenzie, 2011; Koronkowski, Eisenhower, & Marcum, 2016; Malec & Shega, 2015; NCOA, 2017; Phongtankuel et al., 2016; Savvas & Gibson, 2016; Tracy & Morrison, 2013):

- Pain assessment can be disproportionately confounded by cognitive impairment or dysfunction, memory difficulties, age-related changes in vision and hearing, depression, and alcohol or substance abuse.
- Normal age-related physical changes which can affect volume of distribution, plasma concentration, and elimination of medications include decreased renal and hepatic clearance, reduced intravascular volume, decreased total body water, reduced muscle mass, and increased fat-to-lean body mass ratio. These factors must be considered in analgesic selection and dosing.
- The presence of polypharmacy, multiple healthcare providers, multimodal medications or analgesic stacking, multiple diagnosis, complex symptoms from comorbid conditions, and potentially inappropriate medication use may further complicate the pain experience.
- The patient's ability to self-medicate independently and participate in the pain management plan may be affected by functional factors, such as impaired vision, impaired hand dexterity, memory problems, cognitive impairments, as well as place of residence (e.g., nursing home or other care facility).
- Identify the patient's caregiver. The caregiver may be an older person, or the patient may live alone with the caregiver living elsewhere. Evaluate the ability, availability, and desire of the caregiver and of other family and friends to assist with care, administer pain medications, and participate in the pain management plan.

Special Considerations in Those With Impaired Communication

Communication is essential to pain assessment and effective pain management. People who have difficulty self-reporting their pain are at higher risk for inadequate pain control. Impaired communication can have many causes but the primary reasons include language barriers, and the limited ability or inability to communicate verbally. People who may be unable to self-report their pain may include infants and preverbal toddlers, critically ill/unconscious patients, people with intellectual disabilities, older adults with dementia, and patients at the EOL (Herr et al., 2011; McGuire et al., 2016).

The National Council on Interpreting in Health Care (NCIHC) is an organization that promotes language access in healthcare. NCIHC published national standards of practice in September 2005. These standards are a useful resource in addressing communication impairment related to language barriers (NCIHC, 2005). To assess pain when a language barrier exists, it is best to avoid using family members for interpreters as they may filter the information or lack the medical vocabulary to provide the necessary complete information. Nurses also need to be aware of the impact that the patient's religious or cultural background may have upon pain assessment and management (NCCN, 2017).

The American Society for Pain Management Nurses has developed a position paper with clinical practice recommendations for working with people who are unable to self-report pain due to cognitive or physiological issues. Their recommendations are based on the premise that pain assessment is guided by the following hierarchy: (a) self-report, (b) search for potential causes of pain, (c) observe patient behaviors, (d) proxy reporting of pain behaviors by those who know the patient, and (e) attempt an analgesic trial. This useful resource includes specific population clinical practice recommendations (Herr et al., 2011).

Recommended practices for pain assessment and management with people who have communication impairments continue to evolve. Clinicians are advised to stay alert for new developments. In the meantime, the following points may be useful (Herr et al., 2011; McGuire et al., 2016; NCCN, 2017; NCIHC, 2005; Savvas & Gibson, 2016):

- Identify the communication deficit that is impeding the patient's ability to report pain, pain relief, and compliance with the pain management plan.
- Obtain the appropriate pain assessment tool, assure placement for easy clinician/caregiver access (i.e., bedside), and use consistently while caring for the patient.
- If the patient and his or her caretakers do not speak the same language, identify the patient's language and identify available translators. Obtain a pain scale in the patient's language and review it with the patient and translator. It is helpful to write keywords or phrases in both the patient's language and the corresponding translations in the caregiver's language.
- If the patient cannot communicate, it is useful to collaborate with the patient's family and caregivers to determine what behavioral activities may indicate pain for this patient. These behaviors include: grimacing, pacing, restlessness, moaning, lying still, or guarding.
- Document possible pain behaviors and any tools needed for pain assessment in the patient's record to assist other caregivers in providing continuity of care.
- Provide more frequent pain assessments using a valid and reliable tool if a patient is unable to ask for pain medication or avoids asking for pain medication.
- If the patient is to die at home, issues related to impaired communication need to be addressed in the home setting. Family members and other caregivers may need extra education and support. If a language barrier is present, explore the possibility of involving home health aides or nurses who speak the patient's language.

Special Considerations in Pediatric Patients

Although infants, children, and adolescents with many different life-threatening conditions such as sickle cell disease or cystic fibrosis experience pain, most of the work of documenting pain and its management has taken place in the field of oncology. Not so long ago, pain in the dying child was not viewed as a significant problem. Children were not considered to feel pain as intensely as adults and were therefore considered not to need aggressive pain management. Fortunately, the literature on pediatric pain has expanded significantly since the 1970s and pediatric pain is viewed as a specialty in its own right. Nurses have played a significant role in this development with such programs as Pediatric ELNECPPC and Education in Palliative and End-of-Life Care (EPEC; American Association of Colleges of Nursing, 2016; IPPC, 2014). The nurse caring for the dying child needs to be well versed in how to manage pain in children, using a multidimensional approach with an awareness of issues specific to the pediatric population (Collins, Berde, & Frost, 2011; Kars, Grypdonck, & van Delden, 2011; Layman-Goldstein & Kramer, 2015).

Pain assessment is dependent upon a child's chronological age and developmental state. A detailed review of pediatric pain assessment is beyond the scope of the chapter. Readers are directed to other resources when selecting age- and population-specific pediatric pain assessment tools that may be observational or a self-report, depending on the clinical situation and the infant's or child's developmental stage and ability to verbalize (Collins et al., 2011; Crellin, Sullivan, Babl, O'Sullivan, & Hutchinson, 2007; Ghai, Kaur-Makkur, & Wig, 2008).

The WHO three-step analgesic ladder for pain relief in children was modified in 2012 to a two-step ladder when the WHO refined its approach for relief of cancer pain in children. In this revised pharmacological approach, the first step of this ladder is mild pain and the use of non-opioids, such as paracetamol (acetaminophen) and ibuprofen, is indicated. The second step is moderate-to-severe pain and involves the use of low starting doses of "strong" opioids, such as morphine. This medication for persistent pain is administered on a regular schedule with prn doses for breakthrough or intermittent pain. The doses of these medications are adjusted based on reassessment of the individual child and titrated upward until satisfactory analgesia without dose-limiting side effects is achieved. In the original three-step model, codeine, a "weak" opioid, was utilized. By eliminating the "weak opioids" (i.e., codeine and tramadol) used in the earlier version, it was possible to incorporate into the model subsequent research that demonstrated that these medications are to be avoided in children because they have a narrow therapeutic window and variable individual metabolism which pose both safety and efficacy problems (WHO, 2012).

Many of the principles of pain assessment and management reviewed in this chapter can be applied to children.

However, children should not be viewed as mini-adults. Nurses caring for children need to be mindful of several important points (Collins et al., 2011; Layman-Goldstein & Kramer, 2015; Wallace, 2013; Wolfe et al., 2008):

- The child and family is the unit of care. Successful interventions can only happen when parents are included in the assessment and pain management plans. No one knows a child better than his or her parents; therefore, no one is better able to advocate for the child than the parents of that child.
- It is helpful to initiate discussions about pain and to learn the individual child's word for pain.
- Pain assessment is dependent upon the child's age and cognitive developmental stage.
- Developmentally appropriate tools exist to evaluate the child in pain.
- A child's self-report of pain is considered the most reliable and valid indicator for estimate of pain location and intensity.
- Behavioral observation is the primary assessment measure for preverbal or nonverbal children. Observed pain behaviors may include vocalizations, facial expressions, body movements, autonomic responses, or changes in daily activities, usual behaviors, appetite, or sleep.
- The goal of pain management in children is to prevent as much pain as possible and to treat procedural pain aggressively.
- It is important to consider the child's age, developmental level, verbal capabilities, past experiences, cultural factors, type of pain, and context when developing a pain management plan.
- Address family concerns regarding the risk of addiction in the medically ill child.
- The pharmacological management principles—by the ladder, by the clock, by the appropriate route, and by the child—are similar to those used with adults with the exception that the starting doses are determined by chronological age and body weight (milligrams or micrograms per kilogram). The child is frequently assessed and doses are titrated to effect.
- The oral route is the desired route whenever possible. Avoid the rectal route and IM injections. Consider transdermal, IV, and topical routes when the oral route is not possible.

Special Considerations in Those With a History of Substance Use Disorder

The prevalence of substance use disorder (SUD) in the United States is estimated to be 8.4%.

It is a very heterogeneous group with very diverse clinical problems. It includes individuals who are living drug-free lives, those in methadone maintenance programs (MMP), and those who are currently abusing drugs or alcohol. It is not uncommon to find individuals in this group with co-occurring mental disorders and

SUDs, those with addictive disease who also have a concurrent psychiatric illness such as anxiety, depression, bipolar disorder, or schizophrenia (Center for Behavioral Health Statistics and Quality, 2015; Oliver et al., 2012). Although the epidemiology is not well defined, within this population of people with SUD are individuals with significant pain from cancer and other serious illnesses. These individuals are at high risk of undertreatment of their pain. Their treatment needs to address both their chronic pain and their SUD (Kirsh, Compton, Egan-City, & Passik, 2015).

The field of addiction medicine is a developing science based upon recent neuroscience advances that include identification of the brain mechanisms involved with addiction, vulnerability, and nociception (Oliver et al., 2012). SUD is a chronic disease of the brain. Like other chronic diseases, this disease can become worse over time if not addressed. Just as someone who has both cancer and diabetes needs to have both diseases treated simultaneously for optimal outcomes, someone with both cancer and SUD needs both illnesses addressed by the team caring for them (Kirsch et al., 2015).

Often the challenge is to provide humane, high-quality care to people at the EOL who have a history of drug abuse in a societal context that often views addiction from a moral or criminal perspective (Oliver et al., 2012). Pain management for individuals with advanced illness and SUD involves the same principles discussed earlier in this chapter, utilizing multimodal approaches based on a thorough pain assessment of each individual, but also addressing issues specific to addiction. Opioids are to be used for significant pain but with some modifications. Experts advise choosing an opioid prescribed around-the-clock and using long-acting formulations as appropriate. Use of short-acting, prn doses may be limited or even eliminated. Non-opioid adjuvant analgesics and nonpharmacological interventions should be incorporated into the pain management plan whenever appropriate but are not to be a substitute for necessary opioids. Depending on an individual's circumstances, prescribers may need to limit the amount of medications prescribed at any one time to a few days or a week's supply. Pill counts and urine toxicology screening can be utilized to confirm compliance with a pain management plan. Individuals who demonstrate poor compliance are to be referred to an addiction specialist (Kirsch et al., 2015).

Formal involvements by experts from the fields of PC and SUD are working to improve pain management for individuals with advanced disease and SUD. The following points are helpful to keep in mind when working with PC patients with pain who have a history of substance abuse (Blackhall, Alfson, & Barclay, 2013; Childers & Arnold, 2012; Claxton & Arnold, 2011; Compton & Chang, 2017; Kirsh et al., 2015; Oliver et al., 2012; Owen, Burton, Schade, & Passik, 2012; Smith et al., 2009; Walsh & Broglio, 2016):

■ Recognize that addiction is a chronic, relapsing illness, with periods of remissions and exacerbations—and respond with increasing structure and compassion. Relapse often occurs during early abstinence or during periods of increased stress.

■ SUD occurs on a continuum. Identify whether the individual has a far distant history of drug abuse, is in a MMP, or is actively abusing substances.

■ Encourage participation in recovery programs (e.g., 12-step) if the patient is willing and physically able. Consider consultation with an addictions/mental health professional.

■ Patients who are actively abusing substances are the most challenging of the three groups to work with. An interprofessional team that emphasizes clear communication is most effective in addressing the multiple medical, psychosocial, and administrative problems.

■ Treat pain aggressively; poorly treated pain can increase substance abuse behaviors.

■ Use non-opioid analgesics and nonpharmacological measures to their full potential.

■ Patients who have a far distant history of drug abuse or who are in MMP may be reluctant to take opioids because of fear of re-addiction.

■ Individuals with a history of substance abuse, past or present, may be tolerant of opioids and require higher doses of opioids to effectively treat pain as compared to patients without a history of drug abuse.

■ If a patient is currently in MMP, he or she must provide permission to contact the program and coordinate therapy. Some MMP providers wish to remain actively involved at the EOL and others do not.

■ Many MMP patients frequently keep the methadone dose taken for addiction separate from whatever medication they take for pain control. For others, however, it may be useful to incorporate the equianalgesic daily methadone dose into their analgesic regimen, especially at EOL or for those who are unable to swallow.

■ Methadone may be stigmatized as an analgesic in patients who have a history of substance abuse. Patients, their families, and friends may need education about the effectiveness of methadone as an analgesic.

■ Practitioners need to be aware of the need for more frequent dosing of methadone when given for analgesia, usually at least every 6 to 8 hours. Some patients require an every 4-hour schedule for adequate pain control.

■ Formalize a treatment plan and coordinate it with all other health professionals involved. One NP or physician should be identified to write all analgesic orders or prescriptions with a backup plan for coverage. This plan needs to be communicated to all caring for the patient.

■ Consider use of a written opioid agreement with carefully defined patient and provider expectations.

■ Urine drug testing (UDT), if used to demonstrate compliance, should be done at baseline, before prescribing opioids and at random intervals. Use of UDT can help determine if a patient is or is not taking the prescribed medication, or other illicit drugs. The gas chromatography/mass spectrometry is the UDT of choice as it is able to identify specific medications (including semisynthetic opioids), and metabolites, something the dipstick tests are unable to do.

■ Consistent documentation that shows the assessment of the four domains of functioning—pain relief, patient functioning, adverse effects, and drug-related behaviors—is important in the care of all patients receiving chronic opioid therapy, especially those who have a history of SUD.

■ Individuals with a history of SUD frequently have difficulties handling stress and will need extra support during periods of cancer re-staging, disease recurrence, progression of disease, and at the EOL. Psychiatric symptoms and comorbidities such as anxiety, depression, and bipolar disorders are frequently encountered and are to be promptly treated.

Special Considerations in Cancer Survivors

In the United States, the number of cancer survivors has increased from 3 million to over 15 million within the past 45 years (Miller et al., 2016). While improvements in screening and cancer therapies have supported this significant change, cancer survivors are at risk for the chronic effects of the disease and its treatments which can negatively impact their QOL (ASCO, 2016). Approximately one-third to 40% of this population experiences chronic pain (ASCO, 2016; NCCN, 2017). While the literature supports that these patients should receive pain management consistent with the treatment of chronic pain (Glare et al., 2014), recent concerns over the long-term effects of opioid therapy for this population have been questioned. In addition to the CDC guidelines, ASCO (2016) summoned an expert panel and undertook a systematic review to highlight the assessment and management of pain in the cancer survivor. Subsequent recommendations included: ongoing pain screening and evaluation of new pain complaints as a potential cancer recurrence, inclusion of an interdisciplinary approach for those survivors with complicated needs, trials of non-opioid and nondrug therapies, and guidelines for initiating opioid therapy.

While cancer survivors may receive a trial of opioid therapy at the lowest dose for the least amount of time, universal precautions should be implemented to reduce the risk of misuse and abuse (ASCO, 2016). Although the safe use of opioid analgesics is important, these recommendations have the potential for placing cancer survivors at risk for undertreated pain (Fisch & Chang, 2016). Anecdotally, survivors are concerned that their access to opioid therapy will be impacted, as providers may become more unwilling to prescribe opioid analgesics or they may not meet the exemption criteria since they do not have an active cancer diagnosis. For these reasons, nurses must remain vigilant in advocating for appropriate pain management for survivors and other patient populations at risk.

■ THE ROLE OF NURSES IN IMPLEMENTING COMPREHENSIVE PAIN MANAGEMENT

Nurses caring for PC patients have both collaborative and independent functions in implementing a comprehensive pain management plan. First, nurses must be aware of which nonpharmacological interventions they are able to perform. Factors to consider when making this determination include the nurse's scope of practice, education in the use of particular techniques, comfort in teaching or implementing a particular intervention, availability of patient and family educational materials, accessibility and affordability of specific devices, and time available to initiate a particular therapy. Depending on the nurse's practice setting, rehabilitative interventions for pain relief such as the use of superficial heat or cooling, massage, or vibration may require a medical order. Nurses often have some level of expertise in providing many of the psychologically based interventions, such as patient/family education, distraction, and relaxation. Additionally, the nurse can act as an important resource for patients and families, especially when access to other specialists, such as anesthesiologists or psychologists, is needed. Most importantly, the nurse should identify the patient's and family's preferences and advocate for the inclusion of these preferences in the pain management plan (Demir, 2012).

It is important to consider whether a patient or the family has the physical, mental, or emotional energy necessary to participate in a particular treatment. Nonpharmacological interventions that need a high level of patient involvement may not be possible when an individual is debilitated or when the caregiver is totally exhausted from the experience. Assessment needs to include a patient's ability to concentrate and follow directions, level of fatigue, and cognitive status (Sagar, Dryden, & Wong, 2007). Education of the patient, family, and caregivers regarding the non-drug intervention in the pain management plan can elicit cooperation and promote successful use of the intervention. It is important to stress that nonpharmacological interventions are not a replacement for analgesics. These therapies can complement the pharmacological treatment and have benefits that include (a) increasing the individual's sense of control; (b) decreasing the feeling of weakness; (c) improving the activity level and functional capacity; (d) reducing stress and anxiety; (e) reducing pain behavior and pain focus; and (f) reducing analgesic dosage without escalation of pain, thus decreasing the side effects of the treatment (Demir, 2012).

■ CONCLUSIONS

The assessment and management of pain in patients with life-threatening, progressive illness underscores the importance of integrating assessment and treatment strategies to address the needs of the individual patient. From the moment they graduate, nurses are expected to care for those who are seriously ill and dying. The delivery of optimal therapy depends on the patient's medical condition and psychosocial state, the goals of care, the comprehensive assessment of the pain, an understanding of the clinical pharmacology of the analgesic drugs, and the identification of appropriate nonpharmacological interventions. Although the nurse will usually be part of an interprofessional team, he or she will often be the one responsible for assessing pain, administering analgesics, monitoring for adequacy of pain relief and presence of side effects, communicating with other members of the team, and ensuring continuity of pain management across care settings, including at home. These responsibilities cannot be met unless the nurse is knowledgeable in the basic principles of pain assessment and multimodal pain management, and in the recognition of patients who are at risk of inadequate pain assessment and control.

CASE STUDY *Conclusion*

Ms. T. is transitioned to a morphine PCA to manage her pain and is started on an antidepressant to address her mood and anxiety. She is seen by the interdisciplinary team, including social work and pastoral care. Supports are also provided to her husband who pursues treatment of his alcoholism. Once her pain is managed, Ms. T. is able to engage in goals of care conversations and she is agreeable to hospice services. She is transitioned to an inpatient facility and dies soon after.

CASE STUDY

AN INTERPROFESSIONAL PERSPECTIVE

Lauren Koranteng, PharmD, BCPS, CPE
Memorial Sloan Kettering Cancer Center

This case study raises some discussions surrounding opioid-induced constipation, potential drug–herbal interactions, and pharmacological management of depression.

Ms. T's chronic pain was managed on a scheduled opioid in addition to a short-acting opioid and gabapentin, a co-analgesic. Gabapentin is an anticonvulsant that is approved for postherpetic neuralgia and partial onset seizures. It is often used off-label for several indications such as fibromyalgia syndrome and neuropathic pain. It is usually started at doses of 100 to 300 mg orally at bedtime. It has a favorable side effect profile and minimal drug interactions. While it has a minimal side effect profile, it can cause sedation, particularly when used in conjunction with other sedating medications such as opioids, as in Ms. T's case. It is titrated every 3 days until an effective dose is attained. Dose titration may take several weeks to reach higher doses. Additionally, patients with renal impairment issues will require dose reductions.

For patients on scheduled medications, a bowel regimen is required to prevent opioid-induced constipation. Ms. T. was initially started on a bowel regimen using Senna (Sennosides) and Docusate (Docusate Sodium or Docusate Calcium) and it's worth noting that Senna may be titrated up to 68.8 mg a day if needed (usually administered as 4 tablets orally twice daily using the 8.6 mg tablet). Other dosage formulations for Senna that may be considered based on patient preference include the Senna liquid or tea formulations.

The case study also mentions that Ms. T. sought holistic and herbal treatment when she experienced disease recurrence. While it's not clear if she was receiving chemotherapy by her oncology team, it is important to encourage patients to share with the clinical team if they are taking any herbal formulations to ensure that there are no drug–herbal interactions that could compromise treatment.

Lastly, most antidepressants take about 2 to 4 weeks to take effect; therefore, it's very important to take into consideration a patient's prognosis prior to initiating him or her. Additionally, one may consider comorbid conditions that a patient has prior to choosing an agent, as some agents may be effective at targeting other symptoms such as insomnia or poor appetite in addition to treating depression.

Evidence-Based Practice

Brant, J. M., Keller, L., McLeod, K., Yeh, C., & Eaton, L. H. (2017). Chronic and Refractory Pain. *Clinical Journal of Oncology Nursing, 21*(3), 31–53. doi:10.1188/17.CJON.S3.31-53

Methods
As part of the Oncology Nursing Society's Putting Evidence into Practice (PEP) guidelines, the authors undertook a systematic review to explore the evidence for the pharmacological treatment of chronic and refractory cancer pain.

Results
One hundred and eighty-four articles (including systematic reviews, meta-analysis, and clinical guidelines) were reviewed and the evidence was categorized using the PEP classification system created by Mitchell and Friese (n.d.).

Conclusions

The authors' findings include the following:

■ Opioid analgesics remain the foundation for the treatment of cancer-related pain.
■ The use of adjuvant or co-analgesics plays an important role in maximizing pain relief in the cancer population.
■ While the use of herbal supplements and other pharmacological approaches continues to be evaluated for their effectiveness, further research is needed to identify their role in the treatment of cancer pain management.

■ FUTURE RESEARCH RECOMMENDATIONS

Future research recommendations include the identification and treatment of pain syndromes in non-cancer patients; identification of new non-opioid–based drug therapies to treat pain; exploration of the role of marijuana in pain management; the effectiveness of complementary and integrative therapies in treating pain; and the impact of the CDC and CMS opioid guidelines on pain management in the PC patient (Exhibit 20.1).

Exhibit 20.1
Practice Guidelines, Websites, and Other Resources Related to Pain Management

Organizations:

- American Pain Society (APS): www.americanpainsociety.org
- American Society for Pain Management Nursing (ASPMN): www.aspmn.org
- American Society of PeriAnesthesia Nurses (ASPAN): www.aspan.org
- American Chronic Pain Association: www.theacpa.org
- National Cancer Institute (NCI): www.cancer.gov
- Center to Advance Palliative Care (CAPC): www.capc.org
- Hospice and Palliative Nurses Association (HPNA): hpna.advancingexpertcare.org
- American Academy of Hospice and Palliative Medicine (AAHPM): www.aahpm.org
- World Health Organization (WHO) cancer pain ladder: www.who.int/cancer/palliative/painladder/en
- World Health Organization (WHO). (2011). WHO model list of essential medicines: www.who.int/medicines/publications/essentialmedicines/en/
- International Association for the Study of Pain (IASP): www.iasp-pain.org/Organizations?navItemNumber=679
- Oncology Nursing Society (ONS): www.ons.org
- National Comprehensive Cancer Network (NCCN): www.nccn.org

Practice guidelines:

- American College of Critical Care Medicine and Society of Critical Care Medicine Task Force. (2013). Clinical practice guidelines for the management of pain, agitation, and delirium in adult patients in the intensive care unit. *Critical Care Medicine, 41*(1), 263–306. doi:10.1097/CCM.0b013e3182783b72
- American Nurses Association. (2018). *Official ANA position statements.* www.nursingworld.org/practice-policy/nursing-excellence/official-position-statements/
- American Society of Anesthesiologists. (2010). Practice guidelines for chronic pain management: An updated report by the American Society of Anesthesiologists Task Force on Chronic Pain Management and The American Society of Regional Anesthesia and Pain Management. *Anesthesiology, 112*(4), 810–833. doi:10.1097/ALN.0b013e3181c43103
- American Society for Pain Management Nursing. (2018). *Position* papers. www.aspmn.org/Pages/positionstatements.aspx
- The Joint Commission: Pain Management. (2017). www.jointcommission.org/topics/pain_management.aspx
- American Pain Society. (2017). Clinical practice guidelines. http://americanpainsociety.org/education/guidelines/overview
- American Academy of Pain Medicine—Position Statements: www.painmed.org/PatientCenter/position-statements
- Hospice and Palliative Nurses Association (2017). Position Statement: Pain Management. advancingexpertcare.org/wp-content/uploads/2018/02/Pain-Management-at-the-End-of-Life.pdf
- American Society of Clinical Oncology. (2017). Practice and guidelines. www.asco.org/practice-guidelines/cancer-care-initiatives/palliative-care-oncology

Additional websites:

- End-of-Life Nursing Education Consortium (ELNEC): www.aacnnursing.org/ELNEC
- Education in Palliative and End-of-Life Care (EPEC): www.epec.net
- National Institutes of Health (NIH): cancer.gov/cancertopics/pdq/supportivecare/pain/HealthProfessional
- American Nurses Credentialing Center (ANCC): www.nursingworld.org/ancc/
- American Cancer Society (ACS): www.cancer.org
- Palliative Care Network of Wisconsin: www.mypcnow.org/fast-facts
- National Quality Forum: www.qualityforum.org
- City of Hope Pain & Palliative Care Resource Center: prc.coh.org

■ REFERENCES

Abdulla, A., Adams, N., Bone, M., Elliott, A. M., Gaffin, J., Jones, D., ... Schofield, P.; British Geriatric Society. (2013). Guidance on the management of pain in older people. *Age and Ageing, 42*(Suppl. 1), i1–i57. doi:10.1093/ageing/afs200

Adams, R., White, B., & Beckett, C. (2010). The effects of massage therapy on pain management in the acute care setting. *International Journal of Therapeutic Massage and Bodywork, 3*(1), 1–9.

Aitken, E., McColl, G., & Kingsmore, D. (2017). The role of Qutenza® (Topical Capsaicin 8%) in treating neuropathic pain from critical ischemia in patients with end-stage renal disease: An observational cohort study. *Pain Medicine, 18*, 330–340. doi:10.1093/pm/pnw139

Alpert, C. M., Smith, M. A., Hummel, S. L., & Hummel, E. K. (2017). Symptom burden in heart failure: Assessment, impact on outcomes, and management. *Heart Failure Review, 22*, 25–39. doi:10.1007/s10741-016-9581-4

Alsubaie, M., Abbott, R., Dunn, B., Dickens, C., Keil, T. F., Henley, W., & Kuyken, W. (2017). Mechanisms of action in mindfulness-based cognitive therapy (MBCT) and mindfulness-based stress reduction (MBSR) in people with physical and/or psychological conditions: A systematic review. *Clinical Psychology Review, 55*, 74–91. doi:10.1016/j.cpr.2017.04.008

American Association of Colleges of Nursing. (2016). ELNEC fact sheet. Retrieved from http://www.aacn.nche .edu/elnec/about/fact-sheet

American Geriatrics Society. (2009). AGS clinical practice guideline: Pharmacological management of persistent pain in older persons. *Journal of the American Geriatrics Society, 57*(8), 1331–1346. doi:10.1111/j.1532-5415.2009.02376.x

American Geriatrics Society. (2013). American Geriatrics Society 2013 annual scientific meeting. *Journal of the American Geriatrics Society, 61*(S1), ii–vi. doi:10.1111/jgs.12262

American Nurses Association. (2016a). Nurses' roles and responsibilities in providing care and support at the end of life. Retrieved from https://www.nursingworld.org/~4af078/globalassets/docs/ana/ethics/endoflife -positionstatement.pdf

American Nurses Association. (2016b). Therapeutic use of marijuana and related cannabinoids. Retrieved from https://www.nursingworld.org/~4ad4a8/globalassets/docs/ana/therapeutic-use-of-marijuana-and-related -cannabinoids.pdf

American Pain Society. (2008). *Principles of analgesic use in the treatment of acute pain and cancer pain* (5th ed.). Glenview, IL: Author.

American Physical Therapy Association. (2014). *Guide to physical therapist practice* (3rd ed.). Alexandria, VA: Author.

American Society for Pain Management Nursing. (2015). Statement on the use of medical marijuana. Retrieved from http://www.aspmn.org/Documents/Advocacy%20Positions%20Statements/Statement%20on%20the% 20use%20of%20Medical%20Marijuana%206-17-2015%20final.pdf

American Society of Clinical Oncology. (2016). ASCO issues new guideline on chronic pain management in adult cancer survivors. Retrieved from https://www.asco.org/about-asco/press-center/news-releases/ asco-issues-new-guideline-chronic-pain-management-adult-cancer

Amr, M. A., Shams, T., & Al-Wadani, H. (2013). Does haloperidol prophylaxis reduce ketamine-induced emergence delirium in children? *Sultan Qaboos University Medical Journal, 13*(2), 256–262.

Baker, D. W. (2017). History of The Joint Commission's pain standards lessons for today's prescription opioid epidemic. *Journal of the American Medical Association, 317*(11), 1117–1118. doi:10.1001/jama.2017.0935

Ballantyne, J. C., & LaForge, K. S. (2007). Opioid dependence and addiction during opioid treatment of chronic pain. *Pain, 129*(3), 235–255. doi:10.1016/j.pain.2007.03.028

Barathi, B., & Chandra, P. S. (2013). Palliative sedation in advanced cancer patients: Does it shorten survival time? A systematic review. *Indian Journal of Palliative Care, 19*(1), 40–47. doi:10.4103/0973-1075.110236

Barawid, E., Covarrubias, N., Tribuzio, B., & Liao, S. (2015). The benefits of rehabilitation for palliative care patients. *American Journal of Hospice and Palliative Care, 32*, 34–43. doi:10.1177/1049909113514474

Becker, D. E. (2010). Pain management: Part 1: Managing acute and postoperative dental pain. *Anesthesia Progress, 57*(2), 67–79. doi:10.2344/0003-3006-57.2.67

Ben-Arye, E., Shulman, B., Eilon, Y., Woitiz, R., Cherniak, V., Shalom Sharabi, I., ... Admi, H. (2017). Attitudes among nurses toward the integration of complementary medicine into supportive cancer care. *Oncology Nursing Forum, 44*(4), 428–434. doi:10.1188/17.ONF.428-434

Benítez-Rosaria, M. A., Salinas-Martín, A., Aguirre-Jaime, A., Pérez-Méndez, L., & Feria, M. (2009). Morphine-methadone opioid rotation in cancer patients: Analysis of dose ratio predicting factors. *Journal of Symptom Management, 37*(6), 1061–1068. doi:10.1016/j.jpainsymman.2008.05.016

Bennett, M. I., Rayment, C., Hjermstad, M., Aass, N., Caraceni, A., & Kaasa, S. (2012). Prevalence and aetiology of neuropathic pain in cancer patients: A systematic review. *Pain, 153*(2), 359–365. doi:10.1016/j.pain.2011.10.028

Bickel, K., & Arnold, R. (2009). #109 Death rattle and oral secretions. Retrieved from https://www.mypcnow.org/blank-wz9l3

Birthi, P., & Sloan, P. (2013). Interventional treatment of refractory cancer pain. *The Cancer Journal, 19*(5), 390–396. doi:10.1097/PPO.0b013e3182a631a2

Blackhall, L. J., Alfson, E. D., & Barclay, J. S. (2013). Screening for substance use and diversion in Virginia hospices. *Journal of Palliative Medicine, 16*(3), 237–342. doi:10.1089/jpm.2012.0263

Bobb, B. (2016). A review of palliative sedation. *Nursing Clinics of North America, 51*, 449–457. doi:10.1016/j.cnur.2016.05.008

Bockbrader, H. N., Wesche, D., Miller, R., Chapel, S., Janiczek, N., & Burger, P. (2010). A comparison of the pharmacokinetics and pharmacodynamics of pregabalin and gabapentin. *Clinical Pharmacology, 49*(10), 661–669. doi:10.2165/11536200-000000000-00000

Bradt, J., Dileo, C., Magill, L., & Teague, A. (2016). Music interventions for improving psychological and physical outcomes in cancer patients. *Cochrane Database of Systematic Reviews, 15*(8), CD006911. doi:10.1002/14651858.CD006911.pub3

Brant, J. M., Keller, L., McLeod, K., Yeh, C., & Eaton, L. H. (2017). Chronic and refractory pain: A systematic review of pharmacologic management in oncology. *Clinical Journal of Oncology Nursing, 21*(3), 31–53. doi:10.1188/17.CJON.S3.31-53

Bredlau, A. L., Thakur, R., Korones, D. N., & Dworkin, R. H. (2013). Ketamine for pain in adults and children with cancer: A systematic review and synthesis of the literature. *Pain Medicine, 14*, 1505–1517. doi:10.1111/pme.12182

Broglio, K., & Portenoy, R. K. (2016). Pain assessment and management in the last weeks of life. In D. M. F. Savarese (Ed.), *UpToDate.* Retrieved from http://www.uptodate.com/contents/pain-assessment-and-management-in-the-last-weeks-of-life

Brown, S. T., Kirkpatrick, M. K., Swanson, M. S., & McKenzie, I. L. (2011). Pain experience in the elderly. *Pain Management Nursing, 12*(4), 190–196. doi:10.1016/j.pmn.2010.05.004

Brull, R., McCartney, C. J., Chan, V. W., & El-Beheiry, H. (2007). Neurological complications after regional anesthesia: Contemporary estimates of risk. *Anesthesia and Analgesia, 104*(4), 965–974. doi:10.1213/01.ane.0000258740.17193.ec

Buchanan, D. D., & MacIvor, F. J. (2010). A role for intravenous lidocaine in severe cancer-related neuropathic pain at the end-of-life. *Support Care Cancer, 18*(7), 899–901. doi:10.1007/s00520-010-0864-3

Burton, J. H., Harrah, J. D., Germann, C. A., Dillon, D. C. (2008). Does end-tidal carbon dioxide monitoring detect respiratory events prior to current sedation monitoring practices? *Academic Emergency Medicine, 13*(5), 500–504.

Bush, S. H. (2016). Delirium. In S. Yennurajalingam & E. Bruera (Eds.), *Oxford American handbook of hospice and palliative medicine and supportive care* (2nd ed., pp. 153–166). New York, NY: Oxford University Press.

Campbell, C. M., Kipnes, M. S., Stouch, B. C., Brady, K. L., Kelly, M. S., Schmidt, W. K., … Campbell, J. N. (2012). Randomized control trial of topical clonidine for treatment of painful diabetic neuropathy. *Pain, 153*(9), 1815–1823. doi:10.1016/j.pain.2012.04.014

Candy, B., Jones, L., Goodman, M. L., Drake, R., & Tookman, A. (2011). Laxatives or methylnaltrexone for the management of constipation in palliative care patients. *Cochrane Database of Systematic Reviews, 19*(1), CD003448. doi:10.1002/14651858.CD003448.pub3

Carter, B. S., & Brunkhorst, J. (2017). Neonatal pain management. *Seminars in Perinatology, 41*(2), 111–116. doi:10.1053/j.semperi.2016.11.001

Center for Behavioral Health Statistics and Quality. (2015). *Behavioral health trends in the United States: Results from the 2014 National Survey on Drug Use and Health* (HHS Publication No. SMA 15-4927, NSDUH Series H-50). Retrieved from https://www.samhsa.gov/data/sites/default/files/NSDUH-FRR1-2014/NSDUH-FRR1-2014.htm

Centers for Disease Control and Prevention. (2016). CDC guideline for prescribing opioids for chronic pain—United States, 2016. Retrieved from https://www.cdc.gov/mmwr/volumes/65/rr/rr6501e1.htm

Centers for Medicare and Medicaid Services. (2015). Hospital CAHPS (HCAHPS). Retrieved from https://www.cms.gov/Research-Statistics-Data-and-Systems/Research/CAHPS/hcahps1.html

Centers for Medicare and Medicaid Services. (2016). What is a prescriber's role in preventing the diversion of prescription drugs? Retrieved from https://www.cms.gov/Medicare-Medicaid-Coordination/Fraud-Prevention/Medicaid-Integrity-Education/Provider-Education-Toolkits/Downloads/prescriberrole-drugdiversion-factsheet-082914.pdf

Chandok, N., & Watt, K. (2010). Pain management in the cirrhotic patient: The clinical challenge. *Mayo Clinic Proceedings, 85*(5), 451–458. doi:10.4065/mcp.2009.0534

Chau, D. L., Walker, V., Pai, L., & Cho, L. M. (2008). Opiates and elderly: Use and side effects. *Clinical Interventions in Aging, 3*(2), 273–278.

Cherney, N. (2010). Taxonomy of distress: Including spiritual suffering and demoralization. *Supportive Oncology, 8*(1), 13–14.

Cherney, N. (2017). Palliative sedation. In D. M. F. Savarese (Ed.), *UpToDate.* Retrieved from https://www.uptodate.com/contents/palliative-sedation

Cherney, N., & Coyle, N. (1994). Suffering in the advanced cancer patient: A definition and taxonomy. *Journal of Palliative Care, 10*(2), 57–70.

Childers, J. W., & Arnold, R. M. (2012). "I feel uncomfortable 'calling a patient out'": Educational needs of palliative medicine fellows managing opioid misuse. *Journal of Pain and Symptom Management, 43*(2), 253–260. doi:10.1016/j.jpainsymman.2011.03.009

Chou, R., Cruciani, R. A., Fiellin, D. A., Compton, P., Farrar, J. T., Haigney, M. C., … Zeltzer, L. (2014). Methadone safety: A clinical practice guideline from the American Pain Society and College on Problems of Drug

Dependence, in collaboration with the Heart Rhythm Society. *Journal of Pain, 15*(4), 321–337. doi:10.1016/j.jpain.2014.01.494

Chou, R., Peterson, K., & Helfand, M. (2004). Comparative efficacy and safety of skeletal muscle relaxants for spasticity and musculoskeletal conditions: A systematic review. *Journal of Pain and Symptom Management, 28*(2), 140–175. doi:10.1016/j.jpainsymman.2004.05.002.

Cincinnati Children's Hospital Medical Center. (2012). Best evidence statement (BESt). The effects of music therapy on well-being in pediatric patients. Retrieved from https://www.guidelinecentral.com/summaries/best-evidence-statement-best-the-effects-of-music-therapy-on-well-being-in-pediatric-inpatients/

Claxton, R., & Arnold, R. (2011). Screening for opioid misuse and abuse #244. *Journal of Palliative Medicine, 14*(11), 1260–1. doi:10.1089/jpm.2011.9637

Collins, J. C., Berde, C. B., & Frost, J. A. (2011). Pain assessment and management. In J. Wolfe, P. S. Hinds, & B. M. Sourkes (Eds.), *Textbook of interdisciplinary pediatric palliative care* (pp. 284–299). Philadelphia, PA: Elsevier/Sanders.

Coluzzi, P. H., Schwartzberg, L., Conroy, J. D., Charapata, S., Gay, M., Busch, M. A., ... Portenoy, R. K. (2001). Breakthrough cancer pain: a randomized trial comparing oral transmucosal fentanyl citrate (OTFC) and morphine sulfate immediate release (MSIR). *Pain, 91*(1–2):123–30.

Compton, P., & Chang, Y. (2017). Substance abuse and addiction: Implications for pain management in patients with cancer. *Clinical Journal of Oncology Nursing, 21*(2), 203–209. doi:10.1188/17.CJON.203-209

Connors, A. F., Jr., Dawson, N. V., Desbiens, N. A., Fulkerson, W. J., Jr., Goldman, L., Knaus, W. A., ... Ransohoff, D. (1995). A controlled trial to improve care for seriously ill hospitalized patients. *Journal of the American Medical Association, 274*, 1591–1598. doi:10.1001/jama.1995.03530200027032

Cooney, M. F., & Broglio, K. (2017). Acute pain management in opioid-tolerant individuals. *Journal for Nurse Practitioners, 13*(6), 394–399. doi:10.1016/j.nurpra.2017.04.016

Cooney, M. F., Czarnecki, M., Dunwoody, C., Eksterowicz, N., Merkel, S., Oakes, L., & Wuhrman, E. (2013). American Society for Pain Management nursing position statement with clinical practice guidelines: Authorized Agent Controlled Analgesia. *Pain Management Nursing, 14*(3), 176–181. doi:10.1016/j.pmn.2013.07.003

Covington-East, C. (2017). Hospice-appropriate universal precautions for opioid safety. *Journal of Hospice and Palliative Nursing, 19*(3), 256–260. doi:10.1097/NJH.0000000000000339

Coyle, N., & Layman-Goldstein, M. (2007). Pharmacologic management of adult cancer pain. *Oncology, 21*(2), 1–17.

Cramer, H., Lauche, R., Paul, A., Langhorst, J., Kummel, S., & Dobos, G. J. (2015). Hypnosis in breast cancer care: A systematic review of randomized controlled trials. *Integrative Cancer Therapies, 14*(1), 5–15. doi:10.1177/1534735414550035

Crellin, D., Sullivan, T. P., Babl, F. E., O'Sullivan, R., & Hutchinson, A. (2007). Analysis of the validation of existing behavioral pain and distress scales for use in the procedural setting. *Paediatric Anaesthesia, 17*(8), 720–733. doi:10.1111/j.1460-9592.2007.02218.x

Creswell, J. D. (2017). Mindfulness interventions. *Annual Review of Psychology, 68*, 491–516. doi:10.1146/annurev-psych-042716-051139

Cruccu, G., Aziz, T. Z., Garcia-Larrea, L., Hansson, P., Jensen, T. S., Lefaucheur, J. P., ... Taylor, R. S. (2007). EFNS guidelines on neurostimulatory therapy for neuropathic pain. *European Journal of Neurology, 14*, 952–970.

Cruciani, R. A. (2008). Methadone: To EKG or not to EKG—That is still the question. *Journal Pain and Symptom Management, 36*(5), 545–552. doi:10.1016/j.jpainsymman.2007.11.003

Czarnecki, M. L., Turner, H. N., Collins, P. M., Doelkman, D., Wrona, S., & Reynolds, J. (2011). Procedural pain management: A position statement with clinical practice recommendations. *Pain Management Nursing, 2*(2), 95–111. doi:10.1016/j.pmn.2011.02.003

D'Arcy, Y. (2012). Managing end-of-life symptoms. *American Nurse Today, 7*(7), 15–18.

Darwish, M., Kirby, M., Jiang, J. G., Tracewell, W., & Robertson, P., Jr. (2008). Bioequivalence following buccal and sublingual placement of fentanyl buccal tablet 400 mcg in healthy subjects. *Clinical Drug Investigation, 28*(1), 1–7.

Darwish, M., Kirby, M., Robertson, P., Jr., Tracewell, W., & Jiang, J. G. (2007). Absolute and relative bioavailability of fentanyl buccal tablet and oral transmucosal fentanyl citrate. *Journal of Clinical Pharmacology, 47*(3), 343–350. doi:10.1177/0091270006297749

Davison, S., & Hui, D. (2016). Kidney palliative care. In S. Yennurajalingam & E. Bruera (Eds.), *Oxford American handbook of hospice and palliative medicine and supportive care* (2nd ed., pp. 397–406). New York, NY: Oxford University Press.

De Groef, A., Van Kampen, M., Dieltjens, E., Christiaens, M. R., Neven, P., Geraerts, I., & Devoogdt, N. (2015). Effectiveness of postoperative physical therapy for upper-limb impairments after breast cancer treatment: A systematic review. *Archives of Physical Medicine and Rehabilitation, 96*, 1140–1153. doi:10.1016/j.apmr.2015.01.006

Demir, Y. (2012). Non-pharmacological therapies in pain management. In G. B. Racz & C. E. Noe (Eds.), *Pain management—Current issues and opinions*. InTech Open Access Book. Retrieved from http://www.intechopen.com/books/pain-management-current-issues-and-opinions

Deng, G. E., Cassileth, B. R., Cohen, L., Gubili, J., Johnstone, P. A., Kumar, N., ... Tripathy, D. (2007). Integrative Oncology Practice Guidelines. *Society for Integrative Oncology 5*(2):65–84. doi:10.2310/7200.2007.002

Deng, G., Cassileth, B. R., & Simon, Y. K. (2004). Complementary therapies for cancer-related symptoms. *Supportive Oncology, 2*, 419–429.

Deng, G. E., Rausch, S. M., Jones, L. W., Gulati, A., Kumar, N. B., Greenlee, H., ... Cassileth, B. R. (2013). Complementary therapies and integrative medicine in lung cancer. Complementary therapies and integrative medicine. *Chest, 143*(5 Suppl.), e420S–e436S. doi:10.1378/chest.12-2364

Derry, S., Sven-Rice, A., Cole, P., Tan, T., & Moore, R. A. (2013). Topical capsaicin (high concentration) for chronic neuropathic pain in adults. *Cochrane Database of Systematic Reviews, 28*(2), CD007393. doi:10.1002/14651858 .CD007393.pub3

Doran, N. J. (2014). Experiencing wellness within illness: Exploring a mindfulness-based approach to chronic back pain. *Qualitative Health Research, 24*(6), 749–760. doi:10.1177/1049732314529662

Eaton, L. H., Brant, J. M., McLeod, K., & Yeh, C. (2017). Nonpharmacologic pain interventions. *Clinical Journal of Oncology Nursing, 21*(3), 54–70. doi:10.1188/17.CJON.S3.54-70

Education for Physicians on End-of-Life Care. (2017). About us. The EPEC project. Retrieved from http://bioethics. northwestern.edu/programs/epec/about/index.html

Eisenberg, E., Suzan, E., & Pud, D. (2015). Opioid-induced hyperalgesia (OIH): A real clinical problem or just an experimental phenomenon? *Journal of Pain and Symptom Management, 49*(3), 632–636. doi:10.1016/ j.jpainsymman.2014.07.005

Engelman, E., & Marsala, C. (2013). Efficacy of adding clonidine to intrathecal morphine in acute postoperative pain: Meta-analysis. *British Journal of Anaesthesia, 110*(1), 21–27. doi:10.1093/bja/aes344

Ferrell, B. R., & Coyle, N. (2010). *Oxford textbook of palliative care nursing* (3rd ed.). Oxford, NY: Oxford University Press.

Ferrell, B. R., Hanson, J., & Grant, M. (2013). An overview and evaluation of the oncology family caregiver project: Improving quality of life and quality of care for oncology family caregivers. *Psycho-Oncology, 22*(7), 1645–1652. doi:10.1002/pon.3198

Fidman, B., & Nogid, A. (2010). Role of Tapentadol immediate release (Nucynta) in the management of moderate-to-severe pain. *Pharmacy and Therapeutics, 35*(6), 330–333.

Fine, P. G. (2012). Treatment guidelines for the pharmacological management of pain in older persons. *Pain Medicine, 13*(Suppl. 2), S57–S66. doi:10.1111/j.1526-4637.2011.01307.x

Fine, P. G., & Portenoy, R. K. (2011). Strategies for opioid rotation: Decision support in chronic pain management. Retrieved from http://www.medscape.org/viewarticle/717832

Fink, R. M., Gates, R. A., & Montgomery, R. K. (2015). Pain assessment. In B. R. Ferrell, N. Coyle, & J. A. Paice (Eds.), *Oxford textbook of palliative care nursing* (4th ed., pp. 113–134). New York, NY: Oxford University Press.

Fisch, M. J., & Chang, V. T. (2016). Striving for safe, effective affordable care for cancer survivors with chronic pain. Another kind of moonshot. *JAMA Oncology, 2*(7), 862–964. doi:10.1001/jamaoncol.2016.0854

Flory, J. H., Wiesenthal, A. C., Thaler, H. T., Koranteng, L., & Moryl, N. (2016). Methadone use and the risk of hypoglycemia for inpatients with cancer pain. *Journal of Pain and Symptom Management, 51*, 79–87. doi:10.1016/j.jpainsymman.2015.08.003

Ford, A. C., Brenner, D. M., & Schoenfeld, P. S. (2013). Efficacy of pharmacological therapies for the treatment of opioid-induced constipation: Systematic review and meta-analysis. *The American Journal of Gastroenterology, 108*, 1566–1574. doi:10.1038/ajg.2013.169.

Gao, X., Prigerson, H. G., Diamond, E. L., Zhang, B., Wright, A. A., Meyer, F., & Maciejewski, P. K. (2013). Minor cognitive impairments in cancer patients magnify the effect of caregiver preferences on end-of-life care. *Journal of Pain and Symptom Management, 45*(4), 650–659. doi:10.1016/j.jpainsymman.2012.03.003

Gélinas, C., Puntillo, K. A., Levin, P., & Azoulay, E. (2017). The behavior pain assessment tool for critically ill adults: A validation study in 28 countries. *Pain, 158*(5), 811–821. doi:10.1097/j.pain.0000000000000834

Ghai, B., Kaur-Makkar, J., & Wig, J. (2008). Postoperative pain assessment in preverbal children and children with cognitive impairment. *Pediatric Anesthesia, 18*(6), 462–477. doi:10.1111/j.1460-9592.2008.02433.x

Glare, P. A., Davies, P. S., Finlay, E., Gulati, G., Lemanne, D., Moryl, N., & Syrjala, K. L. (2014). Pain in cancer survivors. *Journal of Clinical Oncology, 32*(16), 1739–1747. doi:10.1200/JCO.2013.52.4629

Glod, S. A. (2017). The other victims of the opioid epidemic. *New England Journal of Medicine, 376*, 2101–2102. doi:10.1056/NEJMp1702188

Gordon, D., & Dahl, J. (2011). Fast facts and concepts #95: *Opioid withdrawal*. Retrieved from https://www .mypcnow.org/blank-nonh6

Gordon, D., & Schroeder, M. (2008). Oral transmucosal fentanyl citrate—OTFC (ACTIQ™) #103. *Journal of Palliative Medicine, 11*(4), 633–634. doi:10.1089/jpm.2008.9922

Gowing, L., Farrel, M., Ali, R., & White, J. M. (2009). Alpha (2) adrenergic agonists for the management of opioid withdrawal. *Cochrane Database of Systematic Reviews, 15*(2), CD002024. doi:10.1002/14651858. CD002024.pub3

Greenlee, H., DuPont-Reyes, M. J., Baineaves, L. G., Carlson, L. E., Cohen, M. R., Deng, G., … Tripathy, D. (2017). Clinical practice guidelines on the evidence-based use of integrative therapies during and after breast cancer treatment. *CA: A Cancer Journal for Clinicians, 67*(3), 194–232. doi:10.3322/caac.21397

Greer, J. A., Park, E. R., & Safren, S. A. (2010). Tailoring cognitive-behavioral therapy to treat anxiety comorbid with advanced cancer. *Journal of Cognitive Psychotherapy, 24*(4), 283–313. doi:10.1891/0889-8391.24.4.294

Gutgsell, K. J., Schluchter, M., Margevicius, S., DeGolia, P. A., McLaughlin, B., Harris, M., … Weincek, C. (2013). Music therapy reduces pain in palliative care patient: A randomized controlled trial. *Journal of Pain and Symptom Management, 45*(5), 822–831. doi:10.1016/j.jpainsymman.2012.05.008

Hall, L. M., & O'Lenic, K. (2012). Treatment strategies to overcome end-of-dose failure with oral and transdermal opioids. *Journal of Pharmacy Practice, 25*(5), 503–509. doi:10.1177/0897190010379719

Hansen, A. P., Marcussen, N. S., Klit, H., Andersen, G., Finnerup, N. B., & Jensen, T. S. (2012). Pain following stroke: A prospective study. *European Journal of Pain, 16*(8), 1128–1136. doi:10.1002/j.1532-2149.2012.00123.x

Hara, K., & Sata, T. (2007). The effects of the local anesthetics lidocaine and procaine on glycine and gamma-aminobutyric acid receptors expressed in xenopus oocytes. *Anesthesia and Analgesia, 104*(6), 1434–1439. doi:10.1213/01.ane.0000261509.72234.a6

Hazin, R., & Giles, C. A. (2011). Is there a color line in death? An examination of end-of-life care in the African American community. *Journal of the National Medical Association, 103*(7), 609–613. doi:10.1016/S0027-9684(15)30387-4

Herr, K., Coyne, P. J., McCaffery, M., Manwarren, R., & Merkel, S. (2011). Pain assessment in the patient unable to self-report: Position statement with clinical practice recommendation: American Society of Pain Management Nursing. *Pain Management Nursing, 12*(4), 230–250. doi:10.1016/j.pmn.2011.10.002

Hesselgard, R., Reinstrup, P., Stromblad, L. G., Undén, J., & Romner, B. (2007). Selective dorsal rhizotomy and postoperative pain management. A worldwide survey. *Pediatric Neurosurgery, 43*(2), 107–112. doi:10.1159/000098382

Hospice and Palliative Nurses Association. (2014). Position statement: The use of medical marijuana. Retrieved from http://hpna.advancingexpertcare.org/wp-content/uploads/2015/08/The-Use-of-Medical-Marijuana.pdf

Hospice and Palliative Nurses Association. (2016). Position statement: Palliative sedation. Retrieved from http://advancingexpertcare.org/wp-content/uploads/2016/01/Palliative-Sedation.pdf

Huff, J. S., & Brenner, B. E. (2012). Spinal cord neoplasm. In B. E. Brenner (Ed.), *Medscape*. Retrieved from http://emedicine.medscape.com/article/779872-overview

Huijer, H., Miaskowski, C., Quinn, R., & Twycross, A. (2013). IASP curriculum outline on pain for nursing. Retrieved from http://www.iasppain.org/AM/Template.cfm?Section=Nursing

Hurley, R. W., & Adams, M. C. B. (2009). Sex, gender and pain: An overview of a complex field. *Anesthesia and Analgesia, 107*(1), 309–317. doi:10.1213/01.ane.0b013e31816ba437

Indelicato, R. A. (2006). The advanced practice nurse's role in palliative care and the management of dyspnea. *Medscape*. Retrieved from https://www.medscape.com/viewarticle/551364

Initiative for Pediatric Palliative Care. (2014). Initiative for pediatric palliative care. Retrieved from http://ippcweb.org/about.htm

Institute of Medicine. (2011). *Relieving pain in America: A blueprint for transforming prevention, care, education and research*. Washington, DC: National Academies Press. Retrieved from http://www.nationalacademies.org/hmd/Reports/2011/Relieving-Pain-in-America-A-Blueprint-for-Transforming-Prevention-Care-Education-Research.aspx

Institute of Medicine. (2014). Dying in America: Improving quality and honoring individual preferences near the end of life. Retrieved from http://www.nationalacademies.org/hmd/Reports/2014/Dying-In-America-Improving-Quality-and-Honoring-Individual-Preferences-Near-the-End-of-Life.aspx

International Association for the Study of Pain. (2009). Barriers to cancer pain treatment. Retrieved from https://s3.amazonaws.com/rdcms-iasp/files/production/public/Content/ContentFolders/GlobalYearAgainstPain2/CancerPainFactSheets/Barriers_Final.pdf

International Association for the Study of Pain. (2012). IASP taxonomy. Retrieved from http://www.iasp-pain.org/AM/Template.cfm?Section=Pain_Definitions

Jacox, A., Carr, D. B., Payne, R., Berde, C. B., Breithart, W., Cain, I. M., ... Weissman, D. E. (1994). *Management of cancer pain: AHCPR Publication No. 94–0592*. Rockville, MD: Agency for Healthcare Policy and Research, U.S. Department of Health and Human Services, Public Health Services.

Jefferies, K. (2010). Treatment of neuropathic pain. *Seminars in Neurology, 30*(4), 425–432. doi:10.1055/s-0030-1267286

Jelinek, H. F., & Barnden, R. (2012). Superficial cold and heat application during transcutaneous electrical stimulation may not change perceived sensation of pain. *The Internet Journal of Pain, Symptom Control and Palliative Care, 9*(1), 1–6.

Johannsen, M., Farver, I., Beck, N., & Zachariae, R. (2013). The efficacy of psychosocial interventions for pain in breast cancer patients and survivors: A systematic review and meta-analysis. *Breast Cancer Research and Treatment, 138*, 675–690. doi:10.1007/s10549-013-2503-4

The Joint Commission. (2012). Facts about pain management. Retrieved from https://www.jointcommission.org/topics/pain_management.aspx

The Joint Commission. (2015). Speak up: About your pain. Retrieved from https://www.jointcommission.org/topics/speak_up_pain.aspx

Jonsson, A. C., Lindgren, I., Hallstrom, B., Norrving, B., & Lindgren, A. (2006). Prevalence and intensity of pain after stroke: A population based study focusing on patients' perspectives. *Journal of Neurology, Neurosurgery, and Psychiatry, 77*(5), 590–595. doi:10.1136/jnnp.2005.079145

Kabat-Zinn, J. (2013). *Full catastrophe living: Using the wisdom of your body and mind to face stress, pain, and illness* (2nd ed.). New York, NY: Bantam Books.

Kachnic, L., & Di Biase, S. J. (2013). Radiation therapy for the management of painful bone metastases. In D. M. F. Savarese (Ed.), *UpToDate*. Retrieved from http://www.uptodate.com/contents/radiation-therapy-for-the-management-of-painful-bone-metastases#

Kars, M. C., Grypdonck, M. H., van Delden, J. J. (2011). Being a parent of a child with cancer throughout the end-of-life course. *Oncology Nursing Forum, 38*(4), E260–71. doi:10.1188/11.ONF.E260-E271

Khawam, E. A., Laurencic, G., & Malone, D. A. (2006). Side effects of antidepressants: An overview. *Cleveland Clinic Journal of Medicine, 73*(4), 351–361. doi:10.3949/ccjm.73.4.351

Kemp, D. E., Malhotra, S., Franco, K. N., Tesar, G., & Bronson, D. L. (2013). Heart disease and depression: Don't ignore the relationship. *Cleveland Clinic Journal of Medicine, 70*(9), 745–761. doi:10.3949/ccjm.70.9.745

Kirsh, K. L., Compton, P., Egan-City, K., & Passik, S. D. (2015). Caring for the patient with substance use disorder at the end of life. In B. R. Ferrell, N. Coyle, & J. Paice (Eds.), *Oxford textbook of palliative nursing* (4th ed., pp. 650–660). New York, NY: Oxford University Press.

Knotkova, H., Fine, P. G., & Portney, R. K. (2009). Opioid rotation: The science and limitations of equianalgesic dose table. *Journal of Pain and Symptom Management, 38*(3), 426–439. doi:10.1016/j.jpainsymman.2009.06.001

Koncicki, H. M., Unruh, M., & Schell, J. O. (2017). Pain management in CKD: A guide for nephrology providers. *American Journal of Kidney Diseases, 69*(3), 451–460. doi:10.1053/j.ajkd.2016.08.039

Koronkowski, M., Eisenhower, C., & Marcum, Z. (2016). An update on geriatric medication safety and challenges specific to the care of the older adults. *Annals of Long-Term Care, 24*(3), 37–40.

Koyyalagunta, D., Bruera, E., Aigner, C., Nusrat, H., Driver, L., & Novy, D. (2013). Risk stratification of opioid misuse among patients with cancer pain using the SOAPP-SF. *Pain Medicine, 14,* 667–675. doi:10.1111/pme.12100

Kravitz, K. (2015). Complementary and alternative therapies in palliative care. In B. R. Ferrell, N. Coyle, & J. A. Paice (Ed.), *Oxford textbook of palliative care nursing* (4th ed., pp. 449–462). Oxford, NY: Oxford University Press.

Kullgren, J., Le, V., & Wheeler, W. L. (2013). Incidence of hydromorphone-induced neuroexcitation in hospice patients. *Journal of Palliative Medicine, 16*(10), 1205–1209. doi:10.1089/jpm.2012.0467

Laderman, M., & Martin, L. (2017). Health care providers must act now to address the prescription opioid crisis. *NEJM Catalyst.* Retrieved from http://catalyst.nejm.org/act-now-prescription-opioid-crisis

Latifzai, K., Sites, B. D., & Koval, K. J. (2008). Orthopaedic anesthesia—Part 2. Common techniques of regional anesthesia in orthopaedics. *Bulletin of the NYU Hospital for Joint Diseases, 66*(4), 306–316.

Layman-Goldstein, M., & Coyle, N. (2013). Pain. In C. M. Dahlin & M. T. Lynch (Eds.), *Core curriculum for the advanced practice hospice and palliative registered nurse* (2nd ed.; 77–94). Pittsburgh, PA: Hospice and Palliative Nurses Association.

Layman-Goldstein, M., & Kramer, D. (2015). Pediatric pain: Knowing the child before you. In B. R. Ferrell, N. Coyle, & J. A. Paice (Eds.), *Oxford textbook of palliative nursing* (4th ed., pp. 940–957). New York, NY: Oxford University Press.

Lee, C. A., Kim, H. S., Kim, H. Y., & Lee, G. G. (2016). The effect of intrathecal baclofen single injection on neuropathic pain. *Anesthesiology and Pain Medicine, 11*(4), 399–403. doi:10.17085/apm.2016.11.4.399

Lee, J. H., Kim, T. Y., Lee, H. W., Choi, Y. S., Moon, S. Y., & Cheong, Y. K. (2010). Treatment of intractable hiccups with an oral agent monotherapy of baclofen: A case report. *Korean Journal of Pain, 23*(1), 42–45. doi:10.3344/kjp.2010.23.1.42

Light-McGroary, K., & Goodlin, S. J. (2013). The challenges of understanding and managing pain in the heart failure patient. *Current Opinion in Supportive and Palliative Care, 7*(1), 14–20. doi:10.1097/SPC.0b013e32835c1f2f

Lilly, E. J., & Senderovich, H. (2016). Palliative care in chronic obstructive pulmonary disease. *Journal of Critical Care, 35,* 150–154. doi:10.1016/j.jcrc.2016.05.019

Magill, L. (2009). The meaning of the music in palliative care music therapy as perceived by bereaved caregivers of advanced cancer patients. *American Journal of Hospice and Palliative Care, 26*(1), 33–39. doi:10.1177/1049909108327024

Malec, M., & Shega, J. W. (2015). Pain management in the elderly. *Medical Clinics of North America, 99,* 337–350. doi:10.1016/j.mcna.2014.11.007

Mannino, R., Coyne, P., Swainey, C., Hansen, L. A., & Lyckholm, L. (2006). Methadone for cancer-related neuropathic pain: A review of the literature. *Journal of Opioid Management, 2*(5), 269–276. doi:10.5055/jom.2006.0040

Marhofer, P., & Chan, V. W. (2007). Ultrasound-guided regional anesthesia: Current concepts and future trends. *Anesthesia and Analgesia, 104,* 1265–1269. doi:10.1213/01.ane.0000260614.32794.7b

Marhofer, P., Greher, M., & Kapral, S. (2005). Ultrasound guidance in regional anesthesia. *British Journal of Anaesthesiology, 94*(1), 7–17. doi:10.1093/bja/aei002

McGuire, D. B., Kaiser, K. S., Haisfield-Wolfe, M. E., & Iyamu, F. (2016). Pain assessment in noncommunicative adult palliative care patients. *Nursing Clinics of North America, 51*(3), 397–431. doi:10.1016/j.cnur.2016.05.009

Medici, V., & Meyers, F. J. (2016). Palliative care in end-stage liver disease. In S. Yennurajalingam & E. Bruera (Eds.), *Oxford American handbook of hospice and palliative medicine and supportive care* (2nd ed., pp. 385–384). New York, NY: Oxford University Press.

Melton, L. (2017). Brief introduction to cognitive behavioral therapy for the advanced practitioner in oncology. *Journal of Advanced Practice Oncology, 8*(2), 188–193. doi:10.6004/jadpro.2017.8.2.6

Mercadante, S., Villari, P., Ferrera, P., Casuccio, A., & Gambaro, V. (2007). Opioid plasma concentrations during a switch from transdermal fentanyl to methadone. *Journal of Palliative Medicine, 10*(2), 338–344. doi:10.1089/jpm.2006.0140

Miguel, R. (2000). Interventional treatment of cancer pain: The fourth step in the World Health Organization analgesic ladder? *Cancer Control, 7*(2), 149–156. doi:10.1177/107327480000700205

Miller, K. D., Siegel, R. L., Lin, C. C., Mariotto, A. B., Kramer, J. L., Rowland, J. H., ... Jemel, A. (2016). Cancer treatment and survivorship statistics. *CA: A Cancer Journal for Clinicians, 66,* 271–289. doi:10.3322/caac.21349

Mishra, S., Bhatnagar, S., Goval, G. N., Rana, S. P., & Upadhya, S. P. (2012). A comparative efficacy of amitriptyline, gabapentin, and pregabalin in neuropathic cancer pain: A prospective randomized double-blind placebo-controlled study. *American Journal of Hospice and Palliative Care, 29*(3), 177–182. doi:10.1177/1049909111412539

Mitchell, S. A., & Friese, C. R. (n.d.). ONS PEP (Putting Evidence Into Practice) weight of evidence classification schema. Retrieved from https://www.ons.org/practice-resources/pep/evaluation-process

Moens, K., Higginson, I. J., & Harding, R. (2014). Are there differences in the prevalence of palliative care-related problems in people living with advanced cancer and eight non-cancer conditions? A systematic review. *Journal of Pain and Symptom Management, 48*(4), 660–677. doi:10.1016/j.jpainsymman.2013.11.009

Morisset, V., Davis, J. B., & Tate, S. N. (2013). Mechanism of action of anticonvulsants as analgesic drugs. In S. B. McMahon, M. Koltnenburg, I. Tracey, & D. C. Turk (Eds.), *Wall & Melzack's textbook of pain* (6th ed., pp. 491–499). Philadelphia, PA: Elsevier Saunders.

Moryl, N., Coyle, N., & Foley, K. M. (2008). Managing an acute pain crisis in a patient with advanced cancer: "This is as much of a crisis as a code." *Journal of the American Medical Association, 299*(12), 1457–1467. doi:10.1001/jama.299.12.1457

Motov, S. M. (2008). Is there a limit to the analgesic effect on pain medications? Retrieved from https://www.medscape.com/viewarticle/574279

Moulin, D. E., Clark, A. J., Gilron, I., Ware, M. A., Watson, C. P. N., ...Velly, A. (2007). Pharmacological management of chronic neuropathic pain Consensus statement and guidelines from the Canadian Pain Society. *Pain Research & Management, 12*(1), 13–21.

Music Therapy Association. (2013). What is music therapy? Retrieved from http://www.musictherapy.org

Nahin, R. L., Boineau, R., Khalsa, P. S., Stussman, B. J., & Weber, W. J. (2016). Evidence-based evaluation of complementary health approaches for pain management in the United States. *Mayo Clinic Proceedings, 91*(9), 1292–1306. doi:10.1016/j.mayocp.2016.06.007

National Cancer Institute at the National Institutes of Health. (2012). Pain (PDQ): Pharmacologic management. Retrieved from http://www.cancer.gov/cancertopics/pdq/supportivecare/pain/HealthProfessional/page3

National Cancer Institute at the National Institutes of Health. (2013a). Last days of life. Retrieved from https://www.cancer.gov/about-cancer/advanced-cancer/caregivers/planning/last-days-hp-pdq

National Cancer Institute at the National Institutes of Health. (2013b). Nausea, vomiting (emesis), constipation and bowel obstruction in advanced cancer. Retrieved from http://www.cancer.gov/cancertopics/pdq/supportivecare/nausea/HealthProfessional/page

National Cancer Institute at the National Institutes of Health. (2013c). Pharmacology management. Retrieved from http://www.cancer.gov/cancertopics/pdq/supportivecare/pain/HealthProfessional/page3

National Center for Complementary and Integrative Health. (2016). NCCIH 2016 strategic plan. Retrieved from https://nccih.nih.gov/about/strategic-plans/2016

National Comprehensive Cancer Network. (2017). Adult cancer pain guidelines. Retrieved from https://www.nccn.org/professionals/physician_gls/default.aspx

National Council on Aging. (2017). Facts about healthy aging. Retrieved from https://www.ncoa.org/news/resources-for-reporters/get-the-facts/healthy-aging-facts

National Council on Interpreting in Health Care. (2005). National standards of practice for interpreters in health care. Retrieved from http://www.ncihc.org/assets/documents/publications/NCIHC%20National%20Standards%20of%20Practice.pdf

NIH Consensus Conference Acupuncture. (1998). NIH consensus development panel on acupuncture. *Journal of the American Medical Association, 280*(17), 1518–1524. doi:10.1001/jama.280.17.1518

Nordqvist, C. (2011). Tylenol maximum daily dosage to drop to 3,000 mg per day from 4,000 mg. *Medical News Today*. Retrieved from http://www.medicalnewstoday.com/articles/231915.php

O'Connor, A., Schug, S. A., & Cardwell, S. (2000). A comparison of the efficacy and safety of morphine and pethidine as analgesia for suspected renal colic in the emergency setting. *Journal of Accidents and Emergency Medicine, 17*, 261–264. doi:10.1136/emj.17.4.261

O'Donnell, M. J., Diener, H. C., Sacco, R. L., Panju, A. A., Vinisko, R., & Yusuf, S. (2013). Chronic pain syndromes after ischemic stroke: PRoFESS trial. *Stroke, 44*(5), 1238–1243. doi:10.1161/STROKEAHA.111.671008

Ogawa, K., & Washiyama, K. (2012). Bone target radiotracers for palliative therapy of bone metastases. *Current Medicinal Chemistry, 19*(20), 3290–3300. doi:10.2174/092986712801215865

Ohtake, P. J. (2013). Physical therapy—Key component of the rehabilitation team. Retrieved from http://cirrie.buffalo.edu/encyclopedia/en/article/356

Okamoto, Y., Tsuneto, S., Tanimukai, H., Matsuda, Y., Ohno, Y., Tsugane, M., & Uejima, E. (2013). Can gradual dose titration of ketamine for management of neuropathic pain prevent psychotomimetic effects in patients with advanced cancer? *American Journal of Hospice and Palliative Care, 30*(5), 450–454. doi:10.1177/1049909112454325

Okon, T. R. (2016). Overview of comprehensive patient assessment in palliative care. In D. M. F. Savarese (Ed.), *UpToDate*. Retrieved from http://www.uptodate.com/contents/overview-of-comprehensive-patient-assessment-in-palliative-care

Oliver, J., Coggins, C., Compton, P., Hagan, S., Matteliano, D., Stanton, M., ... Turner, H. N. (2012). American Society for Pain Management Nursing Position Statement: Pain management in patients with substance use disorder. *Pain Management Nursing, 13*(3), 169–183. doi:10.1016/j.pmn.2012.07.001

Owen, G. T., Burton, A. W., Schade, C. M., & Passik, S. (2012). Urine drug testing: Current recommendations and best practices. *Pain Physician, 15*(3 Suppl), ES119–ES133.

Paice, J. A. (2015). Pain at the end of life. In B. R. Ferrell, N. Coyle, & J. A. Paice (Eds.), *Oxford textbook of palliative care nursing* (4th ed., pp. 135–153). New York, NY: Oxford University Press.

Paice, J. A. (2016). Pain. In C. Dahlin, P. J. Coyne, & B. R. Ferrell (Eds.), *Advanced practice palliative nursing* (p. 219–232). New York, NY: Oxford University Press.

Paice, J. A., & Ferrell, B. (2011). The management of cancer pain. *CA: A Cancer Journal for Clinicians, 61*(3), 157–182. doi:10.3322/caac.20112

Paice, J. A., Portenoy, R. K., Lacchetti, C., Campbell, T., Cheville, A., Citron, M., ... Bruera, E. (2016). Management of chronic pain in survivors of adult cancers: American Society of Clinical Oncology clinical practice guideline. *Journal of Clinical Oncology, 34*(27), 3325–3345. doi:10.1200/JCO.2016.68.5206

Palangio, M., Northfelt, D. W., Portenoy, R. K., Brookoff, D., Doyle, R. T., Dornseif, B. E., & Damask, M. C. (2002). Dose conversion and titration with a novel, once-daily, OROS osmotic technology, extended-release hydromorphone formulation in the treatment of chronic malignant or nonmalignant pain. *Journal of Pain Symptom Management, 23*(5), 355–368. doi:10.1016/S0885-3924(02)00390-1

Parker, R., Stein, D. J., & Jelsma, J. (2014). Pain in people living with HIV/AIDS: A systematic review. *Journal of the International AIDS Society, 17*, 18719. doi:10.7448/IAS.17.1.18719

Pasero, C., & McCaffery, M. (2011). *Pain assessment and pharmacologic management*. St. Louis, MO: Mosby Elsevier.

Peppin, J. F., Albrecht, P. J., Argoff, C., Gustorff, B., Pappagallo, M., Rice, F. L., & Wallace, M. S. (2015). Skin matters: A review of topical treatments for chronic pain. Part two: Treatments and applications. *Pain and Therapy, 4*(1), 33–50. doi:10.1007/s40122-015-0032-z

Pergolizzi, J. V., Mercadante, S., Echaburu, A. V., Van den Eynden, B., de Faría Fragoso, R. M., Mordarski, S., … Slama, O. (2009). The role of transdermal buprenorphine in the treatment of cancer pain: An expert panel consensus. *Current Medical Research and Opinion, 25*(6), 1517–1528. doi:10.1185/03007990902920731

Phongtankuel, V., Amorapanth, P. X., & Siegler, E. L. (2016). Pain in the geriatric patient with advanced chronic disease. *Clinics in Geriatric Medicine, 32*(4), 651–661. doi:10.1016/j.cger.2016.06.008

Plonk, W. (2005). Simplified methadone conversion. *Journal of Palliative Medicine, 8*(3), 478–479. doi:10.1177/1049909110373508

Portenoy, R. K., & Ahmed, E. (2014). Principles of opioid use in cancer pain. *Journal of Clinical Oncology, 32*(16), 1662–1670. doi:10.1200/JCO.2013.52.5188

Portenoy, R. K., Ahmed, E., & Keilson, Y. Y. (2015). Cancer pain management: Use of acetaminophen and nonsteroidal anti-inflammatory drugs. In D. M. F. Savarese (Ed.), *UpToDate*. Retrieved from https://www.uptodate.com/contents/cancer-pain-management-use-of-acetaminophen-and-nonsteroidal-antiinflammatory-drugs

Portenoy, R. K., Ahmed, E., & Keilson, Y. Y. (2017). Cancer pain management: Adjuvant analgesics (coanalgesics). In D. M. F. Savarese (Ed.), *UpToDate*. Retrieved from https://www.uptodate.com/contents/cancer-pain-management-adjuvant-analgesics-coanalgesics?source=related_link

Portenoy, R. K., & Copenhaver, D. J. (2017). Cancer pain management: Interventional therapies. In D. M. F. Savarese & M. Crowley (Eds.), *UpToDate*. Retrieved from http://www.uptodate.com/contents/cancer-pain-management-inteventional-therapies

Portenoy, R. K., & Dhingra, L. K. (2015). Assessment of cancer pain. In D. M. F. Savarese & M. Crowley (Eds.), *UpToDate*. Retrieved from http://www.uptodate.com/contents/assessment-of-cancer-pain

Portenoy, R. K., & Koh, M. (2009). Adjuvant analgesic drugs. In E. D. Bruera & R. K. Portenoy (Eds.), *Cancer pain: Assessment and management* (2nd ed., pp. 272–286). Cambridge, NY: Cambridge University Press.

Portenoy, R. K., Mehta, Z., & Ahmed, E. (2017a). Cancer pain management with opioids: Optimizing analgesia. In D. M. F. Savarese (Ed.), *UpToDate*. Retrieved from https://www.uptodate.com/contents/cancer-pain-management-with-opioids-optimizing-analgesia

Portenoy, R. K., Mehta, Z., & Ahmed, E. (2017b). Prevention and management of side effects in patients receiving opiods for chronic pain. In D. M. F. Savarese (Ed.), *UpToDate*. Retrieved from https://www.uptodate.com/contents/prevention-and-management-of-side-effects-in-patients-receiving-opioids-for-chronic-pain?search=Prevention%20and%20management%20of%20side%20effects&source=search_result&selectedTitle=1~150&usage_type=default&display_rank=1

Press, C. D. (2015). Topical anesthesia. Retrieved from http://reference.medscape.com/article/109673-overview

Price, J. R., Hawkins, A. D., & Passik, S. D. (2015). Opioid therapy: Managing risks of abuse, addiction and diversion. In N. Cherney, M. Fallon, S. Kaasa, R. K. Portenoy, & D. C. Currow (Eds.), *Oxford textbook of palliative medicine* (5th ed., pp. 560–566). New York, NY: Oxford University Press.

Reinhard, S. C., Given, B., Petlick, N. H., & Bernis, A. (2008). Supporting family caregivers in providing care. In R. G. Hughes (Ed.), *Patient safety and quality: An evidence-based handbook for nurses* (pp. 41–64). Rockville, MD: Agency for Healthcare Research and Quality.

Riccio, A. I., Wodajo, F. M., & Malawer, M. (2007). Metastatic carcinoma of the long bones. *American Family Physician, 76*(10), 1489–1494.

Rinaldi, R. C., Steindler, E. M., Wilford, B. B., & Goodwin, D. (1988). Clarification and standardization of substance abuse terminology. *Journal of the American Medical Association, 259,* 555–557. doi:10.1001/jama.1988.03720040047025

Rini, C., Vu, M. B., Lerner, H., Bloom, C., Carda-Auten, J., Wood, W. A., … Keefe, F. J. (2017). A qualitative study of patient and provider perspectives on using web-based pain coping skills training to treat persistent cancer pain. *Palliative and Supportive Care, 7,* 1–15. doi:10.1017/S1478951517000086

Risser, A., Donovan, D., Heintzman, J., & Page, T. (2009). NSAID prescribing precautions. *American Family Physician, 80*(15), 1371–1378.

Rosenblatt, L., & Meyer, F. L. (2017). Psychosocial issues in advanced illness. In D. M. F. Savarese (Ed.), *UpToDate*. Retrieved from https://www.uptodate.com/contents/psychosocial-issues-in-advanced-illness

Rosielle, D. A. (2015). Fast facts and concepts #148: The lidocaine patch. Retrieved from https://www.mypcnow.org/blank-nhf6r

Sagar, S. M., Dryden, T., & Wong, R. K. (2007). Massage therapy for cancer patients: A reciprocal relationship between body and mind. *Current Oncology, 14*(2), 45–56. doi:10.3747/co.2007.105

Sartor, O., Coleman, R., Nilsson, S., Heinrich, D., Helle, S. I., O'Sullivan, J. M., … Parker, C. (2014). Effect of radium-223 dichloride on symptomatic skeletal events in patients with castration-resistant prostate cancer and bone metastases: Results from a phase 3, double-blind, randomized trial. *The Lancet Oncology, 15,* 738–746. doi:10.1016/S1470-2045(14)70183-4

Saunders, C. M. (1967). *The management of terminal illness*. London, UK: Hospital Medicine.

Savvas, S. M., & Gibson, S. J. (2016). Overview of pain management in older adults. *Clinics in Geriatric Medicine, 32,* 635–650. doi:10.1016/j.cger.2016.06.005

Sehgal, N., Smith, H., & Manchikanti, L. (2011). Peripherally acting opioids and clinical implications for pain control. *Pain Physician, 5*(14), 249–258.

Sharma, S., Rajagopal, M. R., Palat, G., Singh, C., Haji, A. G., & Jain, D. (2009). A phase II pilot study to evaluate use of intravenous lidocaine for opioid-refractory pain in cancer patients. *Journal of Pain and Symptom Management, 37*(1), 85–93. doi:10.1016/j.jpainsymman.2007.12.023

Sheinfeld Gorin, S., Krebs, P., Badr, H., Janke, E. A., Jim, H. S., Spring, B., … Jacobsen, P. B. (2012). Meta-analysis of psychosocial interventions to reduce pain in patients with cancer. *Journal of Clinical Oncology, 30,* 539–547. doi:10.1200/JCO.2011.37.0437

Simopoulos, T. T., Smith, H. S., Peeters-Asdourian, C., & Stevens, D. S. (2002). Use of meperidine in patient-controlled analgesia and the development of a normeperidine toxic reaction. *Archives of Surgery, 137*(1), 84–88. doi:10.1001/archsurg.137.1.84

Smith, H. S. (2009). Opioid metabolism. *Mayo Clinic Proceedings, 84*(7), 613–624.

Smith, H. S., Kirsh, K. L., & Passik, S. D. (2009). Chronic opioid therapy issues associated with opioid abuse potential. *Journal of Opioid Management, 5*(5), 287–300. doi:10.5055/jom.2009.0029

Soloman, M., Mekhail, M. N., & Mekhail, N. (2010). Radiofrequency treatment in chronic pain. *Neurotherapeutics, 10*(3), 469–474. doi:10.1586/ern.09.153

Spathis, A., & Booth, S. (2008). End of life care in chronic obstructive pulmonary disease: In search of a good death. *International Journal of Chronic Obstructive Pulmonary Disease, 3*(1), 11–29. doi:10.2147/COPD.S698

Strax, T. E., Gonzales, P., & Cuccurullo, P. (2004). Physical modalities, therapeutic exercise, extended bedrest, and aging effects. In P. Cuccurullo (Ed.), *Physical medicine and rehabilitation board review* (pp. 553–584). New York, NY: Demos Medical.

Strouse, T. B., Flanagan, F., Kerrihand, T., Williams, C., & Wolcott, D. L. (2006). Managing cancer pain in a 24-hour outpatient cancer center. *Supportive Oncology, 4*(6), 351–354.

Swegle, J. M., & Logemann, C. (2006). Management of common opioid-induced adverse effects. *American Family Physician, 7*(8), 1347–1354.

Syrjala, K. L., Jensen, M. P., Mendoza, M. E., Yi, J. C., Fisher, H. M., & Keefe, F. J. (2014). Psychological and behavioral approaches to cancer pain management. *Journal of Clinical Oncology, 32*(16), 1703–1711. doi:10.1200/JCO.2013.54.4825

Tacani, P. M., Franceschini, J. P., Tacani, R. E., Machado, A. F., Montezello, D., Góes, J. C., & Marx, A. (2016). Retrospective study of physical therapy modalities applied in head and neck lymphedema treatment. *Head & Neck, 38*, 301–308. doi:10.1002/hed.23899

Tarumi, Y., Wilson, M. P., Szafran, O., & Spooner, G. R. (2013). Randomized, double-blind, placebo-controlled trial of oral docusate in the management of constipation in hospice patients. *Journal of Pain and Symptom Management, 45*(1), 2–13. doi:10.1016/j.jpainsymman.2012.02.008

Tateo, S. (2017). State of the evidence: Cannabinoids and cancer pain—A systematic review. *Journal of the American Association of Nurse Practitioners, 29*, 94–103. doi:10.1002/2327-6924.12422

Thomas Jefferson University. (2016). Thomas Jefferson University announces Center for Medical Cannabis Education and Research. Retrieved from http://www.jefferson.edu/university/news/2016/05/31/thomas-jefferson -university-announces-center-for-medical-cannabi.html

Tracy, B., & Morrison, S. (2013). Pain management in older adults. *Clinical Therapeutics, 35*(11), 1659–1668. doi:10.1016/j.clinthera.2013.09.026

Twycross, R., Prommer, E. E., Mihaly, M., & Wilcock, A. (2012). Fentanyl (transmucosal). *Journal of Pain and Symptom Management, 44*(1), 131–149. doi:10.1016/j.jpainsymman.2012.05.001

U.S. Department of Health and Human Services. (2016). Opioids: The prescription drug and heroin overdose epidemic. Retrieved from https://www.hhs.gov/opioids

U.S. Food and Drug Administration. (2007). Information for healthcare professionals: Fentanyl transdermal system (marketed as Duragesic and generics). Retrieved from https://www.fda.gov/Drugs/DrugSafety/ PostmarketDrugSafetyInformationforPatientsandProviders/ucm114961.htm

U.S. Food and Drug Administration. (2011). FDA limits acetaminophen in prescription combination products: Requires liver toxicity warnings. Retrieved from https://www.fda.gov/Drugs/DrugSafety/ucm239821.htm

Valeberg, B. T., Miaskowski, C., Paul, S. M., & Rustøen, T. (2016). Comparison of oncology patients' and their family caregivers' attitudes and concerns toward pain and pain management. *Cancer Nursing, 39*(4), 328–334. doi:10.1097/NCC.0000000000000319

Vallerand, A. H., Collins-Bohler, D., Templin, T., & Hasenau, S. M. (2007). Knowledge of and barriers to pain management in caregivers of cancer patients receiving homecare. *Cancer Nursing, 30*(1), 31–37. doi:10.1097/00002820-200701000-00006

van den Heuvel, S. A. S., van der Wal, S. E. I., Smedes, L. A., Radema, S. A., van Alfen, N., Vissers, K. C. P., & Steegers, M. A. H. (2017). Intravenous lidocaine: Old-school drug, new purpose—Reduction of intractable pain in patients with chemotherapy induced peripheral neuropathy. *Pain Research and Management, 2017*, 8053474. doi:10.1155/2017/8053474

van Middelkoop, M., Rubinstein, S., Kuijpers, T., Verhagen, A. P., Ostelo, R., Koes, B. W., & van Tulder, M. W. (2011). A systematic review on the effectiveness of physical and rehabilitation interventions for chronic non-specific low back pain. *European Spine Journal, 20*(1), 19–39. doi:10.1007/s00586-010-1518-3

van Tulder, M. W., Touray, T., Furlan, A. D., Solway, S., & Bouter, L. M. (2003). Muscle relaxants for non-specific low back pain. *Cochrane Database of Systematic Reviews*, (2), CD004252. doi:10.1002/14651858.CD004252

Vargas-Schaffer, G. (2010). Is the WHO analgesic ladder still valid? *Canadian Family Physician, 56*, 514–517.

Voelkner, R. (2010). Ethnic shifts raise issues in elder care. *Journal of the American Medical Association, 303*(4), 321. doi:10.1001/jama.2009.1978

Vyvey, M. (2010). Steroids as pain relief adjuvants. *Canadian Family Physician, 56*(12), 1295–1297.

Walbert, T. (2016). Palliative care in end-stage neurological disease. In S. Yennurajalingam & E. Bruera (Eds.), *Oxford American handbook of hospice and palliative medicine and supportive care* (2nd ed., pp. 419–434). New York, NY: Oxford University Press.

Wald, A. (2016). Constipation advances in diagnosis and treatment. *Journal of the American Medical Association, 315*(2), 185–191. doi:10.1001/jama.2015.16994

Walker, P. W., Palla, S., Pei, B., Kaur, G., Zhang, K., Hanohano, J., … Bruera, E. (2008). Switching from methadone to a different opioid: What is the equianalgesic dose ratio? *Journal of Palliative Medicine, 11*(8), 1103–1108. doi:10.1089/jpm.2007.0285

Wallace, J. D. (2013). Pediatrics. In C. M. Dahlin & M. T. Lynch (Eds.), *Core curriculum for the advanced practice hospice and palliative registered nurse* (2nd ed., pp. 481–510). Pittsburgh, PA: Hospice and Palliative Nurses Association.

Walsh, A. F., & Broglio, K. (2016). Pain management in the individual with serious illness and comorbid substance use disorder. *Nursing Clinics of North America, 51*, 433–447. doi:10.1016/j.cnur.2016.05.003

Weinstein, E., & Arnold, R. (2015). Fast facts and concepts #113: Bisphosphonates for bone pain. Retrieved from https://www.mypcnow.org/blank-ux03d

Weissman, D. (2009). Fast facts and concepts #069: Pseudoaddiction. Retrieved from https://www.mypcnow.org/blank-bua5r

Wells, N., Pasero, C., & McCaffery, M. (2008). Improving the quality of care through pain assessment and management. In R. G. Hughes (Ed.), *Patient safety and quality: An evidence-based handbook for nurses* (pp. 34–63). Rockville, MD: Agency for Healthcare Research and Quality.

Wen, H., Schackman, B. R., Aden, B., & Bao, Y. (2017). States with prescription drug monitoring mandates saw a reduction in opioids prescribed to Medicaid enrollees. *Health Affairs, 36*(4), 733–741. doi:10.1377/hlthaff.2016.1141

Wentlandt, K., & Zimmermann, C. (2016). Palliative care in patients with AIDS. In S. Yennurajalingam & E. Bruera (Eds.), *Oxford American handbook of hospice and palliative medicine and supportive care* (2nd ed., pp. 407–418). New York, NY: Oxford University Press.

Weschules, D. J., & Bain, K. T. (2008). A systematic review of opioid conversion rations used with methadone for the treatment of pain. *Pain Medicine, 9*(5), 595–612. doi:10.1111/j.1526-4637.2008.00461.x

Whiting, P. F., Wolff, R. F., Deshpande, S., Di Nisio, M., Duffy, S., Hernandez, A. V., … Kleijnen, J. (2015). Cannabinoids for medical use. A systematic review and meta-analysis. *Journal of the American Medical Association, 313*(24), 2456–2473. doi:10.1001/jama.2015.6358.

Wolanczyk, M. J., Fakhrian, K., & Adamietz, A. A. (2016). Radiotherapy, bisphonates and surgical stabilization of complete or impending pathologic fractures in patients with metastatic bone disease. *Journal of Cancer, 7*(1), 121–124. doi:10.7150/jca.13377

Wolfe, J., Hammel, J. F., Edwards, K. E., Duncan, J., Comeau, M., Breyer, J., … Weeks, J. C. (2008). Easing of suffering in children with cancer at the end of life: Is care changing? *Journal of Clinical Oncology, 26*(10) 1717–1723. doi:10.1200/JCO.2007.14.0277

Wong, A., & Reddy, S. K. (2016). Pain assessment and management. In S. Yennurajalingam & E. Bruera (Eds.), *Oxford American handbook of hospice and palliative medicine and supportive care* (2nd ed., pp. 27–68). New York, NY: Oxford University Press.

Woolf, C. J. (2011). Central sensitization: Implications for the diagnosis and treatment of pain. *Pain, 152*(Suppl. 3), S2–S15. doi:10.1016/j.pain.2010.09.030

World Health Organization. (2010). WHO's pain ladder for adults. Retrieved from http://www.who.int/cancer/palliative/painladder/en

World Health Organization. (2011). WHO model list of essential medicine. Retrieved from http://www.who.int/medicines/publications/essentialmedicines/en/index.html

World Health Organization. (2012). WHO guidelines on the pharmacological treatment of persisting pain in children with medical illnesses. Geneva, Switzerland: Author. Retrieved from http://apps.who.int/iris/bitstream/handle/10665/44540/9789241548120_Guidelines.pdf;jsessionid=E94CB9F2A866D1C6B777E511C2C1E249?sequence=1

Zeppetella, G. (2008). Opioids for cancer breakthrough pain: A pilot study reporting patient assessment of time to meaningful pain relief. *Journal of Pain and Symptom Management, 35*(5), 563–567. doi: 10.1016/j.jpainsymman.2007.06.012

Dyspnea

KEY POINTS

- Dyspnea is a multidimensional symptom; assessment is based on the patient's report.
- Efforts should be made to encourage and promote reporting dyspnea using an appropriate assessment tool, considering age (children and elders may underreport) and the ability to self-report.
- Treatment of the underlying cause(s) does not necessarily mean dyspnea resolution. Improved physiological measures do not always equate to reduction in or elimination of dyspnea.
- Interventions should be directed at more than one dimension of dyspnea; that is, physical (impact or burden), sensory (perception), affective (distress), and social domains.
- Caregivers of patients with dyspnea need to be included in the treatment plan.
- Dyspnea in advanced disease is often prognostic of impending death.

CASE STUDY

I met Dee at her home one Saturday morning; she was 72 years old and living in an apartment with her adult son. She struggled with shortness of breath and other symptoms of chronic obstructive pulmonary disease (COPD), a result of smoking from one to two packs of cigarettes per day since she was in her teens. Despite her dependence on oxygen, she was still smoking but had transitioned primarily to electronic cigarettes. She also suffered with the effects of fibromyalgia and congestive heart failure, namely, fatigue and pain. She was easily stressed, even with the assistance of a walker, when moving from her bedroom to the bathroom, a distance of about 15 feet. Her recovery time lasted from 25 to 45 minutes once she got back to bed. She slept on several pillows to keep her head elevated so she could breathe easier. She reported a dyspnea on exertion rating of 10 (0–10 scale) and from 4 to 6 at rest. Her work of breathing was significant as evidenced by accessory muscle use in her chest, shoulders, and back. Her pain level also scored high, ranging from 6 to 8, primarily in her lower extremities. Dee's legs were swollen, with mild pitting edema bilaterally. Her skin color was dusky, and nailbeds varied from normal to blue tinged. Her son described her as inconsolable at her worst, even with medications. He believed anxiety played a large role, noting that the more anxious she was, the less her medications relieved her symptoms. She did not disagree.

Dee responded well to my questions in the health interview. She acknowledged the severity of her illnesses, though her son reported many extremes, from being able to participate in family events one weekend to nearly dying the next. I noted that Dee was confused at times, often mixing up the past and the present.

Dee's primary care provider had referred her to a home-based palliative care program, the reason for my visit. She was not completely convinced of the need for this program, but her son and other family members felt strongly about it. She also had community services with a home health aide (HHA) for a couple hours each day, Monday through Friday. Since her son had to leave for work in the morning, the HHA came to assist her with personal hygiene and breakfast. Later in the day, her neighbor would come and check on her. She kept her cell phone at her side, a fall alert button on a string around her neck, and the family planned to install a camera that connected to the son's cell phone for virtual observation.

During our discussion, Dee revealed that on a good day, she would sit outside without the oxygen and smoke a traditional cigarette or two. She enjoyed smoking so much that it was worth it to her, especially since she realized her days were numbered. When asked to explain, Dee said she knew her medical problems were not going away and that she would eventually die from one or more of her conditions. We talked about her goals at this stage of her life, especially in relation to her symptom burden. She verbalized a desire to enjoy her family as much as possible. She was clear that she did not want to return to the hospital, even if she was dying. Hospice services were presented as an option, but neither she nor her family were ready to commit to a hospice program on the initial visit. She was, however, willing to sign a do not resuscitate (DNR) form.

We developed a plan of care that included a trial of physical and occupational therapy and adding more hours for the HHA. Education and demonstration regarding energy conservation measures, pacing activities, and breathing techniques were offered. For example, instead of walking to the bathroom at night, I suggested she use a bedside commode so her sleep and rest would not be entirely disrupted. Her medications were adjusted and a low-dose steroid trial was ordered.

■ DYSPNEA

According to the American Thoracic Society's (ATS) 2012 official statement, dyspnea is "a subjective experience of breathing discomfort that consists of qualitatively distinct sensations that vary in intensity (ATS, 2012). The experience derives from interactions among multiple physiological, psychological, social and environmental factors, and may induce secondary physiological and behavioral responses" (Parshall et al., 2012, pp. 436–437). In general, the definition of dyspnea is the sensation of difficulty breathing, including the person's reaction to that sensation. Dyspnea can be acute, chronic, acute on chronic, or terminal (Hutchinson, Pickering, Williams, Bland, & Johnson, 2017; Simon, Higginson, et al., 2013).

Acute or episodic dyspnea consists of high-intensity, time-limited shortness of breath that occurs as an immediate response to an acute physiological or psychological event, seen in such conditions as myocardial infarction (MI), pulmonary emboli, or hyperventilation from an excitatory state. International experts on breathlessness have defined episodic dyspnea as "a severe worsening of breathlessness intensity or unpleasantness beyond usual fluctuations, with or without underlying continuous breathlessness" (Simon, Weingärtner, Higginson, Voltz, & Bausewein, 2014, p. 833). Acute dyspnea may be predictable or unpredictable, depending on the identification of

trigger(s) such as pain, emotions, allergens, or exertion. More than one trigger may be responsible for episodic dyspnea.

Chronic dyspnea is persistent shortness of breath of variable intensity, usually seen in chronic conditions, such as COPD or congestive heart failure (CHF). Acute on chronic dyspnea occurs when high-intensity shortness of breath compounds the usual persistent shortness of breath experienced in chronic conditions (Hutchinson et al., 2017). Terminal dyspnea (constant or episodic) occurs in people with end-stage diseases and is one of the most common symptoms reported in the last 48 hours of life (Hall, Schroder, & Weaver, 2002; Morris & Galicia-Castillo, 2017). In fact, only 11.4% of patients imminently dying report no shortness of breath (Currow et al., 2010).

The sensation of dyspnea often changes over the course of an illness, requiring a variety of different treatment approaches (Freeman, Hirdes, Stolee, Garcia & Smith, 2015; Lanken et al., 2008; Selecky et al., 2005). Bausewein et al. (2010) found four patterns of breathlessness: fluctuating, increasing, stable, and decreasing. For example, patients with COPD experience moderate-to-severe dyspnea that increases over time, while cancer patients report a higher intensity closer to death (Bausewein et al., 2010; Currow et al., 2010; Weingaertner et al., 2014). Dyspnea may also be refractory to treatment, causing both patients and providers to feel powerless over the symptom (Carel, McNaughton, & Dodd, 2015; Weingaertner et al., 2014).

Common descriptions of dyspnea fall into the categories of difficulty with air movement, increased effort, and unsatisfied inspiration (Parshall et al., 2012). Such descriptors include air hunger, choking, smothering, congestion, tightness, suffocation, and strangling as well as emotional responses such as panic, fear, worry, frustration, and an inability to stop thinking about breathing (Dunger et al., 2015, Elia & Thomas, 2008; Schwartzstein, 1999). Clearly, dyspnea is more than "just another symptom" to manage; "it threatens a person's very existence, psychological well-being, and social functioning" (Currow et al., 2011, p. 389).

■ INCIDENCE

Dyspnea is a frequent and devastating symptom that occurs in as many as 62% of older adults and 95% of patients with advanced diseases, primarily those with lung cancer and end-stage heart or lung disease (Carel et al., 2015; Dudgeon, Kristjanson, Sloan, Lertzman, & Clement, 2001; Edmonds, Karlsen, Khan, & Addington-Hall, 2001; Mullerova, Lu, Li, & Tabberer, 2014; Parshall et al., 2012). However, 24% of terminal patients participating in the National Hospice Study reported dyspnea despite the absence of pulmonary or cardiac disease (Reuben & Mor, 1986). In fact, dyspnea occurs in greater than 50% of individuals with breast, lymphoma, genitourinary, and head/neck cancers (Dudgeon et al., 2001). Moreover, 41% of patients in palliative care (PC) experience dyspnea and 46% of those describe the severity as moderate to severe (Charles, Reymond, & Israel, 2008; Cleary & Carbone, 1997; Currow, 2008). Consequently, dyspnea accounts for more than 10% of PC consults and is the fourth most common reason for patients receiving PC to visit the ED (Henson et al., 2015; Kamal et al., 2009).

Intensity of dyspnea on arrival in the ED is predictive of hospital admission (Saracino, Weiland, Jolly, & Dent, 2010; Skaug, Eide, & Gulsvik, 2009). In the case study, Dee is an elder with advanced COPD who has made many trips to the ED, some resulting in hospitalization due to severe dyspnea.

Dyspnea can seriously affect the quality of life (QOL) in those who experience it and may limit activity to the extent that even the slightest exertion may precipitate breathlessness. For example, eating may cause significant respiratory distress, which will impact an individual's nutritional state as well as mobility and functional status. However, in patients with advanced noncardiopulmonary disease, an overall decline in functional status may be the primary reason for shortness of breath (Currow et al., 2010). Regardless, health-related QOL, as measured by the European Organization for Research and Treatment of Cancer Quality of Life Questionnaire—Core 30, decreases significantly over the last 3 months of life, with

an increase from 14% (3 months) to 43% (1 month) of patients reporting difficulty with self-care activities (Elmqvist, Jordhoy, Bjordal, Kaasa, & Jannert, 2009). Dee's shortness of breath was significantly affected by physical activity and exacerbated by anxiety resulting in panic that was not always responsive to medications, rest, or breathing techniques. This led to a loss of independence because she required assistance with nearly all of her activities of daily living.

In the terminal phase of the illness, fear of suffocation may be experienced. The frequency and severity of dyspnea often increases with the progression of disease and/or when death is approaching.

Intensive-care patients at a high risk of dying reported shortness of breath as the most distressing symptom, even when not the most prevalent (Puntillo et al., 2010). Patients with inoperable lung cancer ranked dyspnea as the most distressing symptom, with its prevalence and intensity peaking in the month before death (Tishelman, Petersson, Degner, & Sprangers, 2007). Symptom burden was higher and functional levels lower closer to death. Other contributing factors include a history of or current smoking, environmental exposures, chemotherapy, radiation treatment, Karnofsky less than or equal to 40, cough, pain, anxiety, fatigue, depression, and vital capacity or maximal inspiratory pressure less than 80% predicted (Bruera, Schmitz, Pither, Neumann, & Hanson, 2000; Dudgeon et al., 2001). In COPD and advanced cancer patients, dyspnea is considered a prognostic indicator of decreased survival time, whether alone or in association with other symptoms and/or performance status (Ben-Aharon, Gafter-Gvili, Paul, Leibovici, & Stemmer, 2008; Maltoni et al., 1995; Nishimura, Izumi, Tsukino, & Oga, 2002).

■ MECHANISMS OF DYSPNEA

To understand the complex mechanisms of dyspnea, it may help to review the control of respiration. The respiratory center in the medulla activates the muscles that expand the chest wall, inflate the lungs, and produce ventilation. The process of breathing regulates the oxygen and carbon dioxide balance and hydrogen ion concentration in the blood and body tissues. The automatic regulation of breathing is controlled by chemoreceptors in the blood and brain. Changes in PCO_2 and PO_2 are sensed by central chemoreceptors in the medulla and peripheral chemoreceptors in the carotid and aortic bodies, which send feedback to the brainstem respiratory centers to adjust breathing to maintain blood-gas and acid-base homeostasis (Parshall et al., 2012). All the input returned to the brain from body sensors contributes in some fashion to the individual's perception of dyspnea. Any state of imbalance, such as difficulty breathing, is a threat to homeostasis.

The most recent ATS update concludes: "New evidence reliably associates distinct physiologic mechanisms and afferent pathways with different sensory qualities related to the sensation of dyspnea, namely work/effort, tightness, and air hunger or unsatisfactory inspiration" (Parshall et al., 2012, p. 436). Though the neurophysiology is not well understood, three mechanisms remain dominant and interrelated in the creation of the dyspneic sensation: (a) A conscious awareness of the neuromotor command to the respiratory muscles, that is, cerebral processing, similar to the sensation in exercising muscle; for example, an increased sense of effort experienced with aging, malnutrition, deconditioning, and hypoxemia; (b) Stimulation of the receptors in the airways, lungs, and chest wall, which detect changes in lung volume, stretch, and pressure and are responsible for the feeling of tightness; for example, the sensation of respiratory muscle abnormalities, such as those found in neuromuscular conditions and respiratory muscle fatigue, as well as diseases that inhibit normal airflow and ventilation, such as COPD, asthma, and pulmonary fibrosis. (c) Stimulation of the chemoreceptors; for example, the sensation of blood-gas abnormalities (e.g., hypoxia and hypercapnia) that indirectly trigger ventilation, thereby causing air hunger or unsatisfied inspiration. Moreover, it is likely that more than one mechanism is involved; therefore, the sensations do not occur in isolation and vary in unpleasantness and emotional significance (Parshall et al., 2012).

These mechanisms support the idea that dyspnea is caused by an imbalance or "mismatch" between central respiratory motor activity and feedback from receptors in the airways, lungs, and chest wall. However, psychological, social, spiritual, and environmental factors interact with the physiological ones to produce the subjective sensation of dyspnea. In other words, the sensation of dyspnea is produced by various physiological mechanisms (neural activation); however, the perception of dyspnea is the reaction to the sensation as determined in the cortical and limbic areas of the brain that also subserves interoceptive awareness and nociceptive sensations such as pain (Parshall et al., 2012). Specifically, the right anterior insular cortex supports a representation of visceral responses accessible to emotional awareness, known as interoception (Critchley, Wiens, Rotshtein, Ohman, & Dolan, 2004). Without recognizing all of the components, that is, perception, emotional response, and functional consequences, contributing to the total suffering of dyspnea, successful management is difficult to achieve (Currow, 2008; Zepetella, 1998). Symptom control, therefore, may require more diligence than with other symptoms common in advanced disease (Hayen, Herigstad, & Pattinson, 2013; Williams, 2006).

■ ASSESSMENT

Dyspnea is a personal experience that accounts for a high proportion of disability, impaired QOL, and suffering. Each patient's experience with the symptom is as unique to the person as is the individual's journey with a life-limiting condition (Kamal, Maguire, Wheeler, Currow, & Abernethy, 2011). Thus, a thorough interprofessional assessment includes a careful, comprehensive history to obtain a complete understanding of the patient's experience with dyspnea. Specific information about dyspnea, including its timing, precipitating factors, associated symptoms, alleviating factors, and quality of the symptom, should be assessed. The influences of culture, race, age, and gender should also be taken into account.

Timing

Dyspnea may suddenly appear and just as quickly disappear, with little, if any, explanation (Gysels & Higginson, 2008). Despite the elusive nature of the symptom, the duration, frequency, and onset of dyspnea may provide insight into the etiology and management. For example, dyspnea that comes on suddenly may reflect bronchoconstriction, pulmonary embolism, cardiac ischemia, or abrupt airway occlusion. Chronic dyspnea occurs gradually and is likely to be manifested in slowly progressive disorders such as COPD, interstitial lung disease, or a slow-growing tumor. If the dyspnea occurs more at night, then it may be secondary to the redistribution of fluid in the supine position from diseases such as CHF. Dyspnea can also result from an exacerbation of gastroesophageal reflux disease (GERD), which triggers bronchoconstriction. Assessing whether dyspnea is present with activity and/or at rest offers a better understanding of the severity of the symptom. Dee's breathlessness occurred at rest and worsened with activity; it often appeared due to no apparent reason, making anticipatory planning difficult.

Precipitating Factors

The identification of precipitating factors, or triggers, assists in determining the underlying cause of dyspnea (Hasson et al., 2008; Henoch, Bergman, & Danielson, 2008; Shumway, Wilson, Howard, Parker, & Eliasson, 2008). Exercise or overexertion commonly precipitates dyspnea in most chronic cardiopulmonary conditions, as does a change in position. Often patients with COPD or CHF feel dyspneic when supine, while those with cirrhosis or pneumonectomy may feel the sensation when upright. Anticipation of stressful events is another typical precipitant. Inhalation of allergens (pollen, grass, and weeds), smoke, fumes, and other aerosolized substances may trigger bronchospasm in patients with COPD and asthma. Respiratory infections usually cause an exacerbation of symptoms. Dee elevated the head of her bed, initially with pillows and then using the bed control. She and her caregivers had to be educated on energy conservation and pacing activities as these concepts were new.

Associated Symptoms

Since objective clinical measures are often disconnected from subjective reports, concurrent symptoms can direct strategies for reduction of dyspnea. However, the search for etiology should not take precedence over the symptom itself (Carel et al., 2015). Clutching sternal chest pain is most likely indicative of myocardial ischemia, while brief, sharp lateral chest pain suggests pulmonary embolism, pneumothorax, or pleurisy. Wheezing is usually a sign of asthma, COPD, or CHF. Coughing, if productive, may indicate the presence of an infection, especially if there is a change in color, consistency, or volume of sputum. Nonproductive coughing occurs with rhinitis, reactive airway disease, interstitial fibrosis, GERD, and others. Hemoptysis is most common with tuberculosis, lung cancer, and pulmonary embolism. Weight loss is another problem that occurs often in patients with cancer, cardiopulmonary diseases, and AIDS.

Psychological symptoms are equally as important since anxiety has been found to correlate with the intensity of dyspnea in patients with cancer and lung disease (De Peuter et al., 2004; Smith et al., 2001). Hutchinson et al. (2017) found one-third of patients who presented to the ED with a chief complaint of breathlessness were sent home after anxiety-reduction measures. Tactful questioning and skillful observation may be needed as the patient may not directly admit to anxiety as a symptom. One of every seven patients with dyspnea does not tell anyone about it (Hutchinson et al., 2017). Caregivers can be approached for assistance with this component of the assessment, although they may also suffer from anxiety when the patient is experiencing dyspnea (Freeman, Hirdes, Stolee, & Garcia, 2016; Malik, Gysels, & Higginson, 2013; Mercadante, Masedu, Valenti, Mercadante, & Aielli, 2016).

Alleviating Factors

Pharmacological and nonpharmacological strategies are necessary to relieve dyspnea and associated discomfort. Medications can be prescribed based on the identified etiology of dyspnea, such as cardiac or pulmonary problems or for the symptom alone (Bausewein & Simon, 2013; Chin & Booth, 2016; Kamal, Maguire, Wheeler, Currow, & Abernethy, 2012; Lanken et al., 2008). Bronchodilators relax bronchial smooth muscle and work well in diseases such as COPD and asthma (Williams, 2006). Nitroglycerin is the initial drug of choice for myocardial ischemia, which may cause dyspnea (Spector, Connolly, & Carlson, 2007). Benzodiazepines, as an adjunct to opioids, often provide relaxation by decreasing the anxiety that frequently accompanies shortness of breath (Ekstrom, Bornefalk-Hermansson, Abernethy, & Currow, 2014). Position changes can also offer clues as to etiology. Sitting up in a high Fowler's position or standing may relieve shortness of breath by allowing for better diaphragmatic expansion in the case of pulmonary disease or promoting redistribution of fluid in CHF (Spector et al., 2007).

Quality of Dyspnea

Schwartzstein (1999) documented that dyspnea is composed of many distinct sensations that are distinguishable by patients; patients' descriptive language of dyspnea can lead to a better understanding of management and perhaps etiology (Caroci & Lareau, 2004; Dunger et al., 2015; Hasson et al., 2008; Hechler et al., 2008; Henoch et al., 2008; Mahler & Harver, 2000; Scano, Stendardi, & Grazzini, 2005; Schwartzstein, 1999; Wilcock et al., 2002). It is important to carefully question the patient about the quality and characteristics of the dyspnea experienced. For example, adults with more severe dyspnea may say they have an "urge to breathe," "need more air," or report a "sense of suffocation." Those with neuromuscular or chest wall disease may describe it as "heavy breathing." Still others, especially those with cardiac disease, may call it "chest tightness." Dee described her dyspnea as "taking her breath away."

The assessment should include a thorough review of the patient's past medical history, including all current and recent medications. Some medications become problematic related to drug–drug interactions that occur secondary to multiple prescribers. Beta-blockers, for example, antagonize beta-2 receptors and inhibit their potential bronchodilation effect. An adequate nutritional history is valuable because malnutrition contributes to respiratory muscle fatigue and, thus, promotes dyspnea. Information about exposure to chemicals, smoke, fumes, and other environmental pollutants adds to the data obtained from the history.

Physical Examination

A focused physical examination of the head, neck, and chest will yield specific information about the patient's condition and assist with the identification of treatment options. Inspection should include the color of skin, nails, lips, nutritional state, sternal/spinal deformities, chest shape and movement, breathing rate and rhythm (full minute), capillary refill, the presence/absence of nasal flaring, tracheal deviation, jugular venous distention, costal retractions, accessory muscle use, and clubbing. Other clues include facial/oral expression and inspiration–expiration ratio. Palpation can yield information about tenderness, fremitus, masses, nodes, and crepitus. Percussion of the chest will indicate the degree of resonance, where dull is the consolidation of tissue and tympanic is the presence of air. Auscultation of the lungs will detect adventitious or diminished breath sounds, voice sounds, or pleural friction rubs. Dee's physical exam revealed a barrel chest, taut neck and shoulder muscles, clubbed fingers, and rapid breathing with a prolonged expiratory phase. On percussion, her chest was tympanic, and with auscultation, she had shallow breath sounds with occasional expiratory wheezing.

Diagnostic Tests

Based on the need to determine the underlying cause(s) of dyspnea, several diagnostic tests may be of value. These include chest radiography, computed tomography, spirometry and/or pulmonary function tests, pulse oximetry (preferred) or arterial blood-gas analysis, ECG, electrolyte profile, and complete blood count. Performance of any test should take into consideration the risk/benefit ratio, the patient and his or her family's wishes, the prognosis, and goals of care.

■ MEASUREMENT OF DYSPNEA

Dyspnea is a subjective, multidimensional symptom; therefore, it is important that instruments used to measure it take into account the sensation, the impact of it on QOL (patient and caregivers), and the response to interventions. Although many tools exist, no one tool measures all dimensions of dyspnea. Without a gold standard, clinicians and researchers should choose the appropriate tool based on criteria such as the definition of dyspnea, setting, diagnostic group, disease stage, sensitivity required, and variables involved (Bausewein, Farquhar, Booth, Gysels, & Higginson, 2007; Dorman, Byrne, & Edwards, 2007). In general, the Visual Analog Scale (VAS), Numerical Rating Scale (NRS), or the Modified Borg Scale provides useful assessment data. If there is a specific focus on QOL, multidimensional tools such as the Chronic Respiratory Questionnaire (CRQ) or Lung Cancer Symptom Scale (LCSS) would be best. If the focus is more on the sensation and its impact on function, then the Cancer Dyspnea Scale (CDS) is most appropriate. For patients unable to self-report, the Respiratory Distress Observation Scale (RDOS) assesses objective indicators of dyspnea, such as tachypnea, gasping, use of accessory muscles, anxiety, restlessness, agitation, grimacing, and tachycardia (Campbell, Templin, & Walch, 2010). Researchers should consider using both uni- and multidimensional instruments in order to understand the full impact on the patient and caregivers.

A VAS is recommended due to its ease of use and availability. On either a 100-mm horizontal or vertical line, the anchors "not at all breathless" on the low end and "severely breathless" at the high end represent the extremes of dyspnea (Gift, 1989; Martinez et al., 2000). The VAS can measure even minute changes when used consistently. Another commonly used tool is the Modified Borg Scale, which has the numbers 0 to 10 listed horizontally with descriptors along the line. On both, the patient is asked only to rate the shortness of breath;

no other dimensions are measured. While nonverbal adults can simply point to a number or position, some may find it difficult and need assistance to rate their symptom. For this reason, another choice would be an NRS as patients generally find it easier to verbally pick a number from a simple scale such as 0 to 5. Nevertheless, each of these unidimensional tools is reliable and valid and can be helpful when assessing dyspnea in a variety of settings. All are self-administered and quick, and can be used over the phone. Johnson, Bland, Oxberry, Abernethy, and Currow (2013) reported that a 1-point reduction in intensity is clinically meaningful, thereby emphasizing the importance of repeated measurements. In the case study, we used the NRS due to its ease of use and familiarity with the scale. However, in retrospect, a more comprehensive tool would have been helpful in designing Dee's treatment plan.

For patients with advanced disease, the CDS is a 12-question self-report of shortness of breath that includes aspects of dyspnea such as sense of effort, anxiety, and discomfort, which continue to be validated and evaluated, most recently as an English version in patients with advanced cancer (Henoch, Bergman, & Gaston-Johansson, 2006; Tanaka, Akechi, Okuyama, Nishiwaki, & Uchitomi, 2000). The CRQ has demonstrated validity, reliability, and responsiveness but only in the populations of chronic lung disease and CHF. Further evaluation of these and other tools will benefit the patients, caregivers, and healthcare providers in dyspnea assessment.

Because patients unable to self-report are often undertreated (Campbell, Templin, & Walch, 2009), Campbell et al., Walch (2010) developed the RDOS, an eight-item tool that measures objective indicators for those who cannot communicate their needs. Validity and reliability have been documented in adolescents and adults but require RN assessment (Campbell et al., 2010).

Whichever instrument is used, the patient and family should feel comfortable and encouraged to utilize it in order to evaluate current therapeutic interventions. Consistency over time will maximize the relevance and usefulness of the measurement. It is important to reemphasize that physiological parameters do not always correlate with the degree of dyspnea reported. The patient must remain the singular authority on the symptom, whether verbal or nonverbal.

Gerontological Considerations

Three major factors contribute to the effects of aging on the pulmonary system: an increase in chest wall stiffness, a decline in respiratory muscle strength, and a decrease in lung elasticity (Mahler, Rosiello, & Loke, 1986; Tan et al., 2009; see Table 21.1). Respiratory infections and inhalation of allergens, smoke, fumes, and other aerosolized substances are more likely to result in dyspnea in older adults as aging increases susceptibility to both

TABLE 21.1 Effects of the Aging Process on the Pulmonary System

Structural Changes (Pediatric)	Result (Pediatric)	Structural Changes (Geriatric)	Result (Geriatric)
Upper Airways			
Infants = nasal breathers	Nasal congestion = airway obstruction	Nasal cartilage weakens, causing obstruction	Difficulty breathing through the nose
Large tongue	Easily occludes airway	Nasal blood flow decreases	Drying of secretions; nasal congestion
Narrowed cricoid cartilage	Potential for airway obstruction	Nasal turbinates shrink	Drying of secretions; nasal congestion
Cartilaginous larynx	Susceptible to edema, airway obstruction	Mucus increases in viscosity	Lodges in nasopharynx and stimulates coughing
Large Airways			
Trachea = small diameter (e.g., finger of child)	Easily obstructed	Trachea and large bronchi stiffen	Decreases air exchange
Small Airways			
Diameter increases over time		Diameter decreases	
		Alveolar ducts dilate	
Alveolar surface area increases		Alveolar surface area decreases	
		Combined changes	Increase residual volume
Thoracic Cage			
Thin chest wall	Increases compliance (i.e., retractions)	Ribs decalcify	Affects posture
Cartilaginous ribs	Increases compliance (i.e., retractions)	Costal cartilages calcify	Affects posture
Cartilaginous sternum	Increases compliance (i.e., retractions)	Costovertebral joints stiffen (arthritic changes)	Decreases height
Flattened position of diaphragm	Any impedance affects work of breathing	Dorsal kyphosis occurs	Increases anterior-posterior diameter (barrel shape)
		Combined changes	Decreases vital capacity, increases residual volume
Pulmonary Vasculature			
		Arteries enlarge and thicken (lose distensibility)	Decreases cardiac output during exercise/exertion
Mechanical Changes (Pediatric)	**Result (Pediatric)**	**Mechanical Changes (Geriatric)**	**Result (Geriatric)**
Small Airways			
Potential for premature closing	Grunting generates PEEP and may prevent atelectasis	Premature closure	Air trapping/hyperinflation; impairs gas exchange and mucociliary clearance

(continued)

TABLE 21.1	Effects of the Aging Process on the Pulmonary System (*continued*)		
Respiratory Musculature			
Immature	Easily fatigued	Strength decreases; oxygen needs increase	Muscle fatigue; less reserve
Lung Volumes, Capacities, Flow Rates			
		Forced expiratory volume in 1-second decreases	Increases residual volume
		Forced vital capacity decreases	Increases residual volume
		Functional residual capacity increases	Increases work of breathing
		Diffusing capacity decreases	Impairs gas exchange

PEEP, positive end-expiratory pressure.

Sources: McCaskey, M. S. (2007). Pediatric assessment: The little differences. *Home Healthcare Nurse, 25*(1), 20–24; Sheahan, S. L., & Musialowski, R. (2001). Clinical implications of respiratory system changes in aging. *Journal of Gerontological Nursing, 27*(5), 26–34; quiz 48. doi:10.3928/0098-9134-20010501-08; Tan, M. P., Wynn, N. N., Umerov, M., Henderson, A., Gillham, A., Junejo, S., & Bansal, S. K. (2009). Arm span to height ratio is related to severity of dyspnea, reduced spirometry volumes, and right heart strain. *Chest, 135*(2), 448–454. doi:10.1378/chest.08-1270; Thompson, L. F. (1996). Failure to wean: Exploring the influence of age-related pulmonary changes. *Critical Care Nursing Clinics of North America, 8*(1), 7–16.

infections and allergens due to a diminished immune system (Sheahan & Musialowski, 2001). Other effects of aging include a prevalence of silent GERD and sleep apnea secondary to discoordinated activity of the upper airway muscles and the diaphragm. In a study conducted by Johansson et al. (2012), community-dwelling elders experienced nighttime dyspnea, palpitations, and pain, which significantly affected sleep and indirectly affected the presence of depressive symptoms, regardless of the presence or absence of illness. A recent cardiovascular health study of community-dwelling elders noted five factors strongly associated with moderate-to-severe dyspnea—FEV1 less than the lower limit of normal, ejection fraction of less than 45%, inability to perform a single chair stand, depression, and obesity (BMI ≥ 30)—and five modestly associated additional factors: respiratory muscle weakness, diastolic cardiac dysfunction, grip weakness, anxiety, and use of cardiovascular and psychotropic medications (Miner et al., 2016). Similar findings were reported by Johnson et al. (2017) for dyspneic elders in the last year of life, namely, anxiety, depression, and mobility problems.

Neurologically, age reduces chemoreceptor functioning, causing an inadequate ventilatory response to hypercapnia and acute hypoxia (Thompson, 1996). This makes older adults more sensitive and vulnerable to adverse outcomes from conditions that produce lower oxygen levels, such as pneumonia and COPD. Therefore, in the dyspneic elder, a successful treatment plan may need to include interventions aimed at specific comorbidities, such as renal disease, CHF, or COPD. Miner et al. (2016) described dyspnea as a multifactorial geriatric

health condition requiring systematic evaluation of impairments commonly seen with advancing age. While Johnson et al. (2017) agree with a systematic evaluation, they suggest that dyspnea may be part of a final common pathway near the end of life. In a secondary analysis of community-dwelling elders in the year preceding death, dyspnea restricted activities in more than 50% (*n* = 548) and increased in frequency in the months closer to death, irrespective of cause (Johnson et al., 2017).

For example, in the case of COPD, reduced ventilator capacity from respiratory muscle weakness, increased ventilator demand from anaerobic metabolism, and the presence of psychosocial and environmental factors often increase oxygen requirements (Fried, Vax Fragoso, & Rabow, 2012). Therefore, the elderly with COPD need to be monitored more carefully for the possibility of carbon dioxide retention and subsequent acidosis (Ofir, Laveneziana, Webb, Lam, & O'Donnell, 2008). Ade-Oshifogun (2012) found that dyspnea along with a 6-minute walk distance and diffusion capacities were direct predictors of functional performance in elders with COPD, regardless of truncal obesity. However, the investigator reported an indirect effect of obesity on functional performance due to increased dyspnea, resulting in a recommendation for nurses to consider a weight-loss intervention with obese older adults. In dyspneic elders with advanced non–small cell lung cancer, shortened distance in a 6-minute walk test was an objective predictor of poor response to palliative chemotherapy (Werynska, Porebska, & Brzecka, 2017). In elders with CHF (greater than or equal to 75 years of age), dyspnea is the most frequently self-reported symptom (Goldberg et al., 2010). Dyspnea, along with fatigue, limits activities of daily living, causing dependency and resulting in poor health-related QOL (Falk, Ekman, Anderson, Fu, & Granger, 2013). Elders with advanced COPD describe their lives as fragile and burdensome with frequent exacerbations that are both unpredictable and frightening (Jerpseth, Dahl, Nortvedt, & Halvorsen, 2018). Johansson et al. (2012) found five times the prevalence of sleep-disordered breathing and insomnia among elders with CHF when compared with controls. Renal or hepatic impairment will impact the dosages/frequencies of certain medications for elders with these conditions.

Nursing interventions similar to those offered in pulmonary rehabilitation have been found to help elders focus on attainable goals and learn techniques to enhance their QOL (Booth, Farquhar, Gysels, Bausewein, & Higginson, 2006). Indeed, the nurse may need to utilize person-centered techniques to gain mutual understanding as older patients have more difficulty in detecting and interpreting the symptom of dyspnea (Riegel et al., 2010). In studies of symptom recognition for elders with CHF, elders were twice as likely to report a different level of shortness of breath than the healthcare provider assessed (Barnes et al., 2006; Riegel et al., 2010). The underreporting by dyspneic elders may be explained by the Geriatric Dyspnea Model (GDM; Petersen, vonLeupoldt, & VandenBergh, 2014). The GDM highlights risk factors for reduced perception and report in older age, primarily enhanced affective regulation of dyspnea, and increased motivation to regulate negative experiences. Essentially, elders may become very successful at redirecting attention away from symptoms, such as pain and dyspnea. Lastly, due to the thoracic changes attributable to aging, positioning, as described earlier, becomes a major factor in managing the symptom for the dyspneic elder. Dee definitely underreported, which resulted in a rapid escalation of her symptom when she did report it. She had a strong desire to deny the severity of her condition, especially to her family.

■ PEDIATRIC CONSIDERATIONS

More than 15,000 children and adolescents are diagnosed with cancer each year and nearly 2,000 die from the disease (Ward, DeSantis, Robbins, Kohler & Jemal, 2014), making cancer the leading cause of nonaccidental death in children ages 5 to 14 years (Centers for Disease Control and Prevention [CDC], 2014). Among children ages 1 to 4 years, congenital malformations and chromosomal abnormalities account for the majority of nonaccidental deaths (CDC, 2014). In addition, nearly 27% of children in the United States, approximately 1 in 5, live with chronic conditions that seriously affect daily living and normal childhood activities (Focus for Health, 2017; Rafferty & Sullivan, 2017). The number is expected to grow as chronic illnesses in children doubled

between 1994 and 2006 (Van Cleave, Gortmaker, & Perrin, 2010). Each year over 42,000 children die, many as a result of complex chronic conditions (Lindley, 2017).

In the last year of life, children with complex chronic conditions experienced one to five hospital admissions (totaling 7 to 84 days) and incurred costs up to $410,000 (Ananth, Melvin, Feudtner, Wolfe, & Berry, 2015). Children with three or more chronic conditions spent more than 2 months hospitalized in the year before death. It is not surprising that three-fourths of pediatric deaths occur in hospitals, primarily in the ICU (Davies et al., 2008; Morell et al., 2012). As many as 82% report dyspnea at the end of life, second only to loss of appetite (100%; Hongo et al., 2003) and fatigue (98%; Wolfe et al., 2000). Schindera et al. (2014) studied children with cancer at the end of life and found a diagnosis of leukemia, an increased number of relapses, and intravenous (IV) chemotherapy in the month prior to death strongly associated with severe dyspnea. Two studies over a decade apart asked parents to rate the degree of suffering their child experienced at the end of life (Blume et al., 2014; Wolfe et al., 2000). Both found nearly 50% reported "somewhat," "a lot," or "a great deal" of suffering due to dyspnea. According to the parents, 65% of the children were treated for dyspnea, yet only 16% believed the treatment to be successful even though the symptom is generally considered responsive to treatment (Wolfe et al., 2000).

An additional consequence for undertreatment of dyspnea is long-term parental grief, found to be associated with the severity of dyspnea in children with cancer at the end of life (VanderGeest et al., 2014). However, a collaborative agreement on symptom severity by parents and healthcare professionals improves satisfaction with care as well as parental QOL, even if symptom control is not successful (Vollenbroich et al., 2016). Palliation of dyspnea is complicated by several factors: the child's ability to communicate the degrees of dyspnea and relief, the tension between curative care and PC, and the desire to treat the child as part of the family unit (Robinson, 2012). Mack and Wolfe (2006) describe the tension between curative care and PC as persisting until the end of life in pediatrics, whereas in adult care the focus moves more smoothly to palliation.

The respiratory system in children continues to grow and develop long after birth. Because respiratory function is immature in younger patients, deterioration can occur rapidly when disease is present (McCaskey, 2007). One exception is the neonate, who due to increased chest wall compliance may demonstrate abnormal breathing patterns that are actually adaptive for the condition (Robinson, 2012). Special attention should be given to the possibility of congenital anomalies (cardiac or respiratory) in this circumstance. Another difference in pediatrics is a higher respiratory load detection threshold, meaning children and adolescents require a greater change in stimulus intensity before reporting a change in sensation (Pianosi, Huebner, Zhang, Turchetta, & McGrath, 2015). This finding may be responsible for the effectiveness of pictorial scales (nonlinear) in pediatrics since children and adolescents are less able to distinguish between numerous gradations of sensation, as presented in a numerical instrument (linear; Lands, 2017; Pianosi et al., 2015). Similar to adults, but worth repeating, is the fact that lung function improvement does not necessarily correlate with an improved dyspnea rating (Lands, 2017). Therefore, it may be important for health professionals to pursue additional diagnostic testing despite a decrease in reported dyspnea.

Observation, physical assessment, and a medical history are the tools to evaluate respiratory distress as the pediatric patient is not always able to communicate how he or she feels, especially if very young (Lands, 2017). However, in those who can describe their symptom(s), it is important to use pediatric age-appropriate tools, such as the Wong-Baker Faces or the Dalhousie Dyspnea and Perceived Exertion Scale (Khan, Reddy, & Baptist, 2009; Pianosi et al., 2015). Once a baseline measurement has been obtained, integration of dyspnea management with opioids may be introduced along with other interventions for the child's specific condition as indicated. The initial opioid dose is weight based and may range from 2.1 mg/kg/24 hr to 4.4 mg/kg/24 hr (Hewitt, Goldman, Collins, Childs, & Hain, 2008). A general rule of thumb is to start opioids at one-fourth of that used for pain and increase as needed for good effect (Robinson, 2012). Children with solid tumors outside the central nervous system (CNS) may need increased doses of opioids or multiple different opioids to successfully manage their symptoms (Hewitt et al., 2008). According to parents, nonverbal children with neurological impairment benefited greatly from morphine, that is, looking more relaxed and comfortable, less distressed, and more alert (Hauer, 2015). The experience in the case series reported by Hauer (2015) suggests earlier consideration of symptom treatment, rather than waiting till death is near.

Complementary therapies may also assist with dyspnea management but have not been evaluated in children (Ladas, Post-White, Hawks, & Taromina, 2006). Hypnosis, however, is one therapy that has been tested in children, though the evidence is limited to case series, retrospective studies, and only one small randomized trial (McBride, Vlieger, & Anbar, 2014). Hypnotherapy has been used as both adjunct and primary treatment in hyperventilation, habitual cough, and dyspnea with success. Promoting relaxation through hypnosis may be one of the mechanisms through which dyspnea is reduced. Similarly, a reassurance protocol achieved a reduction in exertional dyspnea in otherwise healthy children (Mahut et al., 2014). The reassurance protocol was similar to that used in pulmonary rehabilitation programs, namely, confidence building, education, and breathing retraining.

The scarcity of research in managing pediatric dyspnea in the palliative setting means that many of the treatments are based more on practical wisdom than published evidence specific to pediatrics (Collins & Fitzgerald, 2006). Consequently, the majority of interventions are similar to those used with the adult population (Craig, Henderson, & Bluebond-Langner, 2015). One therapy not as common in adults is the use of airway clearance techniques to remove excess mucus production or to assist children with ineffective cough ability. The techniques range from postural drainage to the use of mechanical devices. One such option for children with chronic dyspnea is negative pressure ventilation using a cuirass (i.e., "turtle") or a raincoat (poncho-like device, which surrounds the child; Robinson, 2012). Getting a good fit is essential and may prohibit the use of the device.

It is not surprising that one of the greatest fears parents have for their dying child is that he or she will be uncomfortable during the last days of life (Widger & Wilkins, 2004). Yet barriers to quality end-of-life (EOL) care such as prognostic uncertainties and discrepancies in treatment goals between staff and family members prevent dying children from being kept as comfortable as possible (Davies et al., 2008; Vollenbroich et al., 2016). Fewer than 1% of children who need hospice care actually receive it (Mellichamp, 2007). Consequently, health professionals in both Canada and the United States continue to advocate for quality pediatric palliative care (PPC) through improvement of two key components: communication and decision making and pain and symptom management (Jones & Wolfe, 2014). Seeking positive outcomes such as an overall improvement in whole-person and family-centered care, a decreased number of ED visits and hospitalizations, and an increased ability of the patient/family to make informed decisions and set realistic goals remains a key intent of PPC (Liben, Langner, & Bluebond-Langner, 2014). Clarifying the objectives of treatment and frequently revisiting both the child's and the parent's experiences while being sensitive to the burden of treatment and balancing it with the expected outcome for the child are essential interventions for health professionals (Robinson, 2012).

■ TREATMENT AND INTERVENTIONS: NONPHARMACOLOGICAL

Because dyspnea is now recognized as a multidimensional symptom with psychosocial as well as physical components, pulmonary and PC experts are increasingly promoting the use of nonpharmacological interventions along with pharmacological therapies to improve the QOL for patients living with breathlessness (Booth, 2013; Rocker, 2011, 2012). Booth (2013) concluded that focused listening and acknowledgment of both patient's and caregivers' concerns is the most effective way of addressing the dyspneic patient's needs. To assist with ongoing efforts to control the symptom, a classification system for nonpharmacological interventions grouped according to the component affected (i.e., breathing, thinking, and functioning) is under development (Booth, 2013).

Cooling and Vibration

When stimulated, temperature and mechanical receptors of the trigeminal nerve in the cheek and nasopharynx alter feedback to the brain and modify the perception of dyspnea. The use of a fan set on low speed and directed toward the face will stimulate this response (Booth, Moosavi, & Higginson, 2008; Elia & Thomas, 2008). In a study of 50 patients with advanced disease who were not on oxygen, Galbraith, Fagan, Perkins, Lynch, and Booth (2010) demonstrated a significant decrease in dyspnea when air from a handheld electric fan was directed toward the face for 5 minutes. In some patients, the effect continued even after discontinuation of the airflow stimulation. The same intervention demonstrated a significant reduction in dyspnea and respiratory rate in patients with lung cancer when compared to diaphragmatic breathing alone (Puspawati, Sitorus, & Herawati, 2017). Kako et al. (2018) reported similar results with an effect duration of more than 1 hour, although an end point was not evaluated. Cooling the body may have a beneficial effect as well. Simple techniques include applying cool damp cloths to the forehead or chest; offering a cool water sponge bath; or providing a clean, fresh pillow. Altering the environment by circulating cool air with either an air conditioning unit or a ceiling fan, or by placing the patient by an open window, may add an element of comfort (Williams, 2006). Dee always kept her ceiling fan and air conditioning on for better (and cooler) air movement within her room.

Stimulation of the mechanical receptors in the respiratory muscles can alter the sensation of dyspnea, too. This accounts for why chest wall vibration is helpful in some patients (Parshall et al., 2012). An electric massager can be purchased for this use, which also helps with relaxation and relief of pain. Another stimulatory modality, called acu-transcutaneous electrical nerve stimulation (TENS), is showing promise in its over acupoints. A double-blind randomized controlled trial (RCT) showed decreased dyspnea and respiratory rate and increased FEV1 and beta-endorphin in ambulatory patients with COPD during a 45-minute acu-TENS session (Ngai, Jones, Hui-Chan, & Yu, 2011). Further investigation is warranted to evaluate the effects in a PC setting. However, in a Cochrane review both chest wall vibration (CWV) and TENS demonstrated strong evidence for reducing dyspnea (Bausewein, Booth, Gysels, & Higginson, 2008). Similarly, the use of neuromuscular electrical stimulation applied bilaterally to the quadriceps muscles of patients with COPD (twice daily 5 d/wk for 8 weeks) resulted in significant reduction in dyspnea, increased endurance, and improved mechanical efficiency (Vieira et al., 2014).

Breathing Retraining

Diaphragmatic and pursed-lip breathing have been advocated to relieve dyspnea, especially in patients with COPD; however, relief is highly variable. Moreover, patients often resort to rapid, shallow breathing when unobserved. Despite these inconsistencies, both techniques offer an option that has no associated cost, is readily available, and can be easily learned. In some patients, breathing exercises can promote effective lung function, feelings of relaxation, and stress reduction (Cairns, 2012). Families can play an active role in the patient's care by learning these techniques and coaching the patient during daily interactions. Dee was already trained in pursed-lip breathing and naturally resorted to this technique with exertion but not so much at rest.

Positioning

Patients should be assisted to find a position of comfort. The leaning-forward position has been reported to improve overall inspiratory muscle strength, increase diaphragmatic excursion, and decrease abdominal paradoxical breathing as well as reduce dyspnea in patients with COPD (Parshall et al., 2012). While reducing the participation of the chest wall and neck muscles overall, sitting and leaning forward with arms supported on a table facilitates a more focused effort on respiration rather than on maintenance of body posture and/or arm movement (Campbell, 1996; Spector et al., 2007). Dee did not alter her body position much except for elevating the head of her bed, as mentioned earlier.

Optimal comfort as well as ventilation and perfusion may be accomplished by placing the patient's good lung in a dependent position where gravity may assist in perfusing the healthiest area of lung tissue. In some patients, terminal dyspnea may be relieved only by an upright position, where vital capacity is increased because of the lowered diaphragm. The clinician should accept the patient's position of choice, even if it belies traditional thinking.

Energy Conservation

Activities of daily living strain dyspneic patients even if they are passive during the activity. Walking aids, such as a wheeled walker or rollator, allow forward leaning and may decrease the work of breathing and increase confidence. Oxygen consumption is increased with any activity, so it is important to allow for an adequate recovery period. All care should be evaluated with regard to what the patient can tolerate and what is desired. In some cases, the activity or intervention can be modified to accommodate decreased tolerance. For example, a bath and linen change could be stretched out over the course of several hours, focused on face and hands only, or eliminated entirely. As noted earlier, a position of comfort is not only helpful but also critical to accommodating the patient's wants/needs with any required activities. However, if the care is more burdensome than beneficial, it should be reevaluated regarding the merit in continuing it (Ben-Aharon et al., 2008). Dee was instructed on energy conservation and pacing her activities, but this required ongoing review and reinforcement. She continued to insist on walking to the bathroom, even at night, instead of using the bedside commode.

■ COGNITIVE-BEHAVIORAL APPROACHES/ COMPLEMENTARY THERAPIES

Distraction and relaxation strategies are important and useful adjuncts in the treatment of dyspnea. Distraction helps to focus the patient on something other than breathing. Relaxation eases muscular tension, thereby allowing breathing to be less strenuous and more effective. One method, guided imagery, uses mental images to promote relaxation. Other therapeutic activities include mindfulness, stress-reduction techniques, massage, music therapy, Reiki, therapeutic touch, and aromatherapy. Yoga demonstrated a small improvement in dyspnea scores when taught to patients with COPD, though the difference was not statistically significant (Donesky-Cuenco, Nguyen, Paul, & Carrieri-Kohlman, 2009; Melendez, Nguyen, & Carrieri-Kohlman, 2012). In any case, a wide range of alternatives evaluated in a systematic review of 47 RCTs and controlled clinical trials failed to provide enough evidence to yield specific recommendations related to complementary therapies (Bausewein et al., 2008).

Acupuncture and acupressure have emerged as possible options for relief of dyspnea. Acupuncture has already been integrated into PC settings in the United Kingdom (Suzuki et al., 2008). A review of the literature found 27 randomized controlled clinical trials, with 23 reporting statistically significant results for symptoms such as dyspnea, pain, nausea, and vomiting (Standish, Kozak, & Congdon, 2008). Recently, the COPD-acupuncture trial (CAT) found that exertional dyspnea was reduced after the 6-minute walk test in patients with COPD who received acupuncture weekly for 12 sessions compared with a similar group who received placebo (Suzuki et al., 2012). However, the results for dyspnea alone are mixed; thus, the evidence remains low to moderate. More research is needed to evaluate the potential benefits of this modality.

A number of essential oils (highly concentrated plant constituents) are thought to enhance respiration. These oils possess certain qualities such as expectorant, mucolytic, antiallergic, or immune stimulant; some also have antiviral and antibacterial benefits. No randomized controlled clinical trials have been conducted with the specific end point of reduced dyspnea. However, one

randomized, crossover, washout trial was conducted with 50 hospitalized patients with leukemia to determine if aromatherapy improves insomnia and other symptoms (Blackburn et al., 2017). Only sleeplessness demonstrated statistical significance, even though anxiety, dyspnea, and other symptoms showed improvement. Most of the essential oils useful in respiratory conditions come from the bark, leaves, berries, and branches of certain trees. Once properly diluted, essential oils can be applied directly to the skin (check for sensitivity first), in the form of massage, placed on pulse points, or inhaled through the use of a diffuser, aroma lamp, vaporizer, humidifier, or an absorbent material, such as a cotton ball. Hongratanaworakit (2011) found a reduction in autonomic arousal (heart rate, blood pressure) and improved affective scores (relaxed, calm) after blended essential oils were applied topically to the skin when compared with placebo. Oils are non–habit forming and excreted via the kidneys, skin, or lungs. Essential oils that can be used for dyspnea include eucalyptus, peppermint, ginger, hyssop, lavender, bergamot, basil, pine, sandalwood, and cypress. Blends of various oils are commonly used to achieve the maximum effect.

Education of the patient and family on dyspnea management techniques and the basic rationale for each empowers them to take an active role in the treatment plan. Coaching both the patient and the family reinforces these interventions. Mularski et al. (2013) recommend formulating an action plan for crisis episodes and routine practice of "what to do" at each encounter. Active listening and emotional support by the nurse encourages expression of thoughts and feelings and also helps with early identification of potential problems. Benefits have been achieved using a rehabilitative approach that combines breathing retraining, psychosocial support, and help to develop adaptive strategies for breathlessness (Bredin et al., 1999; Corner, Plant, A'Hern, & Bailey, 1996; Hately, Laurence, Scott, Baker, & Thomas, 2003; Wadell et al., 2013). This was clearly found in a systematic review conducted by McCarthy et al. (2015), where 65 RCTs showed strong evidence for pulmonary rehabilitation in the management of COPD. Questions emerging from the analysis include identification of key components, ideal length and location, degree of supervision and intensity of training required, and length of treatment effect. In the case study, every effort was made to include at least one of Dee's caregivers at each visit when teaching relaxation techniques, such as imaging and focused breathing. However, a more formalized action plan with regular practice may have been helpful.

Building on the rehabilitative approach, Higginson et al. (2014) conducted an RCT of an integrated palliative and respiratory care service for patients with advanced disease and refractory breathlessness. Mastery of dyspnea in the intervention group led to increased survival, significant for patients with COPD and interstitial lung disease, but not cancer. Farquhar et al. (2014) found similar results in a mixed-methods RCT that included patients with advanced cancer and their caregivers as recipients of a Breathlessness Intervention Service (BIS). A second mixed-methods RCT by Farquhar et al. (2016) utilizing the BIS for patients with nonmalignant disease and their caregivers demonstrated a positive impact qualitatively but was not statistically significant. Also, the costs were slightly higher in contrast to the study with cancer patients, where the BIS was found to be both clinically effective and cost-effective. Caregiver inclusion in breathlessness programs may help reduce the isolation and burden they experience as well as promote management techniques for symptom relief (Janssen, Wouters, & Spruit, 2015; Malik et al., 2013; Marques et al., 2015).

■ NONINVASIVE POSITIVE PRESSURE VENTILATION

Noninvasive positive pressure ventilation (NIV), often referred to as bilevel positive airway pressure (BiPAP), represents a controversial alternative method to treat dyspnea. While it is widely accepted as a curative intervention, only one study has been conducted on NIV as a comfort measure at the end of life. In a randomized feasibility study, Nava et al. (2013) compared NIV with oxygen therapy in 200 patients with end-stage cancer. Dyspnea decreased more rapidly and the total morphine dose was lower in the NIV group compared with the oxygen group. The most benefit occurred within the first hour of treatment and in hypercapnic patients.

For patients with advanced motor neuron diseases such as amyotrophic lateral sclerosis, NIV is considered the standard of care in the final phase of life (Tripodoro & De Vito, 2008). For patients who choose to forego endotracheal intubation in the presence of respiratory failure, the best candidates for NIV are patients with COPD, cardiogenic pulmonary edema, and immunosuppression (Schettino, Altobelli, & Kacmarek, 2005) with mixed results for patients with advanced cancer (Cuomo et al., 2004). The Society of Critical Care Medicine Task Force on the Palliative Use of NIV developed a framework for using NIV in patients with acute respiratory failure, especially for those patients who decline endotracheal intubation or who are receiving PC (Curtis et al., 2007). The proposed result is a categorical approach using an ethical framework based on the goals of care and informed patient and family preferences.

Frequent, ongoing, and interprofessional patient and family communication is inherent in choosing or continuing NIV as an intervention. Clinical practice guidelines developed in Germany state that success of NIV for PC is measured by an improvement in dyspnea without adverse effects and the ability to communicate with family (Schonhofer et al., 2008). NIV should be discontinued if it is not meeting these goals or causing unnecessary discomfort.

Advantages include a lack of adverse effects when compared to medications, continued patient participation, maintenance of communication, and relief of dyspnea and other symptoms related to hypoxia or hypercarbia. Disadvantages include the cost of equipment, hospice restrictions, lack of hypercarbic effect at the end of life (potential for increased suffering), the potential to decrease the use of analgesics and anxiolytics prematurely, and the question of when/how to discontinue therapy (Booth et al., 2003; Williams, 2006). Adverse effects include facial irritation or discomfort, gastric distention, nasal/oral dryness or congestion, air leaks, failure to ventilate effectively, failure to tolerate, and, rarely, aspiration (Schettino et al., 2005).

As yet, many questions remain about the role of NIV at the end of life. However, if used in conjunction with traditional therapies, it may evolve into an effective tool for relieving dyspnea and improving QOL in terminal patients by reducing the demand on respiratory muscles. At this point, surveys indicate that physicians and respiratory therapists are using NIV in patients with "do not resuscitate" orders but are less inclined to use it for patients choosing comfort measures only (Sinuff et al., 2008). Other technological advances that may be of value for the dyspneic patient include laser therapy and the placement of endobronchial or tracheal stents to facilitate airway dilation, especially with tumor encroachment. In addition, recent case reports have suggested compassionate intubation for refractory dyspnea in cancer patients with extensive pulmonary metastases and/or airway impingement or obstruction (Habashy, Caldwell, & Baker, 2017).

Another advancement is a minimally invasive alternative to the treatment of chronic or recurrent pleural effusion or malignant abdominal ascites, both of which cause dyspnea. This is an indwelling, cuffed, tunneled catheter placed percutaneously in an outpatient setting that facilitates patient-controlled drainage of either pleural or ascitic fluid without requiring hospitalization or office visits (Suzuki et al., 2011; Tapping, Ling, & Razack, 2012). Not only has this device shown substantial relief of dyspnea but it offers the patient a degree of control at the end of life as well (Arber, Clackson, & Dargan, 2013).

■ PHARMACOLOGICAL THERAPIES

Oxygen

Supplemental oxygen depresses the hypoxic drive, thereby reducing ventilation and subsequently relieving dyspnea. This physiologic response occurs at rest and during exertion in patients with a variety of lung diseases. Oxygen should be titrated to the individual's comfort level using the least restrictive device possible (e.g., nasal cannula does not interfere with eating and communication). Humidification is recommended for comfort and to prevent drying of mucous membranes at or above 4 L/minute. Continuous oxygen has proven to be beneficial in two RCTs in patients with COPD experiencing severe hypoxemia (PaO_2 < 55 mmHg or PaO_2 < 59 mmHg in right-sided heart failure or polycythemia; Medical Research Council Working Party, 1981; Nocturnal Oxygen Therapy Trial Group, 1980). However, some people may prefer to use oxygen intermittently although assurance of the immediate availability of oxygen may be of greater importance. Dee was oxygen dependent and had been for several years. She was accustomed to wearing it and rarely took it off. Her son assisted with titration based on her response. Both were instructed to increase the flow of oxygen prior to activities, such as walking, bathing, or eating.

High concentrations of oxygen can be problematic for those with COPD who are carbon dioxide retainers (i.e., their only drive to breathe is the hypoxic drive), but this should not be a major concern in the final hours of life because hypercarbia produces a sedating effect. Other potential adverse effects of oxygen include activity restriction, cumbersome apparatus, fire hazard, cost, psychological dependence, impaired communication, and difficult withdrawal. In contrast, high-flow nasal oxygen (up to 100% FiO_2) may be appropriate for patients with acute hypoxemic respiratory failure as an alternative to intubation. One RCT found the alleviation of dyspnea and improved physiologic parameters in 23 patients with advanced cancer (Hui et al., 2013). These results justify larger RCTs to determine the best candidates and the potential for long-term benefits. However, high-flow oxygen is currently limited to acute care settings due to equipment and cost.

It should be noted that the benefit of oxygen therapy for patients without hypoxemia remains controversial. High-quality evidence (20/22 RCTs) shows that oxygen improves dyspnea during short-term exercise in COPD, while the evidence for patients with COPD at rest, CHF, and cancer (three small studies, one RCT) is weak (Brunnhuber, Nash, Meier, Weissman, & Woodcock, 2008). In fact, one review found oxygen equivalent to room air in patients with cancer (Booth et al., 2008). Clinical recommendations from the Association of Palliative Medicine emphasize tailored individual assessment and patient/family consultation with ongoing supervision to ensure that the goals of care are met (Booth et al., 2003).

Regardless of whether or not oxygen is indicated, it is frequently prescribed for long-term palliative use in patients with refractory dyspnea (Abernethy, Currow, & Frith, 2004; Abernethy et al., 2010; Abernethy, Wheeler, & Currow, 2010; Stringer, McFarlane, & Hernandez, 2004). Currow, Agar, Smith, and Abernethy (2009) studied dyspnea scores on more than 400 patients (a majority had cancer) before and at 1 and 2 weeks after the introduction of palliative oxygen. The investigators found that only one-third of the population ($n = 150$)

experienced an improvement in breathlessness. Predictive characteristics in the responders could not be identified. Overall, there was no clinically significant improvement with palliative oxygen in these subjects. The study authors suggested that, since oxygen is assumed to be beneficial, clinicians need to remember to conduct a reassessment after a week of therapy; if no benefit is perceived, discontinue the oxygen. Alternatively, there are patients as found in this study who may benefit from oxygen that does not meet standard (i.e., Medicare) criteria. For example, in a Cochrane review and meta-analysis by Uronis, McCrory, Samsa, Currow, and Abernethy (2011), 18 studies demonstrated oxygen effectiveness for people mildly hypoxemic or nonhypoxemic with COPD. Yet, in an updated Cochrane review and meta-analysis by Ekstrom, Ahmadi, Bornefalk-Hermansson, Abernethy, and Currow (2016), oxygen was found to relieve breathlessness primarily during exercise in mildly or nonhypoxemic patients with COPD (25 studies). No evidence demonstrated improvement in health-related QOL or benefit in daily life.

Based on the evidence, Abernethy et al. (2010) recommended that if oxygen is prescribed, appropriate patients should have dyspnea scores of 4 points or more on a 0 to 10 NRS; those with scores of greater than or equal to 7 points might be even more likely to experience benefit. The most benefit is likely to be observed in the first 24 hours of therapy with no additional benefit after 3 days. Therefore, a therapeutic trial should last no longer than 72 hours. Furthermore, in patients near death or without signs of respiratory distress, oxygen is not supported (Campbell, Yarandi, & Dove-Medows, 2013). A research agenda has been proposed to determine mechanisms whereby oxygen may help ameliorate dyspnea, define subgroups for whom oxygen therapy may be beneficial, and identify the true role of palliative oxygen, clinically relevant burdens, and drivers for prescribing oxygen (Johnson, Abernethy, & Currow, 2013).

Due to the decrease in airway resistance when helium is inhaled with oxygen, heliox gas mixtures for the relief of dyspnea have stimulated interest in this modality. Heliox reduces dynamic hyperinflation as well as decreases work of breathing in patients with COPD (Chiappa et al., 2009) and improves exercise tolerance in patients with lung cancer (Laude & Ahmedzai, 2007). Ahmedzai, Laude, Robertson, Troy, and Vora (2004) conducted a double-blind RCT of lung cancer patients with promising results, but the effectiveness has not yet been established pending further investigation. Widespread use of heliox may be limited by cost, equipment logistics, geographical availability, and a lack of guidelines for patient selection (Kamal et al., 2012).

Opioids

Opioids reduce dyspnea through a number of mechanisms: decreasing the ventilatory response to hypercapnia and hypoxia, reducing metabolic rate and oxygen consumption, and altering the perception of breathlessness. Furthermore, the cardiovascular effects of vasodilatation and decreased peripheral resistance help to improve oxygen supply and reduce lung congestion.

Despite concerns regarding the use of opioids, morphine therapy forms the basis for treatment of dyspnea at the end of life. One study found that improving the use of opioids is mostly a matter of improving communication and empathy between providers and patients (Bendiane et al., 2005). Opioids are very beneficial for many cardiopulmonary conditions, including lung cancer, CHF, COPD, and interstitial lung disease, as well as neuromuscular and other problems. The strongest evidence is for patients with COPD (12 RCTs), while the weakest is for patients with cancer and CHF (2 RCTs; Ben-Aharon et al., 2008; Brunnhuber et al., 2008; Jennings, Davies, Higgins, Gibbs, & Broadley, 2002; Lorenz et al., 2008; Oxberry et al., 2011). In chronic dyspnea, Currow et al. (2011) found 10 mg of sustained-release oral morphine once daily was safe and effective for 70% of patients ($n = 58$), most of whom suffered from COPD. For the subjects who remained on opioids for the length of the study, benefit was maintained at 3 months.

There is no ceiling dose with opioids, so it is appropriate to titrate morphine to the desired effect, that is, dosing interval and quantity based on frequent symptom assessment and limited only by intolerable side effects. Commonly seen side effects include constipation, nausea and vomiting, urinary retention, altered mental status, and drowsiness; tolerance to all of these side effects, except constipation, usually occurs within a week. A bowel regimen should always be established when opioids are prescribed to prevent constipation. While the most feared opioid-related side effect is respiratory depression, titration for symptoms has not been shown to cause it (Estfan et al., 2007). In fact, respiratory depression appears primarily to be an effect of rapid escalation of the drug (Hallenbeck, 2012). Furthermore, Bengoechea, Gutierrez, Vrotsou, Onaindia, and Lopez (2010) found a longer median survival time for patients with cancer who received at least twice their initial dose of opioids (22 days) than those who did not (9 days).

The oral route of morphine is preferred at the end of life because it is better tolerated, least invasive, and less costly. Other routes, such as sublingual, rectal, IV, subcutaneous, or aerosolized, can be utilized. Furthermore, a pilot study demonstrated relief of dyspnea in patients with advanced emphysema using epidural methadone without adverse effects (Juan et al., 2005). Opioid-naïve adults start with the morphine equivalent of 5 mg orally every 4 hours, and thereafter, increase the dose 30% to 50% daily or more frequently until dyspnea is relieved or sedation or other adverse effects become problematic (Elia & Thomas, 2008; Rousseau, 1997). For those already receiving morphine and experiencing dyspnea as a new symptom, the dose should be increased by 25% to 50% daily for mild-to-moderate dyspnea and

50% to 100% for moderate-to-severe dyspnea and then titrated accordingly (Elia & Thomas, 2008; Rousseau, 1997). Dee started on immediate-release morphine at 5 mg for episodes of dyspnea, as often as needed. A trial of long-acting morphine (30 mg twice daily) was conducted, but her son believed it was too sedating, so it was discontinued. She continued on gabapentin for her fibromyalgia pain with good effect.

While morphine is the primary opioid studied, fentanyl is another opioid under investigation for its potential effect on dyspnea. A randomized, double-blind, crossover clinical trial by Pinna, Bruera, Moralo, Correas, and Vargas (2015) was conducted to evaluate the efficacy of oral transmucosal fentanyl citrate (OTFC) on exertional dyspnea in patients with advanced cancer. In the first visit, 13 patients were assigned to receive either investigational drug or placebo, and vice versa in the second visit. Testing occurred before and after the intervention and included oxygen saturation, distance in a 6-minute walk test, and Edmonton Symptom Assessment score. No differences were noted between the treatments in any of the measures. Hui et al. (2014) found opposite results after conduction of a preliminary, double-blind RCT with subcutaneous fentanyl in 20 patients with cancer. Dyspnea scores, distance walked, and respiratory rate showed significant improvements; however, the placebo arm also demonstrated improvement, though not statistically significant. An exploratory study of IV fentanyl was undertaken to determine the efficacy in hospitalized dyspneic patients with terminal cancer (Pang, Qu, Tan, & Yee, 2016). Of 16 patients, seven responded favorably, reporting less dyspnea, but the results were not significant when compared to the nonresponders. No other measures were taken except categorical dyspnea scores (mild, moderate, severe), self-reported at baseline and again at 24 hours after the fentanyl infusion. Hospitalized patients with cancer were also the subjects for a clinical trial of nebulized inhaled fentanyl, where patient perception, respiratory rate, and oxygen saturation were measured (Coyne, Viswanathan, & Smith, 2002). Twenty-six of 32 patients reported significant improvement in breathing; oxygen saturation and respiratory rate also improved. No adverse events were noted in any of the studies. Lastly, Simon, Koskeroglu, Gaertner, and Voltz (2013) performed a systematic review of the evidence surrounding fentanyl. Of the two RCTs available at the time, one included only two patients and the other failed to demonstrate significance compared with placebo. Therefore, with the exception of Pinna et al. (2015), all the investigators have recommended more research, especially with larger RCTs.

Since opioid receptors have been demonstrated to exist in the airways, nebulized morphine, hydromorphone, or fentanyl can be given in addition to systemic opioids or alone (Coyne, 2003; Shirk, Donahue, & Shirvani, 2006). Some patients experience relief of dyspnea with fewer side effects due to the lack of systemic concentration achieved by inhalation. However, morphine and hydromorphone can cause histamine release leading to bronchoconstriction; thus, the preference by some for fentanyl. Regardless, this method of delivery remains controversial as studies have been conflicting, with nine RCTs demonstrating no symptomatic improvement (Bausewein & Simon, 2014; Ben-Aharon et al., 2008; Jennings, Davies, Higgins, & Broadley, 2001). Nevertheless, commonly used initial doses of preservative-free injectable solution are morphine 2.5 to 10 mg, hydromorphone 0.25 to 1 mg, and fentanyl 25 mg diluted in 2 mL of normal saline (Charles et al., 2008; Ferraresi, 2005).

One protocol recommends nebulized morphine only when intolerable side effects have occurred from systemic administration (Spector, Klein, & Rice-Wiley, 2000). This protocol begins at a conservative dose of 5 mg and titrates up to a maximum of 40 mg every 4 hours; the protocol includes frequent reevaluation of breathlessness. Dyspnea refractory to other routes of administration may justify a trial of nebulized opioids. However, further research is needed to determine what patients may achieve maximum benefit.

Anxiolytics

Although not supported by RCT evidence for frontline therapy (Ben-Aharon, Gafter-Gvili, Leibovici, & Stemmer, 2012; Simon et al., 2016), an anxiolytic may help relieve dyspnea when morphine is not completely effective; anxiety is often one of the dimensions of dyspnea (Navigante, Cerchietti, Castro, Lutteral, & Cabalar, 2006; Reddy, Parsons, Elsayem, Palmer, & Bruera, 2009). Anxiolytics should be considered in combination with opioids and nonpharmacological anxiety-reduction measures as a way to break the anxiety and shortness of breath cycle (Bausewein & Simon, 2013; Clemens & Klaschik, 2011; Elia & Thomas, 2008). Low-dose benzodiazepines and phenothiazines are the categories of anxiolytics most commonly used in the management of dyspnea. These drugs have hypnotic, sedative, anxiolytic, anticonvulsant, and muscle-relaxant actions, thereby achieving control of dyspnea via multiple mechanisms of action. Benzodiazepines depress the hypoxic/hypercapnic ventilatory response as well as alter the emotional response to dyspnea (Parshall et al., 2012). Specifically, they bind to a site on the gamma-aminobutyric acid (GABA) receptor and potentiate the action of GABA, which acts as an inhibitory neurotransmitter in the CNS. One consideration with the use of long-term anxiolytics is the possibility of worsening the respiratory condition through excessive muscle relaxation. Dee had been taking benzodiazepines for years prior to palliative and hospice care. She continued to self-medicate with alprazolam, but its positive effect became less pronounced with disease progression.

Due to the long half-life of oral anxiolytics, some patients are unable to tolerate the side effects of prolonged sedation and cognitive impairment. Nevertheless,

lorazepam 0.5 to 2.0 mg sublingual/oral every 4 to 6 hours as needed or around the clock (ATC) is frequently used (Dahlin, 2006). To break a severe anxiety–dyspnea cycle, the medication can be given as often as hourly until the patient is comfortable (Dahlin, 2006). Side effects include drowsiness, ataxia, reduced psychomotor performance, loss of appetite, and perceptual disturbances. Diazepam, alprazolam, clonazepam, buspirone, and chlorpromazine are considered alternative medications (Allcroft et al., 2013; Elia & Thomas, 2008; Spector et al., 2007).

Subcutaneous midazolam (5 mg every 4 hours) has been reported as a safe and effective adjunct to morphine in advanced cancer patients (Navigante et al., 2006). In this prospective, randomized, single-blind study, dyspneic cancer patients received either (a) ATC morphine with midazolam for breakthrough dyspnea, (b) ATC midazolam with morphine for breakthrough, or (c) ATC morphine plus midazolam with morphine for breakthrough. Dyspnea relief was achieved at the rates of 69%, 46%, and 92%, respectively. Midazolam may be better tolerated than other benzodiazepines due to a shorter half-life (less than 5 hours) and lack of active metabolites. More recently, a study of 63 ambulatory patients with cancer-related dyspnea were randomized to receive either oral morphine or oral midazolam (Navigante, Castro, & Cerchietti, 2010). Patients in both groups had a reduction of dyspnea by at least 50% during the initial phase of the study. For the control of baseline and breakthrough dyspnea, midazolam was superior to morphine in the ambulatory phase of the study. The investigators concluded that oral midazolam could be considered as a first-line option for cancer-related dyspnea in ambulatory patients.

Corticosteroids

Corticosteroids, while controversial in the treatment of dyspnea, may be of value because they reduce inflammation by suppressing the migration of polymorphonuclear leukocytes and reversing the increase in capillary permeability. Euphoria in the form of an overall feeling of well-being and an increase in appetite exhibit as secondary responses. In the lungs, corticosteroids decrease airway inflammation that may be experienced with COPD and radiation or drug-induced pneumonitis, reduce edema associated with tracheal or lung tumors, and increase vital capacity in interstitial disease.

Corticosteroids can improve airway obstruction in cases of carcinomatous lymphangitis or superior vena cava syndrome (Lin, Adelman, & Mehta, 2012). Maeda and Hayakawa (2017) studied more than 50 patients with terminal cancer and found those that responded to corticosteroids had a prolonged survival time compared to patients who did not respond to corticosteroids. The dose and duration of therapy for dexamethasone and prednisone, two commonly used drugs, depend on the patient's condition and response. Starting doses are usually high, and then reduced to a lower maintenance dose. Adverse reactions (such as insomnia, nervousness, delirium, and hyperglycemia) are not unusual; the nurse should monitor the patient closely for any untoward outcomes. Corticosteroids can be given orally, subcutaneously, intramuscularly, intravenously, or by inhalation. Dee benefited greatly from her burst of prednisone, so it was tapered to 10 mg daily and continued until near the end of her life.

Bronchodilators

With substantial evidence from RCTs (Gotfried, Kerwin, Lawrence, Lassen, & Kramer, 2012; Jones, Mahler, Gale, Owen, & Kramer, 2011), a trial of bronchodilator therapy is warranted to relieve dyspnea, especially with COPD, asthma, or other problems associated with reactive airways (Parshall et al., 2012). Beta-2 agonists and anticholinergics cause smooth muscle dilation of the airways, thus removing any impedance to airflow and deflating an overinflated lung. In patients with COPD, both classes of bronchodilators increase the resting inspiratory capacity about 15% above baseline, a change that promotes reduced dyspnea and increased endurance (Mahler & O'Donnell, 2015). Two approved combinations of long-acting beta-2 agonists and long-acting anticholinergics in a single dry powder inhaler have shown significant and clinically meaningful improvement in dyspnea in RCTs (Mahler et al., 2012, 2014). The magnitude of improvement in dyspnea scores was greater than with a single bronchodilator. Bronchodilators also stabilize mast cells and stimulate the respiratory tract cilia to expel mucus. The preferred route is inhaled, either by a metered dose inhaler or by a nebulizer, but the drug is also available in oral preparations. Side effects such as tremors, agitation, and anxiety that may heighten the dyspnea are due to sympathetic stimulation. These potential systemic effects, however, are greater with the oral route. The patient's response should dictate the use of bronchodilators. Initially, Dee often used a bronchodilator/anticholinergic nebulized treatment to ease her breathing several times each day. However, even this therapy became ineffective over time.

Diuretics

Dyspnea may be associated with fluid volume excess, which can be treated with diuretics, such as furosemide, to mobilize edema, normalize blood volume, reduce vascular congestion, and reduce the workload of the heart (Oxberry & Johnson, 2008; Spector et al., 2007). Furosemide inhibits reabsorption of sodium and chloride in the ascending loop of Henle and distal renal tubule, interfering with the chloride-binding cotransport system, thus causing increased excretion of water and electrolytes. Normal doses can be administered orally, subcutaneously, intramuscularly, intravenously, and by inhalation. For conditions where diuresis is urgently needed (e.g., CHF or pulmonary edema), the IV form may be preferred. Other disease states where diuretics may be helpful to relieve dyspnea include pulmonary hypertension and abdominal ascites (Selecky et al., 2005). For the control of dyspnea refractory to standard treatments, inhaled furosemide has been tried. Thus far, a few small trials in patients with COPD show promising results and warrant further investigation (Jensen, Amjadi, Harris-McAllister, Webb, & O'Donnell, 2008; Ong, Kor, Chong, Earnest, & Wang, 2004; Sheikh et al., 2013). Of note, all these studies use nebulized saline as the control arm, which also improved dyspnea scores, thereby indicating a possible role in dyspnea management (Khan & O'Driscoll, 2004; Barbetta, Currow, & Johnson, 2017).

Anticholinergics

The lack of ability to protect one's airway in the final hours of life contributes to the build-up of secretions that lead to what is commonly referred to as the "death rattle" (i.e., noisy breathing). While caregivers consider it to be a disturbing symptom for families and loved ones of the patient, recent studies have found that this is not necessarily the case (Wee, Coleman, Hillier, & Holgate, 2006). In contrast, it does have a negative impact on staff and volunteers working with dying patients, causing them to act without knowing which treatment is the most effective (Wee & Hillier, 2008; Wee et al., 2006). The "death rattle" occurs in 25% to 92% of dying patients, occurs more commonly in men and patients with brain and lung neoplasms, and predicts most will die within 48 hours (Bennett, 1996; Plonk & Arnold, 2005; Wildiers & Menten, 2002). It is caused by the collection of secretions in the bronchi and posterior oropharynx, a decreased ability to swallow, an absent cough reflex, and, in severe cases of cardiopulmonary failure, pulmonary edema (Bickel & Arnold, 2008; Picella, 1997).

Despite the lack of evidence-based guidelines, the standard of care has been to use anticholinergic drugs, namely, scopolamine, hyoscyamine, glycopyrrolate, and atropine (Bickel & Arnold, 2008). The mechanism of action is the blockade of acetylcholine at parasympathetic sites in smooth muscle, secretory glands, and the CNS with the primary clinical effect of inhibition of salivary secretions. Side effects are generally not reported as the patient is unresponsive but may include dry mouth, urinary retention, visual disturbances, and less often confusion.

No controlled studies have determined if anticholinergics are the treatment of choice and, if so, which drug/dosage/route is best (Lokker, VanZuylen, VanderRijt, & VanderHeide, 2014; Wee & Hillier, 2008). Only glycopyrrolate crosses the blood–brain barrier, making it not only more potent but also more erratically and poorly absorbed (Bickel & Arnold, 2008). The scopolamine patch is convenient with the dosage being one to three patches every 3 days (Bickel & Arnold, 2008). Hyoscyamine offers the most flexibility as it comes in short-acting, sustained-released oral tablets and solution (Bickel & Arnold, 2008). Anecdotal and case reports suggest the use of atropine eye drops sublingually as a reasonable alternative, as long as side effects are monitored (e.g., tachycardia; Shinjo & Okada, 2013). Wildiers et al. (2009) compared the effectiveness of atropine, hyoscine, and scopolamine in 333 terminal patients with death rattle. All three medications decreased the intensity of the rattle with no significant differences between them. However, the route of administration was subcutaneous, which may not be practical in the home setting. Treatment was more effective when started as soon as the rattle was detected. Nonpharmacological interventions have not been studied either but include positioning (side-lying or semiprone), gentle oropharyngeal suctioning, postural drainage, and reduced fluid intake (Bickel & Arnold, 2008; Lawrey, 2005; Plonk & Arnold, 2005). Once Dee was transferred to hospice, she was positioned on her side and given atropine ophthalmic drops sublingually every 4 hours to decrease secretions. She suffered no untoward effects from the atropine.

■ CONCLUSION

Dyspnea is a frequent, multidimensional, self-reported symptom that is often underreported or undertreated, resulting in symptom invisibility (Gysels & Higginson, 2008). Individuals with contributory behaviors, such as cigarette smoking, are less apt to seek treatment due to guilt or embarrassment. In addition, children and elders experience age-related symptom differences that magnify underreporting. Healthcare professionals often associate improved physiological parameters with a reduction in dyspnea and consider the symptom managed without continued assessment.

In actuality, dyspnea does not necessarily correlate with disease management. Despite improved lung function, dyspnea may be acute and short lasting or chronic with episodic crises. Furthermore, individual dyspnea trajectories do not match collective disease trajectories (Bausewein et al., 2010). In other words, though a pattern of dyspnea exists in patients with cancer and patients with COPD, individual specificity remains. Overall, the symptom is strongly associated with anxiety and panic, seriously impacting the QOL. Individuals with dyspnea suffer from a loss of independence, decreased mobility, fear, isolation, and helplessness. People living with dyspnea are not the only ones impacted; loved ones and caregivers often suffer from anxiety, fear, and prolonged grief disorder.

Freeman et al. (2015) propose that dyspnea is not inevitable in PC if professionals are diligent in assessing and proactive in managing the symptom using an integrated approach. Thus, all aspects of the symptom should be addressed, the underlying condition as well as the affective, sensory, and cognitive dimensions. At the very least, the intensity of dyspnea should be measured before and after interventions using an appropriate tool (Mularski et al., 2013). Treatment typically consists of opioids, anxiolytics, and oxygen in select subgroups. Positioning, energy conservation, crisis-management plans, and complementary therapies add benefit to the treatment plan. Time-limited trials may be most helpful as a variety of interventions are chosen based on patient, caregiver, and provider preferences. Furthermore, an n-of-1 study may be justified when seeking resolution of the symptom (Mularski et al., 2013).

Despite progress made in the treatment and management of dyspnea, too many individuals continue to suffer breathlessness at the end of life (Campbell, 2012). Morris and Galicia-Castillo (2017) found nearly 85% of patients dying in the hospital experienced dyspnea, yet healthcare providers noted only 50% as dyspneic. The ATS concludes that progress in management has not matched the progress in understanding the physiological mechanisms underlying dyspnea (Parshall et al., 2012). Two research areas have been identified: (1) interdisciplinary translational research to connect dyspnea mechanisms with treatments and (2) validated dyspnea measures as patient-reported outcomes in clinical trials. The Hospice and Palliative Nurses Association (HPNA, 2014) has outlined a similar agenda, namely, interventional studies, measurement trials, and assessment of family/caregiver needs.

An international breathlessness interest group met recently to discuss trends in dyspnea research (Chin et al., 2015). Functional brain-imaging techniques are leading future investigations of dyspnea mechanisms. The focus is on neural responses to therapies, as revealed by magneto-encephalography scanning (MEG), and neural involvement with the emotional and mechanical control of breathing, as detected by diffusion tractography. Oxygen and long-acting and nebulized morphine are pharmaceuticals that continue to be studied for the potential benefit in subgroups of people with dyspnea. Banzett & O'Donnell (2014), and others propose a routine assessment of dyspnea in all patients in order to reduce suffering as well as to gain understanding of medical needs (Baker et al., 2013; Baker, DeSanto-Madeya, & Banzett, 2017; Pesola, Forde, & Ahsan, 2017). Indeed, Banzett is calling for dyspnea to be the "first vital sign" and continuing to study objective measurements of dyspnea for use in clinical practice (Chin et al., 2015). Nonpharmacological intervention research includes evaluating the concurrent treatment of symptom clusters, that is, breathlessness, cough, and fatigue, in patients with lung cancer. The Living With Breathlessness study continues to investigate the trajectory of dyspnea in patients with COPD and the educational needs of caregivers, including their preferences for content and delivery modes (Farquhar et al., 2014, 2016). With these and other scientific endeavors designed for larger studies and in different subgroups of patients, the future looks hopeful for a better understanding of the complex symptom of dyspnea.

CASE STUDY *Conclusion*

For about 3 weeks, Dee did well with few, if any, episodes of breathing difficulty that did not respond to recommended interventions. But the effect was short lived as the intensity and frequency of her episodes worsened, usually on the weekends when more family was around. Her son, the primary caregiver, also became increasingly anxious and panicky when she did not respond to treatment. It became clear that a supportive plan of care was more appropriate for Dee and her family. We discussed hospice again; she consented with agreement from her family. Medications were adjusted once again, with scheduled morphine and anxiolytics, now supervised by her son. The hospice chaplain and social worker began working with Dee and her family and physical and occupational therapies were discontinued. Nursing visits were increased to three times weekly, usually Monday, Wednesday, and Friday. The treatment plan was reviewed at each visit and every effort was made to include her son and other family members as available.

One weekend shortly after admission to hospice, Dee's dyspnea was refractory to any interventions. She was started on a morphine subcutaneous infusion and transferred to our hospice house. Anxiolytics were given at least every 4 hours, either subcutaneously or sublingually. Within 24 hours, Dee drifted into a moribund state. Her family was at her bedside, though not all at the same time as there was unresolved conflict between at least two of her grown children. Speaking to each of them individually, they were sad but relieved to see their mother comfortable and no longer struggling. According to them, she died a peaceful death. Bereavement follow-up, including grief support, was conducted by the hospice team.

CASE STUDY

AN INTERPROFESSIONAL PERSPECTIVE

Susan M. Collins, BA, MDiv
Chaplain

Dee's chronic obstructive pulmonary disease is life limiting and makes it difficult to enjoy her life; however, she demonstrates little desire to make changes to improve her QOL. Dee has a fixed belief that her COPD and/or comorbidities will take her life soon.

Dee enjoys smoking and her family, even though family visits tend to be contentious. With the exception of e-cigarettes, she has made no change to her smoking habit of 50-plus years; when she is able, she enjoys going to the porch to smoke. Her life is limited to her two-bedroom apartment, with brief family and HHA visits. Her younger son is the primary decision maker. He is fixed in his approach to her life and treatment options and is satisfied for Dee to stay at home alone for several hours at a time while he is at work with only HHA visits. Both Dee and her son are agreeable to increasing services to the home, but decline placement in a long-term care facility or substantial changes in the home. Her son states there are no financial resources for sitters in the home. A lifetime of decisions contributed to this situation and particular outcome.

At this point, Dee is receiving hospice services, which include the supportive services of spiritual care and social workers. Dee believes she will die soon and her son finds death impossible to accept at this point. It is possible that chaplaincy services will help Dee find some peace at the end of her life. A possible earlier intervention for the patient through the family might have been to have turned to her church's spiritual resources. Ultimately, she did respond to spiritual care interventions provided in her apartment, including receiving the sacraments and prayers with the chaplain while on hospice.

Evidence-Based Practice

Luckett, T., Disler, R., Hosie, A., Johnson, M., Davidson, P., Currow, D., ... Phillips, J. (2016). Content and quality of websites supporting self-management of chronic breathlessness in advanced illness: A systematic review. *Primary Care Respiratory Medicine*, 26(16025), 1–5. doi:10.1038/npjpcrm.2016.25

Purpose

Internet-based health information has the potential to influence patient behavior and relations with health professionals in both positive and negative ways. The aim of this study is to describe the content and quality of websites concerned with self-management of chronic breathlessness, highlight underserved areas to inform future content development, and identify any websites posing safety concerns.

Materials and Methods

Google and YouTube were searched using the five most common search terms for breathlessness: breathless, shortness of breath, dyspnea, wheeze, and difficulty breathing. Websites associated with respiratory-related national associations were also searched. Quality appraisal was undertaken by one reviewer using a tool designed for this purpose (AMA benchmarks). Readability was also assessed using the Flesch–Kincaid Grade-level index.

Results

Seventy-five web pages and 16 videos from 44 Internet sites were included in the review. Most items reviewed did not reveal authorship information (54%–77%) and some were not dated (23%). Reading grade ranged from 5 to 16, with more than half failing to meet recommendations to keep the reading level at or below the eighth grade. Content included structured education, breathing techniques, cognitive symptom management, action planning, use of support services, self-efficacy, lifestyle and environmental factors, EOL considerations, and partnering with healthcare professionals. Additional content based on ATC guidelines identified sites with advice on managing breathlessness crises and using pharmacological and nonpharmacological treatments. Only 7% offered information on monitoring breathlessness. No sites offered advice on goal-setting or unsafe advice.

Conclusion

The majority of the websites originated in the United States and focused on breathing techniques and COPD. More content is needed to support self-management such as goal setting, action planning, problem solving, and monitoring of breathlessness. More websites need to deal with the effects of disease progression, such as worsening breathlessness, decline in function, and EOL concerns. Also, more information is needed for the caregivers, especially related to self-care, changing roles, and increasing care required as EOL nears. Interactive sites should be the goal for future development. Lastly, national associations are encouraged to improve the visibility of their resources and pay more attention to the quality and readability of health information.

■ REFERENCES

Abernethy, A. P., Currow, D. C., & Frith, P. (2004). Prescription of palliative oxygen: A clinician survey of expected benefit and patterns of use. *Journal of Palliative Care, 20,* 303–307.

Abernethy, A. P., McDonald, C. F., Frith, P. A., Clark, K., Herndon, J. E., Marcello, J., … Currow, D. C. (2010). Effect of palliative oxygen versus room air in relief of breathlessness in patients with refractory dyspnoea: A double-blind, randomised controlled trial. *Lancet, 376*(9743), 784–793. doi:10.1016/S0140-6736(10)61115-4

Abernethy, A. P., Wheeler, J. L., & Currow, D. C. (2010). Common approaches to dyspnoea management in advanced life-limiting illness. *Current Opinion in Supportive and Palliative Care, 4*(2), 53–55. doi:10.1097/SPC.0b013e328338f921

Ade-Oshifogun, J. B. (2012). Model of functional performance in obese elderly people with chronic obstructive pulmonary disease. *Journal of Nursing Scholarship, 44*(3), 232–241. doi:10.1111/j.1547-5069.2012.01457.x

Ahmedzai, S. H., Laude, E., Robertson, A., Troy, G., & Vora, V. (2004). A double-blind, randomized, controlled phase II trial of Heliox28 gas mixture in lung cancer patients with dyspnea on exertion. *British Journal of Cancer, 90*(2), 366–371. doi:10.1038/sj.bjc.6601527

Allcroft, P., Margitanovic, V., Greene, A., Agar, M. R., Clark, K., Abernethy, A. P., & Currow, D. C. (2013). The role of benzodiazepines in breathlessness: A single site, open label pilot of sustained release morphine together with clonazepam. *Journal of Palliative Medicine, 16*(7), 741–744. doi:10.1089/jpm.2012.0505

American Thoracic Society. (2012). An Official American Thoracic Society Statement: Update on the Mechanisms, Assessment, and Management of Dyspnea. *American Journal of Respiratory and Critical Care Medicine, 185(4),* 435–452. doi:10.1164/rccm.201111-2042ST

Ananth, P., Melvin, P., Feudtner, C., Wolfe, J., & Berry, J. G. (2015). Hospital use in the last year of life for children with life-threatening complex chronic conditions. *Pediatrics, 136*(5), 938–946. doi:10.1542/peds.2015-0260

Arber, A., Clackson, C., & Dargan, S. (2013). Malignant pleural effusion in the palliative care setting. *International Journal of Palliative Nursing, 19*(7), 316–317. doi:10.12968/ijpn.2013.19.7.320

Baker, K., Barsamian, J., Leone, D., Donovan, B. C., Williams, D., Carnevale, K., … Banzett, R. (2013). Routine dyspnea assessment on unit admission. *American Journal of Nursing, 113*(11), 42–50. doi:10.1097/01.NAJ.0000437112.43059.a0

Baker, K., DeSanto-Madeya, S., & Banzett, R. B. (2017). Routine dyspnea assessment and documentation: Nurses' experience yields wide acceptance. *BMC Nursing, 16,* 3. doi:10.1186/s12912-016-0196-9

Banzett, R. B., & O'Donnell, C. R. (2014). Should we measure dyspnea in everyone? *The European Respiratory Journal, 43*(6), 1547–1550. doi:10.1183/09031936.00031114

Barbetta, C., Currow, D. C., & Johnson, M. J. (2017). Non-opioid medications for the relief of chronic breathlessness: Current evidence. *Expert Review of Respiratory Medicine, 11*(4), 333–341. doi:10.1080/17476348.2017.1305896

Barnes, S., Gott, M., Payne, S., Seamark, D., Parker, C., Gariballa, S., & Small, N. (2006). Communication in heart failure: Perspectives from older people and primary care professionals. *Health and Social Care in the Community, 14*(6), 482–490. doi:10.1111/j.1365-2524.2006.00636.x

Bausewein, C., Booth, S., Gysels, M., & Higginson, I. (2008). Non-pharmacological interventions for breathlessness in advanced stages of malignant and non-malignant diseases. *Cochrane Database of Systematic Reviews,* (2), CD005623. doi:10.1002/14651858.CD005623.pub2

Bausewein, C., Booth, S., Gysels, M., Kuhnbach, R., Haberland, B., & Higginson, I. (2010). Individual breathlessness trajectories do not match summary trajectories in advanced cancer and COPD: Results from a longitudinal study. *Palliative Medicine, 24*(8), 777–786. doi:10.1177/0269216310378785

Bausewein, C., Farquhar, M., Booth, S., Gysels, M., & Higginson, I. J. (2007). Measurement of breathlessness in advanced disease: A systematic review. *Respiratory Medicine, 101*(3), 399–410. doi:10.1016/j.rmed.2006.07.003

Bausewein, C., & Simon, S. T. (2013). Shortness of breath and cough in patients in palliative care. *Deutsches Arzteblatt International, 110*(33–34), 563–572. doi:10.3238/arztebl.2013.0563

Bausewein, C., & Simon, S. T. (2014). Inhaled nebulized and intranasal opioids for the relief of breathlessness. *Current Opinion in Supportive and Palliative Care, 8*(3), 208–212. doi:10.1097/SPC.0000000000000071

Ben-Aharon, I., Gafter-Gvili, A., Leibovici, L., & Stemmer, S. M. (2012). Interventions for alleviating cancer-related dyspnea: A systematic review and meta-analysis. *Acta Oncologica, 51*(8), 996–1008. doi:10.3109/0284186X.2012.709638

Ben-Aharon, I., Gafter-Gvili, A., Paul, M., Leibovici, L., & Stemmer, S. M. (2008). Interventions for alleviating cancer-related dyspnea: A systematic review. *Journal of Clinical Oncology, 26*(14), 2396–2404. doi:10.1200/JCO.2007.15.5796

Bendiane, M. K., Peretti-Watel, P., Pegliasco, H., Favre, R., Galinier, A., Lapiana, J. M., & Obadia, Y. (2005). Morphine prescription to terminally ill patients with lung cancer and dyspnea: French physicians' attitudes. *Journal of Opioid Management, 1*(1), 25–30. doi:10.5055/jom.2005.0008

Bengoechea, I., Gutierrez, S. G., Vrotsou, K., Onaindia, M. J., & Lopez, J. M. Q. (2010). Opioid use at the end of life and survival in a hospital at home unit. *Journal of Palliative Medicine, 13*(9), 1079–1083. doi:10.1089/jpm.2010.0031

Bennett, M. I. (1996). Death rattle: An audit of hyoscine (scopolamine) use and review of management. *Journal of Pain and Symptom Management, 12*(4), 229–233. doi:10.1016/0885-3924(96)00151-0

Bickel, K., & Arnold, R. M. (2008). Death rattle and oral secretions–second edition #109. *Journal of Palliative Medicine, 11*(7), 1040–1041. doi:10.1089/jpm.2008.9865

Blackburn, L., Achor, S., Allen, B., Bauchmire, N., Dunnington, D., Klisovic, R. B., Naber, S. J., … Chipps, E. (2017). The effect of aromatherapy on insomnia and other common symptoms among patients with acute leukemia. *Oncology Nursing Forum, 44*(4), E185–E193. doi:10.1188/17.ONF.E185-E193

Blume, E. D., Balkin, E. M., Aiyagari, R., Ziniel, S., Beke, D. M., Thiagarajan, R., ... Wolfe, J. (2014). Parental perspectives on suffering and quality of life at end-of-life in children with advanced heart disease: An exploratory study. *Pediatric Critical Care Medicine, 15*(4), 336–342. doi:10.1097/PCC.0000000000000072

Booth, C. M., Matukas, L. M., Tomlinson, G. A., Rachlis, A. R., Rose, D. B., Dwosh, H. A., ... Detsky, A. S. (2003). Clinical features and short-term outcomes of 144 patients with SARS in the greater Toronto area. *Journal of the American Medical Association, 289*(21), 2801–2809. doi:10.1001/jama.289.21.JOC30885

Booth, S. (2013). Science supporting the art of medicine: Improving the management of breathlessness. *Palliative Medicine, 27*(6), 483–485. doi:10.1177/0269216313488490

Booth, S., Farquhar, M., Gysels, M., Bausewein, C., & Higginson, I. J. (2006). The impact of a breathlessness intervention service (BIS) on the lives of patients with intractable dyspnea: A qualitative phase 1 study. *Palliative and Supportive Care, 4*(3), 287–293. doi:10.1017/S1478951506060366

Booth, S., Moosavi, S. H., & Higginson, I. J. (2008). The etiology and management of intractable breathlessness in patients with advanced cancer: A systematic review of pharmacological therapy. *Nature Clinical Practice. Oncology, 5*(2), 90–100. doi:10.1038/ncponc1034

Bredin, M., Corner, J., Krishnasamy, M., Plant, H., Bailey, C., & A'Hern, R. (1999). Multicentre randomised controlled trial of nursing intervention for breathlessness in patients with lung cancer. *British Medical Journal, 318*(7188), 901–904. doi:10.1136/bmj.318.7188.901

Bruera, E., Schmitz, B., Pither, J., Neumann, C. M., & Hanson, J. (2000). The frequency and correlates of dyspnea in patients with advanced cancer. *Journal of Pain and Symptom Management, 19*(5), 357–362. doi:10.1016/S0885-3924(00)00126-3

Brunnhuber, K., Nash, S., Meier, D. E., Weissman, D. E., & Woodcock, J. (2008). *Putting evidence into practice: Palliative care* (pp. 1–88). London, UK: BMJ Publishing Group.

Campbell, M. L. (2012). Dyspnea prevalence, trajectories, and measurement in critical care and at life's end. *Current Opinion in Supportive and Palliative Care, 6*(2), 168–171. doi:10.1097/SPC.0b013e328352b67f

Cairns, L. M. (2012). Managing breathlessness in patients with lung cancer. *Nursing Standard, 27*(13), 44–49. doi:10.7748/ns2012.11.27.13.44.c9450

Campbell, M. L. (1996). Managing terminal dyspnea: Caring for the patient who refuses intubation or ventilation. *Dimensions of Critical Care Nursing: DCCN, 15*(1), 4–12; quiz 13.

Campbell, M. L., & Templin, T. N. (2015). Intensity cut-points for the respiratory distress observation scale. *Palliative Medicine, 29*(5), 436–442. doi:10.1177/0269216314564238

Campbell, M. L., Templin, T., & Walch, J. (2009). Patients who are near death are frequently unable to self-report dyspnea. *Journal of Palliative Medicine, 12*(10), 881–884. doi:10.1089/jpm.2009.0082

Campbell, M. L., Templin, T., & Walch, J. (2010). A respiratory distress observation scale for patients unable to self-report dyspnea. *Journal of Palliative Medicine, 13*(3), 285–289. doi:10.1089/jpm.2009.0229

Campbell, M. L., Yarandi, H., & Dove-Medows, E. (2013). Oxygen is nonbenficial for most patients who are near death. *Journal of Pain and Symptom Management, 45*(3), 517–523. doi:10.1016/j.jpainsymman.2012.02.012

Carel, H., McNaughton, J., & Dodd, J. (2015). Invisible suffering: Breathlessness in and beyond the clinic. *Lancet Respiratory Medicine, 3*(4), 278–279. doi:10.1016/S2213-2600(15)00115-0

Caroci, A. D. S., & Lareau, S. C. (2004). Descriptors of dyspnea by patients with chronic obstructive pulmonary disease versus congestive heart failure. *Heart and Lung, 33*(2), 102–110. doi:10.1016/j.hrtlng.2003.11.004

Centers for Disease Control and Prevention. (2014). FastStats: Child health. Retrieved from https://www.cdc.gov/nchs/fastats/child-health.htm

Charles, M. A., Reymond, L., & Israel, F. (2008). Relief of incident dyspnea in palliative cancer patients: A pilot, randomized, controlled trial comparing nebulized hydromorphone, systemic hydromorphone, and nebulized saline. *Journal of Pain and Symptom Management, 36*(1), 29–38. doi:10.1016/j.jpainsymman.2007.08.016

Chiappa, G. R., Queiroga, F., Meda, E., Ferreira, L. F., Diefenthaeler, F., Nunes, M., ... Neder, J. A. (2009). Heliox improves oxygen delivery and utilization during dynamic exercise in patients with chronic obstructive pulmonary disease. *American Journal of Respiratory and Critical Care Medicine, 179*(11), 1004–1010. doi:10.1164/rccm.200811-1793OC

Chin, C., & Booth, S. (2016). Managing breathlessness: A palliative care approach. *Postgraduate Medicine, 92*, 393–400. doi:10.1136/postgradmedj-2015-133578

Chin, C. A., Butcher, H. H., Spathis, A., Ryan, R., Johnson, M., Pattinson, K., ... Booth, S. (2015). What's trending in breathlessness research? Proceedings from the 8th annual meeting of the breathlessness research interest group. *Progress in Palliative Care, 23*(6), 326–330. doi:10.1179/1743291X15Y.0000000005

Cleary, J. F., & Carbone, P. P. (1997). Palliative medicine in the elderly. *Cancer, 80*(7), 1335–1347. doi:10.1002/(SICI)1097-0142(19971001)80:7<1335::AID-CNCR21>3.0.CO;2-7

Clemens, K. E., & Klaschik, E. (2011). Dyspnoea associated with anxiety: Symptomatic therapy with opioids in combination with lorazepam and its effect on ventilation in palliative care patients. *Supportive Care in Cancer, 19*(12), 2027–2033. doi:10.1007/s00520-010-1058-8

Collins, J. J., & Fitzgerald, D. A. (2006). Palliative care and paediatric respiratory medicine. *Paediatric Respiratory Review, 7*(4), 281–287. doi:10.1016/j.prrv.2006.04.001

Corner, J., Plant, H., A'Hern, R., & Bailey, C. (1996). Non-pharmacological intervention for breathlessness in lung cancer. *Palliative Medicine, 10*(4), 299–305. doi:10.1177/026921639601000405

Coyne, P. J. (2003). The use of nebulized fentanyl for the management of dyspnea. *Clinical Journal of Oncology Nursing, 7*(3), 334–335. doi:10.1188/03.CJON.334-336

Coyne, P. J., Viswanathan, R., & Smith, T. J. (2002). Nebulized fentanyl citrate improves patients' perception of breathing, respiratory rate, and oxygen saturation in dyspnea. *Journal of Pain and Symptom Management, 23*(2), 157–160. doi:10.1016/S0885-3924(01)00391-8

Craig, F., Henderson, E. M., & Bluebond-Langner, M. (2015). Management of respiratory symptoms in paediatric palliative care. *Supportive and Palliative Care, 9*(3), 217–226. doi:10.1097/SPC.0000000000000154

Critchley, H. D., Wiens, S., Rotshtein, P., Ohman, A., & Dolan, R. J. (2004). Neural systems supporting interoceptive awareness. *Nature Neuroscience, 7*(2), 189–195. doi:10.1038/nn1176

Cuomo, A., Delmastro, M., Ceriana, P., Nava, S., Conti, G., Antonelli, M., & Iacobone, E. (2004). Noninvasive mechanical ventilation as a palliative treatment of acute respiratory failure in patients with end-stage solid cancer. *Palliative Medicine, 18*(7), 602–610. doi:10.1191/0269216304pm933oa

Currow, D. C. (2008). Managing respiratory symptoms in everyday practice. *Current Opinion in Supportive and Palliative Care, 2*(2), 81–83.

Currow, D. C., Agar, M., Smith, J., & Abernethy, A. P. (2009). Does palliative home oxygen improve dyspnea? A consecutive cohort study. *Palliative Medicine, 23*(4), 309–316. doi:10.1177/0269216309104058

Currow, D. C., McDonald, C., Oaten, S., Kenny, B., Allcroft, P., Frith, P., … Abernethy, A. (2011). Once-daily opioids for chronic dyspnea: A dose increment and pharmacovigilance study. *Journal of Pain and Symptom Management, 42*(3), 388–399. doi:10.1016/j.jpainsymman.2010.11.021

Currow, D. C., Smith, J., Davidson, P. M., Newton, P. J., Agar, M. R., & Abernethy, A. P. (2010). Do the trajectories of dyspnea differ in prevalence and intensity by diagnosis at the end of life? A consecutive cohort study. *Journal of Pain and Symptom Management, 39*(4), 680–690. doi:10.1016/j.jpainsymman.2009.09.017

Curtis, J. R., Cook, D. J., Sinuff, T., White, D. B., Hill, N., Keenan, S. P., … Levy, M. M.; Society of Critical Care Medicine Palliative Noninvasive Positive Ventilation Task Force. (2007). Noninvasive positive pressure ventilation in critical and palliative care settings: Understanding the goals of therapy. *Critical Care Medicine, 35*(3), 932–939. doi:10.1097/01.CCM.0000256725.73993.74

Dahlin, C. (2006). It takes my breath away: End-stage COPD. Part 1: A case study and an overview of COPD. *Home Healthcare Nurse, 24*(3), 148–155; quiz 156.

Davies, B., Sehring, S. A., Partridge, J. C., Cooper, B. A., Hughes, A., Philp, J. C., … Kramer, R. F. (2008). Barriers to palliative care for children: Perceptions of pediatric health care providers. *Pediatrics, 121*(2), 282–288. doi:10.1542/peds.2006-3153

De Peuter, S., Van Diest, I., Lemaigre, V., Verleden, G., Demedts, M., & Van den Bergh, O. (2004). Dyspnea: The role of psychological processes. *Clinical Psychology Review, 24*(5), 557–581. doi:10.1016/j.cpr.2004.05.001

Donesky-Cuenco, D., Nguyen, H. Q., Paul, S., & Carrieri-Kohlman, V. (2009). Yoga therapy decreases dyspnea-related distress and improves functional performance in people with COPD: A pilot study. *Alternative and Complementary Medicine. 15*(3), 225–234. doi:10.1089/acm.2008.0389

Dorman, S., Byrne, A., & Edwards, A. (2007). Which measurement scales should we use to measure breathlessness in palliative care? A systematic review. *Palliative Medicine, 21*(3), 177–191. doi:10.1177/0269216307076398

Dudgeon, D. J., Kristjanson, L., Sloan, J. A., Lertzman, M., & Clement, K. (2001). Dyspnea in cancer patients: Prevalence and associated factors. *Journal of Pain and Symptom Management, 21*(2), 95–102. doi:10.1016/S0885-3924(00)00258-X

Dunger, C., Higginson, I. J., Gysels, M., Booth, S., Simon, S. T., & Bausewein, C. (2015). Breathlessness and crises in the context of advanced illness: A comparison between COPD and lung cancer patients. *Palliative and Supportive Care, 13*(3), 229–237. doi:10.1017/S147895151300120X

Edmonds, P., Karlsen, S., Khan, S., & Addington-Hall, J. (2001). A comparison of the palliative care needs of patients dying from chronic respiratory diseases and lung cancer. *Palliative Medicine, 15*(4), 287–295. doi:10.1191/026921601678320278

Ekstrom, M., Ahmadi, Z., Bornefalk-Hermansson, A., Abernethy, A., & Currow, D. (2016). Oxygen for breathlessness in patients with chronic obstructive pulmonary disease who do not qualify for home oxygen therapy. *Cochrane Database of Systematic Reviews,* (11), CD006429. doi:10.1002/14651858.CD006429.pub3

Ekstrom, M., Bornefalk-Hermansson, A., Abernethy, A. P., & Currow, D. C. (2014). Safety of benzodiazepines and opioids in very severe respiratory disease: National prospective study. *BMJ, 348*, g445. doi:10.1136/bmj.g445

Elia, G., & Thomas, J. (2008). The symptomatic relief of dyspnea. *Current Oncology Reports, 10*(4), 319–325. doi:10.1007/s11912-008-0050-7

Elmqvist, M. A., Jordhoy, M. S., Bjordal, K., Kaasa, S., & Jannert, M. (2009). Health-related quality of life during the last three months of life in patients with advanced cancer. *Supportive Care in Cancer, 17*(2), 191–198. doi:10.1007/s00520-008-0477-2

Estfan, B., Mahmoud, F., Shaheen, P., Davis, M. P., Lasheen, W., Rivera, N., … Rybicki, L. (2007). Respiratory function during parenteral opioid titration for cancer pain. *Palliative Medicine, 21*(2), 81–86. doi:10.1177/0269216307077328

Falk, H. , Ekman, I. , Anderson, R. , Fu, M. & Granger, B. (2013). Older Patients' experiences of heart failure—An Integrative Literature Review. *Journal of Nursing Scholarship, 45*: 247–255. doi:10.1111/jnu.12025

Farquhar, M. C., Prevost, A., T., McCrone, P., Brafman-Price, B., Bentley, A., Higginson, I. J., Todd, C., … Booth, S. (2014). Is specialist breathlessness service more effective and cost-effective for patients with advanced cancer and their carers than standard care? Findings of a mixed-method randomized controlled trial. *BMC Medicine, 12*, 194–214. doi:10.1186/s12916-014-0194-2

Farquhar, M. C., Prevost, A. T., McCrone, P., Brafman-Price, B., Bentley, A., Higginson, I. J., Todd, C. J., … Booth, S. (2016). The clinical and cost effectiveness of a breathlessness intervention service for patients with advanced non-malignant disease and their informal carers: Mixed findings of a mixed method randomized controlled trial. *Trials, 17*, 185–201. doi:10.1186/s13063-016-1304-6

Ferraresi, V. (2005). Inhaled opioids for the treatment of dyspnea. *American Journal of Health-System Pharmacy, 62*(3), 319–320.

Focus for Health. (2017). Chronic illness and the state of our children's health. Retrieved from www.focusforhealth.org/category/chronic-illness

Freeman, S., Hirdes, J. P., Stolee, P., & Garcia, J. (2016). A cross-sectional examination of the association between dyspnea and distress as experienced by palliative home care clients and their informal caregivers. *Journal of Social Work in End-of-Life and Palliative Care, 12*(1–2), 82–103. doi:10.1080/15524256.2016.1156604

Freeman, S., Hirdes, J. P., Stolee, P., Garcia, J., & Smith, T. F. (2015). Correlates and predictors of changes in dyspnea symptoms over time among community-dwelling palliative home care clients. *Journal of Pain and Symptom Management, 50*(6), 793–805. doi:10.1016/j.jpainsymman.2015.06.016

Fried, T. R., Vaz Fragoso, C. A., & Rabow, M. W. (2012). Caring for the older person with chronic obstructive pulmonary disease. *JAMA, 308*(12), 1254–1263. doi:10.1001/jama.2012.12422

Galbraith, S., Fagan, P., Perkins, P., Lynch, A., & Booth, S. (2010). Does the use of a handheld fan improve chronic dyspnea? A randomized, controlled, crossover trial. *Journal of Pain and Symptom Management, 39*(5), 831–838. doi:10.1016/j.jpainsymman.2009.09.024

Gift, A. G. (1989). Clinical measurement of dyspnea. *Dimensions of Critical Care Nursing, 8*(4), 210–216.

Goldberg, R. J., Spencer, F. A., Farmer, C., et al. (2005). Incidence and hospital death rates associated with heart failure: a community-wide perspective. *American Journal of Medicine, 118*, 728–734.

Gotfried, M. H., Kerwin, E. M., Lawrence, D., Lassen, C., & Kramer, B. (2012). Efficacy of indacaterol 75ug once-daily on dyspnea and health status: Results of two double-blind, placebo-controlled 12-week studies. *Journal of Chronic Obstructive Pulmonary Disease, 9*, 629–636. doi:10.3109/15412555.2012.729623

Gysels, M., & Higginson, I. J. (2008). Access to services for patients with chronic obstructive pulmonary disease: The invisibility of breathlessness. *Journal of Pain and Symptom Management, 36*(5), 451–460. doi:10.1016/j.jpainsymman.2007.11.008

Habashy, C., Caldwell, A., & Baker, J. (2017). *Compassionate intubation: Refractory dyspnea at the end of life.* Symposium conducted at the Annual Assembly for Hospice and Palliative Care, Phoenix, AZ.

Hall, P., Schroder, C., & Weaver, L. (2002). The last 48 hours of life in long-term care: A focused chart audit. *Journal of the American Geriatrics Society, 50*(3), 501–506. doi:10.1046/j.1532-5415.2002.50117.x

Hallenbeck, J. (2012). Pathophysiologies of dyspnea explained: Why might opioids relieve dyspnea and not hasten death? *Journal of Palliative Medicine, 15*(8), 848–853. doi:10.1089/jpm.2011.0167

Hasson, F., Spence, A., Waldron, M., Kernohan, G., McLaughlin, D., Watson, B., & Cochrane, B. (2008). I cannot get a breath: Experiences of living with advanced chronic obstructive pulmonary disease. *International Journal of Palliative Nursing, 14*(11), 526–531. doi:10.12968/ijpn.2008.14.11.31756

Hately, J., Laurence, V., Scott, A., Baker, R., & Thomas, P. (2003). Breathlessness clinics within specialist palliative care settings can improve the quality of life and functional capacity of patients with lung cancer. *Palliative Medicine, 17*(5), 410–417. doi:10.1191/0269216303pm752oa

Hauer, J. M. (2015). Treating dyspnea with morphine sulfate in nonverbal children with neurological impairment. *Pediatric Pulmonology, 50*(4), E9–E12. doi:10.1002/ppul.23140

Hayen, A., Herigstad, M., & Pattinson, K. T. S. (2013). Understanding dyspnea as a complex individual experience. *Maturitas, 76*(1), 45–50. doi:10.1016/j.maturitas.2013.06.005

Hechler, T., Blankenburg, M., Friedrichsdorf, S. J., Garske, D., Hübner, B., Menke, A., … Zernikow, B. (2008). Parents' perspective on symptoms, quality of life, characteristics of death and end-of-life decisions for children dying from cancer. *Klinische Pädiatrie, 220*(3), 166–174. doi:10.1055/s-2008-1065347

Henoch, I., Bergman, B., & Danielson, E. (2008). Dyspnea experience and management strategies in patients with lung cancer. *Psycho-Oncology, 17*(7), 709–715. doi:10.1002/pon.1304

Henoch, I., Bergman, B., & Gaston-Johansson, F. (2006). Validation of a Swedish version of the Cancer Dyspnea Scale. *Journal of Pain and Symptom Management, 31*(4), 353–361. doi:10.1016/j.jpainsymman.2006.02.002

Henson, L. A., Gao, W., Higginson, I. J., Smith, M., Davies, J. M., Ellis-Smith, C., & Daveson, B. A. (2015). Emergency department attendance by patients with cancer in their last month of life: A systematic review and meta-analysis. *Journal of Clinical Oncology, 33*(4), 370–376. doi:10.1200/JCO.2014.57.3568

Hewitt, M., Goldman, A., Collins, G. S., Childs, M., & Hain, R. (2008). Opioid use in palliative care of children and young people with cancer. *Journal of Pediatrics, 152*(1), 39–44. doi:10.1016/j.jpeds.2007.07.005

Higginson, I. J., Bausewein, C., Reilly, C. C., Gao, W., Gysels, M., Dzingina, M., McCrone, P., … Moxham, J. (2014). An integrated palliative and respiratory care service for patients with advanced disease and refractory breathlessness: A randomized controlled trial. *Lancet Respiratory Medicine, 2*(12), 979–987. doi:10.1016/S2213-2600(14)70226-7

Hongo, T., Watanabe, C., Okada, S., Inoue, N., Yajima, S., Fujii, Y., & Ohzeki, T. (2003). Analysis of the circumstances at the end of life in children with cancer: Symptoms, suffering and acceptance. *Pediatrics International, 45*(1), 60–64. doi:10.1046/j.1442-200X.2003.01668.x

Hongratanaworakit, T. (2011). Aroma-therapeutic effects of massage blended essential oils on humans. *Natural Product Communications, 6*(8), 1199–1204.

Hospice and Palliative Nurses Association. (2014). HPNA research agenda 2015–2018. Retrieved from http://hpna.advancingexpertcare.org/wp-content/uploads/2015/01/2015-2018-HPNA-Research-Agenda.pdf

Hui, D., Morgado, M., Chisholm, G., Withers, L., Nguyen, Q., Finch, C., … Bruera, E. (2013). High-flow oxygen and bilevel positive airway pressure for persistent dyspnea in patients with advanced cancer: A phase II randomized trial. *Journal of Pain and Symptom Management, 46*(4), 463–473. doi:10.1016/j.jpainsymman.2012.10.284

Hui, D., Xu, A., Chisholm, G., Morgado, M., Reddy, S., & Bruera, E. (2014). Effects of prophylactic subcutaneous fentanyl on exercise-induced breakthrough dyspnea in cancer patients: A preliminary double-blind, randomized, controlled trial. *Journal of Pain and Symptom Management, 47*(2), 209–217. doi:10.1016/j.jpainsymman.2013.03.017

Hutchinson, A., Pickering, A., Williams, P., Bland, J. M., & Johnson, M. J. (2017). Breathlessness and presentation to the emergency department. *BMC Pulmonary Medicine, 17*(1), 53. doi:10.1186/s12890-017-0396-4

Janssen, D. J., Wouters, E. F., & Spruit, M. A. (2015). Psychosocial consequences of living with breathlessness due to advanced disease. *Current Opinion in Supportive and Palliative Care, 9*(3), 232–237. doi:10.1097/SPC.0000000000000146

Jennings, A. L., Davies, A. N., Higgins, J. P., & Broadley, K. (2001). Opioids for the palliation of breathlessness in terminal illness. *Cochrane Database of Systematic Reviews,* (4), CD002066. doi:10.1002/14651858.CD002066

Jennings, A. L., Davies, A. N., Higgins, J. P., Gibbs, J. S., & Broadley, K. (2002). A systematic review of the use of opioids in the management of dyspnea. *Thorax, 57*(11), 939–944. doi:10.1136/thorax.57.11.939

Jensen, D., Amjadi, K., Harris-McAllister, V., Webb, K. A., & O'Donnell, D. E. (2008). Mechanisms of dyspnoea relief and improved exercise endurance after furosemide inhalation in COPD. *Thorax, 63*(7), 606–613. doi:10.1136/thx.2007.085993

Jerpseth, H., Dahl, V., Nortvedt, P., & Halvorsen, K. (2018). Older patients with late-stage COPD: Their illness experiences and involvement in decision-making regarding mechanical ventilation and noninvasive ventilation. *Journal of Clinical Nursing, 27*(3–4), 582–592. doi:10.1111/jocn.13925

Johansson, P., Riegel, B., Svensson, E., Brostrom, A., Alehagen, U., Dahlstrom, U., & Jaarsma, T. (2012). The contribution of heart failure to sleep disturbances and depressive symptoms in older adults. *Journal of Geriatric Psychiatry, 25*(3), 179–187. doi:10.1177/0891988712458366

Johnson, M. J., Abernethy, A. P., & Currow, D. C. (2013). The evidence base for oxygen for chronic refractory breathlessness: Issues, gaps and a future work plan. *Journal of Pain and Symptom Management, 45*(4), 763–775. doi:10.1016/j.jpainsymman.2012.03.017

Johnson, M. J., Bland, J. M., Gahbauer, E. A., Ekstrom, M., Sinnarajah, A., Gill, T. M., & Currow, D. C. (2017). Breathlessness in the elderly during the last year of life sufficient to restrict activity: Prevalence, pattern and associated factors. *Journal of the American Geriatric Society, 64*(1), 73–80. doi:10.1111/jgs.13865

Johnson, M. J., Bland, J. M., Oxberry, S. G., Abernethy, A. P., & Currow, D. C. (2013). Clinically important differences in the intensity of chronic refractory breathlessness. *Journal of Pain and Symptom Management, 46*(6), 957–963. doi:10.1016/j.jpainsymman.2013.01.011

Jones, E., & Wolfe, J. (2014). Is there a "right way" to provide pediatric palliative care? *Journal of Palliative Medicine, 17*(5), 500–501. doi:10.1089/jpm.2014.9432

Jones, P. W., Mahler, D. A., Gale, R., Owen, R., & Kramer, B. (2011). Profiling the effects of indacaterol on dyspnea and health status in patients with COPD. *Respiratory Medicine, 105*(6), 892–899. doi:10.1016/j.rmed.2011.02.013

Juan, G., Ramón, M., Valia, J. C., Cortijo, J., Rubio, E., Morcillo, E., & Calverley, P. (2005). Palliative treatment of dyspnea with epidural methadone in advanced emphysema. *Chest, 128*(5), 3322–3328. doi:10.1378/chest.128.5.3322

Khan, F. I., Reddy, R. C., & Baptist, A. P. (2009). Pediatric Dyspnea Scale for use in hospitalized patients with asthma. *Journal of Allergy and Clinical Immunology, 123*(3), 660–664. doi:10.1016/j.jaci.2008.12.018

Khan, S. Y., & O'Driscoll, B. R. (2004). Is nebulized saline a placebo in COPD? *BMC Pulmonary Medicine, 4*, 9. doi:10.1186/1471-2466-4-9

Kako, J., Morita, T., Yamaguchi, T., Sekimoto, A., Kobayashi, M., Kinoshita, H., … Matsushima, E. (2018). Evaluation of the appropriate washout period following fan therapy for dyspnea in patients with advanced cancer: A pilot study. *American Journal of Hospice and Palliative Medicine, 35*(2), 293–296. doi:10.1177/1049909117707905

Kamal, A. H., Maguire, J. M., Wheeler, J. L., Currow, D. C., & Abernethy, A. P. (2011). Dyspnea review for the palliative care professional: Assessment, burdens, and etiologies. *Journal of Palliative Medicine, 14*(10), 1167–1172. doi:10.1089/jpm.2011.0109

Kamal, A. H., Maguire, J. M., Wheeler, J. L., Currow, D. C., & Abernethy, A. P. (2012). Dyspnea review for the palliative care professional: Treatment goals and therapeutic options. *Journal of Palliative Medicine, 15*(1), 106–114. doi:10.1089/jpm.2011.0110

Kamal, A. H., Swetz, K. M., Liu, H., Ruegg, S. R., Carey, E. C., Whitford, K., … Kaur, J. S. (2009). Survival trends in palliative care patients with cancer: A Mayo clinic 5 year review. *Journal of Clinical Oncology, 27*(15S), 9592. doi:10.1200/jco.2009.27.15s.9592

Ladas, E. J., Post-White, J., Hawks, R., & Taromina, K. (2006). Evidence for symptom management in the child with cancer. *Journal of Pediatric Hematology/Oncology, 28*(9), 601–615. doi:10.1097/01.mph.0000212989.26317.52

Lands, L. C. (2017). Dyspnea in children: What is driving it and how to approach it. *Paediatric Respiratory Reviews, 24*, 29–31. doi:10.1016/j.prrv.2017.03.013

Lanken, P. N., Terry, P. B., Delisser, H. M., Fahy, B. F., Hansen-Flaschen, J., Heffner, J. E., … Yankaskas, J. R.; ATS End-of-Life Care Task Force. (2008). An official American Thoracic Society clinical policy statement: Palliative care for patients with respiratory diseases and critical illnesses. *American Journal of Respiratory and Critical Care Medicine, 177*(8), 912–927. doi:10.1164/rccm.200605-587ST

Laude, E. A., & Ahmedzai, S. H. (2007). Oxygen and helium gas mixtures for dyspnoea. *Current Opinion in Supportive and Palliative Care, 1*(2), 91–95. doi:10.1097/SPC.0b013e3282e1c6f5

Lawrey, H. (2005). Hyoscine vs glycopyrronium for drying respiratory secretions in dying patients. *British Journal of Community Nursing, 10*(9), 421–424, 426.

Liben, S., Langner, R., & Bluebond-Langner, M. (2014). Pediatric palliative care in 2014: Much accomplished, much yet to be done. *Journal of Palliative Care, 30*(4), 311–316.

Lin, R. J., Adelman, R. D., & Mehta, S. S. (2012). Dyspnea in palliative care: Expanding the role of corticosteroids. *Journal of Palliative Medicine, 15*(7), 834–837. doi:10.1089/jpm.2011.0260

Lindley, L. C. (2017). Multiple complex chronic conditions and pediatric hospice utilization among California Medicaid beneficiaries, 2007–2010. *Journal of Palliative Medicine, 20*(3), 241–246. doi:10.1089/jpm.2016.0227

Lokker, M. E., VanZuylen, L., VanderRijt, C. C., & VanderHeide, A. (2014). Prevalence, impact, and treatment of death rattle: A systematic review. *Journal of Pain and Symptom Management, 47*(1), 105–122. doi:10.1016/j.jpainsymman.2013.03.011

Lorenz, K. A., Lynn, J., Dy, S. M., Shugarman, L. R., Wilkinson, A., Mularski, R. A., … Shekelle, P. G. (2008). Evidence for improving palliative care at the end of life: A systematic review. *Annals of Internal Medicine, 148*(2), 147–159. doi:10.7326/0003-4819-148-2-200801150-00010

Mack, J. W., & Wolfe, J. (2006). Early integration of pediatric palliative care: For some children, palliative care starts at diagnosis. *Current Opinion in Pediatrics, 18*(1), 10–14. doi:10.1097/01.mop.0000193266.86129.47

Maeda, T., & Hayakawa, T. (2017). Dyspnea-alleviating and survival-prolonging effects of corticosteroids in patients with terminal cancer. *Progress in Palliative Care, 25*(3), 117–120. doi:10.1080/09699260.2017.1293207

Mahler, D. A., Decramer, M., D'Urzo, A., Worth, H., White, T., Algappan, V. K., … Banerji, D. (2014). Dual bronchodilation with QVA 149 reduces patient-reported dyspnea in COPD: The BLAZE study. *European Respiratory Journal, 43*(6), 1599–1609. doi:10.1183/09031936.00124013

Mahler, D. A., D'Urzo, A., Bateman, E. D., Ozkan, S. A., White, T., Peckitt, C., … Kramer, B. (2012). Concurrent use of indacaterol plus tiotropium in patients with COPD provides superior bronchodilation compared with tiotropium alone: A randomzed, double-blind comparison. *Thorax, 67*(9), 781–788. doi:10.1136/thoraxjnl-2011-201140

Mahler, D. A., & Harver, A. (2000). Do you speak the language of dyspnea? *Chest, 117*(4), 928–929. doi:10.1378/chest.117.4.928

Mahler, D. A., & O'Donnell, D. E. (2015). Recent advances in dyspnea. *Chest, 147*(1), 232–241. doi:10.1378/chest.14-0800

Mahler, D. A., Rosiello, R. A., & Loke, J. (1986). The aging lung. *Clinics in Geriatric Medicine, 2*(2), 215–225.

Mahut, B., Fuchs-Climent, D., Plantier, L., Karila, C., Refabert, L., Chevalier-Bidaud, B., … Delclaux, C. (2014). Cross-sectional assessment of exertional dyspnea in otherwise healthy children. *Pediatric Pulmonology, 49*(8), 772–781. doi:10.1002/ppul.22905

Malik, F. A., Gysels, M., & Higginson, I. J. (2013). Living with breathlessness: A survey of caregivers of breathless patients with lung cancer or heart failure. *Palliative Medicine, 27*(7), 647–656. doi:10.1177/0269216313488812

Maltoni, M., Pirovano, M., Scarpi, E., Marinari, M., Indelli, M., Arnoldi, E., … Amadori, D. (1995). Prediction of survival of patients terminally ill with cancer. Results of an Italian prospective multicentric study. *Cancer, 75*(10), 2613–2622. doi:10.1002/1097-0142(19950515)75:10<2613::AID-CNCR2820751032>3.0.CO;2-1

Marques, A., Gabriel, R., Jacome, C., Cruz, J., Brooks, D., & Figueiredo, D. (2015). Development of a family-based pulmonary rehabilitation program: An exploratory study. *Disability and Rehabilitation, 37*(15), 1340–1346. doi:10.3109/09638288.2014.964376

Martinez, J. A., Straccia, L., Sobrani, E., Silva, G. A., Vianna, E. O., & Filho, J. T. (2000). Dyspnea scales in the assessment of illiterate patients with chronic obstructive pulmonary disease. *American Journal of the Medical Sciences, 320*(4), 240–243. doi:10.1097/00000441-200010000-00003

McBride, J. J., Vlieger, A. M., & Anbar, R. D. (2014). Hypnosis in paediatric respiratory medicine. *Paediatric Respiratory Reviews, 15*, 82–85. doi:10.1016/j.prrv.2013.09.002

McCarthy, B., Casey, D., Devane, D., Murphy, K., Murphy, E., & Lacasse, Y. (2015). Pulmonary rehabilitation for chronic obstructive pulmonary disease. *Cochrane Database of Systematic Reviews*, (2), CD003793. doi:10.1002/14651858.CD003793.pub3

McCaskey, M. S. (2007). Pediatric assessment: The little differences. *Home Healthcare Nurse, 25*(1), 20–24.

Medical Research Council Working Party. (1981). Long term domiciliary oxygen therapy in chronic hypoxic cor pulmonale complicating chronic bronchitis and emphysema. *Lancet, 1*(8222), 681–686. doi:10.1016/S0140-6736(81)91970-X

Melendez, M., Nguyen, H. Q., & Carrieri-Kohlman, V. (2012). A responder analysis of the effects of yoga for individuals with COPD: Who benefits and how? *International Journal of Yoga Therapy, 22*, 23–36.

Mellichamp, P. (2007). End-of-life care for infants. *Home Healthcare Nurse, 25*(1), 41–44.

Mercadante, S., Masedu, F., Valenti, M., Mercadante, A., & Aielli, F. (2016). The characteristics of advanced cancer patients followed at home, but admitted to the hospital for the last days of life. *Internal and Emergency Medicine, 11*(5), 713–718. doi:10.1007/s11739-016-1402-1

Miner, B., Tinetti, M. E., VanNess, P. H., Han, L., Leo-Summers, L., Newman, A. B., … VazFragoso, C. A. (2016). Dyspnea in community-dwelling older persons: A multifactorial geriatric health condition. *Journal of the American Geriatric Society, 64*(10), 2042–2050. doi:10.1111/jgs.14290

Morell, E., Wolfe, J., Scheurer, M., Thiagarajan, R., Morin, C., Beke, D. M., … Blume, E. D. (2012). Patterns of care at end of life in children with advanced heart disease. *Archives of Pediatrics and Adolescent Medicine, 166*(8), 745–748. doi:10.1001/archpediatrics.2011.1829

Morris, D., & Galicia-Castillo, M. (2017). Dying with dyspnea in the hospital. *American Journal of Hospice and Palliative Medicine, 34*(2), 132–134. doi:10.1177/1049909115604140

Mularski, R. A., Reinke, L. F., Carrieri-Kohlman, V., Fischer, M. D., Campbell, M. L., Rocker, G., … White, D. B. (2013). An official American Thoracic Society workshop report: Assessment and palliative management of dyspnea crisis. *Annals of the American Thoracic Society, 10*(5), S98–S106. doi:10.1513/AnnalsATS.201306-169ST

Mullerova, H., Lu, C., Li, H., & Tabberer, M. (2014). Prevalence and burden of breathlessness in patients with chronic obstructive pulmonary disease managed in primary care. *PLOS ONE, 9*(1), e85540. doi:10.1371/journal.pone.0085540

Nava, S., Ferrer, M., Esquinas, A., Scala, R., Groff, P., Cosentini, R., … Grassi, M. (2013). Palliative use of non-invasive ventilation in end-of-life patients with solid tumors: A randomized feasibility study. *Lancet Oncology, 14*(3), 219–227. doi:10.1016/S1470-2045(13)70009-3

Navigante, A. H., Castro, M. A., & Cerchietti, L. C. (2010). Morphine versus midazolam as upfront therapy to control dyspnea perception in cancer patients while its underlying cause is sought or treated. *Journal of Pain and Symptom Management, 39*(5), 820–830. doi:10.1016/j.jpainsymman.2009.10.003

Navigante, A. H., Cerchietti, L. C., Castro, M. A., Lutteral, M. A., & Cabalar, M. E. (2006). Midazolam as adjunct therapy to morphine in the alleviation of severe dyspnea perception in patients with advanced cancer. *Journal of Pain and Symptom Management, 31*(1), 38–47. doi:10.1016/j.jpainsymman.2005.06.009

Ngai, S. P., Jones, A. Y., Hui-Chan, C. W., & Yu, H. P. M. (2011). Acute effects of acu-TENS on FEV1 and blood beta-endorphin level in chronic obstructive pulmonary disease. *Alternative Therapies in Health and Medicine, 17*(5), 8–13.

Nishimura, K., Izumi, T., Tsukino, M., & Oga, T. (2002). Dyspnea is a better predictor of 5-year survival than airway obstruction in patients with COPD. *Chest, 121*(5), 1434–1440. doi:10.1378/chest.121.5.1434

Nocturnal Oxygen Therapy Trial Group. (1980). Continuous or nocturnal oxygen therapy in hypoxemic chronic obstructive lung disease: A clinical trial. *Annals of Internal Medicine, 93*(3), 391–398. doi:10.7326/0003-4819-93-3-391

Ofir, D., Laveneziana, P., Webb, K. A., Lam, Y. M., & O'Donnell, D. E. (2008). Mechanisms of dyspnea during cycle exercise in symptomatic patients with GOLD stage I chronic obstructive pulmonary disease. *American Journal of Respiratory and Critical Care Medicine, 177*(6), 622–629. doi:10.1164/rccm.200707-1064OC

Ong, K. C., Kor, A. C., Chong, W. F., Earnest, A., & Wang, Y. T. (2004). Effects of inhaled furosemide on exertional dyspnea in COPD. *American Journal of Respiratory and Critical Care Medicine, 169*(9), 1028–1033. doi:10.1164/rccm.200308-1171OC

Oxberry, S. G., & Johnson, M. J. (2008). Review of the evidence for the management of dyspnoea in people with chronic heart failure. *Current Opinion in Supportive and Palliative Care, 2*(2), 84–88. doi:10.1097/SPC.0b013e3282ff122e

Oxberry, S. G., Torgerson, D. J., Bland, J. M., Clark, A. L., Cleland, J. G. F., & Johnson, M. J. (2011). Short-term opioids for breathlessness in stable chronic heart failure: A randomized controlled trial. *European Journal of Heart Failure, 13*(9), 1006–1012. doi:10.1093/eurjhf/hfr068

Pang, G. S., Qu, L. M., Tan, Y. Y., & Yee, A. C. P. (2016). Intravenous fentanyl for dyspnea at the end of life: Lessons for future research in dyspnea. *American Journal of Hospice and Palliative Medicine, 33*(3), 222–227. doi:10.1177/1049909114559769

Parshall, M. B., Schwartzstein, R. M., Adams, L., Banzett, R. B., Manning, H. L., Bourbeau, J., Calverley, P. M. … O'Donnell, D. E. (2012). An official American Thoracic Society statement: Update on the mechanisms, assessment, and management of dyspnea. *American Journal of Respiratory and Critical Care Medicine, 185*(4), 435–452. doi:10.1164/rccm.201111-2042ST

Pesola, G. R., Forde, A. T., & Ahsan, H. (2017). Screening for shortness of breath: Stretching the screening paradigm to tertiary prevention. *American Journal of Public Health, 107*(3), 386–388. doi:10.2105/AJPH.2016.303625

Petersen, S., vonLeupoldt, A., & VandenBergh, O. (2014). Geriatric dyspnea: Doing worse, feeling better. *Ageing Research Reviews, 15,* 94–99. doi:10.1016/j.arr.2014.03.001

Pianosi, P. T., Huebner, M., Zhang, Z., Turchetta, A., & McGrath, P. J. (2015). Dalhousie pictorial scales measuring dyspnea and perceived exertion during exercise for children and adolescents. *Annals of the American Thoracic Society, 12*(5), 718–726. doi:10.1513/AnnalsATS.201410-477OC

Picella, D. V. (1997). Palliative care for the patient with end stage respiratory illness. *Perspectives in Respiratory Nursing: A Publication of the Respiratory Nursing Society, 8*(4), 1, 4, 6.

Pinna, M. A., Bruera, E., Moralo, M. J., Correas, M. A., & Vargas, R. M. (2015). A randomized crossover clinical trial to evaluate the efficacy of oral transmucosal fentanyl citrate in the treatment of dyspnea on exertion in patients with advanced cancer. *American Journal of Hospice and Palliative Care, 32*(3), 298–304. doi:10.1177/1049909113513063

Plonk, W. M., & Arnold, R. M. (2005). Terminal care: The last weeks of life. *Journal of Palliative Medicine, 8*(5), 1042–1054. doi:10.1089/jpm.2005.8.1042

Puntillo, K. A., Arai, S., Cohen, N. H., Gropper, M. A., Neuhaus, J., Paul, S. M., & Miaskowski, C. (2010). Symptoms experienced by intensive care unit patients at high risk of dying. *Critical Care Medicine, 38*(11), 2155–2160. doi:10.1097/CCM.0b013e3181f267ee

Puspawati, N. L. P. D., Sitorus, R., & Herawati, T. (2017). Hand-held fan airflow stimulation relieves dyspnea in lung cancer patients. *Asia-Pacific Journal of Oncology Nursing, 4*(2), 162–167. doi:10.4103/apjon.apjon_14_17

Rafferty, K. A., & Sullivan, S. L. (2017). You know the medicine, I know my kid. *Health Communications, 32*(9), 1151–1160. doi:10.1080/10410236.2016.1214221

Reddy, S. K., Parsons, H. A., Elsayem, A., Palmer, J. L., & Bruera, E. (2009). Characteristics and correlates of dyspnea in patients with advanced cancer. *Journal of Palliative Medicine, 12*(1), 29–36. doi:10.1089/jpm.2008.0158

Reuben, D. B., & Mor, V. (1986). Dyspnea in terminally ill cancer patients. *Chest, 89*(2), 234–236. doi:10.1378/chest.89.2.234

Riegel, B., Dickson, V. V., Cameron, J., Johnson, J. C., Bunker, S., Pate, K., & Worrall-Carter, L. (2010). Symptom recognition in elders with heart failure. *Journal of Nursing Scholarship, 42*(1), 92–100. doi:10.1111/j.1547-5069.2010.01333.x

Robinson, W. M. (2012). Palliation of dyspnea in pediatrics. *Chronic Respiratory Disease, 9*(4), 251–256. doi:10.1177/1479972312452439

Rocker, G. (2011). Dyspnea: Recent insights and innovations. *Progress in Palliative Care, 19*(5), 219–221. doi:10.1179/174329111X13147108047456

Rocker, G. (2012). Palliation of dyspnea. *Chronic Respiratory Disease, 9*(1), 49–50. doi:10.1177/1479972311433420

Rousseau, P. (1997). Management of dyspnea in the dying elderly. *Clinical Geriatrics, 5*(6), 42–48.

Saracino, A., Weiland, T. J., Jolly, B., & Dent, A. W. (2010). Verbal dyspnea score predicts emergency department departure status in patients with shortness of breath. *Emergency Medicine Australasia, 22*(1), 21–29. doi:10.1111/j.1742-6723.2009.01254.x

Scano, G., Stendardi, L., & Grazzini, M. (2005). Understanding dyspnoea by its language. *The European Respiratory Journal, 25*(2), 380–385. doi:10.1183/09031936.05.00059404

Schettino, G., Altobelli, N., & Kacmarek, R. M. (2005). Noninvasive positive pressure ventilation reverses acute respiratory failure in select "do-not-intubate" patients. *Critical Care Medicine, 33*(9), 1976–1982. doi:10.1097/01.CCM.0000178176.51024.82

Schindera, C., Tomlinson, D., Bartels, U., Gillmeister, B., Alli, A., & Sung, L. (2014). Predictors of symptoms and site of death in pediatric palliative patients with cancer at end of life. *American Journal of Hospice and Palliative Medicine, 31*(5), 548–552. doi:10.1177/1049909113497419

Schonhofer, B., Kuhlen, R., Neumann, P., Westhoff, M., Berndt, C., & Sitter, H. (2008). Clinical practice guideline: Non-invasive mechanical ventilation as treatment of acute respiratory failure. *Deutsches Arzteblatt International, 105*(24), 424–433. doi:10.3238/arztebl.2008.0424

Schwartzstein, R. M. (1999). The language of dyspnea: Using verbal clues to the diagnosis. *Journal of Critical Illness, 14*(8), 435–441.

Selecky, P. A., Eliasson, C. A., Hall, R. I., Schneider, R. F., Varkey, B., & McCaffree, D. R. (2005). Palliative and end-of-life care for patients with cardiopulmonary diseases: American College of Chest Physicians position statement. *Chest, 128*(5), 3599–3610. doi:10.1378/chest.128.5.3599

Sheahan, S. L., & Musialowski, R. (2001). Clinical implications of respiratory system changes in aging. *Journal of Gerontological Nursing, 27*(5), 26–34; quiz 48. doi:10.3928/0098-9134-20010501-08

Sheikh Motahar Vahedi, H., Mahshidfar, B., Rabiee, H., Saadat, S., Shokoohi, H., Chardoli, M., & Rahimi-Movaghar, V. (2013). The adjunctive effect of nebulized furosemide in COPD exacerbation: A randomized controlled clinical trial. *Respiratory Care, 58*(11), 1873–1877. doi:10.4187/respcare.02160

Shinjo, T., & Okada, M. (2013). Atropine eyedrops for death rattle in a terminal cancer patient. *Journal of Palliative Medicine, 16*(2), 212–213. doi:10.1089/jpm.2011.0537

Shirk, M. B., Donahue, K. R., & Shirvani, J. (2006). Unlabeled uses of nebulized medications. *American Journal of Health-System Pharmacy, 63*(18), 1704–1716. doi:10.2146/ajhp060015

Shumway, N. M., Wilson, R. L., Howard, R. S., Parker, J. M., & Eliasson, A. H. (2008). Presence and treatment of air hunger in severely ill patients. *Respiratory Medicine, 102*(1), 27–31. doi:10.1016/j.rmed.2007.08.015

Simon, S. T., Higginson, I. J., Benalia, H., Gysels, M., Murtagh, F., Spicer, J., & Bausewein, C. (2013). Episodic and continuous breathlessness: A new categorization of breathlessness. *Journal of Pain and Symptom Management, 45*(6), 1019–1029. doi:10.1016/j.jpainsymman.2012.06.008

Simon, S. T., Higginson, I. J., Booth, S., Harding, R., Weingartner, V., & Bausewein, C. (2016). Benzodiazepines for the relief of breathlessness in advanced malignant and non malignant diseases in adults. *Cochrane Database of Systematic Reviews,* (10), CD007354. doi:10.1002/14651858.CD007354.pub3

Simon, S. T., Koskeroglu, P., Gaertner, J., & Voltz, R. (2013). Fentanyl for the relief of refractory breathlessness: A systematic review. *Journal of Pain and Symptom Management, 46*(6), 874–886. doi:10.1016/j.jpainsymman.2013.02.019

Simon, S. T., Weingärtner, V., Higginson, I. J., Voltz, R., & Bausewein, C. (2014). Definition, categorization, and terminology of episodic breathlessness: Consensus by an international Delphi survey. *Journal of Pain and Symptom Management, 47*(5), 828–838. doi:10.1016/j.jpainsymman.2013.06.013

Sinuff, T., Cook, D. J., Keenan, S. P., Burns, K. E., Adhikari, N. K., Rocker, G. M., ... Hill, N. S. (2008). Noninvasive ventilation for acute respiratory failure near the end of life. *Critical Care Medicine, 36*(3), 789–794. doi:10.1097/CCM.0B013E3181653584

Skaug, K., Eide, G. E., & Gulsvik, A. (2009). Hospitalisation days in patients with lung cancer in a general population. *Respiratory Medicine, 103*(12), 1941–1948. doi:10.1016/j.rmed.2009.05.016

Smith, E. L., Hann, D. M., Ahles, T. A., Furstenberg, C. T., Mitchell, T. A., Meyer, L., ... Hammond, S. (2001). Dyspnea, anxiety, body consciousness, and quality of life in patients with lung cancer. *Journal of Pain and Symptom Management, 21*(4), 323–329. doi:10.1016/S0885-3924(01)00255-X

Spector, N., Connolly, M. A., & Carlson, K. K. (2007). Dyspnea: Applying research to bedside practice. *AACN Advanced Critical Care, 18*(1), 45–58; quiz 59. doi:10.4037/15597768-2007-1006

Spector, N., Klein, D., & Rice-Wiley, L. (2000). Terminally ill patients breathe easier with nebulized morphine. *Nursing Spectrum,* 1–6.

Standish, L. J., Kozak, L., & Congdon, S. (2008). Acupuncture is underutilized in hospice and palliative medicine. *American Journal of Hospice and Palliative Care, 25*(4), 298–308. doi:10.1177/1049909108315916

Stringer, E., McFarlane, C., & Hernandez, P. (2004). Physician practices for prescribing supplemental oxygen in the palliative care setting. *Journal of Palliative Care, 20*(4), 303–307.

Suzuki, K., Servais, E., Rizk, N., Solomon, S., Sima, C. S., Park, B. J., , ... Adusumilli, P. S. (2011). Palliation and pleurodesis in malignant pleural effusion: The role for tunneled pleural catheters. *Journal of Thoracic Oncology, 6*(4), 762–767. doi:10.1097/JTO.0b013e31820d614f

Suzuki, M., Muro, S., Ando, Y., Omori, T., Shiota, T., Endo, K., ... Mishima, M. (2012). A randomized, placebo-controlled trial of acupuncture in patients with chronic obstructive pulmonary disease: The COPD-acupuncture trial. *Archives of Internal Medicine, 172*(11), 878–886. doi:10.1001/archinternmed.2012.1233

Suzuki, M., Namura, K., Ohno, Y., Tanaka, H., Egawa, M., Yokoyama, Y., ... Yano, T. (2008). The effect of acupuncture in the treatment of chronic obstructive pulmonary disease. *Journal of Alternative and Complementary Medicine, 14*(9), 1097–1105. doi:10.1089/acm.2007.0786

Tan, M. P., Wynn, N. N., Umerov, M., Henderson, A., Gillham, A., Junejo, S., & Bansal, S. K. (2009). Arm span to height ratio is related to severity of dyspnea, reduced spirometry volumes, and right heart strain. *Chest, 135*(2), 448–454. doi:10.1378/chest.08-1270

Tanaka, K., Akechi, T., Okuyama, T., Nishiwaki, Y., & Uchitomi, Y. (2000). Development and validation of the Cancer Dyspnoea Scale: A multidimensional, brief, self-rating scale. *British Journal of Cancer, 82*(4), 800–805. doi:10.1054/bjoc.1999.1002

Tapping, C. R., Ling, L., & Razack, A. (2012). PleurX drain use in the management of malignant ascites: Safety, complications, long-term patency and factors predictive of success. *British Journal of Radiology, 85*(1013), 623–628. doi:10.1259/bjr/24538524

Thompson, L. F. (1996). Failure to wean: Exploring the influence of age-related pulmonary changes. *Critical Care Nursing Clinics of North America, 8*(1), 7–16.

Tishelman, C., Petersson, L.-M., Degner, L. F., & Sprangers, M. A. G. (2007). Symptom prevalence, intensity, and distress in patients with inoperable lung cancer in relation to time of death. *Journal of Clinical Oncology, 25*(34), 5381–5389. doi:10.1200/JCO.2006.08.7874

Tripodoro, V. A., & De Vito, E. L. (2008). Management of dyspnea in advanced motor neuron diseases. *Current Opinion in Supportive and Palliative Care, 2*(3), 173–179. doi:10.1097/SPC.0b013e32830c9049

Uronis, H. E., McCrory, D. C., Samsa, G., Currow, D., & Abernethy, A. (2011). Symptomatic oxygen for non-hypoxemic chronic obstructive pulmonary disease. *Cochrane Database of Systematic Reviews*, (6), CD006429. doi:10.1002/14651858.CD006429.pub2

Van Cleave, J., Gortmaker, S. L., & Perrin, J. M. (2010). Dynamics of obesity and chronic health conditions among children and youth. *Journal of the American Medical Association, 303*(7), 623–630. doi:10.1001/jama.2010.104

VanderGeest, I. M. M., Darlington, A.-S. E., Streng, I. C., Michiels, E. M. C., Pieters, R., & Vanden Heuvel-Eibrink, M. M. (2014). Parents' experiences of pediatric palliative care and the impact on long-term parental grief. *Journal of Pain and Symptom Management, 47*(6), 1043–1053. doi:10.1016/j.jpainsymman.2013.07.007

Vieira, P. J., Chiappa, A., M., Cipriano, G., Umpierre, D., Arena, R., & Chiappa, G. R. (2014). Neuromuscular electrical stimulation improves clinical and physiological function in COPD patients. *Respiratory Medicine, 108*(4), 609–620. doi:10.1016/j.rmed.2013.12.013

Vollenbroich, R., Borasio, G. D., Duroux, A., Grasser, M., Brandstatter, M., & Fuhrer, M. (2016). Listening to parents: The role of symptom perception in pediatric palliative home care. *Palliative and Supportive Care, 14*(1), 13–19. doi:10.1017/S1478951515000462

Wadell, K., Webb, K. A., Preston, M. E., Amornputtisathaporn, N., Samis, L., Patelli, J., … O'Donnell, D. E. (2013). Impact of pulmonary rehabilitation on the major dimensions of dyspnea in COPD. *COPD: Journal of Chronic Obstructive Pulmonary Disease, 10*(4), 425–435. doi:10.3109/15412555.2012.758696

Ward, E., DeSantis, C., Robbins, A., Kohler, B., & Jemal, A. (2014). Childhood and adolescent cancer statistics, 2014. *CA: A Cancer Journal for Clinicians, 64*(2), 83–103. doi:10.3322/caac.21219

Wee, B., & Hillier, R. (2008). Interventions for noisy breathing in patients near to death. *Cochrane Database of Systematic Reviews*, (1), CD005177. doi:10.1002/14651858.CD005177.pub2

Wee, B. L., Coleman, P. G., Hillier, R., & Holgate, S. H. (2006). The sound of death rattle I: Are relatives distressed by hearing this sound? *Palliative Medicine, 20*(3), 171–175. doi:10.1191/0269216306pm1137oa

Weingaertner, V., Scheve, C., Gerdes, V., Schwarz-Eywill, M., Prenzel, R., Bausewein, C., … Simon, S. T. (2014). Breathlessness, functional status, distress, and palliative care needs over time in patients with advanced COPD or lung cancer: A cohort study. *Journal of Pain and Symptom Management, 48*(4), 569–581. doi:10.1016/j.jpainsymman.2013.11.011

Werynska, B., Porebska, I., & Brzecka, A. (2017). The evaluation of dyspnea in elderly patients with advanced non-small-cell-lung cancer receiving palliative chemotherapy. *Clinics in Oncology, 2*, 1241–1246.

Widger, K. A., & Wilkins, K. (2004). What are the key components of quality perinatal and pediatric end-of-life care? A literature review. *Journal of Palliative Care, 20*(2), 105–112.

Wilcock, A., Crosby, V., Hughes, A., Fielding, K., Corcoran, R., & Tattersfield, A. E. (2002). Descriptors of breathlessness in patients with cancer and other cardiorespiratory diseases. *Journal of Pain and Symptom Management, 23*(3), 182–189. doi:10.1016/S0885-3924(01)00417-1

Wildiers, H., Dhaenekint, C., Demeulenaere, P., Clement, P. M., Desmet, M., VanNuffelen, R., … Menten, J. (2009). Atropine, hyoscine butylbromide, or scopolamine are equally effective for the treatment of death rattle in terminal care. *Journal of Pain and Symptom Management, 38*(1), 124–133. doi:10.1016/j.jpainsymman.2008.07.007

Wildiers, H., & Menten, J. (2002). Death rattle: Prevalence, prevention and treatment. *Journal of Pain and Symptom Management, 23*(4), 310–317.

Williams, C. M. (2006). Dyspnea. *Cancer Journal, 12*(5), 365–373.

Wolfe, J., Grier, H. E., Klar, N., Levin, S. B., Ellenbogen, J. M., Salem-Schatz, S., … Weeks, J. C. (2000). Symptoms and suffering at the end of life in children with cancer. *New England Journal of Medicine, 342*(5), 326–333. doi:10.1056/NEJM200002033420506

Zepetella, G. (1998). The palliation of dyspnea in terminal disease. *The American Journal of Hospice and Palliative Care, 15*(6), 322–330. doi:10.1177/104990919801500606

Nicole G. Loving & Constance M. Dahlin

Anxiety, Depression, and Delirium

KEY POINTS

- Anxiety, depression, and delirium are common symptoms experienced by patients with serious illness.
- Anxiety manifests itself in four ways: physical symptoms, affective symptoms, behavioral responses, and cognitive responses.
- The patient and the family should be reassured that symptoms of depression and anxiety are effectively treated most of the time with pharmacological and nonpharmacological interventions.
- Effective treatment of anxiety, depression, and delirium necessitates a collaborative effort between the patient, family, and the health team.

CASE STUDY

Paul was a 62-year-old male artist, married to Ellen for 30 years and father of three. He was an avid bicyclist, and he enjoyed reading fiction and helping in his local community garden. Eleven years ago, he was diagnosed with Stage II colorectal cancer, for which treatment included resection and chemotherapy. Two years after treatment and follow-up, Paul was found to be cancer free after treatment and continued to regularly receive cancer screenings with no sign of disease recurrence. In the past month, Ellen noticed that Paul spent less time at work in his studio and more time at home in bed. She initially thought that he was experiencing grief over the loss of the family dog. However, his exhaustion did not seem to improve with rest. Initially, Paul denied that he was feeling anything other than his usual self. However, when he experienced persistent bloating and new abdominal pain, he finally admitted he had not been feeling well for the past 3 months. A follow-up appointment was scheduled with his oncologist. Imaging revealed that the colorectal cancer had returned and had spread to his liver. Paul immediately received weekly chemotherapy infusions that left him feeling ill and exhausted.

Ellen worried about Paul's low spirits and social withdrawal. He spent most of the day sleeping in bed, resulting in night wakefulness. Usually surrounded by people, Paul no longer answered the phone, nor responded to texts or emails. Near to his bed, stacks of books and magazines went unread alongside partially eaten plates of food. In addition to his poor appetite, he experienced intermittent abdominal pain, but he refused to take any opioids and would take only ibuprofen. Paul requested that Ellen not share the news of his recurrence with their children or their friends. Ellen felt increasingly helpless, worried and unsure what to do.

The response to a serious, life-threatening diagnosis results in individual coping methods and adaptive behaviors. Often, a person may develop psychiatric symptoms, including anxiety, depression, and delirium. These symptoms range from mild to severe in nature. There is a strong correlation between symptoms of anxiety, depression, and delirium in patients receiving palliative care for a life-limiting illness (Pasacreta, Minarik, Nield-Anderson, & Paice, 2015). As common transient symptoms, anxiety, depression, and delirium may be acute but self-limiting. However, in more chronic and severe diagnoses, these psychiatric issues may inhibit a person's ability to have meaningful communication with family and friends as part of life closure, cause suffering, and affect quality of life.

Palliative care includes attention to psychiatric symptoms and physical symptoms by the interdisciplinary team. The attention to these symptoms is specified in Domain 3 of the National Consensus Project for Quality Palliative Care, *Clinical Practice Guidelines,* Psychological and Psychiatric Aspects of Care Guideline 3.1, which states, "The interdisciplinary team assesses and addresses psychological and psychiatric aspects of care based upon the best available evidence to maximize patient and family coping and quality of life" (National Consensus Project for Quality Palliative Care, 2013). Nurses are often the first direct care provider to identify these symptoms and collaborate with other disciplines to promote positive coping strategies. The specialty palliative care team can diagnose, manage, and treat symptoms of depression, anxiety, delirium, and cognitive impairment. Such symptoms may be a consequence of the serious illness itself or, among patients with comorbid psychiatric illness, accompany their serious or life-threatening illness (National Consensus Project for Quality Palliative Care, 2013). Moreover, treatment and management is done in partnership with the patient and family using interventions informed by evidence-based practice and may include pharmacological, nonpharmacological, and complementary therapies.

In primary care, anxiety and depression may arise as the presenting precursor to another illness such as heart disease or neurological conditions. In palliative care, anxiety and depression commonly arise from fear of death, loss of independence, fear of being a burden to others, hopelessness, and loneliness, in addition to concern about symptom burden and disease progression (Nelson, 2016). Delirium may develop during the course of serious illness, particularly at the end of life, and it is important to remember that anxiety, confusion, or delirium may be the first sign of a medical problem, particularly in older adults (Hosker & Bennett, 2016). Moreover, these symptoms may be interwoven, making it difficult to differentiate among the three diagnoses. Anxiety may precede depression in the diagnosis of certain medical conditions such as myocardial infarction or dementia. Anxiety and depression may be seen together, perhaps in the setting of a diagnosis of a serious illness such as heart disease, pulmonary disease, or advanced cancer. Delirium may cause anxiety stemming from altered consciousness, confusion, and disorientation. This is particularly true if the delirium waxes and wanes and the patient has a sense of his or her cognitive impairment. Anxiety may result in delirium if the patient's anxiety escalates, and he or she either does not have proper nutrition or overmedicates himself or herself. Additionally, depression may result if a patient understands his or her cognitive deficits. Diagnosis and treatment may be challenging when the person is able to compensate for the cognitive deficits, thereby decreasing the likelihood of detection and treatment.

Historically, it was thought that children experience fewer psychosocial symptoms from a diagnosis of serious illness. However, this has been a grave misperception and their symptoms have been significantly underestimated. More important, it may be difficult to distinguish anxiety and depression from sadness or grief in children. To add to the complexity, there are fewer available mental health specialists to treat children and pediatrics (Goldsmith, Ortiz-Rubio, Staveski, Chan, & Shaw, 2011; Pao & Wiener, 2011). Other populations whose symptoms are underestimated include older patients, who may not be forthcoming with their psychological concerns; patients with preexisting mental health issues; patients with financial or insurance issues; and patients from other cultural backgrounds.

Once a diagnosis is made, treatment issues for psychiatric symptoms related to a specific patient must be considered. In particular, the clinician must consider the patient's age. Older adults and young children may have more pronounced and adverse effects from medications. In addition, older adults may experience diminishing functional and physiological processes, as well as social supports. Successful treatment often includes pharmacological medications, complementary therapy, and mobilization of social support of the patient and family. This chapter addresses the comprehensive patient-centered and family-focused care necessary for effective diagnosis, assessment, and treatment of anxiety, depression, and delirium in the palliative care patient.

■ ANXIETY

Definition

Anxiety is defined as feelings of distress, worry, and tension from a known or unknown stimulus (American Psychiatric Association [APA], 2013). It is a necessary aspect of life as a stimulus for our actions. Anxiety manifests itself in multiple ways, and is either acute or chronic in duration. Acute anxiety is comprised of cognitive, physiological, and behavioral manifestations that are relatively self-limiting and respond to treatment or a change in circumstance. Chronic anxiety is characterized by low-grade distress that interferes with psychosocial functioning due to restlessness or being on edge, difficulty in concentration, irritability, muscle tension, and sleep alterations (APA, 2013). The *Diagnostic and Statistical Manual of Mental Disorders* (5th ed.; *DSM-5;* APA, 2013) includes the diagnosis, *Anxiety Disorder Due to Another Medical Condition*, which relates to a patient with a chronic, progressive, or serious life-threatening illness or injury. This diagnosis states that anxiety in patients with serious illness is related to the circumstances of the direct pathophysiological consequences of a medical condition, not a mental disorder. Furthermore, anxiety can affect the patient's social interactions, occupation, and general functioning (APA, 2013). Patients may also experience anticipatory anxiety, an episode of anxiety prior to an event or a procedure, resulting in acute manifestations and can be very distressing to the patient.

Generalized anxiety disorder (GAD) is defined as chronic uncontrollable nervousness, fearfulness, and sense of worry lasting for 6 months or longer (APA, 2013). Patients may describe a sense of worry, fear, concern, or even foreboding. Although anxiety is a very subjective experience, it is often accompanied by somatic complaints such as tachycardia, fatigue, restlessness, difficulty concentrating, muscle tension, headaches, palpitations, sweating, abdominal discomfort, dizziness, urinary frequency, and sleep disturbances. To confirm a diagnosis of GAD, any of the aforementioned symptoms must be present for at least 6 months and should cause impairment in social or occupational functioning. In the older adults with GAD, there may be a concomitant symptom of agoraphobia, or fear of outside the home, which leads to more social isolation (Irwin & Hirst, 2017).

Anxiety within the pediatric population is common. The challenge is twofold: the anxiety of the child and the child's reaction to the stress and anxiety of the parents, family, and caregivers around him or her (Kane & Himelstein, 2007; Pao & Wiener, 2011). This may be common for children and parents of children with chronic illness or congenital conditions. The symptoms that children experience are related to behavioral issues and the change in their functional abilities, specifically irritability, resistance, and refusal of tests and procedures. Anxiety may affect their routines such as in school or other activities (APA, 2013). Younger children may have worries related to separation, strangers, injuries, and loud noises, while teens may have issues regarding personal appearance, self-worth, and competence (Pao & Wiener, 2011). In addition, worries about being hospitalized, treatment sessions, or the side effects of these activities may occur as well.

Incidence

Anxiety symptoms may develop in any individual diagnosed with a life-limiting illness. The diagnosis, itself, is stress and anxiety provoking. An increased incidence of anxiety has been associated with female gender, young age, and low socioeconomic status, as well as with cancer and chronic diseases (Gatto, Thomas, & Berger, 2016; Zvolensky, Garey, & Bakhshaie, 2017). Furthermore, as a serious illness progresses and a person's physical status declines, anxiety may increase. Cancer-related anxiety is a natural response to the crisis precipitated by such a diagnosis, the threat to life, and the future (Traeger, Greer, Fernandez-Robles, Temel, & Pirl, 2012). Within the pediatric population, there are no prevalent studies related to anxiety at the end of life.

Etiology

Anxiety in patients with a life-limiting illness is common and may have a multitude of causes, including adjustment disorder, panic disorder, GAD, phobia, or agitated depression (Gatto et al., 2016). The etiology of anxiety includes medical conditions such as poorly managed pain, endocrine disorders including hypo- and hyperglycemia, hypo- and hyperthyroidism, Cushing's disease, and carcinoid syndrome. Cardiovascular conditions include myocardial infarctions, angina, congestive heart failure, mitral valve prolapse, and hypovolemia; respiratory conditions include asthma, chronic obstructive pulmonary disease (COPD), pneumonia, pulmonary edema, dyspnea, and hypoxia. Neoplasms and neurological conditions such as akathisia, encephalopathy, seizure disorder, and post-concussion disorders can also contribute to or exacerbate anxiety disorders (Fournier, 2013a; Pasacreta et al., 2015).

Stimulant substances may contribute to anxiety. The most common substance is caffeine. The stimulant ephedrine, stimulant-type drugs such as methylphenidate, and withdrawal from medications such as benzodiazepines, alcohol, and barbiturates may cause anxiety. Psychological distress, including worries about family relationships, family strife, and financial issues, can contribute to feelings of anxiety in seriously ill patients. These worries may be exacerbated by concerns about being or becoming a burden to family members during the course of their illness. Lastly, a previous history or family history of anxiety may be a contributory factor resulting in more pronounced anxiety in older patients as they lose physical functioning. See Table 22.1 for further summary of causative factors and Table 22.2 for emergent conditions disguised as anxiety.

TABLE 22.1 Potential Conditions That Produce or Mimic Anxiety

System/Condition	Examples
Cardiovascular conditions	Angina, congestive heart failure, hypovolemia, mitral valve prolapse, myocardial infarction, paroxysmal atrial tachycardia
Endocrine disorders	Carcinoid syndrome, Cushing's disease, hyperglycemia, hypoglycemia, hyperthyroidism, and hypothyroidism
Immune conditions	AIDS, infections
Metabolic conditions	Anemia, hyperkalemia, hyperthermia, hypoglycemia, and hyponatremia
Respiratory conditions	Asthma, chronic obstructive pulmonary disease, hypoxia, pneumonia, pulmonary edema, and pulmonary embolus
Neurological conditions	Akathisia, encephalopathy, brain lesion, seizure disorders, post-concussion syndrome, vertigo, cerebral vascular accident, and dementia
Cancer	Hormone-producing tumors: pheochromocytoma
Medication and substances	Withdrawal of alcohol, benzodiazepines, nicotine, or sedatives. Use of steroids, stimulants, and neuroleptics such as metoclopramide or prochlorperazine
Pain	Uncontrolled or poorly controlled

Sources: Adapted from Breitbart, W., & Dickerman, A. L. (2017, May 10). Assessment and management of depression in palliative care. Retrieved from https://www.uptodate.com/contents/assessment-and-management-of-depression-in-palliative-care; Fournier, D. (2013a). Anxiety disorders. In T. Buttaro, J. Trybulski, P. Bailey, & J. Sandberg-Cook (Eds.), *Primary care: A collaborative approach* (4th ed., pp. 1344–1351). St. Louis, MI: Elsevier Mosby; Pasacreta, J. V., Minarik, P. A., Nield-Anderson, L., & Paice, J. A. (2015). Anxiety and depression. In B. Ferrell & N. Coyle (Eds.), *Oxford textbook of palliative nursing* (4th ed., pp. 366–385). New York, NY: Oxford University Press.

TABLE 22.2 Emergent Conditions Disguised as Anxiety

- Hypoxia
- Sepsis
- Uncontrolled pain
- Pulmonary embolus
- Impending cardiac or respiratory arrest
- Electrolyte imbalance
- Dehydration

Sources: Adapted from Breitbart, W., & Dickerman, A. L. (2017, May 10). Assessment and management of depression in palliative care. Retrieved from https://www.uptodate.com/contents/assessment-and-management-of-depression-in-palliative-care; Fournier, D. (2013a). Anxiety disorders. In T. Buttaro, J. Trybulski, P. Bailey, & J. Sandberg-Cook (Eds.), *Primary care: A collaborative approach* (4th ed., pp. 1344–1351). St. Louis, MI: Elsevier Mosby.

TABLE 22.3 Four Types of Anxiety Manifestation

Classification	Manifestations
Physical symptoms	Autonomic responses such as tachycardia, tachypnea, diaphoresis, light-headedness, tremors
Affective symptoms	Nervous or restless behaviors such as pacing, picking, frequent movement
Behavioral responses	Avoidance, compulsions
Cognitive responses	Edginess, worry, panic, terror, apprehension, obsession, thoughts of physical or emotional damage to self

Source: Adapted from Irwin, S. A., & Hirst, J. M. (2017, May 10). Overview of anxiety in palliative care. In D. M. F. Savarese & R. Hermann (Eds.), *UpToDate.* Retrieved from http://www.uptodate.com/contents/overview-of-anxiety-in-palliative-care

Cardinal Signs

Anxiety has four types of manifestations: physical symptoms, affective symptoms, behavioral responses, and cognitive responses (Pollack, Otto, Wittmann, & Rosenbaum, 2010), as outlined in Table 22.3. Generalized anxiety can be accompanied by symptoms of depression, panic, and phobias. In the older patient, depression is the most common symptom accompanying anxiety (Rosen, Koretz, & Reuben, 2010). Patients may be observed to experience anxiety-related behaviors such as a tense posture and frequent sighing. Older adults are more likely to minimize emotions and feelings and report somatic complaints (Tabloski, 2014). Moreover, older adults are particularly vulnerable to suicide due to the potentially multiple burdens of pain and suffering, poor prognosis, depression, delirium, loss of control, and lack of social support (Breitbart, Chochinov, & Passik, 2010). In differentiating anxiety from fear, evaluation should explore the known presence of an external threat versus anxiety stemming from an unknown internal stimulus (Traeger et al., 2012). The diagnosis of *Anxiety From Another Medical Condition* is helpful to consider as there are many "unknowns" in chronic progressive conditions and/or serious life-threatening illnesses that cause anxiety including, but not limited to, continued surveillance of the disease, concerns over test results, and the rapidity of the disease progression, particularly into advanced conditions. Finally, the loss of control and the multitude of significant losses throughout the course of serious illness may become major stressors.

Severity

Anxiety, in its mildest form, is a positive form of stress that serves as a motivation to perform various functions in learning, working, and adapting to the ongoing changes in life. Levels of anxiety can be mild (which is considered normal), moderate, severe, and panic (Pasacreta et al., 2015). In its most severe form, anxiety becomes panic, which may result in a form of psychological paralysis and isolation. The person may become paralyzed by fear and be confined to his or her immediate surroundings, such as his or her home or room. Table 22.4 outlines the characteristics of mild anxiety to panic.

Assessment

A history and review of medical conditions for potential causes of anxiety are central to the initial evaluation. The evaluation of the serious illness and its symptom burden is important as well as other comorbid conditions. Predisposing factors should be examined, including a previous history of anxiety or trauma, social isolation, and coping style (Traeger et al., 2012). A thorough discussion of psychosocial situations including living conditions, recent changes in the patient's life, and anticipated life changes is warranted. This conversation can sometimes be more revealing if it includes both the patient and his or her family or friends, as permitted by the patient. An open discussion of fears and concerns of an uncertain illness trajectory may be helpful. This may help in determining whether the anxiety is a secondary response to the following: an organic factor, a primary psychiatric disorder, or reactive or situational-related stress (Traeger et al., 2012). Situational-related stress is common and cannot be

TABLE 22.4	Mild to Severe Anxiety and Its Effects
Mild	Awareness, alert attention for problem solving
Moderate	Perceptual field narrowed, decreased observation, and selective attention
Severe	Reduced perceptual field, scattered, escalated anxiety with inability to attend
Panic	Feelings of awe, dread, fear, panic; inability to focus; no perceptual field

Source: Adapted from Pasacreta, J. V., Minarik, P. A., Nield-Anderson, L., & Paice, J. A. (2015). Anxiety and depression. In B. Ferrell & N. Coyle (Eds.), *Oxford textbook of palliative nursing* (4th ed., pp. 366–385). New York, NY: Oxford University Press.

overemphasized. There are many aspects of care that incur anxiety for patients (whether an adult or child) with a serious diagnosis, including the anxiety about the unknown illness trajectory, consultations with specialists, diagnostic procedures, changes in care needs, moving from one care setting to the next, or changing the care provider. For children, a skilled assessment based on children's concerns and worries may help reveal both parent and child anxiety (Mullaney, 2011; Pao & Wiener, 2011).

Physical Examination

A physical examination may reveal tachycardia, tachypnea, skin changes, tongue changes, rapid speech, restlessness, and tremors. Complete blood panels and metabolic screens can delineate other processes such as infection, cardio-pulmonary conditions, and so on. Further assessment includes ruling out associated conditions. For example, if the patient has tachycardia, a thyroid function panel can rule out hyperthyroidism, an electrocardiogram can rule out dysrhythmias, and a glucose test can rule out hypoglycemia. If the patient is found to have a sore tongue along with anxiety, testing folate levels can rule out nutritional deficiencies. Pulmonary function tests and arterial blood gases can rule out hypoxia and pulmonary disease (Fournier, 2013a). Finally, there may be situations where drug toxicology screening is necessary to rule out for cocaine or amphetamine use, or other medications from which the patient may be in withdrawal.

Assessment Tools

The Anxiety Sensitivity Index (ASI) is a 16-item self-report tool in which responses are rated from 0 to 4. A mean score of 20 and below indicates no anxiety. A mean score in the 20s is common for those with GAD, and a mean score of 35 and above indicates panic disorder (Reiss, Peterson, Gursky, & McNally, 1986). Another commonly used tool is the brief Patient Health Questionnaire for Depression and Anxiety (PHQ-4). If the patient screens positive for the PHQ-4, it is suggested that he or she be assessed for major depression or dysthymia using the American Psychiatric Association *DSM-5* criteria for the disorders, and if major depression is present, the Patient Health Questionnaire (PHQ-9) can be used to monitor depression severity over time (Irwin & Hirst, 2017). Other tools include the Hospital Anxiety and Depression Scale, which is a self-report measure of 10 questions, and the Visual Analog Scale or the Distress Inventory Scale (Sheldon, Swanson, Dolce, Marsh, & Summers, 2008).

There are several tools to assess anxiety in well children; however, none have been tested in chronically ill or terminally ill children. Two self-report measures are the Spence Children's Anxiety Scale and the Screen for

Child Anxiety–Related Emotional Disorders. One interview that may help is the Anxiety Disorders Interview Schedule for Children (Kersun & Shemesh, 2007). The questionnaire is comprised of a series of semi-structured questions answered by child and parent self-report. These questions review lifetime and current anxiety, as well as mood. For children younger than 8 years, the questions are usually answered by their caregivers; however, developmentally appropriate assessments in younger children have been reported.

Management

Nurses may be the first to identify anxiety for many patients. A collaborative interdisciplinary team approach is helpful in the treatment of anxiety for patients experiencing serious life-limiting illness. Treatment of anxiety is most successful when psychosocial and psychoeducational interventions are combined with pharmacological interventions (Blatt, 2012; Braun, Pirl, & Greenberg, 2010). Often a medication and dietary review may reveal substances and medications used to manage disease-related symptoms, such as steroids or stimulants, which increase anxiety, but are essential to disease management. In this situation, the times of medication administration may need to be changed to promote sleep.

■ **Pharmacological.** In general, there is a lack of evidence to draw a conclusion about the effectiveness of drug therapy for symptoms of anxiety in adult palliative care patients (Salt, Mulvaney, & Preston, 2017). In a younger, healthier population, selective serotonin reuptake inhibitors (SSRIs) are the first drug of choice for the treatment of anxiety disorders as this class of medication has proven to be effective in addressing panic, GAD, posttraumatic stress disorder, and obsessive–compulsive disorder (Gatto et al., 2016). Tricyclic antidepressants (TCAs) can also be effective and have the benefit of being inexpensive and serving as an adjuvant for neuropathic pain. Because benzodiazepines have a rapid onset, they are commonly used to treat acute anxiety. However, this class of medication has been associated with many adverse events in the medically ill and caution is advised in their use (Irwin & Hirst, 2017).

In older and geriatric populations, it is important to consider medication, dosages, and dose titrations because of the potential of paradoxical responses to certain medications. In addition, it is important to be mindful of the patient's prognosis and his or her insurance coverage for medications. Antidepressant therapies are indicated if prognosis extends beyond 2 months. If time is shorter, benzodiazepines can be prescribed for rapid relief of acute anxiety symptoms. However, due to their long half-life, these medications can cause adverse drug effects, including confusion and worsening anxiety. Due to its shorter half-life, lorazepam is the recommended benzodiazepine of choice with older populations. It has a double result in both relief of nausea and reduction of panic attacks. Very short-acting benzodiazepines, like oxazepam or alprazolam, are not recommended and should be avoided because of the association with a significant risk for rebound anxiety and withdrawal syndromes (Irwin & Hirst, 2017). Generally, tricyclics and beta-adrenergic agents are not well tolerated in older populations, though a trial may be warranted if other medications do not offer relief. If insomnia and anxiety together are symptoms, temazepam 15 to 30 mg at bedtime may be helpful, and patients with decreased hepatic function may do better with temazepam and lorazepam as these medications do not have active metabolites. Drug-induced anxiety may be caused by neuroleptic medications such as haloperidol, and hydroxyzine can cause anticholinergic side effects and delirium. For patients with generalized anxiety and a history of substance abuse, buspirone may be useful. For patients with severe respiratory function, low dose antihistamines may be helpful, and for terminally ill patients with dyspnea, opioids are indicated. For patients for whom anxiety mostly affects the ability to go to sleep and/or stay asleep, but not their daily routine, there may be situations where hypnotics are used to help them either on a short-term or long-term basis. The use of these medications should be carefully monitored (Gatto et al., 2016). See Table 22.5 for drugs and dosages.

In children, benzodiazepines are the medication of choice. The short-acting agent lorazepam is helpful for procedures. Clonazepam and diazepam are helpful long-acting agents, although diazepam's half-life may affect other medications (Mullaney, 2011; Pao & Wiener, 2011). Dosing is based on weight (Mullaney, 2011; Pao & Wiener, 2011). Lorazepam is calculated at 0.025 mg/kg/24-hr dose with a maximum of 2 mg/dose. Diazepam is calculated at 0.01 to 0.02 mg/kg/24 hr with a maximum dose of about 10 mg/d. Clonazepam is calculated at 0.01 mg/kg/24 hr with a maximum initial dose of 0.05 mg/kg/d.

■ **Nonpharmacological.** To manage anxiety, a range of psychosocial strategies are beneficial. When possible, it is helpful to work with patients over time to promote the acknowledgment of their anxiety about their disease, treatment, symptoms, and future. The nurse can reduce general anxiety by offering the patient and family information about the clinical encounter. This includes the process or procedure of home visits, office visits, or the schedule of the day on an acute care or facility unit; preparation and information about tests and procedures; and identification of health procedures. Patients diagnosed with a serious illness may have fears and concerns about dying and the dying process. The process of inquiring about such fears helps to normalize their presence, and addressing them is helpful, particularly in developing an individualized care plan. Discussion of

TABLE 22.5 Medications to Treat Anxiety	
Medication Class	**Range**
Adults	
Benzodiazepines	
Short acting:	
Lorazepam (Ativan)	0.25–5 mg TID
Temazepam (Restoril)	15–30 mg at bedtime
Antipsychotics/Neuroleptics	
Haloperidol (Haldol)	0.5–2 mg q2–12 hr
Olanzapine (Zyprexa, Zydis)	5–15 mg daily
Risperidone	1–3 mg daily
Quetiapine	25–200 mg daily
Azapirones	
Buspirone (BuSpar)	5–20 mg TID
Children	
Benzodiazepines	
Lorazepam (Ativan)	Younger children: 0.025–0.05 mg/kg every 4–6 hr Adolescents above 12 years: 1–2 mg every 8 hr
Clonazepam (Klonipin)	Younger children: 0.01–0.03 mg/kg every 24 hr Adolescents above 12 years: 0.5–1.5 mg every 24 hr
Diazepam (Valium)	Younger children: 0.08–0.12 mg/kg every 8–12 hr Adolescents above 12 years: 5 mg every 8 hr

TID, three times a day.

Sources: Adapted from Blatt, L. (2012). Psychosocial issues. In C. Dahlin & M. Lynch (Eds.), *Core curriculum for the advanced practice hospice and palliative registered nurse* (2nd ed., pp. 187–224). Pittsburgh, PA: Hospice and Palliative Nurses Association; Mullaney, E. (2011). Symptom management in pediatric palliative care. In G. Santucci (Ed.), *HPNA core curriculum for the pediatric hospice and palliative nurse* (pp. 67–106). Pittsburgh, PA: Hospice and Palliative Nurses Association; Pao, M., & Wiener, E. (2011). Psychological symptoms. In J. Wolfe, P. Hinds, & B. Sourkes (Eds.), *Interdisciplinary pediatric palliative care* (pp. 229–238). Philadelphia, PA: Elsevier Saunders; Pasacreta, J. V., Minarik, P. A., Nield-Anderson, L., & Paice, J. A. (2015). Anxiety and depression. In B. Ferrell & N. Coyle (Eds.), *Oxford textbook of palliative nursing* (4th ed., pp. 366–385). New York, NY: Oxford University Press.

values, preferences, and beliefs in the form of advance care planning may be helpful to patients and families to promote proactive planning and provide patients some control in their care. Additionally, interventions such as cognitive behavioral therapy, relaxation training, and supportive counseling may be helpful (Traeger et al.,

2012). Providing structure and predictability can help to allay fears and can take place in the form of future appointments and symptom management (Bakitas, Dahlin, & Bishop, 2017). Offering summary information at the end of every visit about progress and future events may alleviate any surprises and assure the patient and provider share a mutual understanding. If appropriate, encourage patient participation in his or her care. One helpful intervention for pediatric patients is bibliotherapy, which is the use of literature and storytelling to allow children to tell their version of the situation. By using a book to stimulate thought or create a unique story, the child has assistance to review the situation, foster emotional responsiveness, discuss psychological reactions, and consider coping strategies (Pao & Wiener, 2011). Animal therapy is also quite effective in relieving stress as the animal reduces the threatening feelings by offering a social connection and unconditional love (Pao & Wiener, 2011).

Dietary modifications, stress management, and psychotherapy are examples of nonpharmacological treatment that can benefit anxiety. Nutritional assessment includes evaluating the diet for caffeine and alcohol (Blatt, 2012). Sometimes, simply decreasing the daily intake of caffeine (present in all forms of tea, coffee, and chocolate) is helpful, although in many cases, caffeine needs to be eliminated. If this is the case, weaning off caffeine in a planned process helps to avoid common withdrawal symptoms of headache, nausea, and general malaise. In addition, a review of over-the-counter medications for coughs and colds should include eliminating ephedrine. High alcohol intake is common in anxious patients, and it may worsen anxiety because it affects sleep and cognition. Alcohol is commonly consumed as beer, wine, or hard liquors, but is also present in cough medicines and mouthwashes. Reduction or elimination of alcohol intake entirely may be helpful in the management of anxiety. Finally, nicotine may contribute to anxiety, and patients may require smoking cessation programs and/or smoking substitutes, such as nicotine patches and gums, to successfully quit smoking.

Stress management can include exercise programs, breathing exercises, relaxation techniques, massage, touch, distraction, music therapy, and visualization. Guided imagery and hypnosis may offer the patient more control in everyday life and in stressful situations (Plaskota et al., 2012). Some hospitals, healthcare systems, and insurance plans offer exercise programs or gym reimbursement. Many Young Women's Christian Associations/Young Men's Christian Associations (YWCA/YMCAs) offer gentle exercise programs or special programs directed at keeping people of various ages healthy, and provide discounts or subsidies for patients who need financial assistance. Shopping malls may offer patients the opportunity to walk in a safe, weather-friendly environment often at off-hours to allow patients to avoid crowds. For patients in assisted living or skilled nursing facilities, physical therapists (PTs) can often help promote gentle exercise.

Massage therapy can be an effective method to help patients relax. Of course, the patient must be assessed regarding his or her comfort with physical touch and any conditions or injuries that would preclude massage. Some older adults may not have experience with formal massage and may be uncomfortable with such intimate touch. Often patients may receive modified massages from healthcare personnel in various settings, such as outpatient oncology settings, hospitals, skilled facilities, or day care centers.

Distraction can be used to manage anxiety, and it may occur in many forms including watching television; listening to the radio; reading digital devices, books, and newspapers; participating in arts and crafts; and performing hobbies. It is important to assess how the patient spends his or her time and what activities are distracting and helpful for him or her. Music therapy has been shown to be effective in anxiety, as it can reduce pain, promote physical comfort, and induce relaxation (Meghani, Tracy, Hadidi, & Lindquist, 2017).

Evaluating a patient's environment may be very important, as patients may worry about aspects of their living situation, particularly navigating stairs and bathroom areas. PTs and occupational therapists (OTs) can assist with home-safety evaluations, and social workers can assist with issues of personal safety. In the case of older adults, social workers evaluate situations of potential abuse and neglect, transportation, or lack of access to good nutrition. Too often, the patient loses control over his or her life as the disease, treatments, or side effects interrupt daily routines. Facilitating the patients' control in the details and planning their day decreases anxiety. This includes their self-care, meals, healthcare appointments, and other activities that can help them feel less anxious.

Psychotherapy may include counseling, spiritual care, and cognitive behavioral therapy. Counseling generally includes exploration of specific fears and conversations about those fears. Spiritual care interventions focus on existential fears around death and dying by offering supportive exploration and guidance (Borneman, 2012). Cognitive behavioral therapy focuses on restructuring the issues using various techniques over a discrete period of time.

For children, stress and anxiety management may be developed into more structured programs. Children may need specially trained pediatric practitioners to assist with these areas. Anxiety can be managed with a variety of therapies including expressive therapy (art, music, and journaling), touch therapy, and talk therapy (Mullaney, 2011). Art and music therapy may promote a release in anxiety from tactile and intellectual stimulation. Other therapeutic activities include sports, music, or, for younger children, play therapy activities with child life specialists. Adherence to routines and schedules helps reduce stress and normalize their illness. Of particular importance is attendance at school and related activities since these activities play a major role in the context of their daily routine and social networks (Mullaney, 2011). Parents may need to participate with the child so they may experience anxiety reduction together. This is important if the child appears to be reactive to the parent's or guardian's anxiety.

Dependent, Independent, and Collaborative Interventions

Treatment of anxiety for a patient with a life-threatening illness requires a collaborative approach by an interprofessional team. The nurse has a role in assuring team communication within the plan of care. Specifically, the team needs to review the patient history and medications and then determine symptom management together. Since treatment usually requires psychological support and medication management, clear delineation of roles should be clarified for the patient and his or her family. This provides consistent direction and support to the patient and family without provoking further anxiety. A physician or an advanced practice registered nurse can diagnose and treat anxiety, as well as provide medications and psychological support. A social worker can be quite effective in assessing the living conditions and the family dynamics that affect anxiety, as well as offering both counseling and stress management techniques. An OT or PT can assess in-home safety and teach the family safe transfers to promote mastery in the delivery of care in the home. A pharmacist can examine a medication regimen for polypharmacy. A common observation for nurses working with patients is that the anxiety can be easily absorbed. Therefore, anxious patients and families can make the nurse feel anxious or frustrated. Therefore, the nurse needs time and distance to dispense or relieve himself or herself of the anxiety of the patient and family.

Family Concerns and Considerations

Education for the family and caregiver is important as this information may promote early recognition of symptoms and can help the patient utilize both medications and complementary strategies to manage anxiety. The patient and family should also understand that in some cases, long-term use of medication to treat anxiety may be necessary. These medications may cause some or all of the following side effects to greater or lesser degrees: daytime somnolence, confusion, unsteady stance or gait, paradoxical effects, memory disturbance, depression, withdrawal, abuse, dependence, and respiratory problems. Safety may be an issue, and prior to starting any medications, the prevention or management of potential medication side effects should be discussed. The patient and family may need to discuss the risk–benefit ratio of interventions, particularly if medication side effects are debilitating and worse than the anxiety itself.

Medication information is imperative, as prescription medications as well as over-the-counter medications can cause anxiety, particularly in older populations. A careful review of each medication, its intent, and its dosage can help decrease confusion and improve compliance. A medication box prefilled by family or healthcare personnel with medication in the correct time slots can be tremendously helpful in ensuring correct medication dosage and timing. In addition, a patient or family member can keep a diary of medications, dosages, and time of administration. In creating medication schedules it is best to work around previous rituals such as mealtime and other activities of daily living, with particular attention paid to sleep schedules. Stress management techniques that can be utilized by both the patient and the family should be offered. For older adults, these interventions may include promoting control over their environment (e.g., simple planning of daily activities, toileting, mealtimes, and visiting times). All patients and family members can benefit from a periodic review of anxiety-related symptoms and their management and prevention. Dealing with persistent anxiety can be difficult, so it is important to encourage time for ventilation of feelings and concerns regarding the illness experience. Education is particularly important in terms of how to diffuse anxiety and suggestions for helpful behaviors or strategies that patients and family members can follow to de-escalate stress.

Care should be taken to simplify the day by not overbooking activities for the seriously ill patient. In addition, the nurse can provide information to prepare the patient for any treatment, change in plans, or visitation by other medical personnel; this can greatly help decrease anxiety because the patient will know what to expect and can control the schedule. Concurrently, an appropriate sleep rest schedule should be planned to reduce anxiety and stress secondary to fatigue and exhaustion. All persons involved with the anxious patient need to show patience, speak calmly, and provide any direct care as gently as possible. This is particularly true when the patient has hearing or vision deficits or cognitive impairments. In settings outside the hospital, education regarding medications can allay anxiety and fears, particularly in the home or assisted living facility. With a careful review, patients may understand the appropriate use of each medication. In addition, realistic schedules can be created to apply when there is no 24-hour nursing support for medication regimens that include steroids or diuretics and antianxiety medications.

■ DEPRESSION

When dealing with a serious illness, it is common for patients to experience psychological distress in response to their serious or life-threatening diagnosis. For many years, grief and depression were considered to be normal coping mechanisms in the process of accepting a terminal illness (Block, 2000; Breitbart & Dickerman, 2017), so the treatment of depression was not prioritized. The thought was that treatment would interfere with the natural dying process and the emotional work of dying. It is now understood that not treating depression can interfere with a patient's ability to bring closure to his or her end-of-life issues and concerns.

Depression can be challenging to identify in patients with comorbid conditions, including cardiovascular disease, neurological conditions, autoimmune diseases, and endocrine disorders (Pasacreta et al., 2015). Specifically in cancer, depressive symptoms can mimic symptoms caused by the immunological, chemotherapeutic, and radiotherapeutic treatments; loss of appetite from chemotherapy; fatigue induced by the metabolic changes in cancer; and lack of sleep from compliance with continuous pain- and symptom-medication regimens (Breitbart & Dickerman, 2017).

Depression in children may be complex to assess and manage due to the potential challenges associated with their developmental stages (APA, 2013). Moreover, children may exhibit more irritability and withdrawal due to the consequences of the illness. Their depression may stem from the social issues related to being ill, such as being different from their friends and losing connection with their communities within and around school. Depression may result from changes in the routines of school and afterschool activities. Treating depression in children is further complicated as they may understand their illness through their continued repeated interactions within a healthcare system, rather than understanding the illness itself (Pao & Wiener, 2011). They may also pick up on behaviors and attitudes from their parents, so it is important to assess the family system (Pao & Wiener, 2011). While there have been no specific studies conducted on depression in dying children, a recent study showed that children with acute lymphoblastic leukemia have a higher-than-expected risk for anxiety and depression at 1 month post diagnosis and the risk of depression persists up to 1 year post diagnosis (Myers et al., 2014).

Depression in the older adult may be masked by the normal aging processes that include age-related changes in energy, sleep–wake cycles, diminishing appetite, and the ability to continue previous pursuits (Derby, 2012; Pasacreta et al., 2015). Specific to the older patient, the diagnosis of depression may be difficult secondary to the misperception that older adults experience depression as a normal part of the aging process. Many older adults do not perceive they are depressed; they may be of a generation in which psychological problems were not discussed or admitted.

Further complicating the diagnosis and treatment of depression in seriously ill adult and pediatric patients is inadequate healthcare provider knowledge regarding the treatment of depression (Breitbart & Dickerman, 2017). A thorough assessment requires sufficient time to assess and interview a patient more extensively than a cursory initial evaluation or a comparatively brief follow-up visit. Effective treatment and management require a time commitment that involves working on psychological issues, prescribing psychotropic agents, and monitoring the potential side effects of such agents. Under the time constraints common in healthcare, the necessary time to perform a complete assessment may feel overwhelming to the novice clinician. Ageist attitudes on the part of the prescribing clinician can also affect the treatment for older and younger patients. Clinicians can struggle to understand the complex interrelatedness of a serious illness and the related physical and psychosocial aspects. Some clinicians express feelings of hopelessness around the treatment of life-limiting illness and feel that depression cannot be well treated (Block, 2000). Furthermore, healthcare professionals, including nurses, may believe that by asking about depression, they add to the patient's psychological distress. Clinicians may feel unprepared and overwhelmed by the responsibility of caring for patients with life-threatening illnesses, which is why it is important to involve the resources of the interdisciplinary team. Finally, it is worth noting that for some patients with serious and life-limiting illness, total alleviation of their depression may not be possible.

Definition

Depression is a mood disorder with both psychological and somatic symptoms that alter mood, affect, and personality (APA, 2013). It is a compilation of signs and symptoms that are not considered to be a normal reaction to daily life occurrences. According to the *DSM-5*, depression is defined as a loss of interest or pleasure in nearly all activities (anhedonia) for 2 weeks or longer without improvement. In addition, four or more symptoms are present from the following list: changes in appetite; sleep, weight, or psychomotor activity; decreased energy; feelings of worthlessness or guilt; difficulty thinking, concentrating, or making decisions; or recurrent thoughts of death, suicidal ideation, or attempts at such (APA, 2013). If sufficient criteria are not met for the diagnosis of major depression, patients can be classified as having situational depression, or "adjustment disorder" with depressive features, which may or may not improve as the patient adapts to the reality of the illness (Breitbart & Dickerman, 2017). Depression can be persistent and last indefinitely if left untreated. Symptoms of chronic depression can include inconsistent memory or complaints of memory loss, increased speech latency, and an irritable affect (Chovan, 2016).

Like anxiety, the most recent *DSM-5* recognizes an aspect of depression named *Depressive Disorder Due to Another Medical Condition*, which relates to the patient with a chronic, progressive, or serious life-threatening illness (APA, 2013). Depressive disorder is related to the circumstances of the direct pathophysiological consequences of a medical condition and is not explained by a mental disorder, and it affects the social interaction of the patient (APA, 2013). For patients with chronic, progressive, or serious life-threatening illnesses or injuries in the context of life changes and adaptations resulting from these conditions that alter quality of life, disease and the associated treatment and side effects alone may result in many of the criteria listed in this depression profile (APA, 2013).

Incidence

Depression is common in patients with cancer, with an estimate that 10% to 25% of patients are affected at any given time. Depression may increase with disease progression and in certain types of cancer, including pancreatic, lung, and head and neck cancers; it is also seen in human immunodeficiency virus and acquired immunodeficiency disease syndrome (HIV/AIDS) and coronary artery disease (CAD; Breitbart & Dickerman, 2017; Chovan, 2016). Depression is a major health problem and the most common psychiatric disorder secondary to the events that occur later in life, but it may be overlooked and/or mistaken for dementia in older populations. Most studies on depression look at prevalence rather than incidence.

The incidence of depression in children is less understood because of the absence of large generalized studies to evaluate depressive symptoms in children. Moreover, children have unique ways of coping that are age dependent. More often than not, disruptions in routines, relationships, physical condition, and, for teenagers, loss of independence can be risk factors for depression, along with the adult reports of low self-esteem, guilt, hopelessness, and suicidal ideation (Kersun & Shemesh, 2007; Pao & Wiener, 2011).

Etiology

The etiology of depression is multifactorial and falls into the following overlapping four categories: physical, psychological, social, and biological (see Table 22.6). It is postulated that depression may be caused by deficiencies in serotonin, norepinephrine, and prolactin, as well as abnormal cortisol and dopamine levels. Additionally, there may be factors secondary to certain medical conditions that are associated with depression (see Table 22.7). Physical factors encompass medical conditions, specific diseases, medication effects, and sensory deprivation from loss of vision or hearing. Medications that may cause side effects that mimic depressive symptoms include chemotherapeutic agents, opioids, and glucocorticoids (Marks & Heinrich, 2013). Psychological issues that may precipitate depression cover a wide spectrum, including unresolved conflicts,

TABLE 22.6	Etiology of Depression for Adults and Children
Category	Examples
Physical	Medical conditions including cardiac disease, cerebrovascular disease, autoimmune disease, and endocrine, liver, and renal failure; specific disease relationships; medication effects; symptom related, such as pain or sleep disturbances; treatment effects, such as radiation sensory deprivation
Psychological	Memory loss, unresolved conflict, loss of independence, change in living situation, financial consequences from illness, poor coping and substance abuse
Social	Changes in body image, loss of independence, loss of family and friends, loss of community such as school-related activities, isolation, loss of employment, previous conflicted relationships
Biological	Family history, previous episodes of depression, neurotransmission deficiencies (serotonin, norepinephrine, dopamine, cortisol, prolactin), central nervous effects of cytokine

Source: Adapted from Pasacreta, J. V., Minarik, P. A., Nield-Anderson, L., & Paice, J. A. (2015). Anxiety and depression. In B. Ferrell & N. Coyle (Eds.), *Oxford textbook of palliative nursing* (4th ed., pp. 366–385). New York, NY: Oxford University Press.

TABLE 22.7	Medical Conditions Associated With Depression
Category	Examples
Endocrine disorders	Hypothyroidism, hyperparathyroidism, diabetes, Cushing's syndrome, Addison's syndrome
Cardiovascular conditions	Congestive heart failure, myocardial infarction, cardiac arrhythmias, stroke
Neurological conditions	Cerebral vascular accident, anoxia, Huntington's disease, Alzheimer's disease, dementia, multiple sclerosis, post-concussion syndrome, myasthenia gravis, narcolepsy, subarachnoid hemorrhage, Parkinson's disease
Immune and rheumatological disorders	HIV/AIDS, rheumatoid arthritis, polyarthritis nodosa, lupus
Cancer	Pancreatic, brain, lung, hematologic, head and neck, CNS
Other	Chronic pain syndrome, alcoholism, anemia

CNS, central nervous system.

Sources: Adapted from Breitbart, W., & Dickerman, A. L. (2017, May 10). Assessment and management of depression in palliative care. In D. M. F. Savarese & D. Solomon (Eds.), *UpToDate*. Retrieved from https://www.uptodate.com/contents/assessment-and-management-of-depression-in-palliative-care; Chovan, J. (2016). Depression and suicide. In C. Dahlin, P. Coyne, & B. Ferrell (Eds.), *Advanced practice palliative nursing* (pp. 321–330). New York, NY: Oxford University Press; Pasacreta, J. V., Minarik, P. A., Nield-Anderson, L., & Paice, J. A. (2015). Anxiety and depression.In B. Ferrell & N. Coyle (Eds.), *Oxford textbook of palliative nursing* (4th ed., pp. 366–385). New York, NY: Oxford University Press.

memory loss, loss of independence, change in living situations, and possible financial consequences incurred from a life-limiting illness (Pasacreta et al., 2015). When a person has a serious illness, the loss of his or her social network may cause depression. Patients may not have the energy to participate in hobbies or activities or may want to be private about visible aspects of their condition. Biological factors of depression include family history of depression or other mental illness, prior episodes of depression, neurotransmission deficiencies, and central nervous effects of cytokines. Family history may increase the risk of depression by a factor of 1.5 to 3, and 50% of people with depression have recurrence. Other mental disorders may accompany depression, including somatoform disorders (Blatt, 2012).

For children and adolescents with serious illness, the loss of independence and the loss of school and related community can be difficult (Mullaney, 2011). Young children may experience loss of teachers, friends, sports, afterschool activities, and other social interactions. Coping with the debilitating physical aspects of having a life-limiting illness may also cause depression, including pain and exhaustion. Other triggers include loss of routines and, more importantly, changes in body image. Older children may be embarrassed about the

disease or condition and treatment-related changes in their physical appearance (Mullaney, 2011).

Cardinal Signs of Depression

Depression may affect all aspects of a patient's life. This is because depression may play a role in other conditions, such as pain, confusion, agitation, anxiety, or irritability. As previously stated, contrary to public knowledge, depression is *not* a normal part of aging. However, as part of aging, the older adult may develop physical symptoms that mimic depression rather than changes in emotional affect (Derby, 2012). For that reason alone, it is suggested that the clinician assess cognitive mood symptoms rather than neurovegetative symptoms (Breitbart & Dickerson, 2017). Patients may present with a dysphoric mood or lack of pleasure. Other signs include poor permanal hygiene and grooming; slow thought processes and speech; sadness, tearfulness, hopelessness, helplessness, worthlessness, and social withdrawal; changes in sleep patterns and appetite; fatigue; behavioral slowing; and complaints of diminished ability to think (Pasacreta et al., 2015).

Signs of depression in children manifest as somatic complaints, periods of anger, and other behaviors as well as sadness or melancholy. For teenagers and young adults, depression may be manifested by low self-esteem, guilt, and hopelessness. Patients of all ages may express recurrent thoughts of worthlessness, excessive or inappropriate guilt, and a sense of being a burden (Derby, 2012; Pao & Wiener, 2011).

Patients with dementia manifest depression differently from the person whose cognitive function is intact. More peripheral symptoms may have been seen in older adults with altered cognition such as loss of interest and engagement with activities, isolation and social withdrawal, agitation, repetitive vocalization, apathy, insomnia, food refusal, and/or resisting care (Pattanayak & Sagar, 2011). Depression in this population may lead to increased dependence on activities of daily living and decreased ability to engage in meaningful activities.

Most patients with a life-threatening illness fulfill several of the criteria for depression under DSM-5 (APA, 2013). The challenge lies in differentiating depression from grief (Block, 2000; Chovan, 2016). Grief is the normal response to a loss, injury, insult, illness deprivation, or disenfranchisement that is usually proportionate to the disruption caused by the loss (Jacobsen, Zhang, Block, Maciejewski, & Prigerson, 2010). To differentiate between grief and depression in the patient with a serious illness, the clinician must perform a thorough interview that examines how the patient has coped with past crises to assess resiliency. Evaluation of the somatic distress the patient is experiencing includes hopelessness or helplessness, whether he or she has retained a capacity for joy and whether he or she looks to the future. If the patient can still experience joy, if he or she can look forward to the future, and if the symptoms come in wavelike fashion, the patient is likely experiencing grief rather than depression (Block, 2000).

Severe Depression and Suicide

Depression in its most severe form puts a person at a risk for suicide. The rate of suicide increases with age, with suicide being the third leading cause of death for older adults. One out of five suicides involves a person of 65 years or older. Recent studies have found that having five or more health systems affected by disease was a predictor of suicide (Almedia et al., 2016). Suicidal behavior in the older adult differs from that of a younger person in that the elder person is less likely to express suicidal ideation and more likely to utilize lethal methods. In children and teenagers, depression may be subtle and may include passive thoughts such as being tired of fighting or feeling like it would be okay not to wake up from sleep (Pao & Wiener, 2011). Suicidal ideation is a psychiatric emergency and warrants immediate

assessment. Lack of a previous suicide attempt may not be significant in assessing suicidal risk because the majority of older patients who commit suicide have no prior suicidal behaviors. Many older people who commit suicide have been found to have the most treatable types of depression if they had received appropriate interventions (U.S. Preventive Services Task Force, 2016).

The risk for suicide in the general population includes prior psychiatric diagnosis, including previous depression, family history of suicide, poor social support with isolation, delirium, fatigue, advanced illness with disfiguring disease or surgery, substance or alcohol abuse, poorly controlled pain, increasing age, and lack of control with hopelessness (Braun et al., 2010). Because there are no specific pediatric and teen suicide assessments, they should be screened as adults (Pao & Wiener, 2011). Assessment and evaluation of the following areas is essential for determining suicide potential: strong character; fear of dependence on and/or being a burden on others; refusal of assistance; fear of financial issues related to treatment; unrelieved severe pain; poor functional status; and previous psychiatric distress. Other factors include retirement, recent change in housing, changes in health, history of poor interpersonal relationships, and a terminal diagnosis. For teenagers, the loss of social relationships with the school community, such as loss of relationships due to healthcare treatments, as well as an inability to attend school, activities, or sports, are of particular significance.

When suicidal ideation is detected, it can be an emotional time for the clinician. In a nonjudgmental manner, the clinician must evaluate for the severity of the suicidal ideation (Box 22.1). This includes a review of the presence of suicidal thoughts, any details of a suicide plan, the seriousness of the intent, the patient's social supports, and the degree of the patient's impulsivity (APA, 2016).

In addition, the clinician should assess the history, determine the degree of intent, and evaluate the existence and quality of internal and external controls. This may include a safety assessment of the home to check for firearms, weapons, and alcohol along with the presence of multiple medications. If possible, the clinician should initiate a safety plan with family and friends. This usually consists of a safety contract with the patient and ensuring the patient is not left alone. Of utmost importance is consultation with mental health or

Box 22.1
Suicidal Ideation Questions

Would you prefer that death would come sooner rather than later?
Have you thought that it would be a relief to die sooner?
Have you thought about ending your life or killing yourself?
Have you thought about what method you would use?
(Blatt, 2012)

psychiatric providers for assistance and an evaluation plan (Chovan, 2016).

Assessment

Assessment of depression includes both cognitive and physical assessments. It is imperative that the palliative care clinician normalize depression by first performing a depression screen and evaluating risk factors, which include many of the aspects of disease progression. In particular, this includes past history of psychiatric disorders and substance abuse. The clinician should monitor for changes in life circumstances, function, medications, and comorbid conditions. Cultural assessment should be incorporated since there are racial, religious, and ethnic variances in the expression of depression. Education includes normalization that depression often occurs in serious illness but can be well managed. Psychosocial assessment includes assessment of various domains of life (see Table 22.8).

A thorough physical assessment of the patient includes laboratory testing to rule out other conditions, if appropriate. Prior to proceeding, it is important to consider whether the collection of blood tests presents an undue burden on the patient and there are plans to treat whatever deficiencies are found. Laboratory studies may include serum electrolytes to rule out dehydration; circulating blood count and hematocrit to rule out anemia; thyroid profile to rule out hypothyroidism; a venereal disease research laboratory (VDRL) screen to rule out an STD; vitamin B_{12}/folate levels to rule out

vitamin deficiencies; liver function tests (LFTs) to rule out liver failure; renal function tests to rule out renal failure; a urinalysis to rule out infections; and an ECG to rule out cardiac issues (see Table 22.9).

Physical assessment includes a general examination of the following areas: cardiopulmonary, gastrointestinal, genitourinary, and neurological. If pain develops, radiological and gastrointestinal studies are indicated to rule out fractures, ulcers, and neoplasms. Complaints of chest pain should be evaluated with an electrocardiogram. Noninvasive cardiovascular studies can rule out myocardial infarctions, congestive heart failure, and arrhythmias. Shortness of breath justifies chest films, pulmonary function test, pulse oximetry, and blood gases to rule out COPD, lung neoplasms, and other pulmonary conditions. Moderate-to-severe constipation can be evaluated with an occult blood test. Barium enema

TABLE 22.8 Depression Assessment Areas

Areas of Psychosocial Assessment for the Patient	
Ability to engage in life	Boredom vs. inability to be active
Interest in the world around them	Lack of interest vs. delight in shock, humor, etc.
Engagement in hobbies	Joy vs. lack of interest
Presence of anhedonia (capacity for pleasure)	Inability to anticipate anything with pleasure
View of life	Feelings of hopelessness vs. optimism and plans for the future
Self-worth	Worthfulness vs. worthlessness, any expressions of guilt or self-recrimination, expression of suicidal ideation

Source: Adapted from Block, S. D. (2000). Assessing and managing depression in the terminally ill patient. ACP-ASIM End-of-Life Care Consensus Panel. American College of Physicians—American Society of Internal Medicine. *Annals of Internal Medicine, 132*(2), 209–218. doi:10.7326/0003-4819-132-3-200002010-00007

TABLE 22.9 Types of Conditions and Treatment of Related Depression

Condition	Class of Medications
Cardiovascular disease	SSRIs: Sertraline, Paroxetine, Fluoxetine, Fluvoxamine, Citalopram
	Dopamine reuptake agents: Bupropion
	SNRIs: Venlafaxine
	5 HT antagonists: Trazodone
Gastrointestinal disease	Tricyclics: Nortriptyline, Desipramine
	Dopamine reuptake agents: Bupropion
	5 HT antagonists: Trazodone
Renal disease	Tricyclics: Nortripyline, Desipramine
	SSRIs: Sertraline, Paroxetine, Fluoxetine, Fluvoxamine, Citalopram
	SNRIs: Venlafaxine
	Noradrenergic agonist: Mirtazapine
Hepatic disease	Tricyclics: Nortriptyline, Desipramine
	SSRIs: Sertraline, Paroxetine, Fluoxetine, Fluvoxamine, Citalopram
	SNRIs: Venlafaxine
	Noradrenergic agonist: Mirtazapine

SNRIs, serotonin noradrenaline reuptake inhibitors; SSRIs, selective serotonin reuptake inhibitors.

Sources: Adapted from Breitbart, W., & Dickerman, A. L. (2017, May 10). Assessment and management of depression in palliative care. In D. M. F. Savarese & D. Solomon (Eds.), *UpToDate.* Retrieved from https://www.uptodate.com/contents/assessment-and-management-of-depression-in-palliative-care; Pasacreta, J. V., Minarik, P. A., Nield-Anderson, L., & Paice, J. A. (2015). Anxiety and depression. In B. Ferrell & N. Coyle (Eds.), *Oxford textbook of palliative nursing* (4th ed., pp. 366–385). New York, NY: Oxford University Press.

and thyroid function test may rule out neoplasms and ineffective thyroid. New neurological changes warrant an electroencephalogram (EEG) with a computerized tomography (CT) scan or magnetic resonance imaging (MRI) to rule out cerebrovascular accidents, tumors, or other brain conditions.

For older adults, there are several considerations in the assessment of depression. One, patients with preexisting neurological conditions such as Alzheimer's dementia or Parkinson's disease may not be able to respond to psychosocial assessment, cognitive testing, or physical examination. Additionally, they may exhibit other signs of depression such as food refusal, agitation, repetitive motions, and withdrawal. In the long-term care setting, this can be misinterpreted as boredom. Two, all too often, symptom complaints are not taken seriously by their healthcare practitioners. Several studies have reported low levels of depression detection in residential care facilities despite the known prevalence of mental health disorders in older adults living in these facilities. Explanations include ageist attitudes, inadequate staff training, and the false attribution of depressive symptoms to normal aging (Azulai & Walsh, 2015). The symptoms of depression can signal a medical condition, and a physical workup may be necessary to find the cause of problems. However, depending on the site of care, the patient's quality of life, and the prognosis of the condition, the extent of a workup needs to be consistent with goals of care. Thus, the benefits and burdens of workup need to be considered.

Assessment Tools

There are multiple evidence-based depression screening tools for the adult patient. Unfortunately, there are no tools specific to children or teenagers. Two common screening tools are the Beck Depression Inventory (BDI) and the Geriatric Depression Scale (GDS). The BDI consists of 21 items with a 4-point scale, although there is a shorter 13-item version (Candilis et al., 1999). This self-report inventory investigates neurovegetative, cognitive, and mood symptoms. This scale is useful in examining psychological symptoms to develop a differential diagnosis of depression within its scoring of 10 (mild depression), 16 (mild-to-moderate depression), 20 (moderate-to-severe depression), and 30 (severe depression; Candilis et al., 1999). The GDS (Appendix 22.1) was specifically developed for use with older adults. The long version is a questionnaire that has 30 questions and takes approximately 10 minutes. A score of 11 or more indicates depression. There is also a briefer 15-item Geriatric Depression Screening Scale (GDSS) in which the patient responds to questions that are scored for specific answers (Yesavage et al., 1982). A newer scale, known as the Terminally Ill Grief or Depression Scale (TIGDS), is a self-report measure that contains preparatory grief and depression subscales (Periyakoil et al., 2005). See Table 22.10 for a review of tools.

TABLE 22.10 Depression Scales

Beck Depression Inventory	Geriatric Depression Scale	Terminally Ill Grief or Depression Scale
21-item questionnaire	30-item scale	42-item scale
Multiple choice	Yes/no format	True/false format
Scale of 11 or higher indicates depression 11–19: mild depression 20–30: moderate depression 31 or higher: severe depression	Scale of 11 or more is positive for depression	Scale of 20 or more is positive for depression

Source: Periyakoil, V. S., Kraemer, H. C., Noda, A., Moos, R., Hallenbeck, J., Webster, M., & Yesavage, J. A. (2005). The development and initial validation of the Terminally Ill Grief or Depression Scale (TIGDS). *International Journal of Methods in Psychiatric Research*, 14(4), 203–212. doi:10.1002/mpr.8

Often asking "Are you depressed?" as suggested by Block (2000) will result in an honest assessment by an adult patient. However, this may not be as appropriate in the older adult population because there may be a generational attitude of denying mental health issues. Many older people are not comfortable expressing emotions or directly answering a question. Rather than asking a single question, there is also a two-question screening assessment recommended by the U.S. Preventive Services Task Force (2016) that includes the following questions: (a) Have you often been bothered by feeling down, depressed, or hopeless? (b) Have you often been bothered by having little pleasure or interest in doing things? Of note, little evidence suggests one assessment tool was more effective than another.

Another measure of depression is the mood of the healthcare provider after an encounter. If a healthcare provider feels down, hopeless, or negative after an encounter or has a desire to avoid the patient, there should be a high index of suspicion for depression and a rapid follow-up depression assessment (Lee, Back, Block, & Stewart, 2002).

■ SEVERE DEPRESSION AND SUICIDE ASSESSMENT

If a patient is severely depressed, a screen for suicidal ideation is imperative. Suicide assessment requires specific questioning. The Suicidal Ideation Screening Questionnaire

(SIS-Q) is a four-item screening tool that examines sleep disturbances, mood disturbances, guilt, and hopelessness. A single positive response to a question correlates with 84% of patients with suicidal ideation and necessitates further assessment (Candilis et al., 1999).

Any question that receives a positive or "yes" answer warrants further questioning, assessment, and immediate intervention with the patient and family (Box 22.2). This must be attended to urgently because there is a significant risk and safety must be assured. The nurse should not leave the patient alone. The nurse must call in a colleague or family to be with the patient while he or she calls the appropriate services within the organization. In the home, it may be the social worker or mental health specialist. In the skilled facility, it may be the psychiatrist or psychiatric nurse. In the hospital, it may be acute psychiatric services. Then the nurse must create a safety plan that the patient contracts to do no self-harm while services are being arranged. The nurse cannot leave the situation until the psychiatric team, social worker, or mental health specialist arrives to take over the care. Refer to the management section that follows for guidance regarding the risk of suicide.

Management

Treatment of depression in patients with serious illness must include management of pain and symptoms to ensure that optimal physical comfort is achieved as it is known that pain and discomfort may increase depression (Block, 2000). A patient's mood may improve simply by treating pain. For patients with altered cognition who are unable to report depression, but appear to have signs and symptoms, a trial of medications is warranted.

For the older adult who often has altered metabolism, it is judicious to use the lowest dose of antidepressants possible and to slowly increase the dose. This dose range may particularly vary in elders who have had a stroke, Parkinson's or Alzheimer's, or other comorbidities and may need longer treatment. Practitioners should be careful not to stop therapy with a specific medication too soon because patients may need a longer time to respond or a higher dose of that medication.

For patients with a prognosis of 1 month or less who are bothered by extreme fatigue, a psychostimulant, such as methylphenidate, may be very helpful. Psychostimulants typically work within 1 to 2 days. If the prognosis is longer than 1 month, one can initiate a psychostimulant to promote an immediate response and simultaneously initiate a longer-acting antidepressant medication (Breitbart & Dickerman, 2017). The effect a patient gets from the psychostimulant can help with predicting how he or she will respond to a longer-term medication. Some clinicians will reduce the dose of the psychostimulant once the antidepressant has been in effect for 1 week (Candy, Jones, Williams, Tookman, & King, 2009).

Overall, there is no one antidepressant that is necessarily more effective than another (APA, 2016; Rayner, Price, Hotopf, & Higginson, 2011). Although the second-generation antidepressants seem to be better tolerated in the well population, it appears that mirtazapine, sertraline, and citalopram are better tolerated in terminally ill people (Breitbart & Dickerman, 2017; Li, Fitzgerald, & Rodin, 2012; Marks & Heinrich, 2013). In older patients, TCAs and SSRIs are roughly equivalent in efficacy (Derby, 2012). However, the older adult tends to tolerate SSRIs better than TCAs. Side effects of TCAs include sedation, confusion, orthostatic hypotension, cardiac arrhythmias, dry mouth, constipation, ataxia, and confusion (Blatt, 2012; Derby, 2012). SSRIs have fewer anticholinergic effects, though other side effects of SSRIs include nausea, anorexia, diarrhea, and insomnia. Consideration of one medication over another may include the treatment of several symptoms (Box 22.3).

The use of herbal medications for treatment has shown no benefit over standard antidepressant therapy. More important is that these herbs (St. John's wort, Kava, and Valerian) may interfere with other medications and foods that may cause serious interactions (Blatt, 2012). Furthermore, these medications do not have FDA approval and their ingredients are not subject to consistent regulation. When St. John's wort is taken in combination with other serotonergic drugs, it can cause serotonin syndrome (Chovan, 2016). However, these medications are often used because patients can easily access them, so it is important to assess for over-the-counter medication use. See Table 22.11 for a review of medications used in treating depression.

Box 22.2
Questions for Determining Suicidal Ideation

1. Often patients develop periods of feeling down; do you have any of those feelings?
2. Have you ever felt life is not worth living?
3. Have you thought about harming yourself? In what way?
4. Are you thinking about suicide or taking your own life?
5. Do you have a plan? What is it?
6. Have you ever attempted suicide? (Chovan, 2016)

Box 22.3
Consideration of Multiple Symptoms and Medication Type

Neuropathic pain and depression—tricyclic medication
Depression, poor sleep, and diminished appetite—mirtazapine
Fatigue, depression, poor appetite, pain—steroid

TABLE 22.11 Medications to Treat Depression in Patients With Serious Illness

Adults		
Medication	**Starting Dose**	**Daily Dose**
Psychostimulants		
Dextroamphetamine	5 mg each morning	5–15 mg each morning and noon
Methylphenidate	2.5–5 mg each morning	5–10 mg each morning and noon—may need to adjust for adults' later sleep cycles
Modafinil	100 mg each morning	200 mg each morning
SSRIs with fewer side effects		
Citalopram	10 mg/d	20–40 mg/d
Sertraline	25 mg/d	50–100 mg/d
Fluoxetine	10 mg/d	20–40 mg/d
Paroxetine	10 mg/d	20–40 mg/d
Fluvoxamine	50 mg/d	50–300 mg/d
SNRIs		
Venlafaxine (extended release)	37.5 mg	37.5–225 mg/d
Duloxetine	10–20 mg/d	20–60 mg/d
Tricyclics with fewer side effects		
Desipramine	10 mg every morning	25–150 mg every morning or in two divided doses
Nortriptyline	10 mg every evening	10–100 mg every evening or in two divided doses
Atypical antidepressants		
Bupropion (sustained release)	75 mg in the morning	150 mg in the morning and mid-afternoon
Trazodone	12.5–25 mg before bedtime	25–100 mg 30–60 min before bedtime
Mirtazapine	7.5 mg every evening	15–60 mg every evening
Children		
Methylphenidate		0.1 mg/kg twice a day—may need to give in afternoons with teens who want to stay up late
Antidepressants		SSRIs—but should consult child psychiatry

SNRIs, serotonin noradrenaline reuptake inhibitors; SSRIs, selective serotonin reuptake inhibitors.

Sources: Compiled from Blatt, L. (2012). Psychosocial issues. In C. Dahlin & M. Lynch (Eds.), *Core curriculum for the advanced practice hospice and palliative registered nurse* (2nd ed., pp. 187–224). Pittsburgh, PA: Hospice and Palliative Nurses Association; Breitbart, W., & Dickerman, A. L. (2017, May 10). Assessment and management of depression in palliative care. In D. M. F. Savarese & D. Solomon (Eds.), *UpToDate.* Retrieved from https://www.uptodate.com/contents/assessment-and-management-of-depression-in-palliative-care; Pao, M., & Wiener, E. (2011). Psychological symptoms. In J. Wolfe, P. Hinds, & B. Sourkes (Eds.), *Interdisciplinary pediatric palliative care* (pp. 229–238). Philadelphia, PA: Elsevier Saunders.; Pasacreta, J. V., Minarik, P. A., Nield-Anderson, L., & Paice, J. A. (2015). Anxiety and depression. In B. Ferrell & N. Coyle (Eds.), *Oxford textbook of palliative nursing* (4th ed., pp. 366–385). New York, NY: Oxford University Press.

One of the challenges in treating terminally ill patients with severe depression and potential suicidality is the question of psychiatric hospitalization. This is a difficult decision, but necessary in extreme cases. Sometimes a patient may require hospitalization to manage depression and maximize quality of life. However, focused attention should be provided to the psychiatric unit to educate about symptoms seen at the end of life. Conversely, a patient may need to be on a medical floor with close

psychiatric supervision to promote optimal management of other symptoms.

There may be situations where electroconvulsive therapy (ECT) is warranted, particularly in patients with underlying psychiatric conditions (Breitbart & Dickerman, 2017). These may include severe depression wherein antidepressant therapy has been unsuccessful. Or it may include situations where there are psychotic features, severe suicidality (i.e., brain tumor with suicidality), severe malnutrition or dehydration in the setting of depression, catatonia, severe mania, or previous response to ECT (Blatt, 2012). The challenge is often whether the patient is ambulatory and has insurance and social supports. Studies evaluating the use of ketamine to treat depression are gaining interest due to the ease of administration, low cost, and rapid onset of action (Feifel, Malcolm, Boggie, & Lee, 2017). Studies evaluating oral ketamine in hospice patients have shown overall improvement in depression and anxiety within a 4-week period with little side effect burden (Jordan et al., 2015). However, for many patients, the side effect of hallucinations is overwhelming. Certainly, more research is needed before ketamine can be recommended.

The treatment of children is more complex due to safety of medications. Therefore, nonpharmacological therapies are encouraged as first-line interventions. However, if unsuccessful, then medications are appropriate. The use of antidepressants in children is not encouraged due to black box warnings from the Food and Drug Administration that these medications could lead to suicide or cause serotonin syndrome (Pao & Wiener, 2011). However, children are still prescribed antidepressants with dosing considerations by height, weight, Tanner development, and severity of diagnosis. Citalopram and fluvoxamine have been used as well as TCAs. Although stimulants have been used in seriously ill adults and in children with attention deficit hyperactivity disorder, their use in the pediatric palliative patient has not been well studied. Therefore, it is necessary to collaborate with child psychiatrist to help with medication use and psychotherapy in children with depression.

■ **Nonpharmacological.** In the last few years, it has been found that early-intervention palliative care reduces depression and improves quality of life in cancer patients (Bakitas et al., 2009; Temel et al., 2010). This may be due to the interprofessional nature of palliative care, which includes counseling, medications, and therapeutic use of self. Current studies continue in other noncancer conditions to see how early-intervention palliative care affects depression and quality of life.

Psychotherapy is the mainstay of nonpharmacological interventions. Psychological counseling may be even more important in older patients since they may not physically tolerate medications (Derby, 2012). Psychotherapy allows the reduction of emotional distress and attention to the individual's strengths and self-worth. Psychotherapy may focus on issues surrounding death and dying, including reminiscence and life review. Cognitive therapy focuses on processing emotions, along with reframing and restructuring events. Clinicians can assist patients to set realistic goals, provide compassionate listening, and validate the patients' feelings. In behavior therapy, clinicians can help patients develop a structure for their day and activities (Pasacreta et al., 2015). This may allow a

sense of making amends, identifying accomplishments, improving interactions, and reducing fears of death.

Music and movement therapy may be helpful in stimulating interaction, providing sensory input, and increasing circulation. Other therapies may include pet therapy, group activities, and sensory stimulation. Music therapy allows a person to access his or her feelings because music can tap into emotions that words are unable to access (Irwin & Hirst, 2017). Pet therapy enhances self-worth and fulfills a need to love and be loved in a safe environment, while simultaneously promoting tactile stimulation. Group activities and sensory stimulation increase contact and response to surroundings, stimulate thought and communication, and encourage interaction with other people.

Dependent, Independent, and Collaborative Interventions

The effective management of depression is best achieved by a team approach. Certain behaviors alone may be difficult to evaluate, but patient case review may assist to prevent and identify problems. Interprofessional team members may interact with the patient in different ways due to their different functions, and in staff conferences, vulnerable patients with a predisposition to depression can be identified.

Each team member plays a valuable role. Physicians and advanced practice providers may prescribe antidepressant medications, and a social worker can provide counseling and assessment of social supports. The family caregiver should be assessed for stress, and finances should be reviewed for potential burden. The chaplain may assess spiritual distress and provide spiritual support (Borneman, 2012). Volunteers add to the web of social support, and rehabilitation therapists can help people function. Seeing the patient across the continuum and working within a collaborative approach may increase the seriously ill patient's response to treatment.

Family Concerns and Considerations

Education is very important in depression and families should understand that depression is not a sign of weakness or failure, but rather it is a medical illness. Families should receive information on the factors that make patients vulnerable (e.g., multiple health problems, untreated pain, discomfort, and multiple losses) and learn about worrisome signs and symptoms, as well as available treatment interventions. A review of depressive symptoms can help the family to recognize depression and may help the patient, particularly the older adult, receive treatment sooner or alleviate suffering. In patients with severe depression, clinicians can assist the family in reviewing patient safety issues for potential suicide, including access to weapons, leftover medications, ability to drive, using machinery, and extreme isolation.

Patient education on medications focuses on the therapy, its goal, and potential side effects. The patient and the family should understand that concurrent use of medications related to serious illness may cause depression or interfere with response to antidepressant medications. A discussion of treatment options in relation to possible side effects is important as side effects can include blurred vision, constipation, dry mouth, urinary retention, excessive perspiration, orthostatic hypotension, fatigue, weakness, drowsiness, tremors, twitching, and hallucinations. Regarding medications and dosages, the family needs to understand that in the older adult population, lower medication doses are initially prescribed because of slower metabolism. The patient and family need to be reminded that it can take 6 to 8 weeks before the full effect of the medication is reached and may need encouragement to continue the medication. Medication education should also include the importance of continuing the medication even when the patient feels better and thinks that the medication can be discontinued.

Most important, the patient and his or her family should be reassured that most of the time, symptoms of depression are effectively managed. They should be reassured that the patient will not be abandoned and that a thoughtful treatment plan will be developed to improve quality of life. In the interim, education about severe depression should include information about support and obtaining emergency care if the depression worsens.

■ DELIRIUM

Delirium is defined as an acute disturbance of consciousness that affects cognition, arousal, and attention. Delirium is also described as a confusional state resulting from a more global impairment in mental function and may also be referred to as confusion, agitation, or terminal agitation. This inconsistency in terminology can make diagnosis and management difficult.

Alterations in thought processes are very common during the last weeks of life. Historically, this confusion and agitation was thought to be a normal part of the dying process and one of the expected stages of dying. Currently, delirium is recognized as a distressing symptom that warrants treatment. Delirium-related behaviors include thrashing, agitation, muscle twitching, tossing or turning, moaning, and talking to the air; it also includes lethargy and listlessness in its quiet forms.

Delirium should be considered an emergent situation, particularly in older populations. Delirium is associated with higher mortality rates when it occurs in older patients, as well as longer hospital admissions, increased costs of care, greater likelihood of being placed outside the home post hospitalization, and decreased functional ability (Breitbart & Alici, 2012). Moreover, patients may be terrified by the experience of hallucinations,

misperceptions, paranoid and psychomotor agitation, and changes in sleep–wake cycles.

Delirium interferes with patient comfort and causes distress for family members. Families may be upset by both the unusual behaviors and the sadness they may feel from the premature loss of their loved one. If confusion is extreme, families may experience subsequent guilt and distress at the necessity for physical or chemical restraint for fall prevention and safety. State-of-the-art palliative care includes aggressive management and treatment of delirium and the promotion of the best quality of life.

Definition

According to the *DSM-5,* delirium is an alteration in attention that includes reduced ability to sustain, direct, focus, or shift attention and diminished awareness or orientation to environment (APA, 2013). The key elements that determine delirium include changes in mental status in a short time, alternations in attention or consciousness, changes in cognition or memory, and a change in cognition from a direct physiological consequence of a medical condition (APA, 2013). This disturbance cannot be better accounted for by a preexisting or evolving dementia.

Incidence

Estimates of delirium prevalence and incidence in palliative care patients ranged from 3% to 45%, increasing to 88% in the weeks or hours before death (Burhenn, 2016). In elderly hospitalized patients, delirium is very common, and its treatment adds costly hospital days and patient and family distress. Patients with a preexisting cognitive impairment, increased age, severe illness, and an active infection are particularly susceptible to delirium. And a series of observational studies found that cancer patients with a decreased performance status, lung cancer, and a shorter time since diagnosis were associated with developing cognitive impairment (Hosker & Bennett, 2016).

Etiology

The precise pathophysiology of delirium is not well understood. However, it is thought to involve neurotransmitters in the cortical and subcortical areas of the brain. Proposed etiologies for delirium include reduced acetylcholinergic signals that can directly affect cognition, as well as excess dopamine signaling and elevated proinflammatory cytokines and anti-inflammatory cytokines (Burhenn, 2016).

Generally, the etiology of delirium is multifactorial and includes the following precipitating factors: medications, polypharmacy, hypoxia, sepsis, hypercalcemia, hepatic and renal dysfunction, electrolyte imbalances, bowel obstruction, urinary tract infection, past psychiatric history, and medication withdrawal. Possible medications contributing to delirium include opioids, TCAs, diphenhydramine, antihistamines, H_2 blockers, analgesics, sedatives, and cardiovascular drugs (Derby, 2012).

Brain involvement may be secondary to metastases, primary cerebral disease, primary cancer, or cardiovascular accident. Systemic causes include organ failure, metabolic disturbances, infection, and toxic effects of substances (Hosker & Bennett, 2016). In pediatric patients, infection appears to be a higher source of etiology than pharmaceutical agents (Goldsmith et al., 2011). Factors specific to the older adult can include preexisting dementia, a fracture, systemic infections, malnutrition, addition of three or more medications, simultaneous use of neuroleptics and narcotics, use of restraints, bladder catheters and iatrogenic events, and overall susceptibility due to lack of resilience (Derby, 2012). See Table 22.12 for a summary of conditions that can cause delirium. It is important to identify the causes of delirium for correct management. A helpful mnemonic to rule out possible causes of delirium is I WATCH DEATH (infections, withdrawal, acute metabolic causes, trauma, CNS pathology, hypoxia, deficiencies, endocrinopathies, acute vascular, toxins or drugs, heavy metals).

Cardinal Signs

Delirium has multiple manifestations, many of which are related to perceptual disturbances, which include misperceptions, illusions, and hallucinations. The cardinal signs of delirium include an acute-onset or fluctuating course in a change of mental status, inattention, and disorganized thinking. Specific symptoms include insomnia during the night and somnolence during the day, nightmares, restlessness, hypersensitivity to light or noise, and emotional lability. Typical early signs of delirium include sundowning (agitation that begins with nightfall and worsens throughout the night), withdrawal, irritability, new forgetfulness or befuddlement, and new onset of incontinence. Later signs include outbursts of anger, hostility, or abusive behavior.

TABLE 22.12 Causes of Delirium

Category/Basis	Examples
Disease process	Primary brain tumor or secondary brain metastasis
Side effects of treatment	Chemotherapy, radiation to the brain
Pain and symptom medications	Corticosteroids, opioids, tricyclic antidepressants, H_2 blockers: cimetidine, ranitidine, anticholinergics, antiemetics, thioridazine, amitriptyline, diphenhydramine, over-the-counter antihistamines, benzodiazepines, sedatives: triazolam, acyclovir, cardiovascular drugs: digitalis, nifedipine, quinidine, beta-blockers
Medication withdrawal	Opioids, benzodiazepines, alcohol
Pain	Uncontrolled pain syndrome, urinary retention, constipation/impaction, obstruction
Metabolic fluctuations	Glucose hypoglycemia, sodium hyponatremia, potassium, calcium
Organ failure	Brain: stroke, seizure, cerebrovascular accidents Kidney: uremia Lungs: hypoxia Heart: hypoxia, CO_2 retention, MI, thyroid or adrenal gland
Infection	CNS: meningitis Urinary tract: urinary tract infection Respiratory tract: pneumonia, generalized sepsis, steroid-induced immunocompromise
Nutritional deficiencies	Thiamine, vitamin B_{12}/folate
Miscellaneous	Sleep deprivation, urinary retention, sensory deprivation, change in environment, immobilization
Past psychiatric history	Depression

CNS, central nervous system; MI, myocardial infarction.

Sources: Compiled from Blatt, L. (2012). Psychosocial issues. In C. Dahlin & M. Lynch (Eds.), *Core curriculum for the advanced practice hospice and palliative registered nurse* (2nd ed., pp. 187–224). Pittsburgh, PA: Hospice and Palliative Nurses Association; Derby, S. (2012). The older adult population. In C. Dahlin & M. Lynch (Eds.), *Core curriculum for the advanced practice hospice and palliative care registered nurse* (2nd ed., pp. 511–528). Pittsburgh, PA: Hospice and Palliative Nurses Association; Dick, K. (2013). Delirium. In T. Buttaro, J. Trybulski, P. Bailey, & J. Sandberg-Cook (Eds.), *Primary care: A collaborative approach* (4th ed., pp. 999–1003). St. Louis, MI: Elsevier Mosby; Hosker, C. M. G., & Bennett, M. I. (2016). Delirium and agitation at the end of life. *British Medical Journal, 353*, i3085. doi:10.1136/bmj.i3085

There are three generally recognized subtypes of delirium: hyperactive, hypoactive, and mixed. Hyperactive delirium is characterized by increased psychomotor activity, mood swings, agitation, hallucinations, and inappropriate behaviors. Hypoactive delirium can be identified by severe lethargy and passivity. Mixed delirium can occur when patients rapidly alternate between hyper- and hypoactive states. Hyperactive delirium is readily apparent and easily recognized. Despite being more frequent than the hyperactive states, hypoactive delirium often goes unrecognized because the patient may be quiet and drowsy, and these symptoms may be mistakenly attributed to sedation from opioids, an obtunded state in the last days of life, or desired comfort, especially if symptom management has been difficult (Burhenn, 2016).

Severity

Delirium appears more severe in the hyperactive form when the patient is more agitated and delusional, causing a risk to his or her safety (e.g., falls, skin abrasion, and bruises from flailing limbs). Behaviors can be aggressive, combative, or physically threatening, resulting in a tendency to place the patient in physical restraints to keep the patient from injuring himself or herself, staff, or family, depending on the site of care. If possible, it is best to avoid restraints in facilities because this can further exacerbate the problem if the patient were to fall. Furthermore, physical restraints may worsen agitation because the patient cannot move and is either scared or frustrated by this.

Hypoactive delirium, though less obvious, is of serious concern and should be just as quickly addressed, though this may be more difficult outside the hospital. In severe cases, the result of hypoactive delirium may be premature death. If pain and symptoms have been difficult to manage, the hypoactive patient will look sedated, and the healthcare team may feel they have finally managed the bothersome symptoms because the patient is very calm and quiet. Unfortunately, the hypoactive delirious patient may be lethargic and unable to communicate his or her confusion and distress. In this situation, prescribed medications will continue to result in the depression of the patient's vital functioning. The consequence is premature death by weeks to months (Breitbart & Alici, 2012).

Assessment

Evaluation of delirium includes several components: history, cognitive assessment, physical exam, and laboratory studies. Because delirium can be confused with dementia or depression, the first step in diagnosing delirium is its proper identification. Assessment challenges are primarily due to the lack of uniformity in labeling delirium. Often,

staff lack knowledge regarding early signs of delirium, particularly at long-term care settings where the assumption may be that all older people get confused at some time. Nonetheless, caregivers and family may offer keen insight on subtle behavior changes.

The DSM-5 defines delirium to include disturbances in consciousness with impaired ability to focus or shift attention and changes in cognition or the development of perceptual disturbance that is not better accounted for by a preexisting established or evolving dementia (APA, 2013). The disturbance fluctuates over a short period of time, and evidence from the history, physical exam, or lab findings reveals the disturbance to be caused by psychological consequences of the general medical condition. Diagnostic studies should be ordered if they are likely to change patient management and are within the patient's goals of care (Bakitas et al., 2017). Other assessment tools to screen for delirium include the Delirium Rating Scale (DRS) and the Confusion Assessment Measure (CAM).

Assessment should first include a history and review of current medical conditions, including disease; disease side effects such as a tumor; and side effects of treatment, such as chemotherapy or radiation. Second, it is essential to review medications used to treat symptoms, like corticosteroids, antibiotics, opioids, anticholinergics, antiemetics, and anticonvulsants, and the possibility of withdrawal from medications like benzodiazepines or alcohol (Francis, 2017). Third, physiological causes must be assessed, including discomfort related to uncontrolled pain, urinary retention, or fecal impaction, as well as metabolic fluctuations in glucose, sodium, potassium, or calcium; organ failure including the kidneys, liver, lungs, heart, brain, thyroid, or adrenal glands; infections of CNS, urinary tract, respiratory tract; and generalized sepsis. Finally, attention should include a review and nutritional deficiencies from thiamine or folate/vitamin B_{12} (Breitbart & Alici, 2012). This is followed by a review of the patient's behavior and sleep cycles from the chart, followed by a review of the complete medication regimen.

A critical element of assessment includes the evaluation of mental status to develop a multidimensional clinical picture, functional performance status, and signs/symptoms. A mental status exam provides a baseline for monitoring the course of cognition and is a source of documentation for reference and repeat evaluations. The key aspects of mental status assessment include general state and appearance, orientation, state of consciousness, short- and long-term memory, language, visuospatial functions, cognitive/executive functions (calculations, abstraction, spelling), insight and judgment, thought control, and mood and affect (M. Folstein, S. Folstein, & McHugh, 1975; Nasreddine et al., 2005).

Physical exam is important to rule out possible reversible and treatable causes of delirium. Vital signs may offer information regarding infection, hypoxemia, and hypoglycemia. Integument inspection may reveal sepsis or cardiac failure from cold, clammy skin, or hot red skin from anticholinergic reactions. The head, eye, ear, neck, and throat exam may reveal signs of scleral icterus from liver failure, constricted pupils from opioids, or dilated pupils from anticholinergic toxicity. The oral exam may reveal nutritional deficiencies, and the chest examination may reveal rales reflective of heart failure or dullness from pneumonia. The abdominal exam may reveal urinary retention, fecal slowing, extremities, Trousseau's sign, thiamine, and liver failure (Fournier, 2013b). Helpful lab data may include glucose level, electrolytes, bilirubin, lactate dehydrogenase, LFTs, urine culture, and oxygen saturation level. See Table 22.13 for a review of important elements to the physical exam for the workup of delirium.

Assessment Tools

There are several tools available to assess mental status, and there is no preferred tool. Clinicians are recommended to use one tool consistently as daily screenings

TABLE 22.13	Delirium-Focused Physical Assessment
System	Signs and Probable Cause
EENT	Chvostek's sign–hypocalcemia Intracranial pressure Sclera icterus–liver failure Constricted pupil–opioid toxicity Dilated pupils–anticholinergic toxicity Smooth, shiny tongue–folate deficiency
Pulmonary	Rales in lungs–heart failure Dullness of percussion–pneumonia
Cardiac	S1 gallop–heart failure
Abdominal	Fecal matter palpable–constipation or impaction Bladder palpable–urinary retention
Extremity	Trousseau's sign–hypocalcemia Tender, swollen calves–thiamine deficiency Asterixis–liver failure
Neurological	Hemiplegia/hemiparesis–stroke Proximal myopathy–corticosteroid toxicity Ataxia, loss of vibration sense–thiamine or vitamin B_{12} deficiency Loss of position sense

EENT, eyes, ears, nose, and throat.

Sources: Compiled from Fournier, D. (2013b). Mood disorders. In T. Buttaro, J. Trybulski, P. Bailey, & J. Sandberg-Cook (Eds.), *Primary care: A collaborative approach* (4th ed., pp. 1328–1344). St. Louis, MI: Elsevier Mosby; Francis, J., Jr. (2017). Delirium and acute confusional states: Prevention, treatment, and prognosis. In J. L. Wilterdink (Ed.), *UpToDate.* Retrieved from https://www.uptodate.com/contents/delirium-and-acute-confusional-states-prevention-treatment-and-prognosis

of patients can increase chances of delirium identification and detection (Hosie, Davidson, Agar, Sanderson, & Phillips, 2012). In any mental status examination, several areas must be assessed: presentation, attention, visuospatial/executive function orientation, memory recall, calculation, abstraction, and language. Until the mid-2000s, the most frequently used assessment tool was the Mini-Mental Status Examination (MMSE). However, the document was copyrighted in 2000, and it is now proprietary (M. Folstein et al., 1975). Although the MMSE continues to be used widely, it is not recommended beyond initial screening (Grassi et al., 2015). The MMSE is a brief 30-item tool that measures cognitive impairment, specifically examining immediate memory, short-term memory, aphasia, apraxia, agnosia, and construction ability, along with concentration and spatial ability. The Montreal Cognitive Assessment (MoCA) is also a brief and potentially useful screening tool with a high sensitivity and specificity for detecting cognitive impairment. It is free to use if credit is given, and access is available on the MoCA website (Nasreddine, 2016). It measures the areas of cognitive function and is available in 36 languages and alternative forms (see Appendix 22.2). It is important to mention that the MoCA is a screen and does not replace a more thorough diagnostic assessment (O'Driscoll & Shaikh, 2017).

The Confusion Assessment Method Diagnostic Algorithm (CAM), the DRS, and the Memorial Delirium Assessment Scale (MDAS) are additional tools that have been found to be reliable methods of evaluating the symptoms of delirium and are frequently used across care settings (see Table 22.14). The CAM and the DRS have pediatric versions (Goldsmith et al., 2011). The CAM assesses nine domains of cognitive functioning: acute changes in mental status with fluctuating course including inattention (e.g., digit span, months backward) or observation; disorganized thinking (e.g., rambling, incoherent speech); altered level of consciousness (e.g., sleepy, stuporous, hypervigilant); disorientation (e.g., not cognizant of location or time); memory impairment (e.g., inability to remember events or instructions); perceptual disturbances (e.g., hallucinations or illusions); psychomotor agitation or retardation (e.g., restlessness or sluggishness); altered sleep–wake cycle (e.g., excessive daytime sleepiness with insomnia at night). The presence of at least the first three elements suggests a diagnosis of delirium. It is available in 12 languages and can be accessed on the Hartford Institute of Geriatric Nursing website, ConsultGeri.org.

The DRS is a 10-item structured interview, with each answer rated on a 0 to 3 scale. It is the most widely used assessment of delirium with the longest history of use in the psychiatric setting, and it is intended to be completed by a trained psychiatric clinician. The Delirium Rating Scale-Revised (DRS–R-98) is a detailed 16-item clinician-rated toll that can rate severity and

TABLE 22.14 Delirium Assessment Scales

Confusion Assessment Method (CAM)	Memorial Delirium Assessment Scale (MDAS)	Montreal Cognitive Assessment (MoCA)
9-item scale	10-item scale	11-item scale
Clinician-rated scale	4-point clinician-rated scale based on severity, 0 (none) to 3 (severe) scoring	Clinician-rated scale
Assesses: (1) acute-onset or fluctuating course, (2) inattention, (3) disorganized thinking, (4) altered level of consciousness	Assesses: awareness, disorientation, short-term memory impairment, impaired digit span, inattention, disorganized thinking, perceptual disturbance, delusions, psychomotor activity, sleep–wake cycle disturbance	Assesses: attention and concentration, executive functions, memory, language, visuoconstructional skills, conceptual thinking, calculations, orientation
Presence of first two features and either features three or four indicates a diagnosis of delirium	Score of 13 or above from a range of 0–30 indicates presence of delirium	A final score of 26 and above is considered normal cognitive functioning

Sources: Compiled from Derby, S. (2012). The older adult population. In C. Dahlin & M. Lynch (Eds.), *Core curriculum for the advanced practice hospice and palliative care registered nurse* (2nd ed., pp. 511–528). Pittsburgh, PA: Hospice and Palliative Nurses Association; Dick, K. (2013). Delirium. In T. Buttaro, J. Trybulski, P. Bailey, & J. Sandberg-Cook (Eds.), *Primary care: A collaborative approach* (4th ed., pp. 999–1003). St. Louis, MI: Elsevier Mosby; Nasreddine, Z. S. (2016, January 23). MoCA Montreal—Cognitive assessment. Retrieved from http://www.mocatest.org/pdf_files/test/MoCA-Test-English_7_1.pdf

track change over time (Hosker & Bennett, 2016). The MDAS (Appendix 22.3) is a 10-item assessment tool that is also used to assess severity. The tool measures awareness and cognitive impairment with attention to memory and psychomotor responses. Each response is rated from 0 to 3; a score of 13 or higher is diagnostic of delirium. It correlates well with the CAM, and the nonclinical staff can administer it in about 5 minutes (Burhenn, 2016).

Management

Depending on the setting and the patient's prognosis, the management of delirium includes a review of whether it is reversible and the benefits and burdens of workup and therapy. This is particularly true for patients being cared for in the home, or a long-term care setting who do not want aggressive therapies or to be transferred to an acute care setting. A stepwise approach is taken regarding the treatment of delirium, and predisposing, precipitating, and environmental factors should be quickly determined (Hosker & Bennett, 2016). Predisposing factors, like visual and audio impairments, should be attended to with glasses and hearing aids. If appropriate, postsurgical considerations should be evaluated. Precipitating factors like constipation and urinary retention should be assessed and treated, and an infectious process and metabolic imbalances should be ruled out as well.

A review of current medications is imperative and the clinician should initiate the discontinuation of problematic medications one by one to determine the causative agent. If complete discontinuation of the offending medication is not appropriate, then decreasing the dose may be helpful. Some patients may be sensitive to medications needed for pain and symptom management, specifically opioids. Therefore, discussion is critical regarding the benefits and burdens of pain and symptom management. An opioid rotation may be necessary. Alcohol or benzodiazepine withdrawal should be considered and an appropriate treatment for this should be initiated.

Any necessary treatments such as respiratory care (i.e., oxygen), wound care, or medications should be administered with appropriate pacing and time to promote rest and sleep. Metabolic fluctuations should be corrected, including hydration if consistent with the patient's and/or surrogate decision maker's goals of care. It may be appropriate to do further workup if delirium overlaps dementia or possible depression. See Table 22.15 to compare differences between depression, delirium, and dementia. Finally, throughout the treatment of delirium, counseling and education is offered to the patient, his or her family, and the support staff, with continual reassessment focusing on determining and reversing any other causes of the delirium as the patient's condition evolves.

■ **Pharmacological Interventions.** Pharmacological interventions will depend upon the suspected etiology and the setting. Neuroleptics are the drug of choice, largely because effective alternatives are not available (Francis, 2017). However, in the long-term care setting, it may be more of a challenge to prescribe as these medications can be interpreted as physical restraint medications, for which facilities must provide significant documentation. Considerable clinical experience has made haloperidol, a potent dopamine blocker, the most common first-line therapy for delirium. However, there is still controversy

TABLE 22.15	Comparison of Depression, Delirium, and Dementia		
	Depression	**Delirium**	**Dementia**
Onset	Coincides with major life changes or with a diagnosis of a serious illness	Acute/abrupt	Insidious—chronic
Course	Diurnal effects—worse in a.m.; usually situational fluctuations	Short diurnal fluctuations worse at night	Long—no diurnal effects Progressive
Progression	Variable—rapid or slow	Slow—uneven	Abrupt
Duration	Persistent—at least 2 weeks	Days to hours—less than 1 month	Months to years
Awareness	Clear	Clear	Reduced
Alertness	Normal	Fluctuates	Generally normal
Attention	Minimal impairment	Impaired	Generally normal
Orientation	Selective orientation	Generally impaired	Possibly impaired
Memory	Selective or patchy impairment	Recent and immediate impairment	Recent memory worse, remote impairment
Thinking	Intact often with sense of hopelessness, or helplessness	Disorganized, distorted, fragmented, incoherent	Difficulty with abstraction, word finding
Perception	Intact except severe cases	Distorted, illusions, hallucinations, paranoia	Misperceptions, usually absent
Psychomotor behavior	Variable—retardation or agitation	Variable—hypokinetic or hyperkinetic	Normal with apraxia
Sleep–wake cycle	Disturbed—early a.m. waking, difficulty falling asleep	Cycle reversed	Fragmented
Affect	Depressed/irritable, withdrawn	Labile mood swings	Variable
Family history	May be positive	Noncontributory	May be positive for dementia of Alzheimer type

Sources: Compiled from Breitbart, W., & Dickerman, A. L. (2017, May 10). Assessment and management of depression in palliative care. In D. M. F. Savarese & D. Solomon (Eds.), *UpToDate*. Retrieved from https://www.uptodate.com/contents/assessment-and-management-of -depression-in-palliative-care; Derby, S. (2012). The older adult population. In C. Dahlin & M. Lynch (Eds.), *Core curriculum for the advanced practice hospice and palliative care registered nurse* (2nd ed., pp. 511–528). Pittsburgh, PA: Hospice and Palliative Nurses Association; Pasacreta, J. V., Minarik, P. A., Nield-Anderson, L., &Paice, J. A. (2015). Anxiety and depression. In B. Ferrell & N. Coyle (Eds.), *Oxford textbook of palliative nursing* (4th ed., pp. 366–385). New York, NY: Oxford University Press.

over its use. Haloperidol is safely used in children and older adults; however, increased risk of extrapyramidal side effects is seen in doses of 4.5 mg/d and above (Burhenn, 2016; Goldsmith et al., 2011). Newer atypical antipsychotic agents such as olanzapine, quetiapine, and risperidone have fewer side effects, and in small studies they appear to have similar efficacy to haloperidol. Historically, chlorpromazine has been used to manage delirium; however, it is very sedating and causes orthostatic hypotension. In the home, chlorpromazine is often used because it is available in oral and rectal forms and may be necessary for agitated delirium where sedation is needed to promote safety for the patient and caregivers. Benzodiazepines may be helpful in cases of sedative drug and alcohol withdrawal, or when neuroleptic drugs are contraindicated. However, caution should be used in older adults as they may not be well tolerated. For patients with brain metastases, a trial of steroids may help manage delirium, though steroids have also been shown to cause psychosis. A recent study using methotrimeprazine in infants and children experiencing delirium appeared to be effective and safe (Grassi et al., 2015). Interestingly, ramelton, a melatonin agonist, has been found to be effective in the prevention and management of delirium, though it has not been studied within the palliative care population (Francis, 2017).

In the targeted management of hypoactive delirium, psychostimulants cannot be recommended for treatment due to the risk of precipitating agitation or worsening psychotic symptoms (Francis, 2017). However, aripiprazole has been successfully used to manage hypoactive delirium with a low side effect burden. Table 22.16

offers suggestions for medications and dosages in the treatment of delirium.

If delirium is intractable despite initial medical management, further action is necessary. The clinician should consult pain service, psychiatry, and other disease-specific specialists to explore any further possible treatment options. If the treatment efforts are unsuccessful, palliative sedation may be necessary. Palliative sedation is the use of a variety of nonopioid medications to place patients in an unconscious state. Palliative sedation necessitates team collaboration and discussion of this procedure. It also often includes an ethics consult, depending on the site of care. Patients, as appropriate, and families will need discussion about the benefits and burdens of this treatment in order to obtain informed consent.

■ **Nonpharmacological Interventions.** Nonpharmacological treatments focus on the creation of a safe environment by reducing stimuli and providing gentle reorientation and reassurance. A basic, but often overlooked, intervention is to make sure patients have access to their hearing aids and vision-correcting glasses. Other strategies include attention to the patient's room and

TABLE 22.16 Treatment of Delirium

Adults	Oral Dose
Typical antipsychotics	
Haloperidol	0.5–5 mg every 2–12 hr (every 4 hr in older adults), PO, SC, IV, IM
Atypical antipsychotics	
Olanzapine	2.5–5 mg every 8–12 hr, PO, ODT, IM
Risperidone	0.25–1 mg every 12–24 hr, PO, ODT
Quetiapine	12.5–100 mg q12–24 hr, PO
Children	**Oral Dose**
Haloperidol	0.01–0.03 mg/kg up to 6 mg/d every 8 hr
Olanzapine	1.25–2.5 mg/d
Risperidone	0.0125–0.25 mg/kg every 6–12 hr
Methotrimeprazine	0.02–0.5 mg/kg/dose, IV, PEG, SC

IM, intramuscular; IV, intravenous; ODT, orally disintegrating tablet; PEG, percutaneous endoscopic gastrostomy; PO, by mouth; SC, subcutaneous.

Sources: Francis, J., Jr. (2017). Delirium and acute confusional states: Prevention, treatment, and prognosis. In J. L. Wilterdink (Ed.), *UpToDate.* Retrieved from https://www.uptodate.com/contents/delirium-and-acute-confusional-states-prevention-treatment-and-prognosis; Mullaney, E. (2011). Symptom management in pediatric palliative care. In G. Santucci (Ed.), *HPNA core curriculum for the pediatric hospice and palliative nurse* (pp. 67–106). Pittsburgh, PA: Hospice and Palliative Nurses Association; Pao, M., & Wiener, E. (2011). Psychological symptoms. In J. Wolfe, P. Hinds, & B. Sourkes (Eds.), *Interdisciplinary pediatric palliative care* (pp. 229–238). Philadelphia, PA: Elsevier Saunders.

climate. Adjusting lighting so that it does not cause harsh images or shadows can prevent misinterpretation of the environment, which can cause hallucinations. Cognitive devices, like calendars or clocks, can cue orientation to time and date, and familiar sounds, smells, and touch may help promote calmness. Personal effects (e.g., lotions, perfumes, foods), as well as family and friends, can provide reorientation and reassurance. Another consideration is assuring sleep. Often in settings outside the home, the patients can become disoriented from interrupted sleep or lack of sleep imposed by facility and hospital schedules.

Consistent nurses and staff caring for the patient can increase familiarity and may be of benefit. In situations when the patient is agitated, family or healthcare providers may need to provide "sitters" to avoid the use of restraints. Restraints are best avoided because confused patients may unintentionally harm themselves by trying to undo restraints or by slipping out of bed. In addition, sitters can help with reorientation, respond to the patient's fear, and watch the patient to prevent falls. However, sitters may need to be reassured and coached about how much interaction to have with the patient if interaction is found to stimulate agitation.

Sleep deprivation and disturbances, which are common in hospital settings, may cause further confusion; therefore, the elimination of both visual and sensory stimuli overnight is paramount. If possible, scheduling medications and vital signs without interruption of sleep during the night can decrease sleep loss. Reduction and elimination of noise pollution such as radios, television, or overhead announcements can also increase rest and promote sleep. Indeed, it may be appropriate to close the patient's door, with frequent monitoring, to induce a restful environment. Good nursing care such as gentle massage, regular toileting, and warm drinks can promote sleep.

Family Concerns and Considerations

Education of the family is a cornerstone in the prevention, management, and treatment of delirium. Education includes the importance of skin care; the use of glasses, hearing aids, and assistive devices when appropriate; and the importance of a well-balanced diet and hydration, if these interventions are not a burden or source of distress to the patient. Families of seriously ill patients need to understand predisposing risk factors that can lead to delirium, including pressure sores, poor nutrition, incontinence, sleep disturbances, and decreased functional ability (Breitbart & Alici, 2012). Other preventive measures include the use of cognitive assistive devices such as glasses and hearing aids, avoiding restraints for confusion, judicious use of urinary catheters, removal of unnecessary tubes (rectal tubes or g-tubes), judicious use or removal of lines (intravenous access, subcutaneous access, etc.), prevention of skin ulcers, and maximal psychosocial support and education to family caregivers. Additionally, assessment of the home environment can be quite revealing, particularly whether the patient has the necessities such as food, finances, and medications.

When a patient becomes delirious at the end of life, ongoing support of the family is important. Delirium may be irreversible due to the various medical conditions the patient is experiencing as well as the dying process itself. When making decisions about treatment, discussions about realistic options should occur within the context of life expectancy and the burden versus the benefit of any treatment intervention. Families often welcome a clear discussion about all the current issues, particularly when a patient is thought to be close to death so they can prepare for the anticipated event.

Gerontological Considerations for Delirium, Depression, and Anxiety

There are many developmental tasks of late adulthood, including role changes related to retirement, widowhood, or caring for a spouse. In addition, there are normal biological changes in physical appearance and function that may result in loss of health and independence. Indeed, the older adult may have a keen sense of his or her mortality and limited life span. In response to such events, individuals cope in many ways. Sometimes, individuals develop psychiatric symptoms, including anxiety, depression, and delirium.

Many seriously ill patients may experience delirium, particularly when hospitalized. In the older adult population, delirium is even more prevalent, particularly for patients with dementia. The aging process makes older patients more susceptible to delirium because of decreased kidney function. Diminished kidney function results in an inability to eliminate toxic substances from the body, decreased ability to metabolize medications, and decreased fluid balance mechanisms. Delirium is a serious prognostic marker for older adults (Grassi et al., 2015).

Older seriously ill adults are vulnerable to depressive symptoms due to effects from multiple comorbidities as well as the adjustment to loss of health and possible loss of an independent living situation. Common depressive symptoms include grief, change in appetite that may cause metabolic imbalances, weight changes, changes in energy/fatigue, changes in sleep, and changes in concentration. Fortunately, once depression has been identified, treatment is usually effective. Treatment focuses on the use of antidepressants within the SSRI class because TCAs may cause orthostatic hypotension and be too sedating.

Loss of control and overall sense of vulnerability may increase the risk of anxiety in the geriatric population. A central challenge in treating anxiety in older patients is that they may have a paradoxical effect to the use of benzodiazepines, which are commonly used to treat anxiety in the general population. Therefore, this class of medication should be used with caution. Medications like trazodone and mirtazepine are generally well tolerated in older patients and may also provide additional symptomatic relief.

Pediatric Considerations for Delirium, Depression, and Anxiety

Anxiety, depression, and delirium present differently in the younger population of seriously ill patients. Indeed, it may be hard to differentiate among sadness, anxiety, depression, and panic. These symptoms can go unrecognized and are often underestimated, necessitating more research in the pediatric population.

Anxiety in terminally ill children may include separation anxiety. In older children and teens, anxiety may exhibit itself as posttraumatic distress disorder over treatment; social phobia over the results of treatment effects, particularly if these effects cause physical abnormalities; and general anxiety regarding the unknown future and living with a life-threatening illness. There are no specific tools for assessing pediatric anxiety; pediatric dosages of benzodiazepines are the first line of short-term therapy (Pao & Wiener, 2011).

Depression manifests itself in younger patients similar to older patients. Changes are seen in appetite and sleep, as well as psychomotor retardation and decreased energy. Grief in children is found to be self-limited and can be improved with reassurance over time. Depression can result from self-blaming and decreased self-worth (Pao & Wiener, 2011). Similarly, there is limited experience in treating depression in children. SSRIs have been found to lead to suicidal risk in healthy children, and no further research has been done in children with life-limiting illnesses. Optimal treatment is best achieved in consultation with a pediatric psychiatrist, who can also help with medication utilization and psychotherapy.

Delirium is difficult to determine in children. Like adults, it can manifest with agitation with loud, angry speech; irritability; and crying with unpurposeful activity (Goldsmith et al., 2011). However, its frequency and prevalence, like many other issues in pediatrics, has not been studied. The usual diagnostic algorithm for delirium is followed in children, beginning with identification of symptoms and consideration of possible causes. Identification of delirium-related symptoms includes changes in sleep, impaired attention, mood lability, and confusion. An initial review of medications includes evaluation for recent changes and side effects of the medications. Further physical assessment includes pain, bladder fullness, and positioning. The child should then be evaluated for medical issues such as increased intracranial pressure, hypoxia, and hypercapnia, along with kidney and liver failure. Additionally, infection should be considered (Goldsmith et al., 2011).

Treatment for agitation and delirium in seriously ill children includes soothing touch and voice. Calm music can help in the acute care setting, long-term care setting, and the home. Familiarity also provides calmness, so bringing objects from home such as pillows, pictures, and blankets may help improve delirium by their touch and smell. It is important to limit television and devices that are visually stimulating. Pharmacological treatment again focuses on sedatives and benzodiazepines, though there is a paucity of research in this area (Goldsmith et al., 2011). Neuroleptics continue to be controversial at this point due to their potent side effect burden. Specialist pediatric palliative care providers should be consulted for pediatric delirium.

■ CONCLUSION

Palliative care uses a holistic and interdisciplinary approach to optimize a seriously ill patient's physical, psychological, spiritual, and emotional well-being. A chronic progressive or serious life-threatening illness is a life crisis. Patients may develop psychiatric symptoms in response to such a diagnosis. Anxiety, depression, and delirium can be difficult disorders to recognize and treat, and these conditions can cause suffering on many levels by reducing both daily functioning and quality of life. In addition, these symptoms may herald a serious illness. It is incumbent upon clinicians to be vigilant for the presence of these disorders. Therefore, a thorough assessment, which requires skill, time, and patience, is essential for diagnosis and management.

Patient and family coping may play a role in anxiety and depression. Social issues such as isolation and lack of family support may affect the patient's anxiety and depression and his or her adherence to treatment. Many seriously ill patients may not want to burden family, friends, or relatives with their daily struggles. Children and teenagers worry about burdening siblings, parents, and grandparents or other relatives assisting in care. Older adults worry about the impact of a chronic progressive or serious life-threatening illness on work, finances, insurance, and the future.

Effective treatment of anxiety, depression, and delirium necessitates a collaborative approach between the patient, family, and healthcare team. It may allow the patient to continue care in his or her setting of choice. The patient may perceive something is wrong but cannot articulate the problem; the family may perceive something is wrong but feels it is part of the disease process. The healthcare provider may not account for the biological or developmental differences in the child or elder in evaluating the problem. These factors make communication and vigilance necessary components to good quality care. A collaborative partnership among the circle of care, which includes the patient, family, caregivers, and the medical team, supports a patient's integrity, independence, and dignity. Moreover, a comprehensive interprofessional approach offers a myriad of interventions and strategies to support the patient and family, offering the most effective management and best outcomes. Nurse are an essential part of care for patients with serious illness and promote quality of life. Understanding these symptoms helps the nurse support the patient and assure attention to the psychological and psychiatric aspects of care.

CASE STUDY *Conclusion*

Another month passed and Paul continued to withdraw from friends and family. Ellen grew increasingly concerned and reached out to Paul's oncologist who recommended that Paul see the palliative care team. Paul was assessed by the palliative advanced practice registered nurse (APRN) and social worker, who inquired about his symptom burden, daily activities, and general well-being. The evaluation revealed that Paul's abdominal pain was poorly controlled and that he was also experiencing extreme chemotherapy-related fatigue. He was not sleeping well because of pain and because he often woke up in the middle of the night worrying about his health. He did not feel like himself and felt depressed over the inability to paint and participate in household and community activities. He was started on a low dose of morphine to manage his abdominal pain as needed, dexamethasone 4 mg twice a day for 2 weeks and citalopram 10 mg daily for his mood. The APRN explained that it may take nearly a month to see improvement in his mood, so he was prescribed a lorazepam 0.5 mg tablet, which is needed to manage anxiety, particularly overnight.

Initially, Ellen had to coax Paul into taking the medication. Within a few days of starting this new regimen, Paul found that his energy had improved and he was not able to go to his studio, but he was able to paint at home. Ellen was pleased with Paul's improvement but worried when he began getting up late at night, walking around the house, and going outside. Ellen would try and coax Paul back to bed, but he would not follow her direction. He seemed increasingly agitated the more she tried to assist him. She called the palliative care APRN and explained Paul's state. After reviewing Paul's medication, it became apparent that he was taking the second dose of dexamethasone late in the evening before bed, with the lorazepam to help him sleep. This made him delirious. Paul was instructed to take his second dose of dexamethasone in the early afternoon, and Ellen was advised to help Paul to establish a consistent bedtime routine that included toileting and assuring that his glasses were readily available so he could see the clock at bedside if he woke up in the middle of the night. In addition to working closely with the palliative APRN, Ellen also benefited from monthly conversations with the palliative care team social worker who put her in touch with a caregiver support group.

CASE STUDY

AN INTERPROFESSIONAL PERSPECTIVE

Elissa Kozlov, PhD
Clinical Psychologist
Weill Cornell Medical College

This case highlights many of the challenges of assessing and treating psychological distress in patients with advanced illness including: (a) differentiating which symptoms are a result of a medical condition versus a psychological condition, (b) issues of polypharmacy and delirium when treating psychological symptoms pharmacologically, and (c) caregiver distress.

Paul's symptoms of depression are challenging to differentiate from his symptoms of physical illness and its treatment. For example, Paul's weekly chemotherapy left him feeling ill and exhausted, so he understandably was spending more time resting in bed. Fatigue can be a symptom of depression, but it is also a common side effect of chemotherapy. Furthermore, experiencing physical symptoms such as fatigue and pain can cause or exacerbate psychological symptoms.

One of the clear indications that Paul's mood and behaviors were likely related to his depression rather than to side effects of chemotherapy was that he was withdrawing from activities that did not require physical effort. For example, while he may not have felt physically well enough to go to his studio and paint, there was likely no medical reason preventing him from connecting with his friends and family, reading books and magazines, responding to texts or emails, and answering the phone. Paul was likely experiencing anhedonia—a loss of interest in pleasurable experiences—which is a hallmark symptom of depression. Paul also displayed other symptoms of depression, which can help an assessor better understand and diagnose depression, including low mood, fatigue, and difficulty sleeping at night due partially to worrying.

In many cases, it may be nonpathological or appropriate for patients to report some degree of sadness and worry in the face of medical issues. One important way to differentiate normal versus nonnormal psychological symptoms is the degree of impairment the psychological symptoms are causing in daily life. For example, in Paul's case, his depression was causing him to withdraw from his friends, family, and activities he usually enjoys, and it was severe enough that his wife was worried. Furthermore, his anxiety was interfering with his ability to sleep at night, which likely compounded his difficulties during the day. Paul's level of impairment resulting from his psychological symptoms indicated that he was suffering from clinically significant depression and anxiety.

Paul's palliative care assessment revealed uncontrolled pain and untreated depression with anxiety symptoms, all of which were treated pharmacologically and resulted in episodes of delirium caused by his multiple medications. While depression and anxiety can be treated pharmacologically, there are also highly effective nonpharmacological options that do not carry a risk of polypharmacy and delirium that Paul could have been offered, including cognitive behavioral therapy (CBT), a type of psychotherapy that is especially effective for managing depression and anxiety. Because Paul was spending so much time in bed not engaging in meaningful activities, he likely would have benefited from working with a psychotherapist trained in CBT, which can be highly effective at providing adults with advanced illness the coping skills and strategies needed to continue to pursue a value-driven, meaningful life even in the face of challenging physical symptoms. It may also have been helpful for Paul to speak with a psychotherapist more generally about the worries that kept him up at night and to learn some relaxation and meditation skills as well as sleep hygiene techniques (e.g., staying out of his bed during the day, limiting his number of naps, and establishing regular sleep and wake times) to help him sleep soundly at night or return to sleep after awakening.

Lastly, it is important to discuss Ellen's role as caregiver for Paul, as she reported psychological difficulty in managing Paul's illness. Caregiver distress should be a part of any palliative care assessment because caregivers are not only deserving of their own line of support, but also helping caregivers impacts a patient's well-being. It was clear from this case study that Ellen was struggling with psychological symptoms of her own. There are several good options to help caregivers manage their emotions and new responsibilities including support groups and individual psychotherapy. Additionally, there are screening tools that can be highly effective at detecting caregiver distress, such as the Zarit Caregiver Burden Scale.

Evidence-Based Practice

Greenlee, H., DuPont-Reyes, M. J., Balneaves, L. G., Carlson, L. E., Cohen, M. R., Deng, G., … Tripathy, D. (2017). Clinical practice guidelines on the evidence-based use of integrative therapies during and after breast cancer treatment. *CA: A Cancer Journal for Clinicians*, 67(3), 194–232. doi:10.3322/caac.21397

Research Problem

Patients with breast cancer often use complementary therapies during cancer treatment and to manage treatment-related side effects; however, evidence to support the use of these therapies is limited.

Methodology

The researchers conducted a systematic literature review of peer-reviewed randomized controlled trials from 1990 through 2015. In order for the trials to be selected for inclusion, they must have been published, available in English, included more than 50% of patients with breast cancer, and used an integrative therapy as an intervention during standard treatment. Grades of evidence were determined for each therapy reflective of clinical outcomes. Grades were created from a modified version of the U.S. Preventive Services Task Force grading system.

Findings

Meditation and yoga are recommended to improve quality of life and physical functioning. Music therapy, meditation, stress management, and yoga are recommended for anxiety and stress reduction. Meditation, relaxation, yoga, massage, and music therapy are recommended for depression and mood disorders. Acupressure and acupuncture are recommended for reducing chemotherapy-induced nausea and vomiting. Acetyl-L-carnitine is not recommended to prevent chemotherapy-induced peripheral neuropathy due to possibility of harm. No strong evidence supports the use of ingested dietary supplements to manage breast cancer treatment–related side effects.

Limitations

Challenges to these studies include the inability to blind participants to most of the integrative modalities studied, because most measures are subjective and therefore are susceptible to suggestive biases in which patients perceive benefit to an intervention simply because they are receiving it. Many of the trials did not report toxicities or adverse events from both integrative and conventional therapies systematically. Studies also rarely tested interventions in economically and culturally diverse patient populations.

Implications
There is a growing body of evidence supporting the use of integrative and complementary therapies, especially mind–body therapies, as effective supportive care strategies during breast cancer treatment. However, billions of dollars are spent each year on complementary and integrative health therapies with unknown benefits. Researching these therapies could save significant healthcare spending and resources, and direct patients to treatments with known benefits and better safety profiles.

■ REFERENCES

American Psychiatric Association. (2013). *Diagnostic and statistical manual of mental disorders* (5th ed.). Arlington, VA: American Psychiatric Publishing.

American Psychiatric Association. (2016). *Practice guideline for the psychiatric evaluation of adults* (3rd ed.). Arlington, VA: Author. Retrieved from http://psychiatryonline.org/doi/pdf/10.1176/appi.books.9780890426760

Bakitas, M., Dahlin, C., & Bishop, P. (2017). Palliative and end of life care. In T. Buttaro, J. Trybulski, P. Bailey, & J. Sandberg-Cook (Eds.), *Primary care: A collaborative approach* (5th ed., pp. 94–108). St. Louis, MI: Elsevier Mosby.

Bakitas, M., Lyons, K. D., Hegel, M. T., Balan, S., Brokaw, F. C., Seville, J., ... Ahles, T. A. (2009). Effects of a palliative care intervention on clinical outcomes in patients with advanced cancer: The Project ENABLE II randomized controlled trial. *Journal of the American Medical Association, 302*(7), 741–749. doi:10.1001/jama.2009.1198

Blatt, L. (2012). Psychosocial issues. In C. Dahlin & M. Lynch (Eds.), *Core curriculum for the advanced practice hospice and palliative registered nurse* (2nd ed., pp. 187–224). Pittsburgh, PA: Hospice and Palliative Nurses Association.

Block, S. D. (2000). Assessing and managing depression in the terminally ill patient. ACP-ASIM End-of-Life Care Consensus Panel. American College of Physicians—American Society of Internal Medicine. *Annals of Internal Medicine, 132*(2), 209–218. doi:10.7326/0003-4819-132-3-200002010-00007

Borneman, T. (2012). Spiritual concerns. In C. Dahlin & M. Lynch (Eds.), *Core curriculum for the advanced practice hospice and palliative registered nurse* (2nd ed., pp. 173–186). Pittsburgh, PA: Hospice and Palliative Nurses Association.

Braun, I., Pirl, W., & Greenberg, D. (2010). Patients with cancer. In T. Stern, G. Fricchione, N. Cassem, M. Jellinek, & J. Rosenbaum (Eds.), *Massachusetts General Hospital handbook of general hospital psychiatry* (6th ed., pp. 371–382). Philadelphia, PA: Elsevier Saunders.

Breitbart, W., & Alici, Y. (2012). Evidence-based treatment of delirium in patients with cancer. *Journal of Clinical Oncology, 30*(11), 1206–1214. doi:10.1200/JCO.2011.39.8784

Breitbart, W., Chochinov, H. M., & Passik, S. D. (2010). Psychiatric symptoms in palliative medicine. In G. Hanks, N. Cherny, N. Christaskis, M. Fallon, S. Kaasa, & R. Portenoy (Eds.), *Oxford textbook of palliative medicine* (4th ed., pp. 1453–1482). New York, NY: Oxford University Press.

Breitbart, W., & Dickerman, A. L. (2017). Assessment and management of depression in palliative care. In D. M. F. Savarese & D. Solomon (Eds.), *UpToDate*. Retrieved from https://www.uptodate.com/contents/assessment-and-management-of-depression-in-palliative-care

Burhenn, P. S. (2016). Delirium. In C. Dahlin, P. Coyne, & B. Ferrell (Eds.), *Advanced practice palliative nursing* (pp. 311–320). New York, NY: Oxford University Press.

Candilis, P. J., McLean, R. Y., Otto, M. W., Manfro, G. G., Worthington, J. J., Penava, S. J., ... Pollack, M. H. (1999). Quality of life in patients with panic disorder. *Journal of Nervous and Mental Disease, 187*, 429–434.

Candy, B., Jones, L., Williams, R., Tookman, A., & King, M. (2009). Psychostimulants for depression. *Cochrane Database of Systematic Reviews, (2)*, 1469–1493. doi:10.1002/14651858.CD006722.pub2

Chovan, J. (2016). Depression and suicide. In C. Dahlin, P. Coyne, & B. Ferrell (Eds.), *Advanced practice palliative nursing* (pp. 321–330). New York, NY: Oxford University Press.

Derby, S. (2012). The older adult population. In C. Dahlin & M. Lynch (Eds.), *Core curriculum for the advanced practice hospice and palliative care registered nurse* (2nd ed., pp. 511–528). Pittsburgh, PA: Hospice and Palliative Nurses Association.

Dick, K. (2013). Delirium. In T. Buttaro, J. Trybulski, P. Bailey, & J. Sandberg-Cook (Eds.), *Primary care: A collaborative approach* (4th ed., pp. 999–1003). St. Louis, MI: Elsevier Mosby.

Feifel, D., Malcolm, B., Boggie, D., & Lee, K. (2017). Low-dose ketamine for treatment resistant depression in an academic clinical practice setting. *Journal of Affective Disorders, 221,* 283–288.

Folstein, M. F., Folstein, S. E., & McHugh, P. R. (1975). "Mini-Mental State." A practical method for grading the cognitive state of patients for the clinician. *Journal of Psychiatric Research, 12*(3), 189–198. doi:10.1016/0022-3956(75)90026-6

Fournier, D. (2013a). Anxiety disorders. In T. Buttaro, J. Trybulski, P. Bailey, & J. Sandberg-Cook (Eds.), *Primary care: A collaborative approach* (4th ed., pp. 1344–1351). St. Louis, MI: Elsevier Mosby.

Fournier, D. (2013b). Mood disorders. In T. Buttaro, J. Trybulski, P. Bailey, & J. Sandberg-Cook (Eds.), *Primary care: A collaborative approach* (4th ed., pp. 1328–1344). St. Louis, MI: Elsevier Mosby.

Francis, J., Jr. (2017). Delirium and acute confusional states: Prevention, treatment, and prognosis. In J. L. Wilterdink (Ed.), *UpToDate.* Retrieved from https://www.uptodate.com/contents/delirium-and-acute-confusional -states-prevention-treatment-and-prognosis

Gatto, M., Thomas, P., & Berger, A. (2016). Anxiety. In C, Dahlin, P. Coyne, & B. Ferrell (Eds.), *Advanced practice palliative nursing* (pp. 301–310). New York, NY: Oxford University Press.

Goldsmith, M., Ortiz-Rubio, P., Staveski, S., Chan, M., & Shaw, R. (2011). Delirium. In J. Wolfe, P. Hinds, & B. Sourkes (Eds.), *Interdisciplinary pediatric palliative care* (pp. 251–265). Philadelphia, PA: Elsevier Saunders.

Grassi, L., Caraceni, A., Mitchell, A. J., Nanni, M. G., Bernardi, M. A., Caruso, R., & Riba, M. (2015). Management of delirium in palliative care: A review. *Current Psychiatry Reports, 17*(3), 550. doi:10.1007/s11920-015-0550-8

Hosie, A., Davidson, P. M., Agar, M., Sanderson, C. R., & Phillips, J. (2012). Delirium prevalence, incidence, and implications for screening in specialist palliative care inpatient settings: A systematic review. *Palliative Medicine, 27*(6), 486–498. doi:10.1177/0269216312457214

Hosker, C. M. G., & Bennett, M. I. (2016). Delirium and agitation at the end of life. *British Medical Journal, 353,* i3085. doi:10.1136/bmj.i3085

Irwin, S. A., & Hirst, J. M. (2017, May 10). Overview of anxiety in palliative care. In D. M. F. Savarese & R. Hermann (Eds.), *UpToDate.* Retrieved from http://www.uptodate.com/contents/overview-of-anxiety-in-palliative-care

Jacobsen, J. C., Zhang, B., Block, S. D., Maciejewski, P. K., & Prigerson, H. G. (2010). Distinguishing symptoms of grief and depression in a cohort of advanced cancer patients. *Death Studies, 34*(3), 257–273. doi:10.1080/07481180903559303

Jordan, A. E., Malhotra, S., Maree, R. D., Schenker, Y., Arnold, R. A., & Reynolds, C. F. (2015). Depression in older adults: A palliative medicine perspective. *Harvard Review of Psychiatry, 23*(5), 343–353. doi:10.1097/ HRP.0000000000000069

Kane, J. L., & Himelstein, B. (2007). Palliative care in pediatrics. In A. Berger, J. Shuster, & J. Von Roenn (Eds.), *Principles and practice of palliative care and supportive oncology* (3rd ed.). Philadelphia, PA: Lippincott, William, & Wilkins.

Kersun, L. S., & Shemesh, E. (2007). Depression and anxiety in children at the end of life. *Pediatric Clinics of North America, 54*(5), 691–708, xi. doi:10.1016/j.pcl.2007.06.003

Lee, S., Back, A., Block, S., & Stewart, S. (2002). Enhancing physician-patient communication. *Hematology, 1,* 464–478.

Li, M., Fitzgerald, P., & Rodin, G. (2012). Evidence-based treatment of depression in patients with cancer. *Journal of Clinical Oncology, 30*(11), 1187–1196. doi:10.1200/JCO.2011.39.7372

Marks, S., & Heinrich, T. (2013). Assessing and treating depression in palliative care patients. *Current Psychiatry, 12*(8), 35–40.

Meghani, N., Tracy, M. F., Hadidi, N. N., & Lindquist, R. (2017). Part I: The effects of music for the symptom management of anxiety, pain, and insomnia in critically ill patients. *Dimensions of Critical Care Nursing, 36*(4), 234–243. doi:10.1097/DCC.0000000000000254

Mullaney, E. (2011). Symptom management in pediatric palliative care. In G. Santucci (Ed.), *HPNA core curriculum for the pediatric hospice and palliative nurse* (pp. 67–106). Pittsburgh, PA: Hospice and Palliative Nurses Association.

Myers, R. M., Balsamo, L., Lu, X., Devidas, M., Hunger, S. P., Carroll, W. L., … Kadan-Lottick, N. S. (2014). A prospective study of anxiety, depression, and behavioral changes in the first year after a diagnosis of childhood acute lymphoblastic leukemia: A report from the Children's Oncology Group. *Cancer, 120*(9), 1417–1425. doi:10.1002/cncr.28578

Nasreddine, Z. S. (2016, January 23). MoCA Montreal—Cognitive assessment. Retrieved from http://www .mocatest.org/pdf_files/test/MoCA-Test-English_7_1.pdf

Nasreddine, Z. S., Phillips, N. A., Bédirian, V., Charbonneau, S., Whitehead, V., Collin, I., … Chertkow, H. (2005). The Montreal Cognitive Assessment, MoCA: A brief screening tool for mild cognitive impairment. *Journal of the American Geriatrics Society, 53*(4), 695–699. doi:10.1111/j.1532-5415.2005.53221.x

National Consensus Project for Quality Palliative Care. (2013). *Clinical practice guidelines for quality palliative care* (3rd ed.). Pittsburgh, PA: Author.

Nelson, P. (2016). Palliative sedation. In C. Dahlin, P. Coyne, & B. Ferrell (Eds.), *Advanced practice palliative nursing* (pp. 487–495). New York, NY: Oxford University Press.

O'Driscoll, C., & Shaikh, M. (2017). Cross-cultural applicability of the Montreal Cognitive Assessment (MoCA): A systematic review. *Journal of Alzheimer's Disease, 58,* 789–801. doi:10.3233/JAD-161042

Pao, M., & Wiener, E. (2011). Psychological symptoms. In J. Wolfe, P. Hinds, & B. Sourkes (Eds.), *Interdisciplinary pediatric palliative care* (pp. 229–238). Philadelphia, PA: Elsevier Saunders.

Pasacreta, J. V., Minarik, P. A., Nield-Anderson, L., & Paice, J. A. (2015). Anxiety and depression. In B. Ferrell & N. Coyle (Eds.), *Oxford textbook of palliative nursing* (4th ed., pp. 366–385). New York, NY: Oxford University Press.

Pattanayak, R. D., & Sagar, R. (2011). Depression in dementia patients: Issues and challenges for a physician. *Journal of the Association of Physicians of India, 59,* 650–652.

Periyakoil, V. S., Kraemer, H. C., Noda, A., Moos, R., Hallenbeck, J., Webster, M., & Yesavage, J. A. (2005). The development and initial validation of the Terminally Ill Grief or Depression Scale (TIGDS). *International Journal of Methods in Psychiatric Research, 14*(4), 203–212. doi:10.1002/mpr.8

Plaskota, M., Lucas, C., Evans, R., Cook, K., Pizzoferro, K., & Saini, T. (2012). A hypnotherapy intervention for the treatment of anxiety in patients with cancer receiving palliative care. *International Journal of Palliative Nursing, 18*(2), 69–75. doi:10.12968/ijpn.2012.18.2.69

Pollack, M., Otto, M., Wittmann, C., & Rosenbaum, J. (2010). Anxious patients. In T. Stern, G. Fricchione, N. Cassem, M. Jellinek, & J. Rosenbaum (Eds.), *Massachusetts General Hospital handbook of general hospital psychiatry* (6th ed., pp. 133–152). Philadelphia, PA: Elsevier Saunders.

Rayner, L., Price, A., Hotopf, M., & Higginson, I. (2011). The development of evidence-based European guidelines on the management of depression in palliative cancer care. *British Journal of Cancer, 47*, 702–712. doi:10.1016/j.ejca.2010.11.027

Reiss, S., Peterson, R. A., Gursky, D. M., & McNally, R. J. (1986). Anxiety sensitivity, anxiety frequency and the prediction of fearfulness. *Behaviour Research and Therapy, 24*(1), 1–8. doi:10.1016/0005-7967(86)90143-9

Rosen, S., Koretz, B., & Reuben, D. (2010). Presentation of disease in old age. In H. Fillit, K. Rookwood, & K. Woodhouse (Eds.), *Brocklehurst's textbook of geriatric medicine and gerontology* (7th ed., pp. 205–210). Philadelphia, PA: Saunders Elsevier.

Salt, S., Mulvaney, C. A., & Preston, N. J. (2017). Drug therapy for symptoms associated with anxiety in adult palliative care patients (review). *Cochrane Database of Systematic Reviews*, (5), CD004596. doi:10.1002/14651858. CD004596.pub3

Sheldon, L. K., Swanson, S., Dolce, A., Marsh, K., & Summers, J. (2008). Putting evidence into practice: Evidence-based interventions for anxiety. *Clinical Journal of Oncology Nursing, 12*(5), 789–797. doi:10.1188/08.CJON.789-797

Tabloski, P. (2014). Psychological and cognitive function. In P. Tabloski (ed.), *Gerontological nursing* (2nd ed., pp. 200–237). Upper Saddle River, NJ: Pearson.

Temel, J. S., Greer, J. A., Muzikansky, A., Gallagher, E. R., Admane, S., Jackson, V. A., … Lynch, T. J. (2010). Early palliative care for patients with metastatic non-small-cell lung cancer. *New England Journal of Medicine, 363*(8), 733–742. doi:10.1056/NEJMoa1000678

Traeger, L., Greer, J. A., Fernandez-Robles, C., Temel, J. S., & Pirl, W. F. (2012). Evidence-based treatment of anxiety in patients with cancer. *Journal of Clinical Oncology, 30*(11), 1197–1205. doi:10.1200/JCO.2011.39.5632

U.S. Preventive Services Task Force. (2016). Screening for depression in adults. Recommendation statement. Rockville, MD. Retrieved from http://www.uspreventiveservicestaskforce.org/uspstf09/adultdepression/addeprrs.htm

Yesavage, J. A., Brink, T. L., Rose, T. L., Lum, O., Huang, V., Adey, M., & Leirer, V. O. (1982). Development and validation of a geriatric depression screening scale: A preliminary report. *Journal of Psychiatric Research, 17*(1), 37–49. doi:10.1016/0022-3956(82)90033-4

Zvolensky, M. J., Garey, L., & Bakhshaie, J. (2017). Disparities in anxiety and its disorders. *Journal of Anxiety Disorders, 48*, 1–5. doi:10.1016/j.janxdis.2017.05.004

■ **APPENDIX 22.1**

GERIATRIC DEPRESSION SCALE

Choose the best answer for how you felt over the past week.

1. Are you basically satisfied with your life?
   YES   NO
2. Have you dropped many of your activities and interests?   YES   NO
3. Do you feel that your life is empty?
   YES   NO
4. Do you often get bored?   YES   NO
5. Are you hopeful about the future?
   YES   NO
6. Are you bothered by thoughts you can't get out of your head?   YES   NO
7. Are you in good spirits most of the time?
   YES   NO
8. Are you afraid that something bad is going to happen to you?   YES   NO
9. Do you feel happy most of the time?*
   YES   NO
10. Do you often feel helpless?   YES   NO
11. Do you often get restless and fidgety?
    YES   NO
12. Do you prefer to stay at home, rather than going out and doing things?   YES   NO
13. Do you frequently worry about the future?
    YES   NO
14. Do you feel you have more problems with memory than most?   YES   NO
15. Do you think it is wonderful to be alive now?*
    YES   NO
16. Do you often feel downhearted and blue?
    YES   NO
17. Do you feel pretty worthless the way you are now?
    YES   NO

18. Do you worry a lot about the past?
    YES   NO
19. Do you find life very exciting?*   YES   NO
20. Is it hard for you to get started on new projects?
    YES   NO
21. Do you feel full of energy?*   YES   NO
22. Do you feel that your situation is helpless?
    YES   NO
23. Do you think that most people are better off than you are?   YES   NO
24. Do you frequently get upset over little things?
    YES   NO
25. Do you frequently feel like crying?
    YES   NO
26. Do you have trouble concentrating?
    YES   NO
27. Do you enjoy getting up in the morning?*
    YES   NO
28. Do you prefer to avoid social gatherings?
    YES   NO
29. Is it easy for you to make decisions?*
    YES   NO
30. Is your mind as clear as it used to be?*
    YES   NO

Score:
*Nondepressed answers = yes, all others = no

Norms

Normal	5 ± 4
Mildly depressed	15 ± 6
Very depressed	13 ±

Source: Yesavage J. A., Brink, T. L., Rose, T. L., Lum, O., Huang, V., Adey, M., & Leirer, V. O. (1982). Development and validation of a geriatric screening scale: A preliminary report. *Journal of Psychiatric Research, 17,* 37–49. (Reprinted with permission from Pergamon Press PLC, Headington Hill Hall, Oxford OX3 OBW, UK.)

■ **APPENDIX 22.2**

MONTREAL COGNITIVE ASSESSMENT (MOCA)
Version 7.1 Original Version

NAME :
Education :
Sex :

Date of birth :
DATE :

VISUOSPATIAL / EXECUTIVE		POINTS

Copy cube

Draw CLOCK (Ten past eleven)
(3 points)

E
End

A

5

B

2

1
Begin

D

4

3

C

[ ]

[ ]

[ ]
Contour

[ ]
Numbers

[ ]
Hands

__/5

NAMING

[ ]

[ ]

[ ]

__/3

MEMORY			FACE	VELVET	CHURCH	DAISY	RED	No points
Read list of words, subject must repeat them. Do 2 trials, even if 1st trial is successful. Do a recall after 5 minutes.		1st trial						
		2nd trial						

ATTENTION	Read list of digits (1 digit/ sec.).	Subject has to repeat them in the forward order	[ ] 2 1 8 5 4	__/2
		Subject has to repeat them in the backward order	[ ] 7 4 2	

Read list of letters. The subject must tap with his hand at each letter A. No points if ≥ 2 errors
[ ]   F B A C M N A A J K L B A F A K D E A A A J A M O F A A B   __/1

Serial 7 subtraction starting at 100   [ ] 93   [ ] 86   [ ] 79   [ ] 72   [ ] 65
4 or 5 correct subtractions: **3 pts**, 2 or 3 correct: **2 pts**, 1 correct: **1 pt**, 0 correct: **0 pt**   __/3

LANGUAGE	Repeat : I only know that John is the one to help today. [ ] The cat always hid under the couch when dogs were in the room. [ ]	__/2
	Fluency / Name maximum number of words in one minute that begin with the letter F [ ] _____ (N ≥ 11 words)	__/1

ABSTRACTION   Similarity between e.g. banana - orange = fruit   [ ] train – bicycle   [ ] watch - ruler   __/2

DELAYED RECALL	Has to recall words **WITH NO CUE**	FACE [ ]	VELVET [ ]	CHURCH [ ]	DAISY [ ]	RED [ ]	Points for UNCUED recall only	__/5
Optional	Category cue							
	Multiple choice cue							

ORIENTATION   [ ] Date   [ ] Month   [ ] Year   [ ] Day   [ ] Place   [ ] City   __/6

© Z.Nasreddine MD   www.mocatest.org   Normal ≥ 26 / 30   TOTAL   __/30

Administered by: _____   Add 1 point if ≤ 12 yr edu

Source: Montreal Cognitive Assessment. Retrieved from http://www.mocatest.org/pdf_files/test/MoCA-Test-English_7_1.pdf

■ APPENDIX 22.3

MEMORIAL DELIRIUM ASSESSMENT SCALE

INSTRUCTIONS: Rate the severity of the following symptoms of delirium on the basis of current interaction with the subject or assessment of his or her behavior or experience over the past several hours (as indicated in each time).

Item 1: Reduced Level of Consciousness (Awareness)

Rate patient's current awareness of and interaction with the environment (interviewer, other people/objects; for example, ask patients to describe their surroundings).

0: none   Patient is spontaneously fully aware of the environment and interacts appropriately.

1: mild   Patient is unaware of some elements in the environment, or not spontaneously interacting appropriately with the interviewer; becomes fully aware and appropriately interactive when prodded strongly; interview is prolonged but not seriously disrupted.

2: moderate   Patient is unaware of some or all elements in the environment, or not spontaneously interacting with the interviewer; becomes incompletely aware and inappropriately interactive when prodded strongly; interview is prolonged but not seriously disrupted.

3: severe   Patient is unaware of all elements in the environment, with no spontaneous interaction or awareness of the interviewer, so that the interview is difficult to impossible, even with maximal prodding.

Item 2: Disorientation

Rate current state by asking the following 10 orientation items: date, month, day, year, season, floor, name of hospital, city, state, and country.

0: none   Patient knows 9 to 10 items.
1: mild   Patient knows 7 to 8 items.
2: moderate   Patient knows 5 to 6 items.
3: severe   Patient knows no more than 4 items.

Item 3: Short-Term Memory Impairment

Rate current state by using repetition and delayed recall of three words (patient must immediately repeat and recall words five minutes later) after an intervening task. Use alternate sets of three words for successive evaluation (e.g., apple, table, tomorrow, sky, cigar, and justice).

0: none   All three words repeated and recalled.
1: mild   All three repeated, patient fails to recall one.
2: moderate   All three repeated, patient fails to recall two.
3: severe   Patient fails to repeat one or more words.

Item 4: Impaired Digit Span

Rate current performance by asking subjects to repeat first three, four, then five digits forward and then three, then four backward: continue to the next step only if patient succeeds at the previous one.

0: none   Patient can do at least five numbers forward and four backward.
1: mild   Patient can do at least five numbers forward, three backward.
2: moderate   Patient can do four to five numbers forward, cannot do three backward.
3: severe   Patient can do no more than three numbers forward.

Item 5: Reduced Ability to Maintain and Shift Attention

As indicated during the interview by questions needing to be rephrased and/or repeated because patient's attention wanders, patient loses track, patient is distracted by outside stimuli, or patient is overabsorbed in a task.

0: none   None of the above: patient maintains and shifts attention normally.
1: mild   Above attention problems occur once or twice without prolonging the interview.
2: moderate   Above attention problems occur often, prolonging the interview without seriously disrupting it.

Above attention problems occur constantly, disrupting and making the interview difficult to impossible.

Item 6: Disorganized Thinking

Disorganized thinking is indicated during the interview by rambling, irrelevant, or incoherent speech, or by tangential, circumstantial, or faulty reasoning. Ask patient a somewhat complex question (e.g., "Describe your current medical condition.").

0: none   Patient's speech is coherent and goal directed.

1: mild   Patient's speech is slightly difficult to follow; responses to questions are slightly off target but not so much as to prolong the interview. Disorganized thoughts or speech are clearly present, such that interview is prolonged but not disrupted.

3: severe Examination is very difficult or impossible due to disorganized thinking or speech.

Item 7: Perceptual Disturbance

Misperceptions, illusions, or hallucinations inferred from inappropriate behavior during the interview or admitted by subject as well as those elicited from nurse/family/chart accounts of the past several hours or of the time since last examination.

0: none   No misperceptions, illusions, or hallucinations

1: mild   Misperceptions or illusions related to sleep, fleeting hallucinations on one or two occasions without inappropriate behavior

2: moderate Hallucinations or frequent illusions on several occasions with minimal inappropriate behavior that does not disrupt the interview

3: severe Frequent or intense illusions or hallucinations with persistent inappropriate behavior that disrupts the interview or interferes with medical care

Item 8: Delusions

Rate delusions inferred from inappropriate behavior during the interview or admitted by the patient as well as delusions elicited from nurse/family/chart accounts of the past several hours or of the time since the previous examination.

0: none   No evidence of misinterpretations or delusions

1: mild   Misinterpretations or suspiciousness without clear delusional ideas or inappropriate behavior

2: moderate Delusions admitted by the patient or evidenced by his/her behavior that do not or only marginally disrupt the interview or interfere with medical care

3: severe Persistent and/or intense delusions resulting in inappropriate behavior, disrupting the interview or seriously interfering with medical care

Item 9: Decreased or Increased Psychomotor Activity

Rate activity over past several hours as well as activity during interview.

0: none   Normal psychomotor activity

1: mild   Hypoactivity is barely noticeable, expressed as slight slowing of movement. Hyperactivity is barely noticeable or appears as simple restlessness.

2: moderate Hypoactivity is undeniable with marked reduction in number of movements or marked slowness of movement: subject rarely spontaneously moves or speaks. Hyperactivity is undeniable: subject moves almost constantly. In both cases, examination is prolonged as a consequence.

3: severe Hypoactivity is severe; patient does not move or speak without prodding or is catatonic. Hyperactivity is severe; patient is constantly moving, overreacts to stimuli, and requires surveillance and/or restraint. Getting through the exam is difficult or impossible.

Item 10: Sleep–Wake Cycle Disturbance (Disorder of Arousal)

Rate patient's ability to either sleep or stay awake at the appropriate times. Utilize direct observation during the interview as well as reports from nurses, family, patient, or charts describing sleep–wake cycle disturbance over the past several hours or since last examination. Use observations of the previous night for morning evaluations only.

0: none   At night, sleeps well. During the day, has no trouble staying awake.

1: mild   Mild deviation from appropriate sleepfulness and wakefulness states at night, difficulty falling asleep or transient night awakenings, needs medication to sleep well: during the day, reports periods of drowsiness, or during the interview, is drowsy but can easily fully awaken himself or herself.

2: moderate Moderate deviations form appropriate sleepfulness and wakefulness states at night, repeated and prolonged night awakening; during the day, reports of frequent and prolonged napping, or, during the interview, can only be roused to complete wakefulness by strong stimuli.

3: severe   Severe deviations from appropriate sleepfulness and wakefulness states at night, sleeplessness; during the day, patient spends most of the time sleeping, or, during the interview, cannot be roused to full wakefulness by any stimuli.

Source: Reprinted with permission from Breitbart, W., Rosenfeld, B., Roth, A., Smith, M. J., Cohen, K., & Passlk, S. (1997). The Memorial Delirium Assessment Scale. *Journal of Pain and Symptom Management, 13*(3), 128–137, by the U.S. Cancer Pain Relief Committee.

Kristen H. Sorocco & Kristi L. Bratkovich

Posttraumatic Stress Disorder and End-of-Life Care

CHAPTER

23

KEY POINTS

■ There is a high likelihood that anyone who is receiving palliative care has been exposed to a traumatic event during his or her life that may place him or her at risk of posttraumatic stress disorder (PTSD), and life-limiting medical diagnoses have the potential to trigger an increase in PTSD symptoms.

■ PTSD can negatively impact patient–provider communication and lead to increased psychological distress at the end of life.

■ Although evidence-based research is limited, there are a number of approaches to address PTSD at the end of life that bring comfort to both the individual receiving palliative care and his or her family.

CASE STUDY

PALLIATIVE CARE CASE

Jimmy Mac, a 64-year-old American Indian and a Vietnam-era veteran, was brought to the Veterans Administration Medical Center by ambulance for low-back pain and reported an increase in pain over the last 4 months. Prior medical history included stroke, HIV/AIDS, previous L1 to L3 compression fracture, and a history of mental health treatment. He completed 16 weeks of vancomycin for epidural abscesses as well as methicillin-resistant *Staphylococcus aureus* (MRSA) bacteremia. MRI on admission showed an acute compression fracture of L5 vertebral body and stable compression fractures of L1 to L4. He was found to have *Clostridium difficile* and was started on vancomycin. During the admission, he became septic and progressed into respiratory failure and was taken to the ICU. He was found to have bilateral consolidations in his lungs and was placed on an antibiotic regimen, and then he developed persistent diarrhea. By the end of the month, he was short of breath and his hemoglobin had dropped. Adherence to the medical plan of care had been inconsistent over the years and pain has become difficult to manage. Medical providers had difficulty understanding his reasoning for his advance care decision, specifying he wanted all life-sustaining treatments. A palliative care consult was placed.

What details of this case are suggestive of PTSD? What assessment approaches should be used with this patient? What interventions would be appropriate to consider?

The likelihood of being exposed to a traumatic event, such as a natural disaster, child sexual or physical abuse, serious accident, sexual or physical assault, terrorist attack, or combat, increases across a life span. By the time an individual reaches his or her early 20s, there is a high chance that the individual has already experienced a trauma, with prevalence rates as high as 84% among nonclinical college samples (Vrana & Lauterbach, 1994). After experiencing a traumatic event, most people experience stress-related reactions such as fear, sadness, guilt, anger, or sleep problems. For many, stress-related reactions resolve over time, but about 7% of individuals who experience a traumatic event will continue to have difficulty coping with symptoms associated with the event and develop posttraumatic stress disorder (PTSD; Gradus, 2007).

Given the high likelihood that an individual receiving palliative care has experienced a traumatic event during his or her life, it is important to be familiar with how PTSD may impact end-of-life (EOL) care. Treatment of PTSD at the end of life is directly relevant to the recommended competencies and curricular guidelines for EOL nursing care put forth by the American Association of Colleges of Nursing (AACN, 2013). Specifically, this chapter will address AACN competencies related to communication, interprofessional care, and use of evidence-based practices, as well as highlight the importance of assessing for specific mental health disorders such as PTSD in order to allow both the individual and his or her family to receive state-of-the-art EOL care.

The objectives of this chapter are to provide the reader with an overview of PTSD and evidence-based treatments within a palliative care setting. The criteria for PTSD are outlined along with a description of appropriate approaches to assessment. Currently available evidence-based treatments are described and illustrated with case examples. The importance of addressing PTSD in EOL care for both the individual and his or her family is highlighted.

■ DIAGNOSTIC CRITERIA FOR POSTTRAUMATIC STRESS DISORDER

According to the *Diagnostic and Statistical Manual of Mental Disorders* (5th ed.; *DSM-5*; American Psychiatric Association [APA], 2013), a diagnosis of PTSD must involve the "exposure to actual or threatened death, serious injury, or sexual violence." The exposure itself does not always need to be the direct experience of a traumatic event. According to *DSM-5* criteria (APA, 2013), an individual can also develop PTSD by witnessing a traumatic event

in person, learning that the traumatic events occurred to a close family member or friend, or experiencing repeated or extreme exposure to aversive details of the traumatic event. Medical conditions would qualify as traumatic events only if the incidents involved sudden, catastrophic events, such as waking during surgery or anaphylactic shock (APA, 2013). Emotional reactions to the traumatic event, such as fear or helplessness, are no longer part of the diagnostic criteria with the release of the *DSM-5* (APA, 2013).

Following the exposure, the individual must experience one or more symptoms in each of the following symptom clusters (APA, 2013): (a) reexperiencing (e.g., recurrent distressing memories or dreams); (b) avoidance (e.g., evasion of memories or cues related to traumatic event); (c) negative alterations in cognitions or mood (e.g., inability to remember details related to traumatic event, increased negative beliefs, persistent negative mood state); and (d) changes in arousal and reactivity (e.g., irritability, hypervigilance, poor sleep). The reexperiencing and avoidance symptom clusters require a minimum of one symptom in each cluster, while the other symptom clusters require two or more symptoms to be present to meet diagnostic criteria (APA, 2013). The duration of the symptoms must be for a month or longer, cause clinically significant impairment, and cannot be due to substances or another medical condition (APA, 2013). The previous criteria are for children older than 6 years, adolescents, and adults. The *DSM-5* has modified PTSD criteria for children 6 years and younger (APA, 2013).

It is important to note the difference between a medical diagnosis-specific trauma, such as cancer-related posttraumatic stress, and PTSD. The National Cancer Institute defines cancer-related posttraumatic stress as PTSD-like symptoms, with presentations that are less severe and occurring at any time during or after treatment. Although a life-limiting diagnosis and subsequent treatments do not meet *DSM-5*'s criteria for a "trauma" that could lead to the development of PTSD, it is important to note that any PTSD-like symptoms that are interfering in a patient's quality of life (QOL) need to be addressed whether or not they meet full criteria for a diagnosis of PTSD.

Prevalence

Compared to 8% in the general population, PTSD symptoms occur at a significantly higher rate among individuals receiving care in a medical setting for potentially life-threatening illnesses. The prevalence of PTSD among patients treated in an ICU, regardless of diagnosis, was found to be as high as 64% depending upon the method of assessment (Griffiths, Fortune, Barber, & Young, 2007). Similar findings are noted in pediatric patients treated in a pediatric intensive care unit (PICU; Stuber & Shemesh, 2006). Rees, Gledhill, Garralda, and Nadel (2004) found 21% of PICU-discharged children developed PTSD in comparison to a control group of children receiving care on a general pediatric ward.

PTSD symptoms also are more prevalent among medical diagnoses that are potentially life limiting. For example, in comparison to community samples, prevalence rates have been shown to be higher for individuals with cancer (Alter et al., 1996; Amir & Ramati, 2002). According to the National Cancer Institute, posttraumatic stress has been studied among many types of cancers—melanoma, Hodgkin lymphoma, breast cancer, and mixed cancers (NCI, 2015). Studies using *DSM-IV* diagnostic criteria have shown that the prevalence ranges from 3% to 4% in recently diagnosed patients to 35% in patients evaluated after treatment. When subsyndrome prevalence symptom rates are used, the incidence ranges from 20% in patients with early-stage cancer to 80% in those with recurrent cancer.

Impact of Posttraumatic Stress Disorder on End-of-Life Care

The very nature of the symptoms, including hyper-arousal and avoidance, may complicate EOL care. The simple distress associated with being confronted with a life-threatening illness may exacerbate PTSD symptoms and provoke similar responses to the original trauma. Normal life review is an important part of the dying process in order to resolve unfinished business (Feldman & Periyakoil, 2006), but it may also result in symptoms such as intense anxiety, anger, guilt, or sadness due to traumatic memories. As a result, individuals with PTSD may avoid traumatic memories and may be unable to come to terms with unresolved life events.

Avoidance symptoms may also interfere with processes, such as communication with medical providers, which are paramount to successful EOL care. PTSD symptoms can impede the ability for the healthcare practitioner to engage in direct, problem-focused communication regarding the patient's care (Feldman & Periyakoil, 2006). Refusal of care or excessive questioning of providers' actions or distrust of authority may result (Feldman & Periyakoil, 2006). It has been documented that people with PTSD diagnoses tend to have poor medical adherence (Shemesh et al., 2004). In addition, individuals with PTSD may experience decreased social support or a lack of caregivers as a result of social isolation and avoidance.

Impact of Posttraumatic Stress Disorder on the Family

PTSD can negatively impact interpersonal relationships. The National Center for PTSD's website documents that family members themselves may have a number of reactions to the patient having PTSD, including sympathy, negative feelings, avoidance, depression, anger, guilt, or health problems. Research has documented that spouses of veterans have higher rates of caregiver burden and mental health problems themselves (Carlson & Ruzek, 2013). Among the veteran population, those with PTSD are more likely to report marital difficulties and have higher rates of divorce and interpersonal violence. As a result, individuals with severe PTSD in palliative care settings may have very limited social support networks, and existing family relations may be strained.

Family members of critically ill individuals are also susceptible to developing PTSD. Prevalence studies of family members of critically ill patients in France suggest rates may be as high as 33% (Azoulay et al., 2005). Lautrette et al. (2007) documented a reduction in depression, anxiety, and PTSD symptoms through the implementation of family conferences and psycho-education on grief and bereavement in a French population. Curtis et al. (2012) evaluated an interprofessional communication intervention to improve family outcomes in the United States, with qualitative data suggesting positive outcomes.

■ ASSESSMENT OF POSTTRAUMATIC STRESS DISORDER AT END OF LIFE

Accurately assessing symptoms, providing appropriate treatment, monitoring symptom change, communicating, and evaluating the effectiveness of an intervention are all crucial. Assessing for PTSD can pose several daunting challenges. First, the criteria for the diagnoses of PTSD are changing as the field learns more about this syndrome and the numerous ways it can present. This section identifies age-related issues that may impact how PTSD is manifested across the life span, how EOL issues may affect the presentation of PTSD, and what approaches and measures are utilized to assess PTSD.

When determining the most appropriate measure to utilize in assessing PTSD at the end of life, several factors are important to consider. First, due to the varied nature of life-threatening or life-limiting illnesses, the amount of time required to administer the measure is a critical factor. There are numerous measures that vary in the amount of time required to administer, ranging from 5 to 120 minutes. Second, not all measures are written at the same comprehension level; therefore, the reading level of the patient and his or her English-language fluency are important considerations. Third, the clinician needs to evaluate for a single or multiple traumatic events. Another important consideration when assessing patients for PTSD is whether the assessment focuses on determining the specific diagnosis of PTSD or whether the objective is to identify PTSD symptoms. Finally, the level of training and competency of the clinician administering and interpreting the results will impact the validity of the findings.

Key Components to Assess

When assessing for PTSD at the end of life, an evaluation of past traumatic events (e.g., combat, sexual assault, natural disasters, and accidents) is critical. Once the traumatic event(s) are identified, the meaning the patient has attributed to them and how they have coped with these symptoms provides useful information for treatment. Averill and Beck (2000) suggest that the meaning a person attributes to the event and his or her related coping style can influence the severity of the disorder. Also, assessing the influence of various psychosocial factors (e.g., social support, chronic exposure to oppressive conditions, health status, employment status, and activity level) and their effect on PTSD symptoms should be considered. Patients may not offer this information freely, possibly because they may not consider the information relevant to their current circumstances, may not want to discuss the event, or may not remember many aspects of the event (in the case of childhood trauma or dementia). This may be an adaptive process as reflected by Davison et al. (2016), who have broadened our understanding and conceptualization of trauma and the aging process. This group originally brought us the concept of late-onset stress symptomology. Because of Davison et al. (2006), we now have the concept of later-adulthood trauma reengagement (LATR). This reconceptualization is more reflective of normalizing the developmental process that is associated with trauma and the aging process. As people engage with their trauma memories as they age in later life, the developmental task of meaning-making and coherence may facilitate a reworking of their trauma, which may result in more adaptive functioning. On the other hand, patients may not offer information pertaining to traumatic events or their current understanding of these events freely, possibly because they may not consider the information relevant to their current circumstances, may not want to discuss the event, may not remember many aspects of the event (in the case of childhood trauma or dementia), or do not trust the provider. A thorough assessment should focus on the age of onset, duration, severity, and course of symptoms.

There are numerous approaches to the assessment of PTSD or associated symptoms that include chart review, screening measures, interviews, self-report measures, and trauma exposure measures. A comprehensive chart review can be an invaluable tool in assessing a patient for PTSD. The patient's medical illness may inhibit him or her from being able to share his or her mental health history with you. Also, given that avoidance is a core symptom of PTSD, the patient may not readily share this information, even when asked if he or she has a mental health history. A comprehensive chart review can be conducted by evaluating the following: the history of a preexisting mental health diagnosis, the use of prescribed psychotropic medication (past/present), and any documentation pertaining to the patient's mental health. Once the patient's chart has been reviewed, a brief note including the findings from the chart review and a discussion of the clinical implications for EOL care should be documented. After reviewing the mental health history in the medical record, the next phase of assessment is to talk with the patient to discuss his or her symptoms and background to fill in missing data from the chart review. Any of the remaining approaches (screening, interview, self-report, and trauma exposure measure) can be utilized after the chart review has been conducted.

Screening measures are designed to identify people who are at a higher risk for PTSD. A screening measure is useful particularly when there is ease of administration and minimal administration time. A positive screen indicates that further evaluation is warranted in order to determine if a patient's symptoms meet the criteria for a diagnosis of PTSD. When utilizing screening measures, it is important to understand the unique needs of the person who is being assessed. A vital assessment factor is the history of a traumatic event. For example, when working with veterans, it is important to ask, "Did you see combat?" and "Is there anything about your military service that still bothers you?" Also, be aware of culture-specific traumatic events, for example, being separated from family and being placed in an Indian boarding school. The most effective way to screen for PTSD is to ask about current symptoms and past experiences (primary care PTSD screen; Feldman & Periyakoil, 2006).

A clinical interview is considered to be the most comprehensive assessment of PTSD. However, this assessment requires more time and training of the interviewer. The PTSD interview varies in the breadth and depth of information regarding symptom severity and frequency that can be gathered. Assessment measures for PTSD are provided in Table 23.1, with the Clinician-Administered PTSD Scale (CAPS; Blake et al., 1995; Elhai, Gray, Kashdan, & Franklin, 2005) considered the "gold standard" in assessing PTSD due to its quality of psychometric properties and flexibility (Weathers, Keane, & Davidson, 2001). Some of the interview scales designed for assessing PTSD are the CAPS (Blake et al., 1995); PTSD Symptom Scale-Interview Version (PSS-I; Foa & Tolin, 2000); Structured Clinical Interview for DSM-IV PTSD Module (SCID; First, Spitzer, Gibbon, & Williams, 1996); and the Structured Interview for PTSD (SI-PTSD; Davidson, Kudler, & Smith, 1990). When a patient's trauma history is unknown, a trauma exposure measure may be helpful in assessing what traumatic events he or she may have experienced during his or her lifetime. Trauma exposure measures vary with regard to length, types of trauma assessed, and the amount of information gathered about each event. The purpose of the assessment will determine what type of measure is needed.

TABLE 23.1 Assessment Measures for PTSD		
Measure	Time Required (min)	Type
Clinician-Administered PTSD Scale (CAPS)	45	Interview
Structured Interview for PTSD (SI-PTSD)	20–30	Interview
Structured Clinical Interview for *DSM-IV* PTSD Module (SCID)	20–30	Interview
PTSD Symptom Scale-Interview Version (PSS-I)	20–30	Interview
Primary Care PTSD Screen (PC-PTSD)	2–3	Screen
Trauma Screening Questionnaire (TSQ)	2–3	Screen
Short Posttraumatic Stress Disorder Rating Interview (SPRINT)	5	Self-report
Late-Onset Stress Symptomology (LOSS)	20–30	Self-report
PTSD Checklist (PCL)	5	Self-report
Impact of Event Scale (IES)	5	Self-report
Minnesota Multiphasic Personality Inventory (MMPI)	60–120	Self-report

DSM-IV, Diagnostic and Statistical Manual of Mental Disorders, 4th edition; PTSD, posttraumatic stress disorder.

Finally, self-report measures play a vital role in the assessment of PTSD. As with the previously mentioned assessment measures, self-report measures vary in length and the amount of detailed information that is gathered regarding symptoms and their severity. The commonly utilized self-report measures are the three versions of the PTSD Checklist (Weathers, Litz, Herman, Huska, & Keane, 1993): military, civilian, and specific versions (i.e., PCL-M, PCL-C, and PCL-S); SPRINT (Connor & Davidson, 2001); Trauma Screening Questionnaire (Brewin et al., 2002), and late-onset stress symptomology (Davison et al., 2006). Keep in mind that a lower cut-off score is recommended for several of these measures. Specifically, the PCL has a clinically significant cut-off score of 50; however, a score of 42 has been indicated to effectively differentiate older adults with and without PTSD (Cook, Blaustein, Spinazzola, van der Kolk, 2003).

Life-Span Considerations for Pediatric Assessments

According to the National Child Traumatic Stress Network (NCTSN, 2014), child traumatic stress occurs when children and adolescents are exposed to traumatic events or traumatic situations that overwhelm their ability to cope. Symptom presentation will be influenced by age and developmental level. There are a number of reliable and valid assessment measures by trauma type to assess for PTSD in children and adolescents. For a complete listing, please refer to the National Center for PTSD and the NCTSN's websites in the Resources section at the end of this chapter.

Assessment of Older Adults

Due to the dearth of literature pertaining to the assessment of PTSD at the end of life, assessment strategies that are focused on assessing PTSD in older adults may be lacking a vital first step. The patient's ability to contribute to the assessment process, as well as decisions regarding treatment and medication regimens, can be more accurately planned once the patient's cognitive status has been determined (Kaiser et al., 2013). If warning signs suggest a cognitive impairment is present, a Mental Status Examination can help determine if the patient needs to be referred for a neurological examination in the case of suspected dementia or for a medication evaluation if delirium or a medication interaction is suspected (Kaiser et al., 2013).

Comorbid medical and mental health problems also should be evaluated. Older adults are more likely to report physical health symptoms (e.g., pain, sleep issues, gastrointestinal distress, or cognitive difficulties) rather than emotional difficulties (i.e., anxiety or depression). These responses should be further explored to determine whether or not these terms are associated with changes in mood or activities. Furthermore, substance use, abuse, and dependence, as well as suicidal and para-suicidal behaviors, should be evaluated, especially since older veterans are at a higher risk for completed suicide (Zivin et al., 2007).

Finally, a patient's medication adherence needs to be determined. Since avoidance is one component of PTSD (Kaiser et al., 2013), patients who experience PTSD may struggle with treatment adherence (e.g., missing appointments, not refilling medications, etc.). Another important consideration regarding the use of medication is if the patient is taking medication to treat some of his or her PTSD symptoms. If they are currently managing with these symptoms pharmacologically, they may not be evident during the clinical assessment. This is important to be aware of when determining the diagnosis.

■ OVERVIEW OF EVIDENCE-BASED TREATMENTS FOR POSTTRAUMATIC STRESS DISORDER

There are a number of effective treatments for PTSD; clinical practice guidelines by the Institute of Medicine (IOM, 2007) and Veterans Administration/Department of Defense (2010; Department of Veterans Affairs, 2010) conclude that cognitive-behavioral therapies are the most effective treatment for PTSD. Cognitive-behavioral therapies involve a multifaceted approach including psycho-education, anxiety management, exposure, and cognitive restructuring. Cognitive processing therapy (CPT) and prolonged exposure (PE) are the two subtypes of cognitive-behavioral therapies with the most evidence-based research (Hamblen, Schnurr, Rosenberger, & Eftekhari, 2013). Eye movement desensitization and reprocessing (EMDR) has also been recommended by some guidelines. All of these treatment approaches are explained in detail on the website for the National Center for PTSD, but the four main components of each approach are identified in Table 23.2.

The practitioner who treats individuals with PTSD should be trained in a specific approach such as CPT or PE. When this is not possible, therapy should be conducted by a mental health professional who has received training in cognitive-behavioral techniques. Therapists can always utilize peer consultation and supervision to augment their competency level. In general, treatment is administered in a weekly or biweekly basis. The average number of sessions required to complete the treatment is between 8 and 15 sessions, with each session lasting between 60 and 90 minutes (National Center for Posttraumatic Stress Disorder [NCPTSD], 2009b, 2009c). In addition to therapy sessions, the individual should engage in practice assignments outside of the session. Although treatment may be considered time intensive, cognitive-behavioral therapies are very effective in helping individuals to manage their reactions to stressful memories (NCPTSD, 2007).

The most effective classes of medication to treat PTSD symptoms are selective serotonin reuptake inhibitors (SSRIs), which increase the level of serotonin in the brain (NCPTSD, 2007). Low levels of serotonin are correlated with poorer mood states. Both sertraline (Zoloft) and paroxetine (Paxil) are approved by the FDA for the treatment of PTSD (NCPTSD, 2009a). The four most common side effects of these medications are nausea, decreased libido, feeling drowsy or tired, or sleeping too much (NCPTSD, 2009a).

Treatment Approaches for Posttraumatic Stress Disorder in Palliative Care

Although there are several effective evidence-based treatments for PTSD, there are several problems with these standard psychological treatments in a palliative

Individual Therapy Components	Cognitive Processing Therapy	Prolonged Exposure Therapy	Eye Movement Desensitization and Reprocessing
TABLE 23.2 Four Main Components of Each of the Cognitive-Behavioral Treatments Recommended for PTSD			
Component 1	Learning PTSD symptoms and how treatment can help	Education to learn about symptoms and how treatment can help	Identification of a target memory, image, and belief about the trauma
Component 2	Becoming aware of your thoughts and feelings	Breathing retraining to help you relax and manage distress	Desensitization and reprocessing, which involves focusing on mental images while doing eye movements that the therapist has taught the individual receiving therapy
Component 3	Learning skills to challenge your thoughts and feelings (cognitive restructuring)	Real-world practice (in vivo exposure) to reduce distress in safe situations that have been avoided	Installing positive thoughts and images, once the negative images are no longer distressing
Component 4	Understanding the common changes in beliefs that occur after going through trauma	Talking through the trauma (imaginal exposure) to get control of thoughts and feelings related to the trauma	Body scan to focus on tension or unusual sensations in the body to identify any additional issues you may need to address in later sessions

PTSD, posttraumatic stress disorder.

care setting. First, these approaches often are too demanding for individuals receiving palliative care. The manualized treatments require anywhere from 12 to 18 sessions, with each session lasting 60 to 90 minutes. The life expectancy for many individuals receiving hospice care may not be sufficient enough to complete the treatment and the length of sessions may require too much stamina. This may present a problem for the clinician who is considering initial therapy because the completion of treatment is paramount given that the interventions may lead to short-term distress with an increase in symptoms prior to full relief of symptoms (Feldman, 2011).

Second, the current evidence-based treatments that are available are designed for traumas that have ended (Feldman, 2011). If an individual's PTSD is related to his or her medical diagnosis, the trauma is ongoing and requires a different approach to care. Third, existing PTSD treatments do not address EOL issues. Incorporating traumatic events into the life review process is an important aspect of EOL care, particularly if the trauma has not been previously processed. As discussed earlier, PTSD also can have a significant impact on family members. There is little role for family members in existing PTSD treatments. Lastly, for some older adults with cognitive deficits, PTSD treatments may need to be adapted based on the individual's specific neurocognitive deficits (Kaiser et al., 2013).

A Palliative Approach to Posttraumatic Stress Disorder at the End of Life

As a result of these shortcomings related to standard evidence-based treatments for PTSD, a new approach needed to be developed for a palliative care setting. Feldman (2011) proposed a staged, patient-centered model for treating PTSD symptoms at the end of life. Movement from one stage to the other is dictated completely by the individual's palliative care needs, with particular attention to life expectancy as well as the nature and acuity of symptoms. Stages of the model are highlighted in Table 23.3 and each stage is described in detail in the text that follows (Feldman, 2011).

Stage I of the model is designed to palliate immediate discomfort and provide social support. This stage is best suited for palliative care patients who are unable to tolerate time-intensive interventions because of either a short life expectancy or fatigue. Immediate distress is alleviated through emotional support and environmental adaptations, such as the presence of supportive family and other caregivers as well as creating safe and comforting surroundings. Communication techniques that are used during this stage include active listening, reassurance, and mediating discussions with medical providers or family members. Direct assistance with

TABLE 23.3   A Staged Model for Treating PTSD at the EOL
Stage I: Palliate immediate discomfort and provide social supports
Stage II: Provide psycho-education and enhance coping skills
Stage III: Treat specific trauma issues

EOL, end of life; PTSD, posttraumatic stress disorder.

problem solving (such as finding a notary or notifying a family member) and working with healthcare providers and family about how to avoid triggering PTSD symptoms also are important aspects of Stage I (Feldman, 2011).

Providing psycho-education regarding PTSD and enhancing coping strategies is the goal of Stage II. Consistent with a palliative care approach, Stage II is designed to enhance the QOL by helping the individual better manage PTSD symptoms. Education and training on the symptoms of PTSD are given to the patient, family, and interprofessional treatment team members. Evidence-based cognitive-behavioral therapy (CBT) coping strategies, such as relaxation (Goldfried & Davison, 1994), cognitive restructuring (Beck, 1995), and acceptance-based techniques (Hayes, Strosahl, & Wilson, 2003), are taught to the patient. A mental health provider can help match a CBT technique to a particular CBT symptom. For example, relaxation and breathing techniques can help to reduce somatic symptoms of anxiety, and cognitive restructuring assists with distorted thinking regarding either the medical condition or the trauma (Feldman, Sorocco, & Bratkovich, 2014). Problem-solving and communication skills are also often taught during Stage II. A mental health provider often initially teaches the patient these coping skills and then their use can be encouraged by care partners, including family and interprofessional treatment team members.

Stage III involves the treatment of specific trauma issues. The application of specific evidence-based treatment approaches (e.g., CBT) occurs only after consideration is given to the patient's preference, prognosis, energy level, and life expectancy. As part of a palliative care approach to PTSD, a life review–based exposure approach conducted by a mental health practitioner is recommended (Feldman, 2011). A safe environment is established that would allow the individual to share traumatic memories. The patient dictates the pace of the life review sessions, with sessions typically occurring more frequently and for a shorter duration than other previously discussed approaches. During the life review, the therapist places an emphasis on reframing and meaning-making in a semi-structured format through the use of a set of planned questions that promote life review dictated by the pace and content choice of the patient (Feldman, 2011).

Role of Interprofessional Treatment Providers

Nurses and other interprofessional treatment team members play a vital role in the successful implementation of a palliative care approach to manage PTSD symptoms. Prior to the development of the stage-based model to manage PTSD symptoms at the end of life, Feldman and Periyakoil (2006) outlined general considerations for the psychosocial management of PTSD, which included adopting a patient-centered approach, educating the staff, educating the patient, and developing a set of PTSD resources. These recommendations included a focus on communication skills (i.e., active listening, empathy, and respecting the individual's autonomy and staff education; emphasizing how PTSD symptoms influence nursing care). According to the authors of this chapter, these general approaches to the psychosocial management of PTSD at the end of life should be followed by all disciplines regardless of the degree of mental health resources available.

Interprofessional treatment providers can also directly implement portions of the stage-based model to manage PTSD symptoms (Feldman, 2011). For example, in Stages I and II, practitioners outside of mental health should be able to assist in the identification of PTSD symptoms and implement effective environmental interventions. In order to facilitate this, both active and passive approaches to staff education need to be implemented in palliative care settings. An active approach to staff education is to require general training on PTSD symptoms by palliative care staff. Free, online educational resources (see Resources section for listing) are accessible to the general public. Interprofessional treatment practitioners with some expertise in the management of PTSD can educate staff during interprofessional treatment team meetings and even through their charting notes. For example, when a chart review reveals a potential or confirmed diagnosis of PTSD, the provider can alert others to possible symptoms of PTSD and their impact on patient care. An example of this documentation is as follows:

> Clinical literature has documented that veterans with PTSD may have an increase in symptoms when dealing with issues related to palliative care, even if symptoms were well controlled prior to the change in health status. Common PTSD symptoms related to palliative care include: intense anxiety, anger, guilt, or sadness; poor medical adherence; difficulty engaging in direct problem focused communication regarding care; refusal of care or excessive questioning of provider's actions or distrust of authority.

Staff education is the essential component to the implementation of successful interventions to manage PTSD at the end of life.

Pharmacological Approaches to Treat Posttraumatic Stress Disorder at End of Life

Pharmacological approaches to the treatment of PTSD are important to consider in conjunction with psychosocial approaches, particularly when life expectancy is limited (Feldman, 2011). Patient preference regardless of life expectancy may also dictate the use of pharmacological approaches. Therefore, interprofessional practitioners should know that there are two major classes of medications that have been shown to be effective for alleviating symptoms of PTSD. The first major class of drugs is the SSRIs, which have been found to alleviate the avoidance and numbing symptoms associated with PTSD (NCPTSD, 2009a). The second class of medications are tricyclic antidepressants (TCAs), which have been shown to alleviate intrusive symptoms, anxiety, and depressed affect (NCPTSD, 2009a).

In conjunction with SSRIs or TCAs, practitioners may also choose to prescribe other medications such as benzodiazepines. Benzodiazepines can be prescribed in combination with SSRIs in order to alleviate anxiety, panic, and hyperarousal symptoms (NCPTSD, 2009a). It is important to note that benzodiazepines are not recommended for long-term treatment of PTSD because they have not been found to treat the core symptoms of PTSD and have additive properties, although they can be effective for EOL care. Although there is a paucity of research on medication to treat PTSD at the end of life, a more detailed review of pharmacotherapy for PTSD can be found on the National Center for PTSD website.

■ FUTURE DIRECTIONS

The need for additional research on the impact of PTSD and EOL care was recommended more than two decades ago during the National Cancer Institute of Canada Workshop on Symptom Control and Supportive Care in Patients with Advanced Cancer (Breitbart, Bruera, Chochinov, & Lynch, 1995). During this workshop, the panelists recommended the need for prevalence and intervention studies on PTSD among advanced cancer patients. Despite the apparent need, there continue to be very limited data on the prevalence of PTSD and the effectiveness of evidence-based interventions to address PTSD in palliative care patients. For example, PTSD symptoms often influence the perception and experience of pain at the end of life (Chang et al., 2007). Informative and evidence-based websites regarding PTSD symptoms across the life span exist; however, none of them to date include recommendations regarding EOL care. To provide quality palliative care, educating the treatment team members on the management of PTSD at the EOL needs to form a core component of palliative care training. However, with the exception of the End-of-Life Nursing Education Consortium for veterans, PTSD is not even addressed. Regardless of whether or not an individual meets criteria for a PTSD diagnosis or has PTSD-like symptoms as the result of an acute medical procedure, his or her symptoms will need to be palliated. Education and research in the area of PTSD and the end of life is in need of development.

In the absence of current evidence, a possible area to explore in the treatment of PTSD and the end of life may be to consider components of Marsha Linehan's work in dialectical behavior therapy (DBT). This treatment is a combination of behavioral and crisis intervention strategies and its primary tenets are focused on acceptance and tolerance. There are four areas of focus in DBT, which are interpersonal effectiveness, emotion regulation, distress tolerance, and mindfulness. Skills from these modules can be taught to address specific symptoms in a variety of settings, including PTSD symptoms at the end of life. The major tenets of acceptance and tolerance can serve to validate the patient's experiences and symptoms and give them tools to cope with the present. These tools can also be taught to the patient's caregivers, as well as the nurses and interprofessional treatment providers.

CASE STUDY *Conclusion*

Prior to reviewing a chart for mental health issues or directly working with the patient, there are often clues that might suggest a diagnosis of PTSD. Specific to Jimmy Mac, key aspects included basic patient demographics (e.g., Vietnam-era veteran, American Indian), mistrust of the medical system, and poor medical adherence. Jimmy had experienced child abuse, cultural oppression (i.e., being removed from his family and placed in an Indian boarding school), and recurrent combat traumas, resulting in having high levels of mistrust of authority.

Appropriate assessment approaches might include a chart review, an intake interview that would include evaluation of past traumatic events, the meaning of those traumas, and screening measures to identify symptoms in need of intervention. The meaning of specific traumas and how they impacted Jimmy's worldview often helps practitioners involved in his care understand the medical decisions that he makes related to his healthcare. A structured clinical interview is less often used when life expectancy is limited.

The goal of the assessment in palliative care is to identify which symptoms of PTSD are currently distressing to the patient and to determine how to best manage these symptoms to improve the individual's QOL. Appropriate interventions include making sure the interprofessional treatment team is aware of any mental health diagnoses, such as PTSD. Effective communication skills and developing a strong rapport with the individual is vital to build a trusting relationship. Environmental adaptations such as knocking on the door before entering and not abruptly waking patients will help to prevent symptoms related to an exaggerated startle response. Psycho-education and techniques for enhancing coping strategies shall be based on life expectancy and their level of fatigue.

CASE STUDY

AN INTERPROFESSIONAL PERSPECTIVE

Edward J. Gabriel, MPA, EMT-P, CEM, CBCP
Principal Deputy Assistant Secretary for Preparedness and Response
U. S. Department of Health and Human Services

All practitioners and patients are at a risk for developing symptoms of PTSD. As a longtime emergency provider, I know we often do not take enough time to prepare ourselves for the emotional impacts that occur during crisis events. To add to that stress, we all must confront crisis situations knowing that critique, process, and protocol drive our every decision.

As a responder who has been directly involved in some of the most significant disaster and emergency responses in this country, I can tell you that each crisis has had a direct emotional impact on me. During these events, concerns regarding choices that were made, stay in our memories and are continually reviewed and critiqued. Questions such as why

I made "that decision," what about the family, what would I want to happen if it was my family member, what would the patient want, should I follow the standards, will I be sued, and who should I treat first will continually be internally critiqued. As clinicians, we want to provide the best care possible, yet we have internal personal struggles regarding ethical and moral decisions in crisis situations.

In this case study, Jimmy Mac may have PTSD and not be aware of it. The cumulative effects of crisis experiences throughout his life could be taking a toll on him and affect our ability to care for him. The palliative care patient's physical symptoms can often be managed appropriately; however, emotional symptoms may be difficult to recognize if you do not assess for PTSD.

It is important to recognize our own biases and experiences that influence our thoughts, critical thinking, and plan of care. We need to be personally aware of the risk for PTSD and its emotional effects. As we experience unfortunate events and respond to and manage circumstances, we can believe ourselves immune to the effects over time. Of course, this is not the case, and I would suggest that we follow the advice we give to our patients and peers. Look for symptoms, connect with a provider, talk to someone, ask questions, don't overdo it, and take care of ourselves. Remember, we are not invulnerable.

Evidence-Based Practice

Prince-Paul, M., Peereboom, K., & Daly, B. J. (2016). Confronting mortality: Narrative of military veterans enrolled in Home Hospice Care. *Journal of Hospice and Palliative Nursing, 18*(3), 219–226. doi:10.1097/NJH.0000000000000250

Objectives
To advance the understanding and meaning of veterans' life experiences among those enrolled in home hospice care at the end of life.

Methods
Phenomenological, hermeneutic, and qualitative approaches were used to collect interview data from 15 veterans across military branches who had life-limiting illnesses, were enrolled in home hospice, and were without significant cognitive impairment or uncontrolled pain.

Results
Five main themes emerged from the interview data: (1) limited opportunities, (2) broken relationships, (3) obligation, (4) life influence not definition, and (5) lack of fear/ acceptance of death.

Conclusions
EOL care needs to meet the personal needs of each veteran and his or her family. A veteran's military experience may be influential and unique, but not life defining.

■ RESOURCES

National Center for Child Traumatic Stress Network—www.nctsn.org
National Center for PTSD—www.ptsd.va.gov

■ REFERENCES

Alter, C. L., Pelcovitz, D., Axelrod, A., Goldenberg, B., Harris, H., Meyers, B., ... Kaplan, S. (1996). Identification of PTSD in cancer survivors (Research Support, U.S. Govt, P.H.S.). *Psychosomatics, 37*(2), 137–143. doi:10.1016/S0033-3182(96)71580-3

American Association of Colleges of Nursing. (2013). Peaceful death: Recommended competencies and curricular guidelines for end-of-life nursing care. Retrieved from https://files.eric.ed.gov/fulltext/ED453706.pdf

American Psychiatric Association. (2013). *Diagnostic and statistical manual of mental disorders* (5th ed.). Arlington, VA: American Psychiatric Publishing.

Amir, M., & Ramati, A. (2002). Post-traumatic symptoms, emotional distress and quality of life in long-term survivors of breast cancer: A preliminary research. [Multicenter Study]. *Journal of Anxiety Disorders, 16*(2), 195–206. doi:10.1016/S0887-6185(02)00095-6

Averill, P. M., & Beck, J. G. (2000). Posttraumatic stress disorder in older adults: A conceptual review. *Journal of Anxiety Disorders, 14*(2), 133–156. doi:10.1016/S0887-6185(99)00045-6

Azoulay, E., Pochard, F., Kentish-Barnes, N., Chevret, S., Aboab, J., Adrie, C., ... Schlemmer, B. (2005). Risk of post-traumatic stress symptoms in family members of intensive care unit patients. *American Journal of Respiratory and Critical Care Medicine, 171*(9), 987–994. doi:10.1164/rccm.200409-1295OC

Beck, A. (1995). *Cognitive therapy: Basics and beyond.* New York, NY: Guilford Press.

Blake, D. D., Weathers, F. W., Nagy, L. M., Kaloupek, D. G., Gusman, F. D., Charney, D. S., & Keane, T. M. (1995). The development of a Clinician-Administered PTSD Scale. [Review]. *Journal of Traumatic Stress, 8*(1), 75–90. doi:10.1002/jts.2490080106

Breitbart, W., Bruera, E., Chochinov, H., & Lynch, M. (1995). Neuropsychiatric syndromes and psychological symptoms in patients with advanced cancer. *Journal of Pain and Symptom Management, 10*(2), 131–141. doi:10.1016/0885-3924(94)00075-V

Brewin, C. R., Rose, S., Andrews, B., Green, J., Tata, P., McEvedy, C., ... Foa, E. B. (2002). Brief screening instrument for post-traumatic stress disorder. *British Journal of Psychiatry, 181*, 158–162. doi:10.1192/bjp.181.2.158

Carlson, E. B., & Ruzek, J. (2013). *PTSD and the family.* VA National Center for PTSD. Washington, DC: U.S. Department of Veterans Affairs.

Chang, V. T., Sorger, B., Rosenfeld, K. E., Lorenz, K. A., Bailey, A. F., Bui, T., ... Montagnini, M. (2007). Pain and palliative medicine. *Journal of Rehabilitation Research and Development, 44*(2), 279–294. doi:10.1682/JRRD.2006.06.0067

Connor, K. M., & Davidson, J. R. (2001). SPRINT: A brief global assessment of post-traumatic stress disorder. *International Clinical Psychopharmacology, 16*(5), 279–284.

Cook, A., Blaustein, M., Spinazolla, J., van der Kolk, B. (2003). *Complex trauma in children and adolescents.* White paper from the national child traumatic stress network complex trauma task force. Los Angeles, CA: National Center for Child Traumatic Stress.

Curtis, J. R., Ciechanowski, P. S., Downey, L., Gold, J., Nielsen, E. L., Shannon, S. E., ... Engelberg, R. A. (2012). Development and evaluation of an interprofessional communication intervention to improve family outcomes in the ICU. *Contemporary Clinical Trials, 33*(6), 1245–1254. doi:10.1016/j.cct.2012.06.010

Davidson, J. R. T., Kudler, H. S., & Smith, R. D. (1990). Assessment and pharmacotherapy of posttraumatic stress disorder. In J. E. L. Giller (Ed.), *Biological assessment and treatment of posttraumatic stress disorder* (pp. 205–221). Washington, DC: American Psychiatric Press.

Davison, E. H., Kaiser, A. P., Spiro, A., III, Moye, J., King, L. A., & King, D. W. (2016). From late-onset stress symptomatology to later-adulthood trauma reengagement in aging combat veterans: Taking a broader view. *Gerontologist, 56*(1), 14–21. doi:10.1093/geront/gnv097

Davison, E. H., Pless, A. P., Gugliucci, M. R., King, L. A., King, D. W., Salgado, D. M., ... Bachrach, P. (2006). Late life emergence of early life trauma: The phenomenon of late-onset stress symptomatology among aging combat veterans. *Research on Aging, 28*, 84–114. doi:10.1177/0164027505281560

Department of Veterans Affairs and Department of Defense. (2010). The VA/DoD clinical practice guidelines for management of post-traumatic stress. *Version 2.0–2010.* Washington, DC: Author.

Elhai, J. D., Gray, M. J., Kashdan, T. B., & Franklin, C. L. (2005). Which instruments are most commonly used to assess traumatic event exposure and posttraumatic effects? A survey of traumatic stress professionals. *Journal of Traumatic Stress, 18*(5), 541–545. doi:10.1002/jts.20062

Feldman, D. B. (2011). Posttraumatic stress disorder at the end of life: Extant research and proposed psychosocial treatment approach. *Palliative and Supportive Care, 9*(4), 407–418. doi:10.1017/S1478951511000435

Feldman, D. B., & Periyakoil, V. S. (2006). Posttraumatic stress disorder at the end of life. *Journal of Palliative Medicine, 9*(1), 213–218. doi:10.1089/jpm.2006.9.213

Feldman, D. B., Sorocco, K. H., & Bratkovich, K. L. (2014). Treatment of PTSD at end of life: Application of the Stepwise Psychosocial Palliative Care model. *Palliative and Supportive Care, 12*(3), 233–243. doi:10.1017/S1478951513000370

First, M. B., Spitzer, R. L., Gibbon, M., & Williams, J. B. W. (1996). *Structured Clinical Interview for* DSM-IV *Axis I Disorders, Clinician Version (SCID-CV)*. Washington, DC: American Psychiatric Press.

Foa, E. B., & Tolin, D. F. (2000). Comparison of the PTSD symptom scale-interview version and the clinician-administered PTSD scale. *Journal of Traumatic Stress, 13*(2), 181–191. doi:10.1023/A:1007781909213

Goldfried, M. R., & Davison, G. C. (1994). *Clinical behavior therapy*. New York, NY: John Wiley & Sons.

Gradus, J. L. (2007). Epidemiology of PTSD. National Center for PTSD Website. Retrieved from http://www.ptsd.va.gov/professional/pages/epidemiological-facts-ptsd.asp

Griffiths, J., Fortune, G., Barber, V., & Young, J. D. (2007). The prevalence of post traumatic stress disorder in survivors of ICU treatment: A systematic review. *Intensive Care Medicine, 33*(9), 1506–1518. doi:10.1007/s00134-007-0730-z

Hamblen, J. L., Schnurr, P., Rosenberger, S., & Eftekhari, A. (2013). Overview of psychotherapy for PTSD. Retrieved from https://www.ptsd.va.gov/professional/treatment/overview/overview-treatment-research.asp

Hayes, S. C., Strosahl, K. D., & Wilson, K. G. (2003). *Acceptance and commitment therapy: An experiential approach to behavior change*. New York, NY: Guilford Press.

Institute of Medicine. (2007). *Treatment of posttraumatic stress disorder: An assessment of the evidence*. Washington, DC: National Academies Press.

Kaiser, A. P., Wachen, J. S., Potter, C., Moye, J., Davidson, E., & Hermann, B. (2013, February 27). PTSD assessment and treatment in older adults. Retrieved from https://www.ptsd.va.gov/professional/treatment/older/assessment_tx_older_adults.asp

Lautrette, A., Darmon, M., Megarbane, B., Joly, L. M., Chevret, S., Adrie, C., ... Azoulay, E. (2007). A communication strategy and brochure for relatives of patients dying in the ICU. *New England Journal of Medicine, 356*(5), 469–478. doi:10.1056/NEJMoa063446

National Cancer Institute. (2015, January 7). PDQ® Supportive and Palliative Care Editorial Board. PDQ Cancer-Related Post-Traumatic Stress. Bethesda, MD: Author. Retrieved from https://www.cancer.gov/about-cancer/coping/survivorship/new-normal/ptsd-hp-pdq

National Center for Posttraumatic Stress Disorder. (2007, July 3). Treatment of PTSD. Retrieved from https://www.ptsd.va.gov/public/treatment/therapy-med/treatment-ptsd.asp

National Center for Posttraumatic Stress Disorder. (2009a, May 8). Clinician's guide to medications for PTSD. Retrieved from https://www.ptsd.va.gov/professional/treatment/overview/clinicians-guide-to-medications-for-ptsd.asp

National Center for Posttraumatic Stress Disorder. (2009b, March 12). Cognitive processing therapy. Retrieved from https://www.ptsd.va.gov/public/treatment/therapy-med/cognitive_processing_therapy.asp

National Center for Posttraumatic Stress Disorder. (2009c, June 17). Prolonged exposure therapy. Retrieved from https://www.ptsd.va.gov/public/treatment/therapy-med/prolonged-exposure-therapy.asp

National Child Traumatic Stress Network. (2014, March 31). Defining trauma and child traumatic stress. Retrieved from http://www.nctsn.org/resources/audiences/parents-caregivers/what-is-cts

Prince-Paul, M., Peereboom, K., & Daly, B. J. (2016). Confronting mortality: Narrative of military veterans enrolled in Home Hospice Care. Journal of Hospice and Palliative Nursing, 18(3), 219–226. doi:10.1097/NJH.0000000000000250

Rees, G., Gledhill, J., Garralda, M. E., & Nadel, S. (2004). Psychiatric outcome following pediatric intensive care unit (PICU) admission: A cohort study. *Intensive Care Medicine, 30*, 1607–1614. doi:10.1007/s00134-004-2310-9

Shemesh, E., Yehuda, R., Milo, O., Dinur, I., Rudnick, A., Vered, Z., & Cotter, G. (2004). Posttraumatic stress, nonadherence, and adverse outcome in survivors of a myocardial infarction. *Psychosomatic Medicine, 66*(4), 521–526. doi:10.1097/01.psy.0000126199.05189.86

Stuber, M. L., & Shemesh, E. (2006). Post-traumatic stress response to life-threatening illnesses in children and their parents. *Child and Adolescent Psychiatric Clinics of North America, 15*(3), 597–609. doi:10.1016/j.chc.2006.02.006

Vrana, S., & Lauterbach, D. (1994). Prevalence of traumatic events and post-traumatic psychological symptoms in a nonclinical sample of college students (Comparative Study Research Support, Non-U.S. Gov't Research Support, U.S. Gov't, P.H.S.). *Journal of Traumatic Stress, 7*(2), 289–302.

Weathers, F. W., Keane, T. M., & Davidson, J. R. (2001). Clinician-administered PTSD scale: A review of the first ten years of research. *Depression and Anxiety, 13*(3), 132–156. doi:10.1002/da.1029

Weathers, F. W., Litz, B. T., Herman, D. S., Huska, J. A., & Keane, T. M. (1993, October). *The PTSD checklist (PCL): Reliability, validity, and diagnostic utility*. Paper presented at the 9th Annual Conference of the ISTSS, San Antonio, TX.

Zivin, K., Kim, H. M., McCarthy, J. F., Austin, K. L., Hoggatt, K. J., Walters, H., & Valenstein, M. (2007). Suicide mortality among individuals receiving treatment for depression in the Veterans Affairs Health System: Associations with patient and treatment setting characteristics. *American Journal of Public Health, 97*(12), 2193–2198. doi:10.2105/ajph.2007.115477

Raymond R. Blush III

Gastrointestinal Symptoms

CHAPTER

24

KEY POINTS

- Gastrointestinal (GI) symptomatology is common in patients receiving palliative care; however, research to support evidence-based interventions in this population specifically is insufficient as the pathology that may lead to palliative care services can be broad.
- Assessment of GI symptoms in patients in palliative care should begin with the identification of the underlying cause that is often related to disease pathology and/or treatment.
- Anorexia and subsequent cachexia are common in patients at the end of life with multiple potential and often overlapping causes. An assessment of the impact of these symptoms and a thorough discussion of potential risks and benefits of supplemental nutrition are critical.
- The evidence to support treatment of nausea and vomiting (N&V) in palliative care is predominantly drawn from chemotherapy-induced nausea and vomiting (CINV); however, the mechanisms and pathophysiology of CINV and the N&V of the palliative care population may be very different than with other pathology.
- The diagnosis and treatment of dysphagia is based on the patient's prognosis. With a longer prognosis, medically assisted feeding and hydration may be considered. With a shorter prognosis, the treatment may be different.
- Multiple medications, although primarily opioids, are a principal cause of constipation in the palliative care population.
- Laxatives may be used either as a preventive measure or as a treatment for constipation.
- Signs and symptoms of bowel obstruction are based on the site of the obstruction. In older adults, the signs and symptoms of obstruction may be less apparent than in the younger population.
- The most common cause of diarrhea in palliative care is inappropriate laxative therapy.
- Other clinical conditions include ascites, xerostomia, and pain. Each of these should be addressed based on the cause and indications for symptom management.

CASE STUDY

Three months ago, Mrs. Adams was diagnosed with pancreatic cancer with metastasis to her stomach, liver, and intestines, resulting in a poor prognosis. She is 65 years of age with a history of regular tobacco and alcohol use. There is no family history of cancer, and Mrs. Adams had no significant health history until this new diagnosis. With the involvement of other organs, she made the decision not to have surgery. She is admitted to the medical unit today for severe abdominal pain, constipation, nausea, and vomiting.

Mrs. Adams's daughter is with her today and is concerned that her mother waited too long to come to the hospital for treatment of her symptoms. She states that her appetite has been poor, and she has not been taking the Viokase as prescribed because of her vomiting. Her last bowel movement was 2 days ago, consistent with diarrhea. She states that she has been taking morphine sulfate orally at home and an antiemetic that she cannot remember the name of. The nurse completed the admission assessment and found that Mrs. Adams is jaundiced and has a bruit located in the left upper quadrant. A nasogastric tube has been inserted and is connected to low intermittent wall suction. Breath sounds reveal fine crackles in the bases bilaterally. Notable lab results include Hbg 4.0 g/dL and Hct 13%, Na 133, and K+ 3.4 mEq/L, total bilirubin of 4 mg/dL, amylase 2,500 IU/dL, AST 30 units/L. Arterial blood gas results demonstrate pH of 7.33, $PaCO_2$ 34, and HCO_3 21.

In most countries of the world, sharing meals with others is a social activity. While the primary purpose of a meal may be consumption of food, nutrition socialization with others while eating may be even more important. Communities, organizations, and churches often have events where individuals gather to share a meal. If an individual is unable to share a meal with others due to gastrointestinal (GI) symptoms, the effect on the emotional health of the individual from being socially isolated and unable to participate in such activities may be greater than the physical effects of the symptoms. This can have a notable impact on patients at the end of life with palliative care needs, where social interaction can be as critical to their overall well-being as any medical therapy and intervention.

It is well established that both adult and pediatric patients at the end of life suffer from numerous GI symptoms. For those with cancer, nausea and vomiting (N&V) occurs in nearly 50% and potentially in greater than 90% within the first 24 hours of initiating chemotherapy (Dean, Harris, Regnard, & Hockley, 2006; Gilmore et al., 2014). Individuals with chronic kidney disease often suffer from numerous GI symptoms due to uremia. In particular, they are prone to the development of upper GI symptoms, including erosive gastritis, ulcerative esophagitis, and duodenitis (Thomas et al., 2013). GI symptomatology is also common in HIV/AIDS patients and end-stage heart failure (Dean et al., 2006). Patients suffering from continuous nausea, vomiting, or diarrhea may be precluded from leaving their care setting, whether it is home, assisted living, or a long-term care facility, and may affect their quality of life and the ability to function normally.

The incidence of GI symptoms in children who die of non–cancer-related illness is unknown; however, GI symptomatology in pediatric cancer patients at the end of life is significant. Common GI symptoms include pain, constipation, and N&V. These may be a result of the disease process itself or treatments such as chemotherapeutic agents. In addition, treatment of symptoms with medications such as narcotics can contribute to constipation and N&V. Decreased oral intake, poor hydration, and decreased activity all can contribute to GI

symptoms as well (Klick & Hauer, 2010). This chapter focuses on the cluster of GI symptoms that occurs in the adult and pediatric patient who are under palliative care.

While the identification of the cause of GI symptoms in those involved in palliative care should be directed at specific disease pathology and potential treatment effects, broadly understanding the impact on the individual patient is necessary. Other symptoms to consider include anorexia and cachexia, dyspepsia, constipation and bowel obstruction, diarrhea, and hiccups. There are several suggested ways of assessing and diagnosing the symptomatology that a patient may develop from the side effects of treatment and/or comfort measures. A suggested mnemonic, developed by Esper and Heidrich (2005), gives the caregiver a resource in assessing and managing the multiple symptoms that may be experienced by the patient (Esper & Heidrich, 2005, p. 20). This mnemonic uses RESCUE to address symptoms, allows the clinician to cluster them in both assessment and management approaches, potentially reduces polypharmacy and systemic toxicities, and improves the patient's quality of life.

R—Review the situation
E—Explore findings
S—Strategize a plan of action
C—Carry out the plan
U—Umbrella resources
E—Evaluate and modify as needed

■ ANOREXIA AND CACHEXIA

The definition of anorexia includes both the loss of appetite and the reduction in oral intake, and can significantly impact those at the end of life (Cunningham, 2014). It is a common cause of malnutrition and weight loss in end-of-life patients, impacting overall symptoms and leading to the burden of disease. While exact mechanisms are not entirely known, it is likely multifactorial and related to the impact of the disease as well as treatment and therapies. It can be a part of presenting symptoms, as a result of a therapy or an evidence of a progressive disease, and in conjunction with other overlapping issues. Often anorexia is a precursor to cachexia but may also be a symptom as well. Cachexia is a syndrome where protein and energy balance are effected, leading to a loss of skeletal muscle mass. With progressive disease states, cachexia is generally poorly improved by nutritional support and may suggest an expected survival of less than 3 months. Additionally, anorexia and cachexia have been found present in up to 80% of patients with cancer, with an increase in prevalence as disease states progress (Fearon et al., 2011).

Etiology of Anorexia and Cachexia

Causes of anorexia are multifactorial and may depend on the disease causes as well as the potential treatment and palliative therapies. Oncology patients may develop anorexia from their treatment rather than the cancer itself. Both chemotherapy and radiation therapy cause a variety of side effects that can contribute to anorexia and weight loss, including nausea and vomiting, fatigue, changes in taste perception, and dry mouth. With a decrease in nutritional intake, patients who may already be at an increased risk for nutritional deficits based on their disease states become increasingly more so. With specific regard to cancer patients, recent studies also suggest that antineoplastic agents may be contributing to some of the body composition changes observed in cachexia. Others have observed that cancer patients treated with sorafenib (Nexavar) manifest notable degrees of muscle wasting over time and that this may be an independent rick factor for wasting and nutritional deficiencies (Jatoi, 2015).

Signs and Symptoms

Objectively, patients with anorexia have a loss of appetite with decreased oral intake. Additionally, they often note early satiety as a common issue. This may be related to both liquid and solid food intake. Consideration should be given to the onset of the symptoms. Pathology and treatment might differ in a patient who has these as a presenting complaint of their disease versus those symptoms that begin after treatment has started. Related symptoms may include dysphagia, mucositis, xerostomia, early satiety, nausea, vomiting, constipation or diarrhea, bloating after eating, flatulence, abdominal pain, dysgeusia (taste alteration), dyspnea, and fatigue. Anorexia may also be a symptom of other conditions such as infections, bowel obstructions, and depression, and should always be considered in the palliative care patient. Cachexia is also a common manifestation of anorexia and other related symptoms. It is indicated by more than 5% loss of stable body weight over the previous 6 months; or a body mass index (BMI) less than 20 kg/m^2 and ongoing weight loss of more than 2%; or sarcopenia and ongoing weight loss of more than 2% (Fearon et al., 2011).

Assessment of Anorexia and Cachexia

Several screening tools have been developed to measure the potential impact of malnutrition and identify at-risk patients. While variable in their specific items, each generally has measures that assess food intake patterns, history of unintentional weight loss, mobility, psychosocial stressors, and the possibility of neuropsychological issues like depression and dementia, and establish a patient's BMI (Elia, 2003). These assessments gather information regarding a patient's overall nutritional intake, evaluation of his or her own nutrition-related beliefs, items concerning the patient's concerns and expectation for treatment, self-care behavior, and the impact of the disease state. They may also involve physical examination and diagnostic testing aimed to evaluate ongoing and progressive nutritional status. Patients who have a positive score or those who are identified at risk may be referred to a nutritionist for a comprehensive nutritional assessment and subsequent development of a nutritional plan. Tools such as the Malnutrition Universal Screening Tool (MUST), developed by the British Association for Parenteral and Enteral Nutrition, (BAPEN) Malnutrition Advisory Group, specifically screen for nutritional issues using a multi-symptom inventory paired with serial body weight measurements (Levin, 2012).

The MUST screening tool is a five-step approach to identify adults who are malnourished or at risk of malnutrition, and have unplanned weight loss. It also includes management guidelines that can be used to develop a care plan. It is for use in hospitals, community, and other care settings where patients are acutely ill and there has been or is likely to be no nutritional intake for greater than 5 days (Malnutrition Advisory Group, 2011). Step 1 involves the measurement of a patient's height and weight to calculate a BMI score. This score can either be obtained by measuring the patient's height and weight or, if that is not possible, determined by alternate approaches that estimate the height by using the length of the forearm and weight by the mid–upper arm circumference. Step 2 calculates the percentage of unplanned weight loss and creates a score using tables provided. Step 3 establishes the impact of acute disease and the potential effect on a patient's nutrition. Step 4 then cumulates the scores from Steps 1, 2, and 3 to obtain the overall risk of malnutrition for the patient. With the results of the MUST scoring, management guidelines are suggested that are guided by the assessment of that patient's nutritional status and if he or she is at a low (0), medium (1), or high ($\geq$2) risk for malnutrition. Importantly, the guidelines suggest routine reassessment of patients identified at risk as they move through care settings so that ongoing support can be addressed. The MUST toolkit is available online at the BAPEN website (www.bapen.org.uk/pdfs/must/must-full.pdf).

After establishing the impact of anorexia and the potential rate and severity of weight loss, it is important to identify what steps can be taken to address these concerns. The identification of potentially treatable causes of anorexia such as candidiasis, nausea and vomiting, pain, dyspnea, constipation, and fatigue needs to be addressed. Other medical conditions, including hypogonadism, metabolic dysfunction, and thyroid dysfunction, should be considered as well, either as part of the primary issue or as a result of therapy. Addressing emotional and psychosocial concerns is essential as well. Identification of concerns such as depression, access to care, expectations regarding treatment impact and overall disease progression, and anticipated outcomes for the patient and caretakers is essential (National Comprehensive Cancer Network [NCCN], 2017).

Diagnostic testing may be considered to evaluate the patient with anorexia and cachexia who requires palliative care interventions. Part of this evaluation may be established to identify the underlying pathology of disease. This could include x-rays, CT scans, MRI, ultrasound, and endoscopic imaging. These tools may be used in part to discover the causes of primary disease or for evaluation of anorexia alone and are dictated by the clinical picture and anticipated needs and outcomes. The most helpful laboratory studies in assessing potential malnutrition include hematological studies such as a CBC count with RBC indices to evaluate for anemia. Distinguishing anemias from nutritional deficiencies such as iron, folate, and vitamin B_{12} deficits can be helpful. Measures of protein nutritional status include serum albumin, retinol-binding protein, prealbumin, transferrin, creatinine, and blood urea nitrogen (BUN) levels and may be utilized.

Management of Anorexia and Cachexia

Appropriate identification of the causes of anorexia is necessary before steps to symptom relief can be taken. Management of anorexia should primarily focus on the treatment of potentially reversible causes such as dysphagia, mucositis, candidiasis, pain, constipation, or diarrhea. As anorexia may be a symptom of other clinical conditions such as bowel obstruction, infection, and depression, these should be considered and addressed as well (M. T. Lynch, 2014).

As patients are identified at a high risk for nutritional deficiencies, a prompt evaluation with a nutritional assessment is necessary. Assessment with a nutrition consultant who can address these concerns, including the need for nutritional support, can be essential. Focusing on patient goals and preferences, providing family ways to care for and support the patient, and providing emotional support can be helpful. Also, providing the patient realistic projected outcomes for disease progress can be helpful with regard to nutritional needs. Support to patients with anorexia should primarily be directed at treating underlying causes when appropriate. Being considerate

of the impact of treatment on the symptom of anorexia should be addressed. Likely, there is a balance in the need to offer curative treatment, palliation, and symptom support, each of which needs to be discussed with any patient and their family. Weighing the risks of offering support against the potential benefits is important to discuss in any setting and involves outlining the impact of the disease, the influence of anorexia and possible malnutrition, and anticipated goals and outcomes of the disease state, regardless of the pathology.

■ **Pharmacological Interventions for Anorexia and Cachexia.** The NCCN offers guidelines that suggest evaluation and treatment approaches for numerous conditions where patients may require palliative care. When there are anticipated months to years of life expectancy, mirtazapine 7.5 to 30 mg at bedtime may be helpful. Early satiety may be helped by metoclopramide 5 to 10 mg four times daily 30 minutes before meals and at bedtime, and may offer some relief. Specifically to address anorexia, megestrol 400 to 800 mg daily is used as an appetite stimulant to treat loss of appetite and may be helpful. Patients whose anticipated life expectancy is less than months, and those actively dying, may benefit from enhanced pharmacological therapy. In addition to treatments mentioned, the addition of dexamethasone 4 to 8 mg daily and possibly cannabinoid may offer some benefit (NCCN, 2017).

■ **Nonpharmacological Interventions for Anorexia and Cachexia.** Nonpharmacological interventions to enhance symptoms of anorexia and possible resultant malnutrition focus on methods to support patient nutrition. Interventions range from oral feeding, oral supplemental nutrition, enteral nutrition, parenteral nutrition, and hydration alone. Each should be addressed with consideration to the individual patient, the anticipated outcomes, and goals and preferences. Eating more frequent smaller meals may be more practical and should be encouraged. Personalizing favorite meals and liberalizing the diet may be helpful. Food itself can be pleasing, so as long as it is enjoyable and offers some pleasure to the patient, it should be encouraged. This should be dictated by the specific clinical picture given safety and anticipated outcomes. Table 24.1 outlines symptom management interventions for anorexia and cachexia (M. T. Lynch, 2014).

■ **Family Concerns and Considerations Regarding Anorexia and Cachexia.** Particularly with the possibility of withdrawal of nutritional support when indicated, education and support to the patient and family can be critical. There are several important points to inform the patient and family of concerning progressive disease, including that the absence of thirst and hunger is normal in a dying patient; even if

TABLE 24.1 Symptom Management Interventions for Anorexia/Cachexia

Identification and Management of Contributing Symptoms

Patient and family education	Lack of appetite and weight loss are often linked to complex changes in the body. Patterns of eating and nutritional support will not change the course of the disease but in early stages can improve quality of life and tolerance of cancer-directed therapies.
Psychosocial support	Acknowledge the psychological, social, cultural, and religious impact of eating and weight loss as appropriate for patient and family Refer for social work or psychiatric support if needed
Nutrition counseling	Mouth care Small frequent meals or snacks Largest meal in the morning or when energy is best Pleasant eating environment Use enriched and fortified foods to increase calories and protein Use of commercial oral liquid nutritional supplements Consultation with qualified nutritionist
Artificial hydration and nutrition	Generally not tolerated or beneficial in patients who have end-stage disease. Individualized goals of the therapy need to be considered. May benefit patients with early-stage disease who have temporary limitation in oral nutritional intake (e.g., examples are patients undergoing radiation therapy for head and neck cancers; those with GI malfunctions related to cancer or therapies that have high performance status).

Pharmacology	Prokinetic agent for early satiety: Metoclopramide 10 mg up to four times daily Appetite stimulants: Megestrol acetate is a first-line agent with typical onset of effect in 1 week. Suggested dose is 160–800 mg/d. Corticosteroids: Mechanism of action unknown Also considered first-line treatment for anorexia Optimal drug and dose are not established. Consider dexamethasone 4–8 mg once daily in the morning Cannabinoids: Dronabinol is FDA approved for AIDS-related anorexia in doses of 5–20 mg/daily initial dose. Its use in cancer-related anorexia is under investigation.	Extrapyramidal side effects including akathisia may occur. Side effects of edema and thromboembolic events may limit use in some patients. Beneficial effect is short term, and the risk of side effects including gastric upset, muscle wasting, edema, and immune suppression increases over duration of use. Use for symptom management is usually restricted to short courses of therapy, or for those nearing death. Side effects include sedation, cognitive slowing, and confusion.
	Under study: Mirtazapine, a tetracyclic antidepressant, may improve appetite and weight. Olanzapine, an atypical antipsychotic, may act synergistically with megestrol to reduce anorexia.	

FDA, Food and Drug Administration; GI, gastrointestinal.

Source: Reprinted from Lynch, M. T. (2014). Palliative care at the end of life. *Seminars in Oncology Nursing, 30*(4), 268–279. doi:10.1016/j.soncn.2014.08.009. Copyright (2014), with permission from Elsevier.

nutritional support is offered, it may not be metabolized in a dying patient; and there is inherent risk in offering artificial nutrition in a dying patient that may not be beneficial (i.e., fluid overload, electrolyte abnormalities, aspiration, pain; (NCCN, 2017). Evidence has been routinely suggested that the use of enteral and parenteral nutritional therapies in dying patients may increase suffering, with nausea, abdominal bloating and cramping, and fluid overload (Del Ferraro, Grant, Koczywas, & Dorr-Uyemura, 2012).

CASE STUDY

1. What issues with Mrs. Adams might contribute to her symptoms of anorexia?
2. How might aspects of her diagnosis, treatment, and psychosocial interactions impact her symptoms of anorexia?
3. What measures might you consider to evaluate and address her anorexia?
4. What therapies might you use to offer her improvement in her symptoms and improve her outcomes?

■ NAUSEA AND VOMITING

Nausea and vomiting (N&V) are unpleasant GI symptoms that often are described by patients as more severe and disabling than pain (Chilton & Faull, 2005). Although nausea may occur without vomiting on occasion, they commonly occur together and are discussed in tandem in this chapter. Nausea is a nonobservable subjective symptom involving an unpleasant sensation experienced in the back of the throat and the epigastrium that precedes but may or may not result in vomiting (Rhodes & McDaniel, 2001). Patients will state that they feel as though they are about to vomit or use other descriptors including "sick to the stomach" or "queasy." Vomiting is the forceful expulsion of gastric contents through the oral or nasal cavity, which typically is preceded by nausea (Rhodes & McDaniel, 2001).

Although N&V are primarily associated with chemotherapy in cancer treatment, these symptoms occur in 40% to 70% of all patients in palliative care settings (Dalal, Del Fabbro, & Bruera, 2006). While chemotherapy is also used as a palliative measure in the oncology population, patients with AIDS, heart, renal, and hepatic failure often have nausea during the disease process and at the end of life as well (Barnes et al., 2006; Mannix, 2005).

Most of the literature regarding management and treatment is derived from studying chemotherapy-induced nausea and vomiting (CINV). As this type of N&V differs both in mechanism and in pathophysiology from N&V due to advanced disease, it is important to note that these findings may not be completely applicable to the entire palliative care setting (Tyler, 2000). While there has been growth in the understanding of the etiology of nausea and vomiting in the oncology setting, particularly distinguishing CINV- and radiation-induced nausea and vomiting, little progress has been made in understanding the mechanism and determining the optimal treatment of these symptoms, especially with overlapping conditions (King, 2006).

Etiology of Nausea and Vomiting

N&V involve activities at multiple levels of the nervous system. Two distinct sites in the medulla are critical for the control of emesis: the vomiting center (VC) and the chemoreceptor trigger zone (CTZ; Dalal et al., 2006). The VC is not a discrete anatomical structure but represents an interrelated neural network, including the nucleus tractus solitarius (NTS) and the dorsal motor nucleus of the vagus (DMV). The NTS is where numerous afferent neuronal pathways from these sources converge. Once the NTS receives signals from the various afferent sources, this information is processed and the DMV emits an appropriate vasomotor response (respiratory, salivary, gut, diaphragm, and abdominal muscles), including nausea, retching, or vomiting, depending on the intensity of the signals (Dalal et al., 2006).

Multiple pathways stimulate the VC. Understanding the pathways is necessary to determine the cause and appropriate treatment (King, 2006). The various pathways include (King, 2006):

- Peripheral pathways
  - Vagal afferents
  - Pharyngeal afferents
  - Vestibular system
- Central pathways
  - Midbrain afferents
  - CTZ

Figure 24.1 demonstrates the various pathways and potential factors that may contribute to each.

Table 24.2 lists potential causes and conditions associated with N&V that may occur in patients receiving palliative care. It should be emphasized that if comorbidities exist, the etiology of N&V may be difficult to ascertain. This is particularly an issue in the older adult who may have more than one disease process present. As with the case of chemotherapy, the treatment itself often contributes to the symptoms. Without a clear appreciation of the cause, successful treatment may become even more challenging.

Signs and Symptoms

Nausea is a subjective symptom that a patient experiences, and it is not measurable to the caregiver. Although it is not objective, nausea may produce significant distress

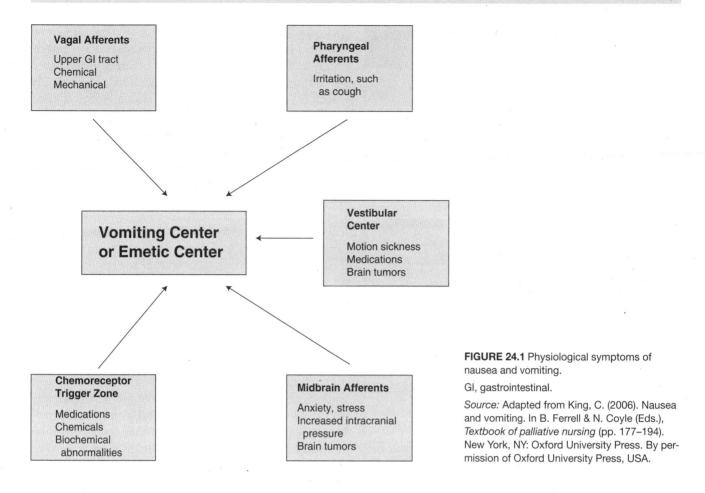

FIGURE 24.1 Physiological symptoms of nausea and vomiting.

GI, gastrointestinal.

Source: Adapted from King, C. (2006). Nausea and vomiting. In B. Ferrell & N. Coyle (Eds.), *Textbook of palliative nursing* (pp. 177–194). New York, NY: Oxford University Press. By permission of Oxford University Press, USA.

for the patient and affect activities of daily living and quality of life. The active process of vomiting not only is discomforting to the patient but also puts him or her at risk for other issues such as dehydration, electrolyte disturbances, and aspiration.

N&V may have accompanying signs and symptoms. With nausea, there may be evidence of increased salivation and swallowing, perspiration, and tachycardia. In patients with N&V triggered by GI tract stasis, there may be accompanying epigastric discomfort, fullness, early satiety, flatulence, acid reflux, hiccups, and large-volume vomitus (possibly projectile). In patients with N&V associated with increased intracranial pressure (ICP), headache and nausea, both diurnal in nature, may occur. Other neurological signs may or may not be present with increased ICP.

Assessment of Nausea and Vomiting

There are a number of factors to consider when assessing N&V in a patient. Some data can be obtained from self-report or from family caregivers, while other information may be objective. Assessment of N&V includes the frequency and duration of symptoms, color, the amount and consistency of vomitus, contributing factors to the N&V, the pattern of the N&V, the presence of abdominal pain, the presence of other abdominal symptoms, and disruption to the patient (e.g., can the patient continue

activities of daily living and other "normal" activities with N&V present?).

Patients should be questioned about the frequency of their bowel movements because in the palliative care population, as with the elderly, chronic constipation is frequently present and may contribute to nausea. In patients with cancer, it is important to obtain details of the sites of the tumor involvement as well. Intraabdominal cancer involvement may lead to nausea with or without vomiting and can often be caused by liver metastasis, bowel obstruction by the tumor, or peritoneal carcinomatosis (Dalal et al., 2006). Unrelieved pain is another common cause of N&V. Pain originating from the GI tract, whether related to luminal disruption or visceral sensitivity, often exacerbates N&V (Kenny, 2007). Narcotics, commonly used in the treatment of pain, are also well established as a cause of N&V (Buenaventura, Adlaka, & Sehgal, 2008).

A large number of medications are associated with nausea; thus, a detailed medication history is necessary. Nausea often accompanies the use of opioids, nonsteroidal anti-inflammatories, anticholinergics, and antibiotics. Many of these are commonly used in treatment and symptom management of a patient in palliative care. Patients with HIV often have nausea as a side effect of the highly active antiretroviral therapy (HAART) drugs. Physiological changes such as decreased renal function, variations in body fat distribution, and alterations in

TABLE 24.2 Causes of Nausea and Vomiting in Palliative Care

Chemoreceptor trigger zone mediated
- ■ Medications
  - ■ Opioids
  - ■ Antibiotics
  - ■ Chemotherapy
  - ■ Corticosteroids
  - ■ Digoxin
  - ■ NSAIDs
  - ■ Iron
- ■ Metabolic
  - ■ Hypercalcemia
  - ■ Hyponatremia
  - ■ Uremia

Midbrain afferents
- ■ Emotional factors
  - ■ Anxiety
  - ■ Fear
  - ■ Pain
- ■ Increased intracranial pressure
- ■ Primary or metastatic brain tumors
- ■ Meningitis

Vagal afferents
- ■ Gastrointestinal distention, stasis, or obstruction
- ■ Constipation
- ■ Gastritis
- ■ External pressure ("squashed stomach syndrome")

Pharyngeal afferents
- ■ Thick sputum
- ■ Oral infection
- ■ Chronic cough
- ■ Unpleasant tastes

Vestibular apparatus
- ■ Motion sickness
- ■ Brain tumors
- ■ Opioids

NSAIDs, nonsteroidal anti-inflammatory drugs.

Source: Adapted from Gullatte, M. M., Kaplow, R., & Heidrich, D. E. (2005). Oncology. In K. K. Kuebler, M. P. Davis, & C. D. Moore (Eds.), *Palliative practices: An interdisciplinary approach* (p. 230). St. Louis, MO: Mosby Elsevier.

hepatic metabolism can lead to higher levels of medications and a greater susceptibility to adverse effects in the geriatric patient (Bishop & Morrison, 2007; Gullatte, Kaplow, & Heidrich, 2005, p. 229). Alterations in or discontinuation of corticosteroids or high-dose progesterone therapy can also lead to N&V due to adrenal insufficiency (Morrow, Hickok, Andrews, & Stern, 2002). Assessing for hypercalcemia, hyponatremia, and SIADH (syndrome of insufficient and diuretic hormone), particularly in cancer patients, is important. High levels of serum calcium and low sodium stimulate the CTZ and may incite N&V (Gullatte et al., 2005).

History should be directed to understand possible causes of the symptoms. Glare, Miller, Nikolova, and Tickoo (2011) offer six such questions and suggested etiology: (a) intermittent nausea associated with early satiety and postprandial fullness or bloating. It is relieved by vomiting that is usually small volume, occasionally forceful, and may contain food. This suggests impaired gastric emptying and is the cause in 35% to 45% of cases. (b) Persistent nausea, aggravated by the sight and smell of food, unrelieved by vomiting. This suggests chemical causes, activating the CTZ. It is found in 30% to 40% of cases. (c) Intermittent nausea associated with abdominal cramping and altered bowel habits. It is relieved by vomiting that may be large in volume and bilious or feculent. This suggests a bowel obstruction and is the cause in 10% to 30% of cases. (d) Early-morning symptoms associated with headache that suggest raised ICP. (e) Nausea aggravated by movement, including motion sickness or even just turning the head. This indicates a vestibular component. (f) N&V associated with anxiety, suggesting a cortical component. The final three occur in less than 15% of patients (Glare et al., 2011).

Assessing the young child for causes of N&V is often more challenging. Although the mentioned assessment guide can be used, very young children may have difficulty differentiating between nausea and pain (Santucci & Mack, 2007). Even older children may have confusion in understanding and describing the difference between nausea, GI reflux symptoms, and pain.

As part of any symptom assessment, it is essential to understand if the patient considers the N&V to affect his or her quality of life or if it is seen merely as a nuisance. To have a clearer understanding of the patient's N&V, an instrument with known reliability and validity should be utilized.

■ **Instruments.** Accurate assessment of signs and symptoms can better determine the pattern of occurrence, if there is one, and the effect of interventions. There are both self-report and observer-report tools, although there is a debate as to which type of tool is best (Saxby, Ackroyd, Callin, Mayland, & Kite, 2007). Some see self-report as essential to determine effective interventions, while others believe that the antiemetic medications given can cause sedation, mood alteration, disorientation, or memory loss, and thus accurate self-report may be affected (Saxby et al., 2007). Many of the specific tools have been validated in chemotherapy outpatient settings, although none have been extensively validated for the assessment of emesis in a palliative care population specifically (Saxby et al., 2007).

Rhodes (1997) suggests the following points when using an instrument to measure N&V: (a) use self-report tools; (b) determine and describe the symptoms; (c) consider the clarity, cultural sensitivity, and understandability of the tool; (d) consider the reliability and validity of the tool; (e) use an instrument in an easy-to-read format; (f) consider the purpose of the tool and the population of patients it caters to; and (g) consider the type of scoring and the ease of scoring.

The tools mentioned in this chapter have limited reliability and validity, specifically to the palliative care setting. As mentioned, much of the focus regarding the assessment of N&V has been directed toward the oncology population and the effects of CINV. The Index of Nausea, Vomiting, and Retching–Revised (INVR-R) instrument measures nausea, vomiting, retching, and the associated perceived patient distress. The tool is an 8-item 5-point Likert-type self-report tool with "check the box inserts." Although it was originally developed for the adult oncology population, it has been demonstrated to have use in other populations also (Rhodes & McDaniel, 1997; Saxby et al., 2007). Of the multiple assessment tools for nausea, vomiting, and retching, the INVR has been shown to be the most reliable (Wood, Chapman, & Eilers, 2011).

A number of other instruments are more global in nature and include examining all symptomatology present. These include the Visual Analog Scale (VAS), the Verbal Categorical Scale (VCS), the Adapted Symptom Distress Scale (SDS-2), and the Edmonton Symptom Assessment Scale (ESAS; Saxby et al., 2007). The use of reliable and valid instruments is necessary to develop evidence-based interventions to assist patients with these symptoms.

Management of Nausea and Vomiting

A thorough evaluation to determine both the etiology of the symptoms and the pathophysiological mechanism by which they are triggered allows directed interventions to begin. Therapy should include not only antiemetics, but also measures to alleviate the cause of the symptoms. Interventions should take into account the symptoms and the central emetogenic pathways involved (Mannix, 2005).

■ Pharmacological Interventions of Nausea and Vomiting.
Although progress has been made in identifying antiemetic agents that alleviate CINV, little work has been accomplished to establish drugs that alleviate the N&V experienced at the end of life specifically. Benze, Geyer, Alt-Epping, and Nauck (2012) reviewed 75 studies to analyze the current evidence for antiemetic treatment with 5-HT$_3$ receptor antagonists, steroids, antihistamines, anticholinergics, somatostatin analogs, benzodiazepines, and cannabinoids in palliative care patients with far advanced cancer not receiving chemotherapy or radiotherapy, AIDS, chronic obstructive pulmonary disease (COPD), progressive heart failure, amyotrophic lateral sclerosis (ALS), or multiple sclerosis (MS). And while the overall strength of evidence is low, and they acknowledge that well-designed studies in palliative care patients are needed to provide evidence-based therapy, there is evidence that several different treatments, often in combination, do offer some beneficial symptom relief (Benze et al., 2012).

Having an understanding of the potential causes of N&V in the palliative care patient is essential in directing the correct therapy toward symptom relief. Different antiemetics act on different parts of the N&V process; therefore, when antiemetics are not prescribed correctly, optimal results will not occur. These sites hold receptors for one or more neurotransmitters, including dopamine type 2 (D$_2$), serotonin types 2 to 4 (5HT$_{2-4}$), histamine type 1 (H$_1$), and acetylcholine (muscarinic receptors type 1 to 5, M1–5). Other receptors such as substance P, cannabinoid type 1 (CB1), and endogenous opioids may also be involved (Glare et al., 2011). Table 24.3 lists examples of medications, site of action, receptors, and comments that may be useful in determining the appropriate antiemetic choice.

Mannix (2005) recommends seven steps in choosing the appropriate antiemetic: (a) identify the cause of the N&V, (b) identify the pathway triggering the vomiting reflex, (c) identify the neurotransmitter receptor involved in the pathway, (d) choose the most potent antagonist to the receptor identified, (e) choose a route of administration that ensures optimal action, (f) titrate the dosage, and (g) if symptoms persist, review the cause (pp. 459–460).

Some antiemetics are not well tolerated in older adults, often as a result of impaired renal or hepatic clearance. Metoclopramide, for example, must be used with caution in older adults as decreased hepatic function increases drug toxicity and increases the incidence of extrapyramidal effects such as tardive dyskinesia (Gridelli, 2004). Although typically the dosage guidelines of the most common 5-HT$_3$ receptor antagonists do not differ, these drugs do vary in terms of receptor selectivity, duration of action, and metabolism (Gridelli, 2004). These differences may have potential clinical implications in older adults and should be considered. As an example, granisetron has a duration of action of 24 hours, while ondansetron's action is 9 hours. Additionally, three of these drugs, dolasetron, palonosetron, and tropisetron, have cardiovascular effects and should not be prescribed to patients of any age with a cardiovascular history (Gridelli, 2004). Regardless of the antiemetic agent, it is imperative to have an understanding of the drug and its properties to ensure a positive effect and prevent potential adverse outcomes.

Drugs from other classifications may be used in palliative care as well. These include corticosteroids, octreotide, cannabinoids, and benzodiazepines. Corticosteroids have intrinsic antiemetic properties and have been known to enhance the effects of other antiemetics (Mannix, 2005). They should be considered cautiously, however, given the potential negative effects of prolonged therapy, including adrenal suppression, increased risk for the development of infection, psychosis, and altered glucose control. There is also evidence that cannabinoids may reduce N&V in CINV. Studies assessing its use in individuals with advanced disease are lacking, and its use is indicated only in patients with symptoms refractory to conventional treatment. With other safe and effective antiemetics available, cannabinoids are not recommended

TABLE 24.3 Receptor-Specific Antiemetics for Use in Palliative Care

Drug	Site	Receptor	Comments
Haloperidol	CTZ	Dopamine antagonist	Use in opioid-induced nausea and chemical and mechanical nausea; use when anxiety symptoms aggravate N&V; may have additive effects with other CNS depressants.
Metoclopramide Cisapride	CTZ GIT	Metoclopramide is a dopamine antagonist at low doses; at doses greater than 120 mg/24 hr, it becomes a 5-HT$_3$ antagonist	Use in gastric stasis, ileus, and chemotherapy; use diphenhydramine to decrease extrapyramidal symptoms; cisapride has potentially fatal cardiac arrhythmias
Phenothiazines (prochlorperazine, chlorpromazine, levomepromazine, thiethylperazine)	CTZ GIT VC	Predominantly as dopamine antagonists	Use in intestinal obstruction, peritoneal irritation, vestibular causes, raised ICP, and nausea of unknown etiology; extrapyramidal effects; not recommended for routine use
Scopolamine	VC	Anticholinergic	Use in intestinal obstruction, increased ICP, and peritoneal irritation; useful if N&V exists with colic
5-HT$_3$ receptor antagonists (ondansetron, granisetron, tropisetron, palonosetron)	CTZ VC GIT	Serotonin antagonist	Use in chemotherapy, abdominal radiation, and postop N&V; safe for children and older adults; effectiveness increased by combining with dexamethasone
Antihistamines (cinnarizine, cyclizine, diphenhydramine, promethazine)	VC	H$_1$ receptor	Use in intestinal obstruction, increased ICP, vestibular causes, and peritoneal irritation; cyclizine is the least sedative

CNS, central nervous system; CTZ, chemoreceptor trigger zone; GIT, gastrointestinal tract; ICP, intracranial pressure; N&V, nausea and vomiting; VC, vomiting center.

Sources: Adapted from Dalal, S., Del Fabbro, E., & Bruera, E. (2006). Symptom control in palliative care—Part I: Oncology as a paradigmatic example. *Journal of Palliative Medicine, 9*(2), 391–408. doi:10.1089/jpm.2006.9.391; Gullatte, M. M., Kaplow, R., & Heidrich, D. E. (2005). Oncology. In K. K. Kuebler, M. P. Davis, & C. D. Moore (Eds.), *Palliative practices: An interdisciplinary approach* (pp. 197–245). St. Louis, MO: Mosby Elsevier; King C. (2001). Nausea and vomiting. In B.R. Ferrell & N. Coyle (Eds.), *Textbook of palliative nursing* (pp. 107–121). New York, NY: Oxford University Press.; Mannix, K. (2005). Palliation of nausea and vomiting. In D. Doyle, G. Hanks, N. Cherny, & K. Calman (Eds.), *Oxford textbook of palliative medicine* (3rd ed., pp. 459–468). New York, NY: Oxford University Press.

as first- or second-line therapy for CINV. Some guidelines recommend pharmaceutical cannabinoids as third-line treatment in the management of breakthrough nausea and vomiting. As there continued to be a lack of RCT data and safety concerns, herbal cannabis is not recommended for CINV and should not be considered in other palliative care settings as a primary treatment strategy (Tafelski, Häuser, & Schäfer, 2016). Benzodiazepines have been used in combination with other antiemetics in chemotherapy. Although they have little antiemetic potency on their own, in combination, they may also reduce anxiety and akathisia (Mannix, 2005). Benzodiazepines should be considered cautiously in elderly patients as there is increasing evidence that they put older patients at risk for cognitive decline and memory impairment, and increased falls and risk of fractures (Salzman & Shader, 2015). Given their limited potential impact on N&V, they should be considered prudently. While the research is ongoing, it seems that the treatment of N&V utilizing multiple therapies is more effective than any one agent alone (Slatkin, 2007).

The NCCN has published guidelines for the treatment of N&V in a palliative care patient. From a treatment perspective, it outlines an approach that titrates and adds therapy based on the patient's symptom response. The algorithm starts with titrating and maximizing oral dopamine receptor antagonists (e.g., prochlorperazine, haloperidol, metoclopramide), then adding 5-HT$_3$ blockers (e.g., ondasetron) as well as possibly anticholinergics (e.g., scopolamine), antihistamines (e.g., meclizine), and cannabinoids. If symptoms persist, the addition of corticosteroids (e.g., dexamethasone) may be beneficial. With continued symptoms, it is recommended that the previous therapy be tried by infusion or the subcutaneous injection route as needed and then to a scheduled approach. With severe protracted symptoms, adding an alternative therapy (e.g., acupressure, hypnosis, cognitive behavioral therapy) may be beneficial (NCCN, 2017).

Medications appropriate for use in the pediatric client include ondansetron, lorazepam, promethazine, dexamethasone, metoclopramide, diphenhydramine, octreotide, meclizine, olanzapine, scopolamine, and hydroxyzine (Hellsten &

Kane, 2006; Hinds, Oakes, Hicks, & Anghelescu, 2005; Santucci & Mack, 2007). As with the adult patient, identification of the possible cause as well as treatment of the source when possible is paramount to symptom control.

■ Nonpharmacological and Complementary Interventions for Nausea and Vomiting.

Often there are adjunct interventions to accompany medications. Establishing a research basis for those interventions is more difficult, although much has been written using anecdotal data. Research studies in the literature are based on patients with CINV and not specifically patients with N&V at the end of life.

Simple self-care strategies may be instituted to control N&V (Table 24.4), which may start with dietary and environmental changes. Avoidance of environmental stimuli, such as sights, sounds, or smells that may initiate nausea, is recommended (Glare et al., 2011). Encouraging the patient to use interventions that have relieved N&V at other times in his or her life, such as during pregnancy, illness, or times of stress, may be helpful. A particular food associated with a positive past experience can be suggested (Enck, 2002). Dietary changes such as drinking clear liquids and eating bland foods may be helpful as well. Minimizing or even eliminating liquids prior to a meal or during a meal may decrease nausea (Kemp, 1999). Patients with advanced disease often have decreased or altered taste (Fearon et al., 2011). When that occurs, they may prefer different foods than what they have previously enjoyed.

Patients and their families should be encouraged to keep a self-care log of symptoms, interventions, and

TABLE 24.4 Self-Care Activities for Nausea and Vomiting
■ Oral hygiene after each emesis
■ Cool, damp washcloth to the forehead, neck, and wrists
■ Eat bland, cool foods
■ Have fresh air with a fan or an open window
■ Limit environmental stimuli that precipitate nausea and vomiting
■ Lie flat for 2 hours after eating
■ Eat small meals
■ Practice relaxation techniques and/or guided imagery
■ Provide distraction

Sources: Adapted from Enck, R. C. (2002). *The medical care of terminally ill patients* (2nd ed.). Baltimore, MD: Johns Hopkins University Press; Glare, P., Miller, J., Nikolova, T., & Tickoo, R. (2011). Treating nausea and vomiting in palliative care: A review. *Clinical Interventions in Aging*, 6, 243–259. doi:10.2147/CIA.S13109; Kemp, C. (1999). *Terminal illness: A guide to nursing care* (2nd ed.). New York, NY: Lippincott; King C. (2001). Nausea and vomiting. In B. R. Ferrell & N. Coyle (Eds.), *Textbook of palliative nursing* (pp. 107–121). New York, NY: Oxford University Press.; Rhodes, V. A., & McDaniel, R. W. (2001). Nausea, vomiting, and retching: Complex problems in palliative care. *CA: A Cancer Journal for Clinicians*, 51(4), 232–248; quiz 249. doi:10.3322/canjclin.51.4.232

responses. The log reinforces interventions that work for the patient and may demonstrate "good days" when the N&V was tolerable. The log can also help the patient feel more in control of his or her life in addition to providing the caregiver with information on which to base interventions.

Music therapy has shown some benefits as an adjunct therapy. Ezzone, Baker, Rosselet, and Terepka (1998) demonstrated that music therapy was a statistically significant adjunct treatment during high-dose chemotherapy to reduce N&V. Relaxation techniques and guided imagery are also complementary therapies that can be used to decrease N&V and reduce anxiety. However, the research basis of these nonpharmacological interventions (Table 24.5) needs to be established to support evidence-based practice. While there is literature that supports the use of some nonpharmacological strategies in controlling N&V, this again is focused primarily on CINV. Tentative recommendations can be made for cognitive distraction, exercise, hypnosis, music therapy, relaxation, and systematic desensitization to CINV (Lotfi-Jam et al., 2008).

Acupuncture and ginger are two common complementary interventions used to manage N&V (Thompson & Zollman, 2005). Acupuncture is an ancient healing art using the insertion of fine gauge needles to palliate symptoms. The needles are inserted into carefully chosen acupuncture points and left in place for up to 20 minutes. Multiple studies have looked at the use of acupuncture/acupressure in patients with CINV and found that evidence supports the addition of electroacupuncture by clinicians competent in its administration (Naeim et al., 2008). It has been shown that the addition of acupuncture has a significantly positive effect on the control of CINV as opposed to antiemetic therapy alone in the pediatric population as well (Genc & Tan, 2015; Gottschling et al., 2008).

Various other alternative therapies have been studied to assess relief from N&V; however, again they tend to focus on CINV, with little evidence that is supportive of their use in other palliative care settings. Herbal interventions such as ginger, lemon, chamomile, and peppermint all have been suggested as adjuncts to traditional treatment. At best, they offer complementary benefit to the traditional and established therapy, as has been described (Tipton et al., 2007).

Family Concerns and Considerations Regarding Nausea and Vomiting

N&V are visible signs of an unhealthy state; as such, family caregivers can be distressed and anxious about their loved one. It is important that the nurse addresses the family's anxiety associated with N&V. Family education is vital to facilitate functioning as a care team member and helping the loved one experience an optimal quality of life.

TABLE 24.5   Nonpharmacological Interventions for Nausea and Vomiting

Behavioral Intervention	Description	Comments
Self-hypnosis	Evolution of physiological state of altered consciousness and total body relaxation. This technique involves a state of intensified attention and receptiveness to an idea	Use to control anticipatory N&V; limited studies, mostly in children and adolescents; easily learned; no side effects; decreases intensity and duration of nausea; decreased frequency, severity, amount, and duration of vomiting
Relaxation	Progressive contraction and relaxation of various muscle groups	Often used with imagery; can use for other stressful situations; easily learned; no side effects; decreases nausea during and after chemotherapy; decreases duration and severity of vomiting; not as effective with anticipatory nausea and vomiting
Biofeedback	Control of specific physiological responses by receiving information about changes in response to induced state of relaxation	Two types of electromyographic and skin temperature; used alone or with relaxation; easily learned; no side effects; decreased nausea during and after chemotherapy; more effective with progressive muscle relaxation
Imagery	Mentally take self away by focusing mind on images of a relaxing place	Most effective when combined with another technique; increases self-control; decreases duration of nausea; decreases perceptions of degree of vomiting; feel more in control, relaxed, and powerful
Distraction	Learn to divert attention from a threatening situation and to relaxing sensations	Can use videos, games, and puzzles; no side effects; decreases anticipatory N&V; decreases post-chemotherapy distress; inexpensive
Desensitization	Three-step process involving relaxation and visualization to decrease sensitization to aversive situations	Inexpensive; easily learned; no side effects; decreases anticipatory N&V

N&V, nausea and vomiting.

Source: Adapted from King, C. R. (1997). Nonpharmacologic management of chemotherapy-induced nausea and vomiting. *Oncology Nursing Forum, 24*(7 Suppl), 41–48.

Families should be taught to systematically assess the patient's N&V. Use of a simple log of what activity the patient is engaging in when the episode of N&V occurs provides evidence to the family and patient when the nausea increased or decreased, and how and when the vomiting occurred as well. The family and healthcare professional can then assess the situation by viewing the log and determine what pharmacological or nonpharmacological interventions may have offered the most relief.

CASE STUDY

1. What specific pathology for Mrs. Adams might be contributing to her symptoms of N&V?
2. Which six questions could you ask to discover suggestive causes of her symptoms of N&V?
3. What therapy (pharmacological and nonpharmacological) could you recommend to help control her symptoms?

■ DYSPHAGIA

Dysphagia suggests the presence of an organic abnormality in the passage of solids or liquids from the oral cavity to the stomach. Patients' complaints range from the inability to initiate a swallow to the sensation of solids or liquids being hindered during their passage through the esophagus into the stomach. Significant symptoms can affect nutrition, lead to aspiration, and reduce quality of life (Hirano & Kahrilas, 2015). Most of the data on the incidence of dysphagia come from clients with head and neck cancer. These clients may suffer from dysphagia in the early, middle, and terminal stages of the disease. One source indicates that 79% of those patients have significant eating problems (Barbour, 1999). In the late stages of MS, dysphagia is reported in 10% to 33% of clients (Dahlin & Goldsmith, 2006). In ALS, 25% of clients present with dysphagia as their initial complaint at diagnosis (Dahlin & Goldsmith, 2006). Sixty-three percent of patients with Parkinson's disease have objective evidence of difficulty with swallowing (Regnard, 2005).

Etiology of Dysphagia

Swallowing is a complex activity that requires intact anatomy, normal mucosa, normal functioning of six cranial nerves and the brainstem, and the coordination of the cortex, limbic system, basal ganglia, cerebellum, brainstem centers involved in respiration, salivation, and motor function of 34 skeletal muscles (Regnard, 2005). Dysphagia may occur as a result of a disruption in any of the four stages of swallowing: oral preparatory stage, oral stage, pharyngeal stage, and esophageal stage.

Both the oral preparatory and the oral stage of swallowing are voluntary actions. In the oral preparatory stage, food is taken into the mouth and saliva helps form a paste bolus. During the oral stage, the bolus is centered and moved to the posterior oropharynx. The pharyngeal phase is not voluntary, but reflexive, as the swallowing reflex carries the food bolus through the pharynx. Peristaltic waves carry the food bolus to the stomach during the esophageal stage (Hirano & Kahrilas, 2015).

Each of the stages of swallowing is affected by aging, and dysphagia is a common complaint of the older adult. The skeletal muscles involved with swallowing may undergo age-related changes of atrophy and weakness that occur in all skeletal muscles (Plahuta & Hamrick-King, 2006). Similarly, there are aging changes that occur in the nerves that innervate the oral region. Each of the stages of swallowing is a precisely timed contraction/relaxation sequence and can be affected by the aging process. The sequence may become desynchronized and the entire process of swallowing may become ineffective (Timiras, 1994).

Hirano and Kahrilas (2015) list the causes of dysphagia commonly seen and suggested in palliative care. They can be distinguished by oropharyngeal and esophageal dysphagia but with similar resultant symptoms, including neoplasm (includes brain tumors, head and neck cancer, and esophageal tumors); progressive neuromuscular diseases such as ALS, Parkinson's disease, and MS; connective tissue disorders like scleroderma; dementia; systemic dysphagia as a result of inflammatory and infectious factors; and general deconditioning that may include multisystem disease and failure, and the side effects of medications and/or polypharmacy (Hirano &

Kahrilas, 2015). Each cause of dysphagia may occur for a different reason. For example, in Parkinson's disease there is disruption in the oral stage of swallowing because of rigidity of the lingual musculature (Dahlin & Goldsmith, 2006). As a result of this rigidity, pharyngeal swallow responses are delayed and aspiration may occur before or during the swallow. Regnard (2005) suggests there is a defect in the nondopaminergic pathway from the medulla and a disturbance of the oral phase due to bradykinesia (p. 468). In head and neck cancers, dysphagia may occur because of the pressure and size of the tumor, or as a result of chemotherapy, radiation, or the surgery itself.

Common side effects of radiation, mucositis and xerostomia, may further exacerbate dysphagia as well as pain on swallowing, dry mouth, anorexia, or anxiety (Baines, 1992; Rudd & Worlding, 2005). Dysphagia may not be a part of the terminal illness itself but may be a result or symptom of other comorbidities. For example, an older adult who is terminally ill with cancer and also has advanced Parkinson's disease or has suffered a previous cerebrovascular accident has issues with dysphagia likely caused by a combination of these diagnoses.

Signs and Symptoms

An initial indication of dysphagia is choking or coughing when eating or drinking. A patient may complain of having the feeling that something is caught in his or her throat. Swallowing can be accompanied by coughing, choking, nasopharyngeal regurgitation, aspiration, and a sensation of residual food remaining in the pharynx. Esophageal dysphagia is distinguished by trouble swallowing several seconds after initiating a swallow and the sensation of food getting stuck in the esophagus. These signs of dysphagia are often accompanied by fear and anxiety on the part of the patient, fear that food may actually be trapped in his or her lungs, and the anxiety that he or she will be unable to breathe because of food "going down the wrong pipe." Some patients exhibit no signs of choking, although food or liquids may be entering the trachea and lung; these patients are known as "silent aspirators." Noting the quality of the patient's voice and whether or not any expressive aphasia or dysphasia is present may provide clues to the nurse that the patient may be aspirating (Easton, 1999).

Depending on the stage of swallowing that is affected, the signs of dysphagia may differ. Table 24.6 outlines characteristics of dysphagia associated with the oral, pharyngeal, and esophageal stages. Each characteristic may have varying degrees of seriousness.

Assessment of Dysphagia

In the terminal stages of illness, it is likely that dysphagia is not a new symptom, but one that has been present for some time and is worsening. In assessment during

TABLE 24.6   Signs and Symptoms of Dysphagia

Oral phase	Drooling
	Pocketing of food
	Excessive chewing
	Facial asymmetry or weakness
	Tongue weakness
	Inability to close lips tightly or move lips
	Weakness or absence of gag reflex
	Weakness or absence of a swallowing reflex
	Nasal drainage due to nasal regurgitation
	Loss of internal or external sensation of the oral cavity or face
Pharyngeal phase	Delayed or absence of swallowing
	Coughing while drinking or eating fluids
	History of aspiration pneumonia
	Wet, gurgling, moist, or nasal voice
	Frequent clearing of throat
	Complaints of burning
Esophageal phase	Burping or substernal distress due to esophageal reflux
	Coughing or wheezing

Source: Adapted from Hickey, J. (1997). Rehabilitation of neuroscience patients. In J. Hickey (Ed.), *The clinical practice of neurological and neurosurgical nursing* (4th ed., p. 255). Philadelphia, PA: Lippincott.

palliative care, the goals of the swallowing evaluation should be clear. Dahlin and Goldsmith (2006, p. 202) list the following goals of assessment:

1. Identify the underlying physiological nature of the disorder
2. Determine whether any short-range interventions can alleviate the dysphagia
3. Collaborate with the patient, family, and caregivers on the safest and most efficacious method of providing nutrition and hydration

Difficulty with specific food consistencies provides the nurse with some assessment data, but may be misleading. Lesions and/or tumors that produce an obstruction generally produce dysphagia for solids first as opposed to liquids. However, clients with neuromuscular disorders may have dysphagia with both solids and liquids (Regnard, 2005).

Castell (1996) suggests that 80% of dysphagia can be diagnosed with a thorough history. Key questions include the following: What type of food causes the symptom? Is the swallowing problem intermittent or progressive? Is heartburn present (Cowely, Diebold, Gross, & Hardin-Fanning, 2006)?

The physical examination involves cognitive, neuromuscular, and respiratory assessment. Cognitive assessment includes interest in eating, ability to focus on and complete a meal, and ability to remember and follow directions for safe eating. Neuromuscular and respiratory assessment includes testing sensory and motor components of the cranial nerves, breath sounds, the strength of cough, and the ability to clear the throat (Cowely et al., 2006). The gag reflex is not a reliable indicator of the patient's ability to swallow (Regnard, 2005). Careful inspection of the mouth and pharynx should evaluate for lesions or evidence of disease that may interfere with swallowing. Missing teeth should also be specifically addressed as it can interfere with chewing and worsen an existing cause of dysphagia. While likely late in a clinical picture, skin changes may suggest a diagnosis of scleroderma and could contribute to dysphagia that is esophageal in origin (Hirano & Kahrilas, 2015). Evaluation of the patient's current medications is an important component of the assessment. Contributing medications to dysphagia are those that decrease saliva, reduce cognition, and decrease the strength of the muscles used in swallowing. Treatment could also potentially be contributing to symptoms of dysphagia. Chemotherapy and radiation commonly lead to mucositis and may be important to consider.

The prognosis of the patient will determine whether a professional swallowing evaluation merits consideration. If the patient's life expectancy is reasonably long and the patient is clearly in distress, a comprehensive evaluation performed by a speech–language pathologist with expertise in swallowing disorders may be indicated. A modified barium swallow is used to radiologically determine the phase of swallowing where the disturbance is occurring and thus to identify potential interventions, as well as evaluating the compensatory mechanisms of the patient (Dahlin & Goldsmith, 2006).

Management of Dysphagia

If the patient has a very short prognosis (days), it may be determined by the patient, family, and caregivers that hydration and/or feeding are not warranted. If the patient has a longer prognosis, medically assisted feeding and hydration may be attempted. Regnard (2005) offers the following factors to help determine the appropriateness of interventions:

1. Anticipated decline of the patient
2. Patient's opinion
3. Opinions of significant others and/or family
4. Opinions of formal caregivers
5. Feasibility/advantages/disadvantages of alternative feeding routes

Transnasal intubation, percutaneous endoscopic gastronomy or jejunostomy, esophagogastroduodenoscopy (EGD), or surgical gastrostomy or jejunostomy may be considered if the prognosis of the patient determines that these interventions will provide optimal palliation. Any surgical intervention must be undertaken with input from the patient and family, and is determined by the overall goals of care.

■ Pharmacological Interventions of Dysphagia.
If dry mouth and/or oral lesions are present and are exacerbating the dysphagia, pharmacological treatment is appropriate. The most common mucosal infection causing oral lesions is candidiasis. Antifungal medications such as nystatin, ketoconazole, miconazole, and fluconazole may be used in treatment (Dahlin & Goldsmith, 2006; Regnard, 2005).

Dry mouth (xerostomia) could occur as a result of prescribed medications, particularly anticholinergics and opiates. These medications may need to be continued if there are limited alternatives to treat other symptoms, making the dry mouth unavoidable. In that case, artificial saliva, such as Salagen or porcine mucin, may be used. Glycerin and lemon should be avoided because glycerin dehydrates the mucosa and lemon affects the salivary glands (Regnard, 2005). A prokinetic agent such as metochlopramide may be prescribed for poor esophageal motility. Proton pump inhibitors (e.g., omeprazole) and H$_2$ blockers (e.g., ranitidine) may be used in patients with gastroesophageal reflux disease to reduce gastric acid secretion and reduce symptoms.

■ Nonpharmacological Interventions of Dysphagia.
After a thorough evaluation of the patient, and once it has been determined that oral intake is appropriate, the guiding principle of management should be optimization of caloric intake while minimizing the effort to obtain it (Dahlin & Goldsmith, 2006). If the degree of dysphagia is minimal, simple positioning may be the primary intervention. Patients should be positioned in an upright, nearly 90° angle, with the head tilted slightly forward and the chin tucked in to prevent food moving to the posterior oropharynx before it is properly chewed. If the patient is unable to hold his or her head

independently, the caregiver can assist the patient in maintaining this position. If the older adult has had a past stroke, pocketing of food on the affected side of the mouth is a common problem. The patient, family, or caregiver can sweep the mouth with a finger after each bite to alleviate this problem.

The American Dietetic Association has published a monograph entitled the National Dysphagia Diet: Standardization for Optimal Care (NDD). This diet aimed to establish standard terminology and practice applications of dietary texture modification in dysphagia management (McCullough, Pelletier, & Steele, 2003). A group consisting of speech–language pathologists (SLPs), dietitians, and food scientists developed a hierarchy of diet levels. Provided here is an example of the different stages of semisolid/solid foods:

- Level I: Dysphagia-pureed (homogeneous, very cohesive, pudding like, requiring very little chewing ability)
- Level II: Dysphagia-mechanical altered (cohesive, moist, semisolid foods, requiring some chewing)
- Level III: Dysphagia-advanced (soft foods that require more chewing ability)
- Level IV: Regular (all foods allowed)

Liquid consistencies included spoon thick, honey like, nectar like, and thin (McCullough et al., 2003).

Simple dietary changes such as providing pureed or blended food may be appropriate. Patients with oropharyngeal dysphagia may require thickened liquids. There are a number of commercial products that are used in rehabilitation facilities (e.g., Thick-it) to address these issues; however, a simple food starch can be used as effectively.

Family Concerns and Considerations Regarding Dysphagia

Positioning techniques that allow the patient to continue oral feeding can be easily explained and taught to the patient and/or his or her family. Dietary changes, such as using thickening agents, if appropriate, should be suggested to the family as well. Any interventions that can be taught to the family or caretakers may increase their feeling of wanting to help the individual.

As described previously, eating is considered a social activity as much as it is a necessity of life. Society has conditioned us to believe that eating wholesome, healthy food will keep us well. As a family member sits by the bedside of his or her loved one and sees that oral intake is impossible due to dysphagia and potential aspiration, feelings of helplessness and anxiety may also occur. Family may feel like they are neglecting their obligation to the person. For both the patient and the family, the act of eating is viewed as compatible with life; the inability to eat is a harbinger of death. Such factors influence decisions regarding feeding at the end of life.

Even if the decision to discontinue oral feeding and initiate alternate feeding methods is made, the decision is not easy. It is clearly difficult to make the initial decision to feed a patient or loved one "artificially," and more difficult if a decision is made to discontinue feedings. The patient and family must be fully aware of the risks and benefits of artificial nutrition and hydration. It is important to inform the patient and family of the natural history of disease and anticipate trajectory as well as the benefits and risks of any intervention. In some cases, more aggressive interventions such as feeding tubes and endoscopies may have a higher risk than the perceived benefit. During this period of time, the support of the nurse to the patient and family is paramount.

CASE STUDY

1. Are there any issues that you think might put Mrs. Adams at risk for dysphagia?
2. Are there physical exam findings that might raise your suspicion for dysphagia or other related issues?

▪ CONSTIPATION

Constipation is often seen in advanced disease related to bowel obstruction, adverse effects from medications, hypercalcemia, dehydration, and inadequate dietary intake (Esper & Heidrich, 2005). Similar to the concept of pain, constipation is a subjective complaint and often undertreated (Economou, 2006). It is a common complaint in all populations and typically refers to persistent, difficult, infrequent, or the sensation of incomplete passage of stool. While there is a wide variation in the "normal" frequency for the passage of stool, anywhere from three times daily to three times weekly, assigning a precise definition can be difficult (Hirano & Kahrilas, 2015). Fundamentally, it is defined by the patient and their perceived alteration in their typical bowel patterns. Constipation is a common cause of morbidity in the palliative care setting and the numbers increase if the patient is treated with opioids. The incidence of constipation in older adults or ill persons may be 20% to 50% (Economou, 2006).

Various tools are available for the assessment of constipation in a palliative care patient, each of which has been designed to evaluate the presence and severity of constipation. Larkin et al. (2008) note that while using them to allow the patient to understand his or her own bowel habits, or when communication between the patient and the clinician may be difficult, their utility in clinical practice is marginal. Four of the most frequently used scales are the Bristol Stool Form Scale, the Constipation Assessment Scale (CAS), the Constipation Visual Analogue Scale, and the Eton Scale Risk Assessment for Constipation (Larkin et al., 2008).

Children are often symptomatic, and their symptoms increase with time, particularly within the terminal phase of illness (Collins, 2005). Constipation in children is distressing, although often more disturbing for the caregiver than the child. Laxative use is generally not recommended in children, and there is inadequate evidence to endorse the use of laxatives to treat constipation in the pediatric population (Pijpers, Tabbers, Benninga, & Berger, 2009). The research recommends a change in dietary intake, fluid intake, and increased mobility as opposed to laxative use (Collins, 2005). If these changes do not help in relieving the constipation, laxatives may be used, but the dosing is difficult to manage due to few resources for pediatric dosing; therefore, they must be approached cautiously.

Etiology of Constipation

Bowel function includes three areas of control: small intestinal motility, colon motility, and defecation (Economou, 2006, p. 220). If any of these processes malfunction or is delayed, it can affect defecation. The small intestine moves contents through in 1 to 2 hours, whereas the colon moves content much slower, in 2 to 3 days. Not eating properly; going without food, fluids, or fiber; a decrease in activity; or even less privacy when using the bathroom can all affect defecation and result in constipation. Other factors that may affect bowel elimination are opioid pain medications; specific cancers, especially those causing luminal obstruction; ascites; confusion; and diuretics (Economou, 2006). Dehydration is a common cause of constipation in the pediatric palliative care population (Dean et al., 2006). Table 24.7 outlines some of the common causes of constipation.

Pharmacological-induced constipation may occur due to the use of opioids to control pain. Opioids affect the small bowel and the colon by binding with the receptors of the smooth muscle, thus affecting contractions and peristalsis of the bowel. Lengthening the time that

TABLE 24.7	Causal and Contributing Factors to Constipation in Palliative Care Patients
Organic Factors	
Pharmacological agents	Antacids, anti-epileptics, anti-emetics (5-HT$_3$ antagonists), antihypertensives, antiparkinsonians, anticholinergics, antidepressants, antitussives, antidiarrheals (when used in excess), cancer chemotherapies (vinca alkaloids), diuretics (when causing dehydration), iron (orally administered), opioid analgesics, neuroleptics
Metabolic disturbances	Dehydration (fever, vomiting, polyuria, poor fluid intake, diuretics), hypercalcemia, hypokalemia, uremia, hypothyroidism, diabetes
Neurological disorders	Cerebral tumours, spinal cord involvement, sacral nerve infiltration, autonomic failure (primary such as Parkinson's disease, multiple sclerosis, motor neuron disease; or secondary to cancer or diabetes)
Structural abnormalities	Pelvic tumor mass, radiation fibrosis, painful anorectal conditions (hemorrhoids, anal fissure, perianal abscess), uncontrolled cancer-related pain or other pain such as movement-related pain or breakthrough pain
Functional Factors	
Diet	Poor appetite and low amounts of food intake, low-fiber diet, poor fluid intake
Environmental	Lack of privacy, comfort or assistance with toileting
Other factors	Advanced age, inactivity, decreased mobility, confined to bed, depression, sedation

Source: Larkin, P. J., Sykes, N. P., Centeno, C., Ellershaw, J. E., Elsner, F., Eugene, B., . . . Zuurmond, W. W. (2008). The management of constipation in palliative care: clinical practice recommendations. *Palliat Med, 22*(7), 796–807. doi:10.1177/0269216308096908.

the contents are in the colon allows more absorption of fluids and electrolytes, which in turn dries out and hardens the stool.

Cimprich (cited in Economou, 2006, p. 220) describes three types of constipation:

1. Primary—generally caused by reduction of fluids and fiber intake, decrease in activity, and lack of privacy.
2. Secondary—related to the pathological changes the patient experiences.
3. Iatrogenically induced—constipation related to pharmacological interventions.

Assessment of Constipation

The patient receiving palliative care has multiple risk factors for constipation and the assessment should begin with a history of the patient's typical GI and bowel habits. Questions to ask include the following: Is the patient able to chew food? Does the patient wear dentures and do they fit properly? What has the patient's bowel pattern been prior to diagnosis? Was there a history of constipation prior to diagnosis? Has the patient been experiencing abdominal cramping, bloating, and N&V? Does the bowel movement feel complete? Does the patient have an urge to defecate or is there straining? Is the patient requiring the use of laxatives and/or enemas? Do they note any rectal bleeding? What pain medication does the patient take? Has there been a change in fluid intake or appetite? Assessment of the cause and severity of constipation and attempting to remove any nonessential constipating med can be important. It is also important

to understand that patients who are constipated can present with a primary complaint of diarrhea. Overflow diarrhea around more formed and impacted stool can lead to symptoms of diarrhea, a syndrome that can be confusing to patients (NCCM, 2017).

The Mansoura Numeroalphabetic Constipation Score (MNCS), Farid Score is a numeric scoring system that has been developed to help define and assess constipation in an attempt to provide a precise definition that can direct proper management. It is a structured score consisting of nine items that is designed to be completed quickly with each question answered by yes or no. Four items were considered as major criteria, with 2 points for each, and five items were considered minor criteria, with 1 point for each. The maximum possible Mansoura score is 13 points, which is then classified into five stages from 0 to D according to the total score. Constipation was defined when the total score is greater than 2. The higher the score, the more severe the constipation. Table 24.8 outlines the major and minor criteria for use with the MNCS (Emile et al., 2015).

Physical examination may reveal normal findings such as abdominal distention, diminished or hypoactive bowel sounds, and palpation of stool in the large intestine. Distention, however, may be associated with obesity, fluid, tumor, or gas. Percussion of the bowel may result in tympani over the abdomen, thus indicating gas in the bowel. Dullness is related to a solid mass, which could be intestinal fluid, tumor, or feces (Economou, 2006). Deep palpation may result in feeling a "sausage like" mass; however, determining if the mass is stool or a tumor is difficult with palpation alone. Sykes (2005) suggests that a fecal mass usually indents

TABLE 24.8 Mansoura Numeroalphabetic Constipation Score, Farid Score	
Item	**Score**
Minor criteria	
1. Dull rectal pain	1 point
2. Need for enemas at least once a week	1 point
3. Need for anal digitation at least once a week	1 point
4. Major straining in less than 25% of bowel action	1 point
5. Sensation of incomplete evacuation	1 point
Major criteria	
1. Major straining in more than 25% of bowel action and/or the time of defecation	2 points
2. Less than three bowel actions per week	2 points
3. Sensation of anal obstruction upon defecation in over 25% of bowel action	2 points
4. Habitual defecation difficulties even with soft or liquid stool	2 points

Source: Adapted from Emile, S., Youssef, M., Thabet, W., Omar, W., Abd El-Hamed, T. M., Elshobaky, A., & Farid, M. (2015). Mansoura numeroalphabetic constipation score in Obstructed Defecation Syndrome (ODS): Validation of a new score. *International Journal of Advanced Research, 3*(10), 264–275.

if the patient can tolerate firm pressure and may give a crepitus-like sensation because of entrapped gas. A fecal mass may also move over time. A digital rectal exam may reveal impaction, impaired sphincter tone, anal fissures, hemorrhoids, tumors, or even a rectocele (Economou, 2006).

▪ **Diagnostic Tests.** Diagnostic tests are used to confirm or determine the extent of bowel dysfunction due to constipation. The need for an extensive workup in palliative care is rare and should be done only when necessary to continue with comfort measures. In the palliative care, patient clinical assessment should consider diseases to which constipation is secondary such as colon cancer, external compression from malignant lesions, postsurgical abnormalities, metabolic conditions such as electrolyte dysfunction, myopathies like scleroderma, and neuropathies such as Parkinson's disease (Bharucha, Pemberton, & Locke, 2013). If indicated, testing may include an upright and flat plate of the abdomen to determine air/fluid levels indicative of a partial or complete intestinal obstruction possibly due to tumor involvement or secondary to fecal impaction. Radiographic examination, MRI, or CT may also be appropriate to assess the abdomen. Laboratory data used to evaluate constipation may include BUN, as an elevation may signify dehydration, and blood glucose levels, as an elevation may indicate a diversion of fluids from the GI tract to the kidneys with excess renal fluid loss (Bisanz, 1997). It is important to note, however, that these laboratory tests are more to assess for issues that may result from constipation as opposed to evaluating for constipation itself.

Management of Constipation

Prevention of constipation is an essential strategy in providing palliative care. A mix of dietary alterations in addition to pharmacological agents may be required. Bulk-forming and stool-softening agents assist with normal peristaltic function (Beckwith, 2000). All patients beginning opioid therapy should be started on a laxative (Beckwith, 2000). Generally, a combination of a stool softener and laxative offers the most relief from constipation.

Each patient reacts differently to constipation and to the treatments used; thus, individual assessments and interventions must be developed. Interventions that work for one patient may not work for the other and, in fact, may change in their efficacy for the individual patient. Increasing fluids as little as 100 mL is an initial intervention. Care needs to be taken in increasing the fiber content. Fiber without increasing fluids absorbs what little fluid the patient may have available and contributes to more constipation (Economou, 2006). Because of the significant increase in fluid intake needed to balance the required ingestion of fiber to prevent constipation in patients that generally are already suffering from limited oral nutrition, it is felt that for reasons of both efficacy and safety, relying on dietary fiber intake alone for the relief of constipation is not suitable in palliative care patients (Larkin et al., 2008). Exercise, if appropriate, can help establish a regular bowel pattern and can help with the overall well-being of the patient.

The goals of treatment of constipation in the palliative care setting should be to reestablish comfortable bowel habits to the satisfaction of the patient, relieve the pain and discomfort caused by constipation and improve the patient's sense of well-being, restore a satisfactory level of independence in relation to bowel habits, consider individual patient preference, and prevent related GI symptoms such as nausea, vomiting, abdominal distention, and pain (Larkin et al., 2008).

■ **Pharmacological Management.** Even with appropriate preventive strategies, most patients with advanced disease will require laxatives (Sykes, 2005). Laxatives are classified by their action:

Bulk laxatives—provide bulk in the intestine, increase mass, and stimulate the bowel (used in mild constipation).
Lubricant laxative—lubricate the stool surface and soften the stool, leading to easier bowel movements.
Surfactant and/or detergent laxative—increase the absorption of water and fats that leads to a softer stool.
Osmotic laxative—used more often in chronic constipation and in patients who have elevated ammonia levels, such as patients with hepatic failure. This form of laxative has an osmotic effect not only on the small bowel but also on the large intestine by increasing the colon volume in a short period of time.

Saline laxative—increase gastric, pancreatic, and small intestine motility along with increasing the bowel secretions to form a stool.
Stimulant laxative—works on the colon, increasing motility and inducing peristalsis (Economou, 2006, pp. 224–225).

Table 24.9 provides a list of stool softeners and laxatives that may be used in palliative care.

NCCM recommends efforts begin with the prevention of constipation with prophylactic medications such as stimulant laxatives and stool softeners. The overall goal should be to have one nonforced bowel movement every 1 to 2 days. Evaluation for fecal impaction can be necessary when patients have subjective complaints of constipation. Ruling out a bowel obstruction is always important and should be considered as a potential diagnosis in this population, especially those on chronic narcotic therapy. If the patient shows evidence of impaction trialing a glycerine suppository and/or mineral oil retention enema may be warranted. The need for manual disimpaction should also be discussed if there is no relief with therapy. Other considerations include tap water or soap suds enemas (NCCN, 2017).

Other approaches to the management of constipation may include injectable methylnaltrexone, which is part

TABLE 24.9 Stool Softeners and Laxatives

Type	Action	Comments
Lubricant softeners: Mineral oil	Penetrates stool and prevents water absorption	Less palatable than some others
Bulk-forming laxatives: Methylcellulose Psyllium Polycarbophil	Resists bacterial breakdown, increasing bulk and shortening transit time	Must maintain fluid intake of 1.5–2 L a day
Emollient/surfactant softeners: Docusate sodium	Increases water penetration	Increased transit time caused by opioids negates action of these laxatives
Osmotic laxatives: Lactulose Sorbitol Glycerin	Creates osmotic gradient in the intestine	High oral doses to be effective may cause bloating, cramping, and diarrhea
Saline laxatives: Magnesium citrate Magnesium hydroxide Sodium bisphosphate/sodium phosphate	Creates immediate osmotic gradient in the intestine	Oral forms are effective in 0.5–3 hours; enemas often effective within 15 minutes
Stimulant laxative: Senna Cascara sagrada Bisacodyl	Stimulates submucosal nerve plexus to increase motility	May cause cramping; often used in combination with a softener

Source: Adapted from Gullatte, M. M., Kaplow, R., & Heidrich, D. E. (2005). Oncology. In K. K. Kuebler, M. P. Davis, & C. D. Moore (Eds.), *Palliative practices: An interdisciplinary approach* (pp. 197–245). St. Louis, MO: Mosby Elsevier.

of the naltrexone molecule. The medication is intended for the treatment of opioid-induced constipation as the medication antagonizes opioid actions at GI mu-opioid receptors but without impairing analgesia mediated by opioids in the central nervous system (CNS). Its use has been studied in both adult and pediatric palliative care settings, and the evidence is promising for the relief of opioid-induced constipation (Bader, Weber, & Becker, 2012; Ford, Brenner, & Schoenfeld, 2013; Yeomanson, Chohan, & Mayer, 2013).

Researchers are investigating the use of erythromycin in patients who do not respond to traditional treatments to relieve constipation. Erythromycin may cause diarrhea in patients who use it as an antibiotic. Management of constipation with rhubarb or constituents of mulberry, which are similar to Senna, can be used by patients who prefer not to use over-the-counter laxatives. These patients need to be cautioned in purchasing herbal remedies and be aware of the side effects or the interaction with other medications they may be taking (Economou, 2006). Medications used in both the prevention and the treatment in the pediatric palliative care population include docusate, lactulose, polyethylene glycol, and Senna (Santucci & Mack, 2007).

It is a fine balance in managing a patient with constipation (Gullatte et al., 2005). The care provider does not want to have the stool so soft that it is leaking continuously. On the other hand, the patient should not suffer from cramping. The need to balance the effect of the stimulant and softener to facilitate bowel movement is contrasted with overachieving their effects and leading to an alteration in the patient's "normal" bowel habits and limit secondary side effects.

Family Concerns and Considerations Related to Constipation

Family concerns regarding constipation can be addressed through education about potential causes and methods of prevention and limiting complications. Special attention should be given to the patient or family preferences with treatment modalities. Comfort level with routes of medication administration should be assessed; in particular, if rectal administration is not something the family is capable of or comfortable with, caregiver assistance should be provided.

Another concern includes dealing with patient privacy and the use of bedpan versus bedside commode. Privacy is a consideration with patients in the hospital and in their homes. Often if sharing a room in the hospital, using a bedside commode can be embarrassing to the patient and his or her family. The smell and noises during defecation may make the patient unable to go. In the home or in the hospital, trying to use the bathroom in front of another person can lead to apprehension, which may add stress and anxiety to the patient. Typically, bedside commodes are better tolerated than bedpans in facilitating a bowel movement when constipation is a concern.

CASE STUDY

1. Describe how Mrs. Adams has a complaint of diarrhea but may be suffering from constipation.
2. What further steps might you take to evaluate her for constipation?
3. If she does have evidence of constipation, suggest pharmacological and nonpharmacological measures you might suggest to help alleviate her symptoms.

■ BOWEL OBSTRUCTION

Bowel obstructions are common in patients with advanced abdominal, pelvic, ovarian, or primary bowel cancer (Chilton & Faull, 2005). An intestinal obstruction is complete or partial occlusion of the lumen or absence of normal propulsion that produces elimination from the GI tract (Economou, 2006; Sykes, 2005). Intestinal obstruction can occur either mechanically from blockage or from intestinal dysmotility when there is no blockage but the passage of normal bowel contents is slowed. Mechanical bowel obstruction may be caused by extrinsic processes such as adhesions and neoplasms; intrinsic abnormalities of the bowel wall like congenital, inflammatory, neoplastic, or traumatic; or intraluminal abnormalities. Functional obstruction, also known as ileus and pseudo-obstruction, can occur when dysmotility prevents intestinal contents from being propelled through the lumen and there is no existing mechanical blockage (Jacobs, 2014).

Etiology of Bowel Obstruction

Bowel obstructions can present in the clinical setting acutely or gradually and intermittently. Bowel obstructions can be due to constipation, adhesions, drugs, benign conditions, and/or progression of tumors in or around the intestine. Electrolyte abnormalities such as hypokalemia and hypercalcemia can lead to ileus or pseudo-obstruction formation as well (Chilton & Faull, 2005).

Signs and Symptoms

The symptoms of acute intestinal obstruction vary by the nature of the underlying disease process, its location in the intestinal lumen, and resultant changes in blood flow. Abdominal distention occurs because of intestinal gas, ingested fluids, and digestive secretions. When the luminal pressure exceeds venous pressure, venous and lymphatic drainage is impeded. Edema can follow, and the bowel wall proximal to the site of blockage may become hypoxemic. Epithelial necrosis can be identified within 12 hours of obstruction (Jacobs, 2014). If the obstruction is in the duodenum, the patient may experience severe vomiting with a large amount of undigested food. Pain or distention is typically not present, and the patient may have a succession splash present in the bowel sounds. If the obstruction is in the small intestine, there may be moderate to severe vomiting. Bowel sounds may be hyperactive with borborygmi, moderate distention is present, and there is pain in the upper and central abdomen that is colicky in nature.

With an obstruction in the large intestine, vomiting is generally a later side effect, borborygmi bowel sounds and severe distention are present, and the colicky pain is in the central to lower abdomen (Economou, 2006). It is important to note that in the older adult, obstruction may present differently. Instead of a "board-like" abdomen, many older adults may have cramps, dehydration, stringy stool or diarrhea, and vague complaints of not feeling well (Amella, 2004). Diagnosis is suspected by clinical symptoms but is confirmed with abdominal radiography. Abdominal CT scan may be useful in evaluating the patient as well (Ripamonti & Mercadante, 2005).

Management of Bowel Obstruction

Bethany Lynch and Juha Sarazine (2006) determined that nurses could improve symptom management and quality of life for patients who are experiencing malignant bowel obstruction by frequent assessments and being aware that patients with intra-abdominal tumors are at the highest risk for bowel obstruction. Physical assessments may reveal dehydration, dry mucosa, tachycardia, and hypotension, all signs of possible bowel obstruction. An examination of the abdomen may reveal distention, pain, and varied bowel sounds. Bowel obstruction from a malignant source is a pivotal point in the patient's illness, and nurses should have an active role in helping the patient through the decisions that need to be made about aggressive treatment or a more palliative approach to the bowel obstruction.

In managing a bowel obstruction, it should be determined if the obstruction is related to an underlying condition, such as a previous history of bowel obstruction, a tumor, or an opioid-induced obstruction or opioid syndrome, which can occur when there is treatment with narcotics. Medical management may offer suitable symptom control. Patients may live for surprisingly long periods of time, taking in small quantities of food and fluid, without the addition of nasogastric tubes or IV fluids (Chilton & Faull, 2005, p. 174).

Octreotide may be an option in early management to prevent an obstruction. Its action slows the irregular and ineffective peristaltic movements of obstruction through reducing activity and balancing out the intestinal movement (Economou, 2006). The use of continuous analgesics, antisecretory drugs, and/or antiemetics may be effective in controlling pain and N&V in patients who are not surgical candidates. Antiemetics that increase GI motility such as metoclopramide may potentially be harmful in complete obstructions although they may be beneficial in the treatment of incomplete obstructions. Corticosteroids may also be useful due to their anti-inflammatory effects on the tumor and bowel wall, indirect pain improvement related to reduced distension, and antiemetic effects (Laval et al., 2014).

Surgical intervention is the primary treatment for a complete bowel obstruction; however, in the palliative care population this is not always an option, and discussion with the patient and family regarding risks, potential benefits, and prognosis of any procedure is necessary. Risk factors for poorer interventional outcomes include ascites, palpable intra-abdominal masses, multiple bowel obstructions, previous abdominal radiation, advanced disease, and overall poor clinical status (NCCN, 2017). Endoscopic interventions such as percutaneous drainage tubes and stent placement may be used. Self-expanding metallic stents can be placed at the gastric outlet, proximal small bowel, and colon instead of surgery and could be an option in high-risk patients with poor postoperative survival (Frago et al., 2014; Ripamonti & Mercadante, 2005). Distinguishing the difference between small versus large bowel obstruction can be helpful as the proposed treatment as interventions can be different.

B. Lynch and Sarazine (2006) note that once a bowel obstruction has occurred, the mean survival of the patient decreases to approximately 3 months in patients who are terminally ill. This sobering fact makes the prevention of constipation and bowel obstruction imperative both for the healthcare team and for patients and their families.

CASE STUDY

1. Describe what aspects of Mrs. Adams's clinical picture has put her at risk for a bowel obstruction.
2. What further steps might you take to evaluate her for an obstruction?
3. If she does have evidence of an obstruction, propose pharmacological and nonpharmacological measures you might suggest to help alleviate her symptoms.

▪ DIARRHEA

Patients dealing with chronic and terminal illness may encounter bouts of diarrhea depending on the treatments they are receiving. Leakage of stool is common in bowel obstructions, and constipation can be over-treated, causing the patient to experience diarrhea. It is also important to consider that diarrhea may also be associated with lactose intolerance, chemotherapy, bowel obstruction, fecal impaction, sphincter incompetence, chronic radiation enteritis, and infection (Abrahm, 1998).

Diarrhea is defined as the passage of frequent stools, typically unformed and at an increased urgency. For adults, stool weight greater than 200 g/d can generally be considered diarrheal (Longo, Fauci, Kasper, Hauser, & Jameson, 2012). Objectively, it is considered more than three unformed stools within a 24-hour period (Sykes, 2005). Although diarrhea occurs less frequently than constipation in the palliative care setting, patients report having acute episodes of diarrhea related to treatments, overeating of fruits and vegetables, and the use of antibiotics. Generally, in episodes lasting a few days, the nurse needs to be aware of complications that can occur, along with the family being aware of potential complications that could result with diarrhea that is left untreated.

Etiology of Diarrhea

There are four mechanisms of diarrhea: secretory, osmotic, hypermotile, and exudative (Economou, 2006). Secretory diarrhea persists with fasting and may be difficult to control because it occurs because of hypersecretion tumors as well as endogenous mediators that affect electrolyte and water transport (Ratnaike, 1999). Enteral feedings, bleeding in the bowel, and lactose intolerance are all related to osmotic diarrhea. Increased intestinal motility in hypermotile diarrhea may result from overgrowth of bacteria; incomplete digestion of fat in the small intestine, causing it to be expelled in stool (steatorrhea); or due to chemotherapeutic agents. Prostaglandins are released secondary to inflammation of the intestinal mucosa in exudative diarrhea, commonly associated with radiation therapy (Economou, 2006).

Assessment of Diarrhea

As with other complications, the initial assessment includes identification of the underlying cause of diarrhea. Specific description of previous bowel habits, along with current symptoms, may help to identify the etiology and appropriate management approaches. Fatty, pale yellow stool that is difficult to control may indicate an etiology of malabsorption. If diarrhea occurs after a period of constipation, fecal impaction should be suspected (Sykes, 2005). Diarrhea that persists beyond 2 to 3 days of fasting may be attributed to osmotic or secretory mechanisms (Economou, 2006).

Varying bowel habits make it difficult to assess diarrhea from the history alone. Typically, the complaint of loose, watery, or frequent stool is indicative of diarrhea. However, some patients describe diarrhea as frequent bowel movements even if consistency remains normal. Although definitions of diarrhea can be imprecise because patterns of bowel elimination can vary from person to person and even from day to day, it is generally agreed that it involves an increase in the number of bowel movements and in the water content or volume of stool (Blush & Matzo, 2012). The most accurate account of diarrhea is obtained from a 24- to 48-hour collection and measurement, although Wadler (2001) states that this type of assessment in clinical practice is rarely a reasonable method of assessment to assess diarrhea. Moreover, there is little need for this type of investigation in the palliative care setting. A more logical and objective approach to assessment would be the criteria for grading the severity of diarrhea instituted by the National Cancer Institute (Table 24.10). Similarly, the NCCN (2017) recommends screening for diarrhea in all palliative care patients and categorizes diarrhea as bowel movements increased above a patient's baseline as follows: Grade 1—increase of less than 4 stools per day above the baseline or mild increase in ostomy output beyond the baseline; Grade 2—increase of 4 to 6 stools per day above the baseline or moderate increase in ostomy output beyond the baseline; Grade 3—increase of greater than 7 stools per day over the baseline, incontinence, indication for hospitalization, severe increase in ostomy output, limited self-care capability, or interference with

	Grade 1	Grade 2	Grade 3	Grade 4
TABLE 24.10 National Cancer Institute Common Toxicity Criteria for Grading Severity of Diarrhea				
Patients without a colostomy	Increase of less than 4 stools per day over pretreatment	Increase of 4–6 stools per day or nocturnal stools	Increase of greater than or equal to 7 stools per day or incontinence or need for parenteral support for dehydration	Physiological consequences requiring intensive care, or hemodynamic collapse
Patients with a colostomy	Mild increase in loose, watery colostomy output compared with pretreatment	Moderate increase in loose, watery colostomy output compared with pretreatment, but not interfering with normal activity	Severe increase in loose, watery colostomy output compared to pretreatment and interfering with daily activity	Physiological consequences requiring intensive care or hemodynamic collapse

Source: Adapted from U.S. Department of Health and Human Services, National Institutes of Health. (2010). *National Cancer Institute: Common terminology criteria for adverse events (CTCAE), Version 4.0.* Bethesda, MD: Author. Retrieved from https://evs.nci.nih.gov/ftp1/CTCAE/CTCAE_4.03/CTCAE_4.03_2010-06-14_QuickReference_8.5x11.pdf

activities of daily living; Grade 4—life-threatening consequences, urgent intervention indicated.

The most common cause of diarrhea in palliative care is an imbalance in laxative therapy (Sykes, 2005). It is also important to review all past, current, and new medications or treatment modalities. Metabolizing capabilities vary in older adults, but generally, this population is more susceptible to medication side effects. The use of laxatives in conjunction with fiber intake should be explored. Antibiotics can also contribute to diarrhea. In the GI tract, microflora produce protective substances deadly to harmful bacteria. Antibiotics can reduce the number of protective native bacteria and allow the proliferation of bacteria such as *Clostridium difficile* and the *Salmonella* species to proliferate, causing diarrhea. Enterotoxin-producing strains of methicillin-resistant *Staphylococcus aureus* (MRSA) have been shown to cause nosocomial diarrhea in patients taking antibiotics (Blush & Matzo, 2012). These should be considered in patients in palliative care settings as clinically appropriate. Additionally, the patient that has abdominal or pelvic radiation may experience diarrhea up to 2 to 3 weeks after completion of treatment (Sykes, 2005).

Chemotherapy can cause diarrhea and should be considered in those patients who are receiving treatment. If this is felt to be a cause, decreasing or delaying the next treatment may be indicated. Radiation-induced diarrhea is a known complication, especially with treatment aimed in the abdomen and pelvis, with up to 80% of patients receiving radiotherapy potentially developing acute radiation-induced diarrhea (Demers, Dagnault, & Desjardins, 2014). Graft versus host disease and other immunotherapy-related colitis can also develop and should be considered.

Psychosocial effects of diarrhea, whether the diarrhea is acute or chronic in nature, must be evaluated. Physical activity may be limited due to dehydration and weakness if it has been an ongoing problem. The inability to control bowel movements can cause depression and insecurity for the older adult (Economou, 2006). Diarrhea may also prevent patients from completing their activities of daily living and cause social isolation.

Management of Diarrhea

Supportive care and medications are typically appropriate for individuals in palliative care. The goal of treatment should be to eliminate the factors that led to the diarrhea, provide dietary intervention, and maintain fluid and electrolyte balance (Economou, 2006).

■ **Pharmacological Interventions.** The antidiarrheal therapies of choice in palliative medicine are anticholinergic agents and opioids.

When patients have developed grade 2 symptoms, initiation of anticholinergic medications such as hyoscyamine or atropine should be considered. Low-dose morphine may also be beneficial (NCCN, 2017).

Loperamide is another option and works through antisecretory and antiperistaltic properties. It promotes the reabsorption of fluid in the colon through its antimotility effects, and it has been shown that its use does not lead to negative outcomes. It is indicated in the adult population, with an initial dose of 4 mg followed by 2-mg doses with each loose stool, not to exceed 16 mg total dose in 24 hours. This agent should be considered in adult patients who are not febrile or have bloody diarrhea. When an infectious etiology is identified, then treatment with appropriate, organism-directed antibiotic is necessary. (Blush & Matzo, 2012).

Secretory diarrhea, specifically with HIV patients, may be treated with octreotide (e.g., Sandostatin) 50 to 200 mg subcutaneously two to three times daily (Levy, 1991). Although costly, octreotide is a somatostatin analogue with the ability to control even the most severe, intractable diarrhea (Doyle, 1994). Reduction in peristalsis and gastric secretions can also be accomplished using anticholinergics such as atropine and scopolamine (Economou, 2006).

Management of diarrhea also includes encouraging the patient and family to omit lactose-containing foods, spicy foods, and foods that contain high quantities of fat from the patient's dietary intake. Foods that can be added or that are tolerated well are potatoes, rice, and macaroni. Patients and families generally require the instruction to not overuse the laxatives that they have been given to control constipation, which can lead to excessive diarrhea.

■ **Nonpharmacological Interventions.** It is important to prevent dehydration and associated complications for patients who are at the end of their lives. With significant diarrhea, dehydration is a concern, and therefore, recommendations for management should have the primary goal as prevention of or adequately rehydrating those with dehydration. Paramount to this goal is the use of an oral rehydration solution (ORS), which is a solution of sugars and salt in water meant to provide caloric, electrolyte, and fluid replacement in those in whom volume depletion is of concern related to diarrhea. There are commercially available mixtures of ORS (e.g., Pedialyte, Gastrolyte) offered in various forms (liquid, oral, tablet), all of which have predetermined concentrations of sodium, potassium, chloride, bicarbonate, and glucose to be given in a mixture of clean water. In addition to these compounds, recommendations are available for making the mixture at home, if necessary. Several recipes are available; an example is mixing one level teaspoon of salt and eight level teaspoons of sugar into 1 L of clean drinking water along with 4 ounces of orange juice ("Solutions," 2009). For those patients in whom parenteral hydration is necessary, the degree of volume deficit as well as specific patient characteristics (e.g., age, previous medical history) should dictate the appropriate selected interventions (Blush & Matzo, 2012).

Along with hydration, nutritional supplementation with continued feedings should be instituted as soon as the patient can tolerate. The use of the "BRAT" diet (bananas, rice, applesauce, and toast) in children and supplementation with items such as salted crackers and soups in adults can provide initial nutritional support until the patient can tolerate advancing his or her diet. As the episode resolves, proteins and fats can be added gradually into the diet (Economou, 2006). There is also evidence that probiotics may be beneficial in the prevention of radiation-induced diarrhea, particularly in those patients who have abdominal or pelvic cancers during the radiotherapy period (Liu, Li, Shu, & Zhan, 2017).

Caregiver Concerns Related to Diarrhea

Incontinence of stool can be a disturbing problem for the patient and the caregiver. Frequent checks and toileting should be made in cases where patients are confused or unable to express when they need to have a bowel movement. Nurses play a significant role in educating caregivers and family members regarding these issues. Care should be taken to prevent skin breakdown, perineal pain, and other complications with infection. Protective ointments and anesthetics can be applied for comfort measures and should be initiated prior to the development of skin problems (Kemp, 1999). It is also helpful to avoid toilet tissue after a few days of diarrhea; a spray bottle of warm water washes or mild skin cleansers may be less painful.

In the pediatric population, oral zinc supplementation has shown to cause a decrease in the duration and severity of acute diarrhea. The benefit of zinc supplementation occurs because of its role in cellular and humoral immune function as well as direct effects on the GI tract with antisecretory processes and transport of fluid and electrolytes across the mucosa (Blush & Matzo, 2012). There are no studies that have looked at this therapy in the palliative care population specifically.

If the etiology of diarrhea is infectious, appropriate contact precautions should be instituted. The potential benefit of antibiotic therapy must be weighed against not only the benefit of therapy but also the possibility of negative outcomes such as growing antibiotic resistance. Patients, family members, and caregivers should be instructed on proper hand-washing techniques and food preparation to prevent the spread of infection. Disposable briefs should be discarded and tied in plastic bags to prevent contamination.

CASE STUDY

1. What aspects of Mrs. Adams's condition put her at risk for the development of diarrhea?
2. Are there further questions you could ask to determine the impact of her diarrhea?
3. What testing might you consider to assess the impact of the diarrhea on her clinical picture?
4. What interventions could you use to help support her symptoms?
5. What patient/family education would help improve her outcomes?

■ OTHER CONDITIONS

Hiccups

Hiccups, also referred to as singultus, are typically an intermittent phenomenon that is annoying, but benign. The exceptions are those termed *persistent* or *protracted*, lasting longer than 48 hours (Dahlin & Goldsmith, 2006). Chronic recurring hiccups can negatively impact advanced conditions by causing dehydration, insomnia, or abdominal muscle pain (Kemp, 1999). Hiccups lasting longer than 1 month are considered intractable (Kolodzik & Eilers, 1991) and can produce exhaustion if sleep is disturbed for an extended period of time (Dahlin & Goldsmith, 2006). Intractable or persistent hiccups are more likely to be associated with anatomical or organic disorders, and may have complications including oxygen desaturation, ventilatory disturbances, and cardiac arrhythmias (Rousseau, 1995).

The characteristic sound of a hiccup is the result of a sudden, involuntary contraction of one or both sides of the diaphragm, causing a sudden inspiratory response and closure of the glottis (Regnard, 2005). The incidence of hiccups in patients with cancer is approximately 10% to 20% (Dahlin & Goldsmith, 2006). Protracted hiccups are 82% more common in males than females (Rousseau, 1995). Children are more at risk than adults.

■ **Etiology of Hiccups.** Although the exact pathophysiology is unknown, common causes of hiccups include esophagitis, gastric distention, diaphragmatic irritation, phrenic nerve irritation, uremia, infection, brain tumor, or possibly something psychogenic in origin (Lewis, 1985). The hiccup reflex is thought to be composed of three parts: an afferent limb (e.g., phrenic nerve, vagus nerve, sympathetic chain), a central mediator, and an efferent limb (e.g., phrenic nerve with accessory connections to the glottis and inspiratory accessory/intercostal muscles; Smith & Busracamwongs, 2003).

The numerous causes for hiccups are described with relationship to the type: benign, persistent (chronic), or intractable. Some of the most common causes of benign hiccups are alcohol intake, emotional stress, sudden excitement, smoking, laughter, gastric distention from carbonated beverages, eating too fast, overeating, and indigestion. Gastric distention is thought to be the most common cause of hiccups in older adults with terminal cancer (Regnard, 2005).

Persistent and intractable hiccups can be classified according to causes from the CNS, diaphragmatic (phrenic nerve) irritation, vagal nerve irritation, drug or toxin induced, postoperative, infectious, metabolic, psychogenic, and idiopathic. CNS causes of hiccups include structural lesions, neoplasms, hydrocephalus, encephalitis, epilepsy, vascular lesions, and head trauma (Kolodzik & Eilers, 1991). Diaphragmatic irritation may result from hernia, organomegaly, esophageal neoplasms, pericarditis, intra-abdominal abscess, and gastroesophageal reflux disease. Irritation of any of the branches of the vagus nerve (auricular, meningeal, pharyngeal, laryngeal, thoracic, and abdominal) may cause intractable or persistent hiccups. Medications such as steroids, chemotherapy, dopamine antagonists, megestrol, methyldopa, nicotine, opioids, and muscle relaxants may contribute to hiccups (Dahlin & Goldsmith, 2006). It is noteworthy that many of these pharmacological agents are used in the treatment of palliative care patients and may provoke their symptoms.

Evidence suggests that there is a correlation between partial pressure of carbon dioxide (pCO_2) and hiccups. A correlation was observed when there was an increase in pCO_2 resulting in a decrease in hiccups. It was also noted that a decrease in pCO_2 was related to increased frequency of hiccups (Dahlin & Goldsmith, 2006).

■ **Assessment of Hiccups.** In obtaining a thorough assessment of symptoms, it is necessary to inquire about the duration, prior episodes, and the impact on activities of daily living. Interference with resting and sleeping may cause a patient to present with symptoms of exhaustion and fatigue. If the hiccups are so severe that eating habits are affected and appetite is diminished, the patient may be dehydrated, thin, and weak, and may even appear cachectic. The already predisposed terminally ill adult may exhibit signs of sepsis or metabolic dysfunction secondary to immunocompromised states. It may be necessary to perform lab work to determine if metabolic dysfunction is the underlying cause of the hiccups (Dahlin & Goldsmith, 2006). These causes are often easily treated and may resolve persistent symptoms. In palliative care, a comprehensive workup to determine the etiology of persistent hiccups is appropriate only if the result assists in identifying an intervention. A chest x-ray may be necessary if mediastinal or pulmonary processes are suspected (Dahlin & Goldsmith, 2006).

■ **Management of Hiccups**
Pharmacological Interventions (Table 24.11). Pharmacological interventions are selected based on the presumed etiology of hiccups. Hiccups are generally preventable or manageable by decreasing gastric distention and resolving esophageal irritation.

Gastric distention is likely to be the focus of an initial treatment approach in palliative care. Among the most effective medications for gastric distention are simethicone and metoclopramide (Reglan). Simethicone 15 to 30 mL is recommended before and after meals and at bedtime. Metoclopramide 10 to 20 mg orally or IV, up to four times a day, can be used alone or in combination with simethicone. Metoclopramide works to decrease gastric distention by increasing overall gastric motility. This medication should be used with caution in older adults. Metoclopramide should not be used concurrently with peppermint water, another alternative treatment, because

---

TABLE 24.11 Pharmacological Treatment Suggestions for Hiccups

Agents to decrease gastric distention
    Simethicone 15–30 mL PO q4h
    Metoclopramide 10–20 mg PO/IV q4–6h (do not use with peppermint water)

Muscle relaxants
    Baclofen 5–10 mg PO q6–12h up to 15–25 mg/d
    Midazolam 5–10 mg

Anticonvulsants
    Gabapentin 300–600 mg PO TID
    Carbamazepine 200 mg PO QD–TID, titrate up as needed
    Valproic acid 5–15 mg/kg/d PO, then increase by 250 mg/wk until hiccups stop

Corticosteroids
    Dexamethasone 40 mg PO QD

Dopamine agonists
    Haloperidol 1–5 mg PO/SQ q12h
    Chlorpromazine 5–50 mg PO/IM/IV q6–8h

Calcium channel blockers/antiarrhythmics
    Phenytoin 200 mg IV, 300 mg PO QD
    Nefopam 10 mg IV QD–QID
    Lidocaine bolus 1 mg/kg/hr IV, then 2 mg/min until hiccups terminate
    Quinidine 200 mg PO
    Nifedipine 10–80 mg PO QD

Other medications
    Mephenesin 1,000 mg PO QD
    Amitriptyline 25–90 mg PO QD
    Methylphenidate 5–20 mg IV, 5–20 mg QD
    Sertraline 50 mg PO QD

IM, intramuscular; PO, by mouth; q4h, every 4 hours; QD, every day; QID, four times a day; SQ, subcutaneous; TID, three times a day.

Source: Adapted from Economou, D. C. (2006). Bowel management: Constipation, diarrhea, obstruction, and ascites. In B. R. Ferrell & N. Coyle (Eds.), *Textbook of palliative nursing* (2nd ed., p. 215). New York, NY: Oxford University Press.

---

of opposing effects on the lower esophageal sphincter (Regnard, 2005). Esophageal disorders or irritation can be treated with peppermint water, which decreases gastric distention that sometimes leads to esophageal irritation.

Chlorpromazine (Thorazine) 25 to 50 mg orally works by reticular formation and hiccup reflex suppression, and may be taken up to three times per day (Kolodzik & Eilers, 1991). It is an option for prophylactic treatment of intractable hiccups. However, due to side effects of CNS depression and postural hypotension, caution should be exercised in older adults (Regnard, 2005).

Haloperidol (Haldol) 3 mg orally at bedtime for acute treatment followed by regular dosing at bedtime for prophylactic management is successful in resistant cases of hiccups (Regnard, 2005). Anticonvulsants such as carbamazepine (Tegretol), phenytoin (Dilantin), and valproic acid (Depakote, Depakene) are most effective when the cause of hiccups is of a central origin (Kolodzik & Eilers, 1991). There has been an increased use of gabapentin in the treatment of hiccups as well (Dahlin & Goldsmith, 2006; Regnard, 2005). The skeletal muscle relaxant

baclofen 5 to 10 mg orally, twice a day, is also effective for treatment of hiccups (Regnard, 2005).

Proton pump inhibitors may be effective in treating hiccups when their origin is related to gastroesophageal reflux disease. Other more novel treatments include nifedepine, midazolam, lidocaine, sertraline, and even dexamethasone, despite being acknowledged as a possible cause (Woelk, 2011). In severe cases, phrenic nerve stimulation may be necessary to improve the patient's quality of life.

Nonpharmacological Interventions (Table 24.12). Determining the underlying cause of hiccups is the primary factor to consider when selecting treatment. This is not always possible, and therefore, the healthcare provider should be most concerned with assessing the overall effect of persistent hiccups on the patient's quality of life. The aggressiveness of treatment depends on how bothersome the hiccups are.

Patients and family members often attempt nonpharmacological measures before they report hiccups to their healthcare provider. Pharyngeal and glottic stimulation

TABLE 24.12 Nonpharmacological Interventions for Hiccups

Respiratory measures
- Breath holding
- Re-breathing in a paper bag
- Diaphragm compression
- Ice application in mouth
- Induction of sneeze or cough with spices or inhalants

Nasal and pharyngeal stimulation
- Nose pressure
- Stimulant inhalation
- Tongue traction
- Drinking from the far side of a glass
- Swallowing sugar
- Eating soft bread
- Soft touch to palate with cotton-tipped applicator
- Lemon wedge with bitters

Miscellaneous vagal stimulation
- Ocular compression
- Digital rectal massage
- Carotid massage

Psychiatric treatments
- Behavioral techniques
- Distraction

Gastric distention relief
- Fasting
- Nasogastric tube to relieve abdominal distention
- Lavage
- Induction of vomiting

Phrenic nerve disruption
- Anesthetic block

Miscellaneous treatments
- Bilateral radial artery compression
- Peppermint water to relax lower esophagus
- Acupuncture

Source: Ferrell, B., & Coyle, N. (2005).*Textbook of Palliative Nursing,* (2 ed.). Oxford: Oxford University Press. Adapted version of Table 10.9 from Economou, D. C. (2006). Bowel management: Constipation, diarrhea, obstruction, and ascites. In B. R. Ferrell & N. Coyle (Eds.), *Textbook of palliative nursing* (2nd ed., p. 214). New York, NY: Oxford University Press.

by drinking a cold liquid or swallowing sugar granules or dry bread have been effective with acute attacks of hiccups. Other anecdotal "cures" include drinking a glass of water upside down, eating a spoonful of peanut butter, chewing on a lemon, and inhaling pepper to induce a sneeze. Although not entirely understood, it is felt these treatments result in either blocking or stimulating the nerves involved in the hiccup action (Woelk, 2011).

Increasing retention of carbon dioxide by rebreathing into a paper bag has also been suggested to relieve an acute attack (Baines, 1992). Digital rectal massage and carotid massage can be used for vagal stimulation (Dahlin & Goldsmith, 2006). Gastric distention can be relieved by

nasogastric tube insertion for decompression or lavage along with induction of vomiting (Lewis, 1985). Collaborative and complementary therapies that may be useful in the management of hiccups include chest physiotherapy to disrupt diaphragmatic spasms (Regnard, 2005). There is anecdotal evidence of uses of oral and intranasal vinegar for relief of persistent hiccups although further studies are necessary (Gonella & Gonella, 2015; Kako, Kobayashi, Kanno, & Tagami, 2017; Kang & Bruera, 2015).

■ **Family Concerns and Considerations Related to Hiccups.** Various treatment benefits, along with medication side effects, are necessary to make an informed decision regarding regimens patients would like to pursue. When hiccups become overly disruptive to daily life, the patient may be willing to explore more aggressive therapies to obtain relief.

Ascites

Ascites can present either centrally, peripherally, or mixed. Central ascites is a condition that is related to a tumor that has invaded the hepatic parenchyma. This type of tumor generally compresses the portal venous and/or lymphatic system (Economou, 2006). Peripheral ascites is associated with tumor cells from the parietal or visceral peritoneum. There is blockage within the peritoneal space, resulting in a marked increase in macrophages causing ascites by increasing capillary permeability (Economou, 2006). The third type is called mixed type and involves both central and peripheral ascites.

■ **Etiology of Ascites.** In chronic liver disease, ascites initially begins as a result of portal hypertension that leads to increased levels of nitric oxide, vasodilatation, sodium retention, and decreased renal function. These lead to elevation of pressure within the portal vein, smooth muscle contraction and fibrosis, and splanchnic arterial vasodilation that results in pooling of blood and an effective loss of circulating volume. This results in compensatory vasoconstriction by antidiuretic hormone release, resulting in renal sodium and water retention (Longo et al., 2012). Other disorders associated with the development of ascites due to increased hydrostatic pressure include congestive heart failure, constrictive pericarditis, and hepatic vein occlusion (Runyon et al., 1992). According to Runyon et al. (1992), tuberculosis, bacterial peritonitis, and malignant disease of the peritoneum may cause ascites, along with the decreased colloid osmotic pressure seen in malnutrition, nephritic syndrome with protein loss, and end-stage liver disease.

■ **Signs and Symptoms of Ascites.** Patients often complain of abdominal bloating and that their clothes no longer fit across their abdomen. Pain is often associated with the bloating and increase in abdominal girth. Some patients may have heartburn, nausea, and a decreased appetite. If the ascites is pronounced, dyspnea may be apparent (Economou, 2006).

■ **Assessment.** The most distressing physical symptom associated with ascites may be abdominal discomfort or pain caused by the distention. Additional complications such as dehydration and electrolyte imbalances should be considered in the older adult. Depending on the extent of fluid present, scrotal edema may occur along with weakened hernial orifices (Heneghan & O'Grady, 2001). Physical mobility may be difficult, especially for patients who are weakened or fatigued secondary to the excess weight and pressure that occurs with ascites.

The most obvious sign of ascites is increased abdominal girth. Patients may complain of bloating, nausea, and decreased appetite. Secondary to increased abdominal pressure, there may be worsening of gastroesophageal reflux or heartburn as well as dyspnea or orthopnea (Economou, 2006; Kichian & Bain, 2005). In the supine position, physical exam may reveal dullness on abdominal percussion in the dependent flank areas as ascitic fluid typically follows gravity. Tympany may be present toward the center of the abdomen. Shifting dullness can be assessed by turning the patient onto one side, noting the dullness of percussion shifts to the dependent side while tympany shifts to the top. Generally about 1,500 mL of fluid is present before dullness occurs with percussion of fluid alone (Cattau, Benjamin, Knuff, & Castell, 1982). A fluid wave test is performed by asking an assistant to press down firmly on the midline of the abdomen (to stop transmission of a wave through fat) while tapping on one flank of the abdomen. This causes an impulse to be transmitted through ascitic fluid that is felt on the other flank; if the impulse is easily palpable, it suggests the presence of ascites. Liver enlargement, tumor, or mass may also be palpable.

■ **Management of Ascites**

Pharmacological Interventions. The use of diuretics to decrease sodium reabsorption and urinary retention, along with increasing urinary excretion, are the primary interventions for ascites. As helpful as diuretic therapy may be, approximately 10% to 20% of patients will not respond to this intervention (Heneghan & O'Grady, 2001). The potassium-sparing agent spironolactone (100–400 mg/d) is the diuretic of choice for ascites; however, it may be necessary to initiate diuresis with a loop diuretic such as furosemide (40 to 80 mg/d; Kichian & Bain, 2005). Sodium and fluid restriction and diuretic are of limited benefit in patients with peripheral ascites. A trial of diuretics and sodium restriction may be of use in individuals with mixed-type ascites (Kichian & Bain, 2005).

Ascitic fluid may be analyzed to determine if albumin replacement is necessary, as well as bacterial infection of the fluid, which may require antibiotic therapy. Practitioner discretion and family requests will determine if antibiotic therapy is appropriate, given the goals of care of patients who are at the end of their lives. However, in patients with elevated ammonia levels, as is common with severe liver disease, as well as in older adults who are infected, confusion and delirium are common and should be considered when discussing treatment options with the patient and family.

Administration of medications to help with diuresis and pain control is a primary intervention with ascites. Treatment for infection or albumin and potassium replacement may also be warranted. Paracentesis or shunt placement and the prevention of infection may be important components of management. Nursing interventions include monitoring the client to promote symptomatic relief and educating the client and family about ascites and the interventions being performed.

If diuresis is accomplished with pharmacological therapy, it is necessary to make urination as easy as possible for the patient and caregivers. This may include urinary catheterization if needed to prevent injury if the patient has difficulty getting out of bed or in patients who are confused and become agitated from urinary distention. Although it is important to monitor for signs and symptoms of urinary tract infection with catheterization, this intervention is usually considered a safe and effective treatment for patients at the end of life.

Nonpharmacological Interventions. The goal of providing palliative care to a client with ascites is to relieve discomfort. The poor prognosis related to ascites lends itself to palliation of symptoms without the expectation of altering patient survival rates. Management of ascites includes sodium restriction to prevent additional fluid retention. Ascites will be decreased from a dietary sodium restriction of 40 to 60 mcg/d, or 1 to 1.5 g of salt without the need for any further interventions (Heneghan & O'Grady, 2001). When there is marked sodium retention, restriction of sodium must be less than 20 mcg/d, a goal that is not only difficult to achieve, but may impair nutritional status (Heneghan & O'Grady, 2001).

Severe ascites requires therapeutic paracentesis alone or in combination with dietary sodium restriction. Symptomatic relief is accomplished with the removal of 5 to 10 L of fluid with each paracentesis (Kichian & Bain, 2005). Following removal of the ascitic fluid, diuretic therapy is often initiated to prevent reaccumulation. While large-volume paracentesis (greater than 5 L) is generally faster and has fewer significant negative outcomes than diuretic therapy, it is not without its complications, one of which is the associated risk of post-paracentesis circulatory dysfunction. In patients who are already at a compromised hemodynamic state because of their underlying diagnoses, performing a large-volume paracentesis can further exacerbate this issue, leading to hemodynamic collapse. Several studies have looked at complementary albumin infusions and found that they are significantly more effective against the prevention of post-paracentesis circulatory dysfunction and hyponatremia than if not instituted (Bernardi, Caraceni, Navickis, &

Wilkes, 2012). One consideration, however, is the benefit of albumin replacement specifically in the palliative care patient where, according to Doyle (1994), it is rarely justified and should be discussed with the patient and family.

Refractory ascites occurs when repeated attempts to restrict sodium and diuretic therapy are both unable to prevent reoccurrence of ascitic fluid. If drainage is frequently required or there is increased discomfort for the client, placement of a shunt may be warranted. Peritoneovenous shunting provides symptom benefit; however, it is not without complications, including shunt occlusion, infection, loculation, and coagulation disorders. In appropriate patients, however, it has been shown to significantly reduce symptoms approximately 70% of the time (Racca et al., 2010). Candidates for shunting include those with abdominal scars preventing serial paracentesis and limited access or distance from a physician able or willing to perform serial paracentesis (Heneghan & O'Grady, 2001).

Comprehensive nursing assessment is essential to identify any complications that may occur with ascitic fluid accumulation. The nurse should observe for signs and symptoms of infection or peritonitis. Monitor the patient for increased shortness of breath or dyspnea and notify the physician if positioning does not relieve dyspnea. With diuresis, older patients are also at an increased risk of dehydration leading to poor nutritional status and skin breakdown. Frequent repositioning is necessary not only for comfort, but also for prevention of pressure ulcers.

Collaborative care may include dietary consultation to aid with planning meals for sodium restriction, and it may also involve frequent discussions with the physician or palliative care team to accomplish symptom relief from refractory ascites.

■ **Family Concerns and Considerations Related to Ascites.** Caregivers will need instruction on positioning. It may be difficult to achieve a comfortable position in which the pressure of ascitic fluid does not inhibit or make breathing more strenuous. Explain the importance of sodium restriction and provide education regarding how this may help to prevent fluid retention and the associated discomfort. If refractory ascites is present, the risks and benefits of paracentesis should be clearly discussed to ensure that informed decisions about management could be made. It is important that patients and caregivers understand the risks associated with reaccumulation of fluid. Having a discussion with the patient and their family regarding the impact of ascites on the overall clinical picture as well as anticipated outcomes of therapy and longevity can also be important.

CASE STUDY

1. What aspects of Mrs. Adams's clinical picture put her at risk for development of ascites?
2. Are there physical exam findings that might raise your concern for the development of ascites and underlying liver pathology?
3. Are there other items you would be looking for when considering a worsening clinical picture?
4. What education would you give to the patient/family about her current and potential clinical outcomes?

Xerostomia

Xerostomia is a subjective feeling of dry mouth, which may or may not be accompanied by decreased saliva flow (DeConno, Sbanotto, Ripamonti, & Ventafridda, 2005). Xerostomia receives little attention, so its prevalence is unable to be estimated.

■ **Etiology of Xerostomia.** A reduction in the salivary production by the parotid, submaxillary, and sublingual glands may occur as a result of radiotherapy, oral surgery, medication side effects, gland obstruction, brain neoplasms, and hypothyroidism. Typical saliva production is 1,000 to 1,500 mL daily (DeConno et al., 2005). It is an important aspect of oral health functioning to protect against bacteria and fungi, facilitate transport of nutrients and digestive enzymes, lubricate the oral cavity, and help with remineralization (Hopcraft & Tan, 2010).

Medications may contribute to xerostomia either indirectly or directly. These may include anticholinergics, anticonvulsants, antidepressants, antihistamines, corticosteroids, opioid analgesics, nonsteroidal anti-inflammatory agents, calcium channel blockers, beta-blockers, and diuretics. Indirect effects involve the impairment of taste sensation, leading to a decreased secretion of saliva. Polypharmacy is common for older adults, especially those who are terminally ill, and may be a contributing factor in the incidence of xerostomia. A study by Davies, Broadley, and Beighton (2001) revealed a positive correlation between the total number of drugs taken and the presence of xerostomia in older adults with cancer.

Oral cancer, chemotherapy or radiotherapy, stomatitis, and oral infections may cause actual erosion of buccal mucosa. Local causes of dehydration, such as oxygen therapy or mouth breathing, may contribute to xerostomia, along with the systemic causes of diarrhea, vomiting, anorexia, and polyuria (Dahlin & Goldsmith, 2006).

■ **Signs and Symptoms of Xerostomia.** Xerostomia is generally considered a subjective sensation; the severity is related to the amount of discomfort or pain that the individual experiences. Symptoms that are most frequently voiced in relation to dry mouth include diminished taste (dysgeusia), difficulty in chewing foods without fluids (dysmasesis), dysphagia, need for fluids during the night, and a burning sensation on the tongue (DeConno et al., 2005).

■ **Assessment of Xerostomia.** Assessment should begin by discussing with the patients the impact of symptoms on their lives. This is especially important to consider in the geriatric population, as they are more likely to be affected by polypharmacy, as well as those patients who are suffering from head and neck pathology. Important questions to ask include the following: Does the patient feel the amount of saliva in his or her mouth seems to be too little, too much, or he or she does not notice it? Do he or she have any difficulty swallowing? Does his or her mouth feel dry when eating a meal? Does he or she sip liquids to aid in swallowing dry food (Hopcraft & Tan, 2010)?

When assessing the oral cavity, inspect the oral mucosa for dryness, cracking, fissures, pale color, ulcerations, and gingivitis (Cooke, Ahmedzai, & Mayberry, 1996). Remove the dentures to inspect for problems that may otherwise be hidden. Structures that should be evaluated on routine examination are the hard and soft palate, pharynx, buccal areas, floor of the mouth, gum and tooth or denture condition, and upper, lower, and sides of the tongue. Also, evaluate the lips for dry, cracked areas or lesions along with the degree of mouth opening.

Xerostomia can be determined at the bedside using a quick and easy test. Following the inspection of the oral cavity, attempt to stick the tongue blade on the top surface of the tongue. If it remains in place, xerostomia is present (Cooke et al., 1996). Another test that can be attempted is the cracker/biscuit test. This involves asking the patient to eat a dry cracker or biscuit, and if he or she is unable to do so, xerostomia is present (Sreebny & Valdini, 1987). It may be difficult to perform this second type of test if patients are limited in their ability to tolerate oral intake. Caution should be used to prevent aspiration.

The Oncology Nursing Society (2002) has a documentation tool for xerostomia and nursing care that assists in making the assessment and documentation standardized. A 0 is recorded for no evidence of dry mouth; 1 = mild dryness, slightly thickened saliva, minimal taste change; 2 = moderate dryness, thick and sticky saliva, markedly altered taste change; 3 = complete mouth dryness; and 4 = actual salivary necrosis. Some evidence supports that understanding the impact of xerostomia can potentially help predict longevity. Matsuo et al. (2016) found that during palliative care, oral complications such as xerostomia appear more frequently when the date to death period is less than 28 days and suggest that these symptoms may be helpful markers when deciding on the proper timing of oral care interventions to diminish oral problems in terminally ill patients.

■ **Management of Xerostomia.** Managing xerostomia is not based on prevention, but on interventions to alleviate this complication from disease. With that in mind, the healthcare team, including the patient and family, concentrates on preventing further complications. A stepped approach is used in the management of xerostomia (Table 24.13).

Pharmacological Interventions. Implications for reversing symptoms accompanying xerostomia include discontinuing or changing medication regimens, when possible. In palliative care, this is rarely a reasonable option when the medications are utilized for pain and symptom management. There are more than 250 medications that can cause xerostomia (Jackson & Chambers, 2000). Options for helping with the symptoms include both pharmacological and nonpharmacological measures (see Table 24.14).

Nonpharmacological Interventions. Independent interventions for prevention of xerostomia include maintenance of good oral hygiene as frequently as every 2 hours and humidifying the air, especially when oxygen is being administered (Ventafridda et al., 1998). Gustatory stimulation can be enhanced using peppermint water or sugarless gum; however, the results from these interventions tend to be short lived (Cooke et al., 1996). Vitamin C and citric acids may be helpful, but have been found to cause a burning sensation, and generally should be avoided if oral lesions are present (Davies, 1997). Acupuncture has been suggested to be an effective intervention in the management of various

TABLE 24.13 Stepwise Process for Managing Xerostomia
■ Treat underlying infections
■ Review and alter current medications
■ Stimulate salivary flow
■ Replace lost secretions with saliva substitutes
■ Protect teeth
■ Rehydrate
■ Modify diet

Source: Adapted from Dahlin, C. M., & Goldsmith, T. (2006). Dysphagia, dry mouth, and hiccups. In B. R. Ferrell & N. Coyle (Eds.), *Textbook of palliative nursing* (2nd ed., p. 210). New York, NY: Oxford University Press.

TABLE 24.14   Review of Interventions of Xerostomia

Intervention	Role/Effect	Benefit	Side Effect
Nonpharmacological			
Peppermint water	Mucous saliva	Inexpensive	Interacts with metoclopramide
Vitamin C	Chemical reduction	Inexpensive Reduces viscosity	Can irritate mouth if sores present
Citric acid/sweets	Mucous saliva	Inexpensive	Can irritate like vitamin C. In sweets, can cause caries
Chewing gum, mints	Watery saliva	Inexpensive More volume Only dentate	No side effects if sugarless; otherwise, can promote caries
Acupuncture	Increased production	Noninvasive	Expensive
Pharmacological			
Pilocarpine	Nonselective muscarinic	Increases saliva production	Sweating, nausea, flushing, and cramping
Bethanechol	M-3 muscarinic	Relieves side effect of TCAs	
Methacholine	Parasympathetic	Increases saliva	Hypotension
Cevimeline	M-1 and M-3 muscarinic agonist	Increases saliva	Fewer effects than pilocarpine
Yohimbine	Blocks alpha-2 adrenoreceptors	Increases saliva	Drowsiness, confusion, atrial fibrillation

TCA, tricyclic antidepressant.

Source: Adapted from Dahlin, C. M., & Goldsmith, T. (2006). Dysphagia, dry mouth, and hiccups. In B. R. Ferrell & N. Coyle (Eds.), *Textbook of palliative nursing* (2nd ed., p. 211). New York, NY: Oxford University Press.

types of xerostomia as well. Evidence demonstrated that twice weekly treatments for 6 weeks increased saliva for up to 1 year (Dahlin & Goldsmith, 2006). Overall, it is felt that the greatest benefit of xerostomia treatment is found in the frequency of use of a product as opposed to the specific product itself (Chilton & Faull, 2005).

■ **CONCLUSION**

GI symptoms are a common symptom in terminal illness. Many patients have described the constant nausea, vomiting, and diarrhea as more disabling and disturbing than pain. GI symptoms affect patients' activities of daily living and influence their quality of life.

Other common GI symptoms in palliative care patients include dysphagia, constipation and bowel obstructions, hiccups, and xerostomia. All of the GI symptoms may be related to the pathology of the diseases as well as treatments. Having an understanding of both is crucial for the nurse caring for patients in this setting.

As in all palliative care, ongoing assessment of the patient is necessary to determine what interventions are working and which need modification. Interventions include pharmacological, nonpharmacological, and complementary therapies. Patient and family input remains the most important data to be considered in the assessment, planning, implementation, and evaluation of interventions in palliative care. Being thoughtful of the goals of treatment and the wishes of the patient and family are essential when caring for patients in palliative care who are suffering from GI symptoms.

CASE STUDY *Conclusion*

Following an abdominal x-ray, the nurse practitioner (NP) requested the family to visit with him. The NP informed Mrs. Adams and her family that the cancer had spread to her spleen. Before the NP could say anything else, Mrs. Adams interrupted him and said, "I have lived a good life and I'm ready to go when God calls me home. What can be done to make me comfortable until that time comes?" The NP explained to Mrs. Adams and her family the options of IV fluids, pain medications, and medications for nausea. Mrs. Adams requested time to be by herself. She called to speak with the NP 30 minutes later. She informed him that she wanted to be made comfortable, needed a do-not-resuscitate order in place, and wanted to remove the nasogastric tube. The family called the remainder of her family and friends, and Mrs. Adams died 72 hours later in her sleep.

CASE STUDY

AN INTERDISCIPLINARY CASE STUDY RESPONSE

Richard A. Snow, DC, DABCA, FASA
Doctor of Chiropractic
Board Certified in Acupuncture

If Mrs. Adams were to come to my office with a diagnosis of cancer, my focus would be to help improve the function of her body. I have found taking this approach along with relief of symptoms will greatly improve quality of life. Mrs. Adams presents with chief complaints of severe abdominal pain, constipation, nausea, and vomiting. I would tend to agree that the nature of the pathology of the disease and the treatments have a direct correlation to all of her symptoms.

I look at each patient through my Western-trained eyes of chiropractic and my Eastern-trained eyes of acupuncture. I first would assess Mrs. Adams by viewing any recent MRIs or other imaging. I would take a full-spine x-ray to analyze any biomechanical dysfunction in her spine that may be interfering with the nervous system. Beyond vitals, I would complete appropriate orthopedic and neurological tests. My assessment from the Eastern approach may include tongue diagnosis, acupuncture energy graph, and auriculotherapy diagnosis. This information along with a history would be used in the analysis to find imbalances or blockages of energy in her acupuncture meridians.

My recommendations for treatment would consist of gentle and very specific chiropractic adjustments to any areas that have a biomechanical dysfunction. This will assist her parasympathetic nervous system to fully engage, allowing for better function of the entire body. I would administer either electro-acupuncture or needle acupuncture.

I would address the chief complaints with the following protocols. For the severe abdominal pain, I would treat the tender points, which are referred to as Ah Shi (trigger) points. The exact location of the pain would determine what acupuncture points I would stimulate. An acupuncture point is a hole where qi and blood can be manipulated in relation to the channel, organ, or body region. There are 361 acupuncture points associated with the 12 regular channels and the governing and controlling vessels (Micozzi, 2015).

Addressing constipation would involve focusing on increasing large intestine function. Large Intestine 4, Large Intestine 11, Spleen 6, and Stomach 25 are powerful points to help with motility of the large intestine (Figures 24.2 and 24.3). My main point for nausea is Pericardium 6. It is wonderful for any nausea symptoms. I would also use Conception Vessel

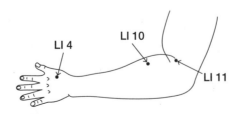

FIGURE 24.2 Large intestine acupuncture points.

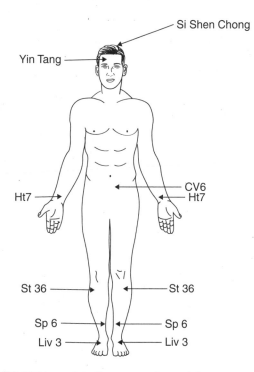

FIGURE 24.3 Large intestine acupuncture points.
CV, conception vessel; Ht, heart; LI, large intestine; Liv, liver;
Sp, spleen; St, stomach.

12, which is located between the xiphoid process and the umbilicus. With regard to the symptom of vomiting, Conception Vessel 12, Stomach 36, and Triple Warmer 5 are great starting points. In Mrs. Adams's conditions, I would also focus on strengthening her overall qi (the body's energy). Conception Vessel 17, Kidney 7, Conception Vessel 6, and specific auriculotherapy points in the ears help to increase the qi. Treatment frequency would be three times per week with reevaluations every 30 days.

Evidence-Based Practice

Levy, M., Smith, T., Alvarez-Perez, A., Back, A., Baker, J. N., Beck, A. C., … Kapo, J. (2016). Palliative care version 1.2016. *Journal of the National Comprehensive Cancer Network, 14*(1), 82–113. doi:10.6004/jnccn.2016.0009

Abstract
The NCCN Guidelines for Palliative Care provide interdisciplinary recommendations on palliative care for patients with cancer. The guidelines are intended to provide guidance to the primary oncology team on the integration of palliative care into oncology. The NCCN Palliative Care Panel's recommendations seek to ensure that each patient experiences the best quality of life possible throughout the illness trajectory. Accordingly, the NCCN Guidelines outline best practices for screening, assessment, palliative care interventions, reassessment, and after-death care.

Nursing Implications

Each patient in a palliative care setting is unique in his or her symptoms and the successful treatment. A treatment that might be effective in treating one issue may not be so in another issue or might potentially impact the onset of additional symptoms. The registered nurses should be thoughtful of these treatment implications as they offer care to their patients in palliative care settings. Having an appreciation of guidelines that help direct therapy can be an important aspect of providing comprehensive care to this patient population.

■ REFERENCES

Abrahm, J. L. (1998). Promoting symptom control in palliative care. *Seminars in Oncology Nursing, 14*(2), 95–109. doi:10.1016/S0749-2081(98)80015-6

Amella, A. (2004). Presentation of illness in older adults. *American Journal of Nursing, 104*(10), 40–51. doi:10.1097/00000446-200410000-00025

Bader, S., Weber, M., & Becker, G. (2012). [Is the pharmacological treatment of constipation in palliative care evidence based? A systematic literature review]. *Schmerz (Berlin, Germany), 26*(5), 568–586. doi:10.1007/s00482-012-1246-1

Baines, M. J. (1992). Symptom management and palliative care. In J. G. Evans & T. F. Williams (Eds.), *Oxford textbook of geriatric medicine* (pp. 685–696). New York, NY: Oxford University Press.

Barbour, L. (1999). Dysphagia. In C. Yarbro, M. Frogge, & M. Goodman (Eds.), *Cancer symptom management* (2nd ed., pp. 209–227). Sudbury, MA: Jones & Bartlett.

Barnes, S., Gott, M., Payne, S., Parker, C., Seamark, D., Gariballa, S., & Small, N. (2006). Prevalence of symptoms in a community-based sample of heart failure patients. *Journal of Pain and Symptom Management, 32*(3), 208–216. doi:10.1016/j.jpainsymman.2006.04.005

Beckwith, M. C. (2000). Constipation in palliative care patients. In A. G. Lipman, K. C. Jackson, & L. S. Tyler (Eds.), *Evidence based symptom control in palliative care* (pp. 147–158). New York, NY: Haworth Press.

Benze, G., Geyer, A., Alt-Epping, B., & Nauck, F. (2012). [Treatment of nausea and vomiting with 5HT3 receptor antagonists, steroids, antihistamines, anticholinergics, somatostatinantagonists, benzodiazepines and cannabinoids in palliative care patients: A systematic review]. *Schmerz (Berlin, Germany), 26*(5), 481–499. doi:10.1007/s00482-012-1235-4

Bernardi, M., Caraceni, P., Navickis, R. J., & Wilkes, M. M. (2012). Albumin infusion in patients undergoing large-volume paracentesis: A meta-analysis of randomized trials. *Hepatology, 55*(4), 1172–1181. doi:10.1002/hep.24786

Bharucha, A., Pemberton, J., & Locke, G. (2013). American Gastroenterological Association technical review on constipation. *Gastroenterology, 144*(1), 218–238. doi:10.1053/j.gastro.2012.10.028

Bisanz, A. (1997). Managing bowel elimination problems in patients with cancer. *Oncology Nursing Forum, 24*(4), 679–686; quiz 687.

Bishop, T. F., & Morrison, R. S. (2007). Geriatric palliative care—Part I: Pain and symptom management. *Clinics in Geriatrics Medicine, 15*(1), 25–32.

Blush, R. R., & Matzo, M. (2012). Acute infectious diarrhea. *The American Journal of Nursing, 112*(8), 65–68. doi:10.1097/01.NAJ.0000418105.99929.4f

Buenaventura, R., Adlaka, R., & Sehgal, N. (2008). Opioid complications and side effects. *Pain Physician, 11,* S105–S120.

Castell, D. O. (1996). The efficient dysphagia work-up. *Emergency Medicine, 58*(2), 73–77.

Cattau, E. L., Benjamin, S. B., Knuff, T. E., & Castell, D. O. (1982). The accuracy of the physical examination in the diagnosis of suspected ascites. *Journal of the American Medical Association, 247*(8), 1164–1166. doi:10.1001/jama.247.8.1164

Chilton, A., & Faull, C. (2005). The management of gastrointestinal symptoms and advanced liver disease. In C. Faull, Y. Carter, & L. Daniels (Eds.), *Handbook of palliative care* (2nd ed., pp. 150–184). Malden, MA: Blackwell.

Collins, J. J. (2005). Symptom control in life-threatening illness. In D. Doyle, G. Hanks, N. Cherney, & K. Calman (Eds.), *Oxford textbook of palliative medicine* (3rd ed., pp. 789–798). New York, NY: Oxford University Press.

Cooke, C., Ahmedzai, S., & Mayberry, J. (1996). Xerostomia—A review. *Palliative Medicine, 10*(4), 284–292. doi:10.1177/026921639601000403

Cowely, J., Diebold, C., Gross, J. C., & Hardin-Fanning, F. (2006). Management of common problems. In K. L. Mauk (Ed.), *Gerontological nursing: Competencies for care* (pp. 475–560). Sudbury, MA: Jones & Bartlett.

Cunningham, R. (2014). The cancer cachexia syndrome. In C. Yarbro, D. Wujcik, & B. Gobel (Eds.), *Cancer symptom management* (pp. 351–368). Burlington, MA: Jones & Bartlett.

Dahlin, C. M., & Goldsmith, T. (2006). Dysphagia, dry mouth, and hiccups. In B. R. Ferrell & N. Coyle (Eds.), *Textbook of palliative nursing* (2nd ed., pp. 195–218). New York, NY: Oxford University Press.

Dalal, S., Del Fabbro, E., & Bruera, E. (2006). Symptom control in palliative care—Part I: Oncology as a paradigmatic example. *Journal of Palliative Medicine, 9*(2), 391–408. doi:10.1089/jpm.2006.9.391

Davies, A. N. (1997). The management of xerostomia: A review. *European Journal of Cancer Care, 6*(3), 209–214. doi:10.1046/j.1365-2354.1997.00036.x

Davies, A. N., Broadley, K., & Beighton, D. (2001). Xerostomia in patients with advanced cancer. *Journal of Pain and Symptom Management, 22*(4), 820–825. doi:10.1016/S0885-3924(01)00318-9

Dean, M., Harris, J., Regnard, C., & Hockley, J. (2006). *Symptom relief in palliative care.* Oxford, UK: Radcliffe.

DeConno, F., Sbanotto, A., Ripamonti, C., & Ventafridda, V. (2005). Mouth care. In D. Doyle, G. Hanks, N. Cherny, & K. Calman (Eds.), *Oxford textbook of palliative medicine* (3rd ed., pp. 673–687). New York, NY: Oxford University Press.

Del Ferraro, C., Grant, M., Koczywas, M., & Dorr-Uyemura, L. (2012). Management of anorexia-cachexia in end stage lung cancer patients. *Journal of Hospice and Palliative Nursing, 14*(6), 397–402. doi:10.1097/NJH.0b013e31825f3470

Demers, M., Dagnault, A., & Desjardins, J. (2014). A randomized double-blind controlled trial: Impact of probiotics on diarrhea in patients treated with pelvic radiation. *Clinical Nutrition, 33*(5), 761–767. doi:10.1016/j.clnu.2013.10.015

Doyle, D. (1994). *Domiciliary palliative care: A handbook for family doctors and community nurses* (Oxford General Practice Series 27). New York, NY: Oxford University Press.

Easton, K. (1999). *Gerontological rehabilitation nursing.* Philadelphia, PA: Saunders.

Economou, D. C. (2006). Bowel management: Constipation, diarrhea, obstruction, and ascites. In B. R. Ferrell & N. Coyle (Eds.), *Textbook of palliative nursing* (2nd ed., pp. 219–238). New York, NY: Oxford University Press.

Elia, M. (2003). *Screening for malnutrition: A multidisciplinary responsibility. Development and use of the Malnutrition Universal Screening Tool ('MUST') for adults.* Redditch, UK: British Association for Parenteral and Enteral Nutrition.

Emile, S., Youssef, M., Thabet, W., Omar, W., Abd El-Hamed, T. M., Elshobaky, A., & Farid, M. (2015). Mansoura numeroalphabetic constipation score in Obstructed Defecation Syndrome (ODS): Validation of a new score. *International Journal of Advanced Research, 3*(10), 264–275.

Enck, R. C. (2002). *The medical care of terminally ill patients* (2nd ed.). Baltimore, MD: Johns Hopkins University Press.

Esper, P., & Heidrich, D. (2005). Symptom clusters in advanced illness. *Seminars in Oncology Nursing, 21*(1), 20–28. doi:10.1053/j.soncn.2004.10.004

Ezzone, S., Baker, C., Rosselet, R., & Terepka, E. (1998). Music as an adjunct to antiemetic therapy. *Oncology Nursing Forum, 10*, 27–35.

Fearon, K., Strasser, F., Anker, S., Bosaeus, I., Bruera, E., Fainsinger, R. L., ... Baracos, V. E. (2011). Definition and classification of cancer cachexia: An international consensus. *The Lancet Oncology, 12*(5), 489–495.

Ford, A. C., Brenner, D. M., & Schoenfeld, P. S. (2013). Efficacy of pharmacological therapies for the treatment of opioid-induced constipation: Systematic review and meta-analysis. *The American Journal of Gastroenterology, 108*(10), 1566–1574. doi:10.1038/ajg.2013.169

Frago, R., Ramirez, E., Millan, M., Kreisler, E., del Valle, E., & Biondo, S. (2014). Current management of acute malignant large bowel obstruction: A systematic review. *The American Journal of Surgery, 207*(1), 127–138. doi:10.1016/j.amjsurg.2013.07.027

Genc, F., & Tan, M. (2015). The effect of acupressure application on chemotherapy-induced nausea, vomiting, and anxiety in patients with breast cancer. *Palliative and Supportive Care, 13*(2), 275–284. doi:10.1017/S1478951514000248

Gilmore, J., Peacock, N., Gu, A., Szabo, S., Rammage, M., Sharpe, J., ... Burke, T. (2014). Antiemetic guideline consistency and incidence of chemotherapy-induced nausea and vomiting in US Community Oncology Practice: INSPIRE study. *Journal of Oncology Practice, 10*(1), 68–74. doi:10.1200/JOP.2012.000816

Glare, P., Miller, J., Nikolova, T., & Tickoo, R. (2011). Treating nausea and vomiting in palliative care: A review. *Clinical Interventions in Aging, 6*, 243–259. doi:10.2147/CIA.S13109

Gonella, S., & Gonella, F. (2015). Use of vinegar to relieve persistent hiccups in an advanced cancer patient. *Journal of Palliative Medicine, 18*(5), 467–470. doi:10.1089/jpm.2014.0391

Gottschling, S., Reindl, T. K., Meyer, S., Berrang, J., Henze, G., Graeber, S., ... Graf, N. (2008). Acupuncture to alleviate chemotherapy-induced nausea and vomiting in pediatric oncology—A randomized multicenter crossover pilot trial. *Klinische Pädiatrie, 220*(6), 365–370. doi:10.1055/s-0028-1086039

Gridelli, C. (2004). Same old story? Do we need to modify our supportive care treatment of elderly cancer patients? Focus on antiemetics. *Drugs & Aging, 21*(13), 825–832. doi:10.2165/00002512-200421130-00001

Gullatte, M. M., Kaplow, R., & Heidrich, D. E. (2005). Oncology. In K. K. Kuebler, M. P. Davis, & C. D. Moore (Eds.), *Palliative practices: An interdisciplinary approach* (pp. 197–245). St. Louis, MO: Mosby Elsevier.

Hellsten, M., & Kane, J. (2006). Pediatric palliative care. In B. Ferrell & N. Coyle (Eds.), *Textbook of palliative nursing* (2nd ed., pp. 895–908). New York, NY: Oxford University Press.

Heneghan, M. A., & O'Grady, J. G. (2001). Palliative care in liver disease. In J. M. Addington-Hall & I. J. Higginson (Eds.), *Palliative care for non-cancer patients* (pp. 82–103). New York, NY: Oxford University Press.

Hickey, J. (1997). Rehabilitation of neuroscience patients. In J. Hickey (Ed.), *The clinical practice of neurological and neurosurgical nursing* (4th ed., p. 255). Philadelphia, PA: Lippincott.

Hinds, P. S., Oakes, L. L., Hicks, J., & Anghelescu, D. L. (2005). End-of-life care for children and adolescents. *Seminars in Oncology Nursing, 21*(1), 53–62. doi:10.1053/j.soncn.2004.10.008

Hirano, I., & Kahrilas, P. (2015). Alterations in gastrointestinal function: Dysphagia. In D. Kasper, A. Fauci, S. Hauser, D. Longo, J. Jameson, & J. Loscalzo (Eds.), *Harrison's principles of internal medicine* (19th ed., Vol. 1, pp. 254–258). New York, NY: McGraw-Hill.

Hopcraft, M. S., & Tan, C. (2010). Xerostomia: An update for clinicians. *Australian Dental Journal, 55*(3), 238–244; quiz 353. doi:10.1111/j.1834-7819.2010.01229.x

Jackson, K. C., & Chambers, M. S. (2000). Oral mucosal problems in palliative care populations. In A. G. Lipman, K. C. Jackson, & L. S. Tyler (Eds.), *Evidence based symptom control in palliative care* (pp. 143–161). New York, NY: Haworth Press.

Jacobs, D. O. (2014). Acute intestinal obstruction. In D. Kasper, A. Fauci, S. Hauser, D. Longo, J. Jameson, & J. Loscalzo (Eds.), *Harrison's principles of internal medicine* (19th ed.). New York, NY: McGraw-Hill Education. Retrieved from https://accessmedicine.mhmedical.com/content.aspx?bookid=1130 & sectionid=79748236

Jatoi, A. (2015, June 1). Anorexia and cachexia. Retrieved from http://www.cancernetwork.com/cancer-management/anorexia-and-cachexia

Kako, J., Kobayashi, M., Kanno, Y., & Tagami, K. (2017). Intranasal vinegar as an effective treatment for persistent hiccups in a patient with advanced cancer undergoing palliative care. *Journal of Pain and Symptom Management, 54*(2), e2–e4. doi:10.1016/j.jpainsymman.2017.02.011

Kang, J. H., & Bruera, E. (2015). Hiccups during chemotherapy: What should we do? *Journal of Palliative Medicine, 18*(7), 572. doi:10.1089/jpm.2015.0106

Kemp, C. (1999). *Terminal illness: A guide to nursing care* (2nd ed.). New York, NY: Lippincott.

Kenny, G. N. C. (2007). Risk factors for postoperative nausea and vomiting. *Anaesthesia, 49*(1), 6–10. doi:10.1111/j.1365-2044.1994.tb03576.x

Kichian, K., & Bain, V. G. (2005). Jaundice, ascites, and hepatic encephalopathy. In D. Doyle, G. Hanks, N. Cherny, & K. Calman (Eds.), *Oxford textbook of palliative medicine* (3rd ed., pp. 507–520). New York, NY: Oxford University Press.

King, C. (2006). Nausea and vomiting. In B. Ferrell & N. Coyle (Eds.), *Textbook of palliative nursing* (pp. 177–194). New York, NY: Oxford University Press.

King, C. R. (1997). Nonpharmacologic management of chemotherapy-induced nausea and vomiting. *Oncology Nursing Forum, 24*(7 Suppl), 41–48.

Klick, J. C., & Hauer, J. (2010). Pediatric palliative care. *Current Problems in Pediatric and Adolescent Health Care, 40*(6), 120–151. doi:10.1016/j.cppeds.2010.05.001

Kolodzik, P. W., & Eilers, M. A. (1991). Hiccups (singultus): Review and approach to management. *Annals of Emergency Medicine, 20*(5), 565–573. doi:10.1016/S0196-0644(05)81620-8

Larkin, P. J., Sykes, N. P., Centeno, C., Ellershaw, J. E., Elsner, F., Eugene, B., & Zuurmond, W. W. (2008). European Consensus Group on Constipation in Palliative Care. The management of constipation in palliative care: Clinical practice recommendations. *Palliative Medicine, 22*(7), 796–807. doi:10.1177/0269216308096908

Laval, G., Marcelin-Benazech, B., Guirimand, F., Chauvenet, L., Copel, L., Durand, A., … Arvieux, C. (2014). Recommendations for bowel obstruction with peritoneal carcinomatosis. *Journal of Pain and Symptom Management, 48*(1), 75–91. doi:10.1016/j.jpainsymman.2013.08.022

Levin, R. (2012). Developing an early intervention model and a "culture of nutrition." In M. Marino & A. Patton (Eds.), *Cancer nutrition services: A practical guide for cancer programs* (pp. 11–15). Rockville, MD: Association of Community Cancer Centers. Retrieved from https://www.accc-cancer.org/docs/docs-imported/publications/pdf/cance-rnutrition-services-a-practical-guide-2012

Levy, M. H. (1991). Constipation and diarrhea in cancer patients. *Cancer Bulletin, 43*, 412–422.

Levy, M. H., Smith, T., Alvarez-Perez, A., Back, A., Baker, J. N., Beck, A. C., … Kapo, J. (2016). Palliative care version 1.2016. *Journal of the National Comprehensive Cancer Network, 14*(1), 82–113. doi:10.6004/jnccn.2016.0009

Lewis, J. H. (1985). Hiccups: Causes and cures. *Journal of Clinical Gastroenterology, 7*(6), 539–552. doi:10.1097/00004836-198512000-00021

Liu, M.-M., Li, S.-T., Shu, Y., & Zhan, H. Q. (2017). Probiotics for prevention of radiation-induced diarrhea: A meta-analysis of randomized controlled trials. *PLOS ONE, 12*(6), e0178870. doi:10.1371/journal.pone.0178870

Longo, D., Fauci, A., Kasper, D., Hauser, S., & Jameson, J. (2012). *Harrison's principles of internal medicine* (18th ed., Vol. 1, pp. 309–316). New York, NY: McGraw-Hill Medical.

Lotfi-Jam, K., Carey, M., Jefford, M., Schofield, P., Charleson, C., & Aranda, S. (2008). Nonpharmacologic strategies for managing common chemotherapy adverse effects: A systematic review. *Journal of Clinical Oncology, 26*(34), 5618–5629. doi:10.1200/JCO.2007.15.9053

Lynch, B., & Sarazine, J. (2006). A guide to understanding malignant bowel obstruction. *International Journal of Palliative Nursing, 12*(4), 164–166, 168–171. doi:10.12968/ijpn.2006.12.4.21013

Lynch, M. T. (2014). Palliative care at the end of life. *Seminars in Oncology Nursing, 30*(4), 268–279. doi:10.1016/j.soncn.2014.08.009

Malnutrition Advisory Group. (2011). Malnutrition universal screening tool. Redditch, UK; British Association for Parenteral and Enteral Nutrition. Retrieved from http://www.bapen.org.uk/pdfs/must/must-full.pdf

Mannix, K. (2005). Palliation of nausea and vomiting. In D. Doyle, G. Hanks, N. Cherny, & K. Calman (Eds.), *Oxford textbook of palliative medicine* (3rd ed., pp. 459–468). New York, NY: Oxford University Press.

Matsuo, K., Watanabe, R., Kanamori, D., Nakagawa, K., Fujii, W., Urasaki, Y., … Higashiguchi, T. (2016). Associations between oral complications and days to death in palliative care patients. *Supportive Care in Cancer, 24*(1), 157–161. doi:10.1007/s00520-015-2759-9

McCullough, G., Pelletier, C., & Steele, C. (2003). National dysphagia diet: What to swallow? *The ASHA Leader, 16*, 27. doi:10.1044/leader.FTR3.08202003.16

Micozzi, M. S. (2015). *Fundamentals of complementary and alternative medicine.* St. Louis, MO: Elsevier Saunders.

Morrow, G. R., Hickok, J. T., Andrews, P. L., & Stern, R. M. (2002). Reduction in serum cortisol after platinum based chemotherapy for cancer: A role for the HPA axis in treatment-related nausea? *Psychophysiology, 39*(4), 491–495. doi:10.1017.S0048577202991195

Naeim, A., Dy, S. M., Lorenz, K. A., Sanati, H., Walling, A., & Asch, S. M. (2008). Evidence-based recommendations for cancer nausea and vomiting. *Journal of Clinical Oncology, 26*(23), 3903–3910. doi:10.1200/JCO.2007.15.9533

National Comprehensive Cancer Network. (2017). NCCN clinical practice guidelines (NCCN Guidelines): Palliative care. Retrieved from https://www.nccn.org/professionals/physician_gls/pdf/palliative.pdf

Oncology Nursing Society. (2002). *Radiation therapy patient care record: A tool for documenting nursing care.* Pittsburgh, PA: Oncology Nursing Society Press.

Pijpers, M. A., Tabbers, M. M., Benninga, M. A., & Berger, M. Y. (2009). Currently recommended treatments of childhood constipation are not evidence based: A systematic literature review on the effect of laxative treatment and dietary measures. *Archives of Disease in Childhood, 94*(2), 117–131. doi:10.1136/adc.2007.127233

Plahuta, J. M., & Hamrick-King, J. (2006). Review of the aging of the physiological systems. In K. L. Mauk (Ed.), *Gerontological nursing: Competencies for care* (pp. 143–264). Sudbury, MA: Jones & Bartlett.

Racca, P., Mussa, B., Ferracini, R., Righi, D., Repetto, L., & Spadi, R. (2010). Palliative techniques and supportive procedures in surgical oncology. In A. Mussa (Ed.), *New technologies in surgical oncology* (pp. 141–150). New York, NY: Springer.

Ratnaike, R. N. (1999). *Diarrhoea and constipation in geriatric practice.* New York, NY: Cambridge University Press.

Regnard, C. (2005). Dysphagia, dyspepsia, and hiccup. In D. Doyle, G. Hanks, N. Cherny, & K. Calman (Eds.), *Oxford textbook of palliative medicine* (3rd ed., pp. 468–483). New York, NY: Oxford University Press.

Rhodes, V. A. (1997). Criteria for assessment of nausea, vomiting, and retching. *Oncology Nursing Forum, 24*(7 Suppl.), 13–19.

Rhodes, V. A., & McDaniel, R. W. (1997). Measuring nausea, vomiting and retching. In M. Frank-Stromberg & S. Olsen (Eds.), *Instruments for clinical health-care research* (2nd ed., pp. 507–517). Sudbury, MA: Jones & Bartlett.

Rhodes, V. A., & McDaniel, R. W. (2001). Nausea, vomiting, and retching: Complex problems in palliative care. *CA: A Cancer Journal for Clinicians, 51*(4), 232–248; quiz 249. doi:10.3322/canjclin.51.4.232

Ripamonti, C., & Mercadante, S. (2005). Pathophysiology and management of malignant bowel obstruction. In D. Doyle, G. Hanks, N. Cherny, & K. Calman (Eds.), *Oxford textbook of palliative medicine* (3rd ed., pp. 496–507). New York, NY: Oxford University Press.

Rousseau, P. (1995). Hiccups. *Southern Medical Journal, 88*(2), 175–181. doi:10.1097/00007611-199502000-00002

Rudd, N., & Worlding, J. (2005). The management of people with advanced head and neck cancers. In C. Faull, Y. Carter, & R. Woof (Eds.), *Handbook of palliative care* (2nd ed., pp. 240–255). Malden, MA: Blackwell Science.

Runyon, B. A., Montano, A. A., Akriviadis, E. A., Antillon, M. R., Irving, M. A., & McHutchison, J. G. (1992). The serum-ascites albumin gradient is superior to the exudate-transudate concept in the differential diagnosis of ascites. *Annals of Internal Medicine, 117*(3), 215–220. doi:10.7326/0003-4819-117-3-215

Salzman, C., & Shader, R. I. (2015). Not again: Benzodiazepines once more under attack. *Journal of Clinical Psychopharmacology, 35*(5), 493–495. doi:10.1097/JCP.0000000000000383

Santucci, G., & Mack, J. W. (2007). Common gastrointestinal symptoms in pediatric palliative care: Nausea, vomiting, constipation, anorexia, cachexia. *Pediatric Clinics of North America, 54*(5), 673–689, x. doi:10.1016/j.pcl.2007.06.001

Saxby, C., Ackroyd, R., Callin, S., Mayland, C., & Kite, S. (2007). How should we measure emesis in palliative care? *Palliative Medicine, 21*(5), 369–383. doi:10.1177/0269216307080173

Slatkin, N. E. (2007). Cannabinoids in the treatment of chemotherapy-induced nausea and vomiting: Beyond prevention of acute emesis. *The Journal of Supportive Oncology, 5*(5 Suppl 3), 1–9.

Smith, H. S., & Busracamwongs, A. (2003). Management of hiccups in the palliative care population. *The American Journal of Hospice & Palliative Care, 20*(2), 149–154. doi:10.1177/104990910302000214

Solutions: The most effective, least expensive way to manage diarrhoeal dehydration. (2009, November 19). Retrieved from http://rehydrate.org/solutions/index.html

Sreebny, L. M., & Valdini, A. (1987). Xerostomia. A neglected symptom. *Archives of Internal Medicine, 147*(7), 1333–1337. doi:10.1001/archinte.147.7.1333

Sykes, N. P. (2005). Constipation and diarrhoea. In D. Doyle, G. W. Hanks, N. Cherney, & K. Calman (Eds.), *Oxford textbook of palliative medicine* (3rd ed., pp. 483–496). New York, NY: Oxford University Press.

Tafelski, S., Häuser, W., & Schäfer, M. (2016). Efficacy, tolerability, and safety of cannabinoids for chemotherapy-induced nausea and vomiting—A systematic review of systematic reviews. *Der Schmerz, 30*(1), 14–24. doi:10.1007/s00482-015-0092-3

Thomas, R., Panackal, C., John, M., Joshi, H., Mathai, S., Kattickaran, J., & Iqbal, M. (2013). Gastrointestinal complications in patients with chronic kidney disease—A 5-year retrospective study from a tertiary referral center. *Renal Failure, 35*(1), 49–55. doi:10.3109/0886022X.2012.731998

Thompson, E., & Zollman, C. (2005). Complementary approaches to palliative care. In C. Faull, Y. Carter, & L. Daniels (Eds.), *Handbook of palliative care* (2nd ed., pp. 437–461). Malden, MA: Blackwell.

Timiras, P. (1994). Aging of the gastrointestinal tract and liver. In P. Timiras (Ed.), *Physiological basis of aging and geriatrics* (pp. 247–257). Boca Raton, FL: CRC Press.

Tipton, J. M., McDaniel, R. W., Barbour, L., Johnston, M. P., Kayne, M., LeRoy, P., & Ripple, M. L. (2007). Putting evidence into practice: Evidence-based interventions to prevent, manage, and treat chemotherapy-induced nausea and vomiting. *Clinical Journal of Oncology Nursing, 11*(1), 69–78. doi:10.1188/07.CJON.69-78

Tyler, L. S. (2000). Nausea and vomiting in palliative care. In A. G. Lipman, K. C. Jackson, & L. S. Tyler (Eds.), *Evidence based symptom control in palliative care* (pp. 163–181). New York, NY: Haworth Press.

Ventafridda, V., Ripamonti, C., Sbanotto, A., & De Conno, F. (1998). Mouth care. In D. Doyle, G. Hanks, & N. MacDonald (Eds.), *Oxford textbook of palliative medicine.* Oxford, UK: Oxford Medical Publications.

Wadler, S. (2001). Treatment guidelines for chemotherapy-induced diarrhea. *Oncology Special Edition, 4,* 81–84.

Woelk, C. J. (2011). Managing hiccups. *Canadian Family Physician, 57*(6), 672–675, e198.

Wood, J. M., Chapman, K., & Eilers, J. (2011). Tools for assessing nausea, vomiting, and retching. *Cancer Nursing, 34*(1), E14–E24. doi:10.1097/NCC.0b013e3181e2cd79

Yeomanson, D., Chohan, O., & Mayer, A. (2013). Paediatric palliative care: Intravenous methylnaltrexone relieves constipation. *BMJ Supportive & Palliative Care, 3*(1), 103–105. doi:10.1136/bmjspcare-2012-000291

Marianne Matzo

Fatigue

KEY POINTS

- Fatigue in older adults may be underreported in patients who believe that fatigue is a normal part of aging.
- COPD-related fatigue is complicated by interactions with other symptoms and is manageable through planned rest periods and treatment of related symptoms and comorbid conditions.
- Patients may need to be evaluated and treated for symptoms of fatigue, including anxiety and depression, before treatment begins.
- Participation in an exercise program that includes a class or short exercise sessions in the home can be effective in reducing symptoms of pain, depression, and fatigue associated with rheumatoid arthritis as has been found in other chronic conditions.
- Quality of life is an important goal of care and an outcome variable in palliative care; it is a priority of patients, families, and health professionals.
- Evaluation of fatigue at the end of life must be targeted to those causes that, if treated, have the best likelihood of improving the quality of life for the patient: anemia, polypharmacy, cognitive function, anxiety and depression, complications of therapies, nutrition, and infection.
- A daily fatigue journal is an important communication tool between the patient and the practitioner that supports counseling for symptom management.

CASE STUDY

Mrs. Dee Ronde is a 37-year-old black female who was diagnosed with a Ewing-type sarcoma in her right thigh 2 months after the birth of her fourth child (who is now 10 months old). Once the diagnosis was made, she had radical surgery on her right thigh, radiation treatment, and three hospitalizations for issues related to wound healing and radiation burns. Three months ago, she was found to have metastasis to her lung; she received radiation treatment to the lung and started on chemotherapy. When she is seen for her first visit in the survivorship clinic at the Cancer Center, she arrives with her husband and is very friendly and talkative to everyone. Alone in the office visit, she breaks down into loud sobs. Through her tears she says that she doesn't understand why she is so tired, and verbalizes that she is a "bad mom" because she does not have the energy to play with her children. She feels guilt that she has missed so much of her newborn's first year because of her frequent hospitalizations.

Dee reports "feeling exhausted with little or no physical or emotional energy for self-care or housekeeping." She states that she has always had a lot of energy, worked out regularly, and enjoys being a mother. She states she has soaking sweats throughout the day, and her grandmother told her she was "going through the change." On assessment, she reports that she has been married for 16 years and that their four children are under the age of 4. She reports that the pain in her surgical site is controlled with her current dose of morphine, but she is not walking or standing straight because of the surgery, and she is having pain from her left hip down her leg which she rates as an 8 out of 10. The morphine does not help this "burning," "shooting" pain.

She says that she "can't seem to get going in the morning," has "difficulty thinking straight and concentrating," and usually does not have the energy to cook, so she "gets a roasted chicken from Sam's and calls it good." Mr. and Mrs. Ronde report that they have no immediate family in the area. At this point Dee sobs even harder stating that she feels like a "burden" asking her husband to open jars and help with the children and that she always did these things for herself. He looks at her puzzled and asks, "How can you be a burden to me? It would be like saying my rib is a burden."

The palliative care nurse practitioner recognizes the cumulative effects of surviving cancer surgery, chemotherapy and radiation, the emotional and existential burdens of diagnosis of life-threatening illness, as well as recovering from childbirth and caring for 4 young children. A complete history, review of systems, physical examination, and laboratory data are warranted to assess the underlying, multidimensional aspects of the fatigue and weakness described by Mrs. Ronde. It is also recognized that depression and fatigue can be correlated in patients with complex chronic medical conditions, to assess Dee's emotional well-being.

Mrs. Ronde has experienced the physical and emotional trauma of surgery, anesthesia, and anesthetics, as well as fatigue induced by chemotherapy and radiation. She became neutropenic and anemic during the chemotherapy regimen and was treated with Procrit and Neulasta. Her fatigue was exacerbated by radiation therapy 2 months ago, which nearly 100% of patients experience toward the end of the cycle and from which few, if any, experience full restoration of energy. Given the extensive history of Mrs. Ronde, and the various etiologies of fatigue and weakness, the palliative care nurse practitioner formed a team in accordance with Dee's goals, preferences, and coexisting symptoms to develop a comprehensive plan of care that conforms to recommended competencies for end-of-life nursing care and guidelines for quality palliative care (National Consensus Project for Quality Palliative Care, 2013). The goals of care will be to focus on evaluating and managing symptoms that exacerbate fatigue, preventing fatigue by managing the activities that increase fatigue, and restoring energy with ultimate improvement in her overall quality of life.

Fatigue is one of the most common symptoms experienced by persons with cancer (Rodrigues, Trufelli, Fonseca, de Paula, & Giglio, 2016), chronic pain (Kirkova, Aktas, Walsh, & Davis, 2011), multiple sclerosis (Veauthier, Hasselmann, Gold, & Paul, 2016), primary biliary cirrhosis (Jopson, Dyson, & Jones, 2016; Silveira et al., 2017), and other incurable, progressive illnesses. Fatigue has a negative influence on the quality of life when associated with medical conditions such as heart failure (Austin, Williams, & Hutchison, 2012) and end-stage renal disease with hemodialysis (Kwok, Yuen, Yong, & Tse, 2016; Picariello, Moss-Morris, Macdougall, Chilcot, & Joseph, 2016), and with inflammatory conditions such as rheumatoid arthritis (Katz et al., 2016) and ankylosing spondylitis (Kvien et al., 2017). The ensuing fatigue affects how patients interact with others and their self-perception, ability to function, and sense

of hopefulness. Its impact compounds the suffering associated with life-threatening illness.

Fatigue is not limited to muscular force or decline in function related to exercise tolerance across age and the length of activity (Cavanaugh, Quigley, Hodgson, Reid, & Behm, 2016; Enoka & Duchateau, 2016), or the emotional exhaustion experienced in relation to work (de Vries et al., 2016; Krabbe, Ellbin, Nilsson, Jonsdottir, & Samuelsson, 2017). Chronic fatigue is an invisible thief that can steal physical and mental abilities, deeply affecting the quality of life and posing great challenges to care providers (Dhillon et al., 2017; Heinrich et al., 2016), including healthcare practitioners and the palliative care team. Like pain, fatigue is what the patient says it is: a subjective experience that must be taken seriously by healthcare practitioners. It is important for the delivery of competent palliative care to recognize the complexity of fatigue as it is related to various disease states, and to understand the patient's experience of fatigue and therapeutic intervention aimed at its management in chronic disease and at the end of life (Anderson et al., 2016).

■ PREVALENCE OF FATIGUE

The overall prevalence of fatigue, generally defined as diminished physical, emotional, and mental energy, is associated with numerous chronic medical conditions (Horneber, Fischer, Dimeo, Rüffer, & Weis, 2012). Generalized muscle fatigue involves changes in muscle force, velocity, and power (Justo et al., 2017), yet its etiology in chronic conditions at the end of life is not clearly understood. Chronic, unrelenting fatigue is a common symptom in patients with chronic disease at the end of life, with a complex array of complaints, including variations in the level of irritability, nighttime sleeplessness, and daytime sleepiness. The clinical definition of fatigue at this stage of life includes lacking physical or mental energy, especially in patients with multiple sclerosis, where fatigue is reported to occur in most patients (Newland, Lunsford, & Flach, 2017). A systematic review of qualitative evidence of adult patients living with heart failure documents that the intensity of fatigue was related to a lower quality of life and that fatigue was persistent in patients when their condition was stable (Schjoedt, Sommer, & Bjerrum, 2016).

Cancer-related fatigue (CRF), though it remains poorly understood, is multidimensional and includes psychosocial factors; side effects of chemotherapy; radiation treatments; medical states that include anemia, malnutrition, and infections; and exacerbation of other symptoms such as depression, sleep disturbance, and chronic pain (Hickman, Barton, & Elkins, 2016). For those with advanced incurable cancer, fatigue is a frequent symptom that is associated with the presence of inflammation, poor quality of sleep, depression/anxiety, and poor quality of life (Rodrigues et al., 2016). The prevalence among cancer patients experiencing CRF ranges from 70% to 100%, depending on the type of treatment, the dose and route of administration, the type and stage of cancer, and the method and timing used to assess fatigue (Holz & Smith, 2017). Fatigue is both physical and cognitive, and the evaluation of symptoms is necessary for effective treatment.

People living with HIV/AIDS should be evaluated for the co-occurrence of fatigue and depression (Byun, Gay, & Lee, 2016; Cook et al., 2016). Fatigue is a common symptom burden for patients with HIV/AIDS. A review of 42 studies relating to HIV therapies finds the prevalence of HIV-related fatigue ranging from 33% to 88% (Jong et al., 2010). In a study investigating a sample of persons with HIV/AIDS using the Functional Assessment of Chronic Illness Therapy-Fatigue (FACIT-F) subscale, the three most frequently reported symptoms—"lack of energy" (65%), "feeling drowsy" (57%), and "difficulty sleeping" (56%)—were all fatigue related (Butt et al., 2013). More specifically, Voss (2005) reported greater intensity of fatigue in HIV/AIDS patients among female (6.3 on a 0–12 scale) participants than among males (5.4 on a 0–12 scale). There are cultural and ethnic differences in the intensity of fatigue among African American, Caucasian, and Hispanic people (Mosack et al., 2016; Nieves-Lugo et al., 2017; Sayegh et al., 2016).

Healthcare practitioners are encouraged to recognize that fatigue does not occur in a vacuum and should be holistically assessed. People should be assessed for energy to perform daily living activities as well as co-occurring symptoms related to chronic medical conditions. The results of a retrospective study of the medical records of 406 consecutive cancer patients who had been referred to a supportive care outpatient center indicated, based on the Edmonton Symptom Assessment Scale (ESAS), that fatigue, pain, anxiety, and depression were the most intense symptoms reported (Yennurajalingam et al., 2011). The authors concluded that the assessment and management of fatigue should be a priority of the palliative consultation team.

■ THE CONCEPT OF FATIGUE

The historical development of the concept of fatigue indicates specific identifying criteria of fatigue: (a) subjective perception, (b) alteration in neuromuscular and metabolic processes, (c) decrease in physical performance, and (d) deterioration in mental and physical activity (Dean & Anderson, 2001). There remains no clear consensus regarding the definition of fatigue or a description of the phenomenon. However, there is an appreciation of the differentiation between "normal" fatigue, from which the majority of the population can recover after a period of rest, and pathologic fatigue, associated with disease or its treatment that is common near the end of life and in patients receiving palliative care. The analysis of pathologic fatigue and weakness, and its etiology, severity, duration, and impact, are important aspects of the conceptual and operational definition of fatigue.

Although no generally accepted standard definition of fatigue has been documented in the literature, it is agreed that fatigue symptoms include a disabling and generalized weakness, leaving the individual with feelings of significant distress or impairment (Bhat & Chokroverty, 2017). There is also agreement that fatigue is subjective, meaning it is described by the individual and, like pain, it is what the individual says it is. Fatigue is also generally accepted as unpleasant, with variation in duration and intensity. Since there are no clear criteria for differences in fatigue, chronic fatigue, and chronic fatigue syndrome (CFS), the duration (6 months) of the condition helps to distinguish its chronicity (Klimas, Broderick, & Fletcher, 2012).

Nurse researchers were viewed as instrumental in laying the foundation of fatigue as a conceptual framework wherein the distinctive characteristics of the acute and chronic conditions were described (Aaronson et al., 1999; Jorgensen, 2008; Piper, 1989). An early definition of fatigue included the influence of circadian rhythm on the feeling of tiredness and the variation in duration and intensity such that it encourages restorative rest or an aversion to activity ensues (Piper, 1989; Piper, Lindsey, & Dodd, 1989). The North American Nursing Diagnosis Association (NANDA) has defined fatigue as "an overwhelming, sustained sense of exhaustion and decreased capacity for physical and mental work at the usual level" (NANDA International, 2011). One of the most comprehensive definitions of fatigue, relevant to palliative care, is "the awareness of a decreased capacity for physical and/or mental activity due to an imbalance in the availability, utilization, and/or restoration of resources needed to perform activity" (Aaronson et al., 1999).

At various points in the course of illness, older adults may interpret fatigue differently. Older adults newly diagnosed with a life-threatening illness may have experienced fatigue as an early indication or warning symptom of the diagnosis. Over the course of treatment(s) for any number of conditions, fatigue may be understood as the side effect of treatment, while for others with recurrence or exacerbation of illness, fatigue is interpreted as the end of a very long struggle.

The concept of fatigue also encompasses emotional, cognitive, and behavioral dimensions. Psychosocial etiologic factors of fatigue across an ethnically diverse population include social adversity, social support, physical inactivity, anxiety, and depression (Bhui et al., 2011). In healthy individuals, overexertion may produce ordinary fatigue, which is relieved relatively quickly by rest; fatigue may also be interpreted as satisfaction given the accomplishment of hard work. However, fatigue associated with illness is perceived as more severe, and comes on after a shorter period of time and with less exertion than ordinary fatigue. It is often described as a general feeling of tiredness or "sapped" energy that occurs on a daily basis and is present intermittently throughout the day or during the evening after a day of normal activities.

Fatigue has been characterized by patients with such descriptors as "worn out, weary, exhausted, sleepiness, low energy, tired, worn down, bone-tired, and rubber knees." In a review and synthesis of qualitative research into patients' experience with CRF, Scott, Lasch, Barsevick, and Piault-Louis (2011) identified several concepts relating to patients' experience of fatigue. These concepts are categorized as the sensation of fatigue, the impact of fatigue, and the effect of fatigue on coping strategies. The sensation of fatigue includes references to low energy level, weakness, or exhaustion. Patients reported the experience of fatigue as overwhelming, all-encompassing, or extraordinarily severe and qualitatively different from tiredness experienced prior to their cancer diagnosis. The impact of the fatigue concept was present in more than 95% of the articles reviewed and included emotional (anger or frustration), physical (out of breath or debilitating), and social (feeling isolated or affecting relationships) aspects. Finally, the effect of fatigue on coping was conceptualized in terms of strategies for living with fatigue, such as increased exercise, eating healthy foods, or planning activities in advance (Scott et al., 2011). Additionally, a relationship between fatigue and multiple psychological and physical characteristics, including physical and psychological symptoms, found primary associations among psychological and physical symptoms of CRF, including feelings of well-being, drowsiness, anorexia, and anxiety (Yennurajalingam et al., 2016). These authors indicate that how fatigue is expressed is important in planning and delivering care for patients with cancer who experience fatigue.

Healthcare practitioners may use terms such as *listless*, *lassitude*, *lethargy*, and *malaise* to describe the fatigue observed in patients. Some practitioners differentiate fatigue from weakness, while others believe that they accompany each other and comprise a syndrome known as asthenia (Al-Osali, Al Qassabi, & Al-Harthi, 2013). Fatigue that persists through resting, is present at awakening, and occurs in the absence of muscle weakness is termed asthenia, and may be considered within the context of clinically chronic and inflammatory conditions previously mentioned involving the nervous system or endocrine system. Asthenia and chronic fatigue are clearly related as unpleasant sensations of whole-body tiredness experienced when an individual's physiological resources are exceeded.

■ MULTIDIMENSIONAL ASPECTS OF FATIGUE

Fatigue is like pain, a multidimensional symptom, a subjective experience associated with diverse etiologies (Al-Osali et al., 2013). The complex phenomenon that is fatigue has physical, emotional, cognitive, and behavioral descriptors to which subgroups are not clearly measurable. The consensus among Chochinov and Breitbart (2012) is that physical etiologies of fatigue in the medically ill older adult include the underlying disease itself, associated treatment of disease (chemotherapy, radiation, surgery, biological response modifiers), co-occurring systemic disorders (anemia, infection, pulmonary disorders, hepatic failure, heart failure, renal failure, malnutrition, neuromuscular and neurogenic disorders), sleep disorders, chronic pain, use of centrally acting drugs, lack of mobility, and lack of exercise. From a physiological perspective, fatigue has been attributed to excessive energy consumption and influenced by events occurring in both the periphery and the central nervous system (CNS; Norheim, Jonsson, & Omdal, 2011).

Independent Categories of Fatigue

Clinical fatigue, classified into independent categories, includes fatigue at rest (asthenia, chronic fatigue), fatigue on physical loading (pathological fatigue, acute fatigue), and fatigue as related to another condition (CRF, treatment-related fatigue) or exacerbation of a condition such as multiple sclerosis (Al-Osali et al., 2013). Fatigue is also linked clinically to metabolic changes such as infection, fever, tissue injury, anemia, hypoxemia, and malnutrition or to conditions involving sleep or mood disorders, including major depression.

In the case of CRF, asthenia, and weakness, three associated physiological mechanisms may affect the CNS or muscles:

1. Direct tumor effects (mechanically by destruction, such as metastasis, or metabolically by lipolytic factors or tumor degradation products);
2. Tumor-induced products (such as tumor necrosis factors [asthenin/cachectin], and other cytokines such as PEG2, interleukin-1 [IL-1], interferon [IF], or IL-6); or
3. Tumor-accompanying factors (cachexia, infection, anemia, hypoxia, neurological disorders, pharmacological side effects, paraneoplastic/metabolic alterations, or dehydration; Neuenschwander & Bruera, 2011).

In cancer populations, there has been a documented relationship between asthenia and cachexia, although one may exist without the other (Tuca, Jimenez-Fonseca, & Gascón, 2013). However, in patients with advanced cancer, both are usually present with asthenia as an epiphenomenon of the cachexia syndrome. In malignancy, changes in carbohydrate, fat, and protein metabolism, as well as direct tumor factors and cytokines previously mentioned, lead to cachexia and the resultant loss of muscle mass. This partially explains cachexia-related asthenia.

Clinical Classification of Fatigue

Research indicates that the mechanisms or pathophysiology of fatigue, weakness, and asthenia differ from one clinical condition to another and are not consistent in the literature. A wide array of immune, inflammatory, oxidative and nitrosative stress (O&NS), bioenergetic, and neurophysiological abnormalities are involved in the etiology in different disease states and may underpin incapacitating fatigue (Morris, Berk, Galecki, Walder, & Maes, 2016). The individual perception of fatigue is multidimensional and may include physical, psychological, and cognitive symptoms, each contributing to the physiological basis for the syndrome (Guerit, 2017).

Fatigue has been classified as either acute physiological, secondary to a medical condition, or chronic (Enoka & Duchateau, 2016). Physiologically, fatigue is classified according to two types: central or peripheral.

Signal, Taylor, and McNair (2008) reviewed central and peripheral influences on neuromuscular fatigue in people after experiencing a cerebrovascular accident (CVA). They reported that patients experience a relatively decreased level of peripheral neuromuscular fatigue and an increased level of central fatigue after suffering a stroke. In central fatigue, the motor pathways in the CNS fail to sustain recruitment and/or frequency of motor units or the generation of descending volleys in the motor cortex due to neurotransmitter modulation (Anish, 2005). Research data suggest that alterations in brain dopamine and 5-HT levels may influence arousal level, sleepiness, mood, and the perception of fatigue. These findings suggest that fatigue can contribute to functional impairment; therefore, the recognition and treatment of fatigue by a palliative care provider is an important consideration. Admittedly, the role of neurotransmitters in the development of central fatigue requires further study of correlates with chronic disease as well as extensive physical exercise (Anish, 2005; Enoka & Duchateau, 2016; Klimas et al., 2012).

In peripheral fatigue, there are metabolic changes in the muscle and a failure in the potential of muscle fiber components, resulting in decreased postural stability (Broxterman, Layec, Hureau, Amann, & Richardson, 2017). This failure to exert effort results from a combined effect of failure in the neural drive, such as fatigue in the mind or CNS, and the failure of neurotransmission in the muscles, though continued research is in progress to understand the mechanisms (Anish, 2005; Kisiel-Sajewicz et al., 2012). Peripheral fatigue has a known association with chronic diseases related to muscle wasting, inflammation, or joint abnormalities, including rheumatoid arthritis and systemic lupus erythematosus, HIV-AIDS, and neurological abnormalities, including Parkinson's disease and post-polio syndrome (Langeskov-Christensen, Bisson, Finlayson, & Dalgas, 2017; Norheim et al., 2011).

Fatigue leads to a decline in mental or intellectual activities and a diminished motivation or capacity to attend (Evans, Boggero, & Segerstrom, 2016). Tartaglia, Narayanan, and Arnold (2008) studied mental fatigue and its impact on motor task impulse activation in patients with multiple sclerosis (MS). They found that MS patients with physical fatigue also experience fatigue for mentally challenging tasks, which can affect motor activities unrelated to age. Similarly, van Kessel et al. (2008) randomized patients with MS into groups for two study treatments: cognitive behavioral therapy (CBT) sessions to address contributory factors related to fatigue, including behavioral, cognitive, emotional, and environmental issues, and relaxation training (RT) sessions, during which relaxation techniques were taught and practiced without advice or strategies for maintaining the practices. Van Kessel et al. reported that both methods result in significant improvements, with the CBT group showing more improvement in fatigue-related impairment, depression and anxiety, and stress level.

■ **Acute (Physiological) Fatigue.** Acute or physiological fatigue is a protective state that is identifiably linked to a single cause, in usually healthy individuals. Acute fatigue is a clinically significant state of tiredness and diminished ability to expend effort as in exercise-induced states (Bower & Lamkin, 2013) to which individuals may recover after a period of restoration. Antecedents to acute fatigue may be associated with physical exertion or lack of sleep that limits the usual activities of daily living (Strahler, Skoluda, Rohleder, & Nater, 2016). Acute fatigue has a rapid onset and short direction, is viewed as normal in the usually healthy person, and can be alleviated by restorative techniques such as rest, diet, exercise, and stress management. Acute fatigue may have immediate effects on activities of daily living and minimal effects on the quality of life.

■ **Chronic Fatigue.** By contrast, chronic fatigue has no known physiological purpose and can occur without any relationship with exertion or activity. Chronic fatigue is commonly associated with severe deconditioning or limited mobility as seen in patients with anemia and diminished aerobic capacity, including those with heart failure, chronic lung conditions, and neurological disorders. Chronic fatigue is frequently experienced by patients with life-threatening illness, is insidious in onset, and persists over time, typically longer than 6 months (Scott et al., 2011). Scott et al. (2011) found patients' conceptualization of chronic fatigue as severe, unrelieved after rest, and having a cognitive, physical, social, and emotional impact. Therefore, chronic fatigue has a significant negative effect on independence, instrumental activities of living, and quality of life (Hughes, Hirsch, Chalder, & Moss-Morris, 2016).

Chronic fatigue syndrome (CFS) is an illness with symptoms of fatigue that are more intense than the feelings experienced by persons who have a difficult workday or who have a stressful interaction. When unexplained fatigue occurs for more than 6 months, and is accompanied by an array of primary symptoms, the Centers for Disease Control and Prevention (CDC) recommends further evaluation and differentiation of CFS from illnesses that may mimic its symptoms (Centers for Disease Control and Prevention, 2012). For example, persons with CFS commonly report impaired cognitive function that lasts more than a day or two, and persons with co-occurring conditions or other illnesses may exhibit psychological problems, including depression, irritability, mood swings, anxiety, and panic attacks (Centers for Disease Control and Prevention, 2012). Symptoms that occur with other disease conditions in which fatigue also occurs signal healthcare professionals to evaluate possible coexistence to determine the level of contribution to functional decline and impairment (Strahler et al., 2016).

■ **Secondary Fatigue.** When a person is experiencing the stress and pathology of chronic disease or cancer, the body reserves can become depleted and ultimately unable to counterbalance the physiological insults. The patient may experience fatigue in association with the advanced stage of chronic disease, as well as concurrent malnutrition, anemia and cachexia, and further deconditioning and weakness. The patient interview should include reviewing the effect of fatigue on lifestyle, the presence of other physical or mental conditions, and possible side effects of medicines or drugs. CRF is reported by nearly 100% of patients undergoing radiation therapy and 95% of those receiving chemotherapy; it is also associated with anemia, cytokine activation, and mood changes, including anxiety and depression (Vardy et al., 2016).

A study of Thai Buddhist patients described consuming concerns about cancer treatment and outcomes that produced uncertainty, fear, weakness, and difficulty sleeping, leading to feelings of fatigue (Lundberg & Rattanasuwan, 2007). Bower et al. (2011) conducted a study of 103 patients with breast cancer who had recently completed treatment of surgery, radiation, or chemotherapy. They revealed symptoms were highest at the end of treatment, with 65% of patients reporting problems with fatigue and sleep and 25% reporting depressive symptoms. Furthermore, an increase in inflammatory markers taken from blood samples suggests that fatigue, sleep disturbance, and depression may stem from biological processes in posttreatment survivors, with inflammatory signaling contributing relatively specifically to fatigue (Bower et al., 2011; Rodrigues et al., 2016). Coexisting symptoms such as nausea and vomiting, inadequate nutrient intake, pain, immobility, loss of muscle mass, infection, metabolic disturbances, shortness of breath, possible gastric obstruction, and anxiety or depression also are associated with the experience of fatigue in the older adult.

The treatment for cancer (surgery, radiation, chemotherapy, bio-therapeutic therapy) can cause feelings of fatigue. The level of role functioning before surgery, preoperative fatigue, state of anxiety, insomnia, and quality of life in most domains have been demonstrated as the strongest predictors for an increase in fatigue following surgery (Rotonda, Guillemin, Bonnetain, Velten, & Conroy, 2013; Vardy et al., 2016). Klampfer (2011) studied patients of colorectal surgery and reported that locally occurring pro-inflammatory cytokines and neopterin may increase postsurgical fatigue; therefore, treating inflammation may reduce the fatigue experienced after a major surgery.

For patients treated with radiotherapy, nearly 100% experience dose-dependent fatigue, which tends to peak toward the end of the cycle. Approximately 95% of patients who receive chemotherapy report that fatigue is one of the worst symptoms they experience within the first 2 weeks after treatment. Bio-therapeutic agents (IFs, ILs) are used as maintenance therapies in older adults, especially those in remission from acute myeloid leukemia. IFs and cytokines can induce dose-related loss of sleep and fatigue through side effects of flu-like symptoms including chills, fever, weakness, and dyspnea (Holliday et al., 2016; Xiao et al., 2016).

Patients with chronic conditions, such as fibromyalgia, may manifest progressive symptoms of psychogenic fatigue, physiological fatigue, pain, depression, sleep disorders, and loss of adaptability. Given the unknown etiology of fibromyalgia, there are limited treatment options for this disease, with relief primarily achieved by the palliation of symptoms. Porter, Jason, Boulton, Bothne, and Coleman (2010) conducted a systematic review and found positive results from treatment with complementary and alternative medicines. The results showed a positive effect in terms of laboratory test results, physical functioning, psychological functioning, and quality of life warranting further investigation. Exercise is also recommended in levels that help sufferers to feel better without initially aiming at training or conditioning (Hoffmann et al., 2016). Older adults who live with chronic conditions like fibromyalgia, rheumatoid arthritis, or CFS should be the recipients of primary and secondary prevention efforts targeted toward comorbid depression and the impact on the overall quality of life and quality of health (Fiest, Currie, Williams, & Wang, 2011; Whitehead, Unahi, Burrell, & Crowe, 2016). Interventions such as psychotherapy and medication management should be initiated to prevent suicidal ideation or attempt.

The causes of HIV-related fatigue are typically connected to physiological and/or psychological factors that influence symptoms associated with fatigue (Barroso et al., 2010). The physiological factors of HIV-related fatigue include hepatic function, thyroid function, HIV viral load, immunologic function, gonadal function, hematologic function, and cellular injury. Psychosocial factors include childhood and adult trauma, anxiety, depression, unemployment, social support, stressful life events, and posttraumatic stress disorder (Barroso et al., 2010). Lofgren et al. (2015) reported that individuals living with HIV reported a high symptom burden, with 77% reporting fatigue. The fatigue experience in patients with HIV/AIDS includes complaints of tiredness and exhaustion, with varying reports that women in some studies experience higher fatigue severity than men (Barroso & Voss, 2013).

■ CORRELATES OF FATIGUE IN SPECIFIC PATIENT POPULATIONS

Fatigue: Pediatric Considerations

For children with advanced cancer, fatigue is the most common symptom reported in the last month of life. The prevalence rate of this symptom is reported as 96%, with nearly 50% reporting as suffering significantly from it (Pan, Wu, & Wen, 2017). In a longitudinal descriptive study, Erickson et al. (2010) found every adolescent cancer patient experienced fatigue during the month

of treatment with variability in severity and duration. Reports of fatigue were independent of chemotherapy agents, doses, and routes of administration and showed an increase in the days immediately following chemotherapy administration (Erickson et al., 2010). In children, as in adults, fatigue typically results in decreased activity, loss of control, and a sense of loneliness and isolation (Olagunju, Sarimiye, Olagunju, Habeebu, & Aina, 2016; Ullrich et al., 2010). Left untreated, fatigue can negatively impact the quality of life and interfere with opportunities for growth and closure at the end of life (Loades & Kagee, 2017).

Assessment of fatigue is dependent on subjective reports of the patient. In children, clinicians may need to rely on the reports of the parents regarding the experience of fatigue. Hockenberry, Hinds, and Barrera (2003) developed a fatigue-rating tool that took into consideration the perspective of the child, parent, and staff. The experience of fatigue by adolescents is expressed as a distressing, dynamic symptom with physical, psychological, and emotional components, while younger children experience fatigue as a physical sensation (Erickson et al., 2010; Hooke, Garwick, & Gross, 2011). Parents and staff share the view that the child's fatigue is manifested by physical, emotional, and mental changes that interfere with the child's ability to participate in activities.

To date there is no evidence to support that interventions aimed at the management of fatigue are any different between children and adults, although there are a few evidence-based studies documenting the efficacy of these interventions in children. However, a recent review and meta-analysis lends support to the idea that exercise interventions may reduce general fatigue in children and adolescents with cancer (Chang, Mu, Jou, Wong, & Chen, 2013). For children, studies are needed regarding the assessment of fatigue in light of developmental stages. Education for children with life-threatening illnesses, their families, and clinicians is needed regarding the recognition and treatment of this symptom in order to lessen the source of suffering.

Fatigue in Older Adults

Fatigue is common in older adults and associated with advanced disease, functional decline, and mortality (Hardy & Studenski, 2010). A review study consisting of a prospective cohort of 495 community-dwelling primary care patients aged 65 years or older found 70% reporting one or more fatigue qualities and 43% reporting feeling tired most of the time. Hardy and Studenski (2010) found these reports to be associated with worse health and functional status.

Fatigue is particularly evident in the older adult in long-term care facilities. In a review of literature related to the unmet symptom needs of residents in long-term care, fatigue was named as one of the more common symptoms in persons with cancer who were not near the end of life (Duncan, Forbes-Thompson, & Bott, 2008). Furthermore, assessment and evaluation of fatigue are not specified in the Minimum Data Set (MDS) required by each nursing home certified by Medicare or Medicaid (Centers for Medicare & Medicaid Services, 2008).

In a study of resident-to-resident aggression among residents of long-term care, researchers conducted 15 focus group interviews with seven residents and 96 staff members in one facility (Rosen et al., 2008). The residents formed one focus group, and staff of differing job levels and responsibilities formed the remaining groups. Although fatigue was named as a nonfrequent trigger or reason for aggression, the research report indicated that fatigue may occur during both public (group) and private (bathroom) activities involving residents, and may also be related to end-of-day staff fatigue (Rosen et al., 2008). Policy recommendations for prevention of resident violence and aggression include specific staff training in geriatrics and long-term care and staff levels that allow sufficient time to attend to the physical and emotional needs of residents. Each study suggests that fatigue may be poorly recognized and undertreated in older people in nursing home facilities.

Palliative treatment of the older adult must encompass the potential for confounding pathology secondary to aging. Clear associations between fatigue and depression (National Institute of Mental Health, 2013), cancer-related treatment modalities (Carlotto, Hogsett, Maiorini, Razulis, & Sonis, 2013; Koll & Dale, 2017), heart failure (Austin et al., 2012), anemia (Balducci, 2010), malnutrition (Tennant, Takacs, Gau, Clark, & Russ, 2012), end-stage renal disease (Hallan & Orth, 2010), and fibromyalgia (Shillam, Dupree Jones, & Miller, 2011) appear in the literature. Healthcare providers, in accordance with the clinical practice guidelines for palliative care (National Consensus Project for Quality Palliative Care, 2013), should regularly and carefully assess symptoms of fatigue and weakness, and the symptoms that frequently accompany these, for all older adult patients and persons near the end of life. Nurses are expected to assess for and recognize the need to treat generally occurring symptoms that may include pain, breathlessness (dyspnea), constipation, anxiety, changes in appetite, nausea, vomiting, changes in sleep pattern, and alterations in cognition and function. Often, the conventional wisdom is that because a person is of advanced age, fatigue is a normal consequence of the aging process.

Many elders and their families erroneously consider fatigue to be an inevitable aspect of aging, and therefore not a symptom to be treated. In fact, older adults may not even report symptoms of weakness and fatigue to their primary care provider. Even for the older adult in palliative care, many causes of fatigue can be successfully treated by examining for and treating the underlying cause. The goal for the healthcare provider related to the symptom of fatigue is to improve the patient's quality of life by treating the symptom and teaching the older adult coping mechanisms and lifestyle changes (Koll & Dale, 2017).

■ **Parkinson's Disease.** A study on the influence of disease severity on fatigue in patients with Parkinson's disease suggests that disease severity directly affects three domains of fatigue: increased levels of general fatigue, physical fatigue and reduced activity, and mental fatigue (van Dijk et al., 2013). In another study, Herlofson, Ongre, Enger, Tysnes, and Larsen (2012) found 55% of patients with Parkinson's disease had clinical significant fatigue in both advanced and early, untreated stages of disease. Additionally, the researchers determined that fatigue was related to, but not causally determined by, depressive symptoms and found no correlation between fatigue and cognitive impairment (Herlofson & Kluger, 2016; Patel, Pahwa, & Lyons, 2017).

■ **Frailty.** Fatigue is commonly included in characterizations of frailty. Evidence exists indicating fatigue and early development of weight loss may be significant predictors of frailty, occurring in up to 80% of transitions to frailty (Liu et al., 2016). Avlund (2010) identifies fatigue without disability as representing an early stage of frailty prior to causing disability. Additionally, both frailty and fatigue are understood to be the result of complex interactions between a multitude of biological, physiological, and psychosocial systems. Avlund (2010) goes on to suggest that placing an emphasis on frailty may result in less attention paid to the individual components of frailty, such as fatigue, which may be an important predictor for practitioners to assess (Alexander, 2016).

■ **Depression.** Depressive symptoms were also associated with baseline frailty in the Women's Health Initiative Observational Study (WHI-OS), and being underweight, overweight, or obese were described as risk factors for frailty, a component of which is poor physical functioning or exhaustion. In a cohort study of older adult women from the WHI-OS, depressive symptoms and antidepressant use were associated with frailty after an initial assessment and a 3-year follow-up (Lakey et al., 2012). The American Psychiatric Association identifies fatigue as a symptom of depression, and depression screening is often measured with criteria that reflect energy level (ability to get going) or the effort required to conduct daily activities (American Psychiatric Association, 2013).

■ **Inflammatory Conditions.** Fatigue is identified by researchers as occurring in patients with inflammatory conditions including biliary cirrhosis (Silveira et al., 2017), rheumatoid arthritis (Katz et al., 2016), and ankylosing spondylitis. Björnsson, Simren, Olsson, and Chapman (2005) studied 96 patients with biliary cirrhosis and a group of matched persons from the general population, patients with functional gastrointestinal disorders, and patients with organic gastrointestinal disorders such as inflammatory bowel disease. They reported that patients with functional gastrointestinal disorders and organic gastrointestinal disorders had higher fatigue scores than persons from the general population and those with biliary cirrhosis. This study validates the necessity to evaluate fatigue in patients with biliary cirrhosis; while present, it may not be related to actual liver function but instead related to the comorbidities including depression, alteration in sleep patterns and quality, or other psychological or psychiatric conditions.

In a study of 68 patients with ankylosing spondylitis, researchers reported an increase in fatigue that was associated with greater disease severity, functional disability, and disease activity (Turan et al., 2007). Repping-Wuts, Fransen, van Achterberg, Bleijenberg, and van Riel (2007) studied a group of 150 patients with rheumatoid arthritis and found that the general health of the patient and the level of disability predicted high scores on measures of fatigue. Severe persistent fatigue was defined as a score of at least 35 at the beginning of the study and after 12 months using the fatigue subscale of the Checklist Individual Strength questionnaire. These two studies underscore the relationships among fatigue, functional disability, and the level of general health. It is therefore important to assess for fatigue and institute measures to reduce its severity in patients with inflammatory conditions such as ankylosing spondylitis and rheumatoid arthritis.

In a randomized controlled study of the effect of exercise on common symptoms in patients with rheumatoid arthritis, 220 patients participated in a guided exercise group, exercised at home with a videotape, or exercised in a control group (Neuberger et al., 2007). All exercises were low impact during which one foot was always in contact with the floor. Findings indicated that fatigue, pain, and depression diminished among participants in the exercise class, whereas participants in the home exercise program experienced no changes (possibly related to less intensity and duration of exercise sessions in the nonguided home exercise participants). Participants who believed that exercise would be beneficial to their overall health tended to exercise more.

■ **Heart Disease.** Patients typically experience increasing fatigue as heart failure progresses, characterized by symptoms of systolic dysfunction and refractory symptoms of dyspnea and fatigue while resting (Austin et al., 2012). However, Austin et al. (2012) found fatigue levels respond positively to cardiac rehabilitation programs and the adoption of a better exercise profile. The breathlessness and dyspnea associated with fatigue may be treated with opioids (narcotic agonist analgesics), which may contribute pharmacologically to the experience of fatigue (Bascom, 2013). Given that fatigue is integral to

the experience of heart failure, interventions are needed to assist patients to cope with the experience of fatigue, such as pacing of activities, relaxation, and restful sleep (Forbush et al., 2017).

While fatigue is just one of several physical symptoms self-reported, it was often associated with dyspnea. Significant measures of physical symptom status in heart failure patients include employment status, patient-perceived control over the management of their condition, anxiety, and depression. In a study of patients with heart failure, a group of 53 older adults completed the fatigue subscale of the Profile of Mood States (Stephen, 2008). Results indicated that, without regard to actual age, older adults who believed that fatigue was related to their aging scored higher on fatigue intensity than older adults who did not believe the relationship. Stephen found that the intensity of fatigue was predicted by the severity of the illness, negative affect (e.g., sadness and depression), perception of health status, satisfaction with life, severity of current co-occurring symptoms, and marital status.

Pulmonary arterial hypertension (PAH) is a chronic, life-threatening illness that primarily affects women. Matura, McDonough, and Carroll (2016) studied symptom severity among young, middle, and older adults with PAH. They found that, for all the age groups, shortness of breath on exertion and fatigue were the two most prevalent symptoms (Matura et al., 2016).

■ **Chronic Obstructive Pulmonary Disease.** A study of 19 women and 17 men with chronic obstructive pulmonary disease (COPD; i.e., not asthma or cancer) were compared with a control group of regional participants statistically matched for sex, marital status, and social support, to explore fatigue and its impact on the daily lives of participants (Theander & Unosson, 2004). Findings indicated that fatigue had a great impact on how participants with COPD felt each day and on their ability to perform daily tasks. Nearly half (44%) of the participants reported that fatigue was experienced daily and was one of their worst symptoms. Participants in this study also reported higher fatigue scores as measured by the Fatigue Impact Scale (FIS; Theander & Unosson, 2004), developed for the assessment of the perceived impact of fatigue on the quality of life of people with a chronic illness (Fisk et al., 1994).

Fatigue and weakness were reported in 96% of patients with COPD near the end of life in a descriptive, retrospective study using informants of the deceased (Elkington, White, Addington-Hall, Higgs, & Edmonds, 2005). The researchers found that accompanying symptoms including low mood, sleep disturbances, anxiety, pain, and breathlessness were frequently among the patients' end-of-life experiences. In a study of persons with moderate to severe COPD, researchers were able to document an association between fatigue and the daily function and activities of persons with COPD (Kapella, Larson, Patel, Covey, & Berry, 2006). The sample of

130 participants reported situation-specific fatigue that was controllable and responsive to planned amounts of rest and sleep. They developed a model describing the direct influence of depressed mood on fatigue and the indirect influence of anxiety and quality of sleep on fatigue, thereby contributing to diminished functional capacity. In a state-of-the-science article examining over 75 articles related to anxiety and depression in patients with COPD, Putman-Casdorph and McCrone (2009) acknowledge the complexity of anxiety and depression and their negative impact on physical performance, compliance with prescribed regimen, symptom burden, and overall quality of life.

■ **Cancer.** The National Comprehensive Cancer Network (NCCN) defines CRF as "a distressing, persistent, subjective sense of tiredness or exhaustion related to cancer or cancer treatment that is not proportional to recent activity and interferes with usual functioning" (National Comprehensive Cancer Network [NCCN], 2013). CRF is influenced and modulated by a number of critical factors, and the mechanism that is both necessary and sufficient to induce development of severe fatigue in patients with cancer has not yet been identified. Specific research efforts to understand the factors that may contribute to CRF development have been made, including studies of the direct effects of tumor burden, the effects of cancer treatment, and other pathophysiological and psychosocial conditions (Filler & Saligan, 2016).

Compared with fatigue reported by healthy people, CRF is described as more distressing, as interfering with usual functioning, and as less likely to be relieved by rest. Most importantly, if left untreated, CRF is a major factor in patient quality-of-life scores (Thiagarajan et al., 2016). Although reported by 60% to 100% of patients undergoing therapy for CRC, fatigue is still considered an underreported symptom for which there are multiple overlapping etiologies, confounding an explanation of its specific pathophysiological mechanisms. CRF may be more prevalent in patients undergoing multimodality treatment such as chemoradiotherapy for rectal carcinoma. CRF may continue for years after treatment is completed, even when the cancer has been cured (Thiagarajan et al., 2016).

CRF has a complex etiology, possibly regulated by physiological, psychological, and situational factors: changes in the production and balance of muscle proteins; glucose, electrolytes, and hormones; a catabolic process resulting from decreased daily energy expenditure and bed rest; and disease-related and treatment-induced anemia. Distinguishing between fatigue and depression is an important aspect of fatigue evaluation (Table 25.1). A complex interplay exists between etiologic factors such as cancer treatment, infection, concomitant medications, and susceptibility of the patient to CRF (Foster et al., 2016).

Multiple risk factors, rather than a single risk factor, appear to put patients with cancer at risk for CRF.

TABLE 25.1   Etiology of Cancer-Related Fatigue

Tumor-Related Causes	Treatment-Related Causes
Disease site	Surgery and postoperative recovery
Paraneoplastic syndrome	Psychological distress
Increased cytokine production	Chemotherapy and chemotherapy effects
Decreased availability of metabolic substrates	Radiotherapy and radiotherapy effects
Cachexia	Anemia
Pain	Pain

Source: Wang, X. S. (2008). Pathophysiology of cancer-related fatigue. *Journal of Oncology Nursing, 12*(5), 11–20. doi:10.1188/08 .CJON.S2.11-20

These risk factors include poor nutrition, sleep disorders, stress, cancer comorbidities (i.e., cardiac, pulmonary, renal, liver, neurological, thyroid, and endocrine, and associated medications), hypoxia, pain, infection, deconditioning, and ongoing therapy. Severe fatigue may be reported by cancer patients even before the start of therapeutic intervention, which might add to the subsequent occurrence of fatigue (Borneman, 2013). In the study of 240 patients with varying forms of cancer, almost one quarter of participants with a diagnosis of cancer reported severe fatigue 1 to 3 years before starting treatment. For example, fatigue was categorized by disease process, and of the 23% participants who complained of severe fatigue, the highest occurrence was in persons with "other" tumors (33%), including gastrointestinal, urogenital, or gynecological. Of participants who reported severe fatigue, 14% were persons with prostate cancer and 20% were persons with breast cancer. Participants with severe fatigue after diagnosis but before therapy also experienced more pain, less physical activity, more sleep disturbance, more depressive feelings, and more anxiety than participants without severe fatigue. The researchers found that although anxiety might be a normal and expected response to a diagnosis of cancer, there was no significant association between the diagnosis of cancer and severe fatigue.

Women diagnosed with breast cancer are known to be fatigued for as long as 5 years following therapeutic intervention including surgery, radiotherapy, and chemotherapy (Peoples et al., 2017). Halkett, Kristjanson, and Lobb (2008) conducted semistructured interviews with 34 patients who discussed their experiences with radiotherapy treatments for breast cancer. They found that fear of fatigue, or "anticipating tiredness" (Halkett, Kristjanson, & Lobb, 2008, p. 881), was often greater than the actual experiences of side effects.

■ FATIGUE AND QUALITY OF LIFE

Regardless of the age of the patient, fatigue has a profound effect on the quality of life. Fatigue is one factor that negatively affects quality of life (Heinrich et al., 2016). Promoting health-related quality of life requires that fatigue must be appropriately assessed and effectively treated (Wang, Huang, Ho, & Chiou, 2016).

■ ASSESSMENT OF FATIGUE

NCCN convened a committee of experts to make recommendations for future studies of CRF. The committee reviewed the current data on the incidence, clinical measurement, and treatment of CRF. The assessment of fatigue is largely derived from self-report questionnaires that address the symptom of fatigue and do not correlate the presence of fatigue with a change in physical activity. The committee noted a strong interaction among fatigue, pain, difficulty sleeping, and distress and recommended that future clinical research address these interactions (Mortimer et al., 2010). As a subjective symptom, practitioners most often rely on the patient's self-report of fatigue to evaluate its severity. However, the assessment of fatigue does include observable characteristics and the impact of the symptom on the quality of life. A comprehensive assessment of fatigue obtained through a health history and review of systems, including fatigue assessment, physical examination, and laboratory data, can assist the practitioner in discriminating between physiological and psychogenic fatigue, depression, and the presence of correctable causes of fatigue (Piper et al., 2008). Appendix 25.1 reviews the characteristics of commonly used fatigue assessment tools.

I. **Health History** should include a medical, psychiatric, family, social, and medication history, which may reveal associated conditions, such as diabetes, hypothyroidism, sleep apnea, anxiety or depressive disorders, inherited metabolic disorders or a history of alcohol or illegal drug use, and the possibility of sexually transmitted infections often associated with fatigue, even in older populations.

II. **Review of Systems** regarding fatigue focuses on changes in other body systems that may indicate potential health problems associated with fatigue, such as respiratory disorders (e.g., dyspnea), cardiac problems, anemia, cancers, depression, or electrolyte disorders. For those patients with chronic, incurable illness, fatigue may also be a side effect of medical treatments, including both prescription and over-the-counter medications. Furthermore, in speaking with the patient, it is important to determine his or her emotional status, particularly whether the person speaks of his/her own death or suicidal ideations.

III. **The Fatigue Assessment** includes questions related to the six dimensions of fatigue (Piper et al., 1998; Appendix 25.2), specifically:

1. **Temporal Dimension,** which includes the assessment of the timing of fatigue (when it occurs), onset (from seconds to years), duration (chronic for more than 6 months), and the pattern (wake-up fatigue, evening fatigue, transient, etc.), and changes in this dimension over time.

2. **Sensory Dimension,** which focuses on how the fatigue feels. For example, is the fatigue localized (e.g., tired eyes, arms, legs) or generalized (e.g., whole-body tiredness, weariness, weakness, lethargy), and what is the intensity or severity of fatigue (using a 0–10 scale)? Additional assessment questions include what exacerbates the fatigue (e.g., pain, nausea, vomiting, environmental heat, or noise)? What helps the patient feel better or alleviates the symptoms (e.g., rest, food, listening to music, etc.)?

3. **Mental/Cognitive Dimension,** which questions the patient's ability to concentrate and focus, attention span, recall, and whether he or she reports being "mentally tired."

4. **Affective/Emotional Dimension,** which assesses the patient's irritability, impatience, mood changes, depression, and the significance of the fatigue.

5. **Behavioral Dimension,** which considers the effect that the fatigue has on the patient's ability to perform activities of daily living (bathing, dressing, cooking, socializing, sexual activity). Family and practitioner observations regarding the patient's posture, gait, appearance (e.g., drooping shoulders), or lack of energy should also be assessed. Acute behavioral manifestations can include a change in alertness, while chronic manifestations may not be obvious to the practitioner because of the ability of many patients to adapt to their fatigue. If the patient also has a dementing illness, the behavioral dimensions may be the only clue that the practitioner has regarding the presence of fatigue.

6. **Physiological Dimension,** which includes biological mechanisms such as laboratory tests, a complete physical examination, and determining if comorbid conditions such as diabetes, cardiac illness, or other disease factors are present.

Table 25.2 offers questions related to the assessment of the pattern of sleep and rest, perceptions/expression of fatigue, and the impact on quality of life.

IV. **Physical Examination** includes the following assessment parameters:
■ Vital signs to determine if fever, low blood pressure, or weak pulse may be the cause of fatigue;
■ General appearance including affect (anxious, depressed, agitated, tearful, angry, or flat), self-care

behaviors, speech patterns, intonation, and general responsiveness;

■ Assessment of cardiac, respiratory, renal, musculoskeletal, and skin status to identify physiological conditions, including signs of infection or dehydration/nutrition that may be associated with fatigue;

■ Appropriate laboratory testing, such as complete blood count and other laboratory studies (electrolytes, blood gases, thyroid function tests, iron profile, and vitamin D_3), which may confirm diseases suspected.

■ MEASURING FATIGUE

Given its subjectivity and the general lack of consensus in the literature regarding a definition of fatigue, the measurement of fatigue remains a challenge. In a study of fatigue in participants with COPD, Theander, Cliffordson, Torstensson, Jakobsson, and Unosson (2007) examined the validity of the FIS and reported reliability coefficients of 0.98 (Cronbach's alpha) and 0.94 test-retest stability, indicating a statistically significant performance. Researchers reported a significant correlation between the level of fatigue and participant reports of fatigue greater than or less than 6 hours daily. The research group then reduced the number of items on the FIS to 25 from the original 40, and psychometric performance was maintained with Cronbach's alpha at 0.96 and test-retest stability at 0.94 for the total scale.

Construct validity is difficult to establish for an instrument since fatigue measure may examine various aspects of fatigue, such as its character, precursors or causes, or the effects of fatigue, and each aspect can be addressed from a physiological, psychosocial, or behavioral perspective (see Appendix 25.1). Significant aspects to assess when measuring fatigue vary among scales and may include combinations of symptoms that are physical, cognitive, affective, or behavioral. Participants in a qualitative investigation of fatigue among working adults described fatigue in characteristic themes that included manifestations in the physical, emotional, and behavioral realms (Aaronson, Pallikkathayil, & Crighton, 2003). For example, objective physical manifestations of fatigue included the signs of slumped shoulders or drawn and slackened face that others can readily see, whereas the subjective physical manifestations of fatigue included symptoms not readily seen by others such as lack of energy and endurance, or weakness (Aaronson et al., 2003). Study participants described emotional, mental, and behavioral symptoms that might also represent depressive symptoms, including sadness, inability to concentrate, and irritability.

As the first characteristic of fatigue, subjective quantification can be measured by the Multidimensional Assessment of Fatigue (MAF) measure (Tack, 1991), which examines the experience of fatigue in the past week and its severity, perceived distress, the timing of fatigue, and interference with activities of daily living (Belza et al., 2001). The MAF provides a Global Fatigue Index (GFI; Appendix 25.3) developed to capture the subjective experience of fatigue for patients with rheumatoid arthritis (Belza, Henke, Yelin, Epstain, & Gillis, 1993) and has been used with multiple patient populations including persons with COPD (Belza et al., 2005; Belza et al., 2001) and older adults. The GFI has also been shown to be a valid and reliable measure of fatigue in community-based patients with HIV (Bormann, Shivley, Smith, & Gifford, 2001; Whitehead, 2009).

As the second characteristic of fatigue, subjective distress can be measured by a single item on the MAF or by the Symptom Distress Scale (SDS; McCorkle & Young, 1978). The SDS was originally developed to contain 10 items on symptoms, which included a single item on fatigue, addressed as "tiredness," in which patients respond to a 5-point semantic differential:

Could not feel more tired   5 4 3 2 1   I am not tired at all

TABLE 25.2 Assessment of Patterns of Sleep/Rest, Perceptions/Expressions of Fatigue, and Impact on Quality of Life

Sleep/Rest Patterns	Perceptions/Expressions of Fatigue	Impact on Quality of Life
Do you nap?	What do you believe is the cause of your fatigue?	Do you feel the quality of your life has changed because of fatigue?
Do you feel rested after a nap?	Are you distressed by fatigue?	Can you work?
Do you have difficulty falling asleep at night or staying asleep?	What do you think is the meaning of this symptom?	Do you socialize?
Has the quality of your sleep at night changed?	Do you feel hopeful?	Has fatigue affected your relationship with others?
How do you feel when you awaken?	Has your appetite changed?	Are you able to enjoy life?
Has your sleeping environment changed?	Do you have other symptoms, such as pain?	Has fatigue affected your outlook?

A more recent version of the SDS is a 13-item self-administered questionnaire that assesses the subjective distress of the patient and demonstrates satisfactory validity and reliability (Cooley et al., 2005). Additionally, significant ($p < .05$) correlation has been found between fatigue and other physical and psychological symptoms, and highlights the potentially confounding relationship between fatigue and these co-occurring symptoms experienced by different clinical populations (Badger, Segrin, & Meek, 2011; Yennurajalingam, Palmer, Zhang, Poulter, & Bruera, 2008).

The third characteristic of fatigue, effect of fatigue on activities of daily living, can be measured by an 11-item subscale of the MAF, which provides a GFI with scores ranging from 1 to 50 indicating *no fatigue* to *severe fatigue* (Belza et al., 2005). The GFI has been shown to be sensitive to changes in the level of fatigue and as such is useful as a monitoring tool for patient response to treatment and rehabilitation. The report of activity interference may provide a more sensitive measure for assessing changes in fatigue or evaluation of the success of an intervention.

The fourth characteristic can be assessed through correlates of fatigue by evaluation of comorbidities and primary conditions, exacerbations, side effects of treatment, and psychosocial factors (Wagner & Cella, 2004). The measurement of comorbidities and primary conditions requires attention to anemias, nutritional status, thyroid function, and infection. Additional correlates affecting fatigue that should be measured include sleep disturbance, changes in function, depression and anxiety, chronic pain, and adjustment to chronic illness. The Profile of Mood States (POMS; McNair, Lorr, & Droppleman, 1996) is also a well-established measure of mood disturbance and includes subscales that measure fatigue and vigor.

These fatigue-rating scales are best used in research studies. A brief visual rating scale is recommended as the most efficient assessment tool for clinical practice (Hinds, Yang, & Gattuso, 2010). The measure may include one or two items that ask the client to rate the severity of fatigue from 1 (no fatigue) to 10 (severe fatigue), and/or the degree to which fatigue prevents or interferes with desired daily activities (degree of impairment from fatigue), also from 1 (no interference) to 10 (severe interference). A cut score of about 5 has been suggested for 10-point scales, or 3 for 4- to 5-point scales, so that persons with at least moderate fatigue will be captured (Butt et al., 2008; Kirsh, Passik, Holtsclaw, Donaghy, & Theobald, 2001; Wagner & Cella, 2004). Clinicians should consistently use the same scale and give the same instructions each time. The patient should be asked to rate his or her fatigue at the time of assessment and in the last 24 hours.

■ MANAGEMENT OF FATIGUE

The goal of the management of fatigue is to achieve the best quality of life that is possible given the patient's specific circumstances. Having the energy to do what is important to the person so that he or she may finalize specific tasks or interact in special relationships is a valuable outcome for treatment. Within the context of palliative care, the management of fatigue must be determined in relation to its ability to protect individuals from activities that may lead to suffering and subsequent detrimental consequences (Radbruch et al., 2008). The impact of fatigue on the quality of life in patients at the end of life must be considered by nurses delivering palliative care.

Interventions for fatigue may focus on treating symptoms that exacerbate fatigue, thereby preventing fatigue from progressing to extreme exhaustion from which there may be no means of recovery (Olson, Krawchuk, & Quddusi, 2007). Nurses may assist patients and families to balance rest with activity and identify those activities that increase fatigue or that restore energy. Interventions for fatigue include nonpharmacological and pharmacological management, and are selected in accordance with the underlying cause of the fatigue. A multistage approach is recommended in the NCCN Cancer-Related Fatigue Guidelines: (a) screening of patients for the presence of fatigue; (b) evaluation of fatigue to determine its intensity or severity and its relationship to the stage of underlying disease processes; (c) management with nonpharmacological and pharmacological interventions; and (d) reevaluation of the patients for improvement, alleviation of symptoms, or worsening of condition followed by effective adjustment of management strategies (NCCN, 2013).

Learning to cope with fatigue is important for promoting quality of life. Energy-conserving strategies may be used to manage and alter the fatigue. Specifically avoid unnecessary or excessive use of energy by pacing yourself and taking extra rest periods; restore energy to avoid further deconditioning and deterioration in physical functioning by keeping the muscles strong through exercising; and continue to be self-reliant by asking for help only when necessary, while taking into account the possibility of escalating fatigue at the end of life (NCCN, 2013). Encourage patients to rejuvenate their energy through relaxation strategies such as "sitting down and resting," "putting your feet up with a cup of tea," and resting before activities by reading, watching television, or taking relaxing baths. In a case report of a retired nurse at the end of life, fatigue was described in association with a myriad of symptoms including anemia, weight loss, loss of interest, social isolation, dyspnea, chronic pain, deconditioning, and medications (Yennurajalingam & Bruera, 2007). This patient refused testing for additional medical information that was not directed at improving her quality of life, an important point that highlights the importance of patient autonomy. It was important to the patient and her palliative care team that her symptoms be evaluated for the purpose of determining which interventions might reduce fatigue, thereby improving her quality of life (Yennurajalingam & Bruera, 2007).

Nonpharmacological Interventions

Nonpharmacological interventions for fatigue include education/cognitive interventions, exercise, energy balance and conservation, and nutritional considerations (Table 25.3). Education/cognitive interventions include preparatory information and anticipatory guidance regarding the likelihood of fatigue as a side effect of many treatment options, the disease itself, or the emotional reaction to the disease. It should be a standard of care that patients are educated about CRF to empower them to anticipate fatigue patterns and apply early home interventions (Borneman, 2013; Ream, 2007).

People are typically comforted to know that fatigue is often an expected outcome with illness, and not a sign of disease progression. An analogy that can be helpful in conceptualizing fatigue is of fatigue as a depletion of a "bank account" of energy. Patients are encouraged to plan the pace of activities for conservation of energy so that there is sufficient energy for selected, though perhaps fewer, activities (Ream, 2007). There is also a recommendation for acupressure or acupuncture for the relief of fatigue as has been demonstrated in patients with end-stage renal disease (Cho & Tsay, 2004; McDougall, 2005).

Patients may be encouraged to keep a daily journal to identify the factors and activities associated with fatigue, energy depletion, and its restoration (Radbruch et al., 2008). The journal could provide a daily entry regarding information learned about engagement in activities, level of energy or fatigue, and impact of treatment on energy or fatigue. Such a journal will also help patients communicate with the healthcare provider regarding various concerns that may be alleviated by effective symptom management. The journal provides the practitioner with objective evidence of how the patient is doing on a day-to-day basis and may then counsel the patient to plan his or her schedule to optimize peak energy times for high-priority tasks. The patient is then encouraged to accept help from available support persons for remaining tasks (Borneman, 2013).

Exercise is an effective intervention for older adults who are fatigued and has been shown to reduce fatigue and increase overall feelings of physical and psychological well-being (Borneman, 2013; Puetz, O'Connor, & Dishman, 2006). Exercise can take place in a structured rehabilitation or physical therapy department, particularly for those who would benefit from rehabilitation therapy for neuro-musculoskeletal deficits and for those who are fatigued due to cardiac or respiratory problems (Cramp & Daniel, 2008; Przybylowski et al., 2007). For others, there may be simply a personal commitment to walk outdoors on a regular basis. Whichever is chosen, the exercise program should be individualized with consideration for the patient's physical condition and other medical problems.

Patients should be instructed not to exercise to exhaustion, but to conduct activities over several days of the week to be most beneficial. Movement can prevent loss of muscle tone that is difficult to regain and helps reduce the incidence of falls. Endorphins are released with even the slightest activity, resulting in increased mood and well-being. Exercise that utilizes the entire body will help maintain tone, strength, and flexibility. Walking, swimming, gardening, or golf are all good considerations; encourage the patient to exercise at least 6 hours before his or her typical bedtime so that the patient will not have difficulty falling asleep.

For patients with progressive illness, Potter, Hami, Bryan, and Quigley (2003) suggest that more appropriate than admitting patients to rehabilitation centers (which have a daily exercise program of 4 hours a day) is admission of these patients to a palliative care unit. On the palliative care unit, the majority of time can be devoted to promoting quality of life and comfort, and the patient does not have to watch others improve dramatically while he or she is just too tired to participate. This approach balances quality of life and the limited amount of therapy, which may be better tolerated.

Energy use and conservation involves finding a balance between rest and exercise that will give patients the most energy to do the things that they would like to do. Sleep disturbances, including insomnia, have been shown to be components of CRF and should be treated (Rao & Cohen, 2004). Although patients may believe that more rest and sleep will increase energy, sleep is not restorative of energy in chronic conditions associated with fatigue. Rao and Cohen suggest that the patient sleep no longer than 8 hours, which establishes a more solid, less-fragmented sleep pattern. Waking up and going to sleep at the same time each day strengthens the circadian cycles, the disruption of which can contribute to depression. Since cancer patients have been shown to have worse sleep quality and more sleep disturbance (Dambrosio & Mazanec, 2013; Fernandes, Stone, Andrews, Morgan, & Sharma, 2006), strategies for establishing rest and sleep patterns may assist in improving sleep quality. Strategies noted by nursing home residents in a study in Taiwan included taking prescribed medicines, lying down, changing position in bed, or taking a walk and thinking pleasant thoughts (Tsai, Wong, & Ku, 2008).

In a review of nonpharmacological management of fatigue in patients with specific autoimmune conditions including MS, systemic lupus erythematosus, and rheumatoid arthritis, recommendations were in the categories of low- to moderate-impact exercise, behavioral therapies (self-help information, readings, life modifications), and physiological treatment of symptoms (Neill, Belan, & Ried, 2006). Additionally, a review of fatigue among health professionals offered several strategies that may also be applicable: encourage individuals to have some exposure to outside light each day, avoid bright light before bedtime, and establish a specific bedtime (with routines to prepare for sleep) and wake time (Borneman, 2013; Owens, 2007). In addition to an established

TABLE 25.3 Pharmacological Therapies for the Treatment of Fatigue

Class of Drug	Examples	Mechanism of Action	Comments
Corticosteroids glucocorticoids	Dexamethasone (4 mg BID) (Yennurajalingam et al., 2013) Prednisone Prednisolone (10–160 mg in 2–3 divided doses 30–45 minutes before meals) Methyl-prednisolone Hydrocortisone	Mechanism of action is unclear. Low dosing recommended. Duration and benefits limited to weeks. May boost appetite and energy; improve activity levels and strength.	May mask the signs of acute infections. Use at the end of life after ruling out other causes of fatigue (National Consensus Project for Quality Palliative Care, 2013) Evidence is inconclusive regarding lessening of fatigue; effectiveness may be short lived (Radbruch et al., 2008).
Stimulants	Methylphenidate (5–20 mg daily or BID) Dextroamphetamine (2.5–5 mg daily or BID) and Pemoline (18.75 mg daily or BID) have been used anecdotally. Modafinil (200 mg in the morning; with titration up to 400 mg daily) Amantadine	Stimulates CNS and respiratory centers, increases appetite and energy levels, improves mood, reduces sedation (Breitbart & Alici, 2008). Inhibits GABA; promotes release of neurotransmitters dopamine, norepinephrine, and serotonin, which promotes wakefulness. Centrally acting: affects cholinergic, dopaminergic, adrenergic, glutamatergic neurotransmission	Titrate to effect. Rapid onset of action, fewer side effects than many antidepressants. May cause agitation (Beers, Berkow, Bogin, Fletcher, & Rahman, 2000). Risk of toxicity increases with dose. No controlled comparisons between efficacies of each of these drugs. Response to one does not predict response to others. Sequential trials to determine the most useful drug is suggested (Breitbart & Alici, 2008). Routine use of stimulants in palliative care is controversial as related to evaluation of evidence, and concerns that fatigue at the end of life may not be responsive (Silveira et al., 2017).
Antidepressant ■ Selective serotonin reuptake inhibitors (SSRIs) ■ Norepinephrine dopamine reuptake inhibitor	Trazodone (25–50 mg at bedtime, increase to 25–50 mg/d as tolerated to a maximum of 300 mg/d; Beers et al., 2000) Paroxetine (20 mg) Fluoxetine (10 mg) Sertraline (25 mg) Bupropion (100 mg daily for 3 days, then 100 mg TID at least 6 hours apart)	Reduces depressive symptoms associated with fatigue. Can improve sleep. Primary choice for treatment of depression in cancer patients. Inhibits serotonin reuptake Acts as a stimulant	Give once daily in the morning. Some SSRIs have long half-lives and should be used cautiously in the terminally ill older adult.
Tricyclic antidepressants	Amitriptyline (10–25 mg qhs) Nortriptyline (25 mg 3–4 times daily)	Block reuptake of various neurotransmitters at the neuronal membrane. Can improve sleep.	Amitriptyline contraindicated in patients on MAOIs or post MI. Use with caution in elders with cardiovascular disease; adverse reaction includes arrhythmias.
Cholinesterase inhibitors	Donepezil (5 mg hs; can increase to 10 mg after 4–6 weeks, maximum dose 23 mg after 3 months)	Reversible acetylcholinesterase inhibitor	
Erythropoietin	150–300 units/kg SQ three times a week	Increases hemoglobin with effects on energy, activity, and overall quality of life while decreasing transfusion requirements (Glaspy, Degos, Dicato, & Demetri, 2002).	Monitor hematocrit and reduce dose if it approaches 36% or increases by greater than 4 points in 2 weeks. Safety concerns associated with higher mortality rates and thromboembolism have resulted in these drugs, which are not recommended in the treatment of CRF (Minton, Richardson, Sharpe, Hotopf, & Stone, 2010)

BID, twice a day; CNS, central nervous system; CRF, chronic renal failure; GABA, gamma-aminobutyric acid; hs, at bedtime; MAOI, monoamine oxidase inhibitor; MI, myocardial infarction; qhs, every day at bed time; SQ, subcutaneous; TID, three times a day.

bedtime, a light bedtime snack and something warm to drink promotes sleep.

Bedtime routines can help the reticular activating system in the brain shut down for about the last half-hour in readying for sleep. Strategies to promote a restful sleep also include the reduction of environmental stimuli (e.g., noise, light), diversional activities to encourage sleep (music, aromatherapy, massage), and the avoidance of alcohol and stimulants (e.g., caffeine, nicotine, steroids). Adjusting the room temperature and humidity, as well as using pillows, may also be helpful in providing support and comfort. Neill, Belan, and Ried (2006) concluded that cooling activities should be tailored to the comfort of the individual and may include cool baths or placing the extremities in cool water. If the patient is unable to fall asleep in 20 minutes, suggest getting out of bed, going into another room to read with a dim light, and returning to bed when he or she gets sleepy.

It is important to acknowledge that fatigue is not a sequestered symptom but one that will affect all aspects of a person's life. As such, patients will need to save their energy and plan for activities that are very important to them. They should be asked what activities they enjoy most and be encouraged to schedule those activities for the time of the day that they have the most energy. Breaks should be scheduled during activities to help restore energy levels, and taking short therapeutic naps (15–20 minutes) between 3 p.m. and 5 p.m. tends to be more restoring than getting into a longer, deeper sleep (Owens, 2007). Energy conservation techniques should be reinforced; for example, do activities sitting down, use a power scooter for grocery shopping, store frequently used items at chest level to avoid bending and stretching, put a terry robe on after the shower instead of using energy to dry off, or wear slip-on shoes. Providing devices such as a raised toilet seat, a reaching device, or a walker can also help conserve energy for people with progressive fatigue.

Patients should also be encouraged to ask for help with specific chores. Some find this type of interdependence as very threatening; try to help them see their energy as something to be "budgeted" and used for something that they enjoy or that is very important for them to do. Jakobsson, Hallberg, and Westergren (2007) studied factors related to quality of life among older adults who were dependent on others for help with daily living and who were in pain. Their findings underscored the importance of evaluating and treating the complexity of accompanying symptoms, including fatigue and depression. The elderly population should be encouraged to feel that they have the option to "spend" their energy on anything that they wish, yet being mindful of their energy as a limited resource. Often reframing their fatigue as one of their resources gives them the enfranchisement that they need to ask for help.

Spending time with family and friends is also very important in promoting a sense of well-being, which may lessen the perception of fatigue. Prioritizing who they would like to visit with can be helpful, as well as planning such visits at a time of day when the patient has the most energy to avoid excessive fatigue. Health professionals may also assist in addressing the negative impact of psychological and social stressors and how to avoid or modify them.

Warth et al. report that while music therapy has been used successfully for over 30 years as part of palliative care programs for severely ill patients, there are few randomized controlled trials studying the effect of music on symptom management. This study compared live music–based relaxation exercises to a control group of verbal relaxation exercises. Music therapy did not differ from control treatment with respect to pain reduction ($F = 0.4$; $p = .53$), but it led to a significantly greater reduction in the fatigue score on the quality-of-life scale ($F = 4.74$; $p = .03$) (Warth, Kesler, Hillecke, & Bardenheuer, 2015).

Nutritional status is also an important consideration; eating low-fat foods and several small meals in a day and avoiding high-sugar foods result in less energy used for digestion. Given that nutrition and hydration are important in preventing fatigue, increasing fluids may be of benefit, unless contraindicated by other medical problems. Protein intake and supplements can also be encouraged if the patient is having trouble with regular food. Recent data suggest that for patients with CFS, equal benefit was experienced from a low-sugar, low-yeast dietary regimen or from a diet of healthy eating, with evidence of decreased fatigue and improved quality of life (Hobday, Thomas, O'Donovan, Murphy, & Pinching, 2008). The healthy-eating control group and the low-sugar, low-yeast treatment group each demonstrated difficulty maintaining compliance with dietary recommendations. Food intake and appetite entries might be a helpful addition to a daily journal for some patients, though food journaling was not found helpful (Hobday et al., 2008). Pharmacological interventions may be necessary to boost appetite and energy.

Pharmacological Management of Fatigue

Palliative care for the fatigued patient is different from the management typically provided for other symptoms. Pharmacological management of other symptoms in palliative care often involves medications that are available to treat the actual cause of the symptom. Yet with fatigue, the cause may not be treatable, and in many cases, medications may not be the primary intervention for this symptom. Furthermore, each medication that the patient receives should be reviewed for its potential for producing sedation and fatigue. Symptoms such as vomiting and pain should be optimally treated as their relief often decreases associated fatigue, thus improving feelings of general well-being. Patients should be made aware that the fatigue experienced with opioid therapy may decrease as tolerance to opioids develops. Optimizing the use of non-opioid analgesics and adjuvant therapies may also reduce fatigue associated with pain management. Treatment of pro-inflammatory cytokines (tumor necrosis factor) has been associated with improvements in symptoms of fatigue.

In addition to treating symptoms such as pain, vomiting, or dyspnea (which may induce fatigue), other medications such as corticosteroids, stimulants, and antidepressants have been of benefit (Table 25.3). There is empirical support for the use of low-dose corticosteroids for patients with fatigue and loss of general feelings of well-being, with recommendations for withdrawal of the medication if improvement does not occur within 5 to 7 days (Ream, 2007; Ream & Stone, 2004). Corticosteroids can improve appetite and elevate mood, resulting in an improved sense of well-being, although the duration of effect may be limited. It must be remembered, however, that corticosteroids may easily be overlooked as a contributor to fatigue (Cornuz, Guessous, & Favrat, 2006). Most commonly, dexamethasone 1 to 2 mg twice daily or prednisone 5 to 10 mg twice daily is prescribed.

In a review of the pharmacological treatment of CRF, the psychostimulant methylphenidate (Ritalin) was found to reduce fatigue over a period of 5 weeks when compared to placebo (Minton, Richardson, Sharpe, Hotopf, & Stone, 2008). Dosing of 10 to 20 mg/d is recommended, based on patient improvement over a period of 2 to 5 weeks (Minton et al., 2008; Ream, 2007). The dose can be gradually increased until favorable effects occur or until toxicities, such as anorexia, insomnia, anxiety, confusion, tremor, or tachycardia, supervene. A randomized, double-blind, placebo-controlled trial indicated that dextroamphetamine produced short-term reduction in fatigue in survivors of breast cancer, patients with advanced cancer, and persons with HIV (Auret, Schug, Bremner, & Bulsara, 2009). Benefits were short lived, however, with no continuation of improvement noted after the duration of the study (8 days). Preliminary data support the use of modafinil to promote wakefulness in persons with advanced cancer, and mixed results have been reported on the use of antidepressants (Breitbart & Alici, 2008). To limit toxicities in the medically ill population, dose escalation should be undertaken with caution, and over longer intervals (Portenoy, 2003).

When fatigue is associated with clinical depression, a trial of an antidepressant drug is appropriate. Depression and CRF may occur as separate conditions and should be treated accordingly (Minton et al., 2008). Antidepressants such as serotonin-specific reuptake inhibitors (SSRIs) have fewer side effects than older antidepressants and are preferred in patients with such chronic conditions as ischemic heart disease, hypertrophic prostatic conditions, or glaucoma that is not controlled (Rao & Cohen, 2004). SSRIs are not associated with food and drug interaction restrictions. A sedating antidepressant can provide peaceful sleep as well as mitigating the depression; potential neurological and cardiac disadvantages may be of a lesser concern for the dying elder or for the palliative care patient at the end of life.

If the patient has had chemotherapy, the fatigue may be a result of anemia or vitamin deficiency. Treatment with recombinant erythropoietin has been shown in randomized studies to increase hemoglobin level, which improves the energy levels and quality of life of patients with CRF (Minton et al., 2008; Ream, 2007), although the impact on the intensity of fatigue may be limited in advanced cancer states (Yennurajalingam et al., 2013). When the hemoglobin level returns to 11 g/dL or 12 g/dL, many of the symptoms of anemia are assuaged.

Treatment may also include addressing such nutrient deficiencies as iron, folate, vitamin B_{12}, or vitamin D_3. Martínez-Alonso, Dusso, Ariza, and Nabal (2016) conducted a cross-sectional study of adults with metastatic cancer to assess the relationship of vitamin D deficiency with health-related quality-of-life issues, fatigue, and physical functioning. They found that among 30 patients in palliative care with advanced solid cancer, 90% were vitamin D deficient. Serum vitamin D concentration was positively correlated with patient-reported absence of fatigue ($s = 0.49$) and physical and functional well-being ($s = 0.44$ and $s = 0.41$, respectively, $p < .01$). Fatigue was the symptom with the highest median impact on their lives and was the only one associated with serum vitamin D ($p = .031$), with lower fatigue in patients with higher vitamin D concentrations. This study indicates that vitamin D supplementation was a potential therapy to enhance the quality of life of patients living with cancer (Martínez-Alonso et al., 2016).

Anemia can also be treated with blood transfusions, but this intervention is not without risks to the patient's health and carries the potential of increasing healthcare costs in the wake of transfusion complications. Risks associated with blood transfusions include systemic infections (e.g., HIV; hepatitis A, B, C) from inadequate screening of the blood supply, acute hemolytic reactions, bacterial contamination, subtle immune modulation, transfusion graft versus host disease, iron overload, and allergic reactions including urticaria and anaphylaxis (Yennurajalingam et al., 2013).

It is important to evaluate the efficacy of both pharmacological and nonpharmacological fatigue interventions on a regular basis. Systematic documentation regarding the assessment, management, and evaluation of the success of the interventions in relieving fatigue is essential to quality care.

■ FATIGUE IN FAMILY CAREGIVERS

Family caregivers are often profoundly fatigued by the stressors inherent in caregiving. Caregivers bear the physical and emotional burden of assisting patients with activities of daily living, as well as with treatments.

They often must assume new roles and responsibilities and at times deal with additional financial distress. As a result, family caregivers may also develop anxiety or depressive disorders associated with fatigue. Severe family fatigue is commonly experienced in four situations: (1) inadequate relief of patient's pain and suffering; (2) inadequate resources to cope with home care; (3) unrealistic expectations of family caregivers of themselves or professional healthcare supports; and (4) emotional distress that persists even when there is adequate relief of patient suffering (Johansen, Cvancarova, & Ruland, 2018; Kim, Shaffer, Carver, & Cannady, 2016; Weiss et al., 2016).

Palliative care practitioners recognize the patient and family as the unit of care, and therefore, assessment and interventions to relieve caregiver burden are essential. Validating the needs and concerns of family caregivers is important. Helping family caregivers to set priorities with regard to competing demands, optimizing stress and coping strategies, encouraging relaxation and rest, while assisting caregivers with respite care are important interventions in preventing or alleviating caregiver fatigue (National Cancer Institute, 2017).

■ CONCLUSION

Healthcare professionals view fatigue as a clue to illness, a side effect of therapeutic intervention, progressive illness, the residual physical change of illness and treatment, or the psychological and emotional strain of illness or caregiving. To the patient and his or her family, fatigue is a symptom that keeps them from moving forward fully with life. Health professionals can be supportive by acknowledging fatigue as real and taking fatigue and its frustrations seriously. Understanding the possible etiology of fatigue and the meaning of the symptom to the patient are important in determining its management. Assisting patients to live fully as they move along the illness trajectory may require the consideration of nonpharmacological as well as pharmacological therapies to comprehensively and effectively treat fatigue. Learning how to prevent fatigue and/or restore energy is important for improving the elder patient's function, his or her ability to socialize, and ultimately the patient's adjustment to a "new normal" baseline as he or she lives with a life-limiting or chronic illness.

CASE STUDY Conclusion

Mrs. Ronde's fatigue was managed through several therapeutic approaches. Laboratory data revealed that Dee's vitamin B_{12} and folate were within normal limits; vitamin D 25-hydroxy (vit D_3) 11.8 ($n = 20–100$); iron 40 ($n = 40–150$); total iron-binding capacity 264 ($n = 250–400$); and iron saturation 11% ($n = 20–55$). The nurse practitioner started her on iron supplements 325 mg BID (with a stool softener to prevent constipation); vitamin D_3 50,000 units weekly for 10 weeks; and venlafaxine 75 mg at bedtime for depression, hot flashes, and neuropathic pain management.

The discussion with Mr. and Mrs. Ronde focused on eating a well-balanced diet and suggesting that perhaps their church members could help with meals a few times a week. Dee agreed that her right leg was weak from surgery and radiation treatment and accepted a referral to physical therapy and cancer rehabilitation with the goal to promote muscle tone, increase endorphin levels, decrease fatigue, and improve mood and sense of well-being. The palliative care nurse helped Ms. Ronde to learn to balance rest with activity, begin to allow her husband to help with household chores, prioritize activities, and carry out activities when she had the greatest energy. Mrs. Ronde was comforted by an understanding that fatigue is a common response to surgery, chemotherapy, and radiation for up to 5 years, rather than considering her fatigue as indicative of disease progression.

Dee's assessment indicated that she was depressed, which exacerbated her perception of fatigue. To treat her depressive symptoms, Dee agreed to a referral to the supportive care psychologist to discuss her feelings and fears (talk therapy). She was counseled regarding strategies to promote a restful night's sleep, including establishing regular bedtime routines and a quiet, relaxing environment. The plan of care involved continual evaluation of the efficacy of such interventions for fatigue. During the follow-up evaluation, Dee expressed a lessening of fatigue, greater sense of control, and improvement in health-related quality of life.

AN INTERDISCIPLINARY CASE STUDY RESPONSE

Kim Hester, DC, FASA
Chiropractor

Mrs. Dee Ronde has had her fourth child within 4 years, the youngest of which is 10 months old. Having four children within that time frame would put pressure on nerves in the spine and affect the elasticity of the ligaments without allowing time for the ligaments to heal. During pregnancy, many women develop low-back pain and sciatica, and chiropractic care would help decrease the stress from the ligaments becoming lax in the pelvic area and spine. Chiropractic care would be needed to restore the proper alignment of the spine and help with the left hip pain (Chan, Tan, Xin, Sudarsanam, & Johnson, 2010).

Additionally, Mrs. Ronde has depleted most of her kidney "Jing." Traditional Chinese Medicine (TCM) expresses that these traits are passed down from one parent to another. Jing means that we all have primordial energy that can be turned into whatever energy is needed in the body (i.e., yin, yang, blood, qi). The problem is that we only get so much "Jing" energy and some people have less than others. People who are born with abundant "Jing" are more able to withstand pain and age well; those with less Jing are just the opposite (Kaptchuk, 2000). This explains why some people abuse their bodies and do just fine while others are delicate and sickly even with good habits. It depends on our abundance of Jing stored in our kidneys.

Jing is stored in the kidneys and is necessary for providing energy. People who abuse their bodies with poor diet and lifestyle habits use more Jing during their lives. People who have healthy diets and habits conserve their Jing.

I believe that Mrs. Dee Ronde has depleted all her Jing from the kidneys due to the many child births she has had over the past 4 years, and her cancer diagnosis and treatment further depleted her. Mrs. Ronde had been experiencing soaking sweats throughout the day, and that is alarming from a TCM standpoint. TCM is a universal law of the yin and the yang, which is an endless cycle. Everything is manifested as (qi) energy. Qi is characterized by five phases: Fire, Earth, Metal, Water, and Wood. The Fire element has the pericardium, heart, small intestine, and triple warmer meridians. The Earth has the stomach and spleen meridians. The Metal element has the lung and large intestine meridians. The Water has the bladder and kidney meridians. The Wood has the liver and gallbladder meridians. The Sheng Cycle consists of these phases in a clockwise manner (Figure 25.1).

Fire creates Earth, Earth is necessary for Fire, and without Earth all other phases would not exist. In the center of the circle is a pentagram representing the Ko Cycle. The Ko Cycle consists of the orderly movement from Fire to Metal to Wood to Earth to Water to Fire in a clockwise pentagram star presentation.

The Sheng Cycle is anabolic and the Ko Cycle is catabolic. The two cycles restrain each other and must be in balance. Mrs. Ronde also has an imbalance at the Water element (i.e., kidneys and bladder); therefore, I would use a Water element as a Chinese formula to put out the Fire she is having with the excessive sweating. The prescription of treatment would be a specific chiropractic adjustment to all areas needed along her spine, acupuncture treatment for balance, and pain management along with a Chinese element Water formula. The nervous system and acupuncture meridians need to be free of any interference for improvement in her health and to eliminate the fatigue. Diet and proper exercise are important and would be monitored throughout her treatment.

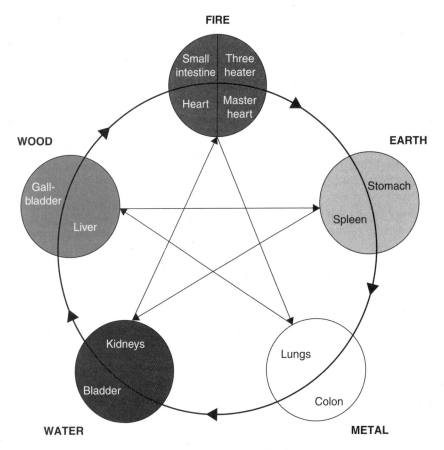

FIGURE 25.1 The Sheng and Ko Cycle.

Evidence-Based Practice

Peters, M. E. W. J., Goedendorp, M. M., Verhagen, C. A. H. H. V. M., Bleijenberg, G., & van der Graaf, W. T. A. (2016). Fatigue and its associated psychosocial factors in cancer patients on active palliative treatment measured over time. *Supportive Care in Cancer, 24*, 1349–1355. doi:10.1007/s00520-015-2909-0

Purpose
Fatigue is a frequently reported symptom by patients with advanced cancer, but hardly any prospective information is available about fatigue while on treatment in the palliative setting. In a previous cross-sectional study, several factors were found to contribute to fatigue in people living with cancer. This study investigated the course of fatigue over time and whether psychosocial factors were associated with fatigue over time.

Methods
Patients on cancer treatment for incurable solid tumors were observed over 6 months. Patients filled in the Individual Strength Check monthly to measure the course of fatigue. Baseline questionnaires were used to measure disease acceptance, anxiety, depressive mood, fatigue catastrophizing, sleeping problems, discrepancies in social support, and self-reported physical activity for their relation with fatigue over time.

Results

At baseline, 137 patients participated; after 6 months, 89 patients participated. The mean duration of participation was 4.9 months. At most time points, fatigue scores were significantly higher in the group dropouts in comparison with the group participating for 6 months (completers). Overall fatigue levels remained stable over time for the majority of participants. In the completers, 42% never experienced severe fatigue, 29% persisted being severely fatigued, and others had either an increasing or a decreasing level. Of the investigated factors, low reported physical activity and nonacceptance of cancer were associated significantly to fatigue.

Conclusions

A substantial number of participants never experienced severe fatigue, and fatigue levels remained stable over time. For those who do experience severe fatigue, nonacceptance of having incurable cancer and low self-reported physical activity may be fatigue-perpetuating factors.

Reprinted by permission from Springer Nature: Peters, M. E. W. J., Goedendorp, M. M., Verhagen, C. A. H. H. V. M., Bleijenberg, G., & van der Graaf, W. T. A. (2016). Fatigue and its associated psychosocial factors in cancer patients on active palliative treatment measured over time. *Supportive Care in Cancer, 24,* 1349–1355.

■ REFERENCES

Aaronson, L. S., Pallikkathayil, L., & Crighton, F. (2003). A qualitative investigation of fatigue among healthy working adults. *Western Journal of Nursing Research, 25*(4), 419–433. doi:10.1177/0193945903025004007

Aaronson, L. S., Teel, C. S., Cassmeyer, V., Neuberger, G. B., Pallikkathayil, L., Pierce, J., … Wingate, A. (1999). State of the science: Defining and measuring fatigue. *Image: Journal of Nursing Scholarship, 31*(1), 45–50. doi:10.1111/j.1547-5069.1999.tb00420.x

Alexander, K. P. (2016). Identifying the frailty phenotype: The evidence for good enough. *American Heart Journal, 182,* 144–145. doi:10.1016/j.ahj.2016.09.005

Al-Osali, M. E. N., Al Qassabi, S. S. A., & Al-Harthi, S. M. (2013). Is the patient fatigued or weak? *Journal of Medicine and Medical Sciences, 4*(7), 258–262.

American Psychiatric Association. (2013). *Diagnostic and statistical manual of mental disorders* (5th ed.). Arlington, VA: American Psychiatric Association.

Anderson, W. G., Puntillo, K., Boyle, D., Barbour, S., Turner, K., Cimino, J., … Pearson, D. (2016). ICU bedside nurses' involvement in palliative care communication: A multicenter survey. *Journal of Pain and Symptom Management, 51*(3), 589–596. e582. doi:10.1016/j.jpainsymman.2015.11.003

Anish, E. J. (2005). Exercise and its effects on the central nervous system. *Current Sports Medicine Reports, 4*(1), 18–23. doi:10.1097/01.CSMR.0000306066.14026.77

Auret, K. A., Schug, S. A., Bremner, A. P., & Bulsara, M. (2009). A randomized, double-blind, placebo-controlled trial assessing the impact of dexamphetamine on fatigue in patients with advanced cancer. *Journal of Pain & Symptom Management, 37*(4), 613–621. doi:10.1016/j.jpainsymman.2008.03.016

Austin, J., Williams, W. R., & Hutchison, S. (2012). Patterns of fatigue in elderly heart failure patients measured by a quality of life scale (Minnesota living with heart failure). *European Journal of Cardiovascular Nursing: Journal of the Working Group on Cardiovascular Nursing of the European Society of Cardiology, 11*(4), 439–444. doi:10.1016/j.ejcnurse.2011.04.002

Avlund, K. (2010). Fatigue in older adults: An early indicator of the aging process? *Aging Clinical and Experimental Research, 22*(2), 100–115. doi:10.1007/bf03324782

Badger, T. A., Segrin, C., & Meek, P. (2011). Development and validation of an instrument for rapidly assessing symptoms: The general symptom distress scale. *Journal of Pain & Symptom Management, 41*(3), 535–548. doi:10.1016/j.jpainsymman.2010.06.011

Balducci, L. (2010). Anemia, fatigue and aging. *Transfusion Clinique Et Biologique: Journal De La Société Française De Transfusion Sanguine, 17*(5–6), 375–381. doi:10.1016/j.tracli.2010.09.169

Barroso, J., Hammill, B. G., Leserman, J., Salahuddin, N., Harmon, J. L., & Pence, B. W. (2010). Physiological and psychosocial factors that predict HIV-related fatigue. *AIDS and Behavior, 14*(6), 1415–1427. doi:10.1007/s10461-010-9691-2

Barroso, J., & Voss, J. G. (2013). Fatigue in HIV and AIDS: An analysis of evidence. *JANAC: Journal of the Association of Nurses in AIDS Care, 24*(1), S5–S14. doi:10.1016/j.jana.2012.07.003

Bascom, P. B. (2013). Dyspnea can be, and should be, effectively palliated with opioids. *Journal of Palliative Medicine, 16*(5), 465. doi:10.1089/jpm.2012.0584

Beers, M. H., Berkow, R., Bogin, R. M., Fletcher, A. J., & Rahman, M. I. (2000). *The Merck manual of geriatrics.* Whitehouse Station, NJ: Merck Research Laboratories.

Belza, B., Henke, C. J., Yelin, E. H., Epstain, W. V., & Gillis, C. L. (1993). Correlates of fatigue in older adults with rheumatoid arthritis. *Nursing Research, 42,* 93–99. doi:10.1097/00006199-199303000-00006

Belza, B., Steele, B. G., Cain, K., Coppersmith, J., Howard, J., & Lakshminarayan, S. (2005). Seattle Obstructive Lung Disease Questionnaire: Sensitivity to outcomes in pulmonary rehabilitation in severe pulmonary illness. *Journal of Cardiopulmonary Rehabilitation, 25*(2), 107–114. doi:10.1097/00008483-200503000-00011

Belza, B., Steele, B. G., Hunziker, J., Lakshminaryan, S., Holt, L., & Buchner, D. M. (2001). Correlates of physical activity in chronic obstructive pulmonary disease. *Nursing Research, 50*(4), 195–202. doi:10.1097/00006199-200107000-00003

Bhat, S., & Chokroverty, S. (2017). Clinical and neurophysiological aspects of fatigue. In S. Chokroverty, & L. Ferini-Strambi (Eds.), *Oxford Textbook of Sleep Disorders*, (pp. 345–359). Oxford, England: Oxford University Press.

Bhui, K. S., Dinos, S., Ashby, D., Nazroo, J., Wessely, S., & White, P. D. (2011). Chronic fatigue syndrome in an ethnically diverse population: The influence of psychosocial adversity and physical inactivity. *BMC Medicine, 9*(1), 26–37. doi:10.1186/1741-7015-9-26

Björnsson, E., Simren, M., Olsson, R., & Chapman, R. W. (2005). Fatigue is not a specific symptom in patients with primary biliary cirrhosis. *European Journal of Gastroenterology & Hepatology, 17*(3), 351–357. doi:10.1097/00042737-200503000-00015

Bormann, J., Shivley, M., Smith, T. L., & Gifford, A. L. (2001). Measurment of fatigue in HIV-positive adults: Reliability and validity of the Global Fatigue Index. *Journal of the Association of Nurses in AIDS Care, 12*(3), 75–83. doi:10.1016/S1055-3290(06)60146-5

Borneman, T. (2013). Assessment and managent of caner-related fatigue. *Journal of Hospice and Palliative Nursing, 15*(2), 77–88. doi:10.1097/NJH.0b013e318286dc19

Bower, J. E., Ganz, P. A., Irwin, M. R., Kwan, L., Breen, E. C., & Cole, S. W. (2011). Inflammation and behavioral symptoms after breast cancer treatment: Do fatigue, depression, and sleep disturbance share a common underlying mechanism? *Journal of Clinical Oncology: Official Journal of the American Society of Clinical Oncology, 29*(26), 3517–3522. doi:10.1200/JCO.2011.36.1154

Bower, J. E., & Lamkin, D. M. (2013). Inflammation and cancer-related fatigue: Mechanisms, contributing factors, and treatment implications. *Brain, Behavior, and Immunity, 30*, S48–S57. doi:10.1016/j.bbi.2012.06.011

Breitbart, W., & Alici, Y. (2008). Pharmacologic treatment options for cancer-related fatigue: Current state of clinical research. *Clinical Journal of Oncology Nursing, 12*(5), 27–36. doi:10.1188/08.CJON.S2.27-36

Broxterman, R. M., Layec, G., Hureau, T. J., Amann, M., & Richardson, R. S. (2017). Skeletal muscle bioenergetics during all-out exercise: Mechanistic insight into the oxygen uptake slow component and neuromuscular fatigue. *Journal of Applied Physiology, 122*(5), 1208–1217. doi:10.1152/japplphysiol.01093.2016

Butt, Z., Lai, J.-S., Rao, D., Heinemann, A. W., Bill, A., & Cella, D. (2013). Measurement of fatigue in cancer, stroke, and HIV using the Functional Assessment of Chronic Illness Therapy—Fatigue (FACIT-F) scale. *Journal of Psychosomatic Research, 74*(1), 64–68. doi:10.1016/j.jpsychores.2012.10.011

Butt, Z., Wagner, L. I., Beaumont, J. L., Paice, J. A., Peterman, A. H., Shevrin, D., … Cella, D. (2008). Use of a single-item screening tool to detect clinically significant fatigue, pain, distress, and anorexia in ambulatory cancer practice. *Journal of Pain & Symptom Management, 35*(1), 20–30. doi:10.1016/j.jpainsymman.2007.02.040

Byun, E., Gay, C. L., & Lee, K. A. (2016). Sleep, fatigue, and problems with cognitive function in adults living with HIV. *Journal of the Association of Nurses in AIDS Care, 27*(1), 5–16. doi:10.1016/j.jana.2015.10.002

Carlotto, A., Hogsett, V., Maiorini, E., Razulis, J., & Sonis, S. (2013). The economic burden of toxicities associated with cancer treatment: Review of the literature and analysis of nausea and vomiting, diarrhoea, oral mucositis and fatigue. *PharmacoEconomics, 31*(9), 753–766. doi:10.1007/s40273-013-0081-2

Cavanaugh, M. T., Quigley, P. J., Hodgson, D. D., Reid, J. C., & Behm, D. G. (2016). Kinesiology tape or compression sleeve applied to the thigh does not improve balance or muscle activation before or following fatigue. *The Journal of Strength & Conditioning Research, 30*(7), 1992–2000. doi:10.1519/JSC.0000000000001297

Cella, M., & Chalder, T. (2010). Measuring fatigue in clinical and community settings. *Journal of Psychosomatic Research, 69*(1), 17–22. doi:10.1016/j.jpsychores.2009.10.007

Centers for Disease Control and Prevention. (2012). Myalgic encephalomyelitis/chronic fatigue syndrome: Symptoms. Atlanta, GA: Department of Health and Human Services. Retrieved from http://www.cdc.gov/cfs/symptoms/index.html

Centers for Medicare & Medicaid Services. (2008). *MDS 3.0 for Nursing Homes*. Baltimore, MD: Department of Health & Human Services. Retrieved from https://www.cms.gov/Medicare/Quality-Initiatives-Patient-Assessment-Instruments/NursingHomeQualityInits/NHQIMDS30.html

Chalder, T., Berelowitz, G., Pawlikowska, T., Watts, L., Wessely, S., Wright, D., & Wallace, E. P. (1993). Development of a fatigue scale. *Journal of Psychosomatic Research, 37*(2), 147–153. doi:10.1016/0022-3999(93)90081-P

Chan, E., Tan, M., Xin, J., Sudarsanam, S., & Johnson, D. E. (2010). Interactions between traditional Chinese medicines and Western therapeutics. *Current Opinion in Drug Discovery and Development, 13*(1), 50–65.

Chang, C.-W., Mu, P.-F., Jou, S.-T., Wong, T.-T., & Chen, Y.-C. (2013). Systematic review and meta-analysis of nonpharmacological interventions for fatigue in children and adolescents with cancer. *Worldviews on Evidence-Based Nursing/Sigma Theta Tau International, Honor Society of Nursing, 10*(4), 208–217. doi:10.1111/wvn.12007

Cho, Y. C., & Tsay, S. L. (2004). The effect of acupressure with massage on fatigue and depression in patients with end-stage renal disease. *Journal of Nursing Research, 12*(1), 51–59. doi:10.1097/01.JNR.0000387488.63438.9a

Chochinov, H. M., & Breitbart, W. (2012). *Handbook of psychiatry in palliative medicine*. New York, NY: Oxford University Press.

Cook, P. F., Hartson, K. R., Schmiege, S. J., Jankowski, C., Starr, W., & Meek, P. (2016). Bidirectional relationships between fatigue and everyday experiences in persons living with HIV. *Research in Nursing & Health, 39*(3), 154–163. doi:10.1002/nur.21718

Cooley, M. E., McCorkle, R., Knafl, G. J., Rimar, J., Barbieri, M. J., Davies, M., & Murren, J. (2005). Comparison of health-related quality of life questionnaires in ambulatory oncology. *Quality of Life Research, 14*(5), 1239–1249. doi:10.1007/s11136-004-5534-9

Cornuz, J., Guessous, I., & Favrat, B. (2006). Fatigue: A practical approach to diagnosis in primary care. *Canadian Medical Association Journal, 174*(6), 765–767. doi:10.1503/cmaj.1031153

Cramp, F., & Daniel, J. (2008). Exercise for the management of cancer-related fatigue in adults. *Cochrane Database of Systematic Reviews,* (2), CD006145. doi:10.1002/14651858.CD006145.pub2

Cuesta-Vargas, A. I., Férnandez-Lao, C., Cantarero-Villanueva, I., Castro-Sánchez, A. M., Fernández-de-Las Peñas, C., Polley, M. J., & Arroyo-Morales, M. (2013). Psychometric properties of the QuickPIPER: A shortened version of the PIPER Fatigue scale. *European Journal of Cancer Care, 22*(2), 245–252. doi:10.1111/ecc.12022

Dagnelie, P. C., Pijls-Johannesma, M. C. G., Pijpe, A., Boumans, B. J. E., Skrabanja, A. T. P., Lambin, P., & Kempen, G. I. J. M. (2006). Psychometric properties of the revised Piper Fatigue Scale in Dutch cancer patients were satisfactory. *Journal of Clinical Epidemiology, 59*(6), 642–649. doi:10.1016/j.jclinepi.2005.09.015

Dambrosio, N. M., & Mazanec, P. (2013). "Nurse, I Can't Sleep": Approaches to management of insomnia in oncology patients. *Journal of Hospice and Palliative Nursing, 15*(5), 267–278. doi:10.1097/NJH.0b013e318296839b

de Vries, J. D., Claessens, B. J., van Hooff, M. L., Geurts, S. A., van den Bossche, S. N., & Kompier, M. A. (2016). Disentangling longitudinal relations between physical activity, work-related fatigue, and task demands. *International Archives of Occupational and Environmental Health, 89*(1), 89.

de Vries, J. D., Michielsen, H., Van Heck, G. L., & Drent, M. (2004). Measuring fatigue in sarcoidosis: The Fatigue Assessment Scale (FAS). *British Journal of Health Psychology, 9*(Pt 3), 279–291. doi:10.1348/1359107041557048

Dean, G. E., & Anderson, P. R. (2001). Fatigue. In B. R. Ferrell & N. Coyle (Eds.), *The textbook of palliative nursing* (pp. 91–100). New York, NY: Oxford University Press.

Dhillon, H., Bell, M., van der Ploeg, H., Turner, J., Kabourakis, M., Spencer, L., … Clarke, S. (2017). Impact of physical activity on fatigue and quality of life in people with advanced lung cancer: A randomised controlled trial. *Annals of Oncology, 28*(8), 1889–1897. doi:10.1093/annonc/mdx205

Duncan, J. G., Forbes-Thompson, S., & Bott, M. J. (2008). Unmet symptom management needs of nursing home residents with cancer. *Cancer Nursing, 31*(4), 265–273. doi:10.1097/01.NCC.0000305738.33958.9f

Elkington, H., White, P., Addington-Hall, J., Higgs, R., & Edmonds, P. (2005). The healthcare needs of chronic obstructive pulmonary disease patients in the last year of life. *Palliative Medicine, 19*(6), 485–491. doi:10.1191/0269216305pm1056oa

Enoka, R. M., & Duchateau, J. (2016). Translating fatigue to human performance. *Medicine and Science in Sports and Exercise, 48*(11), 2228–2238. doi:10.1249/MSS.0000000000000929

Erickson, J. M., Beck, S. L., Christian, B., Dudley, W. N., Hollen, P. J., Albritton, K., … Godder, K. (2010). Patterns of fatigue in adolescents receiving chemotherapy. *Oncology Nursing Forum, 37*(4), 444–455. doi:10.1188/10.ONF.444-455

Evans, D. R., Boggero, I. A., & Segerstrom, S. C. (2016). The nature of self-regulatory fatigue and "ego depletion" lessons from physical fatigue. *Personality and Social Psychology Review, 20*(4), 291–310. doi:10.1177/1088868315597841

Fernandes, R., Stone, P., Andrews, P., Morgan, R., & Sharma, S. (2006). Comparison between fatigue, sleep disturbance, and circadian rhythm in cancer inpatients and healthy volunteers: Evaluation of diagnostic criteria for cancer-related fatigue. *Journal of Pain and Symptom Management, 32*(3), 245–254. doi:10.1016/j.jpainsymman.2006.03.014

Fiest, K. M., Currie, S. R., Williams, J. V. A., & Wang, J. (2011). Chronic conditions and major depression in community-dwelling older adults. *Journal of Affective Disorders, 131*(1–3), 172–178. doi:10.1016/j.jad.2010.11.028

Filler, K., & Saligan, L. N. (2016). Defining cancer-related fatigue for biomarker discovery. *Supportive Care in Cancer: Official Journal of the Multinational Association of Supportive Care in Cancer, 24*(1), 5–7. doi:10.1007/s00520-015-2965-5

Fisk, J. D., Ritvo, P. G., Ross, L., Haase, D. A., Marrie, T. J., & Schlech, W. F. (1994). Measuring the functional impact of fatigue: Initial validation of the Fatigue Impact Scale. *Clinical Infectious Diseases, 18*, S79–S83. doi:10.1093/clinids/18.Supplement_1.S79

Forbush, S., Fisseha, E., Gallagher, R., Hale, L., Malone, S., Patterson, F., … Gehrels, J. (2017). 1067 Sociodemographics, poor overall health, cardiovascular disease, depression, fatigue, and daytime sleepiness associated with social jetlag independent of sleep duration and insomnia. *Journal of Sleep and Sleep Disorders Research, 40*(Suppl. 1), A396–A397. doi:10.1093/sleepj/zsx050.1066

Foster, C., Grimmett, C., May, C. M., Ewings, S., Myall, M., Hulme, C., … Richardson, A. (2016). A web-based intervention (RESTORE) to support self-management of cancer-related fatigue following primary cancer treatment: A multi-centre proof of concept randomised controlled trial. *Supportive Care in Cancer, 24*, 2445–2453. doi:10.1007/s00520-015-3044-7

Glaspy, J., Degos, L., Dicato, M., & Demetri, G. D. (2002). Comparable efficacy of epoetin alfa for anemic cancer patients receiving platinum- and nonplatinum-based chemotherapy: A retrospective subanalysis of two large, community-based trials. *Oncologist, 7*(2), 126–135. doi:10.1634/theoncologist.7-2-126

Guerit, J.-M. (2017). How can clinical neurophysiology help in studying fatigue?. *Clinical Neurophysiology, 47*(2), 85–86. doi:10.1016/j.neucli.2017.03.004

Halkett, G. K., Kristjanson, L. J., & Lobb, E. A. (2008). 'If we get too close to your bones they'll go brittle': Women's initial fears about radiotherapy for early breast cancer. *Psycho-Oncology, 17*(9), 877–884. doi:10.1002/pon.1298

Hallan, S. I., & Orth, S. R. (2010). The conundrum of chronic kidney disease classification and end-stage renal risk prediction in the elderly—What is the right approach? *Nephron Clinical Practice, 116*(4), c307–c316. doi:10.1159/000319166

Hardy, S. E., & Studenski, S. A. (2010). Qualities of fatigue and associated chronic conditions among older adults. *Journal of Pain and Symptom Management, 39*(6), 1033–1042. doi:10.1016/j.jpainsymman.2009.09.026

Heinrich, M., Land, J., McCourt, O., Philpott, S., Paton, B., Beeken, R. J., … D'Sa, S. (2016). *Physical and psychological factors influencing fatigue and quality of life in multiple myeloma survivors: Preliminary results from the mascot lifestyle study.* Poster session presented at ASH 2016 Annual Meeting, San Diego, CA.

Herlofson, K., & Kluger, B. M. (2016). Fatigue in Parkinson's disease. *Journal of the Neurological Sciences, 374,* 38–41. doi:10.1016/j.jns.2016.12.061

Herlofson, K., Ongre, S. O., Enger, L. K., Tysnes, O. B., & Larsen, J. P. (2012). Fatigue in early Parkinson's disease. Minor inconvenience or major distress? *European Journal of Neurology, 19*(7), 963–968. doi:10.1111/j.1468-1331.2012.03663.x

Hickman, K., Barton, D., & Elkins, G. (2016). Cancer-related fatigue. In G. R. Elkins (Ed.), *Handbook of medical and psychological hypnosis: Foundations, applications, and professional issues* (p. 187–192). New York, NY: Springer Publishing.

Hinds, P. S., Yang, J., & Gattuso, J. S. (2010). Psychometric and clinical assessment of the 10-item reduced version of the Fatigue Scale. *Journal of Pain Symptom Management, 39*(3), 572–578. doi:10.1016/j.jpainsymman.2009.07.015

Hobday, R. A., Thomas, S., O'Donovan, A., Murphy, M., & Pinching, A. J. (2008). Dietary intervention in chronic fatigue syndrome. *Journal of Human Nutrition & Dietetics, 21*(2), 141–149. doi:10.1111/j.1365-277x.2008.00857.x

Hockenberry, M. J., Hinds, P. S., & Barrera, P. (2003). Three instruments to assess fatigue in children with cancer: The child, parent, and staff perspectives. *Journal of Pain and Symptom Management, 25*(4), 319–328. doi:10.1016/s0885-3924(02)00680-2

Hoffmann, T. C., Maher, C. G., Briffa, T., Sherrington, C., Bennell, K., Alison, J., ... Glasziou, P. P. (2016). Prescribing exercise interventions for patients with chronic conditions. *Canadian Medical Association Journal, 188*(7), 510–518. doi:10.1503/cmaj.150684

Holliday, E. B., Dieckmann, N. F., McDonald, T. L., Hung, A. Y., Thomas, C. R., & Wood, L. J. (2016). Relationship between fatigue, sleep quality and inflammatory cytokines during external beam radiation therapy for prostate cancer: A prospective study. *Radiotherapy and Oncology, 118*(1), 105–111. doi:10.1016/j.radonc.2015.12.015

Holz, S. A. C., & Smith, S. R. (2017). Cancer-related fatigue: What you need to know. *Archives of Physical Medicine and Rehabilitation, 98*(8), 1717–1718. doi:10.1016/j.apmr.2016.12.020

Hooke, M. C., Garwick, A. W., & Gross, C. R. (2011). Fatigue and physical performance in children and adolescents receiving chemotherapy. *Oncology Nursing Forum, 38*(6), 649–657. doi:10.1188/11.onf.649-657

Horneber, M., Fischer, I., Dimeo, F., Rüffer, J. U., & Weis, J. (2012). Cancer-related fatigue: Epidemiology, pathogenesis, diagnosis, and treatment. *Deutsches Arzteblatt International, 109*(9), 161–171. doi:10.3238/arztebl.2012.0161

Hughes, A., Hirsch, C., Chalder, T., & Moss-Morris, R. (2016). Attentional and interpretive bias towards illness-related information in chronic fatigue syndrome: A systematic review. *British Journal of Health Psychology, 21*(4), 741–763. doi:10.1111/bjhp.12207

Jakobsson, U., Hallberg, I. R., & Westergren, A. (2007). Exploring determinants for quality of life among older people in pain and in need of help for daily living. *Journal of Nursing and Healthcare of Chronic Illness in Association With Journal of Clinical Nursing, 16*(3a), 95–104. doi:10.1111/j.1365-2702.2006.01584.x

Johansen, S., Cvancarova, M., & Ruland, C. (2018). The effect of cancer patients' and their family caregivers' physical and emotional symptoms on caregiver burden. *Cancer Nursing, 41*(2), 91–99. doi:10.1097/ncc.0000000000000493

Jong, E., Oudhoff, L. A., Epskamp, C., Wagener, M. N., van Duijn, M., Fischer, S., & van Gorp, E. C. M. (2010). Predictors and treatment strategies of HIV-related fatigue in the combined antiretroviral therapy era. *AIDS, 24*(10), 1387–1405. doi:10.1097/QAD.0b013e328339d004

Jopson, L., Dyson, J. K., & Jones, D. E. (2016). Understanding and treating fatigue in primary biliary cirrhosis and primary sclerosing cholangitis. *Clinics in Liver Disease, 20*(1), 131–142. doi:10.1016/j.cld.2015.08.007

Jorgensen, R. (2008). Chronic fatigue: An evolutionary concept analysis. *Journal of Advanced Nursing, 63*(2), 199–207. doi:10.1111/j.1365-2648.2008.04649.x

Justo, A. C., Guimarães, F. S., Ferreira, A. S., Soares, M. S., Bunn, P. S., & Lopes, A. J. (2017). Muscle function in women with systemic sclerosis: Association with fatigue and general physical function. *Clinical Biomechanics, 47,* 33–39. doi:10.1016/j.clinbiomech.2017.05.011

Kapella, M. C., Larson, J. L., Patel, M. K., Covey, M. K., & Berry, J. K. (2006). Subjective fatigue, influencing variables, and consequences in chronic obstructive pulmonary disease. *Nursing Research, 55*(1), 10–17. doi:10.1097/00006199-200601000-00002

Kaptchuk, T. J. (2000). *The web that has no weaver: Understanding Chinese medicine.* New York, NY: McGraw-Hill.

Katz, P., Margaretten, M., Trupin, L., Schmajuk, G., Yazdany, J., & Yelin, E. (2016). Role of sleep disturbance, depression, obesity, and physical inactivity in fatigue in rheumatoid arthritis. *Arthritis Care & Research, 68*(1), 81–90. doi:10.1002/acr.22577

Kim, Y., Shaffer, K. M., Carver, C. S., & Cannady, R. S. (2016). Quality of life of family caregivers 8 years after a relative's cancer diagnosis: Follow-up of the National Quality of Life Survey for Caregivers. *Psycho-Oncology, 25*(3), 266–274. doi:10.1002/pon.3843

Kirkova, J., Aktas, A., Walsh, D., & Davis, M. P. (2011). Cancer symptom clusters: Clinical and research methodology. *Journal of Palliative Medicine, 14*(4), 1149–1166. doi:10.1089/jpm.2010.0507

Kirsh, K. L., Passik, S., Holtsclaw, E., Donaghy, K., & Theobald, D. (2001). I get tired for no reason: A single item screening for cancer-related fatigue. *Journal of Pain & Symptom Management, 22*(5), 931–937. doi:10.1016/S0885-3924(01)00350-5

Kisiel-Sajewicz, K., Davis, M. P., Siemionow, V., Seyidova-Khoshknabi, D., Wyant, A., Walsh, D., ... Yue, G. H. (2012). Lack of muscle contractile property changes at the time of perceived physical exhaustion suggests central mechanisms contributing to early motor task failure in patients with cancer-related fatigue. *Journal of Pain and Symptom Management, 44*(3), 351–361. doi:10.1016/j.jpainsymman.2011.08.007

Klampfer, L. (2011). Cytokines, inflammation and colon cancer. *Current Cancer Drug Targets, 11*(4), 451–464. doi:10.2174/156800911795538066

Klimas, N. G., Broderick, G., & Fletcher, M. A. (2012). Biomarkers for chronic fatigue. *Brain, Behavior, and Immunity, 26*(8), 1202–1210. doi:10.1016/j.bbi.2012.06.006

Koll, T. T., & Dale, W. (2017). Evaluation and management of older adults with multimorbidity and cancer: A geriatric perspective on oncology care. In J. R. Burton, A. G. Lee, & J. F. Potter (Eds.), *Geriatrics for specialists* (pp. 317–324). Cham, Switzerland: Springer.

Kos, D., Kerckhofs, E., Carrea, I., Verza, R., Ramos, M., & Jansa, J. (2005). Evaluation of the modified fatigue impact scale in four different European countries. *Multiple Sclerosis, 11*(1), 76–80. doi:10.1191/1352458505ms1117oa

Krabbe, D., Ellbin, S., Nilsson, M., Jonsdottir, I. H., & Samuelsson, H. (2017). Executive function and attention in patients with stress-related exhaustion: Perceived fatigue and effect of distraction. *Stress, 20*(4), 1–30. doi:10.1080/10253890.2017.1336533

Krupp, L. B., LaRocca, N. G., Muir-Nash, J., & Steinberg, A. D. (1989). The fatigue severity scale: Application to patients with multiple sclerosis and systemic lupus erythematosus. *Archives of Neurology, 46*(10), 1121–1123. doi:10.1001/archneur.1989.00520460115022

Kukull, W. A., McCorkle, R., & Driever, M. (1986). Symptom distress, psychosocial variables and survival from lung cancer. *Journal of Psychosocial Oncology, 4*, 91–104. doi:10.1300/J077v04n01_07

Kvien, T., Deodhar, A., Gossec, L., Conaghan, P., Strand, V., Østergaard, M., … Jugl, S. (2017). THU0393 Secukinumab provides sustained reduction in fatigue in patients with ankylosing spondylitis through 3 years: Long-term results of two randomised double-blind placebo-controlled phase 3 studies. *BMJ Journals, 76*(Suppl. 2), 355–356. doi:10.1136/annrheumdis-2017-eular.1839

Kwok, A. O., Yuen, S.-k., Yong, D. S., & Tse, D. M. (2016). The symptoms prevalence, medical interventions, and health care service needs for patients with end-stage renal disease in a renal palliative care program. *American Journal of Hospice and Palliative Medicine, 33*(10), 952–958. doi:10.1177/1049909115598930

Lakey, S. L., LaCroix, A. Z., Gray, S. L., Borson, S., Williams, C. D., Calhoun, D., … Woods, N. F. (2012). Antidepressant use, depressive symptoms, and incident frailty in women aged 65 and older from the women's health initiative observational study. *Journal of the American Geriatrics Society, 60*(5), 854–861. doi:10.1111/j.1532-5415.2012.03940.x

Langeskov-Christensen, M., Bisson, E. J., Finlayson, M. L., & Dalgas, U. (2017). Potential pathophysiological pathways that can explain the positive effects of exercise on fatigue in multiple sclerosis: A scoping review. *Journal of the Neurological Sciences, 373*, 307–320. doi:10.1016/j.jns.2017.01.002

Learmonth, Y. C., Dlugonski, D., Pilutti, L. A., Sandroff, B. M., Klaren, R., & Motl, R. W. (2013). Psychometric properties of the Fatigue Severity Scale and the Modified Fatigue Impact Scale. *Journal of the Neurological Sciences, 331*(1–2), 102–107. doi:10.1016/j.jns.2013.05.023

Liu, T., Tang, Y., Wong, G., Xu, J., Choy, C., & Lum, T. (2016). Differential prediction of global and everyday cognition by physical frailty and chronological age. *The Gerontologist, 56*(Suppl. 3), 248. doi:10.1093/geront/gnw162.1704

Loades, M. E., & Kagee, A. (2017). Exploring our understanding of fatigue among adolescents living with HIV: Highlighting the unknown. *Journal of Health Psychology*, 1359105317710320. doi:10.1177/1359105317710320

Lofgren, S., Friedman, R., Ghermay, R., George, M., Pittman, J. R., Shahane, A., … Marconi, V. C. (2015). Integrating early palliative care for patients with HIV: Provider and patient perceptions of symptoms and need for services. *American Journal of Hospice & Palliative Medicine, 32*(8), 829–834. doi:10.1177/1049909114550391

Lundberg, P. C., & Rattanasuwan, O. (2007). Experiences of fatigue and self-management of Thai Buddhist cancer patients undergoing radiation therapy. *Cancer Nursing, 30*(2), 146–155. doi:10.1097/01.NCC.0000265005.02559.43

Martínez-Alonso, M., Dusso, A., Ariza, G., & Nabal, M. (2016). Vitamin D deficiency and its association with fatigue and quality of life in advanced cancer patients under palliative care: A cross-sectional study. *Palliative Medicine, 30*(1), 89–96. doi:10.1177/0269216315601954

Matura, L. A., McDonough, A., & Carroll, D. L. (2016). Symptom prevalence, symptom severity, and health-related quality of life among young, middle, and older adults with pulmonary arterial hypertension. *American Journal of Hospice & Palliative Medicine, 33*(3), 214–221. doi:10.1177/1049909114554079

McCorkle, R., & Young, K. (1978). Development of a symptom distress scale. *Cancer Nursing, 1*(5), 373–378. doi:10.1097/00002820-197810000-00003

McDougall, G. J. (2005). Research review: The effect of acupressure with massage on fatigue and depression in patients with end-stage renal disease. *Geriatric Nursing, 26*(3), 164–165. doi:10.1016/j.gerinurse.2005.03.008

McNair, D. M., Lorr, M., & Droppleman, L. F. (1996). *Profile of Mood States*, Revised (POMS) (p. 2). San Diego, CA: EdITS/Educational and Industrial Testing Service.

Minton, O., Richardson, A., Sharpe, M., Hotopf, M., & Stone, P. (2008). A systematic review and meta-analysis of the pharmacological treatment of cancer-related fatigue. *Journal of the National Cancer Institute, 100*(16), 1155–1166. doi:10.1093/jnci/djn250

Minton, O., Richardson, A., Sharpe, M., Hotopf, M., & Stone, P. (2010). Drug therapy for the management of cancer-related fatigue. *Cochrane Database of Systematic Reviews, 7*(7): CD006704. doi:10.1002/14651858.CD006704.pub3

Morris, G., Berk, M., Galecki, P., Walder, K., & Maes, M. (2016). The neuro-immune pathophysiology of central and peripheral fatigue in systemic immune-inflammatory and neuro-immune diseases. *Molecular Neurobiology, 53*(2), 1195. doi:10.1007/s12035-015-9090-9

Mortimer, J. E., Barsevick, A. M., Bennett, C. L., Berger, A. M., Cleeland, C., DeVader, S. R., … Rugo, H. S. (2010). Studying cancer-related fatigue: Report of the NCCN scientific research committee. *Journal of the National Comprehensive Cancer Network: JNCCN, 8*(12), 1331–1339. doi:10.6004/jnccn.2010.0101

Mosack, K. E., Rafferty, K. A., Billig, A. K., Wendorf, A. R., Brouwer, A. M., & Stevens, P. (2016). An examination of actor-partner social support effects on HIV-related problems and interpersonal outcomes among a sample of HIV-positive African American dyads. *Cultural Diversity and Ethnic Minority Psychology, 22*(2), 196. doi:10.1037/cdp0000060

NANDA International. (2011). *Nursing diagnoses: Definitions and classification 2012-14.* Oxford, UK: Wiley.

National Cancer Institute. (2017). *PDQ cancer information summaries.* Bethesda, MD: National Cancer Institute.

National Comprehensive Cancer Network. (2013). NCCN clinical practice guidelines in oncology: Cancer-related fatigue. Retrieved from http://www.nccn.org/professionals/physician_gls/pdf/fatigue.pdf

National Consensus Project for Quality Palliative Care. (2013). Clinical practice guidelines for quality palliative care. Retrieved from https://www.nationalcoalitionhpc.org/ncp-guidelines-2013/

National Institute of Mental Health. (2013, August). Depression. Retrieved from http://www.nimh.nih.gov/health/topics/depression/index.shtml

Neill, J., Belan, I., & Ried, K. (2006). Effectiveness of non-pharmacological interventions for fatigue in adults with multiple sclerosis, rheumatoid arthritis, or systemic lupus erythematosus: A systematic review. *Journal of Advanced Nursing, 56*(6), 617–635. doi:10.1111/j.1365-2648.2006.04054.x

Neuberger, G. B., Aaronson, L. S., Gajewski, B., Embretson, S. E., Cagle, P. E., Loudon, J. K., & Miller, P. A. (2007). Predictors of exercise and effects of exercise on symptoms, function, aerobic fitness, and disease outcomes of rheumatoid arthritis. *Arthritis & Rheumatism, 57*(6), 943–952. doi:10.1002/art.22903

Neuenschwander, H., & Bruera, E. (2011). Asthenia. In G. W. C. Hanks (Ed.), *Oxford textbook of palliative medicine* (4th ed., pp. 573–582). Oxford, UK: Oxford University Press.

Newland, P. K., Lunsford, V., & Flach, A. (2017). The interaction of fatigue, physical activity, and health-related quality of life in adults with multiple sclerosis (MS) and cardiovascular disease (CVD). *Applied Nursing Research, 33*, 49–53. doi:10.1016/j.apnr.2016.09.001

Nieves-Lugo, K., del Rio-Gonzalez, A. M., Reisen, C., Poppen, P., Oursler, K. K., & Zea, M. C. (2017). Greater depressive symptoms and higher viral load are associated with poor physical function among Latino men living with HIV. *Journal of the International Association of Providers of AIDS Care (JIAPAC), 16*(1), 30–36. doi:10.1177/2325957416640363

Norheim, K. B., Jonsson, G., & Omdal, R. (2011). Biological mechanisms of chronic fatigue. *Rheumatology, 50*(6), 1009–1018. doi:10.1093/rheumatology/keq454

Olagunju, A. T., Sarimiye, F. O., Olagunju, T. O., Habeebu, M. Y., & Aina, O. F. (2016). Child's symptom burden and depressive symptoms among caregivers of children with cancers: An argument for early integration of pediatric palliative care. *Annals of Palliative Medicine, 5*(3), 157–165. doi:10.21037/apm.2016.04.03

Olson, K., Krawchuk, A., & Quddusi, T. (2007). Fatigue in individuals with advanced cancer in active treatment and palliative settings. *Cancer Nursing, 30*(4), E1–10. doi:10.1097/01.NCC.0000281736.25609.74

Owens, J. A. (2007). Sleep loss and fatigue in healthcare professionals. *Journal of Perinatal & Neonatal Nursing, 21*(2), 92–100. doi:10.1097/01.JPN.0000270624.64584.9d

Paddison, J. S., Booth, R. J., Hill, A. G., & Cameron, L. D. (2006). Comprehensive assessment of peri-operative fatigue: Development of the Identity-Consequence Fatigue Scale. *Journal of Psychosomatic Research, 60*(6), 615–622. doi:10.1016/j.jpsychores.2005.08.008

Paddison, J. S., Effing, T. W., Quinn, S., & Frith, P. A. (2013). Fatigue in COPD: Association with functional status and hospitalisations. The *European Respiratory Journal, 41*(3), 565–570. doi:10.1183/09031936.00021412

Pan, H.-T., Wu, L.-M., & Wen, S.-H. (2017). Quality of life and its predictors among children and adolescents with cancer. *Cancer Nursing, 40*(5), 343–351. doi:10.1097/NCC.0000000000000433

Patel, B., Pahwa, R., & Lyons, K. (2017). Fatigue in Parkinson's disease (P5. 003). *Neurology, 88*(16 Suppl).

Peoples, A. R., Roscoe, J. A., Block, R. C., Heckler, C. E., Ryan, J. L., Mustian, K. M., … Coles, C. (2017). Nausea and disturbed sleep as predictors of cancer-related fatigue in breast cancer patients: A multicenter NCORP study. *Supportive Care in Cancer, 25*(4), 1271–1278. doi:10.1007/s00520-016-3520-8

Peters, M. E. W. J., Goedendorp, M. M., Verhagen, C. A. H. H. V. M., Bleijenberg, G., & van der Graaf, W. T. A. (2016). Fatigue and its associated psychosocial factors in cancer patients on active palliative treatment measured over time. *Supportive Care in Cancer, 24*, 1349–1355. doi:10.1007/s00520-015-2909-0

Picariello, F., Moss-Morris, R., Macdougall, I. C., Chilcot, J. (2016). The role of psychological factors in fatigue among end-stage kidney disease patients: A critical review. *Clinical Kidney Journal, 10*(1), 79–88. doi:10.1093/ckj/sfw113

Piper, B. F. (1989). Fatigue: Current basis of practice. In S. G. Funk, E. M. Funk, Tornquist, E. M., & M. T. Champagne (Eds.), *Key aspects of comfort* (pp. 187–198). New York, NY: Springer Publishing.

Piper, B. F., Borneman, T., Sun, V. C., Koczywas, M., Uman, G., Ferrell, B., & James, R. L. (2008). Cancer-related fatigue: Role of oncology nurses in translating National Comprehensive Cancer Network assessment guidelines into practice. *Clinical Journal of Oncology Nursing, 12*(5), 37–47. doi:10.1188/08.CJON.S2.37-47

Piper, B. F., Dibble, S. L., Dodd, M. J., Weiss, M. C., Slaughter, R. E., & Paul, S. M. (1998). The revised Piper Fatigue Scale: Psychometric evaluation in women with breast cancer. *Oncology Nursing Forum, 25*(4), 677–684.

Piper, B. F., Lindsey, A. M., & Dodd, M. J. (1989). The development of an instrument to measure the subjective dimension of fatigue. In S. G. Funk, E. M. Funk, & M. T. Champagne (Eds.), *Key aspects of comfort* (pp. 199–208). New York, NY: Springer Publishers.

Portenoy, R. (2003). Fatigue. In M. B. Max & J. Lynn (Eds.), *Symptom research: Methods and opportunities.* Bethesda, MD: National Institutes of Health; Department of Health and Human Services.

Porter, N. S., Jason, L. A., Boulton, A., Bothne, N., & Coleman, B. (2010). Alternative medical interventions used in the treatment and management of myalgic encephalomyelitis/chronic fatigue syndrome and fibromyalgia. *The Journal of Alternative and Complementary Medicine, 16*(3), 235–249. doi:10.1089/acm.2008.0376

Potter, J., Hami, F., Bryan, T., & Quigley, C. (2003). Symptoms in 400 patients referred to palliative care services: Prevalence and patterns. *Palliative Medicine, 17*(4), 310–314. doi:10.1191/0269216303pm760oa

Przybylowski, T., Bielicki, P., Kumor, M., Hildebrand, K., Maskey-Warzechowska, M., Korczynski, P., & Chazan, R. (2007). Exercise capacity in patients with obstructive sleep apnea syndrome. *Journal of Physiology & Pharmacology, 58*(Suppl. 5, Pt 2), 563–574.

Puetz, T. W., O'Connor, P. J., & Dishman, R. K. (2006). Effects of chronic exercise on feelings of energy and fatigue: A quantitative synthesis. *Psychological Bulletin, 132*(6), 866–876. doi:10.1037/0033-2909.132.6.866

Putman-Casdorph, H., & McCrone, S. (2009). Chronic obstructive pulmonary disease, anxiety, and depression: State of the science. *Heart & Lung: Journal of Acute & Critical Care, 38*(1), 34–47. doi:10.1016/j.hrtlng.2008.02.005

Quick, M., & Fonteyn, M. (2005). Development and implementation of a clinical survey for cancer-related fatigue assessment. *Clinical Journal of Oncology Nursing, 9*(4), 435–442. doi:10.1188/05.CJON.435-439

Radbruch, L., Strasser, F., Elsner, F., Goncalves, J. F., Loge, J., Kaasa, S., ... Stone, P. (2008). Fatigue in palliative care patients—An EAPC approach. *Palliative Medicine, 22*(1), 13–32. doi:10.1177/0269216307085183

Rao, A., & Cohen, H. J. (2004). Symptom management in the elderly cancer patient: Fatigue, pain, and depression. *Journal of the National Cancer Institute Monographs, 2004*(32), 150–157. doi:10.1093/jncimonographs/lgh031

Ream, E. (2007). Fatigue in patients receiving palliative care. *Nursing Standard, 21*(28), 49. doi:10.7748/ns2007.03.21.28.49.c4536

Ream, E., & Stone, P. (2004). Clinical interventions for fatigue. In J. Armes, M. Krishnasamy, & I. Higginson (Eds.), *Fatigue in cancer* (pp. 255–277). New York, NY: Oxford University Press.

Repping-Wuts, H., Fransen, J., van Achterberg, T., Bleijenberg, G., & van Riel, P. (2007). Persistent severe fatigue in patients with rheumatoid arthritis. *Journal of Nursing and Healthcare of Chronic Illness; Journal of Clinical Nursing, 16*(11c), 377–383. doi:10.1111/j.1365-2702.2007.02082.x

Rodrigues, A. R., Trufelli, D. C., Fonseca, F., de Paula, L. C., & Giglio, A. D. (2016). Fatigue in patients with advanced terminal cancer correlates with inflammation, poor quality of life and sleep, and anxiety/depression. *American Journal of Hospice & Palliative Medicine, 33*(10), 942–947. doi:10.1177/1049909115603055

Rosen, T., Lachs, M. S., Bharucha, A. J., Stevens, S. M., Teresi, J. A., Nebres, F., & Pillemer, K. (2008). Resident-to-resident aggression in long-term care facilities: Insights from focus groups of nursing home residents and staff. *Journal of the American Geriatrics Society, 56*(8), 1398–1408. doi:10.1111/j.1532-5415.2008.01808.x

Rotonda, C., Guillemin, F., Bonnetain, F., Velten, M., & Conroy, T. (2013). Factors associated with fatigue after surgery in women with early-stage invasive breast cancer. *Oncologist, 18*(4), 467–475. doi:10.1634/theoncologist.2012-0300

Sayegh, P., Thaler, N. S., Arentoft, A., Kuhn, T. P., Schonfeld, D., Castellon, S. A., ... Hinkin, C. H. (2016). Medication adherence in HIV-positive African Americans: The roles of age, health beliefs, and sensation seeking. *Cogent Psychology, 3*(1), 1137207. doi:10.1080/23311908.2015.1137207

Schjoedt, I., Sommer, I., & Bjerrum, M. B. (2016). Experiences and management of fatigue in everyday life among adult patients living with heart failure: A systematic review of qualitative evidence. *JBI Database of Systematic Reviews and Implementation Reports, 14*(3), 68–115. doi:10.11124/JBISRIR-2016-2441

Scott, J. A., Lasch, K. E., Barsevick, A. M., & Piault-Louis, E. (2011). Patients' experiences with cancer-related fatigue: A review and synthesis of qualitative research. *Oncology Nursing Forum, 38*(3), E191–203. doi:10.1188/11.ONF.E191-E203

Shillam, C. R., Dupree Jones, K., & Miller, L. (2011). Fibromyalgia symptoms, physical function, and comorbidity in middle-aged and older adults. *Nursing Research, 60*(5), 309–317. doi:10.1097/NNR.0b013e31822bbdfa

Signal, N., Taylor, D., & McNair, P. (2008). Central and peripheral contributions to neuromuscular fatigue in people with stroke. *Physical Therapy Reviews, 13*(4), 249–257. doi:10.1179/174328808X309205

Silveira, M. G., Gossard, A. A., Stahler, A. C., Jorgensen, R. A., Petz, J. L., Ali, A. H., & Lindor, K. D. (2017). A randomized, placebo-controlled clinical trial of efficacy and safety: Modafinil in the treatment of fatigue in patients with primary biliary cirrhosis. *American Journal of Therapeutics, 24*(2), e167-e176. doi:10.1097/MJT.0000000000000387

Stephen, S. A. (2008). Fatigue in older adults with stable heart failure. *Heart & Lung, 37*(2), 122–131. doi:10.1016/j.hrtlng.2007.03.006

Strahler, J., Skoluda, N., Rohleder, N., & Nater, U. M. (2016). Dysregulated stress signal sensitivity and inflammatory disinhibition as a pathophysiological mechanism of stress-related chronic fatigue. *Neuroscience & Biobehavioral Reviews, 68*, 298–318. doi:10.1016/j.neubiorev.2016.05.008

Tack, B. B. (1991). *Dimensions and correlates of fatigue in older adults with rheumatoid arthritis.* (Doctoral disseration). University of California, San Francisco, CA. Retrieved from EBSCOhost ccm database.

Tartaglia, M. C., Narayanan, S., & Arnold, D. L. (2008). Mental fatigue alters the pattern and increases the volume of cerebral activition for a motor task in multiple sclerosis patients with fatigue. *European Journal of Neurology, 15*, 413–419. doi:10.1111/j.1468-1331.2008.02090.x

Tennant, K. F., Takacs, S. E., Gau, J.-T., Clark, B. C., & Russ, D. W. (2012). A preliminary study of symptomatic fatigue in rural older adults. *Aging Clinical and Experimental Research, 24*(4), 324–330. doi:10.3275/8054

Theander, K., Cliffordson, C., Torstensson, O., Jakobsson, P., & Unosson, M. (2007). Fatigue Impact Scale: Its validation in patients with chronic obstructive pulmonary disease. *Psychology, Health & Medicine, 12*(4), 470–484. doi:10.1080/13548500601086771

Theander, K., & Unosson, M. (2004). Fatigue in patients with chronic obstructive pulmonary disease. *Journal of Advanced Nursing, 45*(2), 172–177. doi:10.1046/j.1365-2648.2003.02878.x

Thiagarajan, M., Chan, C. M., Fuang, H. G., Beng, T. S., Atiliyana, M. A., & Yahaya, N. A. (2016). Symptom prevalence and related distress in cancer patients undergoing chemotherapy. *Asian Pacific Journal of Cancer Prevention: APJCP, 17*(1), 171–176. doi:10.7314/apjcp.2016.17.1.171

Tsai, Y. F., Wong, T. K., & Ku, Y. C. (2008). Self-care management of sleep disturbances and risk factors for poor sleep among older residents of Taiwanese nursing homes. *Journal of Clinical Nursing, 17*(9), 1219–1226. doi:10.1111/j.1365-2702.2007.02020.x

Tuca, A., Jimenez-Fonseca, P., & Gascón, P. (2013). Clinical evaluation and optimal management of cancer cachexia. *Critical Reviews in Oncology/Hematology, 88*(3), 625–636. doi:10.1016/j.critrevonc.2013.07.015

Turan, Y., Duruöz, M. T., Bal, S., Guvenc, A., Cerrahoglu, L., & Gurgan, A. (2007). Assessment of fatigue in patients with ankylosing spondylitis *Rheumatology International, 27*, 847–852. doi:10.1007/s00296-0070313-x

Ullrich, C. K., Dussel, V., Hilden, J. M., Sheaffer, J. W., Moore, C. L., Berde, C. B., & Wolfe, J. (2010). Fatigue in children with cancer at the end of life. *Journal of Pain & Symptom Management, 40*(4), 483–494. doi:10.1016/j.jpainsymman.2010.02.020

van Dijk, J. P., Havlikova, E., Rosenberger, J., Nagyova, I., Skorvanek, M., Gdovinova, Z., … Middel, B. (2013). Influence of disease severity on fatigue in patients with Parkinson's disease is mainly mediated by symptoms of depression. *European Neurology, 70*(3–4), 201–209. doi:10.1159/000351779

van Kessel, K., Moss-Morris, R., Willoughby, E., Chalder, T., Johnson, M. H., & Robinson, E. (2008). A randomized controlled trial of cognitive behavior therapy for multiple sclerosis fatigue. *Psychosomatic Medicine, 70*(2), 205–213. doi:10.1097/PSY.0b013e3181643065

Vardy, J. L., Dhillon, H. M., Pond, G. R., Renton, C., Dodd, A., Zhang, H., … Tannock, I. F. (2016). Fatigue in people with localized colorectal cancer who do and do not receive chemotherapy: A longitudinal prospective study. *Annals of Oncology, 27*(9), 1761–1767. doi:10.1093/annonc/mdw252

Veauthier, C., Hasselmann, H., Gold, S. M., & Paul, F. (2016). The Berlin Treatment Algorithm: Recommendations for tailored innovative therapeutic strategies for multiple sclerosis-related fatigue. *The EPMA Journal, 7*, 25. doi:10.1186/s13167-016-0073-3

Voss, J. (2005). Predictors and correlates of fatigue in HIV/AIDS. *Journal of Pain and Symptom Management, 29*(2), 173–184. doi:10.1016/j.jpainsymman.2004.05.006

Wagner, L. I., & Cella, D. (2004). Fatigue and cancer: Causes, prevalence and treatment approaches. *British Journal of Cancer, 91*(5), 822–828. doi:10.1038/sj.bjc.6602012

Wang, T.-C., Huang, J.-L., Ho, W.-C., & Chiou, A.-F. (2016). Effects of a supportive educational nursing care programme on fatigue and quality of life in patients with heart failure: A randomised controlled trial. *European Journal of Cardiovascular Nursing, 15*(2), 157–167. doi:10.1177/1474515115618567

Wang, X. S. (2008). Pathophysiology of cancer-related fatigue. *Journal of Oncology Nursing, 12*(5), 11–20. doi:10.1188/08.CJON.S2.11-20

Warth, M., Kesler, J., Hillecke, T. K., & Bardenheuer, H. J. (2015). Music therapy in palliative care. *Deutsches Arzteblatt International, 112*(46), 788–794. doi:10.3238/arztebl.2015.0788

Weiss, D. M., Northouse, L. L., Duffy, S. A., Ingersoll-Dayton, B., Katapodi, M. C., & LoRusso, P. M. (2016). Qualitative analysis of the experience of mental fatigue of family caregivers of patients with cancer in phase I trials. *Oncology Nursing Forum, 43*(4), E153–E160. doi:10.1188/16.ONF.E153-E160

Whitehead, L. (2009). The measurement of fatigue in chronic illness: A systematic review of unidimensional and multidimensional fatigue measures. *Journal of Pain & Symptom Management, 37*(1), 107–128. doi:10.1016/j.jpainsymman.2007.08.019

Whitehead, L. C., Unahi, K., Burrell, B., & Crowe, M. T. (2016). The experience of fatigue across long-term conditions: A qualitative meta-synthesis. *Journal of Pain and Symptom Management, 52*(1), 131–143. e131. doi:10.1016/j.jpainsymman.2016.02.013

Xiao, C., Beitler, J. J., Higgins, K. A., Conneely, K., Dwivedi, B., Felger, J., … Ong, L. Y. (2016). Fatigue is associated with inflammation in patients with head and neck cancer before and after intensity-modulated radiation therapy. *Brain, Behavior, and Immunity, 52*, 145–152. doi:10.1016/j.bbi.2015.10.016

Yennurajalingam, S., & Bruera, E. (2007). Palliative management of fatigue at the close of life: "It feels like my body is just worn out." *Journal of the American Medical Association, 297*(3), 295–304, E291. doi:10.1001/jama.297.3.295

Yennurajalingam, S., Frisbee-Hume, S., Palmer, J. L., Delgado-Guay, M. O., Bull, J., Phan, A. T., … Bruera, E. (2013). Reduction of cancer-related fatigue with dexamethasone: A double-blind, randomized, placebo-controlled trial in patients with advanced cancer. *Journal of Clinical Oncology: Official Journal of the American Society of Clinical Oncology, 31*(25), 3076–3082. doi:10.1200/JCO.2012.44.4661.

Yennurajalingam, S., Palmer, J. L., Zhang, T., Poulter, V., & Bruera, E. (2008). Association between fatigue and other cancer-related symptoms in patients with advanced cancer. *Supportive Care in Cancer, 16*(10), 1125–1130. doi:10.1007/s00520-008-0466-5

Yennurajalingam, S., Tayjasanant, S., Balachandran, D., Padhye, N. S., Williams, J. L., Liu, D. D., … Bruera, E. (2016). Association between daytime activity, fatigue, sleep, anxiety, depression, and symptom burden in advanced cancer patients: A preliminary report. *Journal of Palliative Medicine, 19*(8), 849–856. doi:10.1089/jpm.2015.0276

Yennurajalingam, S., Urbauer, D. L., Casper, K. L. B., Reyes-Gibby, C. C., Chacko, R., Poulter, V., & Bruera, E. (2011). Impact of a palliative care consultation team on cancer-related symptoms in advanced cancer patients referred to an outpatient supportive care clinic. *Journal of Pain & Symptom Management, 41*(1), 49–56. doi:10.1016/j.jpainsymman.2010.03.017

FATIGUE ASSESSMENT INSTRUMENTS

Instrument	Description	Administration	Validity	Comments
Brief Fatigue Inventory (BFI)	9-Item questionnaire 11-Point Likert Scale Evaluation period: past week, current, past 24 hours, and the impact of fatigue on general activity and mood. Provides a global fatigue score: clinically significant if at least 7.	Self-report Second party (interview) Estimated time for completion: 5 minutes	Validated in men and women Internal reliability verified Test-retest reliability not evaluated Construct verified Convergent: FACT (fatigue and anemia subscales) and POMS (fatigue and vigor subscales) Divergent not evaluated Discriminators: albumin, hemoglobin, and ECOG-PSR	Able to capture physical and psychological aspects. Useful for screening and outcome assessments. Able to distinguish severe fatigue, but less reliable when differentiating mild-to-moderate symptoms.
Cancer Fatigue Scale (CFS)	15-Item questionnaire 5-Point Likert Scale Subscales: physical, affective, cognitive Evaluation period: current	Self-report Second party (interview) Estimated time for completion: 2–3 minutes	Validated in men and women Internal reliability verified Test-retest reliability verified up to 8 days Construct: no healthy controls Convergent: VAS-F and Hospital Anxiety and Depression Scale Divergent: Mini-Mental State Discriminators: ECOG-PSR (physical and affective subscales)	Able to capture physical and psychological aspects. Validation performed in Japanese population, which may affect generalization. Telephone test-retest: lower mean values but retained validity.
Chalder Fatigue Scale; also known as the Fatigue Questionnaire (FQ) (Cella & Chalder, 2010; Chalder et al., 1993).	11-Item scale; originally validated in a general practice setting. Main use has been in the investigation of chronic fatigue syndrome	Self-report Second party (interview) Estimated time for completion: 5 minutes	Validated in 274 adults (aged 18–45 years) in general practice setting. Has also been used in population studies and so has normative data available for comparison with cancer patients.	There is a high degree of internal consistency, and the principal components analysis supported the notion of a two-factor solution (physical and mental fatigue).
Fatigue Assessment Scale (de Vries, Michielsen, Van Heck, & Drent, 2004)	10-Item scale; explores dimensions of fatigue such as mental fitness, energy, ability to perform activities			

(continued)

Instrument	Description	Administration	Validity	Comments
Fatigue Severity Scale (Krupp, LaRocca, Muir-Nash, & Steinberg, 1989)	9-Item scale developed to assess fatigue severity in people with functional disabilities and those with multiple sclerosis			
Fatigue Symptom Inventory (FSI)	14-Item questionnaire 11-Point Likert Scale (12 questions) Remaining questions pertain to number of days/wk (0–7) fatigue is experienced and the pattern of daily fatigue (4-point Likert Scale) Evaluation period: past week, current	Self-report Second party (interview) Estimated time for completion: 5 minutes	Validated in men and women Internal reliability: interference subscale Test-retest reliability: low-to-moderate correlations Construct verified Convergent: POMS-F, SF-36, SLDS-C, and CES-D Divergent: MC-20 Discriminators not evaluated	Similar questions as BFI. Able to capture physical and psychological aspects. Useful for screening and outcome assessments (single assessments only, not repeated measures). Identified a second version of this tool that used a 5-point Likert Scale for the final question pertaining to daily pattern of fatigue.
Functional Assessment of Cancer Therapy-Fatigue (FACT-F) Subscale	27-Item questionnaire 5-Point Likert Scale General cancer assessment tool derived from FACIT database Evaluates physical, functional, emotional, and social well-being (QOL); two questions regarding patient-physician relationships Evaluation period: past week	Self-report Second party (interview) Estimated time for completion: 5 minutes	Validated in men and women Internal reliability verified Test-retest reliability verified Construct: no healthy controls Convergent: POMS, SF-36, SLDS-C, and CES-D Divergent: MC-20 Discriminators: ECOG-PSR	General focus. Useful for screening and outcome assessments.
Functional Assessment of Cancer Therapy-Fatigue (FACT-F) Subscale	13-Item questionnaire administered with FACT-G 5-Point Likert Scale Evaluation period: past week	Self-report Second party (interview) Estimated time for completion: 5–10 minutes	Validated in men and women Internal reliability verified Test-retest reliability: 3–7 days Construct: no healthy controls Convergent: PFS, POMS-F and -V (fatigue and vigor) Divergent: MC-20 Discriminators: hemoglobin and ECOG-PSR	Able to capture physical and psychological aspects. Useful for screening and outcome assessments.

Instrument	Description	Administration	Psychometrics	Comments
Functional Assessment of Cancer Anemia Subscale (FACT-An)	20-Item questionnaire (13 of which are identical to FACT-F administered with FACT-G) 5-Point Likert Scale Assesses symptoms associated with anemia Evaluation period: past week	Self-report Second party (interview) Estimated time for completion: 5–10 minutes	Validated in men and women Internal reliability verified Test-retest reliability: 3–7 days Construct: no healthy controls Convergent: PFS, POMS-F and -V Divergent: MC-20 Discriminators: hemoglobin and ECOG-PSR	Able to capture physical and psychological aspects. Useful for screening and outcome assessments.
Identity-Consequence Fatigue Scale (Paddison, Booth, Hill, & Cameron, 2006)	31 Items in five domains (i.e., vigor, concentration, energy, daily activity, fatigue)			Severe fatigue was associated with a significantly higher risk of hospitalizations for people with COPD (Paddison, Effing, Quinn, & Frith, 2013)
Lee Fatigue Scale (LFS or VAS-F)	18-Item visual analog scale Fatigue subscale: 13 items Energy subscale: 5 items Evaluation period: current	Self-report Second party (interview) Estimated time for completion: less than 5 minutes	Validated in men and women Internal reliability verified Test-retest reliability: limited data Construct verified Convergent: POMS (F and V) and Stanford Sleepiness Scale Divergent not evaluated Discriminators not evaluated	Able to capture physical and psychological aspects. Useful for screening and outcome assessments. Although this tool has been used to assess cancer fatigue, original validation performed in patients with sleep disorders.
Modified Fatigue Impact Scale (MFIS) (Fisk et al., 1994; Kos et al., 2005; Learmonth et al., 2013)	5 Item questionnaire 5-point Likert Scale	Self-report Second party (interview) Estimated time for completion: 5 minutes	Validated in MS patients, Parkinson's patients, and in four European countries.	MFIS is simple, economical, and efficient at capturing the severity and impact of fatigue in MS, primarily the physical nature of fatigue.
Multidimensional Assessment of Fatigue (MAF) Scale (Belza et al., 1993); provides a Global Fatigue Index (Belza et al., 2001).	16-Item questionnaire. 10-point scale for items 1–14; 5-point scale for item 15. 5 dimensions: degree, severity, distress, impact, timing	Self-report. Item 16 is not included in the scoring. Estimated completion time: 10 minutes. Scores range from 1 (no fatigue) to 50 (severe fatigue).	Revision of the Piper Fatigue scale.	Focus is on the type, severity, and distress of fatigue.

(continued)

Instrument	Description	Administration	Validity	Comments
Multidimensional Fatigue Inventory (MFI-20)	20-Item questionnaire 5-Point Likert Scale Scales: general, physical, mental, reduced motivation, reduced activity Evaluation period: past 24 hours	Self-report Second party (interview) Estimated time for completion: 5–10 minutes	Validated in men and women Internal reliability verified Test-retest reliability not evaluated Construct verified Convergent: VAS (single item), BDS and Rhoten Fatigue Scale Divergent not evaluated Discriminators not evaluated	Able to capture physical and psychological aspects. Useful for screening and outcome assessments.
Multidimensional Fatigue Symptom Inventory (MFSI)	Same authors as FSI 83-Item questionnaire 5-Point Likert Scale Rational subscale: global, somatic, affective, cognitive, and behavioral aspects Empirical subscale: general, physical, emotional, mental, aspects; also evaluates vigor Short form (MFSI-SF): developed to evaluate only empiric information Evaluation period: past week	Self-report Second party (interview) Estimated time for completion: 10 minutes	Validated in women Internal reliability: both subscales Test-retest reliability: significant and equivalent correlations noted for both subscales Construct verified Convergent: POMS-F and SF-36 (vitality), STAI, and CES-D Divergent: MC-20 Discriminators: ECOG-PSR	Able to capture physical and psychological aspects. Validation performed in women only, which may affect generalization. Useful for screening, however, may be too long or cumbersome for outcome assessments.
Piper Fatigue Scale (PFS)	27-Item questionnaire 22 Items: 11-point Likert Scale used to estimate fatigue scores 5 Items: open-ended Subscales: behavioral-severity, affective meaning, sensory, and cognitive-mood Evaluation period: current	Self-report Second party (interview) Estimated time for completion: 5 minutes	Validated in women Internal reliability verified Test-retest reliability not evaluated Construct: no healthy controls Convergent: demographic profile (investigator-developed), POMS, and Fatigue Symptom Checklist Divergent: POMS-Vigor Discriminators not evaluated	Able to capture physical and psychological aspects. Useful for screening and outcome assessments. Used clinically to assess CRF in men; however, formal validation efforts have not yet been published.

Instrument	Description	Administration	Validation	Comments
Quick Fatigue Assessment Survey (QFAS) (Quick & Fonteyn, 2005)	17-Item assessment designed for obtaining descriptive data about a patient's cancer-related fatigue. The QFAS identifies the initiation, duration, intensity, and relieving or aggravating factors of the fatigue experience with the use of dichotomous questions, open-ended questions, and ordinal ranking.	Self-report; Second party (interview); Estimated time for completion: 5–10 minutes	Validated in 114 patients from four outpatient oncology clinics; patients aged 22–84 represented a comprehensive sample of the adult oncology population.	The QFAS appears to show promise as a clinically useful technique for obtaining an initial assessment of cancer-related fatigue.
QuickPIPER (Cuesta-Vargas et al., 2013)	15-Item, validated one-dimensional model representing cancer-related fatigue, based on factor analysis testing of the Piper Fatigue Scale-revised (R-PFS)	Self-report questionnaire	111 Breast cancer survivors participated in the prospective, observational study of the QuickPIPER validation.	The 15-item QuickPIPER possesses similar properties to the 22-item R-PFS and offers the important advantage of brevity.
Revised Piper Fatigue Scale (Dagnelie et al., 2006)	22 Items with 10-point numerical rating in four subscales: behavioral/severity; affective meaning; sensory; and cognitive/mood	Self-report questionnaire	Psychometric properties validated in Dutch cancer patients: 16 Males, 13 females with lung cancer; 35 women with breast cancer. Construct validity was established with the MFI; criterion-related validity was moderate with the MFI and the Rotterdam Symptom Checklist (RSCL).	Significantly lower ($p < .01$) scores were found in sensory and cognitive/mood subscales among Dutch Breast cancer patients when compared to the original study population (Piper et al., 1998); no significant differences in behavioral/severity or affective meaning subscales
Profile of Mood States (POMS)	65-Item questionnaire; 5-Point Likert Scale; Subscales: tension-anxiety, anger-hostility, vigor-activity, fatigue-inertia, and confusion-bewilderment; Short form: 30 items (derived from the six subscales); developed for the elderly and individuals with medical disorders or disabilities; Evaluation period: past week	Self-report; Second party (interview); Estimated time for completion: 5–7 minutes (some individuals may require more time)	Validated in men and women; Internal reliability: all subscales; Test-retest reliability: all subscales; Construct verified; Convergent: Hopkins Symptom Distress Scale, Manifest Anxiety Scale, BDS, and Interpersonal Behavior Inventory; Divergent: MC-20; Discriminators not evaluated	Only able to capture psychological aspects. Useful for screening; however, may be too long or cumbersome for outcome assessments. Flexible scoring: entire document or individual subscales.

(continued)

Instrument	Description	Administration	Validity	Comments
Schwartz Cancer Fatigue Scale (SCFS) [original version]	28-Item questionnaire 5-Point Likert Scale Subscales (factors): physical, emotional, cognitive, and temporal Evaluation period: past 2–3 days	Self-report Second party (interview) Estimated time for completion: 5 minutes	Validated in men and women Internal reliability verified Test-retest reliability not evaluated Construct: limited evaluation Convergent: VAS-F Divergent not evaluated Discriminators not evaluated	Able to capture physical and psychological aspects. Described validation under experimental conditions, but validation was not maintained when used in a clinical setting.
Schwartz Cancer Fatigue Scale (SCFS-6) [revised version]	6-Item questionnaire 5-Point Likert Scale Subscales (factors): physical and perceptual Developed because further testing was unable to confirm validation of original version Evaluation period: past 2–3 days	Self-report Second party (interview) Estimated time for completion: 1–2 minutes	Validated in men and women Internal reliability verified Test-retest reliability not evaluated Construct verified Convergent not evaluated Divergent not evaluated Discriminators: limited evaluation	Able to capture physical and psychological aspects. Requires further validation (in the clinical setting). Items are identical to those in POMS. Computerized version has been developed.
Symptom Distress Scale (SDS) (Cooley et al., 2005)	13 Items; 5-point Likert Scale assessment of 11 symptoms (nausea, appetite, insomnia, pain, fatigue, bowel pattern, concentration, cough, appearance, outlook, breathing); and a frequency report for two symptoms (pain, nausea); evaluates feelings on day of administration.	Self-report Estimated completion time: 5 minutes Scores range from 13 (little distress) to 65 (severe symptom distress).	Validity: reported accurately used and completed by over 98% of participants; preferred by participants with lower education when compared with other questionnaires; internal reliability demonstrated by repeated measure (Kukull, McCorkle, & Driever, 1986).	Developed for symptom assessment in adults diagnosed with cancer.

BDS, Beck Depression Scale; BFI, Brief Fatigue Inventory; CES-D, Center for Epidemiological Studies-Depression Scale; COPD, chronic obstructive pulmonary disease; ECOG-PSR, Eastern Collaborative Oncology Group Performance Status Rating; FACIT, Functional Assessment of Chronic Illness Therapy; MC-20, Marlowe-Crowne Social Desirability Scale; MS, multiple sclerosis; PFS, progression-free survival; POMS, problem-oriented medical synopsis; QOL, quality of life; SF-36, Health Outcomes Study Short Form; SLDS-C, Satisfaction With Life Domains Scale-Cancer; STAI, State-Trait Anxiety Inventory; VAS-F; Visual Analog Scale-Fatigue.

■ **APPENDIX 25.2**

PIPER FATIGUE SCALE (PFS)

Directions: Many individuals can experience a sense of unusual or excessive tiredness whenever they become ill, receive treatment, or recover from their illness/treatment. This unusual sense of tiredness is not usually relieved either by a good night's sleep or by rest. Some call this symptom "fatigue" to distinguish it from the usual sense of tiredness.

For each of the following questions, please fill in the space provided for that response that best describes the fatigue you are experiencing now or for today. Please make every effort to answer each question to the best of your ability. If you are not experiencing fatigue now or for today, fill in the circle indicating "0" for your response. Thank you very much!

1. How long have you been feeling fatigue? (Check one response only.)
   - ☐ 1. Not feeling fatigue
   - ☐ 2. Minutes
   - ☐ 3. Hours
   - ☐ 4. Days
   - ☐ 5. Weeks
   - ☐ 6. Months
   - ☐ 7. Other (Please describe)

2. To what degree is the fatigue you are feeling now causing you distress?
   No Distress / A Great Deal — 1 2 3 4 5 6 7 8 9 10

3. To what degree is the fatigue you are feeling now interfering with your ability to complete your work or school activities?
   None / A Great Deal — 1 2 3 4 5 6 7 8 9 10

4. To what degree is the fatigue you are feeling now interfering with your ability to socialize with your friends?
   None / A Great Deal — 1 2 3 4 5 6 7 8 9 10

5. To what degree is the fatigue you are feeling now interfering with your ability to engage in sexual activity?
   None / A Great Deal — 1 2 3 4 5 6 7 8 9 10

6. Overall, how much is the fatigue, which you are now experiencing, interfering with your ability to engage in the kind of activities you enjoy doing?
   None / A Great Deal — 1 2 3 4 5 6 7 8 9 10

7. How would you describe the degree of intensity or severity of the fatigue that you are experiencing now?
   Mild / Severe — 1 2 3 4 5 6 7 8 9 10

8. To what degree would you describe the fatigue that you are experiencing now as being?
   Pleasant / Unpleasant — 1 2 3 4 5 6 7 8 9 10

9. To what degree would you describe the fatigue that you are experiencing now as being?
   Agreeable / Disagreeable — 1 2 3 4 5 6 7 8 9 10

10. To what degree would you describe the fatigue that you are experiencing now as being?
    Protective / Destructive — 1 2 3 4 5 6 7 8 9 10

11. To what degree would you describe the fatigue that you are experiencing now as being?
    Positive / Negative — 1 2 3 4 5 6 7 8 9 10

(continued)

12. To what degree would you describe the fatigue that you are experiencing now as being?
Normal | | | | | | | | | | Abnormal
1 2 3 4 5 6 7 8 9 10

13. To what degree are you now feeling?
Strong | | | | | | | | | | Weak
1 2 3 4 5 6 7 8 9 10

14. To what degree are you now feeling?
Awake | | | | | | | | | | Sleepy
1 2 3 4 5 6 7 8 9 10

15. To what degree are you now feeling?
Lively | | | | | | | | | | Listless
1 2 3 4 5 6 7 8 9 10

16. To what degree are you now feeling?
Refreshed | | | | | | | | | | Tired
1 2 3 4 5 6 7 8 9 10

17. To what degree are you now feeling?
Energetic | | | | | | | | | | Unenergetic
1 2 3 4 5 6 7 8 9 10

18. To what degree are you now feeling?
Patient | | | | | | | | | | Impatient
1 2 3 4 5 6 7 8 9 10

19. To what degree are you now feeling?
Relaxed | | | | | | | | | | A Great Deal
1 2 3 4 5 6 7 8 9 10

20. To what degree are you now feeling?
Exhilarated | | | | | | | | | | Depressed
1 2 3 4 5 6 7 8 9 10

21. To what degree are you now feeling?
Able to Concentrate | | | | | | | | | | Unable to Concentrate
1 2 3 4 5 6 7 8 9 10

22. To what degree are you now feeling?
Able to Remember | | | | | | | | | | Unable to Remember
1 2 3 4 5 6 7 8 9 10

23. To what degree are you now feeling?
Able to Think Clearly | | | | | | | | | | Unable to Think Clearly
1 2 3 4 5 6 7 8 9 10

24. Overall, what do you believe is *most* directly contributing to or causing your fatigue?
_____
_____

25. Overall, the *best* thing you have found to relieve your fatigue is:
_____
_____

(continued)

26. Is there anything else you would like to add that would describe your fatigue better to us?

_____

_____

_____

27. Are you experiencing any other symptoms right now?

_____

_____

_____

Scoring Piper Fatigue Scale (PFS) Survey Results

PFS current format and scoring instructions:

1. The PFS in its current form is composed of 22 numerically scaled, "0" to "10" items that measure four dimensions of subjective fatigue: behavioral/severity (6 items: #2–7); affective meaning (5 items: #8–12); sensory (5 items: #13–17); and cognitive/mood (6 items: #18–23). These 22 items are used to calculate the four subscale/dimensional scores and the total fatigue scores.

2. Five additional items (#1 and #24–27) are not used to calculate subscale or total fatigue scores but are recommended to be kept on the scale as these items furnish rich, qualitative data. Item #1, in particular, gives a categorical way in which to assess the duration of the respondent's fatigue.

3. To score the PFS, add the items contained on each specific subscale together and divide by the number of items on that subscale. This will give you a subscale score that remains on the same "0" to "10" numeric scale. Should you have missing item data, and the respondent has answered at least 75% to 80% of the remaining items on that particular subscale, calculate the subscale mean score based on the number of items answered, and substitute that mean value for the missing item score (mean-item substitution).

4. Recalculate the subscale score. To calculate the total fatigue score, add the 22-item scores together and divide by 22 in order to keep the score on the same numeric "0" to "10" scale.!

Severity Codes:
0	NONE
1–3	MILD
4–6	MODERATE
7–10	SEVERE

Source: Piper, B. F., Dibble, S. L., Dodd, M. J., Weiss, M. C., Slaughter, R. E., & Paul, S. M. (1998). The revised Piper Fatigue Scale: Psychometric evaluation in women with breast cancer. *Oncology Nursing Forum, 25*(4), 677–684.

■ APPENDIX 25.3

GLOBAL FATIGUE INDEX
MULTIDIMENSIONAL ASSESSMENT OF FATIGUE (MAF) SCALE

Fatigue Dimension	Questions	Scoring
Degree	1. To what degree have you experienced fatigue?	1 (not at all)–10 (a great deal)
Severity	2. How severe is the fatigue that you have been experiencing?	1 (not at all)–10 (a great deal)
Distress	3. To what degree has fatigue caused you distress?	1 (not at all)–10 (a great deal)
Impact on Activities of Daily Living (11 items)	4. Household chores?	1 (not at all)–10 (a great deal)
	5. Cook?	1 (not at all)–10 (a great deal)
	6. Bathe or wash?	1 (not at all)–10 (a great deal)
	7. Dress?	1 (not at all)–10 (a great deal)
	8. Work?	1 (not at all)–10 (a great deal)
	9. Visit or socialize with friends or family?	1 (not at all)–10 (a great deal)
	10. Engage in sexual activity?	1 (not at all)–10 (a great deal)
	11. Engage in leisure and recreational activities?	1 (not at all)–10 (a great deal)
	12. Shop and do errands?	1 (not at all)–10 (a great deal)
	13. Walk?	1 (not at all)–10 (a great deal)
	14. Exercise, other than walking?	1 (not at all)–10 (a great deal)
Timing	15. Over the past week, including today, how often have you been fatigued?	0 (hardly any days)–4 (every day)
	16. To what degree has your fatigue changed during the past week?	1 (decreased)–4 (increased)

Scoring: The total score for items 1, 2, and 3. Average items 4–14 (ADLs). Item #15 multiply the score by 2.5. Item 16 is not included in the score. Score ranges from 1 to 50; the higher the score, the greater impairment from fatigue.

Sources: Belza, B., Henke, C. J., Yelin, E. H., Epstain, W. V., & Gillis, C. L. (1993). Correlates of fatigue in older adults with rheumatoid arthritis. *Nursing Research*, *42*, 93–99. doi:10.1097/00006199-199303000-00006; Belza, B., Steele, B. G., Hunziker, J., Lakshminaryan, S., Holt, L., & Buchner, D. M. (2001). Correlates of physical activity in chronic obstructive pulmonary disease. *Nursing Research*, *50*(4), 195–202. doi:10.1097/00006199-200107000-00003

Elizabeth A. Ayello & R. Gary Sibbald

Minimizing Skin Alterations

KEY POINTS

- Skin injury prevention may need to be balanced against the overall goals of care.
- Skin changes, including pressure injuries, are common occurrences during the dying process.
- Wound care should be aimed at improving the patient's quality of life by providing comfort, relieving pain, controlling odor, and containing exudate.

CASE STUDY

Mrs. Rose was an 86-year-old female with a chronic history of right-leg lymphedema and subsequent leg ulcer over the past 17 years. Ten years ago, this ulcer was diagnosed as basal cell carcinoma by biopsy and gradually eroded through the skin and bone. She has had noneffective lympha-press, negative wound pressure therapy, and other advanced therapies through home care. She also had surgical excision and failed skin graft, maximum radiotherapy with recurrence of the tumor around the edges of the wound, use of imiquimod around ulcer edges, and numerous hospitalizations and infections. The leg was unstable and an amputation was recommended, but she would not give her consent for surgery. Her pain level ranged 8–10/10, requiring a formal pain management consultation. The pain was both nociceptive (gnawing, aching) and neuropathic in nature. For the nociceptive pain, acetaminophen was used 500 to 1,000 mg one to three times a day. Occasionally, hydromorphone 1 mg was used for breakthrough pain. However, she took this only rarely as it caused constipation. At night, she took nortriptyline for the burning and stinging to facilitate sleep. She did not tolerate gabapentin due to disorientation. The wound was large and highly exudative with multiple episodes of superficial and deep infection, including *Pseudomonas* and Methicillin-resistant *Staphylococcus aureus* (MRSA). The right-leg fibular and tibial bones had multiple fragments with an unstable foot and exposure of arteries and veins. She could not ambulate and needed to use a pneumatic walker. She moved from her home to a retirement community with a low airflow bed, but developed a coccyx pressure injury secondary to her inability to walk. The injury was treated as a maintenance wound because healing was not expected. An iodine-soaked ribbon gauze was used on the pressure ulcer for bacterial reduction. She consented to an amputation, but died 6 weeks post-op.

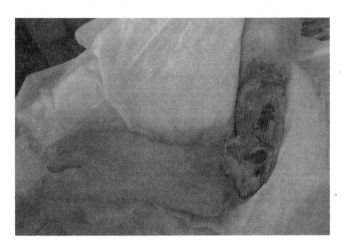 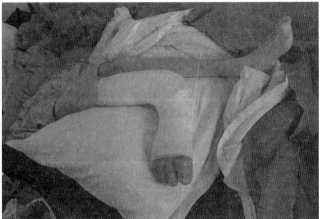

As part of the interprofessional team that cared for Mrs. Rose, how would you have approached the control of the exudate and odor? Did you have any suggestions for the management of her pain?

The Wound Bed Preparation 2015 model can be used as a clinician guide to develop a care plan (Figure 26.1) for a palliative care (PC) patient with an alteration in skin integrity (Sibbald, Elliott, Ayello, & Somayaji, 2016). In this population, wound healing is not often the goal; nonetheless, realistically classifying a wound as healable, maintenance, or non-healable (heal ability) is important. A healable wound has adequate blood supply and the cause can be corrected. A maintenance wound is healable, but either patient factors (unable to tolerate compression bandaging for venous leg edema) or system factors (protective footwear or pressure-relieving devices not covered for patients in the home) are not available. A non-healable wound is a pressure injury with a patient who has a negative protein balance or inadequate blood supply to facilitate healing. Many wounds are treated as maintenance, with important aspects of patient-centered care being focused on in the patient care plan, including wound odor, excessive exudate, superficial critical bacterial colonization (responds to topical antimicrobials), deep/surrounding infection (requires systemic therapy), bleeding, and wound-associated pain. The clinician's role is to advocate that the patient's quality of life (QOL) and comfort supersede care that concentrates on healing outcomes. The prevention of skin injury also needs to be balanced against the overall goals of care. "Strategies used to prevent pressure ulcers in other populations may seem to be in direct conflict with palliative care strategies" (Langemo, 2012, p. 25).

Actual physical examination of the skin is needed to identify patients at risk for skin injury and to initiate prevention protocols. There is, however, no consensus in the literature as to what constitutes a minimum skin assessment. Baranoski and Ayello (2015) have suggested five elements to include in a basic skin assessment: skin temperature, color, moisture, turgor, and whether the skin is intact or has areas of injury, including open areas. In this chapter, several common skin problems will be discussed, including skin tears, pressure injuries formerly known as pressure ulcers, skin tumors, treatment-related skin injuries, peristomal skin, and fistulas (Baranoski & Ayello, 2015).

■ SKIN CHANGES AT LIFE'S END (SCALE)

Despite optimal nursing care, not all pressure injuries at life's end are preventable (Sibbald, Krasner, & Lutz, 2010). An expert group of panelists was assembled to make recommendations for the documentation and treatment of pressure ulcers at life's end. The recommendations are summarized in Table 26.1.

■ PRESSURE INJURIES

In April 2016, the National Pressure Ulcer Advisory Panel (NPUAP) replaced the term *pressure ulcer* with *pressure injury* and revised its definition (Edsberg et al., 2016):

A pressure injury is localized damage to the skin and/or underlying soft tissue usually over a bony prominence or related to a medical or other device. The injury can present as intact skin or an open ulcer and may be painful. The injury occurs as a result of intense and/or prolonged pressure or pressure in combination with shear. The tolerance of soft tissue for pressure and shear may also be affected by microclimate, nutrition, perfusion, comorbidities and condition of the soft tissue (p. 585).

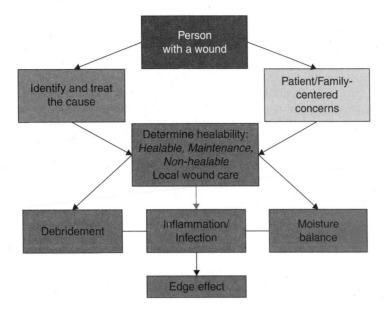

FIGURE 26.1 Wound Bed Preparation Model.

Source: Sibbald, R. G., Elliott, J. A., Ayello, E. A., & Somayaji, R. (2016). Optimizing the moisture management tightrope with Wound Bed Preparation 2015©: Wound care. *Wound Healing Southern Africa, 9*(1), 9–15. doi:10.1097/01.ASW.0000470851.27030.98. Retrieved from https://journals.lww.com/aswcjournal/fulltext/2015/10000/Optimizing_the_Moisture_Management_Tightrope_with.6.aspx

TABLE 26.1 Skin Changes at Life's End (SCALE) Panel Statements	
Statement Number	**Panel Statement**
1	Physiological changes that occur because of the dying process may affect the skin and soft tissues and may manifest as observable (objective) changes in skin color, turgor, or integrity, or as subjective symptoms such as localized pain. These changes can be unavoidable and may occur with the application of appropriate interventions that meet or exceed the standard of care.
2	The plan of care and patient response should be clearly documented and reflected in the entire medical record. Charting by exception is an appropriate method of documentation.
3	Patient-centered concerns should be addressed, including pain and activities of daily living.
4	SCALE is a reflection of compromised skin (reduced soft-tissue perfusion, decreased tolerance to external insults, and impaired removal of metabolic wastes).
5	Expectations regarding the patient's end-of-life goals and concerns should be communicated among the members of the interprofessional team and the patient's circle of care. The discussion should include the potential for SCALE, including other skin changes, skin breakdown, and pressure ulcers.
6	Risk factors, symptoms, and signs associated with SCALE have not been fully elucidated, but may include: ▪ Weakness and progressive limitation of mobility ▪ Suboptimal nutrition, including loss of appetite, weight loss, cachexia and wasting, low serum albumin/ prealbumin level, and low hemoglobin, as well as dehydration ▪ Diminished tissue perfusion, impaired skin oxygenation, decreased local skin temperature, mottled discoloration, and skin necrosis ▪ Loss of skin integrity from any of a number of factors, including equipment or devices, incontinence, chemical irritants, chronic exposure to body fluids, skin tears, pressure, shear, friction, and infections ▪ Impaired immune function
7	A total skin assessment should be performed regularly and all areas of concern documented consistent with the wishes and condition of the patient. Pay special attention to bony prominences and skin areas with underlying cartilage. Areas of special concern include the sacrum, coccyx, ischial tuberosities, trochanters, scapulae, occiput, heels, digits, nose, and ears. Describe the skin or wound abnormality exactly as assessed.

(continued)

Statement Number	Panel Statement
TABLE 26.1	Skin Changes at Life's End (SCALE) Panel Statements *(continued)*
8	Consultation with a qualified healthcare professional is recommended for any skin changes associated with increased pain, signs of infection, or skin breakdown (when the goal may be healing) and whenever the patient's circle of care expresses a significant concern.
9	The probable skin change etiology and goals of care should be determined. Consider the five Ps for determining appropriate intervention strategies: ■ Prevention ■ Prescription (may heal with appropriate treatment) ■ Preservation (maintenance without deterioration) ■ Palliation (provide comfort and care) ■ Preference (patient desires)
10	Patients and concerned individuals should be educated regarding SCALE and the plan of care.

Source: Adapted from Sibbald, R. G., Krasner, D. L., & Lutz, J. (2010). SCALE: Skin changes at life's end: Final consensus statement: October 1, 2009©. *Advances in Skin & Wound Care, 23*(5), 225–236. doi:10.1097/01.ASW.0000363537.75328.36. Retrieved from https://journals.lww.com/aswcjournal/Abstract/2010/05000/SCALE__Skin_Changes_at_Life_s_End__Final_Consensus.9.aspx

TABLE 26.2 Location of Pressure Ulcers Among Deceased Persons

Location	Percentage of Cases	Percentage of Ulcers
Hospital	44.3	44.6
Nursing home	37.8	40.2
Family home	14.2	12

Source: Adapted from Eckman, K. L. (1989). The prevalence of dermal ulcers among persons in the U.S. who have died. *Advances in Skin & Wound Care, 2*(2), 36–39. Retrieved from https://journals.lww.com/aswcjournal/Abstract/1989/05000/THE_PREVALENCE_OF_DERMAL_ULCERS_AMONG_PERSONS_IN.6.aspx

Skin changes do occur at life's end and can be part of the dying process (Sibbald et al., 2010). Eckman (1989) reported the results of a randomized study of 130 funeral homes across the United States. Of the 1,378 deceased persons, one out of four (23.6%) had a pressure injury. The number of wounds ranged from one to 14. Of those with a pressure injury, 31.4% had one pressure injury and 68.6% had more than one pressure injury. Table 26.2 documents the number of cases by location when the location of death was known (Eckman, 1989).

The NPUAP extensively reviewed data and found that, in the United States, the incidence of pressure ulcers in acute care ranged from 2.8% to 9.0%, with a higher incidence in older populations (Pieper, 2012). The incidence in home care was 4.5% to 6.3% (Roca-Biosca, Velasco-Guillén, Rubio-Rico, García-Grau, & Anguera-Saperas, 2012), while for PC, the incidence ranged from 6.5% to 54.7% (Langemo, 2012). In long-term care (LTC), the incidence ranged from 3.6% to 59%, which is a much higher range than the publicly reported Centers for Medicare & Medicaid Services (CMS) minimum data set (MDS) 3.0

for an LTC of 8.20% for the second quarter of 2012 to 7.48% for the first quarter of 2017 (Ayello, 2017; Pieper, 2012). The NPUAP concluded that "significant gaps in knowledge are evident." Table 26.3 summarizes some high points of the NPUAP recommendations and their future research implications (Langemo, 2012).

An earlier study reported data at an even higher PC pressure injury susceptibility rate. Reifsnyder, Hoplamazian, and Maxwell (2004) identified 62.3% of 980 hospice patients were diagnosed with cancer and were at a higher risk of developing a pressure injury as compared to those without cancer. Hanson et al. (1991) reported an incidence of 13% for Stage 1 and 2 pressure injuries. Locations of these pressure injuries were the sacrum (38.4%), elbows (30.7%), and heels (15.4%). Pressure injuries often occurred within 2 weeks of death. Waltman, Bergstrom, Armstrong, Norvell, and Braden (1991) found a higher incidence of pressure injuries in elderly patients with cancer (85%) compared to a matched group without cancer (70%). In this prospective study, the average time to death after developing pressure injuries was 3 weeks.

Kennedy (1989) reported that 56% of patients who died in an intermediate care facility developed a pressure injury within the 6 weeks prior to their death. Furthermore, on her website (www.kennedyterminalulcer.com), Karen Lou Kennedy-Evans has described the following characteristics of the Kennedy terminal ulcer: pear shaped; coccyx or sacrum; red, yellow, or black; sudden onset; and imminent death. Langemo (2012) describes the susceptible patient as follows: "Time in bed increases as their condition deteriorates, which occurs concomitantly as multi-system failure and growing weakness predispose them to risk factors including decreased activity and mobility, depleted nutrition and hydration, incontinence, and changes in sensory perception and consciousness." In a 10-bed PC unit located in an acute care facility, 5% of the patients developed pressure ulcers (Brennan & Trombley, 2010).

TABLE 26.3   NPUAP EPUAP PPPIA Recommendations: Individuals in Palliative Care

Patient and Risk Assessment

1. Complete a comprehensive assessment of the individual. (Strength of Evidence = C; Strength of Recommendation = 2 thumbs up)

1.1. Consider using the Hunters Hill-Marie Curie Centre Risk Assessment Tool, specific to adult individuals in PC. (Strength of Evidence = C; Strength of Recommendation = 1 thumb neutral)

Pressure Redistribution

1. Reposition and turn the individual at periodic intervals, in accordance with the individual's wishes, comfort, and tolerance. (Strength of Evidence = C; Strength of Recommendation = 2 thumbs up)

1.1. Pre-medicate the individual 20 to 30 minutes prior to a scheduled position change for individuals who experience significant pain on movement. (Strength of Evidence = C; Strength of Recommendation = 1 thumb up)

1.2. Consider the individual's choices in turning, including whether she or he has a position of comfort, after explaining the rationale for turning. (Strength of Evidence = C; Strength of Recommendation = 2 thumbs up)

1.3. Consider changing the support surface to improve pressure redistribution and comfort. (Strength of Evidence = C; Strength of Recommendation = 2 thumbs up)

1.4. Strive to reposition an individual receiving PC at least every 4 hours on a pressure redistributing mattress such as viscoelastic foam, or every 2 hours on a regular mattress. (Strength of Evidence = B; Strength of Recommendation = 1 thumb up)

1.5. Document turning and repositioning, as well as the factors influencing these decisions (e.g., individual wishes or medical needs). (Strength of Evidence = C; Strength of Recommendation = 2 thumbs up)

Nutrition and Hydration

Strive to maintain adequate nutrition and hydration compatible with the individual's condition and wishes. Adequate nutritional support is often not attainable when the individual is unable or refuses to eat, based on certain disease states. (Strength of Evidence = C; Strength of Recommendation = 2 thumbs up)

Offer nutritional protein supplements when ulcer healing is the goal. (Strength of Evidence = C; Strength of Recommendation = 2 thumbs up)

Pressure Ulcer Care

1. Set treatment goals consistent with the values and goals of the individual, while considering input from the individual's significant others. (Strength of Evidence = C; Strength of Recommendation = 2 thumbs up)

1.1. Assess the impact of the pressure ulcer on the QOL of the individual and his or her significant others. (Strength of Evidence = C; Strength of Recommendation = 1 thumb up)

1.2. Set a goal to enhance the QOL, even if the pressure ulcer cannot be healed or treatment does not lead to closure/healing. (Strength of Evidence = C; Strength of Recommendation = 1 thumb up)

1.3. Assess the individual initially and at any change in his or her condition to reevaluate the plan of care. (Strength of Evidence = C; Strength of Recommendation = 2 thumbs up)

2. Assess the pressure ulcer initially and with each dressing change, but at least weekly (unless death is imminent), and document findings. (Strength of Evidence = C; Strength of Recommendation = 2 thumbs up)

2.1. Monitor the pressure ulcer in order to continue to meet the goals of comfort and reduction in wound pain, addressing wound symptoms that impact the QOL such as malodor and exudate. (Strength of Evidence = C; Strength of Recommendation = 2 thumbs up)

3. Control wound odor. (Strength of Evidence = C; Strength of Recommendation = 2 thumbs up)

3.1. Manage malodor through regular wound cleansing; assessment and management of infection; and debridement of devitalized tissue, with consideration for the individual's wishes and goals of care. (Strength of Evidence = C; Strength of Recommendation = 2 thumbs up)

3.2. Consider use of topical metronidazole to effectively control pressure ulcer odor associated with anaerobic bacteria and protozoal infections. (Strength of Evidence = C; Strength of Recommendation = 1 thumb up)

3.3. Consider use of charcoal or activated charcoal dressings to help control odor. (Strength of Evidence = C; Strength of Recommendation = 1 thumb up)

3.4. Consider use of external odor absorbers or odor maskers for the room (e.g., activated charcoal, kitty litter, vinegar, vanilla, coffee beans, burning candle, and potpourri). (Strength of Evidence = C; Strength of Recommendation = 1 thumb up)

4. Manage the pressure ulcer and periwound area on a regular basis as consistent with the individual's wishes. (Strength of Evidence = C; Strength of Recommendation = 1 thumb up)

Pain Assessment and Management

1. Do not undertreat pain in individuals receiving PC. (Strength of Evidence = C; Strength of Recommendation = 2 thumbs up)

2. Select a wound dressing that requires less frequent changing and is less likely to cause pain. (Strength of Evidence = C; Strength of Recommendation = 2 thumbs up)

(continued)

TABLE 26.3   NPUAP EPUAP PPPIA Recommendations: Individuals in Palliative Care (*continued*)

Resource Assessment

1. Assess psychosocial resources initially and at routine periods thereafter (psychosocial consultation, social work, etc.). (Strength of Evidence = C; Strength of Recommendation = 1 thumb up)

2. Assess environmental resources (e.g., ventilation, electronic air filters, etc.) initially and at routine periods thereafter. (Strength of Evidence = C; Strength of Recommendation = 1 thumb up)

3. Educate the individual and his or her significant others regarding skin changes at the end of life. (Strength of Evidence = C; Strength of Recommendation = 1 thumb up)

4. Validate that family care providers understand the goals and plan of care. (Strength of Evidence = C; Strength of Recommendation = 2 thumbs up)

Strength of Evidence A	The recommendation is supported by direct scientific evidence from properly designed and implemented controlled trials on pressure ulcers in humans (or humans at risk for pressure ulcers), providing statistical results that consistently support the recommendation (Level 1 studies required).
Strength of Evidence B	The recommendation is supported by direct scientific evidence from properly designed and implemented clinical series on pressure ulcers in humans (or humans at risk for pressure ulcers) providing statistical results that consistently support the recommendation (Level 2, 3, 4, and 5 studies required).
Strength of Evidence C	The recommendation is supported by indirect evidence (e.g., studies in healthy humans, humans with other types of chronic wounds, animal models) and/or expert opinion.

Strengths of Recommendation

👍👍	Strong positive recommendation: definitely do it
👍	Weak positive recommendation: probably do it
✊	No specific recommendation
👎	Weak negative recommendation: probably don't do it
👎👎	Strong negative recommendation: definitely don't do it

EPUAP, European Pressure Ulcer Advisory Panel; NPUAP, National Pressure Ulcer Advisory Panel; PC, palliative care; PPPIA, Pan Pacific Pressure Injury Alliance; QOL, quality of life.

Source: National Pressure Ulcer Advisory Panel, European Pressure Ulcer Advisory Panel and Pan Pacific Pressure Injury Alliance. (2014). *Prevention and treatment of pressure ulcers: Quick reference guide.* Osborne Park, Western Australia: Cambridge Media. Retrieved from https://www.npuap.org/wp-content/uploads/2014/08/Updated-10-16-14-Quick-Reference-Guide-DIGITAL-NPUAP-EPUAP-PPPIA-16Oct2014.pdf © NPUAP EPUAP PPPIA 2014, used with permission.

Preventing Pressure Injuries: Risk Assessment

The European Pressure Ulcer Advisory Panel (EPUAP) and the Pan Pacific Pressure Injury Alliance (PPPIA) in 2014 collaboratively developed a joint international guideline for the prevention and treatment of pressure ulcers (new term for injuries). This guideline outlines evidence-based recommendations for the prevention and treatment of pressure injuries that could be used by healthcare professionals throughout the world. The current use of risk assessment scales to identify patients at risk for pressure injuries is recommended by the 2014 NPUAP–EPUAP Pressure Ulcer Treatment Guidelines. Many pressure risk assessment tools are available, the most commonly used being the Braden Scale (Bergstrom,

TABLE 26.4 Intervals for Pressure Ulcer Risk Assessment

Acute care
Initial assessment on admission
Reassessment every 24–48 hr or whenever the patient's condition changes
Long-term care
Initial assessment on admission
Reassessment weekly for the first 4 wk; then monthly to quarterly or whenever the patient's condition changes
Home healthcare
Initial assessment on admission
Reassessment with every registered nurse visit

Braden, Laguzza, & Holman, 1987), the Waterlow Scale (Waterlow, 1998), the Norton Scale (Norton, McLaren, & Exton-Smith, 1975), and the Hunters Hill-Marie Curie Centre Risk Assessment Tool (Chaplin, 2000), which is specific to palliative patients.

The Braden Scale (Bergstrom et al., 1987) is a widely used risk assessment tool in the United States. This scale has six factor subscales—sensory perception, moisture, activity, mobility, nutrition, and friction/shear—that are ranked to provide a total risk score. One study evaluated the association between the scores of the Waterlow, Braden, and Norton scales and their clinical and social characteristics in critically ill patients (de Azevedo Macena et al., 2017). A cross-sectional study of 78 patients in an adult ICU of a university hospital in northeastern Brazil was conducted from July to December 2015. Data included social and clinical information and the risk factors of the Braden, Norton, and Waterlow scales. Data were analyzed by the descriptive and inferential statistics. Age, use of tobacco, diabetes, and hypertension were associated with the risk of pressure ulcers in patients at an ICU (de Azevedo Macena et al., 2017).

Based on patients on a PC unit in England, a pressure ulcer risk assessment tool was developed and is referred to as the Hunters Hill-Marie Curie Centre (HH-MCC) Pressure Ulcer Risk Assessment Tool; it has two more subscales than the Braden Scale. Both tools have a subscale for sensory/perception, moisture, mobility, activity, and friction/shear. In addition, the HH-MCC Pressure Ulcer Risk Assessment Tool has a subscale for skin condition that is graded on a scale of 1 (*skin condition good*) to 4 (*skin integrity broken*) and also includes weight change patterns in the nutrition subscale. Perhaps one of the biggest differences between this scale and the Braden Scale (low scores are at risk, with 18 being the onset of pressure ulcer risk) is that no impairments have low

subscale numbers, whereas areas of high impairment have the highest numbers. In the HH-MCC Pressure Ulcer Risk Assessment Tool, a total score of 12 or lower means low risk, while scores 13 or higher imply medium risk. There is no ideal ulcer risk assessment tool for all clinical settings, and therefore, the choice should depend on their predictive validity for the patient care setting (Author, 2014).

Prevention Interventions

The Canadian Association of Wound Care concluded that people at the end of life are at risk for pressure injuries: "In many terminally ill patients, multiple factors and co-morbid conditions increase their risk for the development of pressure injuries and need to be identified." Pressure injuries are suggestive of deterioration and are part of the disease trajectory. In many cases, the primary treatment and prevention goal of care is displaced by a greater need for comfort. Some pressure injuries will not heal, and cure is an unrealistic goal; it may, in fact, mark the terminal stage of illness. There are a variety of classifications related to end-of-life wounds and unavoidability of certain pressure ulcers, but a definitive characterization of terminal and unavoidable skin injuries has not been achieved (Levine, 2017). As the number of people living with chronic illness soars, it is increasingly recognized that there are limited benefits of curative treatment. This is where PC offers an alternative to aggressive wound-healing interventions by changing the focus to wound stabilization, symptom management, and patient well-being.

The purpose of performing a risk assessment is to facilitate early identification and initiate preventive interventions (Table 26.4). The goal of reducing risk factors is to prevent pressure injuries. The implementation of prevention strategies is aimed at sparing at-risk older adults' painful and sometimes tiresome treatments. Older adults are considered to be "at risk" when their Braden Scale is 18 or below; intervention protocols have been linked to levels of risk (Prevention Plus, 2016). Attention to an elder's high-risk subscale scores can facilitate pressure injury prevention. Table 26.5 summarizes prevention strategies (Author, 2014).

The NPUAP/EPUAP/PPPIA 2014 Clinical Guideline may need to be modified based on the overall goals of the older adult's care (Author, 2014). For PC patients, following a rigid set time interval for a repositioning schedule may cause the patients undue pain. As the Canadian Association for Wound Care states: "During the time of active dying, the patient's wishes for pain control and comfort may outweigh the desire for pressure injury prevention. Pre-medicating the person with a pressure injury prior to repositioning, respecting the patient's choices in turning schedules and utilizing a support surface may be beneficial. The patient's choices

TABLE 26.5 Pressure Ulcer Prevention Protocol
Inspection and care of skin
Frequency of inspection—daily with documentation ■ Check skin under medical devices ■ Individual bathing—avoid hot water, drying soaps ■ Use emollients to hydrate dry skin ■ Do not massage reddened bony prominences ■ Manage incontinence and protect the skin from exposure to moisture ■ Protect from pressure to vulnerable skin areas such as the sacrum, elbows, greater trochanters, and heels
Mechanical loading and support surfaces
■ Pre-medicate persons who have pain on movement at least 20 min prior to moving them. ■ Individualize the turning and repositioning schedules based on the support surface being used and the person's wishes and choices for a position of comfort, general medical condition, activity and mobility level, care goals, and skin condition. ■ Use transfer devices to lift the person while repositioning rather than dragging. ■ Determine what positions provide comfort; consider the 30° lateral position when in bed. ■ Elevate heels without putting pressure on the Achilles tendon. ■ Use pressure redistribution seat cushions for persons when sitting in a chair/wheelchair. ■ Avoid positioning an individual on any reddened or pressure-discolored areas. ■ Avoid using donut devices.

regarding turning should be respected and include whether they have a 'position of comfort' after an explanation of the rationale for turning" (Author, 2014, p. 59).

Caregivers should negotiate a flexible time interval, premediating prior to repositioning and determining which positions provide the most comfort. Langemo and Black (2010) recommend that a repositioning schedule for patients receiving PC should be flexible and focused around the support surface used, coupled with the preference, needs, and tolerance of the patient. The patient and the family need to clearly understand the implications for skin injury; however, pressure injury prevention strategies in the palliative patient should be tailored to meet the client's wishes and general comfort. This variation in the patient's treatment plan also needs to be documented in the patient's record.

Pressure Injury Location

The sacrum is the number one location for pressure ulcer occurrence in adults; heels are second (VanGilder, MacFarlane, Harrison, Lachenbruch, & Meyer, 2010). For the NICU, pediatric intensive care unit (PICU), and pediatric patients, medical device pressure injuries were more common (VanGilder, Amlung, Harrison, & Meyer, 2009), with the nose being the most common site. In specific PC patients, other sites may be at risk for pressure injury breakdown. For example, elders with chronic obstructive pulmonary disease who are on long-term oxygen therapy are at a higher risk for device-related pressure ulcers. Skin near the ears, mouth, and nose is susceptible to tissue necrosis as a result of increased pressure associated with tubing.

Pressure Injury Staging

Pressure injuries are staged based on the visible assessment of the depth of tissue that has been damaged in the wound bed. Clinicians should use appropriate lighting sources, including natural or halogen lighting, as well as evaluate skin temperature and consistency to detect Stage 1 pressure injuries in clients with darkly pigmented skin.

The 2016 NPUAP pressure injury staging definitions are presented in the following list:

Stage 1 Pressure injury: Non-blanchable erythema of intact skin—Intact skin with a localized area of non-blanchable erythema, which may appear differently in darkly pigmented skin. Presence of blanchable erythema or changes in sensation, temperature, or firmness may precede visual changes. Color changes do not include purple or maroon discoloration; these may indicate deep tissue pressure injury.

Stage 2 Partial-thickness loss of skin with exposed dermis—The wound bed is viable, pink or red, and moist, and may also present as an intact or ruptured serum-filled blister. Adipose (fat) and deeper tissues are not visible. Granulation tissue, slough, and eschar are not present. These injuries commonly result from adverse microclimate and shear in the skin over the pelvis and shear in the heel. This stage should not be used to describe moisture-associated skin damage (MASD), including incontinence-associated dermatitis (IAD), intertriginous dermatitis (ITD), medical adhesive–related skin injury (MARSI), or traumatic wounds (skin tears, burns, abrasions).

Stage 3 Pressure injury: Full-thickness skin loss—Full-thickness loss of skin, in which adipose (fat) is visible in the ulcer and granulation tissue and epiboly (rolled wound edges) are often present. Slough and/or eschar may be visible. The depth of tissue damage varies by anatomical location; areas of significant adiposity can develop deep wounds. Undermining and tunneling may occur. Fascia, muscle, tendon, ligament, cartilage, and/or bone are not exposed. If slough or eschar obscures the extent of tissue loss, this is an unstageable pressure injury.

Stage 4 Pressure injury: Full-thickness skin and tissue loss—Full-thickness skin and tissue loss with exposed or directly palpable fascia, muscle, tendon, ligament, cartilage, or bone in the ulcer. Slough and/or eschar may be visible. Epiboly (rolled edges), undermining, and/or tunneling often occur. Depth varies by anatomical location. If slough or eschar obscures the extent of tissue loss, this is an unstageable pressure injury.

Unstageable pressure injury: Obscured full-thickness skin and tissue loss—Full-thickness skin and tissue loss in which the extent of tissue damage within the ulcer cannot be confirmed because it is obscured by slough or eschar. If slough or eschar is removed, a Stage 3 or Stage 4 pressure injury will be revealed. Stable eschar (i.e., dry, adherent, intact without erythema or fluctuance) on an ischemic limb or the heel(s) should not be removed.

Deep tissue pressure injury (DTPI): Persistent non-blanchable deep red, maroon, or purple discoloration—Intact or non-intact skin with localized area of persistent non-blanchable deep red, maroon, or purple discoloration or epidermal separation revealing a dark wound bed or blood-filled blister. Pain and temperature change often precede skin color changes. Discoloration may appear differently in darkly pigmented skin. This injury results from intense and/or prolonged pressure and shear forces at the bone–muscle interface. The wound may evolve rapidly to reveal the actual extent of tissue injury or may resolve without tissue loss. If necrotic tissue, subcutaneous tissue, granulation tissue, fascia, muscle, or other underlying structures are visible, this indicates a full-thickness pressure injury (unstageable, Stage 3, or Stage 4). Do not use DTPI to describe vascular, traumatic, neuropathic, or dermatologic conditions.

The Centers for Medicare and Medicaid Services (CMS, 2017) stated in its long-term acute care hospital quality reporting program manual:

Skin ulcers that develop in patients who have terminal illness or are at the end of life should be assessed and staged as pressure ulcers until it is determined that the ulcer is part of the dying process (also known as Kennedy ulcers). Kennedy ulcers can develop from 6 weeks to 2 to 3 days before death. These ulcers present as pear-shaped purple areas of skin with irregular borders that are often found in the sacral-coccygeal areas. When an ulcer has been determined to be a Kennedy ulcer, it should not be coded as a pressure ulcer. (p. M-3)

Pressure Injury Treatment

The management of patients on PC with pressure injuries is complex and should focus on a holistic approach. The incorporation of an interprofessional team greatly enhances the provision of optimal care. Naylor (2005) outlined seven principles that should be included in the management of palliative pressure injuries:

1. Correcting or treating the cause of the wound;
2. Preventing the development and/or further breakdown of the wound;
3. Addressing symptoms related to the wound;
4. Having patients (and their circle of care) perform self-assessments;
5. Encouraging independence;
6. Providing psychosocial support;
7. Improving QOL.

Tilley, Lipson, and Ramos (2016) proposed a systematic approach for PC for persons with malignant fungating wounds. They introduced the mnemonic PALCARE, which stands for the following: P—Prognosis, A—Advance care planning, L—Living situation, C—Comprehensive history, A—assessment (comprehensive as well as focused wound assessment), R—Recommendations, E—Education. The NPUAP/EPUAP/PPPIA 2014 pressure injury guideline recommends using normal saline or cleansers that are noncytotoxic to control odor and decrease trauma to the wound (Tilley et al., 2016). Cytotoxic agents are typically not recommended for cleaning of pressure ulcers that are healable. For PC patients, the use of these solutions may be warranted, because the goal is *no longer healing*. The benefits of odor control from these solutions may make them an appropriate choice for persons who are at the end of their lives (e.g., 0.5% acetic acid, povidone iodine, chlorhexidine, or Polyhexamethylene biguanide [PHMB]). Other methods of controlling odor include use of topical metronidazole, activated charcoal dressings, antimicrobial dressings, and external odor absorbers (kitty litter, coffee beans, vinegar, and vanilla; Langemo & Black, 2010).

Pressure injuries may need ongoing debridement of necrotic tissue. Pain associated with debridement is an important component of managing a wound in a palliative patient. Autolytic debridement can be achieved by using calcium alginates, hydrogels, hydrocolloids, films, or other dressings (Choo, Nixon, Nelson, & McGinnis, 2014). Enzymatic debridement may be associated with little pain and can be as effective in the PC setting. Surgical debridement may be best for infected wounds with advancing cellulitis accompanied by appropriate systemic antibiotic coverage to avoid systemic septicemia (Brown, 2013). When comfort is the goal, avoid mechanical debridement accomplished by wet-to-dry dressings because this method is painful and traumatic to the wound bed, often resulting in bleeding of the tissue.

TABLE 26.6   Selected Dressings

Low exudate absorption

Film dressings
- Easily applied
- Can see the wound site
- Waterproof, good for incontinent patients
- Adhesive may cause skin injury during removal (stretch laterally to decrease adhesive bond before lifting off the skin)
- Generally, not recommended for use with infected wounds

Hydrogel dressings
- Available as sheets or gels
- Effective for painful wounds
- High water content, so effective for use in wounds that are dry
- Require a secondary dressing to keep in place

Hydrocolloid dressings
- Available in many shapes and sizes
- Very moldable
- Some are adhesive, some are not
- Can remain in place for many days

Moderate to high exudate absorption

Calcium alginate dressings
- Made from seaweed
- Bio-resorbable, excellent for absorption and autolytic debridement
- Available in sheet (wick laterally) and rope forms (wick vertically)
- Not effective on wounds without enough exudate to convert the fiber to a hydrogel (do not use on dry wounds)
- Be aware that the wound may have the odor of "low tide"
- Switch to another dressing if exudate diminishes, as it can dry out a wound with low exudate
- Requires a secondary dressing to hold in place

Foam dressings
- Very useful for wet, weepy wounds
- Effective for packing deep wounds
- Requires a secondary dressing
- Can be used underneath compression stockings and multiple-layer bandaging systems
- Some have low tack, so they do not "strip" the skin when removed
- Will give a variable amount of moisture back to the wound base and surrounding skin as part of the moisture-balance mechanism. If maceration is associated, consider a superabsorbent dressing instead (e.g., ABD pads or other dressings with absorptive polymer fluid lock dressing similar to diapers)

Negative pressure wound therapy
- Great for wounds with large amounts of exudate
- Requires application technique expertise for placing the specialized foam/dressings into the wound, positioning the tubing, applying the specialized drape, and attaching to the vacuum source
- Some patients report pain with this therapy
- Contraindicated with untreated infection or malignancy in the wound base
- Expensive and may be noisy/disturbing to the palliative patient

Antimicrobial dressings
- Effective for critically colonized/locally infected wounds
- Most require a secondary dressing (not adhesive foams or hydrocolloids)
- No MRI if silver dressings used

Since the discovery of moist wound healing by Winter (1962), many new types of dressings have become available. As a result, dressing selection can be confusing for the clinician. Determination of the most appropriate dressing is a difficult task, and it depends on the characteristics of the wound. In the case of palliative wounds where healing is not the goal, dressing choice should be focused toward those that are nonadherent, absorb exudate well, and require infrequent changing. For many clinicians, the key determining factor is the amount of exudate in the pressure injury wound. For example, wounds with low amounts of exudate can be managed by a dressing with low-absorbent capabilities. If the wound bed were dry, using dressings that add moisture to the wound would be indicated (see Table 26.6 for a brief summary of selected dressings).

Quality-of-Life Issues Including Pressure Ulcer–Associated Pain

Pain is a significant consequence of having a pressure ulcer and affects every aspect of a patient's life (Gorecki et al., 2009). Although they are few in number, some studies have provided clinicians with insights into QOL issues for patients with pressure ulcers and their caregivers (Gorecki et al., 2010). Themes common to both of these studies were pain, lack of knowledge, the meaning of the pressure ulcer, and lifestyle changes imposed by the pressure ulcer (Langemo, 2012).

Acute pain in a person with a pressure injury often indicates extension of the pressure inquiry or secondary complications such as infection, periwound maceration or friction, and shear injury. Wound-associated pain is often due to a combination of nociceptive and neuropathic components. Treatment must consider both the stimulus-dependent nociceptive (gnawing, aching, tender, or throbbing) or the spontaneous neuropathic components (burning, stinging, shooting, and stabbing) that need to be treated differently with a combination of appropriate agents. Nociceptive pain responds to the World Health Organization ladder for cancer pain, including nonsteroidal anti-inflammatory drugs and aspirin progressing to weak and then strong narcotic agents. Short-acting agents should be replaced with long-acting ones with lower doses of short-acting agents for breakthrough. Neuropathic pain is best treated with second-generation tricyclics in a single low nightly dose (e.g., 10–30 mg of nortriptyline or desipramine is preferred over first-generation amitriptyline with lower levels of the critical anti-noradrenalin activity for equal doses). Alternate neuropathic pain choices include antiepileptics, including gabapentin, pregabalin, and carbamazepine.

Total management of skin injuries also requires attention to nutritional needs. Adequate nutrition may be difficult for people experiencing anorexia from cancer or other chronic disease. It also may be inconsistent with their wishes, directives, and the goals of management. The Canadian Nutrition Screening Tool (Laporte et al., 2015) has identified two simple questions, which, if both answered yes and are within the patient's goals of care, should trigger a nutrition consult:

1. Have you lost weight in the past 6 months without trying to lose this weight? (If the patient reports a weight loss but gained it back, consider it as no weight loss.)
2. Have you been eating less than usual for more than a week?

Pressure injuries are a result of unrelieved pressure. Providing an adequate pressure-relieving support cushion, mattress, or bed may greatly decrease the PC patient's pain, prevent skin breakdown, or avoid further tissue destruction in an existing pressure injury. Always check to see if the support surface is "bottoming out" by placing a hand under the support surface. If the patient's bottom can be felt, then the support surface is not adequate. Alternately, the examiner's hand can be placed between the patient and the surface to see if bottoming out occurs (i.e., if the hand can feel the base of the underlying pressure redistributing device). In these cases, a deep foam pressure redistribution static or dynamic support surface should be obtained.

■ SKIN TEARS

The Aging Skin

Aging skin predisposes a patient to skin tears due to many changes that are normal aspects of the aging process. As the skin ages, there is a decrease in the dermal thickness, leading to a thinning of the skin, especially over the legs and forearms. With the decrease in fatty layers and subcutaneous tissues, the bony prominences are less protected and the skin's elastin fibers lose their ability to recoil. Sensation, metabolism, and sweat gland production are also diminished, resulting in dry skin that lacks some of the protection mechanisms. An important change that translates into skin tear injury risk is the decrease in the size of the rete ridges in the basement membrane of the skin. As these ridges become flatter with aging, it becomes easier to accidentally separate the epidermis from the dermis (LeBlanc & Baranoski, 2011; Plikus et al., 2015).

Scope of the Problem

Unlike chronic wounds such as pressure injuries, skin tears are acute wounds and defined by an international consensus panel as "a wound caused by shear, friction and/or blunt force resulting in separation of skin layers. A tear can be partial thickness (separation of the epidermis from the dermis) or full thickness (separation of both the epidermis and dermis from underlying structures)" (LeBlanc & Baranoski, 2011, p. 6). In the United States, CMS data from Section M of the MDS 3.0 Resident Assessment Instrument (RAI) reports a rate of 4.70% for the second quarter of 2012 to 4.57% for the first quarter of 2017 to a high of 5.40% for the third quarter of both 2013 and 2014 in LTC residents (www.cms.gov; Ayello, 2017). Percentage data from undergraduate nursing programs in the United States reveal that 70% taught the prevention of skin tears, 65% taught the common location of skin tears, 26% taught the classification of skin tears, and 60% taught the treatment of skin tears (Ayello, 2017). The International Skin Tear Advisory Panel (ISTAP) developed a simplified and tested skin tear classification system. The panel also provided the best prevention and treatment practices, especially regarding dressing selection. Many useful resources can be downloaded from the ISTAP website (www.skintears.org).

Location and Cause

Eighty percent of skin tears occur on the extensor surface of the upper extremities (arms and hands) over areas of sun damage, which also predisposes these regions to senile purpura (LeBlanc & Baranoski, 2017; Strazzieri-Pulido, Peres, Campanili, & de Gouveia Santos, 2017). Skin tears on the back and buttocks can be mistaken for Stage 2 pressure injuries. For about half of skin tears, there is no apparent cause. When the cause is known, 25% are caused by wheelchair injuries, 25% by accidentally bumping into objects, 18% from transfers, and 12% from falls. Long-term steroid use and decreased hormone levels in older females may also be risk factors for skin tears. Skin tears can also occur in infants and children, especially those who are critically ill or medically compromised (LeBlanc & Baranoski, 2011).

Dependent patients who require total care for all activities of daily living are the most at risk for skin tears. Skin tears occur during routine activities of dressing, bathing, positioning, and transferring. The next most common at-risk areas in independent ambulatory residents were the lower extremities. Last were those slightly impaired residents whose skin tear injuries resulted from hitting furniture or a piece of equipment, such as a wheelchair (LeBlanc & Baranoski, 2011).

The method of skin cleansing and routine bathing practices may affect the occurrence of skin tears. Soap increases skin pH to an alkaline level rather than the normal "acid mantel" of the skin. There is a lower rate of skin tears in long-term residents (34%) who were bathed every other day with emollient soap. Use of the newer no-rinse bathing products (responsible bathing) may also be advantageous. There may also be a decline of skin tears from 23% to 3% in a LTC facility when a no-rinse, one-step bed bath protocol rather than the traditional soap and water was used (LeBlanc & Baranoski, 2017).

Risk factors for skin tears are advanced age, sensory loss, compromised nutrition, history of previous skin tear, cognitive impairment, and dependency. The implementation of a skin tear risk prevention plan of care depends on the number of criteria that a patient meets in a group or a combination of criteria in groups II or III. Additional research with this and most available assessment tools would be valuable in establishing its reliability and validity. Many authors have researched and have come to a consensus on prevention strategies for skin tears (Baranoski & Ayello, 2015; LeBlanc & Baranoski, 2011, 2017).

Classifying Skin Tears

Originally, the Payne-Martin Classification system for assessing skin tears was used to identify the type of skin tear (Payne & Martin, 1993). Although this classification system has been used in some studies, the tool has not been widely used in clinical practice. An international panel proposed the use of a new validated classification system with only three categories (Figure 26.2): Type 1, flap with no skin loss; Type 2, partial flap loss; and Type 3, total flap loss (LeBlanc & Baranoski, 2011, 2017).

Type 1: No skin loss   Type 2: Partial flap loss   Type 3: Total flap loss

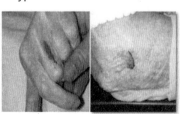 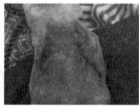 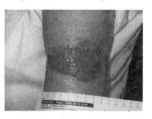

FIGURE 26.2 ISTAP skin tear classification.

ISTAP, International Skin Tear Advisory Panel.

Source: International Skin Tear Advisory Panel (ISTAP). © ISTAP 2013

Linear or flap tear that can be repositioned to cover the wound bed

Partial flap loss that cannot be repositioned to cover the wound bed

Total flap loss exposing entire wound bed

Pathway to Assessment/Treatment of Skin

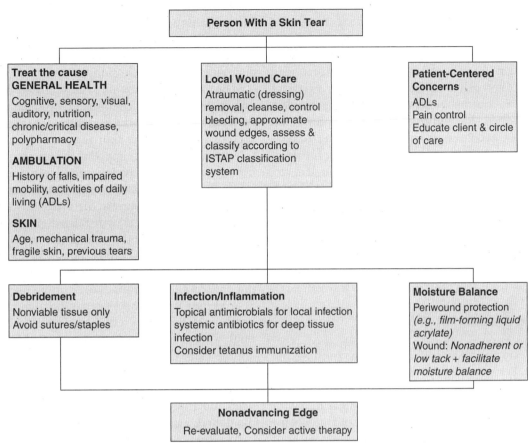

ISTAP, International Skin Tear Advisory Panel.

Plan of Care to Prevent or Treat Skin Tears

Once a patient has been identified as being at risk for developing skin tears, a prevention protocol should be implemented. There is no universal agreement as to the best practice to prevent or treat skin tears in the literature; one example can be found in Appendix 26.1. The Canadian Association of Wound Care released the following guidelines on best practices for skin tears (LeBlanc & Baranoski, 2017).

■ Strategies in Preventing Skin Tears

1. Assess for risk upon admission to nursing home and whenever the individual's condition changes.
2. Implement a systematic prevention protocol.
3. Have individuals at risk wear long sleeves, long pants/trousers, or knee-high socks.
4. Provide shin guards for those individuals who experience repeat skin tears to shins.
5. Ensure safe patient-handling techniques and equipment/environment.
6. Involve individuals and families in preventive strategies.
7. Educate staff and caregivers to ensure proper techniques for providing care without causing skin tears.
8. Consult dietician to ensure adequate nutrition and hydration.
9. Keep skin well lubricated by applying hypoallergenic moisturizer at least two times per day.
10. Protect individuals at high risk from trauma during routine care and from self-injury. (LeBlanc & Baranoski, 2011)

■ Skin Tears Treatment Protocol

1. Gently clean the skin tear with normal saline.
2. Let the area air dry or pat dry carefully.
3. Approximate the skin tear flap.
4. Apply petroleum-based ointment, steri-strips, or a moist nonadherent wound dressing.
5. Calcium alginate dressings facilitate closing in 7 to 10 days.
6. Use caution if using film dressings as skin damage can occur when removing this dressing. Consider using silicone dressings with low tack to avoid tearing the skin.
7. Consider putting an arrow on the dressing to indicate the direction of the skin tear to minimize any further skin injury during dressing removal.
8. Always assess the size of the skin tear; consider doing a wound tracing.
9. Document assessment and treatment findings. For U.S. residents in LTC, this is documented on the MDS RAI in Section M 1040 item G for occurrence of a skin tear and on M 1200 for care interventions.

■ PERISTOMAL (OSTOMY) SKIN

Some patients may require urinary or fecal diversions secondary to the original surgery or because of complications (obstruction from recurrent tumor); this is most commonly seen in patients with colon, rectal, cervical, bladder, or other pelvic malignancies. Once a patient develops an incontinent ostomy, protecting the skin around the stoma—the peristomal skin—and preventing its breakdown becomes an important nursing goal. A wound, ostomy, continence nurse (CWOCN, formerly ET) is an excellent resource in planning and implementing care. The Wound, Ostomy, and Continence Nurses Society (WOCN) has a website and maintains a directory of nurses by geographic area who are available for clinical consults (www.wocn.org). The World Council of Enterostomal Therapists (WCET) has international ostomy guideline recommendations in several languages, which can be found on their website (www.wcetn.org).

Assessing Peristomal Skin

Peristomal skin must be assessed with each pouching system change. Peristomal skin complications are described according to three criteria: discoloration, erosion, and hyperplasia, or raised lesions that can be measured with the size and severity for a maximum score of 5 points for each. Normal peristomal skin should be intact without discoloration and no difference between the peristomal skin and adjacent skin surfaces. Peristomal skin damage has erythema, maceration, denudation, skin rash, ulceration, or blister formation. In darkly pigmented patients, the damaged skin may appear lighter or darker than the surrounding skin.

Protecting the peristomal skin from the damaging effects of urinary or fecal effluent is paramount. The proteolytic enzymes found in the effluent from small bowel stomas can rapidly erode the skin. If the urine from a urinary diversion becomes alkaline, it is more damaging to the skin than normally acidic urine. Large amounts of liquid effluent can result in skin maceration if allowed to pool on the skin surface. The mnemonic "MINDS" can be used to remind clinicians of common peristomal complications: M—mechanical trauma, I—infection, N—noxious chemical and irritants, D—disease of the skin, and S—skin allergens (Doctor & Colibaseanu, 2017).

Maintaining Peristomal Skin Integrity

Maintaining the integrity of peristomal skin can be accomplished, in part, by observing correct pouching principles. Similarly, peristomal skin must be protected from mechanical trauma that can occur from inappropriate cleaning. To avoid skin stripping, use adhesive removers to remove skin barriers and pouching systems. Gently peel the adhesive barriers off the skin by supporting with one hand and then using the adhesive remover as the edge of the barrier that is attached to the skin. Application of skin sealants prior to the application of skin barriers of the pouching system can provide protection to the peristomal skin. Avoid too frequent or unnecessary changing of the pouch–skin barrier.

The nurse should be sure to use the correct products on peristomal skin. Alcohol-based products should never be used, especially if the peristomal skin is denuded. If solvents are used, the skin should be cleaned and the solvent removed before applying the ostomy pouch. Assess for sensitivity to the ostomy products prior to using the product; this includes assessing for latex sensitivity. Skin sealants come in a variety of forms—wipes, gels, and sprays. These products, when dried, provide a thin film to the skin surface, and thus decrease the chance of skin stripping. Some skin sealants contain alcohol and should not be used on denuded skin because they can cause the patient additional pain or burning on application.

A variety of skin barriers can be used to protect the peristomal skin from effluent. These are available as rings, wafers, pastes, and powders. In addition to protecting the skin, they also create a level pouching surface, which can prevent the leakage of effluent underneath the pouch seal in "difficult to fit" stomas. A properly sized and applied skin barrier can protect the skin from the damaging effects of ostomy effluent. Skin barriers vary in their resistance to breakdown by urine or feces. Karaya dissolves with urine, so avoid the use of this product with urinary diversions.

Skin barriers that are powders can be "dusted" onto the denuded skin. Using a skin sealant product over this product can help provide an absorptive protective layer for the peristomal skin. Some companies make products labeled as "no sting" skin barriers that do not cause pain or "burning" when applied to irritated denuded skin.

Selecting the right ostomy pouching system for your patient may require the assistance of the CWOCN (ET) nurse. Pouching systems are provided as one or two pieces. A one-piece system has the skin barrier permanently attached to the ostomy pouch. A two-piece ostomy pouching system has the advantage of the skin barrier remaining on the skin for several days with the ease of snapping the pouch off the skin barrier for emptying of contents. Pouches can be drainable or closed end. There are also pouches specially designed for pediatric patients.

Pouches that are correct for the type of drainage coming from the ostomy should be selected. For example, fecal pouches will not work for urinary diversions. Urinary ostomy pouches have a spout on the bottom for proper emptying of the urine. For fecal pouches, the opening is wide and closed and, in most cases, has a special ostomy clamp. Most modern-day ostomy pouching systems are odor proof when correctly closed and the seal is intact. If there is an unusually large amount of drainage, one of the high-output pouches should be used. Treatments such as chemotherapy or radiation may affect the patient's stool consistency and amount of output. Adjustments in the size of the pouch, more frequent emptying of the pouch, and changes in ostomy irrigations may need to be implemented. It is imperative when selecting the appropriate pouch that it is the correct size for the ostomy stoma. A too large or too small pouch opening size can cause leakage and/or trauma to the stoma.

Total Ostomy Care Management

Care of the older adult patient with an ostomy involves more than just assessing the peristomal skin and pouching system. The elder's emotional and psychosocial acceptance of the stoma is important; for some people, the creation of a diverting ostomy may bring relief from the symptoms of obstruction, but it may also serve as a permanent reminder of the progression of their disease. Supporting the patient to adjust to this change in body image, overcoming concerns about odor, learning new psychomotor self-care skills, and dietary adjustments are just some of the comprehensive care elements that may need to be addressed.

Fistulas

Fistulas are abnormal openings between two organs or an organ and the skin. An internal fistula is inside the body while an abnormal passage between an internal organ or structure and the skin surface, most commonly through the gastrointestinal tract or bladder but sometimes through the vagina or rectum. Fistulas can occur with certain diseases (e.g., malignancies including obstructions, Crohn's disease, or diverticulitis) or from treatment modalities such as radiation or surgery, including postoperative adhesions. A high-output fistula can drain more than 200 mL/24 hours. Assessment of the perifistula skin is critical because irrigation from the effluent can be caustic to the skin and can result in irritation (maceration) and erosion. The perifistula skin should be assessed for signs of fungal infections as well as for redness, papular rash, and satellite lesions.

Identification of the fistula to determine its origin is important for developing the plan for closure (spontaneous [about 50%] or surgical). Goals of fistula management should include maintaining fluid and electrolyte balance (assess for dehydration and metabolic acidosis), protection of the perifistula skin, odor control, effluent containment and measurement, nutritional management, comfort, total parenteral nutrition to meet the nutritional needs, therapeutic communication to respond to the patient's emotional needs from having a foul-smelling fistula, protecting the skin from effluent injury, and eliminating odor.

Women who have had pelvic radiation can develop vaginal fistulas that are often distressing to the patient and challenging to the nurse. Containment of the feces and odor are difficult and require frequent dressing changes. For non-ambulatory patients, containment of the exudate may be obtained with urinary incontinence pouches, commercially available vaginal draining devices, a breast shield, or vaginal diaphragm attached to a male cot catheter.

Management Options

■ **Pouching.** A pouching system may be the primary choice for the management of older adults with odorous fistulas. Using a clear pouch will enable the caregiver or nurse to easily see the type and amount of effluent. Pouching is superior to dressings because it provides better protection to the skin. A pouch with a spout on the bottom works well for fistulas with thin effluent drainage; for thicker drainage, a fecal pouch that can be closed with a clamp is a better choice. Wound management pouches come in a variety of sizes and are useful for treating abdominal fistulas. For patients with odorless fistulas and output (under 100 mL/24 hours), dressings may be used. Preferred absorbent dressings include superabsorbent foams, calcium alginates, or hydrocolloids, which can be selected depending on the exudate. In these cases, the additional use of a petroleum- or zinc-based ointment may protect the perifistula skin from maceration or breakdown. Some patients have such large wounds with enterocutaneous fistulae that the usual commercially available pouches are too small and will not fit.

The more enzymes and liquidity of the fistula output, the greater the need to place additional skin barrier seals around the fistula opening prior to placing a high-output pouch. For older adults who have abdominal fistulas with irregular skin surfaces, skin barrier pastes or strips may need to be placed around the fistula opening to "build up" the skin so the abdominal plane can be "filled in" and then a pouch placed over it. Sometimes, a patient has two fistula openings; if they are close together, one pouch may fit over both fistula orifices. If not, "saddle bagging" two pouches may be the best option.

■ **Tubes and Suction.** Another method is to use drainage tubes, with or without suction. High-output enterocutaneous fistulas can be managed using a Jackson-Pratt (JP) drain tube connected to low-wall suction (60 mmHg of pressure) covered with a saline-soaked gauze and a large surgical plastic drape. When using this technique, be careful in placing the catheter tube so it does not inadvertently cause injury to the tissue.

■ **Trough.** The trough procedure is used for fistulas that are deep within wounds. It is made up of several layers of transparent dressing with an ostomy pouch on the bottom of the wound.

Patient Comfort

Promoting patient comfort is a major priority in caring for a patient with a fistula. The amount of pain or discomfort that a particular management option may cause a patient should influence the decision regarding which management option to select. The goal is to choose the method that will cause the least discomfort and disruption to the patient and caregiver. Medicating the patient prior to removal and application of fistula containment measurements is essential.

■ SKIN DAMAGE FROM RADIATION THERAPY

Radiation therapy damages cellular DNA, resulting in cell death, which is why rapidly dividing cells including skin, hair, or mucosa die after being irradiated. Skin reactions may include erythema or desquamation when dry (flaky, scaly) skin or sweat and sebaceous glands are damaged. Moist blistering, peeling, or sloughing post radiation results from exudate consisting of blood, serum, pus, or a combination of these three elements. Both processes can result in skin ulceration with loss of epidermis and a dermal or deeper base.

While undergoing radiation therapy, care should be taken not to remove any of the treatment field markers on the skin. Avoid activities that could cause mechanical skin damage such as vigorous rubbing, heat, or shaving of the skin in the treatment area. Use of any topical products, such as lotions, creams, or deodorants, is generally discouraged. Any product with metal components or ingredients (e.g., silver or zinc oxide) should not be used during radiation treatment. Patient care goals include keeping the skin intact as well as in correct moisture balance. Products with vitamin A and E or aloe vera gels may be used for treating erythema, although topical steroids should also be considered with the presence of a topical contact irritant dermatitis. Talcum, cornstarch, or baby powder use is controversial as they often contain heavy metals; however, if they are applied, an even layer can be obtained with a cotton ball dabbed on the affected area rather than sprinkling the powder from a container. Sprinkling often leads to local clumping.

■ TUMOR NECROSIS AND SKIN INJURY FROM FECAL INCONTINENCE

Tumor Necrosis and Skin Care

In some people with advanced cancer, the tumor can invade the skin, which results in ulcerated fungating wounds. For example, in people with breast cancer, the tumor can grow outward onto the skin with a blackened cauliflower-like appearance. This results in maceration of the surrounding skin as well as extensive odor from bacterial critical colonization or infection from organisms such as *Pseudomonas aeruginosa*, *Staphylococcus*, *Proteus*, and *Klebsiella* (da Costa Santos, de Mattos Pimenta, & Nobre, 2010). Nodules may enlarge and erupt spontaneously through the abdominal skin in patients with carcinomatosis. While the majority of metastatic skin lesions are found on the anterior trunk, they may also be found on the pelvis, flank, head and neck, and posterior trunk. An assessment of malignant cutaneous wounds include wound depth, color of the wound, drainage, pain, odor, and presence of tunneling or undermining (da Costa Santos et al., 2010).

Management Strategies

In an effort to palliate symptoms, radiation or chemotherapy may be used to shrink the tumors that have grown onto the skin. Patients with malignant wounds report pain, distress from odor and exudate, decreased self-esteem, and poor QOL (Finlayson, Teleni, & McCarthy, 2017). Key symptoms of malignant wounds from a prospective series of 472 cancer patients were studied. Approximately two thirds of the malignant wounds were associated with at least one of these symptoms: pain, mass effect, aesthetic distress, exudate, odor, pruritus, bleeding, and crusting. Management strategies include stabilizing the wounds, preventing new wounds, eliminating odor, controlling pain, infection prophylaxis, absorbent wound dressings, and minimizing dressing changes (Ripley & Collier, 2017).

■ **Cleansing Wounds.** Frequent irrigation of the wound with large amounts of fluid may be important to reduce the bacterial burden on the wound surface. For patients who can get into the shower, cleansing these fungating wounds may provide physical as well as psychological benefits. Instruct the patient not to aim the shower water directly at the wound, but rather above the ulcerated area so the water can trickle down over the wound without undue force. Use of a handheld shower device might be preferred by some patients. For patients who cannot tolerate being showered or where the tissue is very friable, gentle cleaning with saline or commercially available wound cleansers may be substituted (da Costa Santos et al., 2010; Ripley & Collier, 2017).

■ **Managing Wound Exudate.** Management of these wounds can be challenging as they generally have large amounts of exudate because of the tumor's hyperpermeability to fibrinogen and colloids, but primarily due to the secretion of vascular permeability factor by the tumor. There may also be drainage of fecal material in the case of patients with abdominal carcinomatosis. Dressings that are absorbent (foam, calcium alginate, or cotton absorbent dressing pads) should be used. Often there is much necrotic tissue in these wounds and debridement is required. Autolytic debridement techniques including the use of calcium alginate dressings, hydrogel dressings, petroleum-impregnated gauze, or other nonadherent modern dressings are utilized. Picture frame the surrounding fungating wound skin with protective skin barriers, including films and hydrocolloid dressing strips. The use of Montgomery straps to hold the secondary dressing in place will also reduce damage to skin that can be caused by the frequent removal of tape. Dressings in the breast area can be held in place using surgical bras that are stretchy with frontal closure devices (Tilley et al., 2016). Cutting the crotch off mesh underpants and putting this around the chest wall like a tube top can also be done to hold the bulky dressings in place. Mechanical debridement including wet-to-dry dressings should be avoided due to the increased risk of causing more bleeding and increasing pain. The safety of using enzymatic debriding agents in cancer wounds is not yet known (da Costa Santos et al., 2010; Ripley & Collier, 2017).

■ **Controlling Bleeding in Friable Areas.** Bleeding commonly occurs in these types of wounds because tumor cells take over the function of platelets, and the growth and clotting factors that they secrete damage normal tissue. Preventing the dressings from drying out can minimize tissue trauma from the removal of soiled dressings. Calcium alginate dressings or topical thrombin have a hemostatic effect and are a good choice for bleeding wounds. Silver nitrate sticks can be used to control small amounts of blood (Tilley et al., 2016).

■ **Managing Wound Pain.** Pain also results from the tumor growing on the skin and from treatment procedures. Ice packs or topical anesthetic aerosol spray (Hurricane) may alleviate wound pain. Some clinicians have reported using the negative-pressure wound therapy (NPWT) dressing system solely for pain management and comfort of extensive wounds; however, this use is not approved by the Food and Drug Administration and may actually be associated with increased pain in some individuals. Topical extemporaneously compounded opioids or preparations containing amide local anesthetics (lidocaine and prilocaine including EMLA [Eutectic Mixture of Local Anesthetics]) and pyridoxine have also been used to relieve wound pain (Tilley et al., 2016).

■ **Managing Wound Odor.** Odor may be one of the most distressing problems for the patients and their caregivers. There are commercially available wound gel deodorizers; however, some patients may experience burning with the application of these products. The use of Metrogel (1% topical antibiotic wound-deodorizing gel) to control even the most noxious odors has been reported. Metronidazole tablets can be dissolved in normal saline and used to irrigate the wound or can be crushed and sprinkled directly onto the wound bed.

Healthcare professionals should wear a mask to avoid inhaling the particles. Taking metronidazole systemically or using the IV solution as an irrigation solution are alternatives.

The topical application of yogurt or buttermilk has been used to combat extensive odors from tumor necrosis. Antimicrobial cadexomer iodine or silver dressings are also excellent at reducing odor with the added advantage of also controlling the bacterial burden in the surface compartment wound. Another advantage is that some of these dressings can stay in place for up to 7 days, reducing the pain from dressing change. Odor control within the patient's environment may be achieved by utilizing aromatherapy products, such as peppermint oils/sprays or charcoal under the bed.

■ **Quality-of-Life Issues.** Clinicians should be aware of their nonverbal and verbal communication to patients during dressing changes. Patients and/or family members may have difficulty coping with wound odor or appearance, and will look to the clinician to see their reaction. Seeing the extensive death of their own body, coupled with overpowering smells and weeping feces, may be extremely overwhelming to patients. The clinician's resolve to problem solve and provide the patient with the physical comfort from appropriate wound management is vital in helping these patients overcome their (sometimes self-imposed) isolation and hiding.

■ **CONCLUSION**

Focusing on the wound etiology and classifying wounds as healable, maintenance, or palliative (non-healable) can provide realistic expectations for patients, their family unit, and caregivers as well as the healthcare professional team. Local wound care should be aimed at providing comfort, relieving pain, reducing odor, containing exudate, and improving patient's QOL to facilitate the resumption of as many activities of daily living as possible. Local wound care may be aimed at moisture reduction rather than moisture balance, with the antibacterial activity of agents such as acetic acid, povidone iodine, or chlorhexidine and its derivatives viewed as more important than tissue toxicity. Debridement is done to remove slough or devitalized tissue but not to create active bleeding of an acute wound within a chronic wound. It is paramount that the patient's preference be prioritized in the decision-making process and the implementation of realistic treatment care plans.

CASE STUDY *Conclusion*

This case illustrates the importance of a skin biopsy for patients not responding to treatment after approximately 12 weeks. The 8-year delay in diagnosis made the tumor untreatable and was a major contributing factor for Mrs. Rose's death. Remember, within the wound bed preparation, you must identify the correct cause of the wound so the treatment is appropriate.

CASE STUDY

INTERDISCIPLINARY COMMENTARY

Anthony R. Perry, RDN, LD, CDE
Clinical Dietitian/Certified Diabetes Educator
Veterans Affairs Health Care Systems, Oklahoma City, OK

Nutritional concerns are important in this type of situation, with the primary focus being the patient's own goals. Comfort can be provided to some extent with a state of mild dehydration, which would circumvent her already documented constipation and disorientation side effects to medications provided for pain (Schwartz et al., 2014).

A state-of-the-art nutrition assessment should include a nutrition-focused physical exam to determine any protein-calorie malnutrition as well as possible micronutrient deficiencies. Bilateral muscle (temporal, cheek, clavicle area, triceps, calf) and fat (orbital pads) wasting would be addressed with improved intake of both protein and calories. Observation of her tongue, gums, lips, nails, and hair combined with a review of lab work could help rule out low levels of zinc, iron, folate, and B vitamins. Any improvement in wound healing that may simultaneously decrease her level of discomfort would be seen as a benefit.

From personal experience and years of practice, what the patient wants has to be the highest priority; in some cases, this even means providing food sources that wouldn't be considered optimal or the "healthiest" choice. While considering the facility's guidelines, home-cooked foods and splurges (like a chocolate milkshake) might not only boost the patient's spirit but also increase both calories and protein provided. Nutrition supplements are another option to meet caloric needs but may not be the patient's first choice.

Evidence-Based Practice

Reprinted with permission from Finlayson, K., Teleni, L., & McCarthy, A. L. (2017). Topical opioids and antimicrobials for the management of pain, infection, and infection-related odors in malignant wounds: A systematic review. *Oncology Nursing Forum*, 44(5), 626–632. doi:10.1188/17.ONF.626-632

Problem Identification
Patients with malignant wounds report pain, distress from odor and exudate, decreased self-esteem, and poor QOL. This systematic review explores topical opioids, antimicrobials, and odor-reducing agents for preventing or managing malignant wound pain, infection, and odor.

Literature Search
Medline, Embase, the Cochrane Library, CINAHL, and reference lists were searched to identify relevant studies.

Data Evaluation
Eligible study designs included interventions with pre- and postintervention data. Data extraction and risk-of-bias assessments were conducted using the Cochrane approach.

Synthesis
No studies evaluated opioid use. Five studies (four randomized controlled trials) evaluated topical antimicrobials for infection and odor. All studies reported clinically (but generally, not statistically) significant improvements in outcomes.

Conclusions
Although not as prevalent as before, 5% to 10% of tumors, particularly in breast cancer, sarcoma, and melanoma, are expected to fungate. Gaps in the literature exist for use of topical opioids and antimicrobials for managing pain, odor, and infection control in malignant wounds.

Implications for Research
Current recommendations for topical control of malignant wounds are based on case reports and observational studies in patients with breast cancer. Robust, controlled trials of topical opioid and antimicrobial use are warranted in patients with melanoma, breast, or head and neck cancer.

■ REFERENCES

Ayello, E. A. (2017). CMS MDS 3.0 Section M skin conditions in long-term care: Pressure ulcers, skin tears, and moisture-associated skin damage data update. *Advances in Skin & Wound Care, 30*(9), 415–429. doi:10.1097/01.ASW.0000524398.74460.ce

Baranoski, S., & Ayello, E. (2015). *Wound care essentials: Practice principles* (4th ed.). Philadelphia, PA: Lippincott Williams & Wilkins.

Bergstrom, N., Braden, B. J., Laguzza, A., & Holman, V. (1987). The Braden Scale for predicting pressure sore risk. *Nursing Research, 36*(4), 205–210. doi:10.1097/00006199-198707000-00002

Brennan, M., & Trombley, K. (2010). Kennedy Terminal Ulcers—a palliative care unit's experience over a 12-month period of time. *World Council of Enterostomal Therapists Journal, 30*(3), 20–22.

Brown, A. (2013). The role of debridement in the healing process. *Nursing Times, 109*(40), 16–19. Retrieved from https://www.nursingtimes.net/Journals/2013/10/03/d/u/k/The-role-of-debridement-in-the-healing-process-091013.pdf

Centers for Medicare & Medicaid Services. (2017, September 14). Long-term care hospital (LTCH) quality reporting (QRP). Retrieved from https://www.cms.gov/Medicare/Quality-Initiatives-Patient-Assessment-Instruments/LTCH-Quality-Reporting

Chaplin, J. (2000). Pressure sore risk assessment in palliative care. *Journal of Tissue Viability, 10*(1), 27–31. doi:10.1016/S0965-206X(00)80017-0

Choo, J., Nixon, J., Nelson, E. A., & McGinnis, E. (2014). Autolytic debridement for pressure ulcers. *Cochrane Database of Systematic Reviews,* (10), CD011331. doi:10.1002/14651858.CD011331

Cuzzell, J. (2002). Wound assessment and evaluation: Skin tear protocol. [Academic OneFile]. *Dermatology Nursing, 14*(6), 405.

da Costa Santos, C. M., de Mattos Pimenta, C. A., & Nobre, M. R. C. (2010). A systematic review of topical treatments to control the odor of malignant fungating wounds. *Journal of Pain and Symptom Management, 39*(6), 1065–1076. doi:10.1016/j.jpainsymman.2009.11.319

de Azevedo Macena, M. S., da Costa Silva, R. S., Dias Fernandes, M. I. D. C., de Almeida Medeiros, A. B., Batista Lúcio, K. D., & de Carvalho Lira, A. L. B. (2017). Pressure ulcer risk evaluation in critical patients: Clinical and social characteristics. *The Open Nursing Journal, 11*, 91–97. doi:10.2174/1874434601711010091

Doctor, K., & Colibaseanu, D. T. (2017). Peristomal skin complications: Causes, effects, and treatments. *Chronic Wound Care Management and Research, 4*, 1–6. doi:10.2147/CWCMR.S93615

Eckman, K. L. (1989). The prevalence of dermal ulcers among persons in the US who have died. *Advances in Skin & Wound Care, 2*(2), 36–39.

Edsberg, L. E., Black, J. M., Goldberg, M., McNichol, L., Moore, L., & Sieggreen, M. (2016). Revised National Pressure Ulcer Advisory Panel pressure injury staging system: Revised pressure injury staging system. *Journal of Wound, Ostomy and Continence Nursing, 43*(6), 585–597. doi:10.1097/WON.0000000000000281

Finlayson, K., Teleni, L., & McCarthy, A. L. (2017). Topical opioids and antimicrobials for the management of pain, infection, and infection-related odors in malignant wounds: A systematic review. *Oncology Nursing Forum, 44*(5), 626–632. doi:10.1188/17.ONF.626-632

Gorecki, C., Brown, J. M., Nelson, E. A., Briggs, M., Schoonhoven, L., Dealey, C., … Nixon, J. (2009). Impact of pressure ulcers on quality of life in older patients: A systematic review. *Journal of the American Geriatrics Society, 57*(7), 1175–1183. doi:10.1111/j.1532-5415.2009.02307.x

Gorecki, C., Lamping, D. L., Brown, J. M., Madill, A., Firth, J., & Nixon, J. (2010). Development of a conceptual framework of health-related quality of life in pressure ulcers: A patient-focused approach. *International Journal of Nursing Studies, 47*(12), 1525–1534. doi:10.1016/j.ijnurstu.2010.05.014

Hanson, D., Langemo, D. K., Olson, B., Hunter, S., Sauvage, T. R., Burd, C., & Cathcart-Silberberg, T. (1991). The prevalence and incidence of pressure ulcers in the hospice setting: Analysis of two methodologies. *The American Journal of Hospice & Palliative Care, 8*(5), 18–22.

Kennedy, K. L. (1989). The prevalence of pressure ulcers in an intermediate care facility. *Decubitus, 2*(2), 44–45.

Langemo, D. (2012). General principles and approaches to wound prevention and care at end of life: An overview. *Ostomy/Wound Management, 58*(5), 24–26, 28, 30 passim.

Langemo, D. K., & Black, J. (2010). Pressure ulcers in individuals receiving palliative care: A National Pressure Ulcer Advisory Panel White Paper©. *Advances in Skin & Wound Care, 23*(2), 59–72. doi:10.1097/01.ASW.0000363502.84737.c8

Laporte, M., Keller, H. H., Payette, H., Allard, J. P., Duerksen, D. R., Bernier, P., … Teterina, A. (2015). Validity and reliability of the new Canadian Nutrition Screening Tool in the 'real-world' hospital setting. *European Journal of Clinical Nutrition, 69*(5), 558–564. doi:10.1038/ejcn.2014.270

LeBlanc, K., & Baranoski, S. (2011). Skin tears: State of the science: Consensus statements for the prevention, prediction, assessment, and treatment of skin tears©. *Advances in Skin & Wound Care, 24*(9), 2–15. doi:10.1097/01.ASW.0000405316.99011.95. Retrieved from https://journals.lww.com/aswcjournal/fulltext/2011/09001/Skin_Tears__State_of_the_Science__Consensus.1.aspx

LeBlanc, K., & Baranoski, S. (2017). Skin tears: Finally recognized. *Advances in Skin & Wound Care, 30*(2), 62–63. doi:10.1097/01.ASW.0000511435.99585.0d

Levine, J. M. (2017). Unavoidable pressure injuries, terminal ulceration, and skin failure: In search of a unifying classification system. *Advances in Skin & Wound Care, 30*(5), 200–202. doi:10.1097/01.ASW.0000515077.61418.44

National Pressure Ulcer Advisory Panel, European Pressure Ulcer Advisory Panel and Pan Pacific Pressure Injury Alliance. (2014). *Prevention and treatment of pressure ulcers: Quick reference guide.* Osborne Park, Western Australia: Cambridge Media. Retrieved from https://www.npuap.org/wp-content/uploads/2014/08/Updated-10-16-14-Quick-Reference-Guide-DIGITAL-NPUAP-EPUAP-PPPIA-16Oct2014.pdf

Naylor, W. A. (2005). A guide to wound management in palliative care. *International Journal of Palliative Nursing, 11*(11), 572, 574–579.

Norton, D., McLaren, R., & Exton-Smith, A. N. (1975). *An investigation of geriatric nursing problems in hospital* (2nd ed., Vol. 2). New York, NY: Churchill Livingstone.

Payne, R. L., & Martin, M. L. (1993). Defining and classifying skin tears: Need for a common language. *Ostomy/Wound Management, 39*(5), 16–20.

Pieper, B. (2012). *Pressure ulcers: Prevalence, incidence, and implications for the future.* Washington, DC: National Pressure Ulcer Advisory Panel.

Plikus, M. V., Van Spyk, E. N., Pham, K., Geyfman, M., Kumar, V., Takahashi, J. S., & Andersen, B. (2015). The circadian clock in skin: Implications for adult stem cells, tissue regeneration, cancer, aging, and immunity. *Journal of Biological Rhythms, 30*(3), 163–182. doi:10.1177/0748730414563537

Prevention Plus. (2016). Home page. Retrieved from http://www.bradenscale.com

Reifsnyder, J., Hoplamazian, L. M., & Maxwell, T. L. (2004). Preventing & treating pressure ulcers in hospice patients. *Caring, 23*(11), 30–37.

Ripley, K. R., & Collier, M. (2017). Managing tissue viability issues in patients with cancer approaching the end of life. *Nursing Standard, 31*(25), 54–61. doi:10.7748/ns.2017.e10621

Roca-Biosca, A., Velasco-Guillén, M. C., Rubio-Rico, L., García-Grau, N., & Anguera-Saperas, L. (2012). Pressure ulcers in the critical patient: detection of risk factors. *Enfermeria Intensiva, 23*(4), 155–163. doi:10.1016/j.enfi.2012.06.001

Schwartz, D. B., Barrocas, A., Wesley, J. R., Kliger, G., Pontes-Arruda, A., Márquez, H. A., … DiTucci, A. (2014). Gastrostomy tube placement in patients with advanced dementia or near end of life. *Nutrition in Clinical Practice, 29*(6), 829–840. doi:10.1177/0884533614546890

Sibbald, R. G., Elliott, J. A., Ayello, E. A., & Somayaji, R. (2016). Optimizing the moisture management tightrope with wound bed preparation 2015©: Wound care. *Wound Healing Southern Africa, 9*(1), 9–15. doi:10.1097/01.ASW.0000470851.27030.98

Sibbald, R. G., Krasner, D. L., & Lutz, J. (2010). SCALE: Skin Changes at Life's End: Final consensus statement: October 1, 2009©. *Advances in Skin & Wound Care, 23*(5), 225–236. doi:10.1097/01.ASW.0000363537.75328.36

Strazzieri-Pulido, K. C., Peres, G. R. P., Campanili, T. C. G. F., & de Gouveia Santos, V. L. C. (2017). Incidence of skin tears and risk factors: A systematic literature review. *Journal of Wound, Ostomy & Continence Nursing, 44*(1), 29–33. doi:10.1097/WON.0000000000000288

Tilley, C., Lipson, J., & Ramos, M. (2016). Palliative wound care for malignant fungating wounds: Holistic considerations at end-of-life. *Nursing Clinics of North America, 51*(3), 513–531. doi:10.1016/j.cnur.2016.05.006

VanGilder, C., Amlung, S., Harrison, P., & Meyer, S. (2009). Results of the 2008–2009 International Pressure Ulcer Prevalence™ Survey and a 3-year, acute care, unit-specific analysis. *Ostomy/Wound Management*, 55(11), 39–45.

VanGilder, C., MacFarlane, G. D., Harrison, P., Lachenbruch, C., & Meyer, S. (2010). The demographics of suspected deep tissue injury in the United States: An analysis of the international pressure ulcer prevalence survey 2006–2009. *Advances in Skin & Wound Care, 23*(6), 254–261. doi:10.1097/01.ASW.0000363550.82058.7f

Waltman, N. L., Bergstrom, N., Armstrong, N., Norvell, K., & Braden, B. (1991). Nutritional status, pressure sores, and mortality in elderly patients with cancer. *Oncology Nursing Forum, 18*(5), 867–873.

Waterlow, J. (1998). The history and use of the Waterlow card. *Nursing Times, 94*(7), 63–67.

Winter, G. D. (1962). Formation of the scab and the rate of epithelization of superficial wounds in the skin of the young domestic pig. *Nature, 193*, 293–294. doi:10.1038/193293a0

■ **APPENDIX 26.1**

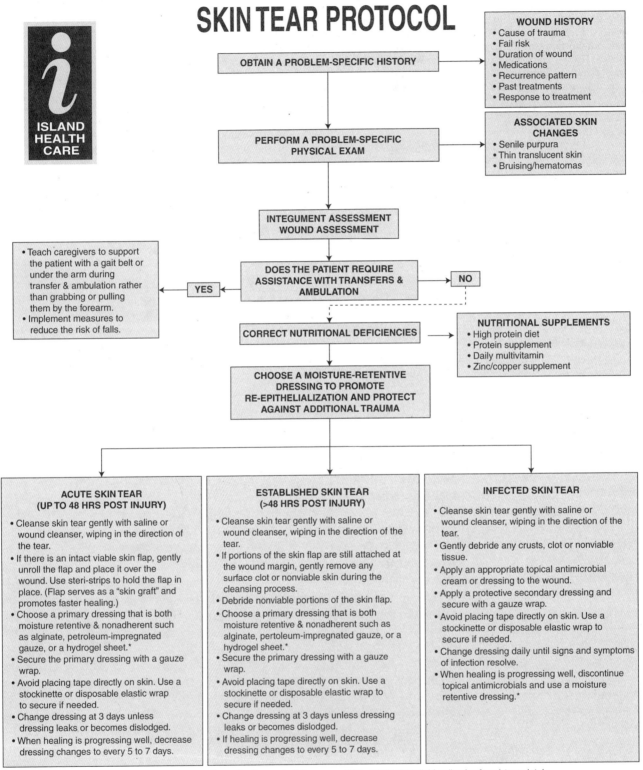

SKIN TEAR PROTOCOL

ISLAND HEALTH CARE

OBTAIN A PROBLEM-SPECIFIC HISTORY

WOUND HISTORY
- Cause of trauma
- Fail risk
- Duration of wound
- Medications
- Recurrence pattern
- Past treatments
- Response to treatment

PERFORM A PROBLEM-SPECIFIC PHYSICAL EXAM

ASSOCIATED SKIN CHANGES
- Senile purpura
- Thin translucent skin
- Bruising/hematomas

INTEGUMENT ASSESSMENT WOUND ASSESSMENT

DOES THE PATIENT REQUIRE ASSISTANCE WITH TRANSFERS & AMBULATION

YES

NO

- Teach caregivers to support the patient with a gait belt or under the arm during transfer & ambulation rather than grabbing or pulling them by the forearm.
- Implement measures to reduce the risk of falls.

CORRECT NUTRITIONAL DEFICIENCIES

NUTRITIONAL SUPPLEMENTS
- High protein diet
- Protein supplement
- Daily multivitamin
- Zinc/copper supplement

CHOOSE A MOISTURE-RETENTIVE DRESSING TO PROMOTE RE-EPITHELIALIZATION AND PROTECT AGAINST ADDITIONAL TRAUMA

ACUTE SKIN TEAR (UP TO 48 HRS POST INJURY)
- Cleanse skin tear gently with saline or wound cleanser, wiping in the direction of the tear.
- If there is an intact viable skin flap, gently unroll the flap and place it over the wound. Use steri-strips to hold the flap in place. (Flap serves as a "skin graft" and promotes faster healing.)
- Choose a primary dressing that is both moisture retentive & nonadherent such as alginate, petroleum-impregnated gauze, or a hydrogel sheet.*
- Secure the primary dressing with a gauze wrap.
- Avoid placing tape directly on skin. Use a stockinette or disposable elastic wrap to secure if needed.
- Change dressing at 3 days unless dressing leaks or becomes dislodged.
- When healing is progressing well, decrease dressing changes to every 5 to 7 days.

ESTABLISHED SKIN TEAR (>48 HRS POST INJURY)
- Cleanse skin tear gently with saline or wound cleanser, wiping in the direction of the tear.
- If portions of the skin flap are still attached at the wound margin, gently remove any surface clot or nonviable skin during the cleansing process.
- Debride nonviable portions of the skin flap.
- Choose a primary dressing that is both moisture retentive & nonadherent such as alginate, petroleum-impregnated gauze, or a hydrogel sheet.*
- Secure the primary dressing with a gauze wrap.
- Avoid placing tape directly on skin. Use a stockinette or disposable elastic wrap to secure if needed.
- Change dressing at 3 days unless dressing leaks or becomes dislodged.
- If healing is progressing well, decrease dressing changes to every 5 to 7 days.

INFECTED SKIN TEAR
- Cleanse skin tear gently with saline or wound cleanser, wiping in the direction of the tear.
- Gently debride any crusts, clot or nonviable tissue.
- Apply an appropriate topical antimicrobial cream or dressing to the wound.
- Apply a protective secondary dressing and secure with a gauze wrap.
- Avoid placing tape directly on skin. Use a stockinette or disposable elastic wrap to secure if needed.
- Change dressing daily until signs and symptoms of infection resolve.
- When healing is progressing well, discontinue topical antimicrobials and use a moisture retentive dressing.*

Note(*): Some patients may benefit from the use of an adhesive product (transparent film, thin hydrocolloid, adhesive foam) to maintain dressing integrity. Adhesive dressings can cause reinjury and should be used with caution.

Source: Cuzzell, J. (2002). Wound assessment and evaluation: Skin tear protocol. [Academic OneFile]. *Dermatology Nursing, 14*(6), 405.

Marianne Matzo & Jane A. Hill

Peri-Death Nursing Care

KEY POINTS

- Nurses caring for a patient who is near death should be aware of the patient's and family's physical and emotional experiences during the dying experience.
- Special considerations for children and elderly patients who cannot make their own decisions should be addressed with the family.
- Families should be informed of the physical processes that occur during the dying process and the nursing interventions and activities that occur after death.
- Nurses should engage in a discussion with families about the options for organ donation, autopsy, and various postmortem responsibilities, rights, and rituals appropriate to the culture, and assist them with accessing resources.
- Nursing interventions do not terminate with a patient's death and should include bereavement care and assistance with accessing appropriate resources.

CASE STUDY

Ellen Owens was a 69-year-old female who had been diagnosed with breast cancer 5 years ago, and despite surgery, chemotherapy, and radiation, she developed metastatic lesions to her liver, bones, and brain. She agreed to additional radiation and chemotherapy for 3 months, but her response CT scan documented that the tumors had shrunk minimally; in fact, there were additional tumors throughout her body. The oncologist told her there were no other recommended treatment options, and she was given a prognosis of 6 weeks to 2 months of life.

Ms. Owens was the only adopted child of older parents who were both deceased. Ms. Owens had extended family on the West Coast, but she lived in the Midwest, in the home that had belonged to her parents. The individuals who represented her family were those with whom she had developed friendships through her faith activities. Many of those friends transported her to her appointments, brought food, shared meals, and stayed with her overnight and through the day to allow her to stay in her home. Ms. Owens appointed one of those longtime friends to be her power of attorney (POA) and another to be durable medical POA. She had previously developed her will and her advance directive, and had requested a do-not-resuscitate order from her physician. She planned her end of life just as she had lived her life: everything in order, and no questions left unanswered. The only variable that she could not control was exactly when the end of her life would come, but she took faith that her careful planning and relationships with her friends would result in the peaceful ending that she planned for.

As an experiential process, dying and death for the individual, his or her family, and the healthcare practitioner can be one of the most profound and significant events experienced in one's lifetime. The last hours of life are conceptualized as the peri-death period, which specifically encompasses the symptoms and experiences right before death occurs, the actual death, and the care of the body after death. This time requires intensive holistic nursing care.

The purpose of this chapter is to relate the role of the nurse during the peri-death period and convey the core knowledge necessary for nurses to help facilitate a "good" death. The information in this chapter should be considered a requirement for nurses educated at a basic level. The role of the advanced practice nurse regarding peri-death nursing includes mentoring and modeling appropriate behaviors for the novice nurse, as well as directing symptom management. Additionally, the role includes supporting the novice nurse through the dying experience and support of the family during the decision-making process regarding autopsy and funeral arrangements.

■ PERI-DEATH 1: SYMPTOMS AND EXPERIENCES BEFORE DEATH

The peri-death period often begins with a preparation phase, the hallmark of which is the realization or acknowledgment that death is inevitable and temporally near. The patient and family members begin to prepare for the death. Similarly, the preparation phase for the terminally ill person is also a time when patients and families have many decisions to make regarding home or hospital care, hospice referral, advance directives, and do-not-resuscitate orders.

The patient may be so uncomfortable with the physical (e.g., pain, dyspnea, fatigue) and emotional (e.g., depression, dependency) aspects of dying that he or she may feel ready for life to end. This sense of readiness may be in tension with a reluctance to die based on fear of the unknown and concern for how the family will cope after the death. Family members are confronted with their role in the dying process, the prospect of losing their loved one, and the conflicts that arise from these and other issues. The patient's role within the family may change as the family learns how to provide care.

The peri-death period often brings the surrogate decision maker's role to the forefront when decisions for the dying patient must be accomplished. Conflicts frequently exist between healthcare providers and surrogates related to the healthcare decisions for the dying patient. Pizzo (2016) suggests that how patients communicate choices about medical care and preferences could result in interventions that will ultimately impact how and where we will die.

Any, all, or none of the following symptoms may occur during the final stages of the dying process. In-depth nursing interventions for the person with advanced disease can be found in the previous chapters of this book. The focus here is on the physiological changes that occur as death is imminent and the nursing interventions that are appropriate at this time.

Pain

Pain is typically a major source of suffering that adversely impacts a patient's quality of life in the peri-death period (Hackett, Godfrey, & Bennett, 2016). As the body begins to shut down and die, the need for pain medication may change or decrease. The World Health Organization's pain ladder (2013) is a simple tool to determine what medications should be used. The liver conjugates these drugs and active metabolites remain in the body, exerting a pharmacological effect until they are cleared by the kidneys. As the body is dying, renal and hepatic function is compromised and the drugs are cleared from the system very slowly. This results in an increase in serum opioid concentrations, which causes increased drowsiness or mild confusion. A nursing priority should be to keep the patient pain free and comfortable but with the understanding that the dosage to accomplish this may be considerably less than what had been previously needed for effective pain management.

Patients, healthcare providers, and family need an understanding of the importance and value of pain management during the dying process. Pain management has improved; the prevalence of inadequate pain management at the end of life remains a key issue (Bailey et al., 2012). The patient may seek pain relief or may view pain as a way to atone for sins and refuse to be medicated. There may be gaps between a patient's preferred level of comfort and how a patient describes suffering. Healthcare providers must help alleviate that suffering, but examine the survival potential, risks, and benefits of therapy (Strand, Feely, Kramer, Moeschler, & Swetz, 2016). Identifying the appropriate dose and frequency can be challenging and may require creativity (McPherson, Kim, & Walker, 2012). Like the nurse, the family may fear being the person to give the "last dose" of morphine before the patient dies. Not adequately medicating for pain, though, can interfere with the memories that the family will carry with them for the rest of their lives. They will remember the death of their loved one as a time of agony and pain rather than a time that could have been used for conversations that are more meaningful and memorable.

The role of the nurse in the management of pain and other distressing symptoms is to assess the level of pain the patient is having and the patient and family's attitudes toward pain. The assessment must be based on an informed understanding of the patient's values and goals, and assure patients and families that comfort and alleviation of pain is a priority. Many providers will prescribe only the dosage of medication needed to relieve intractable pain by reducing awareness of the distressing symptom, which may induce an unconscious state (Strand et al., 2016).

Given that pain medications typically cause constipation, nurses must be vigilant in assessing for constipation. Caregivers should be encouraged to continue prophylaxis bowel regimens to prevent or alleviate its associated discomfort. Additionally, there are medications available to minimize opioid-induced constipation (OIC). Other nonpharmacological interventions that alleviate pain are a calm environment, soothing music, and aromatherapy. Simple human touch or therapeutically intended touch, such as Reiki or therapeutic touch, can relieve stress, be a source of comfort or support, and overcome fear of abandonment.

Anorexia and Dehydration

As patients approach the end of life, they may say they are not hungry, which is a normal predeath finding. Decreased eating results in a metabolic imbalance whereby the energy a patient takes in does not cover the energy he or she expends, resulting in a state of dehydration. Although healthy people who are experiencing dehydration will report pain, abdominal cramps, nausea, vomiting, and dry mouth, patients who are terminally ill do not report such symptoms. At the end of life, patients typically complain only of having a dry mouth, which is often unrelated to hydration status and most often is the result of medication side effects, increased respiration, or mouth breathing.

Food represents more than nutrition to many families and may have symbolic importance. It can have a vital role in helping them to maintain hope and providing comfort to the patient (Hospice and Palliative Nursing Association [HPNA], 2012). However, Lembeck, Pameijer, and Westcott (2016) indicate that "there are cases in which the burdens of artificial nutrition and hydration outweigh the benefits and possibly prolong the patient's suffering" (p. 1132). In many cases, artificial hydration and nutrition provide an opportunity to "do something" at a time when the mistaken perception is that there is little else the nurse can do for them. A patient's right to refuse nutrition has been supported with legal opinions (Soriano & Lagman, 2012), but the family's choice to provide food should be respected (Somers, Grey, & Satkoske, 2016) and balanced with the patient's autonomy (HPNA, 2012).

IV fluids are sometimes given to reverse delirium for a person who is actively dying (Emanuel, Ferris, von Gutten, & von Roenn, 2008). While IV fluids may alleviate symptoms, HPNA (2012) recommends a time-limited trial for IV fluid infusions. IV fluids increase urinary output, which may require a Foley catheter. It may increase respiratory secretions and increase cough

as well as increase gastrointestinal fluids, leading to abdominal distention, nausea, or vomiting. Increasing the intravascular volume in the presence of decreasing renal function can further result in peripheral edema and increase the incidence of decubitus ulcers. Pain can result from the IV site and restraints may become necessary to prevent the patient from removing the tubing. The presence of the IV may act as a physical barrier to the family and may be a cause of anxiety to them. In essence, artificial nutrition and hydration at this stage may lead to symptoms of congestive heart failure, increased tracheal and bronchial secretions, pleural effusions, nausea and vomiting, painful edema, and diarrhea rather than improving symptoms or prolonging life (HPNA, 2012).

The decision to withhold or withdraw life-sustaining treatments is considered to be ethically and legally equivalent (Somers et al., 2016). A patient's right to refuse nutrition has been supported with legal opinions (Soriano & Lagman, 2012) and the Patient Self-Determination Act. There are many benefits to the patient in not utilizing artificial food and fluids as death nears. With calorie deprivation comes an increased production of ketones, which results in an elevation of naturally occurring opioid peptides or endorphins that provide analgesia. An electrolyte imbalance, if present, will also result in increased analgesia. Decreased fluid intake will result in fewer pulmonary fluids, which eases respiration, lessens coughing, and reduces the drowning sensations. If a tumor is present, dehydration may make it smaller in size by reducing the edematous layer around the tumor, resulting in less pressure and pain. Discontinuing total parenteral nutrition can reduce the burden of sepsis, while stopping tube feedings can reduce diarrhea (American Academy of Hospice and Palliative Medicine, 2013). While IV fluids may alleviate symptoms, time-limited trials are recommended. Whatever the decision, nurses should discuss end-of-life (EOL) choices related to patient goals and values (HPNA, 2012).

Nursing interventions focus on meticulous mouth, nasal, and conjunctival care to alleviate mouth dryness and prevent sores, dental problems, infections, and discomfort. Scrupulous cleaning and moistening of the mouth can be one of the most important interventions to prevent suffering in a patient nearing death. The benefits are doubled in preserving a patient's dignity with fresh breath and communication with family members during the process (Croyère, Belloir, Chantier, & McEvan, 2012; Emanuel et al., 2008; Field & Cassel, 1997). The mouth and teeth can be cleaned with a soft-bristled toothbrush or sponge-covered oral swabs. To maintain moisture in mucosal membranes, the mouth should be rinsed frequently with water. A spray bottle can be used to mist the mouth often; a room humidifier is also very helpful. Commercial salivary substitutes or supplements such as Salivart, Oral Balance, Salagen, and MoiStir, or a baking soda mouthwash (one teaspoon salt, one teaspoon baking soda, and one quart tepid water), can also help keep the patient comfortable. Chamomile tea is also very soothing and can be used to clean the mouth or offered to the patient to sip on. EOL halitosis is a frequent phenomenon; two drops of essential peppermint oil in one ounce of purified drinking water can be used on a toothette when providing oral care. It is not an immediate cure for halitosis, but with multiple uses can refresh breath and leave a pleasant taste and aroma for the patient. Generously applying lip lubricant can prevent dry, chapped lips and alleviate associated discomfort. Avoid petroleum-based products if the patient is on oxygen. Ophthalmic lubricating gel or artificial tears can be used to hydrate conjunctiva.

Family members should be shown how to give good mouth, nasal, and conjunctival care and be supported by the nurse in their efforts. It is essential for everyone involved in the care of the patient to realize that not providing food and fluids is not the same as not caring for the patient, only that the concentration of care is on meeting the needs of the dying person and providing comprehensive symptom management (Emanuel et al., 2008).

If the patient is experiencing oral pain, morphine or morphine elixir can be used if the pain is severe or during mouth care and meals. Topical agents for mouth pain include Viscous Xylocaine 2% solution, 5 to 15 mL, swish and spit every 2 to 4 hours as needed. KBX solution (Kaopectate, Benadryl, Xylocaine viscous in equal parts), 5 to 15 mL, swish for 1 minute, then spit or swallow every 2 to 4 hours as needed, may also be ordered. Xylocaine provides topical anesthesia; Benadryl is a short-acting anesthetic; and Kaopectate (Mylanta may be substituted) serves as an alkalizing agent (Gates & Fink, 1997; Schaefer et al., 2008).

If the patient is still sipping fluids, encourage those fluids that contain salt to help prevent electrolyte imbalance. Fluids such as bullion soup, tomato juice, or sports drinks such as Gatorade may be well tolerated. Avoid citrus juices or foods that may irritate the mouth, as well as temperature extremes of foods. It is important not to force food or fluids at this point and to support the family, who may have a difficult time accepting the patient's refusal to eat or drink. Families can be reminded that even in the case of acute illness, such as the flu, food and fluids can create additional distress.

As death approaches, patients often lose their ability to swallow due to weakness or a decrease in neurological function. The gag reflex may diminish and secretions will tend to accumulate in the tracheobronchial tree. Positioning is important to prevent the accumulation of secretions in the back of the throat and upper airways (Ferrell, Virani, & Grant, 1999). This phenomenon, known as a death rattle, is experienced by approximately half of the patients who are dying and usually becomes audible within 24 to 48 hours before death (Campbell, 2015). Historically, anticholinergic interventions such as atropine 1% ophthalmic solution can be administered sublingually, and scopolamine transdermal patches have been used to decrease secretion production and the occurrence of the "death rattle," but there is no evidence that supports that these interventions are superior to placebos (Campbell, 2015). Although not distressing to the patient, this sound can be very upsetting to the family (McPherson et al., 2012). Oropharyngeal suctioning is not recommended as it is frequently ineffective and may stimulate the patient and distress the family even more (Emanuel et al., 2008).

Weakness and Fatigue

Fatigue is a primary complaint of patients in the last hours and days of life. The tiredness may be a result of both the disease and the treatment for the disease, as well as malnutrition and disrupted sleep patterns. Fatigue may interfere with a person's ability to move, bathe, or go to the toilet (Emanuel et al., 2008; Field & Cassel, 1997).

The nurse should be aware that while the patient is at a high risk for a pressure ulcer, turning and positioning should be done as frequently as possible but only as often as comfort permits. Bony prominences should be padded and supported if this is comfortable for the patient. If any of these interventions result in increased pain or suffering, they should not be implemented. Initially, this may be difficult for the novice nurse to support, as it is contrary to the basic nursing skills they have been taught. When a patient is actively dying, intervention goals should focus on comfort; any intervention that compromises this goal should be discontinued.

Dyspnea

Dyspnea is common, and can be the most distressing symptom experienced at the end of life. It results from the lungs' inability to function in proportion to the metabolic demands of the body and may be indicative of significant neurological compromise. Dyspnea can be described by patients in many ways, including a sensation of being "suffocated" or that of "impending death" (Baldwin & Cox, 2016). When a person has trouble breathing, there must be either an increase in ventilation or a decrease in activity. Terminal dyspnea occurs in as many as 75% of patients in the peri-death period. Changes in respiration are normal and should be anticipated prior to death. Physiologically increased carbon dioxide in the blood stimulates respiration. During the peri-death period, increased pulmonary congestion and poor gas exchange result in a rise in carbon dioxide levels, but the brain is less responsive to this signal (Pitorak, 2003). The breathing pattern can become irregular and include shallow breathing alternating with apnea lasting 5 to 60 seconds (Cheyne–Stokes breathing; Emanuel et al., 2008).

Families should be warned that dyspnea and loud respirations are a possibility during the peri-death period. Patients may fear they will suffocate while they are dying and families fear they will have to watch their loved one struggle to breathe. Nurses should educate the patient and family regarding what they can expect and give assurances that medications will be used to effectively palliate these symptoms (Baldwin & Cox, 2016; Emanuel et al., 2008). A valid and reliable tool for measuring respiratory distress (The Respiratory Distress Observation Scale [RDOS]) was reported by Campbell, Templin, and Walch (2010), and can be used when a patient cannot self-report (Baldwin & Cox, 2016).

Nursing interventions include positioning the patient on his or her side, semi-prone, or in brief Trendelenburg, to prevent the accumulation of secretions in the back of the throat and upper airways. For opioid-naive patients, low-dose opiates, such as morphine 5 mg PO every 4 hours, can alleviate the sensation of breathlessness. If morphine is already being used for pain, an increase of 2.5 mg times the regular dose is generally effective. Oxygen is typically effective only if the dyspnea is secondary to hypoxia (e.g., COPD, pulmonary fibrosis), although it may provide a placebo effect (Baldwin & Cox, 2016). A fan blowing a gentle breeze toward the patient's face can also be very effective. Suctioning is usually not recommended as it may incidentally increase secretion production. Emotion-focused interventions such as relaxation techniques, prayer and meditation, and distraction may alleviate the anxiety often associated with dyspnea (Horn, 1992; Spector, Connolly, & Carlson, 2007).

Multisystem Failure

As the body is shutting down, there is a decrease in blood perfusion and a resulting shutdown of the major organs (e.g., renal and hepatic). Decreased cardiac output and intravascular volume result in tachycardia and hypotension. Additionally, the body will conserve blood volume for vital organs, which results in peripheral cooling (as the body conserves heat) and peripheral and central cyanosis. The skin may therefore become mottled and discolored, which is normal before death and a sign that it is imminent. Mottling is typically seen on the earlobes and the soles of the feet before other areas.

Urine output is greatly diminished and there can be a loss of sphincter control, resulting in urinary or fecal incontinence. It may be a good idea to insert a urinary catheter to reduce the need for frequent bedding changes and to prevent skin breakdown. The catheter also helps the continent patient conserve energy by removing the need to use a bedpan or urinal.

Neurological dysfunction is a result of multiple, concurrent, and nonreversible organ failure as a result of infections, nutritional deficits, neurological disorders, electrolyte imbalances, and medications (Chirco, Dunn, & Robinson, 2011). Consequently, the patient may experience reduced cerebral perfusion, hypoxemia, metabolic imbalances, acidosis, accumulation of toxins from renal and hepatic failure, and sepsis (Ferrell et al., 1999). The net effect of these changes may be a decreased level of consciousness or terminal delirium.

Terminal Delirium

Individuals at the end of life can manifest symptoms of end-stage multiorgan failure and other irreversible factors that result in a disturbance of fluctuating consciousness, cognition, and perception known as delirium, but it is often underdiagnosed in the terminally ill (Candy et al., 2012; Hosker & Bennett, 2016). Hosker and Bennett also indicate that delirium can be classified into three subtypes: hyperactive (restless and agitated), hypoactive (drowsy and inactive), and a combination of these two. These are typical symptoms that are indicative that the patient is close to death. Additionally, confusion, a mental state in which a person reacts inappropriately to his or her environment because he or she is confounded or disoriented, may be the side effect of medications or caused by the dying process itself (Chirco et al., 2011; Field & Cassel, 1997). Anxiety is the biological and emotional reaction to stressful situations, including the approach of death.

The patient may experience dread, danger, or tension with somatic complaints that include shortness of breath, nausea, or diarrhea (Field & Cassel, 1997). Moaning and grimacing can accompany agitation and restlessness and may be misinterpreted by the nurse as pain (Ferrell et al., 1999). Uncontrollable pain is not likely to develop during the last hours of life if not previously present (Emanuel et al., 2008). The patient may be restless and make repetitive motions (e.g., pulling on clothing or the sheets). The underlying cause of the restlessness may be opioid toxicity, metabolic disorders and lowered seizure threshold, or full bladder or bowel (Bush, Kanji, & Pereira, 2014; Candy et al., 2012).

Nursing interventions to manage terminal delirium should focus on the treatment of the underlying physical cause if it is practical and possible. Nonpharmacological interventions are preferred, but are not always possible. Antianxiety agents such as benzodiazepines (lorazepam, diazepam, alprazolam) and neuroleptics (Haldol) for drug toxicity can help to quiet distressing symptoms. Barbiturates or propofol have been suggested, as have other antiepileptics such as IV phenytoin, phenobarbital, or carbamazepine (Candy et al., 2012; Emanuel et al., 2008). Second-generation antipsychotics, risperidone and olanzapine, are equally effective (Campbell, 2015).

The family is in need of education and support regarding the cause and the irreversible nature of the behavior. Maintaining a calm environment, spiritual comfort, and emotional support is vital at this time. The family can be advised to continue to talk to the patient and calm the patient with their words. Light massage of the arms, back, or forehead can be very soothing. Soft music and low lights can also be effective. It may be suggested that the number of people in the room be decreased if there is a lot of activity. Refraining from asking the patient many questions can diminish agitation.

Eventually the patient's level of consciousness will decrease and he or she may even become unable to be aroused. This is typically a very upsetting time for families because the patient may seem unresponsive and withdrawn, but it is a normal aspect of the dying process. At this time, the patient is starting to "let go" in preparation for death and is detaching from relationships and the physical environment. A patient may ask to be with only one person toward the end or seem distracted from the family. Reassure the family that this is not a personal rejection, only another aspect of the dying process. A dying person may talk about seeing people who have already died or talk about taking a trip with a long-deceased relative. Patients may describe feeling separate from their body. This is a normal experience and is not considered a hallucination.

Even if the patient is unresponsive, encourage family members to talk with him or her. Assume that the patient hears everything; this is the time for loved ones to say "good-bye," "I'm sorry," "I love you," or "thank you." The patient may have difficulty letting go and the nurse may need to encourage the family to give the patient permission to die. Encourage the family to show affection to the patient, touch the patient, and let the patient know he or she will be missed.

Affirming Life and Maintaining Hope

Two very important goals of PC nursing are to help patients live until they die and to encourage hope. First, the nurse can help patients live until they die by encouraging socialization, listening, being honest, and helping them finish any unfinished business. The nurse can also help families find meaning in the situation. Dialogues about death with healthcare professionals, families, and friends can benefit all involved (Nedjat-Haiem, Carrion, Ell, & Mishra, 2017; Revier, Meiers, & Herth, 2012; Wasserman, 2008). By offering patients choices regarding routines, food, and activities, nurses promote continued independence and the ability to help maintain control over their lives. Of course, the degree of independence depends on patients' energy level and ability (Birchenall & Streight, 1997; Kastbom, Milberg, & Karlsson, 2017). Furthermore, patients' wishes should be respected even if those wishes are inconsistent with the family's or healthcare provider's values.

Second, hope is an important component of the emotional stages of dying and death. It has been a factor in helping the patient and family continue through the difficult months and years leading up to the death. Hope is what maintains a person's spirit and helps the person to go on; as the person is dying, *what* he or she hopes for may change, but it does not go away. There

may be hope for the miracle of a complete cure; it is not acceptable for the nurse to take this hope away or to tell the patient and family to be realistic. It may be dying a good death that has different meaning for each client (Tan & Manca, 2013). Their hopes may change from that of cure to the hope for a full night's sleep, a visit from an important person, or less pain. Persons with hope have been found to live longer and have a greater QOL than those who are hopeless (Birchenall & Streight, 1997). Benzein and Saveman (2008) posit that patients who told their story were able to relieve an unrecognized burden. What is important for the nurse is to be present for the patient and family wherever he or she is in this process and support the feelings that are experienced. The rights of dying can be found in Table 27.1. Listening and caring for their needs are important nursing functions at this time of life.

Palliative Care for the Aged and Individuals With Dementia

The National Academy of Social Insurance (2017) predicts that the Medicare-eligible population will approach 80 million Americans by the year 2030, with a projected cost of 5.1% of the gross domestic product. This will continue to create significant challenges for current hospice, palliative care, and EOL care practices and providers.

Although the body of research regarding EOL care continues to grow, information about the very old or individuals with dementia is more in its infancy. These individuals have unique issues in that they may lose some of their capacity to make decisions or choose to designate surrogates to make those decisions for them. Research indicates surrogate decision making encourages the surrogate to "exercise considerable discretion in the decision making" (Berger, DeRenzo, & Schwartz, 2008, p. 48).

Individuals with dementia often enter an EOL stage without acknowledgment by the family or caregivers, which may lead to inappropriate care during the end stages of dementia (Peacock, 2013). A patient with progressive dementia has the potential for an extended life unless complicating conditions develop (Zerwekh, 2006). One effort to enhance EOL practices for individuals with dementia includes the *Palliative Excellence in Alzheimer Care Efforts* (PEACE) program offered by the University of Chicago (promotingexcellence.org).

Decision making for family members can be compounded by ambivalence, struggles with opposing beliefs, and moral issues. Family members may require additional conversations, and interventions by healthcare workers, to help resolve those conflicts (Peacock, 2013). Advance directives and living wills may create as many problems as they solve as the patient's priorities in the context of aging rather than a specific illness may be more tenuous (Berger et al., 2008).

TABLE 27.1 The Dying Person's Bill of Rights
■ I have the right to be treated as a living human being until I die.
■ I have the right to maintain a sense of hopefulness, however changing its focus may be.
■ I have the right to be cared for by those who can maintain a sense of hopefulness, however challenging this might be.
■ I have the right to express my feelings and emotions about my approaching death, in my own way.
■ I have the right to participate in decisions concerning my care.
■ I have the right to expect continuing medical and nursing attention even though "cure" goals must be changed to "comfort" goals.
■ I have the right not to die alone.
■ I have the right to be free from pain.
■ I have the right to have my questions answered honestly.
■ I have the right not to be deceived.
■ I have the right to have help from and for my family accepting my death.
■ I have the right to die in peace and dignity.
■ I have the right to retain my individuality and not be judged for my decisions, which may be contrary to the beliefs of others.
■ I have the right to discuss and enlarge my religious and/or spiritual experiences, regardless of what they may mean to others.
■ I have the right to expect that the sanctity of the human body will be respected after death.
■ I have the right to be cared for by caring, sensitive, knowledgeable people who will attempt to understand my needs and will be able to gain some satisfaction in helping me face my death.

Note: This Bill of Rights was created at a workshop on "the terminally ill patient and the helping person" in Lansing, Michigan, sponsored by the Southwestern Michigan In-Service Education Council and conducted by Amelia J. Barbus, associate professor of nursing, Wayne State University, in 1975.

Source: Reproduced with permission from Sorrentino, S. A. (1999). *Assisting with patient care*. St. Louis, MO: Mosby.

Special Considerations Related to the Dying Child

Palliative care for the child encompasses a holistic approach to physical, psychological, and spiritual care. Consideration for both the dying child and his or her family supporting optimal functioning until the time of death is a vital role for the nurse (National Hospice and Palliative Care Organization [NHPCO], 2009). Ethical considerations have a significant role in decisions related to a dying child. Identifying if, when, and how much to tell a child about his or her impending death is an important decision for the family. Talking with children about impending death demands an understanding of the child's perception of death based on previous experiences and developmental stage (NHPCO, 2009).

Children are often very perceptive and may know far more than adults assume. Offering time for discussion related to death and the dying process helps the child recognize that he or she will not be alone in the process and will be loved and remembered. EOL communication will not typically send a dying child into a deep depression. Attempts to protect children from knowledge about their impending

death place barriers between them and the people who can best help them understand and deal with their experience. Honest and accurate information about a child's impending death can address separation issues in young children, fears, phobias, and regression in school-age children; emotional lability in preadolescents; and anger, insecurity, and body image in older adolescents (NHPCO, 2009).

Children experience a variety of symptoms in the dying process that may be similar to or different from those of adults, but discomfort, seizure management, pain in nonverbal patients, and feeding issues are most common. These symptoms may be a result of the disease process, previous treatment history, or side effects of palliative medication. It is important to assess the onset of those symptoms, severity, duration, and the impact those symptoms have on the child's comfort. This requires extensive investigation and developmentally appropriate interventions and strategies to identify and manage those symptoms. Physical signs and symptoms that occur in children as death approaches include sleeping more, decreased appetite, and less fluid intake. The urine frequency and output will diminish and breathing may become slow and shallow, with occasional deep sighs.

There may be some gasping and periods of apnea. The skin may be cool to the touch and appear pale, grayish-blue.

Nurses should help families understand what they see may be different from what the child experiences. If the families are given the opportunity to care for the child, utilizing what they feel is best for the child, a gift of confidence is given to the family. Basic caring—bathing, holding, dressing—becomes significantly important during the peri-death period (Emanuel et al., 2008). Caring for the child does not stop at the time of death. Families may choose to engage in the same activities as if the child were alive and should be encouraged if cultural and religious values allow it.

Family Support During the Last Hours of Life

Supporting the family during the last hours of the patient's life is an important nursing role. When possible, one nurse should be assigned to be with the family through the last phase of life. Enough time with the dying person should be given to the family so that they have the opportunity to resolve any final interpersonal issues. If the death is occurring at home, the family should have access to a Symptom Relief Kit with detailed, easy-to-understand instructions for its use (Appendix 27.1). Depending on cultural and religious considerations, the family should be afforded privacy and clergy support. The primary nurse should communicate with the family regarding what they can expect the dying process to be like and how they will know when the person has died.

Many people have not been with someone who is actively dying and do not know what to expect. Even though no two deaths are alike, it helps to give significant others an idea of what the final stage of life may be like and the symptoms they may see during this period. Table 27.2, which shows the final stages of dying, is an information sheet written for the general population regarding the dying process and is a good handout for students.

Palliative Sedation

Sedation for the imminently dying is an intervention to relieve intractable symptoms of patients who are suffering at the end of their life. In contrast to ordinary sedation, which is used to treat specific symptoms, medical use of palliative sedation involves use of sedative medications, within a proportionate approach, to relieve suffering from refractory symptoms when other therapies do not relieve those symptoms (Maltoni, Scarpi, & Nanni, 2013; Strand et al., 2016), by reducing the level of consciousness, but not to intentionally end life. This intervention should occur only when the symptoms or suffering cannot be relieved in any other way. Maltoni et al. (2013) posit palliative sedation as a gradual process of titrating medications to obtain symptom relief.

One of the forms of palliative sedation includes deep continuous sedation (DCS), which is generally used to manage refractory symptoms in late stages of disease. This should not be confused with euthanasia.

Indications for terminal sedation are uncontrolled physical suffering such as intractable pain, dyspnea, seizures, or delirium. Table 27.3 offers general guidelines for terminal sedation, and Table 27.4 lists medications and guidelines for their use in sedating an imminently dying patient. The level of sedation that eliminates objective signs of discomfort is maintained until the elder dies; death will typically occur within hours or days of the initiation of sedation (Quill & Byock, 2000). There is no literature to support the belief that imminently dying patients die quicker when sedated to control intractable symptoms (Maltoni et al., 2013). Panke (2003) suggests that patients with unrelieved symptoms may die sooner secondary to "increased physiologic stress, diminished immunocompetence, decreased mobility, increased risk of thromboembolism and pneumonia, increased difficulty breathing, and greater myocardial oxygen requirements" (p. 31).

Terminal sedation requires participation of the entire healthcare team for monitoring the patient and the support of his or her family. The sedation is maintained by continuous subcutaneous or IV infusion. Opioids that have already been initiated for pain and other symptoms should be continued to prevent unobservable pain or opioid withdrawal, but opioids should not be used to maintain the sedation itself (Quill & Byock, 2000).

Ventilator Release

Withdrawal of mechanical ventilation and removal of the endotracheal (ET) tube (terminal extubation) occurs in clinical situations where prior attempts to wean the patient have not been successful, in cases of futility, when the family decides that continued intubation is a burden and source of suffering for the patient, and when the QOL is unacceptable. There is no universally accepted protocol for release from the ventilator in the case of terminal extubation (Cook & Rocker, 2014). There is a paucity of research evidence to guide terminal extubation so clinicians are often left with only their personal values and beliefs, family preferences, and staff input to guide clinical practice (Billings, 2012). In the case of terminal extubation where the patient is not expected to survive, the clinical obligation and priority should be comfort and to prevent suffering for the patient and his or her family (Matzo & Orwig, 2013).

Cook and Rocker (2014) encourage clinicians to consider discontinuation of other therapies prior to terminating ventilation (e.g., renal replacement therapy, inotropes, or vasopressors). It is important for the clinician and family to discuss weaning a patient from mechanical ventilation versus abrupt discontinuation and extubation. Providing cautions and considerations for each of these situations is as important as sustaining

TABLE 27.2 Final Stages: The Dying Process

When a person enters the final stage of the dying process, two different dynamics are at work. Physically, the body begins the final process of shutting down, which will end when all the physical systems cease to function. Usually this is an orderly, progressive series of physical changes—the ways the body prepares itself to stop. The most appropriate kinds of responses are comfort-enhancing measures.

The other dynamic of the dying process is emotional and spiritual. The "spirit" of the dying person begins the final process of release from the body, its immediate environment, and all attachments. This release follows its own priorities, which may include the resolution of whatever is *unfinished* of a practical nature and exercising permission from family members to "let go." The most appropriate kinds of responses are those that support and encourage this release and transition.

When a person's body is ready and wanting to stop, but the person is still unresolved or not reconciled about an important issue or relationship, the person may linger in order to finish whatever needs finishing. On the other hand, when a person is emotionally/spiritually resolved and ready for this release, but his/her body has not completed its final physical process, the person will continue to live until the physical shutdown is completed.

The experience we call "death" occurs when the body and the spirit complete the process of shutting down, reconciling, and finishing. These processes need to happen in a way appropriate and unique to the values, beliefs, and lifestyle of the dying person. The following are offered to help you understand the natural kinds of things that may happen and how you can respond appropriately. Not all these signs and symptoms occur with every person, nor do they occur in this particular sequence. Each person is unique and needs full acceptance, support, and comfort. The following signs and symptoms are indicative of how the body prepares itself for the final stage of life:

Coolness: The hands, arms, feet, and legs may be increasingly cool. The color of the skin may change. The underside of the body may become darker and the skin mottled or discolored, a normal indication that the circulation of blood is decreasing to the body's extremities and being reserved for the most vital organs. Keep the person warm with a nonelectric blanket.

Sleeping: The person may spend an increasing amount of time sleeping and may appear to be uncommunicative or unresponsive and, at times, difficult to arouse. This is due in part to changes in the metabolism. Sit with your loved one and speak softly and naturally. Plan to spend time when the person seems most alert and awake. Try not to talk as if the person were not there. Speak directly as you normally would, even though there may be no response. Never assume the person cannot hear; hearing is the last of the senses to be lost.

Fluid and food decrease: The person may have a decrease in appetite and thirst, wanting little or no food or fluid. The body will naturally begin to conserve energy that would be expended on these tasks. Do not try to force food or drink into the person. If the person is able to swallow, fluids may be given in small amounts by syringe. Glycerin swabs may help keep the mouth and lips moist and comfortable. A cool, moist washcloth on the forehead may also increase physical comfort.

Incontinence: Control of urine and/or bowels may be lost as the muscles in that area begin to relax. Discuss with your hospice nurse what can be done to keep your loved one clean and comfortable. If it would make the person more comfortable, the nurse may suggest a catheter to drain the bladder. The person's normal urine output may decrease and become dark due to the decrease in circulation through the kidneys.

Congestion: The person may have gurgling sounds coming from the chest. These sounds may become very loud. This is due to the decrease in fluid intake and the inability to cough up normal secretions. The sound of the congestion does not indicate the onset of severe or new pain. Suctioning usually increases the secretions. The nurse or home health aide can show you how to keep the mouth clean with "touthettes."

Breathing pattern change: The person's regular breathing pattern may change and become irregular—shallow breaths with periods of no breathing for a few seconds up to a full minute. This is called Cheyne–Stokes breathing. The person may also experience periods of rapid shallow panting. Elevating the head and/or turning on one side may bring comfort.

Disorientation: The person may seem to be confused about the time, place, and identity of people, including those close and familiar. This is due in part to metabolism changes. Identify yourself by name before you speak; speak softly, clearly, and truthfully when you need to communicate.

Restlessness: The person may make restless and repetitive motions, such as pulling at bed linen or clothing. This is due to the decrease in oxygen circulation to the brain and to metabolism changes. Do not interfere with or try to restrain such motions. To have a calming effect, speak in a quiet, natural way; lightly massage the forehead, back, or arms; read to the person, or play some soothing music. Try to decrease the number of people around the person.

(continued)

TABLE 27.2   Final Stages: The Dying Process (*continued*)
Withdrawal: The person may seem unresponsive, withdrawn, or in a comatose-like state. This indicates preparation for release, a detaching from surroundings and relationships, and a beginning of letting go. Because hearing remains almost all the way to the end, now is the time to say whatever you need to say that will help the person let go. The person may want to be only with a very few or even just one person. If you are not part of this inner circle at the end, it means you have already fulfilled your tasks, and it is time for you to say good-bye.
Vision-like experiences: The person may speak or claim to have spoken to persons who have already died, or to see places not presently accessible or visible. This means the person is beginning to detach from this life and is preparing for the transition. Do not contradict, explain, or argue about what the person claims to have seen or heard. Affirm the experiences. They are normal and natural.
Letting go: The person may continue to perform repetitive and restless tasks. This may indicate that something is still unresolved or unfinished. The hospice team can assist you in identifying what may be happening and help the person find release from tension or fear. As hard as it might be, you need to give the person permission to let go.
Saying good-bye: When the person is ready to die, and you are able to let go, saying good-bye is your final gift of love. It achieves closure and makes the final release possible. It may be helpful to hold or touch and say the things you want to say. It may be as simple (or as complicated) as saying "I love you." It may include saying, "I'm sorry for whatever I've done to cause any tensions or difficulty." You may also want to say "Thank you." Tears are a normal and natural part of saying good-bye. They are a natural expression of your sadness and loss. It is all right to say, "I will miss you so much."
Although you may be prepared for the dying process, you may not be prepared for the actual moment. It may be helpful for you and your family to think about and discuss what you would do if you were alone when the death occurs. The death of a hospice patient is expected and is not an emergency. Nothing must be done immediately. The signs of death include: ■ No heartbeat ■ Release of bowel and bladder ■ No response ■ Eyelids slightly open ■ Pupils enlarged ■ Eyes fixed on a certain spot ■ No blinking ■ Jaw relaxed and mouth slightly open
You may now notify a hospice nurse or the on-call nurse of the death. The nurse will make the pronouncement and notify the physician. The body does not have to be moved until you are ready. The nurse can call the funeral home, but you or a member of your family will probably need to speak with the funeral director.

Source: Adapted from the Visiting Nurses Association of Manchester and Southern New Hampshire, Manchester, NH.

and initiating the appropriate medications and doses to ensure the patient is comfortable.

Post-extubation stridor (PES) has been documented as occurring in 22% of patients who have been intubated for more than 24 hours, likely secondary to airway inflammation and edema (Cheng et al., 2011). One study documented that the incidence of PES can be reduced with one dose (40 mg) of methylprednisolone (Cheng et al., 2011). An observational study documented that in cases of withdrawal of life support in the ICU, extubating intubated patients before death was associated with higher family satisfaction with care ($p = .009$; Gerstel, Engelberg, Koepsell, & Curtis, 2008) but did not test protocols for extubation.

Billings (2012) proposed that the humane response in this situation is to offer "preemptive high doses of opioids and sedatives for anesthesia, or at least deep sedations to assure comfort" (p. 628). We suggest that in addition to premedication and in the absence of clinical indicators to the contrary (i.e., in the case of burns,

airway trauma, or intubation for greater than 14 days, all of which increase the risk of stridor), extubation be included as part of a humane response. It must be emphasized that the discontinuation of mechanical ventilation with or without the removal of the ET tube can and should be done in a way that optimizes symptom management, respects patient and family desires, and acknowledges local culture and practice (Matzo & Orwig, 2013). Table 27.5 offers an order set to guide terminal extubation.

■ PERI-DEATH 2: DEATH

Signs of Death

Signs of death include cessation of a heartbeat and respiration, release of bowel and bladder, eyelids slightly open and not blinking, the eyes glaze, and pupils fixed

TABLE 27.3 General Guidelines for Terminal Sedation

Guideline Domain	Terminal Sedation
Palliative care	Must be available, in place, and unable to adequately relieve current suffering.
Usual patient characteristics	Severe, immediate, or otherwise unrelievable symptoms (e.g., pain, shortness of breath, nausea, vomiting, seizures, delirium) or to prevent severe suffering (e.g., suffocation sensation when mechanical ventilation is discontinued).
Terminal prognosis	Usually days to weeks.
Patient-informed consent	Patient should be competent and fully informed or noncompetent with severe, otherwise irreversible suffering (clinician should use advance directive or consensus about patient wishes and best interests).
Family participation in decision	Clinician should strongly encourage input from and consensus of immediate family members.
Incompetent patient	Can be used for severe, persistent suffering with the informed consent of the patient's designated proxy and family members. If no surrogate is available, team members and consultants should agree that no other acceptable palliative therapies are available.
Second opinion(s)	Should be obtained from an expert in palliative care and a mental health expert (if uncertainty exists about patient's mental capacity).
Healthcare practitioner participation in decision	Input from staff involved in immediate patient care activities is encouraged; physician and staff consent is required for their own participation.

Source: Adapted from Quill, T. E., & Byock, I. R. (2000). Responding to intractable terminal suffering: The role of terminal sedation and voluntary refusal of food and fluids. *Annals of Internal Medicine, 132*(5), 408–414. doi:10.7326/0003-4819-132-5-200003070-00012

TABLE 27.4 Medications Used in Terminal Sedation

Medication	Type	Usual Starting Dosage	Usual Maintenance Dosage	Route
Midazolam	Rapid, short-acting benzodiazepine	0.5–1.5 mg/hr after bolus of 0.5 mg	30–100 mg/d	Intravenous or subcutaneous
Lorazepam	Benzodiazepine	1–4 mg every 4–6 hr orally or dissolved buccally; infusion of 0.5–1.0 mg/hr intravenously	4–40 mg/d	Oral, buccal, subcutaneous, or intravenous
Propofol	General anesthetic; ultra-rapid onset and elimination	5–10 mg/hr; bolus doses of 20–50 mg may be administered for urgent sedation, but continuous infusion is required	10–200 mg/d	Intravenous
Thiopental	Ultrashort-acting barbiturate	5–7 mg/kg of body weight to induce unconsciousness	Initial rate may range from 20–80 mg/hr; average maintenance rates range between 70 and 180 mg/hr	Intravenous
Pentobarbital	Long-acting barbiturate	2–3 mg/kg, slow infusion, to induce unconsciousness	1 mg/hr, increasing as needed to maintain sedation	Intravenous
Phenobarbital	Long-acting barbiturate	200 mg loading dose, repeated every 10–15 min until patient is comfortable	Approximately 50 mg/hr	Intravenous or subcutaneous

Note: Goal of treatment is to relieve suffering by inducing sedation. Dosage should be increased by approximately 30% every hour until sedation is achieved. Once the desired level of sedation is achieved, infusion is usually maintained at that level as long as the patient seems comfortable. If symptoms return, dosages should be increased in 30% increments until sedation is achieved. The ranges noted are representative. Individual patients may require lower or higher doses to achieve the desired goal. Previous doses of opioids and other symptom-relieving medications should be continued.

Source: Adapted from Quill, T. E., & Byock, I. R. (2000). Responding to intractable terminal suffering: The role of terminal sedation and voluntary refusal of food and fluids. *Annals of Internal Medicine, 132*(5), 408–414. doi:10.7326/0003-4819-132-5-200003070-00012

TABLE 27.5 Extubation Orders

Date/time:

1) Diagnosis:

2) Code status:

3) Lab/radiology:

  ( ) Discontinue all previous routine and daily orders
  ( ) Other: _____

4) Respiratory therapy:

  ( ) Notify respiratory therapist for extubation and/or discontinuation of ventilator or BiPAP
    at date/time: _____
  ( ) ET tube and oral/pharyngeal suctioning prior to extubation

  Following extubation or discontinuation of ventilator/BiPAP:

  ( ) Room air
  ( ) O_2 at _____L/min via _____
  ( ) Titrate to comfort

**If the patient has an implanted defibrillator, notify Cardiac Cath Lab for deactivation prior to extubation (may also use magnet to deactivate)

5) Nursing:

  ( ) Notify chaplain and social work/case manager of extubation date/time
  ( ) Discontinue continuous monitoring just prior to extubation:
  ( ) Cardiac
  ( ) Pulse oximetry
  ( ) Arterial line
  ( ) Swan–Ganz catheter
  ( ) Discontinue routine vital signs
  ( ) Vital signs PRN per family request
  ( ) Vital signs every _____ hours
  ( ) Comfort level check and documentation every 15 min for the first hour after extubation and then every hour (pain, dyspnea, nausea, coping, fears, mental/spiritual status, etc.)
  ( ) Discontinue sequential stockings
  ( ) Place NG to suction
  ( ) Discontinue NG/Dobhoff and remove tubing
  ( ) Discontinue tube feeding and/or TPN
  ( ) Wash face and hands, comb hair, put glasses on if available
  ( ) Change top sheet and remove all soiled pads and linens

6) Current medications:

  ( ) Discontinue the following medications:

  _____
  _____
  _____
  _____
  _____

7) Premedications: Give 15 min prior to extubation.

  ( ) Lorazepam (Ativan) _____ mg IV × 1
  ( ) Morphine sulfate _____ mg IV × 1

8) Opioids:

  ( ) Morphine sulfate _____ mg ( ) IV or for pain or dyspnea

9) Anxiety:

  ( ) Lorazepam (Ativan) 1–2 mg IV every 15 min for anxiety/restlessness

(continued)

TABLE 27.5 Extubation Orders (*continued*)
10) Secretions: **Choose one:** ( ) Scopolamine transdermally 1.5 mg patch(es); apply _____ patch(es) now and change every 72 hr ( ) Hyoscyamine 0.125 mg orally/sublingually every ____ hour(s)
11) IV fluids: ( ) Change IV maintenance fluid rate to TKO ( ) Discontinue IV fluids ( ) Other: _____
12) If patient is in a critical care unit and survives post-extubation/discontinuation of ventilator/BiPAP for greater than 2 hr, notify the palliative care team and arrange transfer to the palliative care unit.
13) Notification: ( ) Notify attending and all consultants of change in the plan of care.

BiPAP, bilevel positive airway pressure; ET, endotracheal, NG, nasogastric; PRN, when necessary; TKO, to keep open; TPN, total parenteral nutrition.

and dilated. There is a drop in body temperature and, as the blood settles, the body color turns to a waxen pallor, the jaw is relaxed and slightly open, and there is no response from the patient. These signs do not occur in sequence, and it may take a few minutes for the body to completely stop (Ferrell et al., 1999; Green & Green, 2006). If the death occurs at home, the family should be told that it is not considered an emergency but be given a number to call to inform hospice staff or their physician of the death. The body does not have to be moved immediately, so the family should not feel rushed or pressured to act.

When Death Has Occurred

Post-death nursing care involves preparing the body for the morgue or funeral home and helping the family through decisions regarding autopsy and burial. When death has occurred, the blood will begin to pool in the areas of the body closest to the ground; if the corpse was supine this would be the back and buttocks. A purple-red discoloration of the skin is evident and results from the blood accumulating in the dependent vessels; this is called *livor mortis*. The body begins to cool, and this fall in body temperature after death is called *algor mortis* (Kastenbaum & Kastenbaum, 1989; Pattison, 2008). Initially, at the time of death, the muscles in the body relax, but within 2 to 6 hours, *rigor mortis* begins. Rigor mortis is the stiffening of all muscle groups beginning with the eyelids, neck, and jaw. During the next 4 to 6 hours, it will spread to the other muscles, including the internal organs. Rigor mortis will usually last between 24 and 48 hours depending on the ambient temperature. After this time, the muscles relax and secondary flaccidity develops (Beattie, 2006; Iserson, 2001).

Care of the body by the nurse should include closing the eyes, inserting dentures and closing the mouth, and elevating the head of the bed so that the blood does not drain into the face and discolor it. Any IV or catheter can be removed at this time, and the physical environment should be straightened. Removal of tubes and equipment is dependent on institutional protocol. Follow the agency protocol regarding jewelry; if there is a wedding ring, secure it on the finger with tape. The body should be bathed in plain water and dried; a bed protector should be placed under the body. If there are dressings on wounds, they should be replaced with clean ones. The hair should be combed, the extremities straightened, and the right great toe tied with an identification tag (Pattison, 2008; Sorrentino, 1999).

If the family wants to participate in the preparation of the deceased for the funeral home, they should be encouraged to do so. The family should also be offered the opportunity to bathe and dress the body if they wish. Some people find comfort in giving the last bath and it helps them to believe that no one else will touch the body in this way again.

When the body and the room have been prepared, family and those close to the patient can be encouraged to say a final good-bye. Within the confines of cultural, personal, and religious practices, the family can be invited to touch or hold the person's body and to take the time they need. This time spent with the deceased can help to promote the transition from acute grief to a new stage of the grieving process (Ferrell et al., 1999; Pattison, 2008). Accepting the reality of the death is considered one of the first tasks of mourning necessary for working through the grief (Worden, 1992). Seeing the dead body helps the bereaved see the reality of the death and to say good-bye. The body should not be transported to the morgue or mortuary until the family is prepared and they have given their permission. The family's wishes should be respected regarding their presence during the removal of the body (Beattie, 2006).

When the family has given permission for the body to be moved, the nurse should follow the institutional protocol regarding shrouding the body. If a person has died at home and it is an expected death, the undertaker is called and they remove the body as it is. In a hospital or nursing home setting, the body is wrapped in a shroud or body bag. The shroud should be secured with safety pins or ties and a second identification tag attached to the shroud or body bag. The body is then taken to the morgue (Beattie, 2006; Sorrentino, 1999).

The nurse can offer help with making personal phone calls to give the family time to become accustomed to the immediate loss. The physician should be notified of the death and the nurse should be certain to follow agency protocol regarding the removal of medications and equipment. If the family wishes, support from their clergy or bereavement professionals can be offered.

In many states, the nurse can sign the death certificate if the death occurs in the hospital or nursing home or at the family home if hospice is involved. Once the death certificate is signed, the family can contact the mortuary and the body can be transported to the funeral home or crematorium. If the nurse or physician is unwilling to sign the death certificate because of a suspicious nature of the death, the medical examiner is called and he or she assumes responsibility for the body (Iserson, 2001). If the death is sudden and unexpected or if it occurs at home, the medical examiner must be notified and he or she will decide if an autopsy is required.

The next of kin may request an autopsy even if the medical examiner declines to do one. The nurse should be available to educate the family about the autopsy and assist them in their decision-making process. An autopsy will help determine the cause of death, but the family may be charged a fee for this service, ranging from $100.00 to $7,500.00 depending on case load and facility costs (Sanchez, 2017). This cost is not covered under Medicare, Medicaid, or most insurance plans. Autopsies also serve other purposes, as shown in Table 27.6.

The word *autopsy* comes from the Greek *autopsia*, which means seeing with one's own eyes. Pathologists, who are physicians specialized in human anatomy, perform an autopsy. Organs are removed and inspected, and body fluids are analyzed. There are three degrees of autopsy: complete, limited, and selective. A complete autopsy exposes all body cavities (including the head) for examination; limited autopsy usually excludes the head; and selective autopsy involves examination of only one or more organs specific to the nature of the illness (Iserson, 2001).

If the deceased has requested that his or her organs be donated, the nurse is often the person responsible for notifying the proper agencies for organ and tissue harvesting. Organ donation is the practice of giving a part of the deceased body for transplantation into another person. Persons designate this wish to donate organs

TABLE 27.6   The Benefits of Autopsies
■ Discover new or elucidate uncommon diseases
■ Help explain unknown or unanticipated medical complications
■ Assist in the development and quality assurance of technology, procedures, and therapies
■ Help educate medical students and help continue physician education
■ Provide a source of organs and tissues for medical and scientific purposes
■ Classify and help explain sudden, unexpected, and/or unnatural deaths
■ Identify infectious and contagious diseases
■ Identify and help monitor occupational and environmental health hazards
■ Help with quality control and risk assessment in hospital practices
■ Provide materials and hypotheses for research
■ Help improve accuracy and usefulness of vital statistics
■ Assist in the grieving process
■ Provide a vehicle for organ or tissue contribution
■ Help discover contagious diseases within the family
■ Assist in genetic counseling and identification of family health risks
■ Provide information for insurance/death benefits

Source: Adapted from Iserson, K. V. (2001). *Death to dust: What happens to dead bodies?* Tucson, AZ: Galen Press.

by signing the back of their driver's license, indicating their preferences; by specifying organ donation in an advance directive; or by filling out an organ donor card. Organ donor cards can be ordered from the United Network for Organ Sharing (UNOS; 804-782-4800 or www.unos.org). Persons younger than 18 years of age generally must have the consent of parents or guardians to sign an organ donor card. The Anatomical Gift Act of 2006 has been adopted by many states. Specifics of the act can be found at www.uniformlaws.org/Act .aspx?title=Anatomical%20Gift%20Act%20(2006).

Some states will record the intent to donate an organ in a donor registry, which is a central repository of information regarding the intent to donate. When a potential donor is identified, the donor registry is contacted to determine the person's intent. Complete information on organ donation and times required for specific organ removal can be found at the *Organ Procurement and Transplantation Network* (OPTN) web page at optn. transplant.hrsa.gov (OPTN, 2013). Based on data retrieved in May 2017, the OPTN indicates that more than 118,000 individuals have registered for transplants in the United States. Depending on what organ is being donated, the time for organ removal varies.

Once the organs are removed from the body, it is ready for embalming or cremation. Embalming is the process by which the corpse is preserved and prepared for viewing; it is common for health reasons and protects mourners from being in the presence of a decaying body, but is not legally required, even if it is to be viewed (Shannon, 2006). "Basically, the embalmer is a creator of illusions—of pleasant illusions which banish the traces of suffering and death and present the deceased in an attitude of normal, restful sleep. In the practice of embalming, this illusion is called a 'memory picture.'" (Strub & Frederick, 1967, p. 133). There are four embalming methods that all involve the injection of chemicals to preserve the body. Arterial embalming injects the chemicals into the blood vessels; cavity embalming injects the chest and abdomen; hypodermic embalming injects under the skin; and surface embalming is the application of chemicals in gel or liquid form to the body surface (Iserson, 2001; Mayer & Taylor, 2005). The size of the body, age, water content, temperature, decomposition, condition of the body's blood vessels, and premortem medication regime (e.g., gentamycin inactivates embalming fluid) will dictate the types, solution strengths, and injection rates of the embalming chemicals.

There are a number of different embalming formulations on the market, with an intent to reduce environmental hazards (Brenner, 2014). Embalmers inject these chemicals into the body using a centrifugal pump that pushes the fluids into the body with 5 to 10 psi of pressure. At the same time, blood and fluid are drained from the body by gravity or electrical aspirators. The embalmer will look for evidence that the chemicals have reached the hands and face and facilitate this process by massaging and repositioning the corpse. When the embalming fluid reaches the hands, they are placed in their final position over the chest or abdomen and the fingers are held together by using cyanoacrylate (e.g., Super Glue). The muscles will gradually harden over the 8- to 12-hour period following the embalming; once they are set, the body's position will not be able to be moved.

If there is going to be a viewing at the funeral home, the body is prepared with the use of cosmetics. The hair is styled and the deceased is dressed. The body is then "casketed" in the coffin; typically, the right shoulder is lower than the left so the body does not look like it is flat on its back. Cost of these services (including burial) is approximately $10,000, with prices increasing depending on the type of casket purchased.

Cremation is a popular, less-expensive (direct cremation, the most basic cremation service, can cost less than $1,000, although there are also funeral homes that offer the service for $4,000–$8,000) alternative to embalming and burial that dates back to prehistoric times. Our primitive ancestors believed they could return to their bodies and harm the living and therefore feared the dead; destroying the corpse removed that danger. Ancient civilizations believed that cremation would provide the dead with heat and warmth in the next world and protect the body from mutilation by animals or other humans. Native Americans believe that souls are conveyed to paradise by means of fire.

Cremation is a process to reduce the "corpse and its container to ashes and small bone fragments" (Iserson, 2001, p. 236). The first crematory was built in the United States in 1876 in Pennsylvania. At that time, decomposing bodies were leaking into the water systems and the thought was that there could be a more sanitary way to manage the dead.

Temperatures between 1,400°F and 1,800°F are used to burn the body, which evaporates water (70%–80% of nonbone tissue), burns soft tissue, and reduces the average-sized adult to 4 to 8 pounds of ash (cremains). It takes about 2 to 3 hours to cremate a body, and what is left are gray ash and bone fragments. The cremains are then processed through an electric grinder to pulverize the bone fragments into an even consistency.

Prosthetic devices do not burn (e.g., dental gold, metal plates, and screws) and are removed with a magnet from the ashes. Pacemakers with lithium batteries will explode when burned and are removed before cremation. The body does not have to be embalmed before cremation nor does the family need to purchase a coffin. The only requirement is that the body be burned in a combustible container (e.g., cardboard or particleboard). Typically, there is a 24- to 48-hour waiting period after the death before cremation can legally take place.

Crematories are the facilities that contain the oven or retorts where the cremation will take place. It is becoming increasingly common for funeral homes to build crematories on the site and to offer a wide range of disposal options. There are no local, state, or federal laws that require a body to be cremated in a casket, but some facilities may require a container of some sort (Harris, 2007).

A newer method of cremation (available since 2003) is water-based cremation called alkaline hydrolysis, which was originally used by the Mayo Clinic as an environmentally friendly way to dispose of bodies that had been used for research. This cremation process takes place in a Resomator, a stainless-steel chamber that holds a combination of water, potassium hydroxide, and heat. The Resomator dissolves the body to white fragments that are then pulverized into a fine powder and the water waste is discarded into the wastewater treatment system. The cost is approximately the same as cremation by fire.

Some cemeteries will have a columbarium for the interment of the urn containing the cremains. Memorial gardens are also available for the ashes to be scattered or buried and give visitors a place to visit or place a marker. Some people will divide the cremains to bury, scatter, keep in an urn, share among family members, or even wear in specially designed jewelry. The cremains can be made into a diamond or sent up in a rocket.

■ PERI-DEATH RELIGIOUS AND CULTURAL RITUALS

Nursing care does not stop when a patient dies. There is tremendous variability around the world regarding the care of dead bodies and funeral practices. In India, there are funeral pyres; there are second burial rites by Indonesian hill tribes; and there is a pervasiveness of embalming practices in the United States (Quested & Rudge, 2003). Throughout the dying process, and particularly at the very end of life, the nurse must be aware of cultural and religious values, practices, and traditions of the patient and the family. Customs and rituals have tremendous significance in the healing process following death, and the grief response is often structured by these rituals. The nurse's role is to help the family carry out the rites and practices that provide solace and support. The nurse should be open minded and understanding of the physical, psychosocial, and spiritual needs of the dying patient and his or her family and offer them respect and privacy (Purnell & Paulanka, 2008).

Rituals and customs vary based on a person's faith background or culture. For those of the Roman Catholic faith, priests will offer the Sacrament of the Anointing of the Sick, which in the past was called Extreme Unction or the Last Rites. The sacrament is for those who are seriously ill. The family, friends, and priest gather at the bedside to pray for healing. If it is God's will that the person not recover from his or her illness, then the prayer is that God will accompany the dying person toward the rewards of heaven (Green & Green, 2006; Miller, 1993). The nurse can ask the family if they would like the priest to be called. The priest would hear the patient's confession of sins, absolve the individual, and offer the Sacrament of the Sick. The comfort this ritual can bring to the dying Catholic and his or her family cannot be underestimated.

The preference of the Catholic Church is that the body of the deceased be present for the funeral rites; masses with cremated remains present can be performed. When cremated remains are present, they must be contained in a "worthy vessel," placed on a table, or in the place normally occupied by the casket, and must be covered with a pall, that is, a heavy drape or cloth. The prayer of committal would read "earthly remains" in place of "body" (Green & Green, 2006).

Catholic burial practice calls for the cremains to be buried in an urn within a consecrated grave or placed inside a mausoleum. Keeping ashes at home or scattering them on land or sea, even where legal, is inappropriate to the church's deep reverence for the body as a place where the soul has resided (Serratelli, 2017). The Catholic Church recommends burial or inurnment (placing the cremains in an urn) in a Catholic cemetery. Throughout the history of the church, the Catholic cemetery has served as a visible sign of the faith community: a statement of continued belief in that everlasting life, even in death (Archdiocese of Chicago, 2008).

In the Church of Jesus Christ of Latter-Day Saints (Mormons), church members of the same gender who have permission to be admitted into the temple are the ones who dress deceased members. The body is dressed in white undergarments that are covered by a robe, cap, and apron. Prior to burial, a white cap is placed on a deceased man, and a deceased woman's face is veiled (Green & Green, 2006; Iserson, 2001).

A Hindu who is dying may also request holy rites before death; readings and hymns from holy books are also comforting. Some may wish to lie on the floor to symbolize their closeness to the earth. A Hindu priest would administer the holy rites, which may include tying a thread around the wrists or neck of the dying person, sprinkling blessed water from the Ganges, or placing a sacred *tulsi* leaf in the dying person's mouth. Some Hindus may wish to return to India to die, especially to the holy city of Banaras. Many believe that to die in Banaras ensures a rebirth in heaven or even a release from continued rebirth. At a minimum, a Hindu will request to die at home because death in the hospital is very distressing. Only another Hindu should touch the dead body; if it is necessary for a non-Hindu to touch it, disposable gloves should be worn. Sacred threads, jewelry, and other religious objects should not be removed. The body should not be washed but only wrapped in a plain sheet. Washing of the body is a part of the funeral rite and is typically carried out only by family members; a mixture of milk and yogurt is used to cleanse the body. In India, a funeral takes place within 24 hours; adult Hindus are cremated, although young children and infants may be buried (Green, 1989a, 1989b, 1989c; Green & Green, 2006).

The dying person of the Muslim faith may wish to lie or sit facing Mecca. If it is possible, the bed should be positioned to accommodate this wish. Those of Islamic faith believe the body belongs to God, so reasons for autopsies must be clear and legitimate. Likewise, organ donation and cremation are not acceptable. In Iran, embalming is not practiced, and a person is immediately placed in a casket if he or she has died during the day. If death occurs at night, a copy of the Qur'an should be placed on the chest of the deceased and a lighted candle at the head (Iserson, 2001; Purnell & Paulanka, 2008); the body is watched during the night by a person reading the Qur'an.

Following the death, non-Muslims should wear gloves when touching the body. If there is no family available to carry out postmortem care, the nurse should wear gloves in administering care of the body. However, the body is not washed and hair and nails are not cut; the eyes are closed. According to Green and Green (2006), the normal Muslim procedure is that the body is straightened immediately after death. This is done by flexing the elbows, shoulders, knees, and hips first, before straightening them. This is thought to ensure that the body does not stiffen, thus facilitating its washing and shrouding. Turn the head toward the right shoulder. This is so the body can be buried with the face toward Mecca.

The body is then covered with a sheet that cloaks the whole body until a Muslim is available to perform the ritual bath. The ritual bath includes washing the body three times, first with lotus water, and then camphor water, and last with plain water (Iserson, 2001). This bathing is done from head to toe and front to back. All body orifices are closed and packed with cotton (to prevent body-fluid leakage that is considered unclean). Prayers from the Qur'an are read (especially verses of hope and acceptance) and the body is wrapped in a special cotton shroud. This shroud is made from three pieces of white unsewn cloth, 9 yards long, which are wrapped above, below, and around the midsection. Muslims are buried in a brick- or cement-lined grave with the head facing east toward Mecca. In Iran, the body is buried directly in the earth with the shroud removed from the face and one side of the face turned to be in contact with the earth (Purnell & Paulanka, 2008).

When those of the Jewish faith are dying, they may want to hear or recite special prayers, such as the *Shema*, which confirms one's belief in one God; or psalms, in particular Psalm 23 ("The Lord is my Shepherd"). Jews also have a personal confession prayer called *Viddui*, which is said by the dying person or by another individual when death is imminent (Purnell & Paulanka, 2008). Observant Jews are often buried in shrouds called *takhrikhim*. These are plain white cotton garments that are generally hand sewn and made without buttons, zippers, or fasteners of any kind and cover the entire body (Hill & Daniels, 2007).

The person may also wish to hold the written prayer in his or her hand (Green, 1989d). A relative remains with the dying person to ensure the soul does not leave the body when she or he is alone; it is a sign of disrespect to leave the body alone. Even after death, the body is not left alone until the funeral, so that the body is not left defenseless (Purnell & Paulanka, 2008). The eyes should be closed after death, preferably by a child of the deceased; the body should be covered and left untouched (Green, 1989d). Autopsies are not permitted, although organ transplants are. The body should be handled as little as possible by non-Jews, and burial should take place within 24 hours. Burial is usually only delayed for the Sabbath. Embalming and cosmetics are not part of traditional practice. Orthodox Jews are always buried, although Jews who are more liberal may select cremation.

The body is wrapped in a shroud and a prayer shawl. The casket is made of wood, so that the body and the casket decay at the same rate. There is no wake or viewing of the body. At the funeral, the *Kaddish*, the *prayer* for the dead, is said, which praises God and reaffirms faith (Purnell & Paulanka, 2008).

For those who are Buddhist, an important consideration is the state of mind at the time of death; dying thoughts and desires are crucial in determining the next rebirth of the deceased. A Buddhist monk or minister should be notified at the time of death to offer chant verses to the dead and the family. Buddhists may be cremated because Buddha was cremated (Purnell & Paulanka, 2008). The length of time between death and burial can vary between 3 and 7 days depending on the Buddhist tradition. Family members plan the burial; the tradition is to wear white to the funeral.

In terms of differences based on cultural backgrounds, Cuban Americans who are dying are usually attended by large groups of family and friends. Depending on their religious affiliation, a Catholic priest, Protestant minister, rabbi, or *santero* may be called to perform death rites. For followers of *santero*, these rites may include animal sacrifice, ceremonial displays, and chants (Purnell & Paulanka, 2008). After the death, candles are lit to light the path of the spirit to the afterlife. Burial is the common custom although there is no restriction to cremation.

African Americans generally prefer to have people with terminal illness cared for in the home, but prefer death to occur in the hospital for fear of bad luck being brought to the home. Family members and extended family stay by the bedside of the dying patient as they believe God is ultimately in control of outcomes. Grief is expressed openly and publicly. Autopsy is acceptable, although organ donation is not typical. Death does not end the connection to the family (American Geriatrics Society, 2004; Purnell & Paulanka, 2008).

Mexican Americans may take turns sitting vigil over the dying person; dying in a hospital is not desirable because the spirit may become lost. Spiritual amulets, rosary beads, or other religious artifacts are kept near the patient. Typically, organ donation or autopsy is not allowed. When death occurs, family and friends will often come long distances for the funeral. A *velorio* is a festive watch of the deceased body before burial. Traditional families may exhibit hyperkinetic shaking and seizure-like activity called *ataque de nervios*, which is a way to release emotions related to grieving. The family may erect altars in their homes in honor of the anniversary of their relative's death and may include candles, decorations, and having the deceased's favorite meal at a graveside picnic (Purnell & Paulanka, 1998).

Native Americans have different traditions in each tribe. There is a belief that the spirit of the deceased remains where the person has died; therefore, family may not want the person to die at home. At the same time, it is considered inappropriate for the person to die alone. If the person dies at home, the house must be abandoned or a ceremony is held to cleanse it. Families gather together at the time of death and material possessions are dispersed. When a person dies, a cleansing ceremony is performed or else the spirit of the deceased may try to take over someone else's spirit. Those who work with the dead also must have a ceremonial cleansing to protect themselves from the dead person's spirit. No embalming is done; the deceased are buried in sacred ground with their shoes on the wrong feet, rings on their index fingers, and with many gifts surrounding them; or the body is cremated (Purnell & Paulanka, 2008).

For Appalachians, a death is an important event, even for extended family. The funeral is a significant social occasion and family and friends will come great distances to attend. The body is displayed for long periods of time so that all can see the body who wish to. The deceased is buried in his or her best clothes and some people have custom-made clothes for burial. At the funeral home, personal possessions are displayed and it is common to bury these items with the person. Gravesites are typically on hillsides because of the fear they will be flooded out in low-lying areas (Purnell & Paulanka, 2008).

Subgroups from China, Vietnam, Laos, Thailand, and Burma together are called the Hmong. The Hmong believe that proper burial and worship of the dead and other ancestors directly affects the safety, health, and prosperity of the family. The belief is that the spiritual world coexists with the physical world and that the spirits are able to influence human life. The preference is to die at home because they believe their soul will wander for all of eternity without a resting place if they were to die elsewhere. Some groups believe that death should take place in the hospital so as not to bring bad luck into the home. Autopsy and cremation are acceptable practices to some families. For these groups, burial occurs in the afternoon.

The Chinese will place a coin in the deceased's mouth so that the deceased has money to pay anyone who interferes in the journey. Additionally, symbolic money may be burned to signify the transmission of wealth to the celestial bank, and has recently translated to burning symbolic paper items, which includes houses, cell phones, and cars (Chung & Wegars, 2005). In northern China, the body is placed in burial clothes, and an unpadded quilt is used as a shroud. The face is covered with cloth or paper and the feet are tied with colored string. The wife or oldest son wipes the eyes of the deceased with cotton floss before the coffin is closed. Instead of being buried immediately after the funeral, the body may be stored so that a husband and wife can be buried together (Iserson, 2001).

The Japanese bathe their dead, shave some of the hair, and dress the person in white. The deceased wears a ceremonial hat or triangular piece of white paper tied to the forehead and may also include white socks and white gloves. Special favorite items may be placed in the coffin (Green & Green, 2006). Koreans use perfume to wash the body and dress the body in silk or hemp clothes tied in seven places that correlate with the seven stars in the Ursa Major constellation (Iserson, 2001).

Literature related to Wiccans, Pagans, and Nature Spiritualists (WPNS) and EOL preferences is extremely limited. The passage from this life is generally referred to as "into the Summerland." It is important to include priests, priestesses, and death midwives in the dying process to provide herbal therapies and complementary care. In preparation for death, Pagans may perform rituals or prayers in a circle surrounding the patient. Individuals may sing, pray, or chant, focusing energy on the patient. Alternative healing methods include the use of crystals and stones, Reiki, sound healing, massage, music, and color therapy. Generally, the patient's coven, priest, priestess, or chosen family member will administer last rites. The death midwife may help the family with cleansing, anointing, and dressing the body (Smith-Stoner & Young, 2007).

■ PERI-DEATH 3: FUNERALS AS A CEREMONY OF DEATH

Across cultures, people accept a responsibility to care for, respect, and honor their dead. The funeral can serve to dispose of the dead body, transmit the body to the afterlife, and enable the bereaved community and family to adjust to their new role in society (Brooks-Gordon, Ebetehaj, Herring, Johnson, & Richards, 2007). For most ethnic groups and religious groups, the process of physically preparing the body for the funeral and burial is handled by persons outside the family, but includes some form of preparation for the afterlife. The undertaker—a person who "undertook" the responsibility to keep the body safe and make the funeral arrangements—has been a part of society since ancient times. The general public interchangeably refers to the person who prepares the body for burial and conducts all aspects of the funeral service as the undertaker, mortician, embalmer, or funeral director (Green & Green, 2006; Iserson, 2001).

In modern society, funeral directors may coordinate all the details of the funeral for the family, but are also expected to manage the survivors' distress. They supervise the preparation of the body for viewing or burial, oversee embalming procedures if embalming is desired, coordinate cremation planning, instruct and support the pallbearers, arrange the transportation of the family and the deceased to the cemetery, place death notices in the newspaper, and otherwise facilitate the family's burial decisions (Habenstein & Lamers, 2007; Iserson, 2001; National Funeral Directors Association [NFDA], 2008).

The funeral director may orchestrate all aspects of the funeral, but it is not mandated (NFDA, 2008). Those who work in the funeral industry know that the funeral must be perfectly organized and executed because they will not get a second chance to make things right. It was originally believed that the funeral held merely theological value, but for many people the funeral is one of the first steps of successful grieving. The funeral is "*of the person who has died....* It is *for* those who survive" (Raether, 1993, p. 211).

For families that have a wake, this is the first component of post-death ritual. It may be one of the few times the entire family will reassemble for an event. It is a time for family and friends to view the dead body and to pay their final respects. Seeing the dead body emphasizes the fact that the person is dead; declining to see the body may delay grieving. "I was recently again reminded of how valuable and legitimate a funeral service can be. I accompanied a friend to the funeral of his mother. She had died of a chronic and wasting illness and I had been present at her deathbed. My friend experienced a deep and profound consolation seeing his mother with the lines of suffering erased from her face and lying at peace" (Raether, 1993, p. 211).

The second component of post-death rituals is the funeral. It is a ceremonial service typically consisting of music, prayers, poetry, and eulogies, and it may be part of a funeral Mass, where Communion is celebrated. Some people will plan their funerals before they die, which can be comforting to those who are dying as well as their families (Raether, 1993; Shannon, 2006).

The committal service is the concluding funeral rite. It is the final act of caring for the deceased and is celebrated at the grave, tomb, or crematorium and has seen little change during the past century. The changes that have occurred reflect compassion for the bereaved (Habenstein & Lamers, 2007). This service is a "symbolic demonstration that the kind of relationship which has existed between the mourner and the deceased is now at an end" (Raether, 1993, p. 212).

Seven specific therapeutic values have been assigned to the funeral process as delineated by Raether (1993, p. 209). First, the "therapy of direct expression" denotes that the funeral furnishes the setting and opportunity for the bereaved to express their grief physically. Funerals offer "therapy of language" by providing the bereaved an opportunity to talk about what has happened, voice their feelings, and begin to feel relief in the telling.

The "therapy of sharing" is the coming together of the family and significant others to provide emotional and physical support to each other. Time spent with the bereaved is an important aspect of burying the dead. Immersion in the many aspects of the funeral process also encompasses the "therapy of activity." The routine of greeting mourners at the funeral home or interacting with those who offer their sympathy prevents the bereaved from withdrawing and focuses their energy in the immediate post-death period. The funeral also provides the "therapy of ceremony," which is both glorifying and ennobling. The liturgical aspect of the funeral ceremony

encompasses the views of the meaning of life and the nature of life hereafter. Given that accepting the reality of the death is difficult for many people, the "therapy of viewing" establishes a final and amended view of the deceased. This revised image replaces those composed during the illness or at the time of death and may bring comfort to the mourner. Finally, the "therapy of suffering" addresses the guilt that mourners may be experiencing and provides the occasion to verbalize what had been left unsaid previously.

Another important aspect of the post-death experience for the bereaved is the formation of a new identity within their community. The role of widow, of no longer having a child, or of one who has lost a parent brings with it a change in how the bereaved interact and correspond to society at large. Social groups may shrink, volunteer opportunities may be lost, and favorite activities may be forfeited due to the loss of the deceased. Nurses need to be aware of the difficulties inherent in these role shifts and offer alternatives and community-support referrals during this transitional stage.

Analyses of the Peri-Death Experience

As with any application of the nursing process, the nurse should evaluate the effectiveness of the interventions that have been utilized. In the case of peri-death nursing, there is no way to obtain objective data from the older adult who has just died to determine the efficacy of care. Although family members can be surveyed regarding their experiences, they can truly only report their perceptions as viewed through their own lens. In reality, guilt, remorse, or grief may cloud this lens. The National Hospice and Palliative Care Organization (NHPCO, 2018) provides an online survey entitled *Family Evaluation of Palliative Care,* designed to give providers feedback about the family's perceptions of care.

Bainbridge, Brazil, Ploeg, Krueger, and Taniguchi (2016) suggest healthcare integration as a means of evaluating palliative care outcomes. The *Patient Outcome Domains* within the framework include "satisfaction with domains of care and access." This framework includes measurements within (a) availability of care, (b) free flow and accessibility of information, (c) physical care, (d) pain and symptom management, (e) psychosocial care, and (f) management of expected death. Healthcare providers who can perform a retrospective review of patient care using this framework are able to examine areas where improvements can occur and enhance palliative care interventions.

■ CONCLUSION

When the nurse is providing EOL care, the focus of care is the patient and his or her family. Family-centered care continues after the death of the patient. The goal of post-death nursing care is to promote optimal adjustment and to help the family and significant others with the tasks of bereavement (see Chapter 11). Bereavement is an important developmental stage; the nurse should provide interventions that offer the opportunity for healing and growth, a redefinition of self, and opportunities to make new plans. Follow-up with the family is important during the bereavement period. The nurse should encourage memorial rituals commemorating the deceased's life and death. Unique opportunities exist in peri-death nursing to support the dying patient and the patient's family in making what is a painful and difficult process one that is also priceless.

CASE STUDY *Conclusion*

Ms. Owens shared meals and memories with friends until the last 10 days of her life. She would often doze midway through her conversations, but resumed her thoughts with little prompting. The hospice team provided her with long- and short-acting morphine to manage her cancer-related pain and dexamethasone for the capsular pain secondary to the liver metastasis that allowed her to be comfortable. She had identified her favorite nightgowns and removed herself from her bed to the living room couch. She said this was where she had felt the most comfortable as the disease had progressed. She eventually drifted into a semi-unconscious state that lasted 3 days prior to her death. She died a peaceful death in her home, with a friend beside her.

CASE STUDY

AN INTERDISCIPLINARY COMMENTARY

Linda Edmondson, LCSW
Oklahoma City, OK

When I first read this case study I found myself rereading it to be sure that I had not missed where the oncologist made a recommendation for hospice care. But in this case study, as in real life, even though the oncologist said there were no more treatment options and gave a prognosis of only 6 weeks to 2 months, there was no recommendation for a hospice referral for Ms. Owens. When there are no further treatment options and expected prognosis is weeks to months, a reasonable expectation is that hospice be part of the revised plan of care. No one should ever say, "There is nothing more we can do," when palliative care and hospice are options. Hospice can provide pain management, durable medical equipment, assistance with bathing and activities of daily livings (ADLs), and other services, but not 24/7 care. It is a 100% covered service under Medicare.

Ms. Owens was fortunate to have many devoted friends who helped her remain in her home. She had named one of her friends as a POA for financial decisions and another as her durable power of attorney for healthcare (DPOAHC). These are two distinct roles that are often confused. A simple POA is in effect only while both parties are capacitated. The durable POA will continue even after Ms. Owens becomes incapacitated and unable to make decisions for herself. Ideally, both legal documents and an advance directive should name the same person as the agent/proxy.

In the conclusion to the case study, the services of a hospice team are mentioned, so Ms. Owens obtained that service without a referral from her oncologist. Although a physician order is required to begin hospice, the initial request is often made by the patient, his or her family, or friends. Her friends remained with her as primary caregivers until her peaceful death at home. The hospice staff would certainly have informed her friends what to do as death approached and occurred. An expected death at home usually can be handled without any involvement from a medical examiner or law enforcement authorities. The hospice would know what the practice is in its jurisdiction. Ms. Owens's dying days seemed to have led to what could be called "a good death."

Evidence-Based Practice

Shifrin, M. M. (2016). An evidence-based practice approach to end-of-life nursing education in intensive care units. *Journal of Hospice and Palliative Nursing, 18*(4), 342–348. doi:10.1097/NJH.0000000000000254

Objectives
EOL educational initiatives have resulted in increased awareness regarding the complexity of issues at the end of life and have improved interdisciplinary collaboration and communication. Integration of palliative care into the ICU has resulted in multiple benefits for patients, families, healthcare providers, and healthcare organizations. These include improved symptom assessment and patient comfort, decreased conflict over goals of care, decreased use of nonbeneficial treatments, and decreased ICU length of stay.

Methods/Needs Assessment/Setting
A needs assessment at a 1,019-bed academic, tertiary care hospital in the southeastern United States identified that RNs employed in the organization's ICUs have a wide range of educational preparation and exposure to caring for patients at the end of life. Nurse educators and RNs employed in the six adult ICUs identified several barriers to ICU EOL education. These included a limited number of educational offerings, educational offerings that were scheduled at times or locations inconvenient for RNs, educational offerings that were either too short or too long in duration, and educational content that was not directly relevant to the management of ICU patients at the end of life. Nurse educators and RNs expressed particular interest in educational content related to EOL symptom recognition, both nonpharmacological and pharmacological symptom management, ventilator weaning and compassionate endotracheal extubation, and communication strategies.

Participants
Participants included full- and part-time ICU RNs with an active state license who was employed at the project site during the time of the project and who voluntarily participated. Recruitment occurred using posters, organizational emails, and verbal reminders.

Measurements
The author created a 20-question multiple-choice assessment tool, titled Nursing Management at the End of Life, for outcome evaluation. The assessment tool was administered as both the pretest and the posttest in a pen-and-paper format.

Results
Before the educational sessions, scores on the pretest ranged from 60% to 100% (mean, 79.4%). After the educational intervention, the mean posttest scores ranged from 90% to 100% (mean, 96.7%). A 2-tailed paired t test demonstrated a significant increase in mean scores from the pretest to posttest ($p < .001$). Before the educational intervention, 59% ($n = 27$) of participants reached the established benchmark score of 80% or higher on the pretest. After the educational intervention, 100% ($n = 46$) of participants achieved or exceeded the established benchmark score of 80% on the posttest.

Conclusions

The ICU nursing management of patients at the end of life is challenging on many fronts and is particularly difficult for RNs in ICUs who are trained to aggressively restore patient health to a pre-illness state. Increasing human longevity and comorbid states have led ICU RNs to incorporate the management of EOL patients into their practice. The literature indicates that a lack of nursing education is a primary barrier to ICU EOL care. However, increasing nursing knowledge can contribute to overcoming this deficit. This EBP change project demonstrated that educational intervention resulted in increased knowledge on EOL care in ICUs. Our results mirror those found in the current literature and reinforce the necessity of ongoing EOL education for RNs. Further study of the impact of educational interventions on improving EOL care is needed to evaluate the application to clinical care (Shifrin, 2016, pp. 346–347).

Evidence-Based Practice

Nedjat-Haiem, F. R., Carrion, I. V., Ell, K., & Mishra, S. I. (2017). Exploring healthcare providers' views about initiating end-of-life care communication. *American Journal of Hospice and Palliative Medicine, 34*(4), 308–317. doi:10.1177/1049909115627773

Objectives

To examine healthcare providers' perceptions of both medical and nonmedical providers' roles and responsibilities for initiating EOL care communication with seriously ill patients and their families. A number of healthcare provider types across various disciplines are considered.

Methods, Settings, and Participants

Using semi-structured qualitative interviews with physicians, nurses, social workers, and chaplains working in two large medical centers in Los Angeles, California, we asked providers to describe their roles, define who they thought should be most responsible for initiating EOL discussions, and explain how much of a role they personally had in EOL decision-making discussions with their patients. The study is a part of a larger study on participants' experiences with barriers that limit EOL care communication and factors that hinder transitions at the end of life, and explored the overall importance of engaging in EOL care communication with vulnerable populations.

Results

Three overarching themes describe providers' roles and responsibilities for initiating EOL care communication with seriously ill patients and their families: (1) theme 1: providers' roles for engaging in EOL discussions, (2) theme 2: the responsibility of physicians for initiating and leading discussions, and (3) theme 3: the need for team co-management in patient care.

Conclusions

This study uniquely highlights the interaction among healthcare disciplines, the demands of each discipline, and the interrelatedness that takes place when communicating EOL care and decisions. Healthcare providers are committed to assisting patients and improving the patients' quality of life. However, initiating communication about EOL care is challenging and often difficult for all disciplines. Given the significance and the perceived consequences of the task, it is often avoided. The avoidance of EOL communication has many inherited negative outcomes for patients, their families, and the overall healthcare system. Future studies will address the role of gender, age, ethnicity, and culture in providers' views in initiating EOL communication. This study explored and examined the perceptions of EOL communication among healthcare providers. It also enables healthcare providers to evaluate their practice and interventions in order to increase EOL communication with patients and their families (Nedjat-Haiem et al., 2017, p. 316).

■ REFERENCES

American Academy of Hospice and Palliative Medicine. (2013). Statement on artificial nutrition and hydration near the end of life. Retrieved from http://aahpm.org/positions/anh

American Geriatrics Society. (2004). Older African Americans. In *Doorway thoughts: Cross-cultural health care for older adults* (Vol. 1, pp. 43–53). Sudbury, MA: Jones & Bartlett.

Archdiocese of Chicago. (2008). Catholic cemeteries. Retrieved from http://www.catholiccemeterieschicago.org/sacredplaces.php

Bailey, F. A., Williams, B. R., Goode, P. S., Woodby, L. L., Redden, D. T., Johnson T. M., II, … Burgio, K. L. (2012). Opioid pain medication orders and administration in the last days of life. *Journal of Pain and Symptom Management, 44*(5), 681–691. doi:10.1016/j.jpainsymman.2011.11.006

Bainbridge, D., Brazil, K., Ploeg, J., Krueger, P., & Taniguchi, A. (2016). Measuring healthcare integration: Operationalization of a framework for a systems evaluation of palliative care structures, processes, and outcomes. *Palliative Medicine, 30*(6), 567–579. doi:10.1177/0269216315619862

Baldwin, J., & Cox, J. (2016). Treating dyspnea: Is oxygen therapy the best option for all patients? *Medical Clinics of North America, 100*, 1123–1130. doi:10.1016/j.mcna.2016.04.018

Beattie, S. (2006). Hands-on help. Surgical drains. *RN, 69*(12), 20ac1–20ac4.

Benzein, E. G., & Saveman, B. I. (2008). Health-promoting conversations about hope and suffering with couples in palliative care. *International Journal of Palliative Nursing, 14*(9), 439–445. doi:10.12968/ijpn.2008.14.9.31124

Berger, J. T., DeRenzo, E. G., & Schwartz, J. (2008). Surrogate decision making: Reconciling ethical theory and clinical practice. *Annals of Internal Medicine, 149*(1), 48–53. doi:10.7326/0003-4819-149-1-200807010-00010

Billings, J. A. (2012). Human terminal extubation reconsidered: The role for preemptive analgesia and sedation. *Critical Care Medicine, 40*(2), 625–630. doi:10.1097/CCM.0b013e318228235d

Birchenall, J., & Streight, E. (1997). *Home care aide*. St. Louis, MO: Mosby.

Brenner, E. (2014). Human body preservation: Old and new techniques. *Journal of Anatomy, 224*(3), 316–344. doi:10.1111/joa.12160

Brooks-Gordon, B., Ebetehaj, F., Herring, J., Johnson, M., & Richards, M. (2007). *Death rites & rights*. London, UK: Hart.

Bush, S. H., Kanji, S., & Pereira, J. L. (2014). Treating an established episode of delirium in palliative care: Expert opinion and review of the current evidence base with recommendations for future development. *Journal of Pain and Symptom Management, 48*, 231–248. doi:10.1016/j.jpainsymman.2013.07.018

Campbell, M. L. (2015). Caring for dying patients in the intensive care unit: Managing pain dyspnea, anxiety, delirium, and death rattle. *AACN Advanced Critical Care, 26*(2), 110–120. doi:10.1097/NCI.0000000000000077

Campbell, M. L., Templin, T., & Walch, J. (2010). A respiratory distress observation scale for patients unable to self-report dyspnea. *Journal of Palliative Medicine, 13*(3), 285–290. doi:10.1089/jpm.2009.0229

Candy, B., Jackson, K. C., Jones, L., Leurent, B., Tookman, A., & King, M. (2012). Drug therapy for delirium in terminally ill adult patients. *Cochrane Database of Systematic Reviews*, (11), CD004770. doi:10.1002/14651858.CD004770.pub2

Cheng, K. C., Chen, C. M., Tan, C. K., Chen, H. M., Lu, C. L., & Zhang, H. (2011). Methylprednisolone reduces the rates of postextubation stridor and reintubation associated with attenuated cytokine responses in critically ill patients. *Minerva Anestesiologica, 77*(5), 503–509.

Chirco, N., Dunn, K. S., & Robinson, S. G. (2011). The trajectory of terminal delirium at the end of life. *Journal of Hospice and Palliative Nursing, 13*(6), 411–418. doi:10.1097/NJH.0b013e3182271a6c

Chung, S. F., & Wegars, P. (2005). *Chinese-American death rituals: Respecting the ancestors*. Lanham, MD: AltaMira Press.

Cook, D., & Rocker, G. (2014). Dying with dignity in the intensive care unit. *New England Journal of Medicine, 370*(26), 2506–2514. doi:10.1056/NEJMra1208795

Croyère, N., Belloir, M., Chantier, L., & McEvan, L. (2012). Oral care in nursing practice: A pragmatic representation. *International Journal of Palliative Nursing, 18*(9), 435–440. doi:10.12968/ijpn.2012.18.9.435

Emanuel, L., Ferris, F. D., von Gunten, C. F., & von Roenn, J. H. (2008). The last hours of living: Practical advice for clinicians [Electronic Version]. EPEC-O: Education in palliative and end-of-life care for oncology. (Module 6): Last hours of living The EPEC Project, Chicago, IL, 2005, 18.

Ferrell, B., Virani, R., & Grant, M. (1999). Analysis of end-of-life content in nursing textbooks. *Oncology Nursing Forum, 26*(5), 869–876.

Field, M., & Cassel, C. (1997). *Approaching death: Improving care at the end of life.* Washington, DC: National Academies Press.

Gates, R. A., & Fink, R. M. (1997). *Oncology nursing secrets.* St. Louis, MO: Mosby.

Gerstel, E., Engelberg, R. A., Koepsell, T., & Curtis, J. R. (2008). Duration of withdrawal of life support in the intensive care unit and association with family satisfaction. *American Journal of Respiratory and Critical Care Medicine, 178*(8), 798–804. doi:10.1164/rccm.200711-1617OC

Green, J. (1989a). Death with dignity: Baha'i Faith. *Nursing Times, 85*(10), 50–51.

Green, J. (1989b). Death with dignity: Buddhism. *Nursing Times, 85*(9), 40–41.

Green, J. (1989c). Death with dignity: Hinduism. *Nursing Times, 85*(6), 50–51.

Green, J. (1989d). Death with dignity: Judaism. *Nursing Times, 85*(8), 65.

Green, J., & Green, M. (2006). *Dealing with death* (2nd ed.). London, UK: Jessica Kingsley.

Habenstein, R. W., & Lamers, W. M. (2007). *The history of American funeral directing* (6th ed.). Brookfield, WI: National Funeral Directors Association.

Hackett, J., Godfrey, M., & Bennett, M. I. (2016). Patient and caregiver perspectives on managing pain in advanced cancer: A qualitative longitudinal study. *Palliative Medicine, 30*(8), 711–719. doi:10.1177/0269216316628407

Harris, M. (2007). *Grave matters: A journey through the modern funeral industry to a natural way of burial.* New York, NY: Scribner.

Hill, J., & Daniels, P. (2007). *Life events and rites of passage.* Detroit, MI: Omnigraphics.

Horn, L. W. (1992, March/April). Terminal dyspnea: A hospice approach. *American Journal of Hospice and Palliative Care, 9*(2), 24–32. doi:10.1177/104990919200900206

Hosker, C. M. G., & Bennett, M. I. (2016). Delirium and agitation at the end of life. *BMJ, 353.* doi:10.1136/bmj.i3085

Hospice and Palliative Nursing Association. (2012). Artificial nutrition and hydration in advanced illness. *Journal of Hospice and Palliative Nursing, 14*(3), 173–176. doi:10.1097/NJH.0b013e31824d1143

Iserson, K. V. (2001). *Death to dust: What happens to dead bodies?* Tucson, AZ: Galen Press.

Kastbom, L., Milberg, A., & Karlsson, M. (2017). A good death from the perspective of palliative cancer patients. *Supportive Care Cancer, 25,* 933–939. doi:10.1007/s00520-016-3483-9

Kastenbaum, R., & Kastenbaum, B. (Eds.) (1989). *Encyclopedia of death.* Phoenix, AZ: Oryx Press.

Lembeck, M. E., Pameijer, C. R., & Westcott, A. M. (2016). The role of intravenous fluids and enteral or parenteral nutrition in patients with life-limiting illness. *Medical Clinics of North America, 100,* 1131–1141. doi:10.1016/j.mcna.2016.04.019

Maltoni, M., Scarpi, E., & Nanni, O. (2013). Palliative sedation in end-of-life care. *Current Opinion in Oncology, 25*(4), 360–367. doi:10.1097/CCO.0b013e3283622c47

Matzo, M., & Orwig, S. R. (2013). 50 shades of gray. *Journal of Palliative Medicine, 16*(8), 833–835. doi:10.1089/jpm.2013.0185

Mayer, R. G., & Taylor, J. (2005). *Embalming: History, theory and practice* (4th ed.). New York, NY: McGraw-Hill.

McPherson, M. L., Kim, M., & Walker, K. A. (2012). 50 practical medication tips at end of life. *Journal of Supportive Oncology, 10*(6), 222–229. doi:10.1016/j.suponc.2012.08.002

Miller, E. J. (1993). A Roman Catholic view of death. In K. Doka & J. D. Morgan (Eds.), *Death and spirituality* (pp. 33–50). Amityville, NY: Baywood.

National Academy of Social Insurance. (2017). The future of Medicare. Retrieved from https://www.nasi.org/learn/medicare/future-medicare

National Funeral Directors Association. (2008). Facts and statistics. Retrieved from http://www.nfda.org

National Hospice and Palliative Care Organization. (2009). Standards of practice for pediatric palliative care and hospice. Retrieved from http://www.nhpco.org/sites/default/files/public/quality/Ped_Pall_Care%20_Standard.pdf.pdf

National Hospice and Palliative Care Organization. (2018). Family Evaluation of Palliative Care. Alexandria, VA: Author. Retrieved from https://www.nhpco.org/fepc-survey-materials

Nedjat-Haiem, F. R., Carrion, I. V., Ell, K., & Mishra, S. I. (2017). Exploring health care providers' views about initiating end-of-life care communication. *American Journal of Hospice and Palliative Medicine, 34*(4), 308–317. doi:10.1177/1049909115627773

Organ Procurement and Transplantation Network. (2013). Retrieved from http://optn.transplant.hrsa.gov

Panke, J. (2003). Difficulties in managing pain at the end of life. *Journal of Hospice and Palliative Nursing, 5*(2), 83–90. doi:10.1097/00129191-200304000-00014

Pattison, N. (2008). Care of patients who have died. *Nursing Standard, 22*(28), 42–48. doi:10.7748/ns2008.03.22.28.42.c6434

Peacock, S. C. (2013). The experience of providing end-of-life care to a relative with advanced dementia: An integrative review. *Palliative and Supportive Care, 11*(2), 155–168. doi:10.1017/S1478951512000831

Pitorak, E. F. (2003). Care at the time of death: How nurses can make the last hours of life a richer, more comfortable experience. *American Journal of Nursing, 103*(7), 42–52. doi:10.1097/00000446-200307000-00019

Pizzo, P. A. (2016). Thoughts about *Dying in America*: Enhancing the impact of one's life journey and legacy by also planning for the end of life. *Proceedings of the National Academy of Sciences, 113*(46), 12908–12912. doi:10.1073/pnas.1614266113

Purnell, L. D., & Paulanka, B. J. (1998). *Transcultural health care: A culturally competent approach* (2nd ed.). Philadelphia, PA: Davis.

Purnell, L. D., & Paulanka, B. J. (2008). *Transcultural health care: A culturally competent approach* (3rd ed.). Philadelphia, PA: F. A. Davis.

Quested, B., & Rudge, T. (2003). Nursing care of dead bodies: A discursive analysis of last offices. *Journal of Advanced Nursing, 41*(6), 553–560. doi:10.1046/j.1365-2648.2003.02567.x

Quill, T. E., & Byock, I. R. (2000). Responding to intractable terminal suffering: The role of terminal sedation and voluntary refusal of food and fluids. *Annals of Internal Medicine, 132*(5), 408–414. doi:10.7326/0003-4819-132-5-200003070-00012

Raether, H. C. (1993). Rituals, beliefs, and grief. In K. Doka & J. D. Morgan (Eds.), *Death and spirituality* (pp. 207–216). Amityville, NY: Baywood.

Revier, S. S., Meiers, S. J., & Herth, K. (2012). The lived experience of hope in family caregivers caring for a terminally ill loved one. *Journal of Hospice and Palliative Nursing, 14*(6), 438–446. doi:10.1097/NJH.0b013e318257f8d4

Sanchez, H. (2017). Autopsy rate and physician attitudes toward autopsy. Retrieved from http://emedicine .medscape.com/article/1705948-overview

Schaefer, E. T., Fitzgerald, J. F., Molleston, J. P., Croffie, J. M., Pfefferkorn, M. D., Corkins, M. R., … Gupta, S. K. (2008). Comparison of oral prednisone and topical fluticasone in the treatment of eosinophilic esophagitis: A randomized trial in children. *Clinical Gastroenterology and Hepatology, 6*(2), 165–173. doi:10.1016/j.cgh.2007.11.008

Serratelli, A. (2017). Catholic burial practices: Respecting the person, body and soul. *Catholic News Agency.* Retrieved from http://www.catholicnewsagency.com/column/catholic-burial-practices-respecting-the-person-body-and-soul-3683

Shannon, J. B. (2006). *Death and dying sourcebook* (2nd ed.). Detroit, MI: Omnigraphics.

Shifrin, M. M. (2016). An evidence-based practice approach to end-of-life nursing education in intensive care units. *Journal of Hospice and Palliative Nursing, 18*(4), 342–348. doi:10.1097/NJH.0000000000000254

Smith-Stoner, M. R., & Young, N. C. (2007). Spiritual needs of Wiccan, Pagan, and Nature Spiritualists at end of life. *Journal of Hospice and Palliative Nursing, 9*(5), 279–286. doi:10.1097/01.NJH.0000289658.93666.70

Somers, E., Grey, C., & Satkoske, V. (2016). Withholding versus withdrawing treatment: Artificial nutrition and hydration as a model. *Current Opinion in Supportive and Palliative Care, 10*(3), 208–213. doi:10.1097/SPC.0000000000000225

Soriano, M. A., & Lagman, R. (2012). When the patient says no. *American Journal of Hospice and Palliative Care, 29*(5), 401–404. doi:10.1177/1049909111421163

Sorrentino, S. A. (1999). *Assisting with patient care.* St. Louis, MO: Mosby.

Spector, N., Connolly, M. A., & Carlson, K. K. (2007). Dyspnea: Applying research to bedside practice. *AACN Advanced Critical Care, 18*(1), 45–58; quiz 59. doi:10.4037/15597768-2007-1006

Strand, J. J., Feely, M. A., Kramer, N. M., Moeschler, S. M., & Swetz, K. M. (2016). Palliative sedation and what constitutes active dying: A case of severe progressive dystonia and intractable pain. *American Journal of Hospice and Palliative Medicine, 33*(4), 363–368. doi:10.1177/1049909114561997

Strub, C. G., & Frederick, L. G. (1967). *The principles and practice of embalming.* Dallas, TX: Frederick.

Tan, A., & Manca, D. (2013). Finding common ground to achieve a "good death": family physicians working with substitute decision-makers of dying patients. A qualitative grounded theory study. *BMC Family Practice, 14*(1), 14. doi:10.1186/1471-2296-14-14

Wasserman, L. S. (2008). Respectful death: A model for end-of-life care. *Clinical Journal of Oncology Nursing, 12*(4), 621–626. doi:10.1188/08.CJON.621-626

Worden, W. (1992). *Grief counseling and grief therapy* (2nd ed.). London, UK: Routledge.

World Health Organization. (2013). WHO's cancer pain ladder for adults. Retrieved from http://www.who.int/cancer/palliative/painladder/en/index.html

Zerwekh, J. V. (2006). *Nursing care at the end of life: Palliative care for patients and families.* Philadelphia, PA: F. A. Davis.

■ **APPENDIX 27.1**

SYMPTOM RELIEF KIT

Information for Healthcare Provider:

■ For *pain or dyspnea*: Morphine solution: 0.25 to 0.5 mL (20 mg/mL solution) PO/SL q 2 PRN. May increase up to 1 to 2 mL q 1 to 2 hours, PRN as directed by the healthcare provider.

■ For loud, *wet respirations or excessive secretions*: Hyoscyamine (Levsin) 0.125 mg (one to two tablets) PO/SL q 6 hours PRN.

■ For *unrelieved respiratory fluid accumulation*: Furosemide (Lasix) 40 mg IV/IM/PO/SC. May repeat.

■ For *nausea or vomiting*: Prochlorperazine 25 mg suppository PR q 8 hours PRN.

■ For severe agitation or restlessness:
   ■ If client is in pain, treat accordingly.

■ If client is constipated or having urinary retention, take appropriate action.

■ If agitation persists, administer pentobarbital suppository PR q 6 hours PRN.

■ **Liquid morphine:** For pain or difficulty breathing. Given by mouth.

■ **Three kinds of suppositories in four differently labeled bags:**
   ■ **Prochlorperazine** (the active ingredient in Compazine): For nausea with or without vomiting.
   ■ **Pentobarbital:** For severe agitation or seizures; will make the patient very sleepy.
   ■ **Acetaminophen:** For high fevers.

■ **Levsin** tablets: For noisy, wet, "gurgly" breathing sounds. Can help to dry up secretions.

■ **Furosemide (Lasix):** For severe difficulty breathing because of fluid buildup. The nurse will visit and give this medicine to the patient if you have not been taught how to give "shots."

Information for Patients and Families

The Symptom Relief Kit is designed to help you cope with physical problems that might unexpectedly arise. If you feel that you need to use this kit, call the hospice nurse first.

Symptom	Drug	How to Use It
Unrelieved pain	Morphine solution	1–2 mL in the mouth, under the tongue, every 2–3 hr as needed.
Unrelieved shortness of breath	Morphine solution	0.25–0.5 mL in the mouth, under the tongue, every 2 hr as needed.
Nausea and vomiting	Prochlorperazine suppository	One suppository inserted into the rectum every 8 hr as needed.
Severe agitation and restlessness	Pentobarbital suppository	One suppository inserted into the rectum every 4–6 hr as needed.
Wet, "gurgly" breathing	Levsin tablets	One or two in the mouth or under the tongue every 4–6 hr as needed.
Unrelieved accumulation and respiratory distress	Furosemide injection	Inject 40–80 mg as instructed by the nurse.
Fever	Acetaminophen suppository	One suppository inserted into the rectum every 4 hr as needed.

Note: Clients taking opioids for pain will need to increase their usual morphine dose (for breakthrough pain) for effective treatment of dyspnea.

Source: Adapted from the VNA Home Health and Hospice Services, Manchester, NH.

Index